D1117607

Nurse's Guide to Drugs™

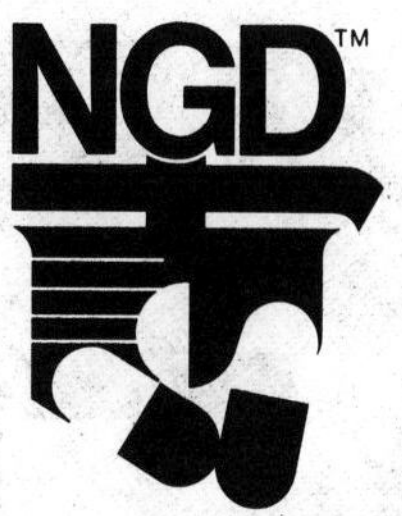

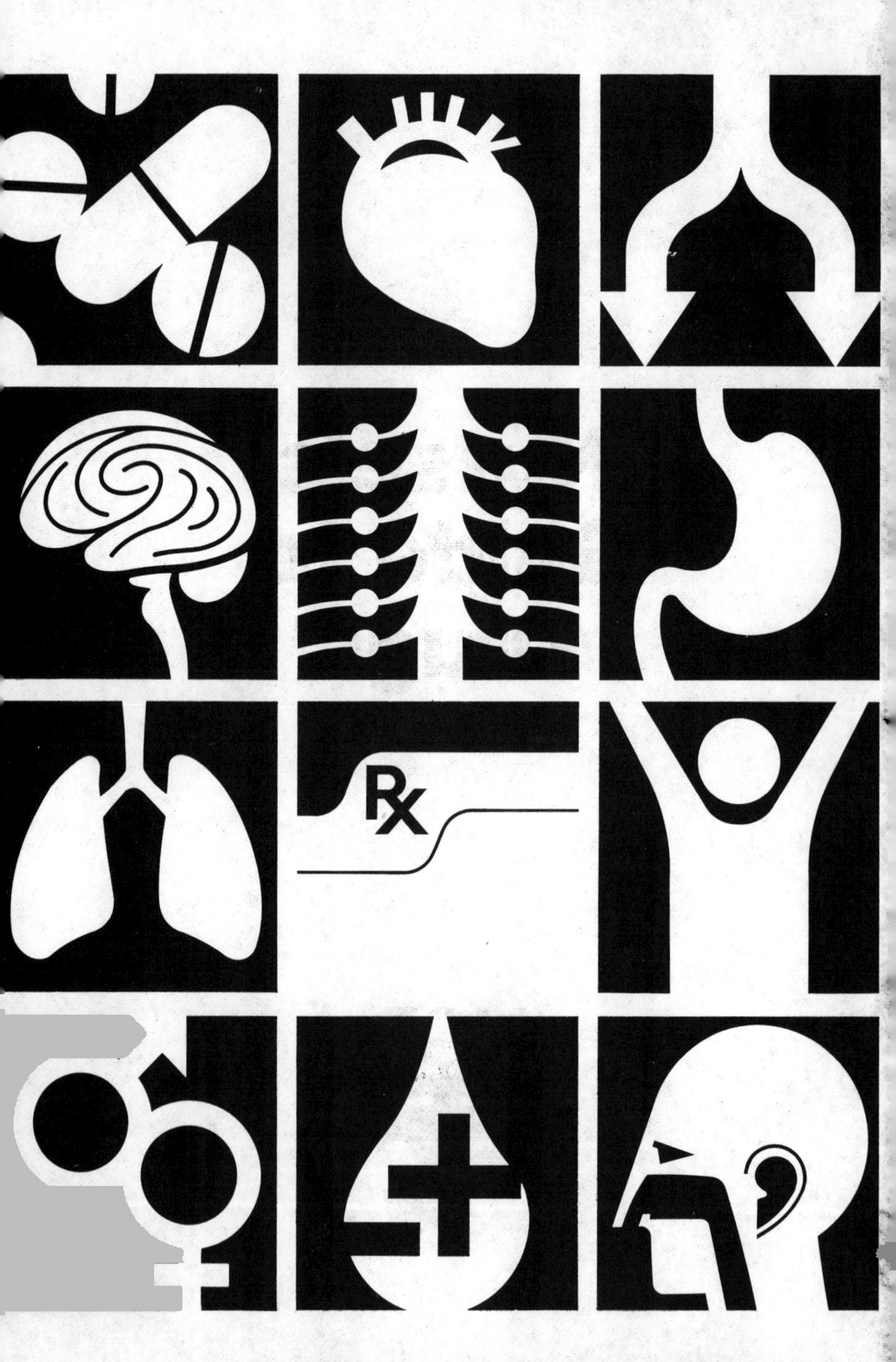
Rx

Nurse's Guide to Drugs™

NURSING80 BOOKS
INTERMED COMMUNICATIONS, INC.
HORSHAM, PENNSYLVANIA

NURSING80 BOOKS
PUBLISHER: Eugene W. Jackson
Graphics Director: John Isely
General Manager: T. A. Temple

NURSE'S REFERENCE LIBRARY
Editorial Director: Helen Hamilton
Clinical Director: Minnie Rose, RN, BSN, MEd
Developmental Editor: Barbara McVan, RN
Production Manager: Bernie Haas

Editorial Staff for this volume
Pharmacy Editor: Larry N. Gever, PharmD
Editors: Jean Robinson, Avery Rome, Elaine Schott-Jones
Assistant Editors: Jean Axelrod, Saretta Berlin, Lisa Z. Cohen, Louise Lux-Sions, Laura Musmanno-Albert, Sanford Robinson, Norman Rudnick, Frank Wilson
Copy Editors: Kathi Foster, Patricia Hamilton, Barbara Hodgson
Indexer: Vonda Heller
Researchers: Carole Gan, June Gomez, Helen O'Connor, Sallie J. Rosenfeld
Designers: Maggie Moyer, Robert Perry
Artists: Diane Fox, Bob Jackson, Sandra Simms
Typography Manager: David C. Kosten
Typography Assistant: Diane Paluba
Production Assistant: Thom Staudenmeyer

Pharmacy Consultants
Leigh Hopkins, PharmD, *Assistant Director Pharmacy Service, Thomas Jefferson University Hospital, Philadelphia, Pennsylvania*
John A. Romankiewicz, PharmD, *Assistant Apothecary-in-Chief, New York Hospital, New York, N.Y., and Instructor, Pharmacology, Cornell University Medical College, Ithaca, N.Y.*

Clinical Consultants
Carolyn Holt, RN, BSEd, *Coordinator, Nursing Staff Development, Columbus-Cuneo-Cabrini Medical Center, Chicago, Illinois*
Despina Seremelis, RN, BSN, *Staff Nurse, Temple University Hospital, Philadelphia, Pa.*

Pharmacy Reviewers
Richard Bailey, RPh, *Clinical Pharmacy Service, Temple University Hospital, Philadelphia, Pennsylvania*
Michael R. Cohen, BS, RPh, *Assistant Director, Department of Pharmacy, Temple University Hospital, Philadelphia, Pennsylvania*
Frank Williams, PharmD, *Temple University Hospital, Philadelphia, Pennsylvania*

Nurse Specialist Consultants
Nancy Burns, RN, MSN, *Assistant Professor, University of Texas School of Nursing, Arlington, Texas*
Jeanne Dupont, RN, *Head Nurse, Emergency Department, Massachusetts Eye and Ear Infirmary, Boston, Massachusetts*
Margarethe Hawken, RN, MA, CNRN, *Clinical Nurse Specialist in Neurology and Epilepsy, Seattle Veterans' Administration Medical Center, Seattle, Washington*
Kathleen M. Hawkins, RN, *Clinical Nurse Specialist in Dermatology, University of Colorado Health Sciences Center, Denver, Colorado*
Gail D'Onofrio Long, RN, MS, *Clinical Nurse Specialist in Medical Intensive Care and Coronary Care, University Hospital, Boston, Massachusetts*
Elizabeth A. Phillips, RN, BA, *Instructor in Nursing, St. Francis Medical Center School of Nursing, Trenton, New Jersey*
Paula Brammer Vetter, RN, BSN, *Clinical Instructor in Coronary Intensive Care, Cleveland Clinic Hospital, Cleveland, Ohio*

Library of Congress Cataloging in Publication Data:
Main entry under title:

NURSE'S GUIDE TO DRUGS
(Nurse's reference library)
"*Nursing80* books."
Includes index.
1. Drugs. 2. Pharmacology. 3. Nursing. I. Series.
[DNLM: 1. Drugs—Nursing texts. 2. Drug therapy—Nursing texts. QV55.3 N979]
RM300.N87 615'.1 79-15265
ISBN 0-916730-14-X

Contents

Section IX

Fluid and Electrolyte Balance

Section X

Blood

Section XI

Antineoplastics

Section XII

Eye, Ear, Nose, and Throat

Section XIII

Skin and Mucous Membranes

Contributors

Richard Bailey, BS, Clinical Pharmacy Service, Temple University Hospital, Philadelphia, Pennsylvania

Marquette L. Cannon, PharmD, Assistant Professor of Clinical Pharmacy, Temple University School of Pharmacy, Philadelphia, Pennsylvania

Peter W. Chan, PharmD, Clinical Pharmacist in Ophthalmology, Alcon Laboratories, Inc., Philadelphia, Pennsylvania

Michael R. Cohen, BS, RPH, Assistant Director, Department of Pharmacy, Temple University Hospital, Philadelphia, Pennsylvania

Judith Hopfer Deglin, PharmD, Assistant Professor of Clinical Pharmacy, West Virginia University School of Pharmacy, Morgantown, West Virginia

Betty H. Dennis, MS, Assistant Professor of Clinical Pharmacy, University of North Carolina School of Pharmacy, Chapel Hill, North Carolina

Dina Dichek, BS, Pharmacist, Oakville-Trafalgar Memorial Hospital, Oakville, Ontario, Canada

Teresa P. Dowling, PharmD, Assistant Professor of Clinical Pharmacy, Philadelphia College of Pharmacy and Science, Philadelphia, Pennsylvania

Dan R. Ford, PharmD, Nuclear Pharmacist, National Radiopharmaceutical Company, Houston, Texas

Bruce M. Frey, PharmD, Clinical Pharmacist in Pediatrics, Thomas Jefferson University Hospital, Philadelphia, Pennsylvania

Lee Gardner, PharmD, Clinical Pharmacist, Kino Community Hospital, Tucson, Arizona

Marie Gardner, PharmD, Clinical Pharmacist, Tucson General Hospital, Tucson, Arizona

Philip P. Gerbino, PharmD, Associate Professor of Clinical Pharmacy, Philadelphia College of Pharmacy and Science, Philadelphia, Pennsylvania

Larry N. Gever, PharmD, Clinical Pharmacist, Thomas Jefferson University Hospital, Philadelphia, Pennsylvania

Patricia J. Hedrick, PharmD, Clinical Pharmacist, University of Illinois Hospital, Chicago

James R. Hildebrand, PharmD, Clinical Pharmacist, Thomas Jefferson University Hospital, Philadelphia, Pennsylvania

Arthur I. Jacknowitz, PharmD, Director, Drug Information Center, West Virginia University School of Pharmacy, Morgantown, West Virginia

Sandra G. Jue, PharmD, Clinical Pharmacist, Veterans Administration Medical Center, Boise, Idaho

Barbara H. Korberly, PharmD, Assistant Professor of Clinical Pharmacy, Philadelphia College of Pharmacy and Science, Philadelphia, Pennsylvania

Sheldon M. Leiman, BS, Assistant Director, Department of Pharmacy, Temple University Hospital, Philadelphia, Pennsylvania

Lauren F. McKaig, BS, Tutor in Clinical Pharmacy, Sunnybrook Medical Centre, University of Toronto, Toronto, Ontario, Canada

Kathryn Murphy, MSN, Instructor, Nursing of Children, University of Pennsylvania, Philadelphia, Pennsylvania

David W. Newton, PhD, Associate Professor of Pharmaceutics, Massachusetts College of Pharmacy and Allied Health Sciences, Boston, Massachusetts

Gerald N. Rotenberg, BS, FACA, Editor, Compendium of Pharmaceuticals and Specialties, Canadian Pharmaceutical Association, Toronto, Ontario, Canada

George David Rudd, MS, Assistant Professor of Clinical Pharmacy, University of North Carolina School of Pharmacy, Chapel Hill, North Carolina

Joel Shuster, PharmD, Clinical Pharmacist in Psychiatry, Thomas Jefferson University Hospital, Philadelphia, Pennsylvania

Jamshid B. Tehrani, PhD, Pharmacist Manager, Skin and Cancer Pharmacy, Temple University Hospital, Philadelphia, Pennsylvania

C. Wayne Weart, PharmD, Associate Professor of Pharmacy and Family Practice, Medical University of South Carolina, Charleston

Frank F. Williams, PharmD, Drug Information Pharmacist, Temple University Hospital, Philadelphia, Pennsylvania

Foreword

A MAJOR RESPONSIBILITY in primary nursing care is the dispensing of medication—an everyday part of the nurse's job. As the member of the health-care team physically and legally responsible for administering many drugs, you need to know a great deal about pharmacology: drug toxicities, untoward effects, drug interactions, and dosage peculiarities—starting dose, maximum dose, best route of administration and so on. To make the matter more complex, the very number of drugs you can be expected to administer during ordinary duty is seemingly endless, each with its own special peculiarities and hazards. How to deal with such massively complex and ever-changing data? Obviously, a dependable reference work on drug therapy is indispensable.

The 1979 NURSE'S GUIDE TO DRUGS was compiled to meet this need. Like the first edition, the 1980 NURSE'S GUIDE TO DRUGS contains over 1,000 drug entries. Each entry reflects the fruitful collaboration of clinical pharmacists and nurses to give you pharmacologically accurate information that focuses clearly on what you need to know. And, its comprehensive content is organized in a format that makes this information easy to find. For example, its index makes each drug accessible by both generic and trade names. Drugs are grouped into 16 major sections, depending on their clinical use; their class pharmacology is summarized at the beginning of each section. In tables that follow, each drug is identified by both generic and trade names and is described in tabular form that summarizes: explicit dosage instruction for approved indications, side effects, clinically significant interactions, and nursing considerations. Under nursing considerations are included contraindications, special cautions and hazards, suggestions for administration and patient comfort, and instructions for proper storage and preparation. A special section in the appendices includes specific instruction for managing drugs that produce acute toxicity (narcotics and digitalis, for example). The information includes what symptoms to look for; how to confirm toxicity; and finally, how to manage such toxicity once it has occurred. For added convenience, this book contains special sections on patient teaching, anatomy, physiology, and other selected supplementary information.

I believe that all nurses will find this drug reference a valuable daily resource. As a quick, clear, and reliable source of drug information, it should help you dispel any uncertainty you may have while dispensing drugs. When certainty about drugs replaces uncertainty, you can proceed with confidence and concentrate more totally on patient care.

—LUTHER CHRISTMAN, *Dean*
Rush College of Nursing
Rush University
Chicago, Illinois

Rx

General Information

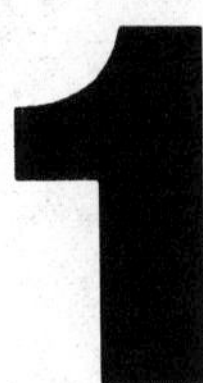

How to use Nurse's Guide to Drugs

Nurse's Guide to Drugs is meant to fill a very special need. It represents a joint effort by pharmacists and nurses to provide the nursing profession with drug information that focuses directly on what nurses need to know. With this in mind, it emphasizes clinical aspects, not pharmacology and does not attempt to replace detailed pharmacology texts. For the same reason, the information is arranged in a format designed to make it readily accessible.

Introductory information

Following this chapter are three other preliminary chapters. Chapters 2 and 3 summarize the nursing implications of drug therapy in adults and children. Chapter 4 explains, in a general way, how drugs work. It also tells about side effects and adverse reactions, and gives general guidelines about drug use in pregnancy and the presence of drugs in breast milk.

In the remaining chapters—except for Chapter 67, which explains the nursing implications of chemotherapy—all drugs are classified according to their common, approved therapeutic use. Each chapter has two parts. The first, an introductory section, summarizes the known pharmacology of the drugs in that chapter. Specifically, this part of the chapter briefly answers the following questions:

- What are the principal therapeutic uses of these drugs?
- Is their mechanism of action known? If so, what is it?
- How are these drugs absorbed, distributed, and excreted?
- How long do they take to act, and how long do their effects last?
- Finally, what are the principal combination products in which these drugs are commonly found?

Tabular information

The second part of each chapter consists of tabular information divided into five columns: *In the first column:* an alphabetic list of drugs by generic name, immediately followed by an alphabetic list of brand names. (Occasionally, a combination product appears in the tables under the head of its major ingredient.) Brands available in both the United States and Canada are designated with a diamond (♦); those available *only* in Canada with a double diamond (♦♦). A brand name with no symbol after it is available only in the United States. If a drug is a controlled substance, that too is clearly indicated (example: Controlled substance Schedule II).

In the second column: major indications and specific dosage instructions for adults and children, as applicable. Children's doses are usually indicated in terms of mg/Kg/day. Dosage instructions reflect current clinical trends in therapeutics and can't be considered an absolute and universal recommendation. For individual application, dosage instructions must be considered in context with the patient's clinical condition.

In the third column: a list of each drug's commonly observed side effects (and rare ones, if hazardous). Side effects are grouped according to the body system in which they appear.

In the fourth column: each drug's confirmed, *clinically significant* interactions with other drugs, including additive effects, potentiated effects, and antagonistic effects. Also included are specific suggestions for dealing with dangerous drug interaction (for example, reducing doses, or monitoring certain lab tests). Drug interactions are listed under the drug that is adversely affected. For example, magnesium trisilicate, an ingredient in antacids, interacts with tetracycline to cause decreased absorption of tetracycline. Therefore, this interaction is listed under tetracycline. To check on the possible effects of using two or more drugs simultaneously, refer to the interaction entry for *each* of the drugs in question.

In the fifth column: nursing considerations starting with contraindications and precautions, followed by monitoring techniques and suggestions for prevention and treatment of side effects. Also included in this column are suggestions for promoting patient comfort, for patient teaching, and for preparing, administering, and storing each drug.

Appendices

Seven appendices offer useful supplementary information. This information includes detailed information on the recognition and management of acute toxicity; a chart that shows compatibility of intravenous solutions; a table of equivalents (conversions); a nomogram for estimating surface area in children—an essential for calculating accurate pediatric doses; an explanation and list of controlled substances; and a list of abbreviations used throughout the book. Finally, a comprehensive index lists each drug alphabetically by both generic and brand name and lists the subject of illustrations and teaching tips. Drugs that do not appear in the index are mainly fillers, preservatives, and drugs that are not used alone.

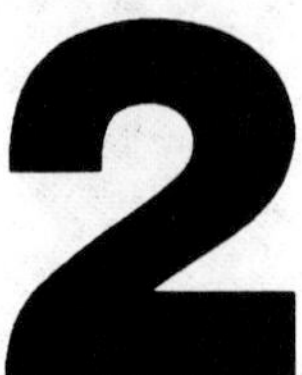

Nursing implications of drug therapy in adults

Since the nurse is the member of the health care team most frequently responsible for administering prescribed medication, her knowledge of drug therapy and administration must be thorough and up-to-date. What follows is a list of key points to keep in mind.

I. General considerations

- No medicine, not even a placebo, should ever be administered to a patient except on doctor's orders. Nevertheless, every nurse should make a point of knowing how a given drug can be expected to act, as well as whatever unpleasant or harmful side effects it can have.
- Before administering a drug in a nonunit dose system, read the label on the bottle three times (when taking it from the shelf, when preparing the dose, and when returning it to the shelf). Remember that the names of different drugs often have similar spellings. If the bottle is without a label, throw it away or return it to the pharmacy. Never give a patient anything found in an unlabeled bottle.
- If you are working with a unit dose system, with doses prepared by pharmacy and placed in patient bins on a drug cart, compare the label on the dose against the medication record. Hand the labeled dose of oral medication to the patient for opening at the time of administration (whenever possible). After observing the patient take the drug(s), return to the medication administration record and sign off the dose as given. Make certain that you check the patient's wristband for proper identification before giving any drug; then address the patient by name.
- Be on guard against interruptions while you are preparing a dose of medication. If you have any doubt whatsoever regarding a dose you have calculated, double-check with the pharmacist or with a knowledgeable nurse. Generally, it is best if the nurse who prepares a dose of medication also administers and records it (except in a unit dose system).
- Always be sure to replace the cap on any bottle of medication you open. Make sure, too, that it is tightly shut. Do not leave any bottles of medication lying about, and never leave medications at a patient's bedside, except—on doctor's orders—antacids, anticholinesterase medications, nonnarcotic cough syrups, inhalants, various lotions and ointments, and nitroglycerin.
- When storing drugs, keep preparations designed for external use only separate and distinct from those designed for internal use. Insist that the pharmacist affix "external use only" labels on drug containers. Keep narcotics and other controlled drugs under double lock.
- Should a patient express doubt or concern as to the particular medication you are about to give him, always recheck, just in case a mistake has been made. After all, there is *no* margin for error when it comes to administering drugs. Always go out of your way, therefore, to make absolutely certain that the *right* dose of the *right* medication is given to the

right patient at the *right* time by the *right* route.

• Should a patient refuse to take his medication, try to find out why he refuses. Report the matter to the team leader and the pharmacist, and make a note in the patient's record as to why he refused. Discard the medication (except under a unit dose system; in that case, return the medication in its wrapper or container, along with proper documentation, to the pharmacy). Should a patient vomit shortly after taking oral medication, determine what the medication was, then notify the doctor. Do not give the patient another dose of the medication in question unless the doctor orders it.

• Doses of medication should always be administered within 30 minutes of the time officially prescribed. Be especially punctual when administering antibiotics, chemotherapeutic agents, and anticholinesterase agents, as it is essential that a particular level of such drugs be maintained in the bloodstream. Should any dose of medication not be given as scheduled, the reason should be recorded in the nurse's notes and reported to the pharmacist.

• When administering drugs p.r.n., always determine that enough time has passed since the last dose.

• Chart fluids given with medication on intake and output record.

• Do not give medication that is discolored or in which a precipitate has formed unless the manufacturer's instructions indicate that doing so is not harmful.

• Provide privacy as needed when administering certain medications (suppositories, retention enemas, etc.).

• Keep accurate records of all doses of medication administered. Also note the patient's reactions to medications, and in the case of narcotics, routinely record the patient's pulse and respiration as well.

• Do not hold tablets or capsules in your hands.

• Discard needles and syringes into proper containers.

• Store drugs as recommended.

• Never borrow a medication intended for one patient to give to another patient. There may be a good reason why a patient's medication is missing (mistranscription on nursing record, order clarification in process, pharmacy never received original order are some possibilities). Borrowing often leads to medication error.

• If more than one or two dosage units (tablets, capsules, or ampules) are needed to prepare a single dose, something might be wrong! Unless you are absolutely familiar with this need—check with a pharmacist before preparing dose. If large numbers of tablets or capsules are found to be necessary, the pharmacist might be able to prepare a dosage form that would be more convenient to the patient.

• Wash your hands thoroughly before preparing or administering any medication.

II. Specific precautions for certain drugs

• *Digitalis preparations.* Before giving a patient any digitalis preparation, note his pulse rate; if the apical pulse is abnormally fast or slow for that patient, or has changed drastically since the previous dose, notify the doctor.

• *Heparin.* When administering heparin subcutaneously, make sure that 0.1 cubic centimeters of air is in the syringe before you inject. This clears the heparin from the syringe and helps prevent it from leaking into tissue, thus avoiding localized hemorrhaging. You can reduce the possibility of hematoma by injecting heparin into the subcutaneous tissues of the abdomen above the iliac crest. *Do not* check for insertion into a vein by drawing back the plunger; doing so will make the needle waver and precipitate a hematoma. For the same reason, never massage the injection site; doing so could rupture capillaries.

• *Insulin.* Administration of insulin requires a definite plan for rotation of injection sites. The arms, thighs, abdomen, and buttocks together provide at least 56 different injection sites (see illustration,p. 625).But care must be taken that the same site is not used more than once every two months; otherwise, changes brought about in the fatty tissue can make the absorption of insulin more difficult.

If called upon to mix regular insulin with a longer-acting type, draw up the regular insulin first; that way you avoid contaminating it with the insoluble longer-acting type. Regular insulin should always be maintained in pure solution, so that, in the event of an emergency, it can be given I.V.

• *Narcotics.* Before administering narcotics, always check and record the patient's respiration. Narcotics tend to depress the respiratory center, and a respiratory rate of 12 or below is too low for safe administration of narcotic drugs. Also check and record the patient's pulse; it is an indicator of pain, and it's important to know how the patient's pulse and respiration rates correlate.

• *Paraldehyde.* Always administer parenteral paraldehyde with a glass syringe; it interacts chemically with plastic. For the same reason, never administer oral paraldehyde in a Styrofoam cup.

III. Oral medications

• Always read the instructions on a bottle of medicine carefully, and follow them to the letter.

• When pouring liquid medicine, pour with the label side up, so that none of the liquid spills over and obscures the instructions written on the label. Also, when you've finished pouring, wipe the mouth of the bottle.

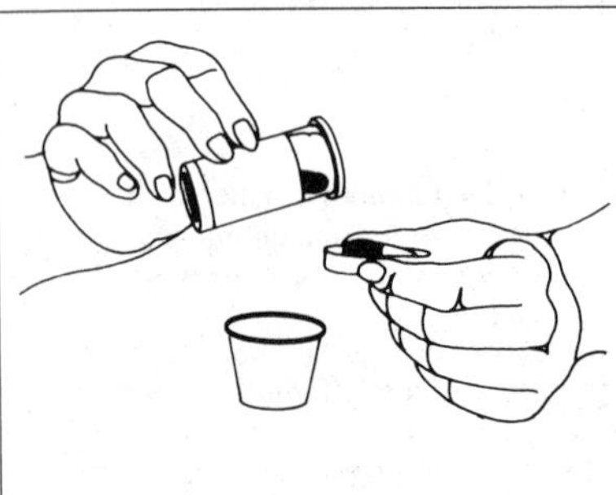

To prevent contamination and insure proper drainage, always pour tablets into their container's cap before placing them in the patient's medication cup.

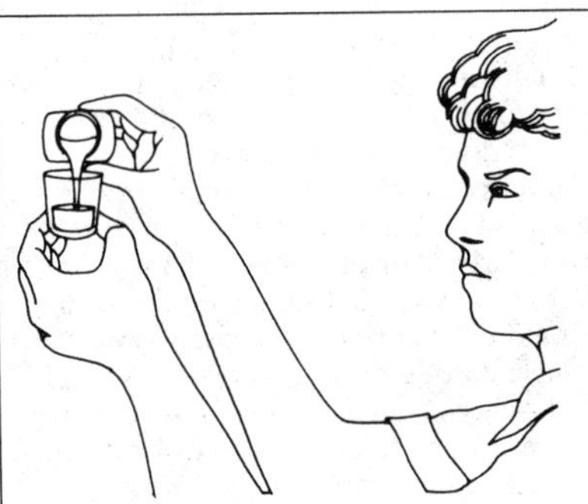

When pouring liquid medication, hold a graduated container at eye level, using the bottom of the meniscus as your measuring guide.

- To insure accuracy when using a graduated medicine cup, hold it at eye level.
- If a dose of medication is to be measured in drops, use a medicine dropper held at a 90° angle.
- Do not break tablets unless they are scored.
- Do not give enteric-coated tablets with milk or antacids. Higher pH causes these tablets to dissolve prematurely in the stomach.
- Instruct the patient not to chew, crush, dissolve, or tamper with enteric-coated tablets or sustained-action medication.
- Should a patient have difficulty swallowing a pill, have him place it far back in his mouth, since stimulating the back of the tongue activates the swallowing mechanism.
- Provide the patient with water or another suitable liquid, and stay with him while he takes the medication.
- Diluting a drug usually makes it more palatable and may promote absorption. Dilute liquid medications—except cough syrups, oils, and antacids—with water or juice, unless contraindicated (check information on label to determine how compatible the medication is with various juices). Use water only for diluting medications for diabetics and for patients on potassium restriction.

IV. Parenteral medications

- The term parenteral, when applied to the administration of drugs, refers to the introduction of drugs into the body by means of injection into the upper layers of the skin, the subcutaneous tissue, the muscles, or the veins.

Intradermal

- Intradermal injections are those made into the upper layers of the skin. Drugs are administered in this way as skin tests.
- The medial surface of the forearm is perhaps the most commonly used site for intradermal injection. Use a tuberculin syringe with a fine, short, 26-gauge needle. Cleanse the area, hold the syringe at a 15° angle, and make sure the tip of the needle enters just under the outer layer of the skin. If done properly, a small bleb should form. No more than 0.1 ml should be injected.

Subcutaneous

- Subcutaneous injections are those made beneath the skin. Drugs administered this way are absorbed into the system more slowly than those administered intramuscularly or intravenously. Only nonirritating drugs should be injected subcutaneously, and the amount injected should never exceed 2 ml. Use a hypodermic syringe with a 25-gauge needle.

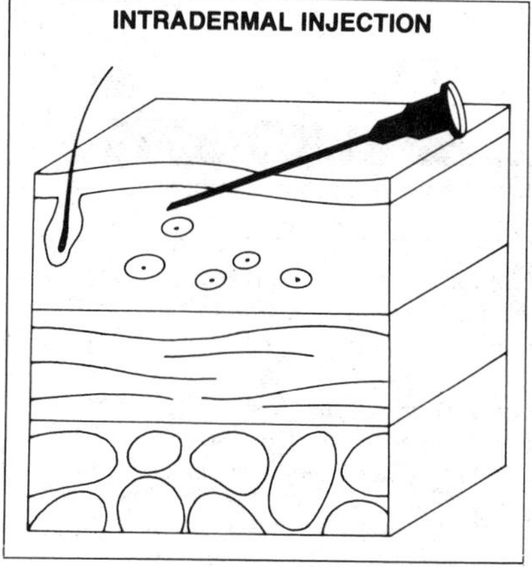

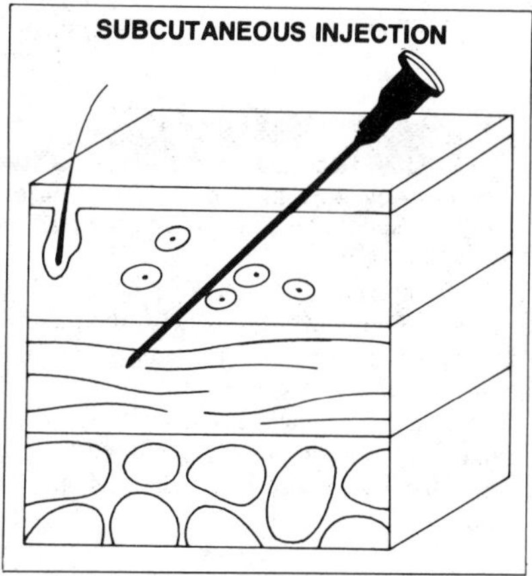

• Any body surface area where there is loose connective tissue that is located away from the large blood vessels and large muscle groups may be used as a site for subcutaneous injection. Favored areas include the outer surface of the upper arm and the anterior and lateral surfaces of the thigh.
• Clean the injection site with an alcohol sponge beforehand, using a circular motion and moving from the center outward.
• To prevent the needle from entering the muscle, insert it at a 45° angle, and hold the tissue surrounding the injection site in cushion fashion. Release the tissue as soon as the needle is inserted; otherwise, pressure against the nerve endings will cause pain.
• Take care that the needle does not enter a blood vessel; if it does, the solution will be absorbed into the patient's system immediately, and this could prove dangerous. Prevent this by pulling back gently on the plunger after the needle is inserted; if blood appears, withdraw the needle, prepare another dose—using another syringe and needle—then insert it again at a different angle and site. Test again, and if no blood appears, slowly inject the solution.
• Withdraw the needle quickly; this prevents the tissue from pulling, which causes pain. Gentle massage of the injection site with an alcohol sponge stimulates the circulation in the area and facilitates the distribution and absorption of the solution into the system.
• Record each injection site and work out a plan for rotation.

Intramuscular

• An intramuscular injection introduces into muscular tissue a medicinal solution that is then absorbed into the bloodstream.
• Any body surface area with a significant amount of muscular tissue and located away from large blood vessels and nerves may serve as sites for intramuscular injection. Favored areas include the mid-deltoid area, the gluteus medius, the ventrogluteal area, and the vastus lateralis.
• When injecting into the gluteal region, take care to avoid injecting the needle into either

VENTROGLUTEAL INJECTION

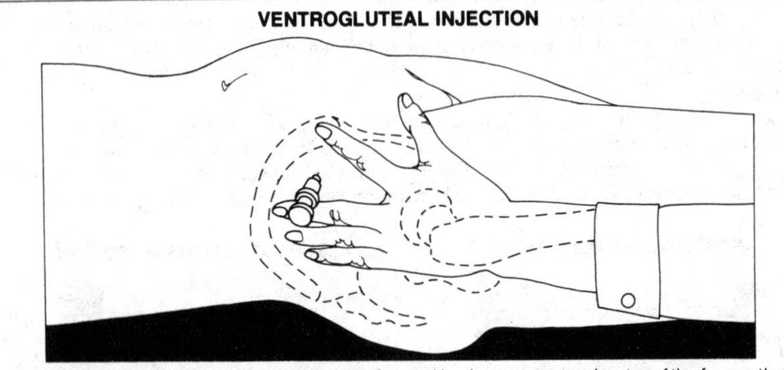

Inject the patient within the triangular area formed by the greater trochanter of the femur, the anterior superior iliac spine and the iliac crest.

the sciatic nerve or the superior gluteal artery. Have the patient lie on his stomach with his toes pointing inward; this helps the muscles relax and provides maximum exposure.
• Injecting a needle into a tense muscle causes pain. Have the patient relax beforehand by taking several slow, deep breaths.
• Ordinarily, a 1½-inch, 21-gauge needle is used for I.M. injections. A shorter needle should be used if the patient is thin, and a longer one if he is obese. The viscosity of the solution itself must also be taken into consideration when determining what gauge needle to use.

• After drawing up the medication into the syringe, draw up approximately 0.2 or 0.3 ml of air into the syringe as well. The air bubble clears the needle after the drug is injected and prevents leakage into subcutaneous tissue.
• Clean the injection site beforehand, using a circular motion and moving from the center outward. Insert the needle at a 90° angle.
• Take care that the needle does not enter a blood vessel; if it does, the solution will be absorbed more rapidly than intended. To prevent this, pull back gently on the plunger after the needle is inserted; if blood appears, withdraw the needle, prepare another dose—using another syringe and needle—then insert it again at a different angle and site. Test again, and if no blood appears, slowly inject the solution.
• Withdraw the needle quickly; this prevents the tissue from pulling, which causes pain. Gentle massage of the injection site with an alcohol sponge stimulates the circulation in the area and facilitates distribution and absorption of the solution into the system.
• When injecting substances that stain or are irritating, use the Z-track method. Use a needle that is 2 inches long. In addition to the medication, draw up approximately 0.2 of air into the syringe. Then change the needle. Before injecting laterally displace the subcutaneous tissue at the injection site (when using this technique, always inject into the gluteus medius). Upon completing the injection, wait 10 seconds before withdrawing the needle. This delay, the air bubble, and the relaxation of the laterally displaced tissue upon its release, together help ensure that the needle track is properly sealed off. Do not massage the injection site after the needle is withdrawn. Doing so can cause the solution to back into the subcutaneous tissue.
• Record each injection site and work out a plan for rotation.

Intravenous

• Intravenous therapy involves introducing medication or other parenteral fluids into a patient's vein. A bolus injection introduces a concentrated amount of solution all at once.

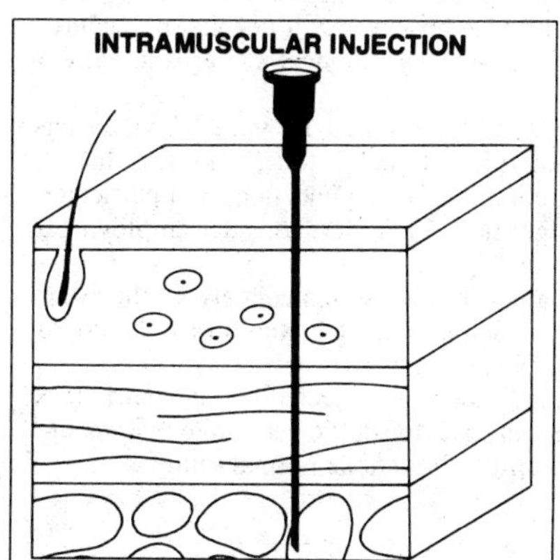

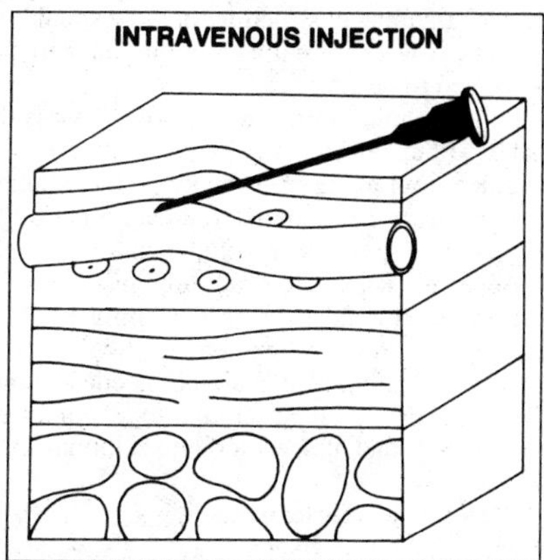

An intravenous infusion introduces a large amount of fluid over an extended period. Intravenous infusions are used to maintain or replace the body's water, electrolytes, and calories; to restore the body's acid/base balance; to replenish blood volume; and to provide access for the administration of various medications.
• Substances injected intravenously are absorbed into the system immediately. Take special care to prevent or recognize toxic reactions or shock caused by introducing too much solution too quickly or by allergic reactions. The patient's condition, age, the type of fluid or drug being administered, the size of the administration set, and the viscosity of the

liquid itself, are the principal factors determining the rate of flow, which should (for accuracy) be measured in microdrops (requiring a special solution set), and strictly in accordance with the doctor's instructions.

• Dilute the medication according to directions, but use an unopened, sterile vial of diluent, since diluent used previously for other drugs may well have been contaminated by them. Most drugs prove irritating to the vessel walls, but proper dilution can at least keep such irritation to a minimum. Unit doses are best diluted and prepared by the pharmacist.

• Before administering any medication intravenously, take into consideration the possibility of drug incompatibilities. Clean the injection site with an alcohol sponge before inserting the needle or catheter, using a circular motion and moving from the center outward.

• I.V. tubing and dressings should be changed daily. Apply antimicrobial ointment to the injection site. Record on the I.V. dressing and on the patient's chart the catheter type and the date the needle or catheter was inserted.

• To administer small amounts (150 ml or less) of I.V. solution or diluted medication, a volume-control I.V. set may be used. Such sets should be changed daily, and the date and time of change should be recorded. Only one medication may be administered via a single volume-control set.

• Another method is the piggyback technique, which uses minibottles or minibags. Pharmacy prepares a single dose in a 100- to 250-ml bottle. The bottle is attached to a solution set before administration and the line cleared of air. This set is "piggybacked" by needle into a primary line.

• Supplemental drugs may be administered with a needle and syringe into the injection device on the tubing, which should be flushed with 10 ml of sterile normal saline solution immediately before and after each such injection. Make sure also that supplemental drugs are administered only one at a time.

• Should the flow of solution stop, first check for signs of infiltration. Then try to determine if the tubing is in any way defective. Also, by holding the bottle below the level of the needle, anything obstructing the flow should be dislodged backward. If hospital procedure permits, irrigate the catheter with 1 ml sterile normal saline solution. If a filter is in place, it may need to be changed.

• Before administering an I.V. bolus, assess the patient's tolerance. How are his vital signs? Is his output sufficient? Administer slowly. A good rule of thumb is to take not less than 1 minute (but make sure you know the administration rate before injecting). If a particular drug needs to be administered over a period longer than 5 minutes, consider employing a piggyback infusion, or a volume-control set infusion.

• Adverse reactions to drugs administered I.V. can occur almost immediately. In the event such a reaction does occur, discontinue administration immediately and notify the doctor. Emergency drugs and equipment should be available at all times.

• When additional fluids are not needed, some medications are injected into a heparin lock, a catheter or cannula inserted into a vein for that purpose. Flush the heparin lock immediately before and after with dilute solutions of heparin and/or sterile normal saline.

V. Ophthalmic medications

• First, wash your hands.

• To instill eyedrops, position the patient with his head back and his eyes open. Pull the lower eyelid down in such a way as to form a small pocket with the lid. Have the patient roll his eyes upward, then squeeze one drop of medication onto the lining of the lid. (If more than one drop needs to be administered, have the patient blink before instilling the second. Do not be concerned about the part of the dose lost in tears.) The medication should be aimed at the lower conjunctiva and not at the cornea, which is very sensitive. Also, do not touch any part of the eye with the eyedropper. Have the patient close his eyes immediately upon your releasing his eyelid, then gently blot away any excess medication with a tissue or a cotton ball.

• To instill eye ointments, first cleanse the patient's eyelids with a saline or other irrigating solution. Take care not to contaminate the applicator. Squeeze a small amount of medication onto the lining of the lower lid. Release the eyelid, have the patient close his eyes, and gently blot away any excess medication. See p. 811 for further instuctions.

VI. Ear drops

• Always administer drops at room temperature, since cold drops can cause severe pain. Have the patient lie on his side; gently pull the pinna up and back; instill the drops. Have the patient remain lying on his side for several minutes longer. See p. 850 for futher instructions.

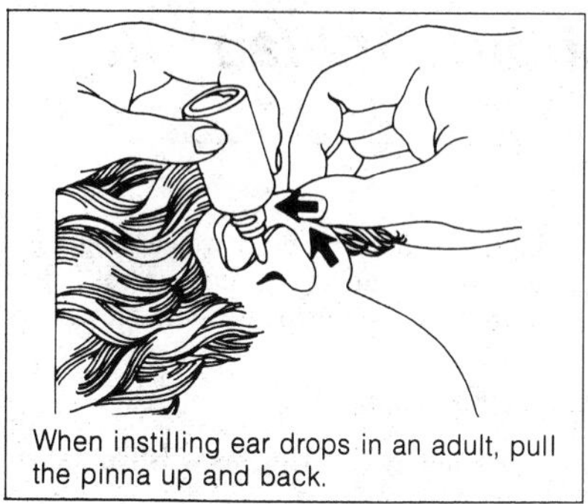

When instilling ear drops in an adult, pull the pinna up and back.

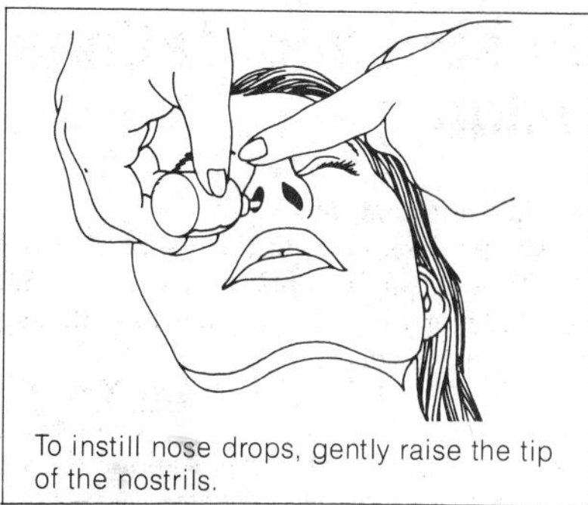

To instill nose drops, gently raise the tip of the nostrils.

VII. Nose drops

• Medication is absorbed into the nostrils more easily if the patient tilts his head backward. Gently raise the tip of the nostril and instill the drops. Make sure that the dropper does not come into contact with the nasal mucosa.

VIII. Topical drugs and suppositories

• Liquid and semisolid topicals should be applied strictly according to the directions on the label and the doctor's directions.

• To administer a rectal suppository, first lubricate the tip of the suppository with a small amount of water-soluble jelly. Have the patient lie on his left side. Insert the suppository with a gloved hand, then press downward on the buttocks for a few moments until the urge to expel subsides. Instruct the patient about the purpose of the suppository.

• To administer a vaginal suppository, first have the patient assume the lithotomy position. Lubricate the tip of the suppository with a small amount of water-soluble jelly or water, then insert it into the vagina with a gloved hand or applicator. Have the patient remain with her hips elevated for about 5 minutes.

• When administering a urethral suppository, first cleanse the perineal area thoroughly, then insert the suppository using standard sterile procedures.

• Sublingual tablets should be placed under the patient's tongue, where the rich supply of blood facilitates absorption. Ask the patient not to drink fluids or swallow excessively until the drug is completely absorbed.

IX. Instructing the patient

• Patients have a right to know what drugs they are receiving. Warn them beforehand as to possible side effects and possible allergic reactions. Moreover, inform patients who do experience adverse reactions how to prevent another such reaction to future doses. Prepare patients who are being discharged and their families by telling them everything they need to know about taking their medication at home.

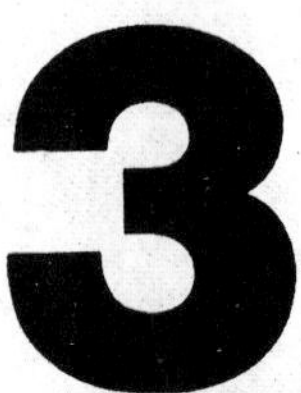

Nursing implications of drug therapy in children

General considerations

• Pediatric doses of medication should be calculated in terms of either body weight (mg/Kg/day) or body surface area ($mg/m^2/day$). If information concerning a given dose is not available in mg/Kg, and you question the dose prescribed, the following formula may be used to double-check:

$$\frac{\text{adult dose X child's age (in years)}}{\text{child's age} + 12} = \text{dose}$$

• Before giving any child medication, verify his identification by checking his wristband. Do not simply ask the child his name.

• The doctor's accountability for the doses of medication he prescribes does not relieve the nurse of her responsibility for knowing whether or not a particular dose of medication she administers is safe. Especially make sure to double-check with another nurse regarding doses of insulin, anticoagulants, or digitalis preparations.

• Positive reinforcement invariably proves more effective in dealing with children than threats or bribes. Allow a child to express his fears, but encourage him to overcome them, and praise him when he does.

• Meticulously record the number and the size of every dose of medication you administer, as well as the time at which each was administered.

Oral medications

• Infants should always be given oral medication in liquid form, if available. First, measure the dose with a tuberculin syringe or oral syringe. Then, lift the infant's head to prevent aspiration, and press down on his chin to open his mouth. Administer the medication in small amounts with a plastic dropper or syringe, aiming the fluid at the inside of the cheek. You may also place the medication in a nipple and allow the child to suck the contents; or you can add the medication to small amounts of food, provided the drug's absorption into the system will not be affected. Remember, too, that certain drugs, such as antibiotics, cannot be administered immediately after meals.

• If the child is a toddler, provide him with a simple explanation of what is going to happen. To increase his cooperation, try to think of choices you can offer the child. Enlist the parent's help in gaining the child's cooperation, or in restraining him only if necessary and only if, in your judgment, the parent will not become upset and aggravate the situation.
If the drug is in tablet form, you may crush the tablets—provided they are not enteric-coated or timed-release—and dissolve them in a small amount of syrup. Don't mix medication with food, however; doing so may cause a child to start refusing his meals. Also, use a calibrated medication cup, since it's easier for a small child to drink a liquid than to take it from a spoon.

• Have a school-age child place the tablet or capsule on the back of his tongue and swallow it with water or juice.

Intravenous

- Accurately record the solution, the rate, and the amount of I.V. fluid administered.
- In infants, the easiest place to insert an I.V. needle or catheter, and the place where it is least likely to be dislodged, is in the vein located in the temporal region of the skull.
- As little as 10 cc of air, introduced into the bloodstream, can prove fatal. So take care to ensure that the I.V. tubing is free of air. First, attach the tubing and the graduated chamber to the bottle of fluid. Next, hang the bottle on an I.V. pole, approximately 18 to 24 inches above the vein. Open the clamp and let the fluid fill both chamber and tubing. This should eliminate any air bubbles. In addition, to prevent accidental dripping into the chamber, be certain that the flow clamp opening between the bottle and the graduated chamber or drip regulator is completely shut.
- Since the tubing is heavy enough to dislodge the needle, anchor the tubing in such a way as to keep it from pulling. Place a shield over the injection site to protect the needle further from accidental dislodgement: Take a paper cup, cut the top off, and cut a hole on both sides, so the tubing can fit through. If the needle is inserted into an arm vein, use an armboard for added support. Make sure the drip regulator is out of the child's reach and that he cannot dislodge the needle by moving his extremities. You may do this by placing a clip or tab of adhesive tape below the regulator; this will prevent it from slipping down the tubing, into the child's reach. Restrain the child only when absolutely necessary—that is, when all else fails. Try padding the area well, and place a mitt or nylon hose over his hands first. Watch the child closely. If a child must be restrained at night to prevent pulling at the I.V. in his sleep, explain to him—if he is old enough to understand—why this is so, and that the restraint will be removed in the morning.
- Because of their smaller size, infants or children who are given too much I.V. fluid too quickly can experience a fatal coronary episode. Pressure, the size of the tubing, and the viscosity of the liquid itself are the principal factors determining the rate of flow, which should be regulated in terms of microdrips (1 drop: 1/60 ml) and strictly in accordance with the doctor's instructions. Check the rate of flow and the child's reaction at least once every hour—and more frequently than that at the start of an infusion and when infusing medication—and carefully record both intake and output. Adjust the rate of flow while the child is quiet, because crying tends to constrict the blood vessels, and the rate of flow is likely to increase when the crying stops.
- To infuse small amounts of fluid more precisely, use a mechanical infusion pump. The amount of fluid infused should be checked at least once every hour. Mechanical infusion devices are by no means fail-safe. Bear in mind, too, that they continue to pump even if the needle becomes dislodged.
- When the amount of fluid prescribed has been administered, stop the flow by closing the clamp nearest the needle. When removing the needle, be especially careful; otherwise, tissue may be damaged in the process. Moreover, any skin puncture can admit bacteria into

the system and lead to infection. Hold the needle firmly with one hand, and with the other carefully remove the adhesive tape. Then, while holding a sterile cotton sponge over the injection site, slowly pull the needle out. Make sure the hub of the needle stays flush with the skin, and avoid dragging the needle against the vein's posterior wall. Exert pressure on the injection site until whatever bleeding occurs subsides.

- Reassess the child's fluid balance at least once every four hours. In particular, be alert for signs of *fluid overload* or *dehydration*. Symptoms of fluid overload include fine rales, edema, rapid pulse, hypertension, rising urine output, and falling urine specific gravity. Symptoms of dehydration include depressed fontanels, dry mucous membranes, poor skin turgor, falling urine output, and rising specific gravity.
- Should the rate of flow become slower than what was ordered, assess the child's ability to tolerate an increased rate, then consult with the doctor as to the advisability of gradually infusing the additional amount over several hours. Do not attempt to catch up by rapidly increasing the rate of flow, and *never* increase the rate if the glucose concentration of the infusion is greater than 5%.
- Before administering any medication intravenously, always examine the injection site for signs of infiltration or infection. Be especially careful in dealing with infants, because they can't tell you if they feel pain at the site of injection. Be careful, too, with peripheral infusions of substances that are irritating, such as levarterenol.
- If using a catheter, tape it securely, but don't obscure the site so much that subsequent assessment is made difficult.
- Change the solution, the graduated chamber, and the tubing every day.

Intramuscular

- In children under the age of two, use one of the vastus lateralis muscles as the site of injection. In children over age two, use either the ventrogluteal area or the gluteus medius.
- In determining what size needle to use, consider the child's age, his nutritional status, muscle mass, and the viscosity of the drug. When injecting less than 1 ml, use a tuberculin syringe for greater accuracy. Record the injection sites, and use them subsequently in rotation.
- Never tell a child that an injection he is about to receive won't hurt; if it does, he'll never

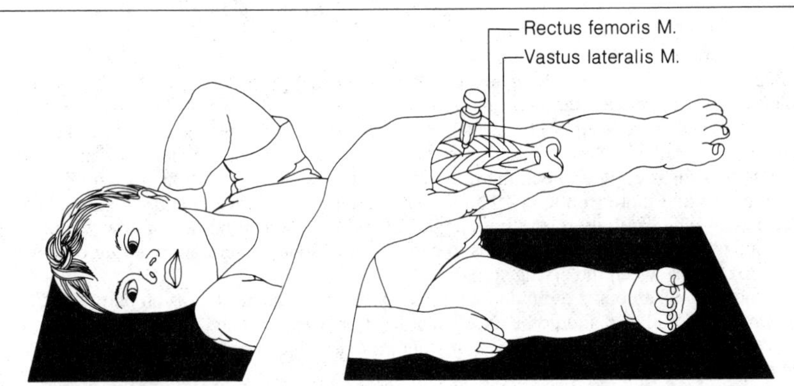

To give an I.M. injection to an infant or child under 2 years, use the vastus lateralis. The major muscle of the quadriceps femoris group in the anterolateral thigh, it's better developed and thus a superior choice over the gluteal group.

trust you again. Tell him instead that you know the injection is probably going to hurt at least a bit, but that it will help him to get well. Restrain even the most cooperative child, but praise, rock, and reassure him afterward.

• To keep the child's initial reaction when the needle is inserted to a minimum, stimulate peripheral nerves by gently tapping the injection site several times with your fingers before you give an injection.

• Clean the injection site beforehand with an alcohol sponge, using a circular motion and moving from the center outward.

Subcutaneous

• Subcutaneous injections are commonly used for administering insulin and heparin to children, but the details of administration are essentially the same as for adults, except for dosage.

Ear drops

• Always use warm drops; cold drops can cause severe pain. If the child is younger than three years, pull the pinna down and back; if he is over three years old, pull the pinna up and back.

Rectal suppositories

• Lubricate the tip of the suppository with a small amount of water-soluble jelly; insert the suppository, then press downward on the buttocks for a few moments until the urge to expel subsides. In preschool children, a certain amount of distraction may prove helpful also.

Nasal drops

• Medication is absorbed into the nares more easily if the head is hyperextended. Make sure that the dropper does not come into contact with the nasal mucosa, since microorganisms can spread as a result.

• A congested nose can interfere with an infant's ability to suck. For this reason, decongestant nose drops should be instilled 20 minutes before feeding time.

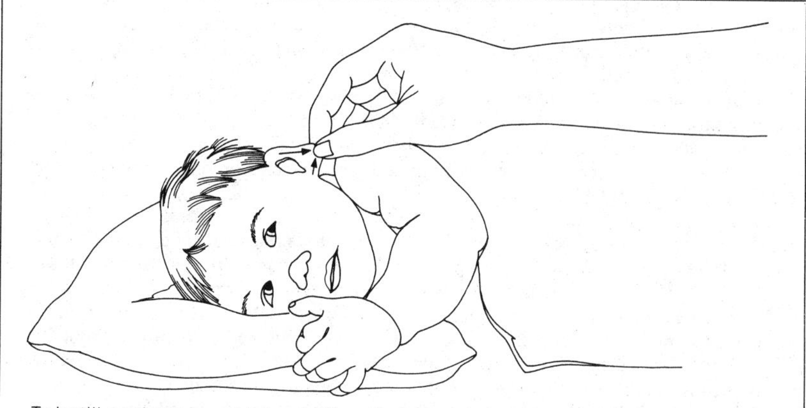

To instill eardrops in a child under 3, pull pinna down and back. After the drops, if the child has any pain, notify the doctor.

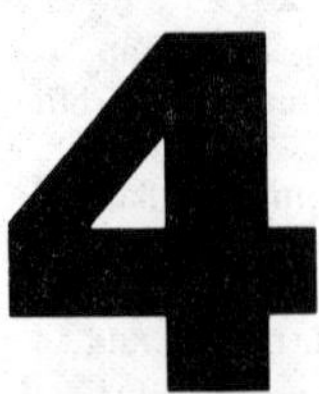

Drug actions, reactions, and interactions explained

Administration of any drug provokes a series of events within the body. The first event, when a drug combines with cell drug receptors, is known as the drug action. What follows as a result of this action of the drug is known as the drug effect. Depending upon the number of different cellular drug receptors affected by a given drug, a drug effect can be local or systemic, or both. For example, the antipeptic ulcer drug Tagamet (cimetidine) acts solely by blocking histamine receptor cells in the small intestine and the stomach. This is known as a local drug effect because the drug action is sharply limited to one area and does not spread to other parts of the body. On the other hand, Benadryl (diphenhydramine) produces a systemic effect, in that it blocks histamine receptors in widespread areas of the body. In other words, local drug effects are specific to a limited number of organ systems, whereas systemic drug effects are generalized and affect different and diverse organ systems.

Three factors modify drug action

1. Absorption

Before a drug can act within the body, it must be absorbed into the bloodstream—usually after oral administration, the most frequently used route. Before a drug contained in a tablet or capsule can be absorbed, the dosage form must disintegrate, that is, break into smaller particles. Then, these smaller particles can dissolve in gastric juices. Only after so dissolving can a drug be absorbed into the bloodstream. Once absorbed and circulating in the bloodstream, it is said to be bioavailable, or ready to produce a drug effect. Of course, whether such absorption is complete or partial depends on several factors: the physiochemical effects of the drug, the formulation of the drug product, its interactions with other substances in the gastrointestinal tract, and various patient characteristics. These same factors also determine the speed of absorption. Thus, oral solutions and elixirs, which bypass the need for disintegration and dissolution, are usually absorbed more rapidly. Drugs administered intramuscularly must first be absorbed through the muscle, into the bloodstream. Rectal suppositories must dissolve to be absorbed through the rectal mucosa. Of course, drugs administered intravenously are placed directly into the circulation and are completely and immediately bioavailable.

2. Distribution

After absorption, a drug moves from the bloodstream into various fluids and tissues within the body; this is distribution. Individual patient variations can greatly alter the amount of drug that is distributed throughout the body. For example, in an edematous patient, a given dose must be distributed to a larger volume than in a nonedematous patient; the amount of drug must sometimes be increased to account for this. Remember, the dosage should be decreased when the edema is corrected. Conversely, in an extremely dehydrated patient, the drug will be distributed to a much smaller volume, so the dose must then be decreased. The total area to which a drug is distributed is known as volume of distribution. Patients who are particularly obese may present another problem when considering drug distribution. Some drugs—such as digoxin, gentamicin, and tobramycin—are not well distributed to fatty tissue. Therefore, dosing based on actual body weight may lead to overdose and serious toxicity. In some cases, dosing must be based on lean body weight, which may be estimated from actuarial tables that give average weight range for height.

3. Metabolism and excretion (drug elimination)

Most drugs are metabolized in the liver and excreted by the kidneys. Hepatic diseases may affect one or more of the metabolic functions of the liver. Therefore, in patients with hepatic disease, the metabolism of a drug may be increased, decreased, or unchanged. Clearly, all patients with hepatic disease must be monitored closely for drug effect and toxicity. Some drugs (digoxin, gentamicin) are eliminated almost unchanged by the kidneys. For safe use of such drugs, renal function must be adequate or the drug will accumulate, producing toxic effects. Some drugs can alter the effect and excretion of other drugs. For example, they can stimulate hepatic metabolizing enzymes to speed up the rate of metabolism and change the drug effect. Or, they can block or promote renal excretion of other drugs, causing them to accumulate and enhance their effects, or causing them to be too rapidly excreted and so diminish their effects. Some slight elimination takes place by way of perspiration, saliva, breast milk, and so on. (Certain volatile anesthetics, however—halothane, for instance—are eliminated primarily by exhalation.)

The rate at which a drug is metabolized varies with the individual. In some patients, drugs are metabolized so quickly that their serum and tissue levels prove therapeutically inadequate. In others, the rate of metabolism is so slow that ordinary doses can produce toxic results.

Other modifying factors

An important factor that influences a drug's action and effect is its *binding to plasma proteins,* especially albumin, and other tissue components. Because only free, unbound drug can act in the body, such binding greatly influences effectiveness and duration of effect. The *patient's age* is another important factor. Elderly patients usually have decreased hepatic function, less muscle mass, and diminished renal function. Consequently, lower doses and sometimes longer dosage intervals are needed to avoid toxicity in the elderly. With similar consequences, neonates have underdeveloped metabolic enzyme systems and depressed renal function. They need highly individualized dosage and careful monitoring. *Underlying disease* can also markedly affect drug action and effect. For example, acidosis may cause insulin resistance. Genetic diseases such as glucose-6-phosphate dehydrogenase (G-6-PD) deficiency and hepatic porphyria may turn drugs into toxins, with serious consequences. Patients with G-6-PD deficiency may develop hemolytic anemia when given aspirin, sulfonamides, or any of a number of drugs. A genetically susceptible patient can develop an acute porphyria attack if given a barbiturate. Also, patients who have highly active hepatic enzyme systems (for example, rapid acetylators), when treated with isoniazid, can develop hepatitis from the rapid intrahepatic buildup of a toxic metabolite.

Things to consider about administration

1. Dosage forms do matter. Some tablets and capsules are too large to be readily swallowed by very ill patients. You may then request an oral solution or elixir of the same drug, but bear in mind that because a liquid is more easily and completely absorbed, it produces higher serum levels than a tablet. When a potentially toxic drug is given, the increased amount absorbed could cause toxicity. One example of this is digoxin tablets versus digoxin elixir. Sometimes a change in dosage form requires a change in dose.

2. Routes of administration are not therapeutically interchangeable. For example, phenytoin (Dilantin) is readily absorbed orally but is slowly and erratically absorbed intramuscularly. On the other hand, carbenicillin must be given parenterally because oral administration yields inadequate serum levels to treat systemic infections. However, it can be given orally to treat urinary tract infections because it concentrates in the urine.

3. The timing of drug administration can be important. Sometimes giving an oral drug during or shortly after mealtime decreases the amount of drug absorbed. This is not clinically significant with most drugs and may in fact be desirable with irritating drugs such as aspirin or phenylbutazone. But penicillins and tetracyclines should not be scheduled for administration at mealtimes because certain foods can inactivate them. If in doubt about the effect of food on a certain drug, check with a pharmacist.

4. Consider the patient's age, height, and weight. The doctor will need this information when calculating the dose for many drugs. It should be accurately recorded on the patient's chart. This chart should also include current laboratory data, especially renal and hepatic function studies, so the doctor can consider them and adapt dosage as needed.

5. Watch for metabolic changes. Monitor for any physiologic change that might alter drug effect. Examples: depressed respiratory function and the development of acidosis or alkalosis.

6. Know the patient's history. Whenever possible, obtain a comprehensive family history from the patient or his family. Ask about past reactions to drugs, possible genetic traits that might alter drug response, and the current use of other drugs. Multiple drug therapy can dramatically change the effects of many drugs. These are known as drug interactions.

Drug interactions

When one drug administered in combination with or shortly after another drug alters the effect of one or both drugs, this is known as a drug interaction. Usually, the effect of one drug is increased or decreased. For instance, one drug may inhibit or stimulate the metabolism or excretion of the other; or it may release another from plasma protein-binding sites, freeing it for further action.

Combination therapy is based upon drug interaction. One drug, for example, may be given in order to potentiate another. Probenecid, which blocks the excretion of penicillin, is sometimes given with penicillin to maintain adequate serum levels of penicillin for a longer period. Often two drugs with similar action are given together precisely because of the additive effect that results. Aspirin and codeine, for instance, both analgesics, are often given in combination because together they provide greater relief from pain than either alone.

Drug interactions are sometimes used to prevent or antagonize certain side effects. Hydrochlorothiazide and spironolactone, both diuretics, are often administered in combination, because the former is potassium-depleting, while the latter is potassium-sparing.

But not all drug interactions are beneficial. Multiple drugs can interact to produce effects that are often undesirable and sometimes hazardous. (These interactions are summarized in the tabular section of each chapter.)

Harmful drug interactions decrease efficiency or increase toxicity. A hypertensive patient well controlled with guanethidine may see his blood pressure rise to its former high level if he takes the antidepressant amitriptyline (Elavil) at the same time. Such a drug effect is known as antagonism. Drug combinations that produce these effects when used together should be avoided if possible. Another kind of inhibiting effect occurs when a tetracycline drug is administered concomitantly with calcium- or magnesium-containing drugs or foods (i.e., antacids or milk). These combine with tetracycline in the gastrointestinal tract and cause inadequate absorption of tetracycline.

Side effects

Any drug effect other than what is therapeutically intended can be called a side effect. It may be expected and benign, or unexpected and potentially harmful. For example, during hay fever season, a patient may have to contend with the drowsiness caused by chlorpheniramine to get relief from hay fever symptoms. In such a case, the dose may be adjusted up or down to balance therapeutic effect with side effect.

A side effect may be tolerated for a necessary therapeutic effect or it may be hazardous and unacceptable, and require discontinuation of the drug. Some side effects subside with continued use. As an example, the drowsiness associated with methyldopa (Aldomet) and the orthostatic hypotension associated with prazosin (Minipress) usually subside after several days, as the patient develops a tolerance to these effects. But many side effects are dose-related and lessen or disappear only if dosage is reduced. Although most side effects are not therapeutically desirable, an occasional one can be put to clinical use. An outstanding example of this is the drowsiness associated with diphenhydramine (Benadryl), which makes it clinically useful as a mild hypnotic.

Hypersensitivity, a term sometimes used interchangeably with drug allergy, is the result of an antigen-antibody immune reaction that occurs in the body when a drug is introduced into a susceptible patient. One of the most dangerous of all drug hypersensitivities is penicillin allergy. In its severest form, penicillin anaphylaxis can rapidly become fatal.

Rarely, idiosyncratic reactions occur. These are highly unpredictable, individual, and unusual. Probably the best known idiosyncratic drug reaction is the aplastic anemia caused by the antibiotic chloramphenicol (Chloromycetin). This reaction appears in only 1 out of 40,000 patients, but when it does it is often fatal. A more common idiosyncratic reaction is extreme sensitivity to very low doses of a drug, or insensitivity to much higher than normally tolerated doses.

To deal with side effects correctly, you need to be alert to even minor changes in the patient's clinical status. Such minor changes may be an early warning of pending toxicity. Listen to the patient's complaints about his reactions to a drug, and consider each complaint objectively. You may be able to reduce undesirable side effects in several ways. Obviously, dosage reduction often helps. But often so does a simple rescheduling of the same dose. For example, Sudafed (pseudoephedrine) may produce stimulation that will be no problem if it's given early in the day; similarly, the drowsiness that occurs with antihistamines or tranquilizers can be totally harmless if the dose is given at bedtime. Most important, patients need to be told what side effects to expect so they won't become worried or even stop taking the drug on their own. Of course, patients should report any unusual or unexpected side effects to the doctor.

Recognizing drug allergies or serious idiosyncratic reactions can sometimes be lifesaving. Ask each patient about drugs he is taking or has taken in the past and what, if any, unusual effects he experienced from taking them. If a patient claims to be allergic to a drug, ask him to tell you exactly what happens when he takes it. He may be calling a harmless side effect such as upset stomach an allergic reaction, or he may have a true tendency to anaphylaxis. In either case, you and the doctor need to know this. Of course, you must record and report any clinical changes throughout the patient's hospital stay. If you suspect a hazardous side effect, withhold the drug until you can check with the pharmacist and the doctor.

Toxic reactions

Chronic drug toxicities are generally due to cumulative effect and the resulting buildup of the drug in the body. These effects may be extensions of the desired therapeutic effect. For example, guanethidine-induced norepinephrine depletion produces a desired antihypertensive effect, but in larger doses, this same biochemical action often produces orthostatic hypotension.

Drug toxicities usually occur when serum drug levels rise due to impaired metabolism or excretion. For example, blood levels of theophylline rise when hepatic dysfunction impairs metabolism of the drug. Similarly, digoxin toxicity can follow impaired renal function because digoxin is eliminated from the body almost exclusively by the kidneys (via glomerular filtration). Of course, toxic blood levels also follow excessive dosage. Aspirin tinnitus (ringing in ears) is usually a sign that the safe dose has been exceeded.

Most drug toxicity is predictable and dose-related; fortunately, most drug toxicity is also readily reversible upon dosage adjustment. So it's essential to monitor patients carefully for physiological changes that might alter drug effect. Watch especially for impaired hepatic and renal function. Warn the patient about signs of pending toxicity, and tell him what to do if a toxic reaction occurs. Also, be sure to emphasize the importance of taking a drug exactly as prescribed. Warn the patient about serious problems that could arise if he changes the dose or the schedule for taking it. For detailed management of drug toxicity, see Appendices.

Drugs and pregnancy

Ever since the thalidomide tragedy of the late 1950s—when thousands of malformed infants were born after their mothers used this mild sedative-hypnotic during pregnancy—use of drugs during pregnancy has been a source of serious medical concern and controversy. To identify drugs that may cause such teratogenic effects, preclinical drug studies always include tests on pregnant laboratory animals. These tests do point out gross teratogenicity but do not clearly establish safety. Because different species react to drugs in different ways, animal studies do not rule out possible teratogenic effects in humans. For example, the preliminary studies on thalidomide gave no warning of teratogenic effects, and it was subsequently released for general use in Europe.

To prevent such tragedies, just about every drug now carries a special warning on the official package insert. Such warnings state that safety in human pregnancy has not been established and use of the drug in pregnancy requires the expected therapeutic benefit be weighed against possible hazard to mother and child. With the exception of vitamins and minerals, no drug is approved caveat-free for use in pregnancy. Even Bendectin (a combination of the antihistamine doxylamine and the vitamin pyridoxine), for which nausea and vomiting of pregnancy is an official indication, carries a warning for cautious use during pregnancy.

What about the placental barrier? Once thought to protect the fetus from drug effects, the placenta isn't actually much of a barrier at all. Except for drugs with exceptionally large molecular structure, almost every drug administered to a pregnant woman crosses the placenta and enters the fetal circulation. An example of such large molecular size is heparin, the injectable anticoagulant. Theoretically, then, heparin could be used in a pregnant woman without fear of harming the fetus—but even heparin carries warning for cautious use in pregnancy. Conversely, just because a drug crosses the placenta doesn't necessarily mean it's harmful to the fetus.

Actually, only one factor—stage of fetal development—seems clearly related to exagerrated risk during pregnancy. During two stages of pregnancy—the first and the third trimesters—the fetus is especially vulnerable to damage from maternal use of drugs. During these times, *all* drugs should be given with extreme caution. The most sensitive period for drug-induced fetal malformation is the first trimester, when fetal organs are differentiating (organogenesis). During this time, *all* drugs should be withheld unless doing so would jeopardize the mother's health. Theoretically, during this sensitive time, even aspirin could harm the fetus. So, strongly advise your patients to avoid *all* self-prescribed drugs during early pregnancy.

The other time of special fetal sensitivity to drugs is the last trimester. The reason? At birth, when separated from his mother, the newborn must rely on his own metabolism to eliminate any remaining drug. Because his detoxifying systems are not fully developed, any residual drug may take a long time to be metabolized—and thus may induce prolonged toxic reactions. Consequently, drugs should be used only when absolutely necessary during the last 3 months of pregnancy.

Of course, in many circumstances, pregnant women must continue to take certain drugs. For example, an epileptic woman who is well controlled with an anticonvulsant should continue to take it even during pregnancy. Or a pregnant woman with a bacterial infection must receive antibiotics. In such cases, the potential risk to the fetus is overbalanced by the mother's need.

Following these general guidelines can prevent indiscriminate and potentially harmful use of drugs in pregnancy:

- Before a drug is prescribed for a woman of childbearing age, she should be asked the date of her last menstrual period and whether there is a possibility she is pregnant.
- Especially during the first and the third trimesters, a pregnant patient should avoid *all* drugs except those *essential* to maintain the pregnancy or maternal health.
- Topical drugs are not exempt from the warning against indiscriminate use during pregnancy. Many topically applied drugs can be absorbed in large enough amounts to be harmful to the fetus.
- When a pregnant patient needs *any* drug, the doctor should prescribe the *safest* possible drug in the *lowest* possible dose to minimize any harmful effect to the fetus.
- Every pregnant patient should check with her doctor before taking *any* drug.

Drugs and lactation

Most drugs a nursing mother takes do appear in breast milk. Drug levels in breast milk tend to be high when blood levels are high—generally, shortly after taking each dose. Therefore, the mother should be advised to breast-feed *before* taking medication not *after*.

Nevertheless, with very few exceptions, a mother who wishes to breast-feed may continue to do so with her doctor's permission. The exceptions: Breast-feeding should be temporarily interrupted and replaced with bottle-feeding when the mother must take...

- tetracyclines
- chloramphenicol
- sulfonamides (during first 2 weeks postpartum)
- oral anticoagulants
- iodine-containing drugs
- antineoplastics
- propylthiouracil.

To protect her infant, a nursing mother should avoid taking drugs indiscriminately. If she needs to take a drug to maintain her own health, she should first check with her doctor to be sure of taking the safest drug at the safest dose.

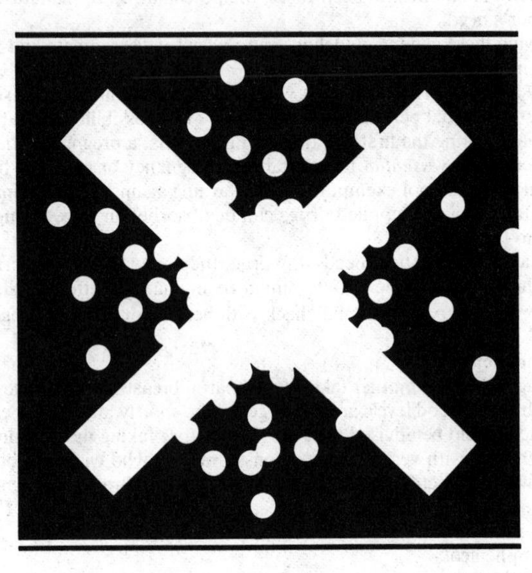

Infection and Infestation

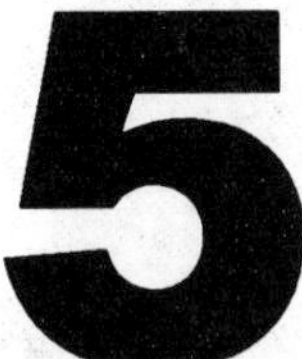

Amebicides and trichomonacides

carbarsone
chloroquine hydrochloride
chloroquine phosphate
diiodohydroxyquin
emetine hydrochloride
metronidazole
paromomycin sulfate

Amebicides and trichomonacides cure or control diseases caused by amebic or trichomonad infestation.

Major uses

• To treat patients with intestinal and extraintestinal amebic infestations or trichomoniasis.

Mechanism of action

• Carbarsone is an organic arsenic derivative with amebicidal activity in the intestinal lumen believed to be due to inhibition of sulfhydryl enzymes.
• Chloroquine is mainly an antimalarial. Its mechanism of action as an amebicide is unknown, but it is useful in the treatment of extraintestinal amebiasis.
• Diiodohydroxyquin is an iodide possessing amebicidal activity within the intestinal lumen. Its precise mechanism of action is unknown.
• Emetine is a tissue amebicide which acts on the intestinal wall and extraintestinal sites such as liver and lungs.
• Metronidazole is a direct-acting trichomonacide and amebicide. It works at both intestinal and extraintestinal sites.
• Paromomycin is an aminoglycoside antibiotic which acts as an amebicidal agent in intestinal sites, effective either in the presence or absence of bacteria.

Absorption, distribution, and excretion

• Carbarsone is readily absorbed from the gastrointestinal tract after oral and rectal administration and is excreted slowly in urine. The drug may accumulate, causing toxicity.
• Chloroquine is almost completely absorbed in the small intestine following oral administration. Approximately 55% is bound to plasma proteins; high concentrations are found in body tissues. It is excreted slowly in urine; small amounts are detectable sometimes for years after therapy.
• Diiodohydroxyquin is poorly absorbed from the gastrointestinal tract; most of it is excreted in the stool.
• Emetine is absorbed from parenteral sites, slowly detoxified by the liver, and primarily excreted by the kidneys. It is detectable in urine 40 to 60 days after treatment.
• Metronidazole is well absorbed after oral administration, primarily in the small intestine,

with peak levels after 1 to 2 hours. Limited data suggests wide distribution with significant concentration in many tissues, abscesses, bile and cerebrospinal fluid. From 60% to 70% is excreted in the urine unchanged; the remainder is probably metabolized by the liver.
• Paromomycin is poorly absorbed from the GI tract after oral administration. Almost all the drug is excreted unchanged in the stool.

Combination products
None.

HOW TO ENFORCE AMEBIASIS PRECAUTIONS

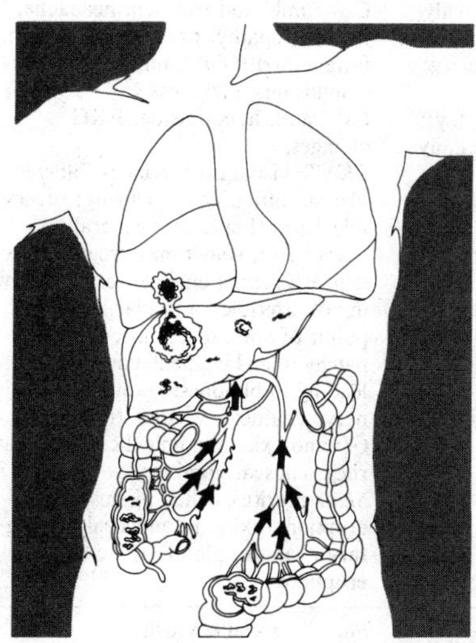

Amebic invasion of intestinal mucosa occurs most commonly in the cecum and rectosigmoid area. Once carried into the bloodstream, it may cause infections anywhere in the body. For example, metastasis through the diaphragm may result in a secondary lung abscess formation.

To avoid spreading amebal infection, have all nurses and visitors in contact with the patient wear a gown and gloves, and wash their hands on entering and leaving the room. Private rooms, however, are only necessary for children or confused patients. Masks are not needed at all.

Remember to disinfect or discard articles contaminated with urine and feces. Exercise extreme caution in the handling and disposing of stool specimens.

NAME	INDICATIONS & DOSAGE	SIDE EFFECTS
carbarsone	*Intestinal amebiasis—* **Adults:** 250 mg P.O. b.i.d. or t.i.d. for 10 days. Rectal (as retention enema): 2 g dissolved in 200 ml warm 2% sodium bicarbonate solution, every other night for 5 doses. Discontinue oral therapy when enema is given. **Children:** average total dose is 75 mg/Kg P.O. daily in 3 divided doses over 10-day period. Recommended total varies according to age—2 to 4 years, 2 g total; 5 to 8 years, 3 g total; 9 to 12 years, 4 g total; and over 12, 5 g total.	*Blood:* agranulocytosis. *CNS:* neuritis, convulsions. *EENT:* sore throat, retinal edema, visual disturbances. *GI:* epigastric pain and burning, irritation, nausea, hepatitis, vomiting, diarrhea, anorexia, constipation, increased motility, abdominal cramps. *GU:* polyuria, albuminuria. *Skin:* eruptions, exfoliative dermatitis, pruritus. *Other:* edema of wrists, ankles, and knees; weight loss; kidney damage; hepatitis; hepatomegaly; splenomegaly; jaundice; hemorrhagic encephalitis.
chloroquine hydrochloride Aralen HC1 **chloroquine phosphate** Aralen Phosphate•, Chlorocon Roquine	*Extraintestinal amebiasis—* **Adults:** 160 to 200 mg chloroquine (hydrochloride) base, I.M. daily for no more than 10 or 12 days. As soon as possible, substitute 1 g (600 mg base) chloroquine phosphate P.O. daily for 2 days; then 500 mg (300 mg base) daily for at least 2 to 3 weeks. Treatment is usually combined with an effective intestinal amebicide.	*Blood:* agranulocytosis, blood dyscrasias. *CNS:* mild and transient headache, neuromyopathy, psychic stimulation, fatigue, irritability, nightmares, convulsions, dizziness. *CV* (rare): hypotension, EKG changes. *EENT:* visual disturbances (blurred vision; difficulty in focusing; reversible corneal changes; generally irreversible, sometimes progressive or delayed, retinal changes, e.g., narrowing of arterioles; macular lesions; pallor of optic disc; optic atrophy; patchy retinal pigmentation, often leading to blindness; ototoxicity; nerve deafness, vertigo, tinnitus. *GI:* anorexia, abdominal cramps, diarrhea, nausea, vomiting. *Skin:* pruritus, lichen planus-like eruptions, skin and mucosal pigmentary changes, pleomorphic skin eruptions.
diiodohydroxyquin Gynovules••, Inserfem, Yodoxin	*Intestinal amebiasis—* **Adults:** 630 to 650 mg P.O. t.i.d. for 20 days. Total daily dose should not exceed 2 g. **Children:** usual dose: 30 to 40 mg/Kg of body weight daily in 2 to 3 divided doses for 20 days. Additional courses of	*Blood:* agranulocytosis. *CNS:* neurotoxicity, dysesthesia, weakness, vertigo, malaise, headache, agitation, retrograde amnesia, atoxia, peripheral neuropathy. *EENT:* optic neuritis, optic atrophy, loss of vision. *GI:* anorexia, nausea, vomiting,

• Also available in Canada.
•• Available in Canada only.
Unmarked trade names available in United States only.

INTERACTIONS	NURSING CONSIDERATIONS
None significant.	• Contraindicated as initial treatment in patients with liver or kidney disease; in patients with contracted visual or color fields; and in patients with known hypersensitivity or intolerance to any arsenical treatment. • Don't exceed recommended dose; toxicity may result. If second treatment is needed, allow at least 10 days between courses. • Divide carbarsone capsule to obtain required dose. Give in ½ glass orange juice or milk, in small amount of 1% sodium bicarbonate solution, or in jelly or other food. • Discontinue upon first sign of intolerance or toxicity. Fatal exfoliative dermatitis and hemorrhagic encephalitis have been reported. • Tell patient to report any unusual symptoms, even post-treatment. • Liver function tests should precede therapy. Careful inspection of skin, vision testing, and palpation of liver and spleen should be repeated regularly. • Monitor intake/output. Notify doctor of number, frequency, and character of stools. • Give a cleansing enema before giving carbarsone enema. • Deliver stool specimen to lab promptly; movements of parasites are seen only when stool is warm. Amebic cysts in stool indicate need for additional therapy. Stool specimen should be studied 1 week after stopping therapy and monthly for 1 year. To help prevent reinfestation, instruct patient in correct hygiene.
None significant.	• Contraindicated in patients with retinal or visual field changes, porphyria. Use with extreme caution in presence of severe GI, neurologic, or blood disorders. Drug concentrates in liver; use cautiously in patients with hepatic disease or alcoholism. Use with caution in patients with G-6-PD deficiency or psoriasis; drug may exacerbate these conditions. • Complete blood cell counts, including liver function studies, should be made periodically during prolonged therapy; if severe blood disorder appears which is not attributable to disease under treatment, drug may need to be discontinued. • Overdosage can quickly lead to toxic symptoms: headache, drowsiness, visual disturbances, cardiovascular collapse and convulsions, followed by sudden and early respiratory and cardiac arrest. Children are extremely susceptible to toxicity; avoid long-term treatment. • Baseline and periodic ophthalmologic examinations needed. Report blurred vision, increased sensitivity to light, or muscle weakness. Check periodically for muscular weakness after long-term use. Audiometric exams recommended before, during, and after therapy, especially if long term. • Give drug immediately before or after meals on same day each week. • To avoid exacerbated drug-induced dermatoses, warn patient to avoid excessive exposure to sun. • Each ml parenteral solution containing 50 mg dihydrochloride salt = 40 mg chloroquine base; each 500 mg tablet phosphate = 300 mg base.
None significant.	• Contraindicated in patients with known hypersensitivity to 8-hydroxyquinoline derivatives or iodine-containing preparations. Diiodohydroxyquin causes hepatic damage in such patients. Also contraindicated in patients with hepatic or renal disease, or preexisting optic neuropathy. • Patient should have periodic ophthalmologic examinations during treatment. • Give after meals. Crush tablets and mix with applesauce or chocolate syrup.

(continued on following page)

NAME	INDICATIONS & DOSAGE	SIDE EFFECTS
diiodohydroxyquin *(continued)*	diiodohydroxyquin therapy should not be repeated before a resting interval of 2 to 3 weeks.	abdominal cramps, diarrhea, increased motility, constipation, epigastric burning and pain, gastritis, anal irritation and itching. *Skin:* pruritus, hives, papular and pustular eruptions, urticaria, discoloration of hair and nails. *Other:* thyroid enlargement, fever, chills, generalized furunculosis, hair loss.
emetine hydrochloride	*Acute fulminating amebic dysentery—* **Adults:** 1 mg/Kg daily up to 65 mg daily (1 or 2 doses) deep S.C. or I.M. 3 to 5 days to control symptoms. Give another antiamebic drug simultaneously. **Children over 8:** no more than 20 mg daily deep S.C. or I.M. for 3 to 5 days. **Children under 8:** no more than 10 mg daily for 3 to 5 days. *Amebic hepatitis and abscess—* **Adults:** 65 mg daily (1 or 2 doses) deep S.C. or I.M. for 10 days. **Children over 8:** no more than 20 mg daily for 10 days. **Children under 8:** no more than 10 mg daily for 10 days.	*CNS:* dizziness, headache, mild sensory disturbances, central or peripheral nerve function changes, neuromuscular symptoms (weakness, aching, stiffness, tenderness, pain, tremors). *CV:* acute toxicity—can occur at any dose (hypotension, tachycardia, precordial pain, dyspnea, EKG abnormalities, gallop rhythm, cardiac dilatation, severe acute degenerative myocarditis, pericarditis, congestive failure, death). *GI:* nausea, vomiting, diarrhea, abdominal cramps, loss of sense of taste. *Local:* skeletal muscle stiffness, aching, tenderness, muscle weakness at injection site. *Metabolic:* decreased serum potassium levels. *Skin:* eczematous, urticarial purpuric lesions. *Other:* edema.
metronidazole Flagyl♦, Neo-Tric♦♦, Novonidazol♦♦, Trikacide♦♦	*Amebic liver abscess—* **Adults:** 500 to 750 mg P.O. t.i.d. for 5 to 10 days. **Children:** 35 to 50 mg/Kg daily (in 3 doses) for 10 days. *Intestinal amebiasis—* **Adults:** 750 mg P.O. t.i.d. for 5 to 10 days. **Children:** 35 to 50 mg/Kg daily (in 3 doses) for 10 days. Follow this therapy with oral diiodohydroxyquin.	*Blood:* leukopenia, neutropenia, dyscrasias. *CNS:* vertigo, headache, ataxia, incoordination, confusion, irritability, depression, restlessness, weakness, fatigue, drowsiness, insomnia, sensory neuropathy, paresthesias of the extremities, psychic stimulation, neuromyopathy. *CV:* EKG change (flattened T wave). *EENT:* blurred vision, difficulty in focusing, nasal congestion.

INTERACTIONS	NURSING CONSIDERATIONS
	• Record intake/output, and color and amount of stool. Send warm specimens to lab frequently. • Watch for diarrhea during the first 2 to 3 days of treatment. Notify doctor if it continues past 3 days. • Advise patient not to discontinue the medication prematurely. Tell him to notify doctor if skin rash occurs.
None significant.	• Contraindicated in patients with heart or kidney disease, except those with amebic abscess or hepatitis not controlled by chloroquine; patients who have received a course of emetine less than 6 to 8 weeks previously; children, except for severe dysentery unresponsive to other amebicides; and in those with polyneuropathy or muscle disease. Use with caution in aged or debilitated patients, patients with hypotension, or those about to undergo surgery. • Record pulse rate and blood pressure 2 to 3 times daily. Discontinue use if drug produces tachycardia, precipitous fall in blood pressure, neuromuscular symptoms, marked gastrointestinal effects, or considerable weakness. Weakness and muscle symptoms usually precede more serious symptoms and serve as a guide for avoiding toxicity. • Don't exceed recommended dose or extend therapy beyond 10 days. Patient confined to bed during treatment and for several days thereafter. • Drug may alter EKG tracings for 6 weeks. EKG should be taken before therapy, after fifth dose, upon completion, and 1 week after therapy. Patterns can resemble those of myocardial infarction. First and most consistent change is T wave inversion. • Deep S.C. administration is preferred; I.M. acceptable, but I.V. route is dangerous and contraindicated. Injections cause necrosis and edema. Rotate sites and apply warm soaks. • Record intake/output; odor and consistency of stools; and presence of mucus, blood, or other foreign matter. Send warm specimens to lab frequently. Repeat fecal examinations at 3-month intervals to assure elimination of amebae. Patients with acute amebic dysentery often become asymptomatic carriers. Check family members and suspected contacts. • Suspect emetine-induced reaction if stools increase in number following initial relief of diarrhea. • To help prevent reinfection instruct patient in correct hygiene. • Drug is very irritating. Avoid contact with eyes and mucous membranes. • Restoration of body fluids and nutrients is an important adjunct to therapy.
Alcohol: disulfiram-like reaction (nausea, vomiting, headache, cramps, flushing). Don't use together. *Disulfiram:* acute psychoses and confusional states. Don't use together.	*Warning:* This drug has been shown to be carcinogenic in mice and possibly rats. Unnecessary use should be avoided. • Contraindicated in patients with a history of blood dyscrasia or CNS disorder, and in patients with retinal or visual field changes. Use with caution in patients with hepatic disease or alcoholism; in conjunction with known hepatotoxic drugs. • Tell patients to avoid alcohol or alcohol-containing medications. • Give with meals to minimize GI distress. • Tell patients metallic taste and dark or reddish-brown urine are possible. • Record number and character of stools when used in the treatment of amebiasis. Metronidazole should be used only after *Trichomonas vaginalis* has been confirmed by wet smear or culture or *Entamoeba histolytica*

(continued on following page)

NAME	INDICATIONS & DOSAGE	SIDE EFFECTS
metronidazole *(continued)*	*Trichomoniasis—* **Adults** (both male and female): 250 mg P.O. t.i.d. for 7 days or 2 g P.O. in single dose; 4 to 6 weeks should elapse between courses of therapy. *Refractory trichomoniasis—* **Women:** 250 mg P.O. b.i.d. for 10 days and 500 mg suppository placed high in vagina daily for 10 days.	*GI:* abdominal cramping, stomatitis, nausea, vomiting, anorexia, epigastric distress, diarrhea, constipation. *GU:* darkened urine, polyuria, dysuria, pyuria, incontinence, cystitis, decreased libido, dyspareunia, dryness of vagina and vulva, sense of pelvic pressure. *Skin:* pruritus, flushing. *Other:* overgrowth of nonsusceptible organisms, especially *Candida,* (glossitis, furry tongue), dry mouth, metallic taste, proctitis, fever.
paromomycin sulfate Humatin	*Intestinal amebiasis, acute and chronic—* **Adults and children:** 25 to 35 mg/Kg daily P.O. in 3 doses for 5 to 10 days after meals.	*Blood:* eosinophilia. *CNS:* headache, vertigo. *EENT:* ototoxicity. *GI:* anorexia, nausea, vomiting, epigastric pain and burning, abdominal cramps, diarrhea, constipation, increased motility, steatorrhea, pruritus ani, malabsorption syndrome. *GU:* hematuria, nephrotoxicity. *Skin:* rash, exanthema, pruritus. *Other:* overgrowth of nonsusceptible organisms.

INTERACTIONS	NURSING CONSIDERATIONS
	has been identified. Asymptomatic sexual partners of patients being treated for *Trichomonas vaginalis* infection should be treated simultaneously to avoid reinfection. Instruct patient in correct hygiene. • Has been used to treat anaerobic infections.
None significant.	• Contraindicated in impaired renal function or intestinal obstruction. Use with caution in ulcerative lesions of the bowel to avoid inadvertent absorption and resulting renal toxicity. Poorly absorbed orally but will accumulate with renal impairment or ulcerative lesions. • Ask about history of sensitivity to this drug before giving first dose. • Administer after meals. • Emphasize personal hygiene, particularly handwashing before eating and after defecation. • Criterion of cure is absence of amebae in stools examined weekly for 6 weeks after treatment and thereafter at monthly intervals for 2 years. Examine feces of family members or suspected contacts. • Avoid high doses or prolonged therapy. • Watch for signs of superinfection (continued fever and other signs of new infections, especially monilial infections).

Anthelmintics

antimony potassium tartrate
diethylcarbamazine citrate
gentian violet
mebendazole
piperazine
pyrantel pamoate
pyrvinium pamoate
thiabendazole

Anthelmintics are used to treat infestations of various worms. The spectrum of activity varies according to the drug.

Major uses

• Eradication of various species of worms.

Mechanism of action

• Diethylcarbamazine appears to sensitize the worms to phagocytosis by the reticuloendothelial system.
• Mebendazole appears to cause selective and irreversible inhibition of glucose uptake and other nutrients in susceptible helminths.
• Piperazine blocks acetylcholine, causing the worm to be paralyzed and then expelled by normal peristalsis.
• Pyrantel is probably effective due to neuromuscular blocking action.
• Pyrvinium, a cynanine dye, appears to destroy parasites by preventing them from using exogenous carbohydrates.
• Mechanism of action of other anthelmintics is unknown.

Absorption, distribution, and excretion

• Piperazine is readily absorbed from the GI tract.
• Pyrantel is metabolized partially in the liver, and the rest is excreted unchanged in the urine and feces. There appears to be large individual differences in rate of excretion.
• Thiabendazole is rapidly absorbed from the GI tract. Most of the drug disappears from plasma within 8 hours. It is almost completely metabolized and excreted in the urine.
• Other anthelmintics appear to be poorly absorbed from the GI tract and are mainly excreted in the feces.

• Diethylcarbamazine is readily absorbed from the GI tract, distributed to all body tissues except fat, and totally excreted within 48 hours in urine.

Onset and duration
• Most anthelmintics are of rapid onset and short duration.

Combination products
None.

THREE PARASITE WORMS

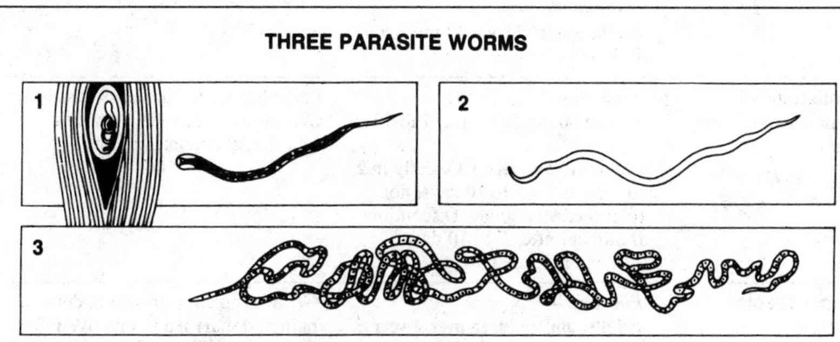

1. Greatly enlarged trichina (right); trichina lodged in muscle fiber (left).
2. Roundworms live both in human beings and animals, causing a variety of symptoms, including anemia, diarrhea, weight loss, and colicky pains.
3. A tapeworm has a flattened body made up of block-like segments. Since it has no mouth, it absorbs its food from the intestine of its host. Tapeworms vary in size from less than one inch with three or four segments to thirty feet long with thousands of segments.

NAME	INDICATIONS & DOSAGE	SIDE EFFECTS
antimony potassium tartrate (not commercially available; must be compounded)	*Schistosoma japonicum*— **Adults:** initially, 8 ml of 0.05% solution in sterile water for injection or 5% dextrose given slow I.V. Increase each subsequent dose 4 ml until 11th day, when 28 ml are given. Give 28 ml on alternate days until a total of 500 ml (2.5 g).	*Blood:* thrombocytopenia. *CV:* hypotension, syncope, bradycardia, EKG changes. *GI:* nausea, vomiting, diarrhea, colic, hepatic necrosis. *Other:* dyspnea, severe arthralgia, albuminuria, fever, dermatitis.
diethylcarbamazine citrate Hetrazan	*Ascariasis (roundworm)*— **Adults:** 13 mg/Kg P.O. daily for 7 days. **Children:** 6 to 10 mg/Kg P.O. t.i.d. for 7 to 10 days. *Loiasis, dipetalonemiasis, onchocerciasis, Bancroftian or Malayan filariasis*— **Adults and children:** 2 mg/Kg P.O. t.i.d. for 3 to 4 weeks. Repeat if necessary. *Tropical (pulmonary) eosinophilia*— **Adults and children:** 13 mg/Kg P.O. daily for 4 to 7 days.	*CNS:* headache, malaise, weakness, lassitude, syncope. *CV:* tachycardia, tachypnea, hypotension, leukocytosis, eosinophilia. *GI:* anorexia, nausea, vomiting. *Skin:* pruritus, dermatitis, bullous eruptions. *Other:* arthralgia, myalgia, joint pain, swelling and edema of face and skin, severe pedal edema, fever, lymphadenitis, sweating, cough.
gentian violet Jayne's P-W Vermifuge	*Pinworms*— **Adults:** 60 mg P.O. t.i.d. 7 to 10 days. **Children:** 2 mg/Kg P.O. daily in 2 to 3 doses for 8 to 10 days, not to exceed 90 mg/day. Discontinue treatment after 7 to 10 days. Resume if needed.	*CNS:* headache, dizziness, lassitude. *GI:* nausea, diarrhea, vomiting (purple), abdominal cramps.
mebendazole Vermox•	*Pinworm*— **Adults, and children over 2 years:** 100 mg P.O. as a single dose. If infestation persists 3 weeks later, repeat treatment. *Roundworm, whipworm, hookworm*— **Adults, and children over 2 years:** 100 mg P.O. b.i.d. for 3 days. If infestation persists 3 weeks later, repeat treatment.	*GI:* occasional, transient abdominal pain and diarrhea in massive infestation and expulsion of worms.
piperazine adipate Entacyl•• **piperazine citrate** Antepar•, Bryrel, Multifuge, Pin-Tega Tabs, Pipril, Ta-Verm, Vermago	*Pinworm*— **Adults and children:** 65 mg/Kg P.O. daily 7 to 8 days. Maximum daily dose is 2.5 g. *Roundworm*— **Adults:** 3.5 g P.O. in single doses for 2 consecutive days. **Children:** 75 mg/Kg P.O. daily in	*CNS:* ataxia, tremors, choreiform movements, muscular weakness, myoclonus, hyporeflexia, paresthesias, convulsions, sense of detachment, EEG abnormalities, memory defect, headache, vertigo. *EENT:* nystagmus, blurred vision, paralytic strabismus, cataracts with

• Also available in Canada.
•• Available in Canada only.
Unmarked trade names available in United States only.

INTERACTIONS	NURSING CONSIDERATIONS
None significant.	• Not for use in other worm infestations; toxicity with this agent is high. • Solutions must be freshly prepared. • Doses should be given 2 hours after a light meal. • Patient should lie down for 1 hour after treatment. • Antiemetics should not be given, since they mask nausea and vomiting, which are signs of hepatic toxicity. • Extravasation may cause painful cellulitis. • Treatment of choice for *Schistosoma japonicum*.
None significant.	• Use with caution in patients with hypertension; severe hepatic, renal, or cardiac disease; and in children under 1 year of age. Treat patients with recent history of malaria with an antimalarial agent first to prevent relapse in nonsymptomatic malarial infections. • Administer carefully to avoid or control allergic or other untoward reactions. Minimize allergic reactions by giving with corticosteroids, antihistamines, or aspirin. • Inform patient that side effects will usually be minor and transient. • Instruct patient in good hygiene. • Give immediately after meals. Drug has sweet but unpleasant taste.
None significant.	• Use with caution in patients with cardiac, hepatic, renal, or GI disease. • Tablets must be taken whole with water. Give with meals. • Patient should abstain from alcohol during treatment. • If nausea and vomiting occur, stop treatment for 1 to 2 days; resume at reduced dosage and notify doctor. Warn that skin, clothing, vomitus, and feces will be stained purple. • Instruct patient in good hygiene.
None significant.	• Tablets may be chewed, swallowed, or crushed and mixed with food. • No dietary restrictions, laxatives, or enemas necessary. • To avoid reinfestation, wash perianal area daily. Change undergarments and bedclothes daily. Wash hands and clean fingernails after bowel movements and before meals. Treat all family members.
None significant.	• Contraindicated in patients with hepatic and/or renal impairment, or convulsive disorders. Use with caution in patients with severe malnutrition or anemia. • Discontinue if CNS or significant GI reactions occur. • Because of potential neurotoxicity, avoid prolonged or repeated treatment, especially in children. • No dietary restrictions, laxatives, or enemas necessary. • May be taken with food.

(continued on following page)

NAME	INDICATIONS & DOSAGE	SIDE EFFECTS
piperazine *(continued)* **piperazine phosphate** Antepar phosphate, Piperaval **piperazine tartrate** Razine Tartrate	single dose for 2 consecutive days. Maximum daily dose: 3.5 g.	visual impairment, lacrimation, rhinorrhea, difficulty in focusing. *GI:* nausea, vomiting, diarrhea, abdominal cramps. *Skin:* urticaria, photodermatitis, erythema multiforme, purpura, eczematous skin reactions. *Other:* arthralgia, fever, bronchospasm.
pyrantel pamoate Antiminth, Combantrin••	*Roundworm and pinworm—* **Adults, and children over 2 years:** single dose of 11 mg/Kg P.O. Maximum dose 1 g. For pinworm, dose should be repeated in 2 weeks.	*CNS:* headache, dizziness, drowsiness, insomnia. *GI:* anorexia, nausea, vomiting, gastralgia, cramps, diarrhea, tenesmus. *Skin:* rashes. *Other:* transient elevation of SGOT, fever, weakness.
pyrvinium pamoate Pamovin••, Povan, Pyr-Pam••, Vanquin••	*Pinworm—* **Adults and children:** 5 mg/Kg P.O. single dose (maximum 350 mg). Repeat in 2 weeks if needed.	*GI:* nausea, vomiting, cramping, diarrhea (vomiting more common with suspension than with tablets). *Skin:* photosensitivity, erythema multiforme.
thiabendazole Mintezol•	*Systemic infestation with pinworm, roundworm, threadworm, whipworm, cutaneous larva migrans, and trichinosis—* **Adults or children over 70 Kg:** 1.5 g P.O. **Adults or children under 70 Kg:** 25 mg/Kg P.O. in 2 doses daily. Maximum dose is 3 g daily. *Cutaneous infestations—larva migrans (creeping eruption)—* **Adults and children:** dose depends on patient's weight. 70 Kg or over, 1.5 g P.O./dose; under 70 Kg, 4.6 mg/Kg/dose. 2 doses daily for 2 successive days. If active lesions still present 2 days after therapy, give second course. *Pinworm—*2 doses daily for 1 day; repeat in 7 days. *Roundworm, threadworm, whipworm—*2 doses daily for 2 successive days. *Trichinosis—*2 doses daily for 2 to 4 successive days	*CNS:* impaired mental alertness, impaired physical coordination, drowsiness, giddiness, headache, dizziness. *GI:* anorexia, nausea, vomiting, diarrhea, epigastric distress. *Skin:* rash, pruritus, erythema multiforme. *Other:* lymphadenopathy, fever, flush, chills.

INTERACTIONS	NURSING CONSIDERATIONS
	• To avoid reinfestation, wash perianal area daily. Change undergarments and bedclothes daily. Wash hands and clean fingernails before meals and after bowel movements. Treat all family members. • Protect from air, light, and moisture.
None significant.	• Use cautiously in severe malnutrition or anemia, or in liver dysfunction. Treat for anemia, dehydration, or malnutrition before giving drug. • No dietary restrictions, laxatives, or enemas necessary. • May be taken with food. Shake well before pouring. • To avoid reinfestation, wash perianal area daily. Change undergarments and bedclothes daily. Wash hands and clean fingernails before meals and after bowel movements. Treat all family members. • Protect from light. Store below 30° C. (86° F.).
None significant.	• Safe use with children who weigh less than 80 lbs. not established. • Swallow tablets whole to avoid staining teeth. May be taken with food. • Warn that drug stains materials, skin, vomitus, and stools bright red. • No dietary restrictions, laxatives, or enemas necessary. • To avoid reinfestation, wash perianal area daily. Change undergarments and bedclothes daily. Wash hands and clean fingernails before meals and after bowel movements. Treat all family members. • Protect from light.
None significant.	• Use with caution in patients with hepatic or renal dysfunction, severe malnutrition, anemia, and with patients who are vomiting. Supportive therapy indicated for anemic, dehydrated, or malnourished patients. In children under 15 Kg, weigh benefits against risks. • Warn that medication may cause drowsiness and dizziness. • Give after meals. Shake suspension before measuring; chew tablets before swallowing. • Laxatives, enemas, and diet restrictions not needed. • To avoid reinfestation, wash perianal area daily. Change undergarments and bedclothes daily. Wash hands and clean fingernails before meals and after bowel movements. Treat all family members.

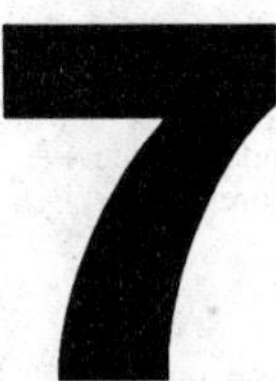

Antifungals

amphotericin B
flucytosine
griseofulvin microsize
griseofulvin ultramicrosize
miconazole
nystatin

The antifungal drugs have fungistatic and/or fungicidal properties which make them effective in treating a variety of mycotic diseases.

Major uses

- To treat systemic fungal infections and meningitis.
- To treat severe fungal infections caused by *Candida* and *Cryptococcus* organisms.
- To treat ringworm infection of the skin, hair, nails.
- To treat monilial infections of the oral cavity (thrush) and of the vaginal and intestinal tracts.
- To treat infections by yeasts.

Mechanism of action

- Amphotericin B, miconazole, and nystatin probably act by binding to sterols in the fungus cell membrane, altering its permeability and allowing the leakage of intracellular components.
- Flucytosine appears to penetrate fungal cells, where it is converted to fluorouracil, a known metabolic antagonist.
- Griseofulvin arrests fungal cell activity by disrupting its mitotic spindle structure.

Absorption, distribution, and excretion

- Amphotericin B is poorly absorbed from GI tract; serum concentrations represent less than 10% of the administered dose with 90% bound to serum proteins. It does not diffuse well into body cavities, eyes, or cerebrospinal fluid. It is slowly excreted by the kidneys. Serum half-life is 24 hours.
- Flucytosine is rapidly absorbed from GI tract, reaching peak levels in about 6 hours. About 90% is excreted unchanged in the urine. It has a half-life of 2.5 to 6 hours in patients with normal renal function; up to 200 hours in those with renal impairment. Approximately 60% to 80% of serum level is found in cerebrospinal fluid.
- Absorption of griseofulvin varies. It is almost completely absorbed through duodenum in ultramicrosize formulation; invariably and unpredictably absorbed in microsize formulation, but administration with a high-fat meal may enhance absorption. Drug concentrates in skin, hair, nails, liver, fat, and skeletal muscles, with highest concentration in outermost horny layer of skin, lowest in deep layers. Does not penetrate keratin tissue well when applied topically. Metabolized in liver, excreted in urine and feces mostly as inactive metabolite and unchanged drug; also excreted in perspiration.
- Miconazole is poorly absorbed from the GI tract; rapidly metabolized in the liver; and excreted mainly as inactive metabolites. Its half-life of up to 24 hours does not increase in renal impairment. Miconazole penetrates into joints.
- Oral absorption of nystatin is negligible; is not absorbed through intact skin or mucous membranes; no measurable blood levels at therapeutic doses; excreted unchanged into stool.

Onset and duration

- Following intravenous infusion of 30 mg amphotericin B, average peak serum level of 1 mcg/ml were observed. Immediately after infusion, no more than 10% of dose appears in serum. Amphotericin B can be detected in blood and urine 4 weeks after therapy is discontinued.
- Flucytosine is well absorbed from GI tract, reaching peak serum levels of 30 to 45 mcg/ml within 6 hours of single 2 g oral dose in patients with normal renal function.
- With intravenous injection of 9 mg/Kg miconazole, blood levels are at least 1 mcg/ml. Rapid fall in blood levels occurs within 30 minutes.
- Griseofulvin reaches peak plasma levels in 4 hours and is undetectable in skin 2 days after drug is discontinued and in plasma after 4 days. Drug levels in skin are higher in warm climates.
- Nystatin products vary in onset and duration.

Combination products

ACHROSTATIN-V: nystatin 250,000 units and tetracycline HC1 250 mg.
COMYCIN: nystatin 250,000 units and tetracycline phosphate complex (equivalent to tetracycline HC1) 250 mg.
DECLOSTATIN TABS: nystatin 500,000 units and demeclocycline HC1 300 mg.
DECLOSTATIN CAPS: nystatin 250,000 units and demeclocycline HC1 150 mg.
MYSTECLIN-F CAPS: tetracycline HC1 250 mg and amphotericin B 50 mg.
MYSTECLIN-F125 CAPS: tetracycline HC1 125 mg and amphotericin B 25 mg.
MYSTECLIN-F SYRUP: tetracycline HCl 125 mg and amphotericin B 25 mg.
TERRASTATIN CAPS: nystatin 250,000 units and oxytetracycline 250 mg.
TETRASTATIN CAPS: nystatin 250,000 units and tetracycline HC1 250 mg.

PATIENT TEACHING AID — HOW TO INSTILL VAGINAL OINTMENT

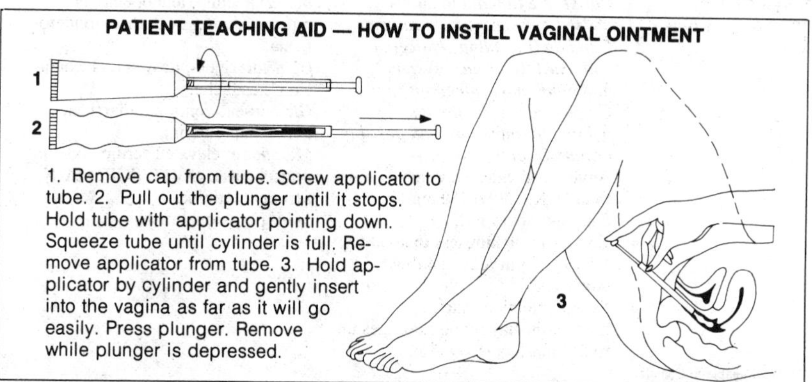

1. Remove cap from tube. Screw applicator to tube. 2. Pull out the plunger until it stops. Hold tube with applicator pointing down. Squeeze tube until cylinder is full. Remove applicator from tube. 3. Hold applicator by cylinder and gently insert into the vagina as far as it will go easily. Press plunger. Remove while plunger is depressed.

NAME	INDICATIONS & DOSAGE	SIDE EFFECTS
amphotericin B Fungizone◆	*Systemic fungal infections (histoplasmosis, coccidioidomycosis, blastomycosis, cryptococcosis, disseminated moniliasis, aspergillosis, phycomycosis), meningitis—* **Adults and children:** initially, 1 mg in 250 ml of 5% dextrose infused over 2 to 4 hours; or 0.25 mg/Kg daily by slow infusion over 6 hours. Increase gradually as patient tolerance develops to maximum 1.0 mg/Kg daily. Therapy must not exceed 1.5 mg/Kg. If drug is discontinued for a week or more, administration must resume with initial dose and again increase gradually. Topical (3% cream, lotion, ointment): apply liberally and rub well into affected area b.i.d. to q.i.d. Intrathecal: 25 mcg (0.1 ml of the reconstituted injection) diluted with 10 to 20 ml of cerebrospinal fluid and administered by barbotage 2 or 3 times weekly. Initial dose should not exceed 50 mcg. *Coccidioidal arthritis:* **Adults:** 5 to 15 mg intra-articular into joint spaces.	*Blood:* normochromic, normocytic anemia. *CNS:* headache, peripheral neuropathy; with intrathecal administration—peripheral nerve pain, paresthesias. *CV:* thrombophlebitis. *GI:* anorexia, weight loss, nausea, vomiting, dyspepsia, diarrhea, epigastric cramps. *GU:* abnormal renal function with hypokalemia, azotemia, hyposthenuria, renal tubular acidosis, nephrocalcinosis; with large doses—permanent renal impairment, anuria, oliguria. *Local:* burning, stinging, irritation, tissue damage with extravasation. *Other:* arthralgia, myalgia, muscle weakness secondary to hypokalemia, fever, chills, pain at site of injection, malaise, generalized pain.
flucytosine Ancobon, Ancotil◆◆	*For severe fungal infections caused by susceptible strains of Candida (including septicemia, endocarditis, urinary system and pulmonary infections) and Cryptococcus (meningitis, pulmonary infection, and possibly urinary tract infections)—* **Adults, and children weighing more than 50 Kg:** 50 to 150 mg/Kg daily q 6 hours P.O. **Children weighing less than 50 Kg:** 1.5 to 4.5 g/m^2/day in 4 divided doses P.O. Severe infections such as meningitis may require dosages up to 250 mg/Kg.	*Blood:* anemia, leukopenia, bone marrow depression, thrombocytopenia. *CNS:* dizziness, drowsiness, confusion, headache. *GI:* nausea, vomiting, diarrhea, abdominal bloating. *Metabolic:* elevated serum alkaline phosphatase, SGOT, SGPT, BUN, serum creatinine. *Skin:* occasional rash.

◆ Also available in Canada.
◆◆ Available in Canada only.
Unmarked trade names available in United States only.

INTERACTIONS	NURSING CONSIDERATIONS
None significant.	• Use cautiously in patients with impaired renal function. • Use parenterally only in hospitalized patients, under close supervision, when diagnosis of potentially fatal fungal infection has been confirmed. • Monitor vital signs; fever may appear 1 to 2 hours after start of I.V. infusion and should subside within 4 hours of discontinuation. • Monitor intake/output; report change in appearance or volume. Renal damage usually reversible if drug stopped at first sign of dysfunction. • Perform liver and renal function tests weekly. If BUN exceeds 40 mg/100 ml, or if serum creatinine exceeds 3 mg/100 ml, doctor may reduce or stop drug until renal function improves. Monitor CBC weekly. Stop drug if elevated Bromsulphalein, alkaline phosphatase, or bilirubin. • Monitor potassium levels closely. Report any signs of hypokalemia. Check calcium and magnesium levels periodically. • Potentially ototoxic; report any hearing loss, tinnitus, dizziness. • In the dry state, store at 2° to 8° C. (35.6° to 46.4° F.). Protect from light. Expires 2 years after date of manufacture. Reconstitute with 10 ml sterile water only. Mixing with solutions containing sodium chloride, other electrolytes, or bacteriostatic agents such as benzyl alcohol causes precipitation. Do not use if solution contains precipitate or foreign matter. Use aseptic technique. • Appears to be compatible with limited amounts of heparin sodium, hydrocortisone sodium succinate, and methylprednisolone sodium succinate. • Reconstituted solution is stable for 1 week under refrigeration or 24 hours at room temperature. Protect from light. Wrap bottle and tubing in aluminum foil. • Recommended infusion solution is 10 mg/100 ml of 5% dextrose in water. • Severity of some side effects can be reduced by premedication with aspirin, antihistamines, antiemetics, or small doses of corticosteroids; addition of phosphate buffer and heparin to the solution; and alternate-day dose schedule. For severe reactions, drug may have to be stopped for varying periods. • For I.V. infusion, an in-line membrane with mean pore diameter larger than 1 micron can be used. Infuse very slowly; rapid infusion may result in cardiovascular collapse. Warn of discomfort at infusion site. • Antibiotics should be given separately; don't mix or piggyback with amphotericin. • Advise patient that several months of therapy may be needed to assure adequate response. • Topical preparations may stain clothing.
None significant.	• Use with extreme caution in patients with impaired liver or renal function, or bone marrow depression. • Hematologic, and renal and liver function studies should precede therapy and should be repeated at frequent intervals thereafter. Before treatment, susceptibility tests should establish that organism is flucytosine sensitive. Tests should be repeated weekly to monitor drug resistance. • Flucytosine is well absorbed from the GI tract. Nausea, vomiting, stomach upset are reduced if capsules are given over a 15-minute period. • Monitor intake and output; report any marked change. • Serum level assays of drug should be performed regularly to maintain flucytosine at therapeutic level (25 to 120 mcg/ml). • Drug is often combined with amphotericin B; use may be synergistic; but may increase toxic effects. • Store in light-resistant containers. • Inform patient that adequate response may take weeks or months.

NAME	INDICATIONS & DOSAGE	SIDE EFFECTS
griseofulvin microsize Fulvicin-U/F♦, Grifulvin V, Grisactin, Grisovin-FP♦♦, Grisowen	*Ringworm infections of skin, hair, nails (tinea corporis, tinea pedis, tinea cruris, tinea barbae, tinea capitis, and tinea unguium) when caused by Trichophyton, Microsporum, or Epidermophyton—* **Adults:** 500 mg P.O. daily in single or divided doses. Severe infections may require up to 1 g daily. **Children over 50 lbs.:** 250 to 500 mg P.O. daily. **Children 30 to 50 lbs.:** 125 to 250 mg daily (approximately 5 mg griseofulvin microsize/lb. daily).	*Blood:* leukopenia, granulocytopenia (requires discontinuation of drug). *CNS:* headaches (in early stages of treatment), fatigue with large doses, occasional mental confusion, impaired performance of routine activities, psychotic symptoms. *GI:* nausea, vomiting, excessive thirst, flatulence, diarrhea. *Metabolic:* porphyria. *Skin:* rash, urticaria, photosensitive reactions (may aggravate lupus erythematosus). *Other:* estrogen-like effects in children, oral thrush.
griseofulvin ultramicrosize Fulvicin P/G, Gris-PEG	**Adults:** 125 mg tablet, P.O. b.i.d. or 250 mg daily. Resistant fungal infections of tinea pedis and tinea unguium may require divided daily dose of 500 mg. **Children over 50 lbs.:** 125 mg to 250 mg daily, P.O. **Children 30 to 50 lbs.:** 62.5 mg to 125 mg daily, P.O.	
miconazole Monistat I.V.	*Treatment of systemic fungal infections (coccidioidomycosis, candidiasis, cryptococcosis, paracoccidioidomycosis), chronic mucocutaneous candidiasis—* **Adults:** 200 to 3,600 mg per day. Doses may vary with diagnosis and with infective agent. May divide daily dose over 3 infusions, 200 to 1,200 mg per infusion. Repeated courses may be needed due to relapse or reinfection. **Children:** 20 to 40 mg/Kg per day. Do not exceed 15 mg/Kg per infusion.	*Blood:* transient decreases in hematocrit, thrombocytopenia. *CNS:* dizziness, drowsiness. *GI:* nausea, vomiting, diarrhea. *Metabolic:* transient decrease in serum sodium. *Skin:* pruritic rash. *Other:* phlebitis at site of injection.
nystatin Mycostatin♦, Nadostine♦♦, Nilstat♦, O-V Statin	*Gastrointestinal infections—* **Adults:** 500,000 to 1,000,000 units as oral tablets, t.i.d. *Treatment of oral, vaginal, and intestinal infections caused by Candida albicans (Monilia) and other Candida species—* **Adults:** 400,000 to 600,000 units oral suspension q.i.d. for oral candidiasis. **Children, and infants over 3 months:** 250,000 to 500,000 units oral suspension q.i.d.	*GI:* transient nausea, vomiting, diarrhea (usually with large oral dosage).

INTERACTIONS	NURSING CONSIDERATIONS
Barbiturates: decreased griseofulvin absorption. Divide into 3 doses of griseofulvin per day.	• Contraindicated in patients with porphyria or hepatocellular failure. Since griseofulvin is a penicillin derivative, cross sensitivity is possible. Use cautiously in penicillin-sensitive patients. Use only when topical treatment fails to arrest mycotic disease. • Blood studies, and renal and liver function tests should be repeated regularly. • Advise patient that a long period of treatment may be needed to control infection and prevent relapse, even if symptoms abate in first few days of therapy. Tell patient to keep skin clean and dry, and to maintain good hygiene. Caution him to avoid intense sunlight. • Most effectively absorbed and causes least GI distress when given after high-fat meal. • Effective treatment of tinea pedis may require concomitant use of topical agent. • Diagnosis of infecting organism should be verified in lab. Continue drug until clinical and laboratory examination confirm complete eradication. • Because griseofulvin ultramicrosize is dispersed in polyethylene glycol (PEG), it is absorbed more rapidly and completely than microsize preparations and is effective at one half the usual griseofulvin dose.
None significant.	• Rapid injection of undiluted miconazole may produce arrhythmia. • Premedication with antiemetic may lessen nausea and vomiting. • Avoid administration at mealtime in order to lessen GI side effects. • Lesser incidence and severity of side effects with this drug may offer a significant advantage over other antifungals. • In treatment of fungal meningitis and urinary bladder infections, must be supplemented with intrathecal administration and bladder irrigation. • Intravenous infusion should be given over 30 to 60 minutes. • Inform patient that adequate response may take weeks or months. • Transient elevations in serum cholesterol and triglycerides may be due to castor oil vehicle.
None significant.	• Nystatin is virtually nontoxic and nonsensitizing when used orally, vaginally, topically; but advise patient to report any redness, swelling, or irritation. • Vaginal tablets can be used by pregnant women up to 6 weeks before term to prevent thrush in newborn. Continue therapy during menstruation. Instruct patient to wash applicator thoroughly after use. • Explain that use of antibiotics, birth control pills, and corticosteroids; diabetes; pregnancy; reinfection by sexual partner; and tight-fitting panty hose are predisposing factors for vaginal infection and should be considered in management program. • For treatment of oral candidiasis (thrush), tell patient to hold suspension in mouth for several minutes before swallowing. For treatment in infants, swab medication on oral mucosa. Patient should observe good mouth

(continued on following page)

NAME	INDICATIONS & DOSAGE	SIDE EFFECTS
nystatin *(continued)*	**Newborn and premature infants:** 100,000 units oral suspension q.i.d. *Vaginal infections—* **Women:** 100,000 units, as vaginal tablets, inserted high into vagina, daily or b.i.d. for 14 days.	

INTERACTIONS	NURSING CONSIDERATIONS
	hygiene. Tell patient overuse of mouthwash or poorly fitting dentures, especially in older patients, may alter flora and promote infection. • Advise patient to continue medication for 1 to 2 weeks after symptomatic improvement to ensure against reinfection. Consult doctor for exact length of therapy. • Instruct patient in careful hygiene for affected areas. • Store in tightly closed, light-resistant containers in cool place. Check expiration date. • Not effective against systemic infections.

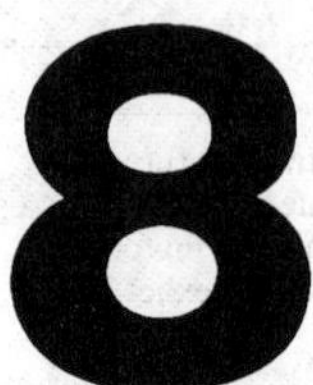

Antimalarials

amodiaquine hydrochloride
chloroquine hydrochloride
chloroquine phosphate
hydroxychloroquine sulfate
primaquine phosphate
pyrimethamine
quinine sulfate

Quinine, the bitter alkaloid obtained from the bark of the cinchona tree, and its synthetic substitutes are used for both prophylaxis and treatment of malaria.

Major uses

- To provide suppressive treatment and treatment of acute attacks of malaria due to *Plasmodium vivax, Plasmodium malariae, Plasmodium ovale,* and certain strains of *Plasmodium falciparum*.
- Certain compounds also used in treating lupus erythematosus, rheumatoid arthritis, tapeworm, and giardiasis (see Chapter 6, Anthelmintics), and extraintestinal amebiasis (see also Chapter 5, Amebicides and Trichomonacides).

Mechanism of action

- Exact mechanism of action of quinine is unknown, but it is often referred to as a generalized protoplasmic poison.
- The 4-aminoquinoline compounds (amodiaquine, chloroquine, hydroxychloroquine) bind to and alter the properties of both microbial and mammalian DNA.
- Primaquine phosphate is a gametocytocidal drug which destroys exoerythrocytic forms and will prevent a delayed primary attack.
- Pyrimethamine exerts its antimalarial effect by inhibiting the reduction of folic acid.

Absorption, distribution, and excretion

- Quinine is rapidly and completely absorbed, is highly protein-bound, and is excreted mostly as inactive metabolites.
- 4-aminoquinoline compounds are rapidly absorbed from the GI tract. They are bound to serum proteins and achieve very high levels in liver, spleen, kidneys, and lungs. They are metabolized and slowly excreted in the urine for years after treatment.
- Primaquine is readily absorbed after oral administration, rapidly metabolized with only a small amount of the unchanged drug excreted.
- Pyrimethamine is completely and regularly absorbed from the GI tract. It is metabolized and excreted in urine and is also excreted in the milk of lactating females.

Onset and duration

- Maximum plasma level reached within 1 to 2 hours.
- Still identifiable in the urine months later.

Combination products

ARALEN PHOSPHATE WITH PRIMAQUINE PHOSPHATE: chloroquine phosphate 500 mg and primaquine phosphate 79 mg.
QUINAMM: quinine sulfate 260 mg and aminophylline 195 mg.

MALARIA FACTS

Even though malaria is rare outside of Asia, Africa, and South America, you can't rule out the possibility of dealing with it in one of your patients. Here are some facts to bring your knowledge about malaria up to date.

- In the United States, malaria carriers are visitors from malarial areas (Africa, Central and South America, and Southeast Asia) and armed forces personnel (especially Viet Nam veterans).
- Malaria is caused by: a protozoa introduced into the human body through the bite of an infected anopheles mosquito; transfusion of blood from an infected donor; or usage of a common syringe by drug addicts.
- The incubation period is usually 10 to 35 days,followed by a short 2- to 3-day prodome of irregular low-grade fever, malaise, headache, and myalgia.
- Attempts to induce immunity with vaccines have failed. Preventive measures include: control of mosquito breeding places; use of residual insecticide sprays in homes and public buildings; screens on windows and doors; mosquito netting where screens are unsuitable; personal use of mosquito repellents; and wearing sufficient clothing, particularly after sundown, to protect as much skin as possible against mosquito bites.
- Disqualify from blood donation for three years persons on suppressive antimalarial therapy and those exposed to malaria (anyone who has visited a region where malaria is prevalent).
- Recognize malaria by periodic attacks of chills and fever without apparent cause, especially with spleen enlargement, in a person who has been in a malarious area within the year.
- Other malarial symptoms to look for: headache, nausea, and vomiting.
- To diagnose malaria, a blood smear should be taken, checking for hepatosplenomegaly cells and Kupffer's cells distended with parasites. Since intensity of the parasites often varies, more than one blood smear is required.

NAME	INDICATIONS & DOSAGE	SIDE EFFECTS
amodiaquine hydrochloride Camoquin HCl	*Suppressive prophylaxis and treatment of acute attacks of malaria due to P. vivax, P. malariae, P. ovale, and susceptible strains of P. falciparum—* **Adults:** (for suppression) single dose of 300 to 600 mg P.O. weekly, preferably on same day of week; (for acute attacks) 600 mg P.O. initially, then 300 mg at 6, 24, and 48 hours. **Children:** (for suppression) 5 mg/Kg P.O. weekly, preferably on same day of week; (for acute attacks) 10 mg/Kg P.O. divided into 3 doses at 12-hour intervals.	*Blood:* blood dyscrasias (agranulocytosis, leukopenia, pancytopenia). *CNS:* mild and transient headache, neuromyopathy, polyneuritis, psychic stimulation, fatigue, irritability, nightmares, convulsions, dizziness, toxic psychosis. *CV* (rare): hypotension, EKG changes. *EENT:* visual disturbances (blurred vision; difficulty in focusing; reversible corneal changes; generally irreversible, sometimes progressive or delayed, retinal changes, e.g., narrowing of arterioles; macular lesions; pallor of optic disc; optic atrophy; patchy retinal pigmentation, often leading to blindness); ototoxicity, nerve deafness, tinnitus, labyrinthitis. *GI:* anorexia, abdominal cramps, diarrhea, nausea, vomiting, toxic hepatitis. *Skin:* pruritus, lichen planus-like eruptions, skin and mucosal pigmentary changes, pleomorphic skin eruptions.
chloroquine hydrochloride Aralen HCl, Roquine **chloroquine phosphate** Aralen Phosphate♦, Chlorocon	*Suppressive prophylaxis and treatment of acute attacks of malaria due to P. vivax, P. malariae, P. ovale, and susceptible strains of P. falciparum—* **Adults:** initially, 600 mg P.O., then 300 mg P.O. at 6, 24, and 48 hours. Or 160 to 200 mg I.M. initially; repeat in 6 hours if needed. Switch to oral therapy as soon as possible. **Children:** initially, 10 mg (base)/Kg P.O., then 5 mg (base)/Kg dose P.O. at 6, 24, and 48 hours (do not exceed adult dose). Or 5 mg (base)/Kg I.M. initially; repeat in 6 hours if needed. Switch to oral therapy as soon as possible. *Malaria suppressive treatment—* **Adults and children:** 5 mg (base)/Kg P.O. (not to exceed 300 mg) weekly on same day of the week (begin 2 weeks before entering endemic area and continue for 8 weeks after it). If treatment begins after exposure, double the initial dose (600 mg for adults, 10 mg/Kg for children) in 2 divided doses, P.O. 6 hours apart.	*Blood:* agranulocytosis, blood dyscrasias. *CNS:* mild and transient headache, neuromyopathy, psychic stimulation, fatigue, irritability, nightmares, convulsions, dizziness. *CV* (rare): hypotension, EKG changes. *EENT:* visual disturbances (blurred vision; difficulty in focusing; reversible corneal changes; generally irreversible, sometimes progressive or delayed, retinal changes, e.g., narrowing of arterioles; macular lesions; pallor of optic disc; optic atrophy; patchy retinal pigmentation, often leading to blindness); ototoxicity; nerve deafness, vertigo, tinnitus. *GI:* anorexia, abdominal cramps, diarrhea, nausea, vomiting. *Skin:* pruritus, lichen planus-like eruptions, skin and mucosal pigmentary changes, pleomorphic skin eruptions.

♦ Also available in Canada.
♦♦ Available in Canada only.
Unmarked trade names available in United States only.

INTERACTIONS	NURSING CONSIDERATIONS
None significant.	• Contraindicated in patients with retinal or visual field changes, porphyria, severe hepatic disease. Use with extreme caution in presence of severe GI, neurologic, or blood disorders. Use with caution in patients with G-6-PD deficiency or psoriasis; drug may exacerbate these conditions. • Complete blood cell counts, including liver function studies, should be made periodically during prolonged therapy; if severe blood disorder appears which is not attributable to disease under treatment, drug may need to be discontinued. • Overdosage can quickly lead to toxic symptoms: headache, drowsiness, visual disturbances, cardiovascular collapse and convulsions, followed by sudden and early respiratory and cardiac arrest. Children are extremely susceptible to toxicity; avoid long-term treatment. • Baseline and periodic ophthalmologic examinations needed. Report blurred vision, increased sensitivity to light, or muscle weakness. Check periodically for muscular weakness after long-term use. Audiometric exams recommended before, during, and after therapy, especially if long term. • Give immediately before or after meals on same day each week. • To avoid exacerbated drug-induced dermatoses, warn patient to avoid excessive exposure to sun.
None significant.	• Contraindicated in patients with retinal or visual field changes, porphyria. Use with extreme caution in presence of severe GI, neurologic, or blood disorders. Drug concentrates in liver; use cautiously in patients with hepatic disease or alcoholism. Use with caution in patients with G-6-PD deficiency or psoriasis; drug may exacerbate these conditions. • Complete blood cell counts, including liver function studies, should be made periodically during prolonged therapy; if severe blood disorder appears which is not attributable to disease under treatment, drug may need to be discontinued. • Overdosage can quickly lead to toxic symptoms: headache, drowsiness, visual disturbances, cardiovascular collapse and convulsions, followed by sudden and early respiratory and cardiac arrest. Children are extremely susceptible to toxicity; avoid long-term treatment. • Baseline and periodic ophthalmologic examinations needed. Report blurred vision, increased sensitivity to light, or muscle weakness. Check periodically for muscular weakness after long-term use. Audiometric exams recommended before, during, and after therapy, especially if long term. • Give drug immediately before or after meals on same day each week. • To avoid exacerbated drug-induced dermatoses, warn patient to avoid excessive exposure to sun. • Each ml parenteral solution containing 50 mg dihydrochloride salt = 40 mg chloroquine base; each 500 mg tablet phosphate = 300 mg base.

NAME	INDICATIONS & DOSAGE	SIDE EFFECTS
hydroxychloroquine sulfate Plaquenil Sulfate♦	*Suppressive prophylaxis of attacks of malaria due to P. vivax, P. malariae, P. ovale, and susceptible strains of P. falciparum—* **Adults and children:** for suppression: 5 mg (base)/Kg body weight P.O. (not to exceed 300 mg) weekly on same day of the week (begin 2 weeks prior to and continue for 8 weeks after leaving endemic area). If not started prior to exposure, double initial dose (600 mg for adults, 10 mg/Kg for children) in 2 divided doses P.O. 6 hours apart. *Treatment of acute malarial attacks—* **Adults, and children over 15 years:** initially, 800 mg (sulfate) P.O., then 400 mg after 6 to 8 hours, then 400 mg daily for 2 days (total 2 g sulfate salt). **Children 11 to 15 years:** 600 mg (sulfate) P.O. stat, then 200 mg 8 hours later, then 200 mg 24 hours later (total 1 g sulfate salt). **Children 6 to 10 years:** 400 mg (sulfate) P.O. stat, then 2 doses of 200 mg at 8-hour intervals (total 800 mg sulfate salt). **Children 2 to 5 years:** 400 mg (sulfate) P.O. stat, then 200 mg 8 hours later (total 600 mg sulfate salt). **Children under 1 year:** 100 mg (sulfate) P.O. stat; then 3 doses of 100 mg 6 to 9 hours apart (total 400 mg sulfate salt). *Lupus erythematosus (chronic discoid and systemic)—* **Adults:** 400 mg P.O. daily or b.i.d., continued for several weeks or months, depending on response. Prolonged maintenance—200 to 400 mg P.O. daily. *Rheumatoid arthritis—* **Adults:** initially, 400 to 600 mg P.O. daily. When good response occurs (usually in 4 to 12 weeks), cut dosage in half.	*Blood:* dyscrasias (agranulocytosis, leukopenia, thrombocytopenia, aplastic anemia). *CNS:* irritability, nightmares, ataxia, convulsions, psychic stimulation, toxic psychosis, vertigo, tinnitus, nystagmus, lassitude, fatigue, dizziness. *CV* (rare): hypotension, EKG changes. *EENT:* visual disturbances (blurred vision; difficulty in focusing, reversible corneal changes; generally irreversible, sometimes progressive or delayed, retinal changes, e.g., narrowing of arterioles; macular lesions; pallor of optic disc; optic atrophy; patchy retinal pigmentation, often leading to blindness); ototoxicity, irreversible nerve deafness, tinnitus, labyrinthitis. *GI:* anorexia, abdominal cramps, diarrhea, nausea, vomiting. *Skin:* pruritus, lichen planus-like eruptions, skin and mucosal pigmentary changes, pleomorphic skin eruptions, bleaching of hair. *Other:* weight loss, skeletal muscle weakness, hypoactive deep tendon reflexes.

INTERACTIONS	NURSING CONSIDERATIONS
None significant.	• Contraindicated in patients with retinal or visual field changes, porphyria. Use with extreme caution in presence of severe GI, neurologic, or blood disorders. Drug concentrates in the liver; use cautiously in patients with hepatic disease or alcoholism. Use with caution in patients with G-6-PD deficiency or psoriasis; drug may exacerbate these conditions. • Complete blood cell counts, including liver function studies, should be made periodically during prolonged therapy; if severe blood disorder appears which is not attributable to disease under treatment, consider discontinuing. • Overdosage can quickly lead to toxic symptoms: headache, drowsiness, visual disturbances, cardiovascular collapse and convulsions, followed by sudden and early respiratory and cardiac arrest. Children are extremely susceptible to toxicity; avoid long-term treatment. • Baseline and periodic ophthalmologic examinations needed. Report blurred vision, increased sensitivity to light, or muscle weakness. Check periodically for muscular weakness after long-term use. Audiometric exams recommended before, during, and after therapy, especially if long-term. • Give drug immediately before or after meals on same day of each week. • 100 mg sulfate salt = 77.5 mg hydroxychloroquine base.

NAME	INDICATIONS & DOSAGE	SIDE EFFECTS
primaquine phosphate	*Radical cure of relapsing vivax malaria, eliminating symptoms and infection completely; prevention of relapse—* **Adults:** 15 to 30 mg (base) P.O. daily for 14 days. (26.3-mg tablet = 15 mg of base)	*Blood:* leukopenia, hemolytic anemia in G-6-PD deficiency, methemoglobinemia in NADH methemoglobin reductase deficiency, leukocytosis, acute intravascular hemolysis, mild anemia, granulocytopenia, agranulocytosis. *EENT:* disturbances of visual accommodation. *GI:* nausea, vomiting, epigastric distress, abdominal cramps. *Skin:* urticaria.
pyrimethamine Daraprim◆	*Malaria prophylaxis and transmission control—* **Adults, and children over 10:** 25 mg P.O. weekly. **Children 4 to 10 years old:** 12.5 mg P.O. weekly. **Children under 4:** 6.25 mg P.O. weekly. Continue in all age groups at least 10 weeks after leaving endemic areas. *Acute attacks of malaria—* not recommended alone in nonimmune persons; use with faster-acting antimalarials, as chloroquine, for 2 days to initiate transmission control and suppressive cure. **Adults, and children over 15:** 25 mg P.O. daily for 2 days. **Children under 15:** 12.5 mg P.O. daily for 2 days. *Toxoplasmosis—* **Adults:** 75 mg P.O. daily for 1 to 3 days, then 25 mg P.O. daily for 3 to 4 weeks; during same time give l g sulfadiazine P.O. q 6 hours. Stop therapy with both drugs for 1 week. Then give 25 mg pyrimethamine P.O. daily for 3 to 4 weeks, along with 1 g sulfadiazine P.O. q 6 hours. **Children:** 1 mg/Kg P.O., then 0.5 mg daily for 3 to 4 weeks, along with 100 mg sulfadiazine/Kg P.O. daily, divided q 6 hours. Stop therapy with both drugs for 1 week. Then give 0.5 mg pyrimethamine P.O. daily for 3 to 4 more weeks, along with 100 mg sulfadiazine/Kg P.O. daily divided q 6 hours.	*Blood:* megaloblastic anemia, bone marrow depression, leukopenia, thrombocytopenia, pancytopenia. *CNS:* stimulation and convulsions (acute toxicity). *GI:* anorexia, vomiting, diarrhea, atrophic glossitis. *Skin:* rashes.

INTERACTIONS	NURSING CONSIDERATIONS
None significant.	• Contraindicated in patients with lupus erythematosus and rheumatoid arthritis; in patients taking bone marrow depressants and potentially hemolytic drugs. • Use with a fast-acting blood schizonticide, such as amodiaquine or chloroquine. Use full dose to reduce possibility of drug-resistant strains. • Caucasians taking more than 30 mg daily, dark-skinned patients taking more than 15 mg (base) daily, and patients with severe anemia or suspected sensitivity should have frequent blood studies and urine examinations. Sudden fall in hemoglobin concentration, erythrocyte or leukocyte count, or marked darkening of the urine suggests impending hemolytic reactions. • Observe closely for tolerance in patients with previous idiosyncrasy (manifested by hemolytic anemia, methemoglobinemia, or leukopenia); family or personal history of favism; erythrocytic G-6-PD deficiency of NADH methemoglobin reductase deficiency. • Administer drug with meals or with antacids.
Folic acid and para-aminobenzoic acid: decreased antitoxoplasmic effects. May require dosage adjustment.	• Contraindicated in chloroguanide-resistant malaria. Use cautiously in patients with convulsive disorders; smaller doses may be needed. Also use cautiously following treatment with chloroguanide. • Dosages required to treat toxoplasmosis approach toxic levels. Twice-weekly blood counts, including platelets, are required. If signs of folic or folinic acid deficiency develop, dosage should be reduced or discontinued while patient receives parenteral folinic acid (leucovorin) until blood counts become normal. • Do not exceed recommended dosage. • Give with meals to minimize GI distress.

NAME	INDICATIONS & DOSAGE	SIDE EFFECTS
quinine sulfate Coco-Quinine	*Malaria, principally vivax: radical cure, relapsing vivax*— **Adults:** 300 to 600 mg P.O. concurrently with 30 mg pamaquine or 5 mg primaquine q 8 hours for 14 days. *Acute attacks of vivax malaria*— **Adults:** 1 g P.O. q 8 hours for 3 doses, followed by 600 mg q 8 hours for 5 to 6 days. *For malaria suppression*—300 mg to 1 g P.O. daily; 300 to 600 mg in 100 to 200 ml sterile H_2O, I.V. infused slowly over 30 minutes; or 600 mg to 1 g I.M. in 5 to 10 ml sterile 0.9% saline q 8 hours until oral dosage is feasible.	*Blood:* hemolytic anemia, thrombocytopenia, agranulocytosis, hypoprothrombinemia. *CNS:* severe headache, apprehension, excitement, confusion, delirium, syncope, hypothermia, convulsions (with toxic doses). *CV:* decreased blood pressure, cardiovascular collapse with overdosage or rapid I.V. administration. *EENT:* altered color perception, photophobia, blurred vision, night blindness, amblyopia, scotomata, diplopia, mydriasis, optic atrophy, tinnitus, impaired hearing. *GI:* epigastric distress, diarrhea, nausea, vomiting. *GU:* renal tubular damage, anuria. *Local:* thrombosis at infusion site. *Skin:* rashes, pruritus. *Other:* asthma, flushing.

INTERACTIONS	NURSING CONSIDERATIONS
Sodium bicarbonate: elevated quinine levels. Use together cautiously.	• Contraindicated in patients with G-6-PD deficiency. Use with caution in patients with cardiovascular conditions. • Discontinue if any signs of idiosyncrasy or toxicity occur. • I.V. therapy must be used cautiously, as marked fall in blood pressure often follows. Monitor blood pressure frequently. • I.V. route is preferred to I.M. route. Avoid extravasation. • Has been used as a treatment for nocturnal leg cramps.

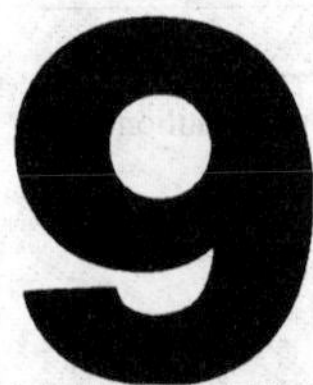

Antituberculars and antileprotics

capreomycin sulfate
cycloserine
dapsone
ethambutol hydrochloride
ethionamide
isoniazid
para-aminosalicylates
pyrazinamide
rifampin
streptomycin sulfate
sulfoxone sodium

The following drugs have a bacteriostatic and/or a bactericidal effect on growing tubercle bacilli: para-aminosalicylates, capreomycin sulfate, cycloserine, ethambutol hydrochloride, ethionamide, isoniazid, pyrazinamide, rifampin, and streptomycin sulfate. Dapsone and sulfoxone sodium have a bacteriostatic effect on *Mycobacterium leprae* (leprosy).

Major uses

- To prevent or treat all forms of tuberculosis.
- To treat all forms of leprosy.

Mechanism of action

- These drugs are thought to exert their antibacterial effect by inhibiting DNA and protein synthesis in susceptible organisms.

Absorption, distribution, and excretion

- Capreomycin sulfate is not significantly absorbed with oral dosage. Given I.M., it quickly reaches peak serum levels and is excreted in the urine essentially unchanged.
- Cycloserine is rapidly absorbed orally and distributed throughout body fluids and tissues, including the cerebrospinal fluid. It is partially metabolized and excreted in the urine.
- Of the sulfones, sulfoxone sodium is hydrolyzed and absorbed mainly as its active parent compound, dapsone. Dapsone is almost completely absorbed, metabolized, and slowly excreted in the urine.
- Ethambutol is absorbed from the GI tract (75% to 80%); distribution is unknown. The drug is detoxified in the liver. Most is recovered from the urine unchanged and as much as 25% from the feces.
- Given orally, ethionamide is rapidly and widely distributed, with significant levels in the cerebrospinal fluid. Most of the drug is metabolized slowly and is subsequently excreted in the urine.
- Isoniazid is readily absorbed from the gastrointestinal tract and injection sites, diffusing into all body fluids, tissues, and excreta. It also crosses the placental barrier and passes into the breast milk in concentrations attained in plasma. About half the drug is metabolized in the liver and is excreted, along with approximately 40% of unchanged drug, in the urine.
- Pyrazinamide is well absorbed from the GI tract and is widely distributed, metabolized,

and excreted in the urine.
• Rifampin is well absorbed and widely distributed, partially metabolized in the liver, crosses placental barrier, and is excreted as metabolites and unchanged drug in the urine and feces.
• All salicylates are readily absorbed from the GI tract, distributed throughout most body fluids and tissues, and excreted in the urine as metabolites and free acid.
• Streptomycin is well absorbed and widely distributed in most body tissue after I.M. injection, crosses placental barrier, and is rapidly excreted in the urine.

Onset and duration
• Capreomycin sulfate reaches peak serum levels in 1 to 2 hours; duration is about 24 hours.
• Cycloserine peaks in 4 to 8 hours; duration is about 12 hours.
• Ethambutol reaches peak levels in 2 to 4 hours; duration is about 24 hours.
• Ethionamide produces peak levels in 3 hours; is metabolized slowly, producing prolonged blood levels.
• Isoniazid peaks within 1 to 2 hours and declines to about 50% within 50 minutes in rapid isoniazid inactivators and within 3 hours in slow isoniazid inactivators.
• Pyrazinamide peaks in 2 hours; duration is about 15 hours.
• Rifampin peaks within 1½ to 4 hours; duration is about 24 hours.
• Salicylates peak within 1 hour; duration is about 10 to 12 hours.
• Streptomycin peaks within 30 minutes to 2 hours; duration is about 8 to 12 hours.
• Sulfoxone sodium peaks rapidly; duration is about 8 hours.
• Dapsone peaks within 1 to 3 hours; duration is about 8 to 12 days.

Combination products
CALPAS-INAH-6: calcium aminosalicylate 0.5 g, isoniazid 20 mg, and pyridoxine HC1 1 mg.
CALPAS ISOXINE: calcium p-aminosalicylate 0.55 g, isoniazid 12.5 mg, and vitamin B-6 2 mg.
CALPAS ISOXONE S: calcium p-aminosalicylate 0.55 g, isoniazid 25 mg, and vitamin B-6 3 mg.
DI-ISOPACIN: buffered aminosalicylic acid 750 mg and isoniazid 25 mg.
DOUBLE-ISOPACIN: sodium para-aminosalicylate 1 g and isoniazid 25 mg.
ISOPACIN: sodium para-aminosalicylate 500 mg and isoniazid 12.5 mg.
NEMASOL-INH-20 BUFFERED♦: buffered p-aminosalicylic acid 0.5 g and isoniazid 20 mg.
RIFAMATE: isoniazid 150 mg and rifampin 300 mg.
RIMACTIAID: isoniazid 100 mg and pyridoxine HCl 5 mg.
TEEBACONIN AND VITAMIN B-6: isoniazid 100 mg and pyridoxine HCl 5 mg.
TRINIAD PLUS 30: isoniazid 300 mg and pyridoxine HCl 30 mg.
UNIAD-PLUS 5: isoniazid 100 mg and pyridoxine HCl 5 mg.

NAME	INDICATIONS & DOSAGE	SIDE EFFECTS
capreomycin sulfate Capastat Sulfate	*Adjunctive treatment in pulmonary tuberculosis—* **Adults:** 15 mg/Kg/day up to 1 g I.M. daily injected deeply into large muscle mass for 60 to 120 days; then 1 g 2 to 3 times weekly for a period of 18 to 24 months. Maximum dose should not exceed 20 mg/Kg daily. Must be given in conjunction with another antitubercular drug but *not* streptomycin sulfate.	*Blood:* eosinophilia, leukocytosis, leukopenia, hypokalemia. *CNS:* headache. *EENT:* ototoxicity (tinnitus, vertigo, hearing loss). *GU:* nephrotoxicity (elevated BUN and nonprotein nitrogen, proteinuria, casts, red blood cells, leukocytes; tubular necrosis, decreased creatinine clearance). *Local:* pain, induration, excessive bleeding and sterile abscesses at injection site. *Other:* abnormal liver function tests, hypersensitivity.
cycloserine Seromycin	*Adjunctive treatment in pulmonary or extrapulmonary tuberculosis—* **Adults:** initially, 250 mg P.O. every 12 hours for 2 weeks; then, if blood levels are below 25 to 30 mcg/ml and there are no clinical signs of toxicity, dose is increased to 250 mg P.O. q 8 hours for 2 weeks. If optimum blood levels are still not achieved, and there are no signs of clinical toxicity, then dose is increased to 250 mg P.O. q 6 hours. Maximum dose 1 g/day. If CNS toxicity occurs, drug is discontinued for 1 week, then resumed at 250 mg daily for 2 weeks. If no serious toxic effects occur, dose is increased by 250 mg increments every 10 days until blood level of 25 to 30 mcg/ml is obtained.	*Blood:* elevated serum transaminase. *CNS:* drowsiness, headache, tremor, dysarthia, vertigo, confusion, loss of memory, possibly suicidal tendencies, hyperirritability, paresthesias, paresis, hyperreflexia, convulsions, coma. *Other:* hypersensitivity (allergic dermatitis).
dapsone Avlosulfon♦	*Lepromatous and tuberculoid leprosy—* **Adults:** 100 mg P.O. 2 times a week for 4 weeks; increased to 200 mg 2 times a week for 4 weeks; then 300 mg 2 times a week for 4 weeks and 400 mg 2 times a week thereafter. **Children:** reduced dosage, but not necessarily by body weight; usually approximately ½ of adult dose using same schedule. *Alternate dosage schedule—* **Adults:** 50 mg P.O. daily. **Children:** 25 mg P.O. daily. A 1-week rest period from therapy every 2 months is recommended.	*Blood:* anemia, especially hemolytic; methemoglobinemia, possible leukopenia. *CNS:* psychosis, headache, dizziness, lethargy, severe malaise, paresthesias. *EENT:* tinnitus, allergic rhinitis. *GI:* anorexia, abdominal pain, nausea, vomiting. *Skin:* allergic dermatitis (generalized or fixed maculopapular rash). *Other:* hepatitis, drug fever.

♦ Also available in Canada.
♦♦ Available in Canada only.
Unmarked trade names available in United States only.

INTERACTIONS	NURSING CONSIDERATIONS
None significant.	• Contraindicated in patients receiving other ototoxic or nephrotoxic drugs. Use cautiously in patients with impaired renal function, history of allergies, or hearing impairment. • Drug is never given I.V.; may cause neuromuscular blockade. • Evaluate patient's hearing before and during therapy. Notify doctor if patient complains of tinnitus, vertigo, hearing impairment. • Monitor renal function (output, specific gravity, blood urea nitrogen, urinalysis, serum creatinine) before and during therapy; notify doctor of decreasing renal function. Dose must be reduced in renal impairment. • Monitor serum potassium levels and liver function periodically. • Reconstituted solutions can be stored for 48 hours at room temperature or 14 days if refrigerated. Straw- or dark-colored solution does not indicate a loss in potency.
Isoniazid: monitor for CNS toxicity (dizziness or drowsiness).	• Contraindicated in patients with seizure disorders, depression or severe anxiety, severe renal insufficiency, or chronic alcoholism. Use cautiously in patients with impaired renal function; reduced dosage required. • Obtain specimen for culture and sensitivity tests before therapy begins. • Cycloserine blood levels should be obtained at least weekly. Toxic reactions may occur with blood levels above 30 mcg/ml. • Pyridoxine, anticonvulsants, tranquilizers, or sedatives may help to relieve side effects. • Observe for personality changes. • Monitor hematologic, renal, and liver function studies. • Instruct patient to take drug exactly as prescribed; warn against discontinuing use without doctor's advice.
Probenecid: elevated levels of dapsone. Use together with extreme caution.	• Contraindicated in renal amyloidosis. Use cautiously in chronic renal, hepatic, or cardiovascular disease; refractory types of anemia. • Therapy should be interrupted if generalized, diffuse dermatitis occurs. • Dapsone dosage should be reduced or temporarily discontinued if hemoglobin falls below 9 g/100 ml; if leukocyte count falls below 5,000; if erythrocyte count falls below 2.5 million; or if it remains persistently low. • Patient should receive hematinics during dapsone therapy. • Antihistamines may help to combat dapsone-induced allergic dermatitis. • Erythema nodosum type of "lepra reaction" may occur during therapy as a result of *Mycobacterium leprae* bacilli (malaise, fever, painful inflammatory induration in the skin and mucosa, iritis, neuritis). In severe cases, therapy should be stopped and glucocorticoids given cautiously. • Twice-a-week dosage schedule reduces toxic effects. • Monitor CBC frequently.

NAME	INDICATIONS & DOSAGE	SIDE EFFECTS
ethambutol hydrochloride Etibi◆◆, Myambutol◆	*Adjunctive treatment in pulmonary tuberculosis—* **Adults, and children over 13 years:** initial treatment for patients who have not received previous antitubercular therapy 15 mg/Kg P.O. daily single dose. Re-treatment: 25 mg/Kg P.O. daily single dose for 60 days with at least 1 other antitubercular drug; then decrease to 15 mg/Kg P.O. daily single dose.	*Blood:* elevated serum uric acid. *CNS:* headache, dizziness, mental confusion, possible hallucinations, peripheral neuritis (numbness and tingling of extremities). *EENT:* optic neuritis (vision loss and loss of color discrimination, especially red and green). *GI:* anorexia, nausea, vomiting, abdominal pain. *Skin:* dermatitis, pruritis. *Other:* anaphylactoid reactions, joint pain, fever, malaise, abnormal liver function tests, bloody sputum.
ethionamide Trecator SC	*Adjunctive treatment in pulmonary or extrapulmonary tuberculosis (when primary therapy with streptomycin, isoniazid, and aminosalicylic acid cannot be used or has failed)—* **Adults:** 500 mg to 1 g P.O. daily in divided doses. Concomitant administration of other effective antitubercular drugs and pyridoxine recommended.	*Blood:* thrombocytopenia. *CNS:* peripheral neuritis, psychic disturbances (especially mental depression). *CV:* postural hypotension. *GI:* anorexia, metallic taste in mouth, nausea, vomiting, sialorrhea, epigastric distress, diarrhea, stomatitis. *GU:* gynecomastia, impotence. *Skin:* rash. *Other:* jaundice, hepatitis, elevated serum transaminase, weight loss.
isoniazid (INH) Hyzyd, Isotamine◆◆, Laniazid, Niconyl, Nydrazid, Rimifon◆◆, Rolazid, Teebaconin	*Primary treatment against actively growing tubercle bacilli—* **Adults:** 5 mg/Kg P.O. or I.M. daily single dose, up to 300 mg/day, continued for 18 months to 2 years. **Infants and children:** 10 to 20 mg/Kg P.O. or I.M. daily single dose, up to 300 to 500 mg/day, continued for 18 months to 2 years. Concomitant administration of at least 1 other effective antitubercular drug is recommended. *Preventive therapy against tubercle bacilli of those closely exposed or those with positive skin test whose chest X-ray and bacteriological studies are consistent with nonprogressive tuberculous disease—* **Adults:** 300 mg P.O. daily single dose, continued for 1 year. **Infants and children:** 10 mg/Kg P.O. daily single dose, up to 300 mg/day, continued for 1 year.	*Blood:* agranulocytosis, hemolytic or aplastic anemia, eosinophilia, leukopenia, neutropenia, thrombocytopenia, methemoglobinemia, pyridoxine-responsive hypochromic anemia. *CNS:* peripheral neuropathy (especially in the malnourished, alcoholics, diabetics, and slow inactivators), usually preceded by paresthesias of hands and feet. *GI:* nausea, vomiting, epigastric distress, constipation, dryness of the mouth. *GU:* gynecomastia. *Local:* irritation at the injection site. *Metabolic:* hyperglycemia, metabolic acidosis. *Other:* rheumatic and systemic lupus erythematosus-like syndromes; hepatitis, occasionally severe and sometimes fatal, especially in the elderly; pyridoxine deficiency; hypersensitivity (fever, rash, lymphadenopathy, vasculitis).

INTERACTIONS	NURSING CONSIDERATIONS
None significant.	• Contraindicated in patients with optic neuritis, and children under 13. Use cautiously in patients with impaired renal function, cataracts, recurrent eye inflammations, gout, and diabetic retinopathy. • Dose must be reduced in renal impairment. • Perform visual acuity tests before and during therapy. • Monitor renal, hematopoietic, and hepatic functions in long-term use. • Observe patient for symptoms of gout. • Instruct patient to take this drug exactly as prescribed; warn against discontinuing use without doctor's advice. • Monitor serum uric acid.
None significant.	• Contraindicated in patients with severe hepatic damage. Use cautiously in patients with diabetes mellitus. • Optimum dosage for children not yet established but used in children if spread of disease is imminent and when other treatments have failed. • Culture and sensitivity tests should be performed before starting therapy. • Stop drug if skin rash occurs; may progress to exfoliative dermatitis. • Monitor hepatic, hematopoietic, and renal function. • Give with meals or antacids to minimize GI effects. • Patient may require antiemetic. • Pyridoxine may be ordered to prevent neuropathy. • Instruct patient to take this drug exactly as prescribed; warn against discontinuing drug without doctor's advice. • Avoid excess alcohol ingestion.
Aluminum-containing antacids and laxatives: may decrease the rate and amount of isoniazid absorbed. Give isoniazid at least 1 hour before antacid or laxative. *Disulfiram:* neurologic symptoms, including changes in behavior and coordination, may develop with concomitant isoniazid use. Avoid concomitant use.	• Contraindicated in patients with acute liver disease, or isoniazid-associated liver damage. Use cautiously in patients with chronic non-isoniazid-associated hepatic disease, seizure disorders, severe renal impairment, chronic alcoholism; in elderly patients; in slow acetylator phenotypes (approximately 50% of Blacks and Caucasians). • Monitor liver function if clinical signs of hepatic dysfunction occur during therapy. Tell patient to notify doctor immediately if symptoms of liver impairment occur (loss of appetite, fatigue, malaise, jaundice, dark urine). • Alcohol may be associated with increased incidence of isoniazid-related hepatitis. Discourage use. • Pyridoxine may be given to prevent peripheral neuropathy, especially in malnourished patients. • Instruct patient to take this drug exactly as prescribed; warn against discontinuing drug without doctor's advice. • Store drug at room temperature. • Avoid excessive laxative use.

NAME	INDICATIONS & DOSAGE	SIDE EFFECTS
para-aminosalicylates		*Blood:* leukopenia, agranulocytosis, eosinophilia, thrombocytopenia, hemolytic anemia, hypokalemia. *CNS:* encephalopathy. *CV:* vasculitis. *GI:* nausea, vomiting, diarrhea, abdominal pain. *GU:* albuminuria, hematuria, crystalluria. *Metabolic:* goiter, with or without myxedema; acidosis. *Skin:* rash. *Other:* infectious mononucleosis-like syndrome, fever, jaundice, hepatitis, lymphadenopathy.
calcium aminosalicylate Teebacin Calcium	*Adjunctive treatment in pulmonary or extrapulmonary tuberculosis—* **Adults:** 13 to 15 g P.O. daily, divided in 2 or 3 doses. **Children:** 375 mg/Kg P.O. daily, divided in 3 or 4 doses.	
para-aminosalicylic acid PAS, Nemasol Sodium••	*Treatment of tuberculosis—* **Adults:** 10 to 12 g P.O. daily, divided in 2 or 3 doses. **Children:** 300 mg/Kg P.O. daily, divided in 3 or 4 doses.	
potassium aminosalicylate Teebacin Kalium	*Treatment of tuberculosis—* **Adults:** 12.5 to 15 g P.O. daily, divided in 3 or 4 doses. **Children:** 375 mg/Kg P.O. daily, divided in 3 or 4 doses.	
sodium aminosalicylate Parasal Sodium, Pasdium, Teebacin	*Treatment of tuberculosis—* **Adults:** 14 to 16 g P.O. daily, divided in 3 or 4 doses. **Children:** 375 mg/Kg P.O. daily, divided in 3 or 4 doses.	
pyrazinamide Tebrazid••	*Hospitalized patients seriously ill with tuberculosis (when primary and secondary antitubercular drugs cannot be used or have failed)—* **Adults:** 25 to 35 mg/Kg P.O. daily, divided in 3 to 4 doses. Maximum dose 3 g daily.	*Blood:* hemolytic anemia, hyperuricemia, possible bleeding tendency due to altered clotting mechanism or vascular integrity. *GI:* anorexia, nausea, vomiting. *GU:* dysuria. *Metabolic:* interference with control in diabetes mellitus. *Other:* fatal hemoptysis, hepatitis, malaise, fever, arthralgia.
rifampin Rifadin•, Rimactane•	*Primary treatment in pulmonary tuberculosis—* **Adults:** 600 mg P.O. daily single dose 1 hour before or 2 hours after meals. **Children over 5 years:** 10 to 20 mg/Kg P.O. daily single dose 1 hour before or 2 hours after meals. Maximum dose 600 mg daily. Concomitant administration of other effective antitubercular drugs is recommended. *Meningococcal carriers—* **Adults:** 600 mg P.O. daily for 4 days.	*Blood:* eosinophilia, thrombocytopenia, transient leukopenia, hemolytic anemia, decreased hemoglobin, elevated BUN and serum uric acid. *CNS:* headache, fatigue, drowsiness, ataxia, dizziness, mental confusion, generalized numbness. *EENT:* visual disturbances, exudative conjunctivitis. *GI:* epigastric distress, anorexia, nausea, vomiting, abdominal pain, diarrhea, flatulence, sore mouth and tongue. *GU:* menstrual disturbances. *Skin:* pruritus, urticaria, rash.

INTERACTIONS	NURSING CONSIDERATIONS
Ascorbic acid, ammonium chloride: made urine acid, increased possibility of para-aminosalicylic acid crystalluria due to acidification. Avoid if possible. *Probenecid:* may increase levels of para-aminosalicylic acid. Use together cautiously. *Rifampin:* para-aminosalicylic acid may interfere with absorption of rifampin. Give these drugs 8 to 12 hours apart. *Diphenhydramine:* inhibits PAS absorption. Monitor for decreased PAS effect.	• Use cautiously in patients with impaired renal function, decreased hepatic function, and gastric ulcers. • Sodium aminosalicylate should not be given to patients on sodium-restricted diets. A 15 g dose provides 1.6 g sodium. • Give with meals or antacid to reduce gastrointestinal distress. Tell patient to swallow enteric-coated tablets whole and not with antacids. • Monitor renal, hematopoietic, hepatic functions, and serum electrolytes. • Tell patient to notify doctor immediately if symptoms of hepatic impairment (loss of appetite, fatigue, malaise, jaundice, dark urine), fever, sore throat, or skin rash occur. • Instruct patient to take any of these drugs exactly as prescribed; warn against discontinuing drug without doctor's advice. • Protect from water, heat, sun. If drug turns brown or purple, don't use. • Concomitant administration of at least 1 other effective antitubercular drug is recommended.
None significant.	• Contraindicated in patients with severe liver disease. Use cautiously in patients with diabetes mellitus or gout. • Nearly 100% excreted in urine; reduced dose needed in renal impairment. • Perform liver function studies and examination for jaundice, liver tenderness or enlargement before and frequently during therapy. • Watch closely for signs of gout and of liver impairment (loss of appetite, fatigue, malaise, jaundice, dark urine, liver tenderness). Call doctor at once. • Report hemoptysis. • Monitor hematopoietic studies and serum uric acid levels. • Due to serious hepatotoxic effects, this drug is not recommended for initial therapy or long-term use. • When used with surgical management of tuberculosis, start pyrazinamide 1 to 2 weeks preop and continue for 4 to 6 weeks postop.
Aminosalicylic acid: may interfere with absorption of rifampin. Give these drugs 8 to 12 hours apart. *Probenecid:* may increase rifampin levels. Use cautiously.	• Contraindicated in children under 5. Use cautiously in patients with liver disease or in those receiving other hepatotoxic drugs. • Monitor liver function, hematopoietic studies, and serum uric acid levels. • Warn patient about drowsiness and the possibility of red-orange discoloration of urine, feces, saliva, sweat, sputum, and tears. • Tell patient to take this drug exactly as prescribed and to report side effects. Warn against discontinuing use without doctor's advice. • Give 1 hour before or 2 hours after meals for optimal absorption.

(continued on following page)

NAME	INDICATIONS & DOSAGE	SIDE EFFECTS
rifampin *(continued)*	**Children over 5 years:** 10 to 20 mg/Kg/day P.O., not to exceed 600 mg/day.	*Other:* serious hepatotoxicity as well as transient abnormalities in liver function tests; red-orange color of urine, feces, saliva, sweat, sputum, and tears.
streptomycin sulfate	*Primary treatment in tuberculosis—* **Adults:** with normal renal function, 1 g I.M. daily every 12 hours injected deeply into upper outer quadrant of buttocks. **Children:** with normal renal function, 20 mg/Kg daily in divided doses injected deeply into large muscle mass. Give concurrently with other antitubercular agents, but not with capreomycin, and continue until sputum specimen becomes negative.	*Blood:* eosinophilia, leukopenia, neutropenia, pancytopenia, hemolytic anemia. *CNS:* transient paresthesias, especially circumoral; lassitude. *CV:* myocarditis. *EENT:* ototoxicity (damage to vestibular and auditory portions of 8th cranial nerve, severe headache, nausea, vomiting, vertigo, ataxia, tinnitus, roaring and sense of fullness in the ears, hearing loss), optic nerve dysfunction (blurred vision, amblyopia). *GI:* stomatitis, nausea. *GU:* nephrotoxicity (transient proteinuria, increase in blood urea nitrogen and serum creatinine levels); nephrotoxicity less common than with other aminoglycosides. *Local:* pain, irritation at injection site. *Other:* hypersensitivity (rash, fever, urticaria, pruritus, angioneurotic edema), overgrowth of nonsusceptible organisms, hepatotoxicity, respiratory depression, lymphadenopathy, joint pains, muscle weakness, systemic lupus erythematosus syndrome.
sulfoxone sodium Diasone Sodium♦	*Lepromatous and tuberculoid leprosy—* **Adults:** 330 mg P.O. daily for 1 week; if no toxic side effects occur, dosage may be increased to 660 mg P.O. daily for 1 to 3 weeks, then increased to a maximum of 990 mg P.O. daily. **Children 6 to 12 years:** initially, 150 mg P.O. daily; if no toxic side effects occur, dosage may be increased gradually at monthly intervals to a maximum of 450 mg P.O. daily. **Children 4 to 6 years:** initially, 150 mg P.O. daily; if no toxic side effects occur, dosage may be increased gradually at monthly intervals to a maximum of 450 mg P.O. daily. Two-week rest periods from therapy every 2 months are advisable.	*Blood:* possible leukopenia, anemia, especially hemolytic; methemoglobinemia. *CNS:* psychosis, headache, dizziness, lethargy, severe malaise, paresthesias. *EENT:* tinnitus, allergic rhinitis. *GI:* anorexia, abdominal pain, nausea, vomiting. *Skin:* allergic dermatitis (generalized or fixed maculopapular rash). *Other:* hepatitis, drug fever.

INTERACTIONS	NURSING CONSIDERATIONS
Other aminoglycosides, methoxyflurane: may increase streptomycin's ototoxic and nephrotoxic effects. Use cautiously. *Ethacrynic acid, furosemide:* may increase streptomycin's ototoxic effects. Monitor carefully. *Dimenhydrinate:* may mask symptoms of ototoxicity. Use together cautiously.	• Contraindicated in patients with labyrinthine disease; those receiving other ototoxic or nephrotoxic drugs, neuromuscular blocking agents, and general anesthetics. Use cautiously in elderly patients and in those with impaired renal function. • Monitor renal function studies. Reduce dose in renal impairment. • Test patient's hearing before, during, and 6 months after therapy. Notify doctor if patient complains of tinnitus, roaring noises, fullness in ears. • Observe patient for respiratory depression. • Watch for signs of superinfection (continued fever and other signs of new infections, especially of the upper respiratory tract). • Very sensitizing topically. Protect hands when preparing drug. • In primary treatment of tuberculosis, streptomycin is discontinued when sputum becomes negative.
None significant.	• Contraindicated in renal amyloidosis. Use cautiously in chronic renal, hepatic, or cardiovascular disease, or refractory anemias. • Therapy should be interrupted if generalized, diffuse dermatitis occurs. • Sulfoxone sodium should be reduced or temporarily discontinued if hemoglobin falls below 9 g/100 ml; if leukocyte count falls below 5,000; if erythrocyte count falls below 2.5 million; or if it remains persistently low. • Patient should receive hematinics during sulfoxone sodium therapy. • Antihistamines may help combat sulfoxone sodium-induced allergic dermatitis. • Erythema nodosum type of "lepra reaction" may occur during sulfoxone sodium therapy as a result of circulating antigens caused by disintegrating *Mycobacterium leprae* bacilli (malaise, fever, painful areas of inflammatory induration in the skin and mucosa, iritis, neuritis). In severe cases, therapy should be interrupted and glucocorticoids given cautiously. • Monitor CBC frequently. • If drug fever is severe or frequent, interrupt therapy or reduce dosage. • Protect drug from light.

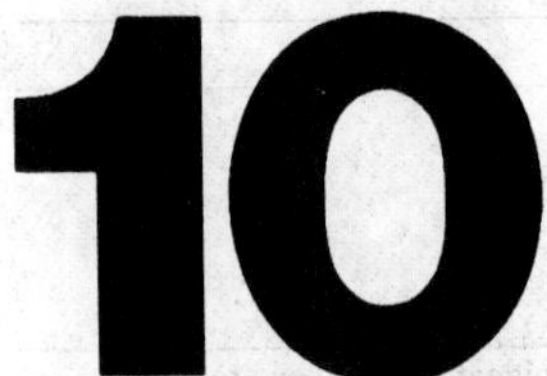

Aminoglycosides

amikacin sulfate	**neomycin sulfate**
gentamicin sulfate	**streptomycin sulfate**
kanamycin sulfate	**tobramycin sulfate**

Aminoglycosides are bactericidal antibiotics with broad-spectrum properties. Their use is generally reserved for life-threatening infections.

Major uses

• To treat infections caused by gram-negative organisms, especially *Enterobacter, Escherichia coli, Klebsiella, Proteus,* and *Pseudomonas aeruginosa*.

• Bowel sterilization prior to GI surgery and in hepatic coma.

Mechanism of action

• Inhibit protein synthesis of the bacterial cells in susceptible organisms.

Absorption, distribution, and excretion

• Not well absorbed from gastrointestinal tract. Aminoglycosides must be given parenterally for systemic effect.

• None penetrates cerebrospinal fluid well.

• All are excreted rapidly in the urine with normal renal function. Toxicity occurs rapidly in impaired renal function.

Onset and duration

• Onset for most of the aminoglycosides is within 1 hour; duration is usually 8 to 12 hours.

Combination products

None.

OTOTOXICITY OF AMINOGLYCOSIDES

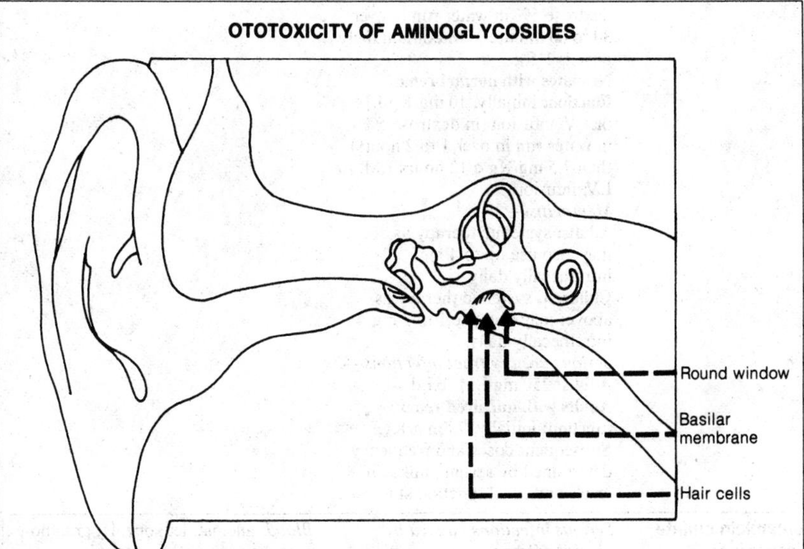

These ototoxic effects primarily occur in the ear labyrinth and sensory hair cells. Ototoxicity may relate to the patient's age; frequency and duration of drug administration; organ system impairment, especially renal function; concomitant use of other ototoxic drugs; and total dose administered.

NAME	INDICATIONS & DOSAGE	SIDE EFFECTS
amikacin sulfate Amikin◆	*Serious infections caused by sensitive Pseudomonas aeruginosa, Escherichia coli, Proteus, Klebsiella, Serratia, Enterobacter, Acinetobacter, Providencia, Citrobacter, Staphylococcus—* **Adults and children with normal renal function:** 15 mg/Kg/day divided q 8 to 12 hours I.M. or I.V. infusion (in 100 to 200 ml dextrose 5% in water run in over 30 to 60 minutes). Maximum daily dose is 1.5 g. **Neonates with normal renal function:** initially, 10 mg/Kg I.M. or I.V. infusion (in dextrose 5% in water run in over 1 to 2 hours), then 7.5 mg/Kg q 12 hours I.M. or I.V. infusion. *Meningitis—* **Adults:** systemic therapy as above; may also use up to 4 mg intrathecally daily. **Children:** systemic therapy as above; may also use 1 to 2 mg intrathecally daily. *Serious urinary tract infections—* **Adults:** 250 mg I.M. b.i.d. **Adults with impaired renal function:** initially, 7.5 mg/Kg. Subsequent doses and frequency determined by serum amikacin levels and renal function studies.	*EENT:* ototoxicity (tinnitus; vertigo; hearing impairment, especially high frequency deafness). *GU:* nephrotoxicity (cells or casts in urine, oliguria, proteinuria, decreased creatinine clearance and specific gravity, increased blood urea nitrogen). *Other:* hypersensitivity, overgrowth of nonsusceptible organisms.
gentamicin sulfate Cidomycin◆◆, Garamycin◆	*Serious infections caused by sensitive Pseudomonas aeruginosa, Escherichia coli, Proteus, Klebsiella, Serratia, Enterobacter, Citrobacter, Staphylococcus—* **Adults with normal renal function:** 3 mg/Kg/day in divided dosage q 8 hours I.M. or I.V. infusion (in 50 to 200 ml of normal saline solution or dextrose 5% in water infused over 30 minutes to 2 hours). For life-threatening infections, patient may receive up to 5 mg/Kg/day in 3 to 4 divided dosages. **Children with normal renal function:** 2 to 2.5 mg/Kg I.M. or I.V. infusion q 8 hours. **Infants and neonates over 1 week with normal renal function:**	*Blood:* anemia, leukopenia, granulocytopenia, thrombocytopenia. *CNS:* headache, lethargy. *EENT:* ototoxicity (tinnitus, vertigo, roaring in the ears, hearing loss). *GI:* nausea, vomiting. *GU:* nephrotoxicity (casts or protein in the urine, oliguria; increased blood urea nitrogen, nonprotein nitrogen, and serum creatinine levels). *Skin:* rash, urticaria. *Other:* hypersensitivity, overgrowth of nonsusceptible organisms, increased serum transaminases.

◆ Also available in Canada.
◆◆ Available in Canada only.
Unmarked trade names available in United States only.

INTERACTIONS	NURSING CONSIDERATIONS
Ethacrynic acid, furosemide: increased ototoxicity. Use cautiously. *Dimenhydrinate:* may mask symptoms of ototoxicity. Use with caution. *Carbenicillin:* amikacin antagonism. Don't mix together in I.V. Schedule 1 hour apart. *Other aminoglycosides, methoxyflurane:* increased ototoxicity and nephrotoxicity. Use together cautiously.	• Use cautiously in patients with impaired renal function; in neonates and infants, elderly patients. • Obtain specimen for culture and sensitivity before first dose. Therapy may begin pending test results. • Weigh patient and obtain baseline renal function studies before therapy begins. • Monitor renal function (output, specific gravity, urinalysis, blood urea nitrogen, creatinine). Notify doctor of decreasing renal function. • Patient should be well hydrated while taking this drug. • Evaluate patient's hearing before and during therapy. Notify doctor if patient complains of tinnitus, vertigo, hearing loss. • Watch for superinfection (continued fever and other signs of new infections, especially of upper respiratory tract). • Usual duration of therapy is 7 to 10 days. If no response after 3 to 5 days, therapy should be stopped and new specimens obtained for culture and sensitivity. • Peak serum levels above 35 mcg/ml are associated with higher incidence of toxicity. • Amikacin is usually reserved for gentamicin-resistant organisms.
Ethacrynic acid, furosemide: increased ototoxicity. Use cautiously. *Dimenhydrinate:* may mask symptoms of ototoxicity. Use with caution. *Carbenicillin:* gentamicin antagonism. Don't mix together in I.V. Schedule 1 hour apart. *Cephalosporins:* increased nephrotoxicity. Use together cautiously. *Other aminoglycosides, methoxyflurane:* increased ototoxicity and nephrotoxicity. Use together cautiously.	• Use cautiously in patients with impaired renal function; in neonates and infants, elderly patients. • Obtain specimen for culture and sensitivity before first dose. Therapy may begin pending test results. • Weigh patient and obtain baseline renal function studies before therapy begins. • Monitor renal function (output, specific gravity, urinalysis, blood urea nitrogen, creatinine). Notify doctor of decreasing renal function. • Patient should be well hydrated while taking this drug. • Evaluate patient's hearing before and during therapy. Notify doctor if patient complains of tinnitus, vertigo, hearing loss. • Watch for superinfection (continued fever and other signs of new infections, especially of upper respiratory tract). • Obtain specimen for gentamicin blood levels ½ hour before and 1 hour after dose. Tell lab if patient is also taking carbenicillin or other antibiotic. • Usual duration of therapy is 7 to 10 days. If no response in 3 to 5 days, therapy should be stopped and new specimens obtained for culture and sensitivity. • Peak serum levels above 12 mcg/ml and trough levels (those drawn ½ hour before next dose) above 2 mcg/ml are associated with higher incidence of toxicity.

(continued on following page)

NAME	INDICATIONS & DOSAGE	SIDE EFFECTS
gentamicin sulfate *(continued)*	2.5 mg/Kg q 8 hours I.M. or I.V. infusion. **Neonates under 1 week:** 2.5 mg/Kg I.V. q 12 hours. For I.V. infusion, dilute in normal saline solution or dextrose 5% in water and infuse over 1 to 2 hours. *Meningitis—* **Adults:** systemic therapy as above; may also use 1 to 2 mg intrathecally daily. **Children:** systemic therapy as above; may also use 0.1 to 1 mg intrathecally. *Endocarditis prophylaxis for GI or GU procedure or surgery—* **Adults:** 1.5 mg/Kg I.M. or I.V. 30 to 60 minutes before procedure or surgery and q 8 hours after for 2 doses. Given with aqueous penicillin G or ampicillin. **Children:** 2 mg/Kg I.M. or I.V. 30 to 60 minutes before procedure or surgery and q 8 hours after for 2 doses. Given with aqueous penicillin G or ampicillin. **Patients with impaired renal function:** initial dose is same as for those with normal renal function. Subsequent doses and frequency determined by renal function tests. *Posthemodialysis to maintain therapeutic blood levels—* **Adults:** 1 to 1.7 mg/Kg I.M. or I.V. infusion after each dialysis. **Children:** 2 mg/Kg I.M. or I.V. infusion after each dialysis.	
kanamycin sulfate Kantrex•	*Adjunctive treatment in hepatic coma—* **Adults:** 8 to 12 g/day P.O. in divided doses. *Preop bowel sterilization—* **Adults:** 1 g P.O. q 1 hour for 4 doses then q 4 hours for 4 doses or 1 g P.O. q 1 hour for 4 doses then q 6 hours for 36 to 72 hours. *Intraperitoneal irrigation—* 500 mg in 20 ml sterile distilled water instilled via catheter into wound after patient fully recovered from anesthesia and neuromuscular blocking agent effects.	*EENT:* with parenteral administration, ototoxicity (high-frequency deafness, an early symptom of hearing impairment; tinnitus and vertigo, symptoms of impending bilateral, irreversible deafness). *GI:* with oral administration, nausea, vomiting, diarrhea. *GU:* with parenteral administration, nephrotoxicity (increased blood urea nitrogen, nonprotein nitrogen, creatinine, oliguria, albuminuria, casts). *Other:* hypersensitivity, overgrowth of nonsusceptible organisms.

INTERACTIONS	NURSING CONSIDERATIONS
	• Hemodialysis (8 hours) removes up to 50% of drug from blood. • Endocarditis prophylaxis is recommended for all patients with rheumatic or congenital heart disease or prosthetic heart valve.
Ethacrynic acid, furosemide: increased ototoxicity. Use cautiously. *Dimenhydrinate:* may mask symptoms of ototoxicity. Use with caution. *Other aminoglycosides, methoxyflurane:* increased ototoxicity and nephrotoxicity. Don't use together.	• Oral use contraindicated in intestinal obstruction; in treatment of systemic infection. Use cautiously in impaired renal function, and the elderly. • Obtain specimen for culture and sensitivity before first dose. Therapy may begin pending test results. • Weigh patient and obtain baseline renal function studies before therapy begins. • Monitor renal function (output, specific gravity, urinalysis, blood urea nitrogen, creatinine). Notify doctor of decreasing renal function. • Patient should be well hydrated while taking this drug. • Evaluate patient's hearing before and during therapy. Notify doctor if patient complains of tinnitus, vertigo, hearing loss. • Watch for superinfection (continued fever and other signs of new infection, especially of upper respiratory tract). • If no response in 3 to 5 days, therapy should be stopped and new specimens obtained for culture and sensitivity.

(continued on following page)

NAME	INDICATIONS & DOSAGE	SIDE EFFECTS
kanamycin sulfate *(continued)*	*Serious infections caused by sensitive Escherichia coli, Proteus, Enterobacter aerogenes, Klebsiella pneumoniae, Serratia marcescens, Acinetobacter—* **Adults and children with normal renal function:** 15 mg/Kg/day divided q 8 to 12 hours deep I.M. into upper outer quadrant of buttocks or I.V. infusion (diluted 500 mg/200 ml of normal saline solution or dextrose 5% in water infused at 60 to 80 drops/minute). Maximum daily dose 1.5 g. **Neonates:** 15 mg/Kg/day I.M. or I.V. divided q 12 hours. *Wound irrigation*—up to 2.5 mg/ml in normal saline irrigation solution.	
neomycin sulfate Mycifradin Sulfate◆, Neobiotic	*Adjunctive treatment in hepatic coma—* **Adults:** 1 to 3 g P.O. q.i.d. for 5 to 6 days; or 200 ml of 1% or 100 ml of 2% solution as enema retained for 20 to 60 minutes q 6 hours. *Infectious diarrhea caused by enteropathogenic Escherichia coli—* **Adults:** 50 mg/Kg/day P.O. in 4 divided doses for 2 to 3 days. **Children:** 50 to 100 mg/Kg/day P.O. divided q 4 to 6 hours for 2 to 3 days. *Suppression of intestinal bacteria preoperatively—* **Adults:** 1 g P.O. q 1 hour for 4 doses, then 1 g q 4 hours for the balance of the 24 hours. **Children:** 40 to 100 mg/Kg/day P.O. divided q 4 to 6 hours. First dose should be preceded by saline cathartic.	*EENT:* ototoxicity (hearing impairment) following prolonged, high-dose therapy in hepatic coma. *GI:* nausea, vomiting, diarrhea, malabsorption syndrome. *GU:* nephrotoxicity (oliguria, casts in urine, albuminuria, azotemia, decreased creatinine clearance) following prolonged high-dose therapy in hepatic coma. *Skin:* rash. *Other:* hypersensitivity, overgrowth of nonsusceptible organisms, respiratory depression.
streptomycin sulfate	*Nonhemolytic streptococcal endocarditis—* **Adults:** 1 g I.M. deep into upper outer quadrant of buttocks q 12 hours for 1 week, then 500 mg I.M. q 12 hours for 1 week with penicillin. *Endocarditis prophylaxis for dental and upper respiratory tract procedures—* **Adults:** 1 g I.M. 30 to 60 minutes	*Blood:* eosinophilia, leukopenia, pancytopenia, hemolytic anemia, thrombocytopenia. *CNS:* circumoral or peripheral paresthesias, muscle weakness. *CV:* myocarditis. *EENT:* ototoxicity (damage to vestibular and auditory portions of 8th cranial nerve, severe headache, nausea, vomiting, vertigo, ataxia, tinnitus, roaring and sense of fullness

INTERACTIONS	NURSING CONSIDERATIONS
	• I.M. route preferred. Use I.V. route only if I.M. route not possible. • Peak serum levels over 30 mcg/ml are associated with increased incidence of toxicity.
Ethacrynic acid, furosemide: increased ototoxicity. Use cautiously. *Dimenhydrinate:* may mask symptoms of ototoxicity. Use with caution. *Other aminoglycosides, methoxyflurane:* increased ototoxicity and nephrotoxicity. Use together cautiously.	• Contraindicated in intestinal obstruction. Use cautiously in patients with impaired renal function, ulcerative bowel lesions, and in elderly patients. • Oral therapy not recommended for systemic infection; parenteral dosage form available for I.M. use but not recommended because of extreme ototoxicity and nephrotoxicity. • Weigh patient and obtain baseline renal function studies before therapy begins. • Monitor renal function (output, specific gravity, urinalysis, blood urea nitrogen, creatinine). Notify doctor of decreasing renal function. • Patient should be well hydrated while taking this drug. • Watch for respiratory depression, especially in renal disease, hypocalcemia, or neuromuscular diseases such as myasthenia gravis. • Evaluate hearing of patient with hepatic or renal disease before and during prolonged therapy. Notify doctor if patient complains of tinnitus, vertigo, hearing loss. Onset of deafness may occur several weeks after drug is stopped. • Watch for superinfection (continued fever and other signs of new infections, especially of upper respiratory tract). • Sometimes used in the treatment of high blood cholesterol. • Nonabsorbable at recommended dosage. However, more than 4 g of neomycin per day may be systemically absorbed and lead to nephrotoxicity.
Dimenhydrinate: may mask symptoms of streptomycin-induced ototoxicity. Use together cautiously. *Ethacrynic acid, furosemide:* increased ototoxicity. Use cautiously. *Other aminoglycosides, methoxyflurane:*	• Contraindicated in labyrinthine disease. Use cautiously in patients with impaired renal function and in the elderly. • Do not give drug I.V. • Obtain specimen for culture and sensitivity before first dose. Therapy may begin pending test results. • Weigh patient and obtain baseline renal function studies before therapy begins. • Monitor renal function (output, specific gravity, urinalysis, blood urea nitrogen, serum creatinine). Notify doctor of decreasing renal function. • Patient should be well hydrated while taking this drug. • Evaluate patient's hearing before, during, and 6 months after therapy.

(continued on following page)

NAME	INDICATIONS & DOSAGE	SIDE EFFECTS
streptomycin sulfate *(continued)*	before procedure. Used with penicillin. **Children:** 20 mg/Kg I.M. 30 to 60 minutes before procedure. Used with penicillin. *Endocarditis prophylaxis for GI or GU procedures or surgery—* **Adults:** 1 g I.M. 30 to 60 minutes before procedure and q 12 hours for 2 doses after. Used with penicillin or ampicillin. **Children:** 20 mg/Kg I.M. 30 to 60 minutes before procedure and q 12 hours for 2 doses after. Used with penicillin or ampicillin. **Patients with impaired renal function:** initial dose is same as for those with normal renal function. Subsequent doses and frequency determined by renal function test results. *Enterococcal endocarditis—* **Adults:** 1 g I.M. q 12 hours for 2 weeks, then 500 mg I.M. q 12 hours for 4 weeks with penicillin. *Tularemia—* **Adults:** 1 to 2 g I.M. daily in divided doses injected deep into upper outer quadrant of buttocks. Continue until patient is afebrile for 5 to 7 days. *Other severe fulminating infections (gram-negative bacillary bacteremia, meningitis, pneumonia, granuloma inguinale, brucellosis, chancroid, urinary tract infections, acute gonorrhea)—* **Adults:** 2 to 4 g I.M. daily in divided doses q 6 to 12 hours injected deep into upper outer quadrant of buttocks. **Children:** 20 to 40 mg/Kg/day I.M. into large muscle mass, divided q 6 to 12 hours.	in the ears, hearing loss). *GU:* nephrotoxicity (transient proteinuria, increased blood urea nitrogen and serum creatinine levels). *Local:* pain, irritation at injection site. *Skin:* exfoliative dermatitis. *Other:* hypersensitivity (rash, fever, urticaria, angioneurotic edema), overgrowth of nonsusceptible organisms, hepatotoxicity, respiratory depression.
tobramycin sulfate Nebcin♦	*Serious infections caused by sensitive strains of Escherichia coli, Proteus, Klebsiella, Enterobacter, Serratia, Staphylococcus aureus, Pseudomonas, Citrobacter, Providencia—*	*Blood:* anemia, thrombocytopenia, granulocytopenia. *CNS:* headache, lethargy. *EENT:* ototoxicity (tinnitus, vertigo, roaring in ears, hearing loss). *GI:* nausea, vomiting. *GU:* nephrotoxicity (increased blood

INTERACTIONS	NURSING CONSIDERATIONS
may increase streptomycin's ototoxic and nephrotoxic effects. Use cautiously.	Notify doctor if patient complains of tinnitus, roaring noises, or fullness in ears. • Watch for superinfection (continued fever and other signs of new infections, especially of upper respiratory tract) and respiratory depression. • When used to treat acute gonorrhea, serological test and dark field examination for syphilis should be done before therapy starts and should be repeated 4 months afterward. Treatment with streptomycin may mask syphilis. • Peak serum concentrations over 25 mcg/ml are associated with increased incidence of toxicity. • Endocarditis prophylaxis is recommended for all patients with rheumatic or congenital heart disease or with prosthetic heart valve. Patients should receive prophylactic antibiotics during GI or GU procedures or surgery, or during upper respiratory tract procedures.
Ethacrynic acid, furosemide: increased ototoxicity. Use cautiously. *Dimenhydrinate:* may mask symptoms of ototoxicity. Use with	• Use cautiously in patients with impaired renal function and in the elderly. • Obtain specimen for culture and sensitivity before first dose. Therapy may begin pending test results. • Weigh patient and obtain baseline renal function studies before starting therapy. • Usual duration of therapy is 7 to 10 days. • Monitor renal function (output, specific gravity, urinalysis, blood urea

(continued on following page)

NAME	INDICATIONS & DOSAGE	SIDE EFFECTS
tobramycin sulfate *(continued)*	**Adults and children with normal renal function:** 3 mg/Kg I.M. or I.V. daily divided q 8 hours. Up to 5 mg/Kg I.M. or I.V. daily divided q 6 to 8 hours for life-threatening infections. **Neonates under 1 week:** up to 4 mg/Kg I.M. or I.V. daily divided q 12 hours. For I.V. use, dilute in 50 to 100 ml normal saline solution or dextrose 5% in water for adults and less volume for children. Infuse over 20 to 60 minutes. **Patients with impaired renal function:** initially, 1 mg/Kg I.M. or I.V. Subsequent doses and frequency determined by renal function study results.	urea nitrogen, nonprotein nitrogen, and serum creatinine, oliguria, proteinuria). *Skin:* rash, itching, urticaria. *Other:* hypersensitivity, overgrowth of nonsusceptible organisms, increased serum transaminases, increased bilirubin, fever.

INTERACTIONS	NURSING CONSIDERATIONS
Carbenicillin: tobramycin antagonism. Don't mix together in I.V. Schedule 1 hour apart. *Cephalosporins:* increased nephrotoxicity. Use together cautiously. *Other aminoglycosides, methoxyflurane:* increased ototoxicity and nephrotoxicity. Use together cautiously.	nitrogen, creatinine). Notify doctor of decreasing renal function. • Patient should be well hydrated while taking this drug. • Evaluate patient's hearing before and during therapy. Notify doctor if patient complains of tinnitus, vertigo, hearing loss. • Watch for superinfection (continued fever and other signs of new infections, especially of upper respiratory tract). • Peak serum levels over 12 mcg/ml are associated with increased incidence of toxicity.

11
Penicillins

amoxicillin trihydrate
ampicillin
ampicillin sodium
carbenicillin disodium
carbenicillin indanyl sodium
cloxacillin sodium
cyclacillin
dicloxacillin sodium
hetacillin
hetacillin potassium
methicillin sodium
nafcillin sodium
oxacillin sodium
penicillin G benzathine
penicillin G potassium
penicillin G procaine
penicillin G sodium
penicillin V
penicillin V potassium
ticarcillin disodium

Penicillins are either broad-spectrum or narrow-spectrum antibiotics, primarily bactericidal, when given in active concentrations.

Major uses

• Highly effective against infections caused by gram-positive cocci, such as *Streptococcus pneumoniae* and nonpenicillinase-producing staphylococci; also effective against some gram-negative cocci, such as *Neisseria meningitides* and *Neisseria gonorrhoeae.* Penicillins are also effective in varying degrees against *Bacillus anthracis, Clostridium perfringens, Treponema pallidum, Actinomyces,* and *Corynebacterium diphtheriae.* Penicillins are not active against viruses, mycobacteria, plasmodia, yeasts, fungi, or rickettsiae.

Mechanism of action

• Thought to exert antibacterial effect on penicillin-sensitive organisms by inhibiting cell wall synthesis during stage of active multiplication.
• More effective against young, rapidly dividing organisms than against mature resting cells that are not in process of cell wall formation.
• A major mechanism in bacterial resistance is the production of penicillinases which convert penicillin to inactive penicilloic acid; however, some penicillins are resistant to these enzymes.

Absorption, distribution, and excretion

• Oral absorption occurs primarily in duodenum, with a small amount stored in stomach. Some penicillins are affected by presence of food in the stomach and the duodenum and therefore are best taken on an empty stomach 30 to 60 minutes before or 2 hours after meals. Parenteral administration results in higher but transient serum levels.
• Widely distributed throughout body fluids in body tissues, including kidneys, liver, lungs, heart, spleen, skin, and intestines. Adequate penetration into cerebrospinal fluid and the brain occurs only with meningeal inflammation. These drugs are excreted primarily unchanged in urine. Penicillins cross placental barrier and are found in amniotic fluid, cord

serum, and human milk. Excretion is delayed in young infants, elderly patients, and in persons with impaired renal function.

Onset and duration

- Peak serum level for oral drugs is usually reached within 1 to 2 hours after administration.
- Duration of action varies but is not sustained unless dosages are frequent.

Combination products

None.

COMBAT SUPERINFECTION

Patients receiving long-term treatment with penicillin or some other broad-spectrum antibiotic are vulnerable to superinfection — a secondary or new infection produced by organism strains insensitive to the antibiotic treatment. They can develop such infection after as few as 4 to 5 days of antibiotic therapy.

Gram-negative bacteria — *Proteus, Pseudomonas* — and *Candida* are traditionally the culprits in superinfection. These bacterial infections may develop from the overgrowth of normally present organisms, from those acquired through other patient and staff contact, or from accidental bacterial contamination during drug injection.

Superinfections commonly involve the mouth, pharynx, or lungs but may spread systemically. Specific organ involvement is usually patterned after those affected by the primary disease.

Remember, superinfection can change a self-limiting disease into a serious, prolonged, or fatal one, so follow these suggestions for avoiding it:

- Use aseptic technique in carrying out patient care. Wash hands frequently — in between treating patients, before and after all procedures.
- Change I.V. tubing, dressing, and solution every 24 hours.
- Keep dressings dry and clean.
- Check I.V. site for signs of phlebitis or infiltration:
  - — swelling at or above infusion site
  - — tenderness
  - — warmth to touch
  - — redness at or around site.
- At the first signs of phlebitis or infection, stop I.V. infusion. Pull and restart I.V. in a completely new site (i.e., opposite arm). Using the same arm could cause trouble with the same problem vein.
- Keep visitors or staff with colds or sore throats away from the patient.

NAME	INDICATIONS & DOSAGE	SIDE EFFECTS
amoxicillin trihydrate Amoxil◆, Larotid, Polymox◆, Robamox, Sumox, Trimox	*Systemic infections caused by susceptible strains of gram-positive and gram-negative organisms—* **Adults:** 750 mg to 1.5 g P.O. daily, divided into doses given q 8 hours. **Children:** 20 to 40 mg/Kg P.O. daily, divided into doses given q 8 hours.	*Blood:* anemia, thrombocytopenia, thrombocytopenic purpura, eosinophilia, leukopenia, agranulocytosis. *GI:* nausea, vomiting, diarrhea. *Other:* hypersensitivity (erythematous maculopapular rash, urticaria, anaphylaxis), overgrowth of nonsusceptible organisms.
ampicillin Amcill◆, Ampilean◆◆, Omnipen, Pen A, Penbritin◆, Pensyn, Roampicillin **ampicillin sodium** Amcill-S, Omnipen-N, Pen A/N, Penbritin-S, Polycillin-N, Princi-pen/N, Totacillin-N	*Systemic infections caused by susceptible strains of gram-positive and gram-negative organisms—* **Adults:** 2 to 4 g P.O. daily, divided into doses given q 6 hours; 2 to 12 g I.M. or I.V. daily, divided into doses given q 6 hours. **Children:** 50 to 100 mg/Kg P.O. daily, divided into doses given q 6 hours; or 100 to 200 mg/Kg I.M. or I.V. daily, divided into doses given q 6 hours. *Meningitis—* **Adults:** 8 to 14 g I.V. drip daily for 3 days, then I.M. divided q 3 to 4 hours. **Children:** up to 300 mg/Kg I.V. drip daily for 3 days, then I.M. divided q 4 hours. *Uncomplicated gonorrhea—* **Adults:** 3.5 g P.O. with 1 g probenecid given as a single dose.	*Blood:* anemia, thrombocytopenia, thrombocytopenic purpura, eosinophilia, leukopenia, agranulocytosis. *GI:* nausea, vomiting, diarrhea, glossitis, stomatitis, black "hairy" tongue. *Other:* hypersensitivity (erythematous maculopapular rash, urticaria, anaphylaxis), overgrowth of nonsusceptible organisms.

◆ Also available in Canada.
◆◆ Available in Canada only.
Unmarked trade names available in United States only.

INTERACTIONS	NURSING CONSIDERATIONS
Probenecid: increased blood levels of penicillin. Probenecid is often used for this purpose. *Chloramphenicol, erythromycin, tetracyclines:* antibiotic antagonism. Give penicillins at least 1 hour before bacteriostatic antibiotics.	• Use cautiously in patients with other drug allergies, especially to cephalosporins (possible cross-allergenicity). • Obtain cultures for sensitivity tests before first dose. Not necessary to wait for results before beginning therapy. • Before giving penicillin, ask patient if he's had any previous allergic reactions to this drug. However, a negative history of penicillin allergy is no guarantee against a future allergic reaction. • Tell patient to take medication exactly as prescribed, even after he feels better. If ordered 4 times a day, be sure to give every 6 hours—even during the night. • Be prepared for possible allergic reaction to this drug. Have available emergency equipment and medications needed for resuscitation. • Give with food to prevent GI distress. • Check CBC and transaminase levels frequently. Drug may cause leukopenia, thrombocytopenia, and elevated SGOT and SGPT. • Large doses may cause increased yeast growths. Report symptoms to doctor. • With prolonged therapy, bacterial and fungal superinfection may occur, especially in the elderly, debilitated, or those with low resistance to infection due to immunosuppressors or irradiation. Close observation is essential. • Check expiration date. Warn patient never to use leftover penicillin for a new illness or to "share" penicillin with family and friends. • Tell patient to call the doctor if rash, fever, or chills develop. A rash is the most common allergic reaction. • Amoxicillin and ampicillin have similar clinical applications. • For symptoms and treatment of anaphylaxis, see p. 1114.
Probenecid: increased blood levels of penicillin. Probenecid is often used for this purpose. *Chloramphenicol, erythromycin, tetracyclines:* antibiotic antagonism. Give penicillins at least 1 hour before bacteriostatic antibiotics.	• Use cautiously in patients with other drug allergies, especially to cephalosporins (possible cross-allergenicity); in patients with mononucleosis; high incidence of maculopapular rash in those receiving ampicillin. • Obtain cultures for sensitivity tests before first dose. Not necessary to wait for results before beginning therapy. • Before giving penicillin, ask patient if he's had any previous allergic reactions to this drug. However, a negative history of penicillin allergy is no guarantee against a future allergic reaction. • Tell patient to take medication exactly as prescribed, even after he feels better. If ordered 4 times a day, be sure to give every 6 hours—even during the night. • Tell the patient to call the doctor if rash, fever, or chills develop. A rash is the most common allergic reaction. • Be prepared for possible allergic reaction to this drug. Have available emergency equipment and medications needed for resuscitation. • When given orally, it may cause GI disturbances. Food may interfere with absorption, so give 1 to 2 hours before meals or 2 to 3 hours after. • Don't give I.M. or I.V. unless infection is severe or patient can't take oral dose. • Check CBC and transaminase levels frequently. Drug may cause leukopenia, thrombocytopenia, and elevated SGOT and SGPT. • When giving I.V., mix with 5% dextrose in water or a saline solution. Don't mix with other drugs, or solutions; they might be incompatible. • Give I.V. intermittently to prevent vein irritation. Change site every 48 hours. • Large doses may cause increased yeast growths. Report symptoms to doctor. • With prolonged therapy, bacterial or fungal superinfection may occur especially in the elderly, debilitated, or those with low resistance to

(continued on following page)

NAME	INDICATIONS & DOSAGE	SIDE EFFECTS
ampicillin **ampicillin sodium** *(continued)*		
carbenicillin disodium Geopen, Pyopen◆	*Systemic infections caused by susceptible strains of gram-positive and especially gram-negative organisms (Proteus, Pseudomonas aeruginosa)*— **Adults:** 30 to 40 g daily I.V. infusion, divided into doses given q 4 to 6 hours. **Children:** 300 to 500 mg/Kg daily I.V. infusion, divided into doses given q 4 to 6 hours. *Urinary tract infections*— **Adults:** 200 mg/Kg daily I.M. or I.V. infusion, divided into doses given q 4 to 6 hours. **Children:** 50 to 200 mg/Kg daily I.M. or I.V. infusion, divided into doses given q 4 to 6 hours.	*Blood:* bleeding with high doses, neutropenia, eosinophilia, leukopenia, thrombocytopenia. *CNS:* convulsions, neuromuscular irritability. *GI:* nausea. *Local:* pain at injection site, vein irritation, phlebitis. *Metabolic:* hypokalemia. *Other:* hypersensitivity (edema, fever, chills, rash, pruritus, urticaria, anaphylaxis), overgrowth of nonsusceptible organisms.
carbenicillin indanyl sodium Geocillin, Geopen Oral◆◆	*Urinary tract infection caused by susceptible strains of gram-negative organisms*— **Adults:** 382 to 764 mg P.O. q.i.d. Not recommended for children.	*Blood:* leukopenia, neutropenia, eosinophilia, anemia, thrombocytopenia. *GI:* furry tongue, dry mouth, nausea, vomiting, diarrhea, flatulence, abdominal cramps, unpleasant taste. *Other:* hypersensitivity (rash, urticaria, pruritus, anaphylaxis), overgrowth of nonsusceptible organisms (vaginitis).

INTERACTIONS	NURSING CONSIDERATIONS
	infection due to immunosuppressors or irradiation. Close observation is essential. • Check expiration date. Warn patient never to use leftover penicillin for a new illness or to "share" penicillin with family and friends. • Initial dilution in vial is stable for 1 hour. Follow manufacturer's direction for stability data when ampicillin is further diluted for I.V. infusion. • For symptoms and treatment of anaphylaxis, see p. 1114.
Probenecid: increased blood levels of penicillin. Probenecid is often used for this purpose. *Gentamicin, tobramycin:* chemically incompatible. Don't mix together in I.V. Give 1 hour apart. *Chloramphenicol, erythromycin, tetracyclines:* antibiotic antagonism. Give penicillins at least 1 hour before bacteriostatic antibiotics.	• Use cautiously in patients with other drug allergies, especially to cephalosporins (possible cross-allergenicity); those with bleeding tendencies, uremia, hypokalemia. Use cautiously in sodium-restricted patients; contains 4.7 mEq sodium/g. • Obtain cultures for sensitivity tests before starting therapy. However, it's not necessary to wait for culture and sensitivity results before beginning therapy. • Before giving penicillin, ask patient if he's had any previous allergic reactions to this drug. However, a negative history of penicillin allergy is no guarantee against a future allergic reaction. • Be prepared for possible allergic reaction to this drug. Have available emergency equipment and medications needed for resuscitation. • Check CBC and transaminase levels frequently. Drug may cause leukopenia, thrombocytopenia, and elevated SGOT and SGPT. • Monitor serum potassium. • If patient has high serum level of this drug, he may have convulsions. Be prepared by keeping side rails up on bed and tongue blade handy. • When giving I.V., mix with 5% dextrose in water or other suitable I.V. fluids. • Give I.V intermittently to prevent vein irritation. Change site every 48 hours. • Large doses may cause increased yeast growths. Report symptoms to doctor. • With prolonged therapy, other superinfections may occur, especially in the elderly, debilitated, or those with low resistance to infection due to immunosuppressors or irradiation. Close observation is essential. • Check expiration date. • For symptoms and treatment of anaphylaxis, see p. 1114.
None significant.	• Use cautiously in patients with other drug allergies, especially to cephalosporins (possible cross-allergenicity). • Obtain cultures for sensitivity tests before starting therapy. • Before giving penicillin, ask patient if he's had any previous allergic reactions to this drug. However, a negative history of penicillin allergy is no guarantee against a future allergic reaction. • Tell patient to take medication exactly as prescribed, even after he feels better. If ordered 4 times a day, be sure to give every 6 hours—even during the night. • Tell patient to call the doctor if he develops rash, fever, or chills. A rash is the most common allergic reaction. • Be prepared for possible allergic reaction to this drug. Have available emergency equipment and medications needed for resuscitation. • When given orally, it may cause GI disturbances. Food may interfere with absorption, so give 1 to 2 hours before meals or 2 to 3 hours after. • Check CBC and transaminase levels frequently. Drug may cause leukopenia, thrombocytopenia, and elevated SGOT and SGPT. • Large doses may cause increased yeast growths. Report symptoms to doctor. • With prolonged therapy, other superinfections may occur, especially in

(continued on following page)

NAME	INDICATIONS & DOSAGE	SIDE EFFECTS
carbenicillin indanyl sodium *(continued)*		
cloxacillin sodium Bactopen♦♦, Clox-apen♦, Novocloxin♦♦, Orbenin♦♦, Tegopen♦	*Systemic infections caused by penicillinase-producing staphylococci*— **Adults:** 2 to 4 g P.O. daily, divided into doses given q 6 hours. **Children:** 50 to 100 mg/Kg P.O. daily, divided into doses given q 6 hours.	*Blood:* eosinophilia. *GI:* nausea, vomiting, epigastric distress, diarrhea. *Other:* hypersensitivity (rash, urticaria, chills, fever, sneezing, wheezing, anaphylaxis), overgrowth of nonsusceptible organisms.
cyclacillin Cyclapen	*Systemic and urinary tract infections caused by susceptible strains of gram-positive and gram-negative organisms*— **Adults:** 250 to 500 mg P.O. q.i.d. in equally spaced doses. **Children:** 50 to 100 mg/Kg/day in equally divided doses.	*Blood:* anemia, thrombocytopenia, thrombocytopenic purpura, leukopenia, neutropenia, eosinophilia. *GI:* nausea, vomiting, diarrhea. *Other:* hypersensitivity (edema, fever, chills, rash, pruritus, urticaria, anaphylaxis), overgrowth of nonsusceptible organisms.

INTERACTIONS	NURSING CONSIDERATIONS
	the elderly, debilitated, or those with low resistance to infection due to immunosuppressors or irradiation. Close observation is essential. • Check expiration date. Warn patient never to use leftover penicillin for a new illness or to "share" penicillin with family and friends. • Use only in patients whose creatinine clearance is 10 ml/minute or more. • Excellent treatment for *Pseudomonas* urinary tract infections in ambulatory patients. • Not effective for any systemic infection because blood levels are nil. • For symptoms and treatment of anaphylaxis, see p. 1114.
Probenecid: increased blood levels of penicillin. Probenecid is often used for this purpose. *Chloramphenicol, erythromycin, tetracyclines:* antibiotic antagonism. Give penicillins at least 1 hour before bacteriostatic antibiotics.	• Use with caution in patients with other drug allergies, especially to cephalosporins (possible cross-allergenicity). • Obtain cultures for sensitivity tests before starting therapy. • Before giving penicillin, ask patient if he's had any previous allergic reactions to this drug. However, a negative history of penicillin allergy is no guarantee against a future allergic reaction. • Tell patient to take medication exactly as prescribed, even if he feels better. If ordered 4 times a day, be sure to give every 6 hours—even during the night. • Tell patient to call the doctor if rash, fever, or chills develop. A rash is the most common allergic reaction. • Be prepared for possible allergic reaction to this drug. Have available emergency equipment and medications needed for resuscitation. • When given orally, it may cause GI disturbances. Food may interfere with absorption, so give 1 to 2 hours before meals or 2 to 3 hours after. • Check CBC and transaminase levels frequently. Drug may cause leukopenia, thrombocytopenia, and elevated SGOT and SGPT. • Large doses may cause increased yeast growths. Report symptoms to doctor. • With prolonged therapy, other superinfections may occur especially in the elderly, debilitated, or those with low resistance to infection due to immunosuppressors or irradiation. Close observation is essential. • Check expiration date. Warn patient never to use leftover penicillin for a new illness or to "share" penicillin with family and friends. • For symptoms and treatment of anaphylaxis, see p. 1114.
Probenecid: increased blood levels of penicillin. Probenecid is often used for this purpose.	• Contraindicated in patients allergic to other penicillins. • Obtain cultures for sensitivity tests before starting therapy. However, it's not necessary to wait for culture and sensitivity results before beginning therapy. • Before giving penicillin, ask patient if he's had any previous hypersensitive reactions to it. However, a negative history of penicillin allergy is no guarantee against a future allergic reaction. • Tell patient he must take all medication exactly as prescribed, for as long as ordered, even after he feels better. • If this drug is ordered 4 times a day, be sure it's given every 6 hours—even during the night. • Be prepared for possible allergic reaction to this drug. Have available emergency equipment and medications needed for resuscitation. • Patients with renal insufficiency should receive less drug. • Large doses of penicillin may cause increased yeast growths. Watch for signs and symptoms and report to doctor. • With prolonged therapy, bacterial and fungal superinfection may occur especially in the elderly, debilitated, or those with low resistance to infection due to immunosuppressors or irradiation. Close observation is essential.

(continued on following page)

NAME	INDICATIONS & DOSAGE	SIDE EFFECTS
cyclacillin *(continued)*		
dicloxacillin sodium Dycill, Dynapen◆, Pathocil, Veracillin	*Systemic infections caused by penicillinase-producing staphylococci—* **Adults:** 1 to 2 g daily P.O. or I.M., divided into doses given q 6 hours. **Children:** 25 to 50 mg/Kg P.O. or I.M. daily, divided into doses given q 6 hours.	*Blood:* eosinophilia. *GI:* nausea, vomiting, epigastric distress, flatulence, diarrhea. *Other:* hypersensitivity (pruritus, urticaria, rash, anaphylaxis), overgrowth of nonsusceptible organisms.
hetacillin Versapen **hetacillin potassium** Versapen K	*Systemic infections caused by susceptible strains of gram-positive and gram-negative organisms—* **Adults:** 225 to 450 mg P.O. q.i.d. **Children:** 22.5 to 45 mg/Kg P.O. daily, divided into doses given q 6 hours. Hetacillin potassium may be given P.O., I.M., or I.V.	*Blood:* thrombocytopenia, thrombocytopenic purpura, eosinophilia, leukopenia, agranulocytosis. *GI:* vomiting, nausea, epigastric distress, diarrhea, glossitis, stomatitis, black hairy tongue. *Local:* vein irritation, phlebitis. *Other:* hypersensitivity (chills, fever, anaphylaxis, maculopapular rash, urticaria), overgrowth of nonsusceptible organisms (oral and rectal moniliasis).

INTERACTIONS	NURSING CONSIDERATIONS
	• Check expiration date before giving this drug. Warn patient never to use leftover penicillin for a new illness or to "share" his penicillin with family and friends. • Tell patient to call the doctor if he develops rash, fever, chills. A rash is the most common allergic reaction. • For symptoms and treatment of anaphylaxis, see p. 1114.
Chloramphenicol, erythromycin, tetracyclines: antibiotic antagonism. Give penicillins at least 1 hour before bacteriostatic antibiotics. *Probenecid:* increased blood levels of penicillin. Probenecid is often used for this purpose.	• Use cautiously in patients allergic to cephalosporins (possible cross-allergenicity). • Obtain cultures for sensitivity tests before starting therapy. • Before giving penicillin, ask patient if he's had any previous allergic reactions to this drug. However, a negative history of penicillin allergy is no guarantee against a future allergic reaction. • Tell patient to take medication exactly as prescribed, even if he feels better. If ordered 4 times a day, be sure to give every 6 hours—even during the night. • Tell patient to call the doctor if rash, fever, or chills develop. A rash is the most common allergic reaction. • Be prepared for possible allergic reaction to this drug. Have available emergency equipment and medications needed for resuscitation. • When given orally, it may cause GI disturbances. Food may interfere with absorption, so give 1 to 2 hours before meals or 2 to 3 hours after. • Don't give I.M. unless infection is severe or patient can't take oral dose. • Check CBC and transaminase levels frequently. Drug may cause leukopenia, thrombocytopenia, and elevated SGOT and SGPT. • Large doses may cause increased yeast growths. Report symptoms to doctor. • With prolonged therapy, other superinfections may occur, especially in the elderly, debilitated, or those with low resistance to infection due to immunosuppressors or irradiation. Close observation is essential. • Check expiration date. Warn patient never to use leftover penicillin for a new illness or to "share" penicillin with family and friends. • For treatment of anaphylaxis, see p. 1114.
Chloramphenicol, erythromycin, tetracyclines: antibiotic antagonism. Give penicillins at least 1 hour before bacteriostatic antibiotics. *Probenecid:* increased blood levels of penicillin. Probenecid is often used for this purpose.	• Contraindicated in patients with mononucleosis. Use cautiously in patients with other drug allergies, especially to cephalosporins (possible cross-allergenicity); gastrointestinal disturbances. • Obtain cultures for sensitivity tests before starting therapy. Not necessary to wait for culture and sensitivity results before beginning therapy. • Before giving penicillin, ask patient if he's had any previous allergic reactions to this drug. However, a negative history of penicillin allergy is no guarantee against a future allergic reaction. • Tell patient to take medication exactly as prescribed, even if he feels better. If ordered 4 times a day, be sure to give every 6 hours—even during the night. • Tell patient to call the doctor if rash, fever, or chills develp. A rash is the most common allergic reaction. • Be prepared for possible allergic reaction to this drug. Have available emergency equipment and medications needed for resuscitation. • When given orally, it may cause GI disturbances. Food may interfere with absorption, so give 1 to 2 hours before meals or 2 to 3 hours after. • Don't give I.M. or I.V. unless infection is severe or patient can't take oral dose. • Check CBC and transaminase levels frequently. Drug may cause leukopenia, thrombocytopenia, and elevated SGOT and SGPT. • When giving I.V., mix with appropriate I.V. solutions.

(continued on following page)

NAME	INDICATIONS & DOSAGE	SIDE EFFECTS
hetacillin **hetacillin potassium** *(continued)*		
methicillin sodium Azapen, Celbenin, Staphcillin◆	*Systemic infections caused by penicillinase-producing staphylococci*— **Adults:** 4 to 12 g I.M. or I.V. daily, divided into doses given q 4 to 6 hours. **Children:** 100 to 200 mg/Kg I.M. or I.V. daily, divided into doses given q 4 to 6 hours.	*Blood:* eosinophilia, hemolytic anemia, transient neutropenia. *CNS:* neuropathy. *GI:* glossitis, stomatitis. *GU:* nephrotoxicity. *Other:* hypersensitivity (chills, fever, edema, rash, urticaria, anaphylaxis), overgrowth of nonsusceptible organisms (oral and rectal monialiasis).
nafcillin sodium Nafcil, Unipen◆	*Systemic infections caused by penicillinase-producing staphylococci*— **Adults:** 2 to 4 g P.O. daily, divided into doses given q 6 hours; 2 to 12 g I.M. or I.V. daily, divided into doses given q 4 to 6 hours. **Children:** 50 to 100 mg/Kg P.O. daily, divided into doses given q 4 to 6 hours; or 100 to 200 mg/Kg I.M. or I.V. daily, divided into doses given q 4 to 6 hours.	*Blood:* transient leukopenia, neutropenia, granulocytopenia, thrombocytopenia with high doses. *GI:* nausea, vomiting, diarrhea. *Other:* hypersensitivity (chills, fever, rash, pruritus, urticaria, anaphylaxis), overgrowth of nonsusceptible organisms.

INTERACTIONS	NURSING CONSIDERATIONS
	• Give I.V. intermittently to prevent vein irritation. Change site every 48 hours. • Large doses may cause increased yeast growths. Report symptoms to doctor. • With prolonged therapy, other superinfections may occur, especially in the elderly, debilitated, or those with low resistance to infection due to immunosuppressors or irradiation. Close observation is essential. • Parenteral hetacillin potassium containing lidocaine is for I.M. injection only. Question patient about possible allergy to lidocaine. • Check expiration date. Warn patient never to use leftover penicillin for a new illness or to "share" penicillin with family and friends. • Very similar to ampicillin. • For treatment of anaphylaxis, see p. 1114.
Chloramphenicol, erythromycin, tetracyclines: antibiotic antagonism. Give penicillins at least 1 hour before bacteriostatic antibiotics. *Probenecid:* increased blood levels of penicillin. Probenecid is often used for this purpose.	• Use cautiously in patients with other drug allergies, especially to cephalosporins (possible cross-allergenicity); those with asthma; and in infants. • Obtain cultures for sensitivity tests before starting therapy. • Before giving penicillin, ask patient if he's had any previous allergic reactions to this drug. However, a negative history of penicillin allergy is no guarantee against a future allergic reaction. • Be prepared for possible allergic reaction to this drug. Have available emergency equipment and medications needed for resuscitation. • If ordered 4 times a day, be sure to give every 6 hours—even during the night. • Check CBC and transaminase levels frequently. Drug may cause leukopenia, thrombocytopenia, and elevated SGOT and SGPT. • If patient has high serum level of this drug, he may have convulsions. Be prepared by keeping side rails up on bed and tongue blade handy. • When giving I.V., mix with a normal saline solution. Don't mix with others because methicillin may be inactivated. Initial dilution must be made with sterile water for injection. • Give I.V. intermittently to prevent vein irritation. Change site every 48 hours. • Large doses may cause increased yeast growths. Report symptoms to doctor. • With prolonged therapy, other superinfections may occur, especially in the elderly, debilitated, or those with low resistance to infection due to immunosuppressors or irradiation. Close observation is essential. • Check expiration date. • For symptoms and treatment of anaphylaxis, see p. 1114.
Chloramphenicol, erythromycin, tetracyclines: antibiotic antagonism. Give penicillins at least 1 hour before bacteriostatic antibiotics. *Probenecid:* increased blood levels of penicillin. Probenecid is often used for this purpose.	• Use cautiously in patients with other drug allergies, especially to cephalosporins (possible cross-allergenicity); and gastrointestinal distress. • Obtain cultures for sensitivity tests before starting therapy. • Before giving penicillin, ask patient if he's had any previous allergic reactions to this drug. However, a negative history of penicillin allergy is no guarantee against a future allergic reaction. • Tell patient to take medication exactly as prescribed, even if he feels better. If ordered 4 times a day, be sure to give every 6 hours—even during the night. • Tell patient to call the doctor if rash, fever, or chills develop. A rash is the most common allergic reaction. • Be prepared for possible allergic reaction to this drug. Have available emergency equipment and medications needed for resuscitation. • When given orally, it may cause GI disturbances. Food may interfere with absorption, so give 1 to 2 hours before meals or 2 to 3 hours after.

(continued on following page)

NAME	INDICATIONS & DOSAGE	SIDE EFFECTS
nafcillin sodium *(continued)*		
oxacillin sodium Bactocill, Prostaphilin◆	*Systemic infections caused by penicillinase-producing staphylococci*— **Adults:** 2 to 4 g P.O. daily, divided into doses given q 6 hours; 2 to 12 g I.M. or I.V. daily, divided into doses given q 4 to 6 hours. **Children:** 50 to 100 mg/Kg P.O. daily, divided into doses given q 6 hours; 100 to 200 mg/Kg I.M. or I.V. daily, divided into doses given q 4 to 6 hours.	*Blood:* granulocytopenia, thrombocytopenia, eosinophilia, hemolytic anemia, transient neutropenia. *CNS:* neuropathy. *GI:* oral lesions. *GU:* nephrotoxicity. *Other:* thrombophlebitis, hypersensitivity (fever, chills, rash, urticaria, anaphylaxis), overgrowth of nonsusceptible organisms (oral and rectal moniliasis).

INTERACTIONS	NURSING CONSIDERATIONS
	• Don't give I.M. or I.V. unless infection is severe or patient can't take oral dose. • Check CBC and transaminase levels frequently. Drug may cause leukopenia, thrombocytopenia, and elevated SGOT and SGPT. • When giving I.V., mix with 5% dextrose in water or a saline solution. Don't mix with others; they might be incompatible. • Give I.V. intermittently to prevent vein irritation. Change site every 48 hours. • Large doses may cause increased yeast growths. Report symptoms to doctor. • With prolonged therapy, other superinfections may occur, especially in the elderly, debilitated, or those with low resistance to infection due to immunosuppressors or irradiation. Close observation is essential. • Check expiration date. Warn patient never to use leftover penicillin for a new illness or to "share" penicillin with family and friends. • For symptoms and treatment of anaphylaxis, see p. 1114.
Probenecid: increased blood levels of penicillin. Probenecid is often used for this purpose. *Sulfamethoxypyridazine:* decreased serum levels of oxacillin. Avoid if possible. *Chloramphenicol, erythromycin, tetracyclines:* antibiotic antagonism. Give penicillins at least 1 hour before bacteriostatic antibiotics.	• Use cautiously in patients with other drug allergies, especially to cephalosporins (possible cross-allergenicity); asthma; and in premature babies, and infants. • Obtain cultures for sensitivity tests before starting therapy. • Before giving penicillin, ask patient if he's had any previous allergic reactions to this drug. However, a negative history of penicillin allergy is no guarantee against a future allergic reaction. • Tell patient essential to take medication exactly as prescribed, even if he feels better. If ordered 4 times a day, be sure to give every 6 hours—even during the night. • Tell patient to call the doctor if rash, fever, or chills develop. A rash is the most common allergic reaction. • Be prepared for possible allergic reaction to this drug. Have available emergency equipment and medications needed for resuscitation. • When given orally, it may cause GI disturbances. Food may interfere with absorption, so give 1 to 2 hours before meals or 2 to 3 hours after. • Don't give I.M. or I.V. unless infection is severe or patient can't take oral dose. • Check CBC and transaminase levels frequently. Drug may cause leukopenia, thrombocytopenia, and elevated SGOT and SGPT. • When giving I.V., mix with 5% dextrose in water or a saline solution. Don't mix with others; they might be incompatible. • Give I.V. intermittently to prevent vein irritation. Change site every 48 hours. • Large doses may cause increased yeast growths. Report symptoms to doctor. • With prolonged therapy, other superinfections may occur, especially in the elderly, debilitated, or those with low resistance to infection due to immunosuppressors or irradiation. Close observation is essential. • Check expiration date. Warn patient never to use leftover penicillin for a new illness or to "share" penicillin with family and friends. • For symptoms and treatment of anaphylaxis, see p. 1114.

NAME	INDICATIONS & DOSAGE	SIDE EFFECTS
penicillin G benzathine Bicillin L-A♦, Megacillin Suspension♦♦, Permanpen	*Congenital syphilis—* **Children under age 2:** 50,000 units/Kg I.M. as a single dose. *Group A streptococcal upper respiratory infections—* **Adults:** 1,200,000 units I.M. in a single injection. **Children over 27 Kg:** 900,000 units I.M. in a single injection. **Children under 27 Kg:** 300,000 to 600,000 units I.M. in a single injection. *Prophylaxis of poststreptococcal rheumatic fever or glomerulonephritis—* **Adults and children:** 1,200,000 units I.M. once a month or 600,000 units twice a month. *Syphilis less than 1 year in duration—* **Adults:** 2,400,000 units I.M. in a single dose. *Syphilis of more than 1 year duration—* **Adults:** 2,400,000 units I.M. weekly for 3 successive weeks.	*Blood:* eosinophilia, hemolytic anemia, thrombocytopenia, leukopenia. *CNS:* neuropathy. *GU:* nephrotoxicity. *Other:* hypersensitivity (maculopapular and exfoliative dermatitis, Jarisch-Herxheimer reaction, laryngeal edema, chills, fever, edema, anaphylaxis).
penicillin G potassium Arcocillin, Biotic-T, Burcillin-G, Cryspen, Deltapen, Falapen♦♦, G-Recillin-T, Hyasorb, Hylenta♦♦, K-Cillin, K-Pen, Ka-Pen♦♦, Lanacillin, Megacillin♦♦, Novopen-G♦, Palocillin, Parcillin, Pensorb, Pentids, P-50♦♦, Pfizerpen	*Moderate to severe systemic infections—* **Adults:** 1.6 to 3.2 million units P.O. daily, divided into doses given q 6 hours (1 mg = 1,600 units); 1.2 to 24 million units I.M. or I.V. daily, divided into doses given q 4 hours. **Children:** 25,000 to 100,000 units/Kg P.O. daily, divided into doses given q 6 hours; or 25,000 to 300,000 units/Kg I.M. or I.V. daily, divided into doses given q 4 hours.	*Blood:* hemolytic anemia, leukopenia, thrombocytopenia. *CNS:* neuropathy, arthralgia, prostration. *Metabolic:* possible severe to fatal potassium poisoning with high doses (hyperreflexia, convulsions, coma). *Other:* hypersensitivity (rash, urticaria, maculopapular eruptions, exfoliative dermatitis, chills, fever, edema, anaphylaxis), overgrowth of nonsusceptible organisms.

INTERACTIONS	NURSING CONSIDERATIONS
Chloramphenicol, erythromycin, tetracyclines: antibiotic antagonism. Give penicillins at least 1 hour before bacteriostatic antibiotics. *Probenecid:* increased blood levels of penicillin. Probenecid is often used for this purpose.	• Use cautiously in patients with other drug allergies, especially to cephalosporins (possible cross-allergenicity). • Obtain cultures for sensitivity tests before starting therapy. Not necessary to wait for culture and sensitivity results before beginning therapy. • Before giving penicillin, ask patient if he's had any previous allergic reactions to this drug. However, a negative history of penicillin allergy is no guarantee against a future allergic reaction. • Tell patient to call the doctor if rash, fever, or chills develop. Fever and eosinophilia are the most common allergic reactions. • Be prepared for possible allergic reaction to this drug. Have available emergency equipment and medications needed for resuscitation. • Check CBC and transaminase levels frequently. Drug may cause leukopenia, thrombocytopenia, and elevated SGOT and SGPT. • Large doses may cause increased yeast growths. Report symptoms to doctor. • Watch closely for fever in first 2 to 4 hours after therapy begins. May indicate Jarisch-Herxheimer reaction in patients with syphilis. • Shake medication well before injection. • Never give I.V. Inadvertent I.V. administration has caused cardiac arrest and death. • Very slow absorption time makes allergic reactions difficult to treat. • Inject deeply into upper outer quadrant of buttocks in adults; in midlateral thigh in infants and small children. • Check expiration date. • For treatment of anaphylaxis, see p. 1114.
Chloramphenicol, erythromycin tetracyclines: antibiotic antagonism. Give penicillins at least 1 hour before bacteriostatic antibiotics. *Probenecid:* increased blood levels of penicillin. Probenecid is often used for this purpose.	• Use cautiously in patients with other drug allergies, especially to cephalosporins (possible cross-allergenicity). • Obtain cultures for sensitivity tests before starting therapy. Not necessary to wait for culture and sensitivity results before beginning therapy. • Before giving penicillin, ask patient if he's had any previous allergic reactions to this drug. However, a negative history of penicillin allergy is no guarantee against a future allergic reaction. • Tell patient to take medication exactly as prescribed, even if he feels better. Give evenly spaced during each 24-hour period. • Tell patient to call the doctor if rash, fever, or chills develop. A rash is the most common allergic reaction. • Be prepared for possible allergic reaction to this drug. Have available emergency equipment and medications needed for resuscitation. • When given orally, it may cause GI disturbances. Food may interfere with absorption, so give 1 to 2 hours before meals or 2 to 3 hours after. • Don't give I.M. or I.V. unless infection is severe or patient can't take oral dose. Extremely painful when given I.M. • Check CBC and transaminase levels frequently. Drug may cause leukopenia, thrombocytopenia, and elevated SGOT and SGPT. • If patient has high serum level of this drug, he may have convulsions. Be prepared by keeping side rails up on bed and tongue blade handy. • When giving I.V., mix with 5% dextrose in water or a saline solution. Don't mix with other solutions; they might be incompatible. • Give I.V. intermittently to prevent vein irritation. Change site every 48 hours. • Large doses may cause increased yeast growths. Report symptoms to doctor. • With prolonged therapy, other superinfections may occur, especially in the elderly, debilitated, or those with low resistance to infection due to

(continued on following page)

NAME	INDICATIONS & DOSAGE	SIDE EFFECTS
penicillin G potassium *(continued)*		
penicillin G procaine Ayercillin♦♦, Crysticillin A.S., Duracillin A.S., Pfizerpen A.S., Tu-Cillin, Wycillin♦	*Moderate to severe systemic infections*— **Adults:** 600,000 to 1.2 million units I.M. daily given as a single dose. **Children:** 300,000 units I.M. daily given as a single dose. *Uncomplicated gonorrhea*— **Adults, and children over 12:** give 1 g probenecid; then 30 minutes later give 4.8 million units of penicillin G procaine I.M., divided into 2 injection sites.	*Blood:* thrombocytopenia, hemolytic anemia, leukopenia. *CNS:* arthralgia. *Other:* hypersensitivity (rash, urticaria, chills, fever, edema, prostration, anaphylaxis), overgrowth of nonsusceptible organisms.
penicillin G sodium Crystapen♦♦	*Moderate to severe systemic infections*— **Adults:** 1.2 to 24 million units daily I.M. or I.V., divided into doses given q 4 hours. **Children:** 25,000 to 300,000 units/Kg daily I.M. or I.V., divided into doses given q 4 hours.	*Blood:* hemolytic anemia, leukopenia, thrombocytopenia. *CNS:* arthralgia, prostration, neuropathy. *CV:* congestive heart failure with high doses. *GU:* nephrotoxicity. *Other:* hypersensitivity (chills, fever, edema, maculopapular rash, exfoliative dermatitis, urticaria, anaphylaxis), overgrowth of nonsusceptible organisms.

INTERACTIONS	NURSING CONSIDERATIONS
	immunosuppressors or irradiation. Close observation is essential. • Monitor serum potassium. • Check expiration date. Warn patient never to use leftover penicillin for a new illness or to "share" penicillin with family and friends. • For treatment of anaphylaxis, see p. 1114.
Chloramphenicol, erythromycin, tetracyclines: antibiotic antagonism. Give penicillins at least 1 hour before bacteriostatic antibiotics. *Probenecid:* increased blood levels of penicillin. Probenecid is often used for this purpose.	• Contraindicated in patients with hypersensitivity to procaine. Use cautiously in patients with other drug allergies, especially to cephalosporins (possible cross-allergenicity), and asthma. • Obtain cultures for sensitivity tests before starting therapy. Not necessary to wait for culture and sensitivity results before beginning therapy. • Before giving penicillin, ask patient if he's had any previous allergic reactions to this drug. However, a negative history of penicillin allergy is no guarantee against a future allergic reaction. • Tell patient to call doctor if rash, fever, or chills develop. A rash is the most common allergic reaction. • Be prepared for possible allergic reaction to this drug. Have available emergency equipment and medications needed for resuscitation. • Check CBC and transaminase levels frequently. Drug may cause leukopenia, thrombocytopenia, and elevated SGOT and SGPT. • Give deep I.M. in upper outer quadrant of buttocks in adults; in midlateral thigh in small children. • Never give I.V. Inadvertent I.V. administration has caused death. • Large doses may cause increased yeast growths. Report symptoms to doctor. • Due to slow absorption rate, allergic reactions are hard to treat. • With prolonged therapy, other superinfections may occur, especially in the elderly, debilitated, or those with low resistance to infection due to immunosuppressors or irradiation. Close observation is essential. • Check expiration date. • For treatment of anaphylaxis, see p. 1114.
Chloramphenicol, erythromycin, tetracyclines: antibiotic antagonism. Give penicillins at least 1 hour before bacteriostatic antibiotics. *Probenecid:* increased blood levels of penicillin. Probenecid is often used for this purpose.	• Contraindicated in patients on sodium restriction. Use cautiously in patients with other drug allergies, especially to cephalosporins (possible cross-allergenicity), and asthma. • Obtain cultures for sensitivity tests before starting therapy. Not necessary to wait for culture and sensitivity results before beginning therapy. • Before giving penicillin, ask patient if he's had any previous allergic reactions to this drug. However, a negative history of penicillin allergy is no guarantee against a future allergic reaction. • Be prepared for possible allergic reaction to this drug. Have available emergency equipment and medications needed for resuscitation. • Check CBC and transaminase levels frequently. Drug may cause leukopenia, thrombocytopenia, and elevated SGOT and SGPT. • If patient has high serum level of this drug, he may have convulsions. Be prepared by keeping side rails up on bed and tongue blade handy. • When giving I.V., mix with 5% dextrose in water or a saline solution. Don't mix with others; they might be incompatible. • Give I.V. intermittently to prevent vein irritation. Change site every 48 hours. • Large doses may cause increased yeast growths. Report symptoms to doctor. • With prolonged therapy, other superinfections may occur, especially in the elderly, debilitated, or those with low resistance to infection due to immunosuppressors or irradiation. Close observation is essential. • Monitor vital signs frequently. • Monitor serum sodium. • Check expiration date. • For treatment of anaphylaxis, see p. 1114.

NAME	INDICATIONS & DOSAGE	SIDE EFFECTS
penicillin V Biotic Powder, Compocillin-V, Ledercillin VK◆, Pfizerpen VK◆, Robicillin-VK, SK-Penicillin VK, Uticillin VK, V-Cillin Drops, V-Pen **penicillin V potassium** Betapen VK, Biotic-V-Powder, Bopen V-K, Cocillin V-K, Compocillin-VK, Dowpen VK, Lanacillin VK, Ledercillin VK◆, LV, Nadopen-V◆◆, Novopen-V◆◆, Penapar VK, Penbec-V◆◆, Pen-Vee-K◆, Pfizerpen VK, PVF K◆◆, Repen-VK, Robicillin VK, Uticillin VK, V-Cillin K◆	*Mild to moderate systemic infections*— **Adults:** 250 to 500 mg (400,000 to 800,000 units) P.O. q 6 hours. **Children:** 15 to 50 mg/Kg (25,000 to 90,000 units/Kg) P.O. daily, divided into doses given q 6 to 8 hours.	*Blood:* eosinophilia, hemolytic anemia, leukopenia, thrombocytopenia. *CNS:* neuropathy. *GI:* epigastric distress, vomiting, diarrhea, nausea, black hairy tongue. *Other:* hypersensitivity (rash, urticaria, chills, fever, edema, anaphylaxis), overgrowth of nonsusceptible organisms.
ticarcillin disodium Ticar	*Severe systemic infections caused by susceptible strains of gram-positive and especially gram-negative organisms (Pseudomonas, Proteus)*— **Adults:** 18 g I.V. or I.M. daily, divided into doses given q 4 to 6 hours. **Children:** 200 to 300 mg/Kg I.V. or I.M. daily, divided into doses given q 4 to 6 hours.	*Blood:* leukopenia, neutropenia, eosinophilia, thrombocytopenia, hemolytic anemia. *CNS:* neuropathy, convulsions, neuromuscular excitability. *GI:* nausea, vomiting. *Local:* pain at injection site, vein irritation, phlebitis. *Metabolic:* hypokalemia. *Other:* hypersensitivity (rash, pruritus, urticaria, chills, fever, edema, anaphylaxis), overgrowth of nonsusceptible organisms.

INTERACTIONS	NURSING CONSIDERATIONS
Chloramphenicol, erythromycin, tetracyclines: antibiotic antagonism. Give penicillins at least 1 hour before bacteriostatic antibiotics. *Neomycin:* decreased absorption of penicillin. Give penicillin by injection. *Probenecid:* increased blood levels of penicillin. Probenecid is often used for this purpose.	• Use cautiously in patients with other drug allergies, especially to cephalosporins (possible cross-allergenicity); asthma; and GI disturbances. • Obtain cultures for sensitivity tests before starting therapy. Not necessary to wait for culture and sensitivity results before beginning therapy. • Before giving penicillin, ask patient if he's had any previous allergic reactions to this drug. However, a negative history of penicillin allergy is no guarantee against a future allergic reaction. • Tell patient to take medication exactly as prescribed, even if he feels better. If ordered 4 times a day, be sure to give every 6 hours—even during the night. • Tell patient to call the doctor if rash, fever, or chills develop. A rash is the most common allergic reaction. • Be prepared for possible allergic reaction to this drug. Have available emergency equipment and medications needed for resuscitation. • When given orally, it may cause GI disturbances. Food may interfere with absorption, so give 1 to 2 hours before meals or 2 to 3 hours after. • Check CBC and transaminase levels frequently. Drug may cause leukopenia, thrombocytopenia, and elevated SGOT and SGPT. • Large doses may cause increased yeast growths. Report symptoms to doctor. • With prolonged therapy, other superinfections may occur, especially in the elderly, debilitated, or those with low resistance to infection due to immunosuppressors or irradiation. Close observation is essential. • Check expiration date. Warn patient never to use leftover penicillin for a new illness or to "share" penicillin with family and friends. • For treatment of anaphylaxis, see p. 1114.
Chloramphenicol, erythromycin, tetracyclines: antibiotic antagonism. Give penicillins at least 1 hour before bacteriostatic antibiotics. *Probenecid:* increased blood levels of penicillin. Probenecid is often used for this purpose. *Gentamicin, tobramycin:* chemically incompatible. Don't mix together in I.V. Give 1 hour apart.	• Use cautiously in patients with other drug allergies, especially to cephalosporins (possible cross-allergenicity); impaired renal function; hemorrhagic conditions; hypokalemia; in sodium-restricted patients (contains 5.2 mEq sodium/g). • Obtain cultures for sensitivity tests before starting therapy. Not necessary to wait for culture and sensitivity results before beginning therapy. • Before giving penicillin, ask patient if he's had any previous allergic reactions to this drug. However, a negative history of penicillin allergy is no guarantee against a future allergic reaction. • Be prepared for possible allergic reaction to this drug. Have available emergency equipment and medications needed for resuscitation. • Check CBC and transaminase levels frequently. Drug may cause leukopenia, thrombocytopenia, and elevated SGOT and SGPT. • If patient has high serum level of this drug, he may develop convulsions. Be prepared by keeping side rails up on bed and tongue blade handy. • When giving I.V., mix with 5% dextrose in water or other suitable I.V. fluids. • Give I.V. intermittently to prevent vein irritation. Change site every 48 hours. • Large doses may cause increased yeast growths. Report symptoms to doctor. • With prolonged therapy, other superinfections may occur, especially in the elderly, debilitated, or those with low resistance to infection due to immunosuppressors or irradiation. Close observation is essential. • Monitor serum sodium and serum potassium. • Check expiration date. • For symptoms and treatment of anaphylaxis, see p. 1114.

12

Cephalosporins

cefaclor
cefadroxil monohydrate
cefamandole naftate
cefazolin sodium
cefoxitin sodium
cephalexin monohydrate
cephaloglycin dihydrate
cephaloridine
cephalothin sodium
cephapirin sodium
cephradine

Cephalosporins are semisynthetic antibiotics structurally related to the penicillins. They all contain 7-aminocephalosporanic acid (B-lactam ring). The cephalosporins are broad-spectrum antibiotics with activity against most gram-positive organisms and some gram-negative organisms.

Major uses

• To treat infections caused by gram-positive cocci (except enterococci), penicillinase-producing staphylococci, some gram-negative bacilli, including *E. coli, Proteus mirabilis,* and *Klebsiella*. These drugs are often used to treat penicillin-allergic patients. However, a small percentage of these patients subsequently develop allergies to cephalosporins.
• Parenteral cephalosporins are used to treat infections of the respiratory tract, skin, soft tissue, genitourinary tract, bones and joints, and septicemia and endocarditis caused by sensitive organisms.
• Oral cephalosporins are used to treat otitis media, infections of the respiratory tract, skin, soft tissue, and genitourinary tract.

Mechanism of action

• Cephalosporins are bactericidal or bacteriostatic, depending on organism susceptibility, dose, serum and tissue concentrations of drug, and rate at which organisms are multiplying. They inhibit cell-wall synthesis at the final step, thereby making the wall less stable osmotically. They are more effective against young, rapidly dividing organisms than against mature, resting cells that are not in process of cell-wall formation.

Absorption, distribution, and excretion

• Of these drugs, cefaclor, cefadroxil, cephalexin, cephaloglycin, and cephradine are given orally because they are well absorbed from the GI tract.
• Cefamandole, cefazolin, cefoxitin, cephaloridine, cephalothin, and cephapirin are not given orally because they are not well absorbed from the GI tract.
• GI absorption of these agents is delayed by the presence of food, resulting in lower and delayed peak serum levels; however, this does not affect the total amount of drug absorbed.

• All drugs in this class are widely distributed throughout body tissues and fluid but enter cerebrospinal fluid in only small amounts.
• Cefaclor, cefadroxil, cefamandole, cefazolin, cefoxitin sodium, cephalexin, cephaloridine, and cephradine are eliminated unchanged in urine and will accumulate in patients with renal insufficiency. Cephaloglycin, cephalothin, and cephapirin are partially metabolized in the liver.

Onset and duration
• Onset and duration depend upon the route of administration, the percentage of drug which is protein-bound, and on renal function.
• Peak serum levels after I.V. administration generally depend upon rate of absorption. They are usually reached after 30 to 60 minutes.
• Duration of action depends upon the half-life of the drug and when the serum level falls below the minimal inhibitory concentration. Protein-bound cephalosporins do not appear to have antibacterial activity.
• The half-life of these drugs in adults with normal renal function and their approximate percentage of protein-binding follow:

cefaclor	29 to 60 minutes	22% to 25%
cefadroxil	72 minutes	0% to 10%
cefamandole	32 to 60 minutes	approximately 70%
cefazolin	69 to 132 minutes	74% to 86%
cefoxitin	41 to 59 minutes	approximately 70%
cephalexin	30 to 72 minutes	6% to 15%
cephaloglycin	90 minutes	0% to 30%
cephaloridine	48 to 108 minutes	0% to 31%
cephalothin	30 to 60 minutes	65% to 80%
cephapirin	21 to 47 minutes	44% to 50%
cephradine	42 to 120 minutes	0% to 20%

Renal impairment prolongs the half-life of these agents. Doses should be adjusted accordingly.

Combination products
None.

NAME	INDICATIONS & DOSAGE	SIDE EFFECTS
cefaclor Ceclor	*Treatment of infections of respiratory or urinary tract, skin and soft tissue, and otitis media due to H. influenzae, Streptococcus pneumoniae and pyogenes, E. coli, P. mirabilis, Klebsiella species, and staphylococci*— **Adults:** 250 to 500 mg P.O. q 8 hours. Total daily dose should not exceed 4 g. **Children:** 20 mg/Kg/day P.O. in divided doses q 8 hours. In more serious infections, 40 mg/Kg/day are recommended, not to exceed 1 g per day.	*Blood:* transient leukopenia, lymphocytosis, anemia, eosinophilia. *CNS:* dizziness, headache, somnolence. *GI:* nausea, vomiting, diarrhea, anorexia, dyspepsia. *GU:* red and white cells in urine, vaginal moniliasis and vaginitis. *Skin:* maculopapular rash, dermatitis. *Other:* elevated transaminases and alkaline phosphatase, hypersensitivity, elevated BUN, fever, edema.
cefadroxil monohydrate Duricef	*Treatment of urinary tract infections caused by E. coli, P. mirabilis and Klebsiella species*— **Adults:** 250 to 1,000 mg q 8 to 12 hours. Not recommended for children.	*Blood:* transient neutropenia, eosinophilia, leukopenia, anemia, agranulocytosis, azotemia. *CNS:* dizziness, headache, malaise, paresthesias. *GI:* nausea, anorexia, vomiting, diarrhea, glossitis, dyspepsia, abdominal cramps, anal pruritus, tenesmus, oral candidiasis (thrush). *GU:* nephrotoxicity, genital pruritus and moniliasis, vaginitis. *Skin:* maculopapular and erythematous rashes, dyspnea, transient elevations of serum transaminases and alkaline phosphatase.
cefamandole naftate Mandol	*Treatment of serious infections of respiratory and genitourinary tract, skin and soft tissue infections, bone and joint infections, bloodstream and peritonitis due to E. coli and other coliform bacteria, S. aureus, (penicillinase and nonpenicillinase producing), S. epidermidis, group A beta-hemolytic streptococci, Klebsiella, H. influenzae, P. mirabilis, and Enterobacter species*— **Adults:** 500 mg to 1 g q 4 to 8 hours. In life-threatening infections up to 2 g q 4 hours may be needed. **Infants and children:** 50 to 100 mg/	*Blood:* transient neutropenia, eosinophilia, hemolytic anemia, leukopenia, thrombocytopenia, azotemia. *CNS:* headache, malaise, paresthesias, dizziness. *GI:* nausea, anorexia, vomiting, diarrhea, glossitis, dyspepsia, abdominal cramps, tenesmus, anal pruritus, oral candidiasis (thrush). *GU:* nephrotoxicity, genital pruritus and moniliasis. *Local:* at injection site—pain, induration, sterile abscesses, temperature elevation, tissue slough; phlebitis and thrombophlebitis with I.V. injection. *Skin:* maculopapular and erythematous rashes, urticaria.

• Also available in Canada.
•• Available in Canada only.
Unmarked trade names available in United States only.

INTERACTIONS	NURSING CONSIDERATIONS
Probenecid: may inhibit excretion and increase blood levels of cefaclor. Use together cautiously.	• Contraindicated in hypersensitivity to other cephalosporins. Use cautiously in impaired renal status and in those with history of sensitivity to penicillin. Ask patient if he's had any reaction to previous cephalosporin or penicillin therapy before administering first dose. • Prolonged use may result in overgrowth of nonsusceptible organisms. Careful observation of patient for superinfection is essential. • Obtain cultures for sensitivity tests before therapy, but therapy may begin pending results of culture and sensitivity tests. • Cefaclor is the newest cephalosporin. • Major clinical use appears to be in treating otitis media caused by *H. influenzae* when resistant to ampicillin or amoxicillin. • Mostly used in ambulatory setting. • Tell patient to take medication as prescribed, even though he may feel better. • Store reconstituted solution in refrigerator. Stable for 14 days if refrigerated. Shake well before using. • Drug may be taken with meals. • Cefaclor is a relatively expensive antibiotic and should only be used when the organism is resistant to other agents.
None significant.	• Contraindicated in hypersensitivity to other cephalosporins. Use cautiously in impaired renal status and in those with history of sensitivity to penicillin. Ask patient if he's had any reaction to previous cephalosporin or penicillin therapy before administering first dose. • Prolonged use may result in overgrowth of nonsusceptible organisms. Careful observation of patient for superinfection is essential. • Obtain cultures for sensitivity tests before therapy, but therapy may begin pending results of cultures and sensitivity tests. • Cefadroxil serum levels are low; used only for urinary tract infections. • If creatinine clearance is below 50 ml/min, dosage interval should be increased so drug doesn't accumulate. • Monitor for signs of renal impairment: appearance of casts in urine, proteinuria, decreased urinary output, increased BUN or serum creatinine, decreased creatinine clearance or urine/plasma creatinine ratio. • Tell patient to take medication as prescribed, even though he may feel better. • Unlike other oral cephalosporins, absorption not delayed by presence of food. • Longer half-life permits twice-daily dosing.
Probenecid: may inhibit excretion and increase blood levels of cefamandole. Use together cautiously.	• Contraindicated in hypersensitivity to other cephalosporins. Use cautiously in impaired renal status and in those with history of sensitivity to penicillin. Ask patient if he's had any reaction to previous cephalosporin or penicillin therapy before administering first dose. • Prolonged use may result in overgrowth of nonsusceptible organisms. Careful observation of patient for superinfection is essential. • Obtain cultures for sensitivity tests before therapy, but therapy may begin pending results of cultures and sensitivity tests. • Cephalosporin of choice for treatment of Enterobacter sepsis. • Not as effective as cefoxitin in treating anaerobic infections. • For most cephalosporin-sensitive organisms, cefamandole offers little advantage over previously available agents. • For I.V. use, reconstitute 1 g with 10 ml of sterile water for injection, 5% dextrose or 0.9% sodium chloride for injection. May be combined with the following intravenous fluids: 0.9% sodium chloride injection, 5% dextrose injection, 10% dextrose injection, 5% dextrose and 0.9% sodium chloride injection, 5% dextrose and 0.45% sodium chloride injection, 5%

(continued on following page)

NAME	INDICATIONS & DOSAGE	SIDE EFFECTS
cefamandole naftate *(continued)*	Kg/day in equally divided doses q 4 to 8 hours. May be increased to total daily dose of 150 mg/Kg (not to exceed maximum adult dose) for severe infections. Total daily dosage is same for I.M. or I.V. administration and depends on susceptibility of organism and severity of infection. In patients with impaired renal function, doses or frequency of administration must be modified according to degree of renal impairment, severity of infection, susceptibility of organism, and serum levels of drug. Should be injected deep I.M. into a large muscle mass, such as gluteus or lateral aspect of thigh.	*Other:* hypersensitivity, dyspnea, transient elevations of serum transaminases and alkaline phosphatase.
cefazolin sodium Ancef◆, Kefzol◆	*Treatment of serious infections of respiratory and genitourinary tracts, skin and soft tissue infections, bone and joint infections, septicemia, and endocarditis due to E. coli, Enterobacteriaceae, enterococci, gonococci, H. influenzae, Klebsiella, P. mirabilis, S. aureus, S. pneumoniae, and group A beta-hemolytic streptococci*— **Adults:** 250 mg I.M. or I.V. q 8 hours to 1 g q 6 hours. **Children over 1 month:** 8 to 16 mg/Kg I.M. or I.V. q 8 hours, or 6 to 12 mg/Kg q 6 hours. Total daily dosage is same for I.M. or I.V. administration and depends on susceptibility of organism and severity of infection. Initial I.V. loading dose (usually 500 mg) recommended. Maximum dose for severe infections: 33 mg/Kg q 8 hours or 25 mg/Kg q 8 hours. In patients with impaired renal function, doses or frequency of administration must be modified according to degree of renal impairment, severity of infection, susceptibility of organism, and serum levels of drug. Should be injected deep I.M. into a large muscle mass, such as gluteus or lateral aspect of thigh.	*Blood:* transient neutropenia, leukopenia, eosinophilia, thrombocythemia, thrombocytopenia, agranulocytosis, azotemia, anemia. *CNS:* dizziness, headache, malaise, paresthesias. *GI:* nausea, anorexia, vomiting, diarrhea, glossitis, dyspepsia, abdominal cramps, anal pruritus, tenesmus, oral candidiasis (thrush). *GU:* nephrotoxicity, genital pruritus and moniliasis, vaginitis. *Local:* at injection site—pain, induration, sterile abscesses, tissue slough; phlebitis and thrombophlebitis with I.V. injection. *Skin:* maculopapular and erythematous rashes, urticaria. *Other:* hypersensitivity, dyspnea, transient elevations of serum transaminases and phosphatase.

INTERACTIONS	NURSING CONSIDERATIONS
	dextrose and 0.2% sodium chloride injection, or sodium lactate injection. • I.M. cefamandole not as painful as cefoxitin. Does not require addition of lidocaine. • After reconstitution, remains stable for 24 hours at room temperature or 96 hours under refrigeration.
Probenecid: may increase blood levels of cephalosporins. Use together cautiously.	• Use cautiously in impaired renal status and in those with history of sensitivity to penicillin. Ask patient if he's had any reaction to previous cephalosporin or penicillin therapy before administering first dose. • Prolonged use may result in overgrowth of nonsusceptible organisms. Watch carefully for superinfection. • Obtain cultures for sensitivity tests before therapy, but therapy may begin pending results of cultures and sensitivity tests. • Excreted in urine; monitor renal function carefully. Watch for signs of impairment: casts in urine, proteinuria, decreased urinary output, increased BUN or serum creatinine, decreased creatinine clearance or urine/plasma creatinine ratio. Cephalosporins may cause falsely elevated BUN and transaminase levels. • Avoid doses greater than 4 g daily in severe renal impairment. • Because of long duration effect, most infections can be treated with a single dose q 8 hours. • For I.M. administration, reconstitute with sterile water, bacteriostatic water, or 0.9% sodium chloride solution as follows: 2 ml to 250 mg vial; 2 ml to 500 mg vial; 2.5 ml to 1 g vial. Shake well until dissolved. Resultant concentration: 125 mg/ml, 225 mg/ml, 330 mg/ml respectively. • Can cause pain and induration when given I.M. • Alternate injection sites if I.V. therapy lasts longer than 3 days. Use of small I.V. needles in the larger available veins may be preferable. • For I.V. administration, reconstituted cefazolin sodium is diluted in 50 to 100 ml of 0.9% sodium chloride injection, 5% or 10% dextrose injection, 5% dextrose in lactated Ringer's, 5% dextrose and 0.9% sodium chloride, 5% dextrose and 0.45% or 0.2% sodium chloride, lactated Ringer's injection, Normosol-M in 5% dextrose in water, Ionosol B with 5% dextrose, or Plasma-lyte with 5% dextrose. • Reconstituted cefazolin sodium is stable for 24 hours at room temperature and for 96 hours under refrigeration. • About 40% to 75% of patients receiving cephalosporins show a false positive direct Coombs' test, but only a few of these indicate hemolytic anemia. • Urine glucose tests with Benedict's Qualitative Reagent, Clinitest, or Fehling's solution may cause false positive reaction during cephalosporin therapy. Clinistix, Diastix, and Tes-Tape are not affected.

NAME	INDICATIONS & DOSAGE	SIDE EFFECTS
cefoxitin sodium Mefoxin	*Treatment of serious infection of respiratory and genitourinary tract, skin and soft tissue infections, bone and joint infections, bloodstream and intra-abdominal infections due to E. coli and other coliform bacteria, S. aureus (penicillinase and non-penicillinase), S. epidermidis, streptococci, Klebsiella, H. influenzae and Bacteroides species, including B. fragilis—* **Adults:** 1 to 2 g q 6 to 8 hours for uncomplicated forms of infection. Up to 12 g per day in life-threatening infections. **Children:** 80 to 160 mg/Kg/day. Total daily dosage is same for I.M. or I.V. administration and depends on susceptibility of organism and severity of infection. In patients with impaired renal function, doses or frequency of administration must be modified according to degree of renal impairment, severity of infection, susceptibility of organism, and serum levels of drug. Should be injected deep I.M. into a large muscle mass such as gluteus or lateral aspect of thigh.	*Blood:* transient neutropenia, eosinophilia, hemolytic anemia, leukopenia, azotemia. *CNS:* headache, malaise, paresthesias, dizziness. *GI:* nausea, anorexia, vomiting, diarrhea, glossitis, dyspepsia, abdominal cramps, tenesmus, anal pruritus, oral candidiasis (thrush). *GU:* nephrotoxicity, genital pruritus and moniliasis. *Local:* at injection site—pain, induration, sterile abscesses, temperature elevation, tissue slough; phlebitis and thrombophlebitis with I.V. injection. *Skin:* maculopapular and erythematous rashes, urticaria. *Other:* hypersensitivity, dyspnea, transient elevations of serum transaminases and alkaline phosphatase.
cephalexin monohydrate Ceporex♦♦, Keflex♦	*Treatment of infections of respiratory or genitourinary tract, skin and soft tissue infections, bone and joint infections, and otitis media due to E. coli and other coliform bacteria; group A beta-hemolytic streptococci, H. influenzae, Klebsiella, P. mirabilis, S. pneumoniae, and staphylococci—* **Adults:** 250 mg to 1 g P.O. q 6 hours. **Children:** 6 to 12 mg/Kg P.O. q 6 hours. Maximum 25 mg/Kg q 6 hours.	*Blood:* transient neutropenia, eosinophilia, leukopenia, thrombocythemia, anemia, thrombocytopenia, agranulocytosis, azotemia. *CNS:* dizziness, headache, malaise, paresthesias. *GI:* nausea, anorexia, vomiting, diarrhea, glossitis, dyspepsia, abdominal cramps, anal pruritus, tenesmus, oral candidiasis (thrush). *GU:* nephrotoxicity, genital pruritus and moniliasis, vaginitis. *Skin:* maculopapular and erythematous rashes, urticaria. *Other:* hypersensitivity, dyspnea, transient elevations of serum transaminases and alkaline phosphatase.

INTERACTIONS	NURSING CONSIDERATIONS
Probenecid: may inhibit excretion and increase blood levels of cefoxitin. Use together cautiously.	• Contraindicated in hypersensitivity to other cephalosporins. Use cautiously in impaired renal status and in those with history of sensitivity to penicillin. Ask patient if he's had any reaction to previous cephalosporin or penicillin therapy before administering first dose. • Prolonged use may result in overgrowth of nonsusceptible organisms. Observe patient for superinfection. • Obtain cultures for sensitivity tests before therapy, but therapy may begin pending results of cultures and sensitivity tests. • A very useful cephalosporin to use when anaerobic or mixed aerobic-anaerobic infection is suspected, especially *Bacteroides fragilis.* • For most cephalosporin sensitive organisms, cefoxitin offers little advantage over previously available agents. • For I.V. use, reconstitute 1 g with at least 10 ml of sterile water for injection, and 2 g with 10 to 20 ml. 5% dextrose and 0.9% sodium chloride for injection can also be used. These primary solutions can be further diluted with the following solutions; Ringer's injection, lactated Ringer's injection, 5% dextrose in lactated Ringer's injection, 5% or 10% invert sugar in water, 10% invert sugar in saline, 5% sodium bicarbonate injection, Aminosol 5% solution, Normosol-M in 5% dextrose in water, Ionosol B with 5% dextrose, Polyonic M 56 in 5% dextrose. • I.M. injection can be reconstituted with 0.5% or 1% lidocaine HC1 (without epinephrine) to minimize pain on injection. • May cause false positive for urine glucose with Clinitest tablets. • May be useful in the treatment of resistant gonorrhea. • First cephalosporin that is a cephamycin derivative. • After reconstitution, remains stable for 24 hours at room temperature or one week under refrigeration.
Probenecid: may increase blood levels of cephalosporins. Use together cautiously.	• Use cautiously in impaired renal status and in those with history of sensitivity to penicillin. Ask patient if he's had any reaction to previous cephalosporin or penicillin therapy before administering first dose. • Prolonged use may result in overgrowth of nonsusceptible organisms. Watch closely for superinfection. • Obtain cultures for sensitivity tests before therapy, but therapy may begin pending results of cultures and sensitivity tests. • Excreted in urine. Monitor renal function carefully. Watch for signs of impairment: casts in urine, proteinuria, decreased urinary output, increased BUN or serum creatinine, decreased creatinine clearance or urine/plasma creatinine ratio. Cephalosporins may cause falsely elevated BUN and transaminase levels. Avoid doses greater than 4 g daily in severe renal impairment. • Tell patient to take medication for as long as ordered, even after he feels better. Group A beta-hemolytic streptococci infections should be treated for a minimum of 10 days. • Preparation of oral suspension: add required amount of water to powder in two portions. Shake well after each addition. After mixing, store in refrigerator. Stable for 14 days without significant loss of potency. Keep tightly closed and shake well before using. • About 40% to 75% of patients receiving cephalosporins show a false positive direct Coombs' test, but only a few of these indicate hemolytic anemia. • Urine glucose tests with Benedict's Qualitative Reagent, Clinitest, or Fehling's solution may give false positive during cephalosporin therapy. Clinistix, Diastix, and Tes-Tape are not affected.

NAME	INDICATIONS & DOSAGE	SIDE EFFECTS
cephaloglycin dihydrate Kafocin	*Treatment of acute and chronic urinary tract infections, including cystitis, pyelitis, pyelonephritis, and "asymptomatic bacteruria" when due to susceptible strains of E. coli, Klebsiella, Enterobacter, Proteus, staphylococci, and enterococci—* **Adults:** 250 mg P.O. q 6 hours. *Severe infections—* **Adults:** 500 mg P.O. q 6 hours.	*Blood:* transient neutropenia, eosinophilia, leukopenia, thrombocythemia, anemia, thrombocytopenia, agranulocytosis, azotemia. *CNS:* dizziness, headache, malaise, paresthesias. *GI:* nausea, anorexia, vomiting, diarrhea, glossitis, dyspepsia, abdominal cramps, anal pruritus, tenesmus, oral candidiasis (thrush). *GU:* nephrotoxicity, genital pruritus and moniliasis, vaginitis. *Skin:* maculopapular and erythematous rashes, urticaria. *Other:* hypersensitivity, serum sickness, rashes, dyspnea, transient elevations of serum transaminases and alkaline phosphatase.
cephaloridine Ceporan♦♦, Loridine♦	*Treatment of serious infections of respiratory tract, genitourinary tract, bones and joints, bloodstream, skin, and soft tissue due to E. coli and other coliform bacteria, gonococci, H. influenzae, Klebsiella, P. mirabilis, pneumococci, staphylococci (coagulase positive and coagulase negative), beta-hemolytic and other streptococci; also, gonorrhea and early syphilis when penicillin is contraindicated—* **Adults:** 250 mg to 1 g I.M. or I.V. q 6 to 12 hours. Not to exceed 4 g daily. **Children:** 7 to 12 mg/Kg I.M. or I.V. q 6 hours. *Severe infections*—up to 25 mg/Kg q 6 hours. Not recommended for children under 1 month or for premature infants. Total daily dosage is same for I.M. or I.V. administration and depends on susceptibility of organism and severity of infection. Initial loading dose (usually 500 mg) recommended. In patients with impaired renal function, doses and frequency of administration must be modified according to degree of renal impairment, severity of infection, susceptibility of causative organism, and serum levels of drug. Should be injected	*Blood:* transient neutropenia, eosinophilia, leukopenia, thrombocythemia, anemia, thrombocytopenia, agranulocytosis, azotemia. *CNS:* headache, malaise, paresthesias. *GI:* nausea, anorexia, vomiting, diarrhea, glossitis, dyspepsia, abdominal cramps, tenesmus, anal pruritus. oral candidiasis (thrush). *GU:* nephrotoxicity (especially in doses greater than 4 g daily or in patients with renal impairment), genital pruritus and moniliasis, vaginitis. *Local:* at injection site—pain, induration, sterile abscesses, tissue slough; phlebitis and thrombophlebitis with I.V. injection. *Other:* hypersensitivity, maculopapular and erythematous rashes, urticaria, dyspnea, transient elevations of serum transaminase and alkaline phosphatase.

INTERACTIONS	NURSING CONSIDERATIONS
Probenecid: may increase blood levels of cephalosporins. Use together cautiously.	• Use cautiously in impaired renal function and in those with history of sensitivity to penicillin. Ask patient if he's had any reaction to previous cephalosporin or penicillin therapy before administering first dose. • Cephaloglycin serum levels are low; used only for urinary tract infections. • Prolonged use may result in overgrowth of nonsusceptible organisms. Watch for superinfection. • Obtain cultures for sensitivity tests before beginning therapy, but therapy may begin pending results of cultures and sensitivity tests. • Excreted unchanged in urine; monitor renal function carefully. Watch for signs of impairment: casts in urine, proteinuria, decreased urinary output, increased BUN or serum creatinine, decreased creatinine clearance or urine/plasma creatinine ratio. Cephalosporins may cause falsely elevated BUN and transaminase levels. • Tell patient to take medication as prescribed, even after he feels better. • About 40% to 75% of patients receiving cephalosporins show a false positive direct Coombs' test, but only a few of these indicate hemolytic anemia. • Urine glucose tests with Benedict's Qualitative Reagent, Clinitest, or Fehling's solution may give false positive during cephalosporin therapy. Clinistix, Diastix, and Tes-Tape are not affected.
Probenecid: may increase blood levels of cephalosporins. Use together cautiously. *Ethacrynic acid, furosemide:* may enhance nephrotoxicity of cephaloridine. Use together cautiously.	• Contraindicated in renal impairment, since drug causes a relatively high incidence of dose-related nephrotoxicity. Use cautiously in patient with history of sensitivity to penicillin. Ask patient if he's had any reaction to previous cephalosporin or penicillin therapy before administering first dose. Safe use not established in patients with proteinuria, falling urinary output, rising BUN or serum creatinine, decreasing creatinine clearance, and those receiving other antibiotics with nephrotoxic potential. • Prolonged use may result in overgrowth of nonsusceptible organisms. Watch for superinfection. • Obtain cultures for sensitivity tests before beginning therapy, but therapy may begin pending results of cultures and sensitivity tests. • Drug causes relatively little pain when given I.M. • When giving this drug I.V., check frequently for vein irritation and phlebitis. Alternate injection sites if I.V. therapy lasts longer than 3 days. Use of small I.V. needles in the larger available veins may be preferable. • Excreted in urine. Monitor renal function carefully. Watch for signs of impairment: casts in urine, proteinuria, decreased creatinine clearance of urine/plasma creatinine ratio. Avoid doses greater than 4 g daily. Monitor BUN and transaminase levels frequently. Can cause transient rise in SGOT, alkaline phosphatase, and BUN, and decreased creatinine clearance. • About 40% to 75% of patients receiving cephalosporins show a false direct Coombs' test, but only a few indicate hemolytic anemia. • Urine glucose tests with Benedict's Qualitative Reagent, Clinitest, or Fehling's solution may give false positive during cephalosporin therapy. Clinistix, Diastix, and Tes-Tape are not affected.

(continued on following page)

NAME	INDICATIONS & DOSAGE	SIDE EFFECTS
cephaloridine *(continued)*	deep I.M. into a large muscle mass, such as gluteus or lateral aspect of thigh. I.V. is preferable in severe or life-threatening infections.	
cephalothin sodium Keflin Neutral♦	*Treatment of serious infections of respiratory, genitourinary, or gastrointestinal tract; skin and soft tissue infections (including peritonitis); bone and joint infections; septicemia; endocarditis; and meningitis due to E. coli and other coliform bacteria, Enterobacteriaceae, enterococci, gonococci, group A beta-hemolytic streptococci, H. influenzae, Klebsiella, P. mirabilis, Salmonella, S. aureus, Shigella, S. pneumoniae, staphylococci, and S. viridens*— **Adults:** 500 mg to 1 g I.M. or I.V. (or intraperitoneally) q 4 to 6 hours; in life-threatening infections, up to 2 g q 4 hours. **Children:** 14 to 27 mg/Kg I.V. q 4 hours, or 20 to 40 mg/Kg q 6 hours; dose should be proportionately less in accordance with age, weight, and severity of infection. Initial I.V. loading dose (usually 1 to 2 g) is advised, especially when renal function is reduced. Dosage schedule is determined by degree of renal impairment, severity of infection, and susceptibility of causative organism. Should be injected deep I.M. into a large muscle mass, such as gluteus or lateral aspect of thigh. I.V. route is preferable in severe or life-threatening infections.	*Blood:* transient neutropenia, eosinophilia, hemolytic anemia, leukopenia, thrombocythemia, thrombocytopenia, agranulocytosis, azotemia. *CNS:* headache, malaise, paresthesias, dizziness. *GI:* nausea, anorexia, vomiting, diarrhea, glossitis, dyspepsia, abdominal cramps, tenesmus, anal pruritus, oral candidiasis (thrush). *GU:* nephrotoxicity, genital pruritus and moniliasis. *Local:* at injection site—pain, induration, sterile abscesses, temperature elevation, tissue slough; phlebitis and thrombophlebitis with I.V. injection. *Skin:* maculopapular and erythematous rashes, urticaria. *Other:* hypersensitivity, dyspnea, transient elevations of serum transaminases and alkaline phosphatase.
cephapirin sodium Cefadyl♦	*Serious infections of respiratory, genitourinary, or gastrointestinal tract; skin and soft tissue infections; bone and joint infections (including osteomyelitis); septicemia; endocarditis due to S. pneumoniae, E. coli, group A beta-hemolytic streptococci, H. influenzae, Klebsiella, P. mirabilis, S. aureus, and S. viridens*—	*Blood:* transient neutropenia, eosinophilia, anemia, leukopenia, thrombocythemia, thrombocytopenia, azotemia, agranulocytosis. *CNS:* dizziness, headache, malaise, paresthesias. *GI:* nausea, anorexia, vomiting, diarrhea, glossitis, dyspepsia, abdominal cramps, tenesmus, anal pruritus, oral candidiasis (thrush). *GU:* nephrotoxicity, genital pruritus

INTERACTIONS	NURSING CONSIDERATIONS
Probenecid: may increase blood levels of cephalosporins. Use together cautiously.	• Use cautiously in impaired renal functions and in those with history of sensitivity to penicillin. Ask patient if he's had any reaction to previous cephalosporin or penicillin therapy before administering first dose. • Obtain cultures for sensitivity tests before beginning therapy, but therapy may begin pending results of cultures and sensitivity tests. • Prolonged use may result in overgrowth of nonsusceptible organisms. Watch for superinfection. • This drug causes severe pain when given I.M.; avoid this route if possible. • When giving this drug I.V., check frequently for vein irritation and phlebitis. Alternate injection sites if I.V. therapy lasts longer than 3 days. Use of small I.V. needles in the larger available veins may be preferable. • Excreted in urine; monitor renal function carefully. Watch for signs of impairment: casts in urine, proteinuria, decreased urinary output, increased BUN or serum creatinine, decreased creatinine clearance of urine/plasma creatinine ratio. Cephalosporins may cause falsely elevated BUN, transaminase, or 17-ketosteroid levels. Avoid doses greater than 4 g daily in severe renal impairment. • For I.M. administration, reconstitute each gram of cephalothin sodium with 4 ml of sterile water for injection, providing 500 mg in each 2.2 ml. If vial contents do not dissolve completely, an additional 0.2 to 0.4 ml diluent may be added and contents warmed slightly. • For I.V. administration, dilute contents of 4 g vial with at least 20 ml of sterile water for injection, 5% dextrose injection, or 0.9% sodium chloride injection and add to one of following I.V. solutions: acetated Ringer's injection; 5% dextrose injection; 5% dextrose in lactated Ringer's injection; Ionosol B in 5% dextrose in water; lactated Ringer's injection; Normosol-N in 5% dextrose in water; Plasma-Lyte injection; Plasma-Lyte-N injection in 5% dextrose; Ringer's injection or 0.9% sodium chloride injection. Choose solution and fluid volume according to patient's fluid and electrolyte status. • About 40% to 75% of patients receiving cephalosporins show a false positive direct Coombs' test, but only a few of these indicate hemolytic anemia. • Urine glucose tests with Benedict's Qualitative Reagent, Clinitest, or Fehling's solution may give false positive during cephalosporin therapy. Clinistix, Diastix, and Tes-Tape are not affected.
Probenecid: may increase blood levels of cephalosporins. Use together cautiously.	• Use cautiously in impaired renal function and in those with a history of sensitivity to penicillin. Ask patient if he's had any reaction to previous cephalosporin or penicillin therapy before administering first dose. • Prolonged use may result in overgrowth of nonsusceptible organisms. Watch for superinfection. • Obtain cultures for sensitivity tests before beginning therapy, but therapy may begin pending results of cultures and sensitivity tests. • Excreted in urine; monitor renal function carefully. Watch for signs of impairment: casts in urine, proteinuria, decreased urinary output, increased BUN or serum creatinine, decreased creatinine clearance or urine/plasma creatinine ratio. Cephalosporins may cause falsely elevated BUN and

(continued on following page)

NAME	INDICATIONS & DOSAGE	SIDE EFFECTS
cephapirin sodium *(continued)*	**Adults:** 500 mg to 1 g I.V. or I.M. q 4 to 6 hours up to 12 g daily. **Children over 3 months:** 10 to 20 mg/Kg I.V. or I.M. q 6 hours; dose depends on age, weight, and severity of infection. Should be injected deep I.M. into a large muscle mass, such as gluteus or lateral aspect of thigh. Depending upon causative organism and severity of infection, patients with reduced renal function may be treated adequately with a lower dose (7.5 to 15 mg/Kg q 12 hours). Patients with severely reduced renal function and who are to be dialyzed should receive same dose just before dialysis and q 12 hours thereafter.	and moniliasis, vaginitis. *Local:* at injection site—pain, induration, sterile abscesses, tissue slough; phlebitis and thrombophlebitis with I.V. injection. *Skin:* maculopapular and erythematous rashes, urticaria. *Other:* hypersensitivity, dyspnea; transient elevations of serum transaminases and alkaline phosphatase.
cephradine Anspor, Velosef♦	*Serious infection of respiratory, genitourinary, or gastrointestinal tract; skin and soft tissue infections; bone and joint infections; septicemia; endocarditis; and otitis media due to E. coli and other coliform bacteria, group A beta-hemolytic streptococci, H. influenzae, Klebsiella, P. mirabilis, S. aureus, S. pneumoniae, staphylococci, and S. viridens—* **Adults:** 500 mg to 1 g I.M. or I.V. q 6 hours; do not exceed 8 g daily or 250 to 500 mg P.O. q 6 hours. Severe or chronic infections may require larger and/or more frequent doses (up to 1 g P.O. q 6 hours). **Children over 1 year:** 6 to 12 mg/Kg P.O. q 6 hours. 12 to 25 mg/Kg I.M. or I.V., q 6 hours.	*Blood:* transient neutropenia, eosinophilia, anemia, leukopenia, thrombocythemia, thrombocytopenia, agranulocytosis, azotemia. *CNS:* dizziness, headache, malaise, paresthesias. *GI:* nausea, anorexia, vomiting, heartburn, glossitis, dyspepsia, abdominal cramping, diarrhea, tenesmus, anal pruritus, oral candidiasis (thrush). *GU:* nephrotoxicity, genital pruritus and moniliasis, vaginitis. *Local:* at injection site—pain, induration, sterile abscesses, tissue slough; phlebitis and thrombophlebitis with I.V. injection. *Skin:* maculopapular and erythematous rashes, urticaria. *Other:* hypersensitivity.

INTERACTIONS	NURSING CONSIDERATIONS
	transaminase levels. Avoid doses greater than 4 g daily in severe renal impairment. • This drug can cause pain when given I.M. • For I.M. administration, reconstitute 1 g vial with 2 ml sterile water for injection or bacteriostatic water for injection so that 1.2 ml contains 500 mg of cephapirin. • When giving this drug I.V., check frequently for vein irritation and phlebitis. Alternate injection sites if I.V. therapy lasts longer than 3 days. Use of small I.V. needles in the larger available veins may be preferable. • Prepare I.V. infusion using dextrose injection, sodium chloride injection, or bacteriostatic water for injection, as diluent: 20 ml yields 1 g per 10 ml; 50 ml yields 1 g per 25 ml; 100 ml yields 1 g per 50 ml. • I.V. infusion with Y-tube: during infusion of cephapirin solution it is desirable to stop other solution. Check volume of cephapirin solution carefully so that calculated dose is infused. When Y-tube is used, dilute 4 g vial with 40 ml of diluent. • Compatible with following infusion solutions: sodium chloride injection; 5% dextrose in water; sodium lactate injection; 5% dextrose in normal saline; 10% invert sugar in normal saline; 10% invert sugar in water; 5% dextrose and 0.2% sodium chloride injection; lactated Ringer's with 5% dextrose; 5% dextrose and 0.45% sodium chloride injection; Ringer's injection; lactated Ringer's; 10% dextrose injection; sterile water for injection; 20% dextrose injection; 5% sodium chloride in water; and 5% dextrose in Ringer's injection. • Reconstituted cephapirin is stable and compatible for 10 days under refrigeration and for 24 hours at room temperature. • About 40% to 75% of patients receiving cephalosporins show a false positive direct Coombs' test, but only a few indicate hemolytic anemia. • Urine glucose tests with Benedict's Qualitative Reagent, Clinitest, or Fehling's solution may give false positive during cephalosporin therapy. Clinistix, Diastix, and Tes-Tape are not affected.
Probenecid: may increase blood levels of cephalosporins. Use together cautiously.	• Use cautiously in impaired renal function and in those with a history of sensitivity to penicillin. Ask patient if he's had any reaction to previous cephalosporin or penicillin therapy before administering first dose. • Obtain cultures for sensitivity tests before beginning therapy, but therapy may begin pending results of cultures and sensitivity tests. • Prolonged use may result in overgrowth of nonsusceptible organisms. Watch for superinfection. • Excreted in urine; monitor renal function carefully. Watch for signs of impairment: casts in urine, proteinuria, decreased urinary output, increased BUN or serum creatinine, decreased creatinine clearance or urine/plasma creatinine ratio. Avoid doses greater than 4 g daily in severe renal impairment. Cephalosporins may cause falsely elevated BUN and transaminase levels. • I.M. injection painful. • When giving this drug I.V., check frequently for vein irritation and phlebitis. Alternate injection sites if I.V. therapy lasts longer than 3 days. Use of small I.V. needles in the larger available veins may be preferable. • Tell patient to take medication for as long as ordered, even after he feels well. Group A beta-hemolytic streptococci infections should be treated for a minimum of 10 days. • For I.M. administration, reconstitute with sterile water for injection or with bacteriostatic water for injection as follows: 1.2 ml to 250 mg vial; 2 ml

(continued on following page)

NAME	INDICATIONS & DOSAGE	SIDE EFFECTS
cephradine *(continued)*	*Otitis media—* 19 to 25 mg/Kg P.O. q 6 hours. Do not exceed 4 g daily. All patients, regardless of age and weight: larger doses (up to 1 g q.i.d.) may be given for severe or chronic infections. Parenteral therapy may be followed by oral. Injections should be given deep I.M. into a large muscle mass, such as gluteus or lateral aspect of thigh.	

INTERACTIONS	NURSING CONSIDERATIONS
	to 500 mg vial; 4 ml to 1 g vial. I.M. solutions must be used within 2 hours if kept at room temperature and within 24 hours if refrigerated. Solutions may vary in color from light straw to yellow without affecting potency. • Suitable I.V. infusion solutions for Velosef are 5% or 10% dextrose injection, sodium chloride injection, sodium lactate injection (n/y sodium lactate), dextrose and sodium chloride injection (5%:0.9% or 5%:0.45%), 10% invert sugar in water for injection, Normosol-R, and Ionosol B with dextrose 5%. Do not use lactated Ringer's injection. Velosef solutions for I.V. injection retain full potency for 10 hours at room temperature or 48 hours under refrigeration. For prolonged infusions, replace the infusion every 10 hours with a freshly prepared solution. Combining Velosef for injection with other antibiotics is not recommended. Protect powder and reconstituted solutions of Velosef for injection from concentrated light or direct sunlight. • For I.V. administration, reconstitute with sterile water for injection or suitable infusion solution as follows: 10 ml to 1 g vial, 20 ml to 2 g bottle, or 40 ml to 4 g bottle. The 2 g and 4 g I.V. bottles are designed to be suspended from an I.V. stand. They may be infused directly from bottle after adding suitable I.V. infusion solution as follows: 40 ml to 2 g bottle, and 80 ml to 4 g bottle. • About 40% to 75% of patients receiving cephalosporins show a false positive direct Coombs' test, but only a few indicate hemolytic anemia. • Urine glucose tests with Benedict's Qualitative Reagent, Clinitest, or Fehling's solution may give false positive during cephalosporin therapy. Clinistix, Diastix, and Tes-Tape are not affected.

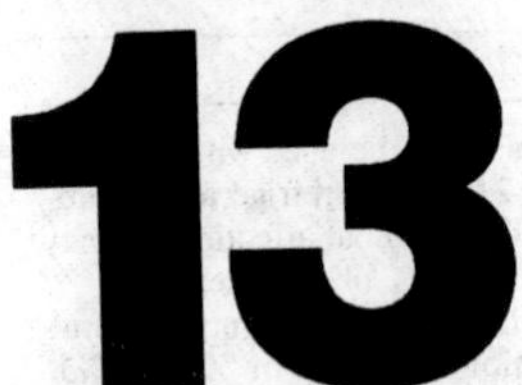

Tetracyclines

chlortetracycline hydrochloride
demeclocycline hydrochloride
doxycycline hyclate
methacycline hydrochloride
minocycline hydrochloride
oxytetracycline hydrochloride
tetracycline hydrochloride
tetracycline phosphate complex

Tetracyclines are broad-spectrum antibiotics, primarily bacteriostatic.

Major uses

- Effective against many gram-positive organisms that are resistant to penicillin.
- Moderately effective against gram-negative rods.
- Effective in some anaerobic infections.
- Alternative agents in treatment of both gonorrhea and syphilis.

Mechanism of action

- Thought to exert antibacterial effect by inhibiting protein synthesis in microorganisms.

Absorption, distribution, and excretion

- Readily absorbed after oral administration.
- Intramuscular administration produces lower blood levels than oral administration. Local anesthetic agents are added to intramuscular preparations; be sure no hypersensitivity to these agents exists before administering.
- Intravenous administration may be used to produce rapid, high blood levels, but be sure to dilute the dose and give it slowly; phlebitis of the injected vein is common. Avoid extravasation.
- Widely distributed in body tissue and fluids. Cross placental barrier.
- Tetracyclines are concentrated by the liver in bile and are excreted in high concentration in the urine and feces.

Onset and duration

- Peak levels after oral administration occur in 2 to 4 hours.

- Serum levels of 1 to 3 mcg/ml persist for 6 hours or longer. Most prolonged levels with doxycycline and minocycline.
- Intramuscular administration gives peak levels after 1 hour, with detectable amounts of drug in serum up to 12 hours.
- Poor absorption from gastrointestinal tract, erratic excretion, and persistently high blood levels in infants; for these reasons and the possibility of adverse effects on teeth and bones, tetracyclines are not recommended for use in infants.

Combination products

MYSTECLIN-F 125: tetracycline 125 mg and amphotericin B 25 mg.
MYSTECLIN-F: tetracycline 250 mg and amphotericin B 50 mg.
MYSTECLIN-F SYRUP: tetracycline 125 mg and amphotericin B 25 mg per 5 ml.
For additional combinations, see Chapter 15, Urinary Tract Germicides.

PATIENT TEACHING AID—TETRACYCLINE FOR TRAVELER'S DIARRHEA

Dear Patient:

If you're traveling abroad, whether it be Mexico, Europe, or Africa, watch the water; watch the salads; watch the fruits; watch the altitude; and when all else fails—take tetracycline. Your doctor can order it for you before you leave.

A one-time oral dose (2.5 g) of tetracycline is a proven cure for *shigella,* a cause of turista, traveler's diarrhea. Your symptoms—diarrhea, fever, abdominal pain, and nausea—can be cleared in 24 to 48 hours. If *shigella* is the culprit, avoid taking antimotility drugs such as Lomotil. These will delay elimination of the infecting organism.

Don't, however, share the tetracycline with children 8 years or younger. It can permanently discolor their teeth.

NAME	INDICATIONS & DOSAGE	SIDE EFFECTS
chlortetracycline hydrochloride Aureomycin•	*Infections caused by susceptible gram-negative and gram-positive organisms, trachoma, amebiasis (with amebicide)—* **Adults:** 250 mg P.O. q 6 hours; up to 2 g daily in divided dosages; 250 to 500 mg I.V. q 6 to 12 hours at a rate not exceeding 20 mg/minute. **Children over 8 years:** 20 to 50 mg/Kg P.O. daily, divided q 6 hours; or 10 to 20 mg/Kg I.V. daily, divided q 12 hours at a rate not exceeding 20 mg/minute. *Brucellosis—* **Adults:** 500 mg P.O. q.i.d. for 3 weeks with streptomycin 1 g I.M. twice daily for 1 week, then once daily the second week. *Syphilis in patients allergic to penicillin—* **Adults:** 500 mg P.O. q.i.d. for 15 days. *Gonorrhea in patients allergic to penicillin—* **Adults:** 1.5 g P.O. initially, then 500 mg P.O. q 6 hours for 4 days (total 9.5 g). Inadequately absorbed by intramuscular route.	*Blood:* hemolytic anemia, thrombocytopenia, neutropenia, eosinophilia. *CNS:* dizziness, headache. *CV:* pericarditis. *EENT:* dysphagia, glossitis, black hairy tongue. *GI:* anorexia, nausea, vomiting, diarrhea, enterocolitis, inflammatory lesions in anogenital region. *Metabolic:* increased BUN. *Skin:* maculopapular and erythematous rashes, photosensitivity, increased pigmentation, urticaria. *Other:* anaphylaxis, anaphylactoid purpura, exacerbation of systemic lupus erythematosus, angioneurotic edema.
demeclocycline hydrochloride Declomycin•, Ledermycin	*Infections caused by susceptible gram-negative and gram-positive organisms, trachoma, amebiasis (with amebecide)—* **Adults:** 150 mg P.O. q 6 hours or 300 mg P.O. q 12 hours. **Children over 8 years:** 6 to 12 mg/Kg P.O. daily, divided q 6 to 12 hours. *Gonorrhea—* **Adults:** 600 mg P.O. initially, then 300 mg P.O. q 12 hours for 4 days (total 3 g).	*Blood:* hemolytic anemia, thrombocytopenia, neutropenia, eosinophilia. *CV:* pericarditis. *EENT:* dysphagia, glossitis. *GI:* anorexia, nausea, vomiting, diarrhea, enterocolitis, inflammatory lesions in anogenital region. *Metabolic:* increased BUN. *Skin:* maculopapular and erythematous rashes, photosensitivity, increased pigmentation, urticaria. *Other:* anaphylaxis, anaphylactoid purpura, angioneurotic edema, exacerbation of systemic lupus erythematosus, diabetes insipidus syndrome (polyuria, polydipsia, weakness).

• Also available in Canada.
•• Available in Canada only.
Unmarked trade names available in United States only.

INTERACTIONS	NURSING CONSIDERATIONS
Antacids (including $NaHCO_3$) and laxatives containing aluminum, calcium, and magnesium; food, milk, or other dairy products: decreased antibiotic absorption. Give antibiotic 1 hour before or 2 hours after any of the above. *Ferrous sulfate and other iron products, zinc:* decreased antibiotic absorption. Give chlortetracycline 3 hours after or 2 hours before iron administration. *Methoxyflurane:* may cause severe nephrotoxicity with tetracyclines. Monitor carefully.	• Use with extreme caution in impaired renal or hepatic function. Use of these drugs during last half of pregnancy and in children younger than age 8 may cause permanent discoloration of teeth, enamel defects, and retardation of bone growth. • Patient may develop thrombophlebitis with I.V. administration. • Obtain cultures before starting therapy. • Check expiration date. Outdated or deteriorated chlortetracycline may cause nephrotoxicity. • Do not expose these drugs to light or heat; store in tight containers. • Watch for overgrowth of nonsensitive organisms. Check patient's tongue for monilia organisms. Stress good oral hygiene. If superinfection occurs, drug should be discontinued. • Observe patient for diarrhea. • Warn patient to avoid direct sunlight and ultraviolet light. Photosensitivity persists for some time after discontinuation of drug. • Effectiveness is reduced if tetracyclines are taken with milk or dairy products, food, antacids, or iron products. Explain this to patient. Tell patient to take each dose with a full glass of water on an empty stomach, at least 1 hour before meals or 2 hours afterward. Give at least 1 hour before bedtime to prevent esophagitis. • Tell patient to take medication exactly as prescribed, even after he feels better. Treat streptococcal infections for at least 10 days. • Use diluent without preservatives to reconstitute injection. Use immediately after reconstitution. Complete infusion within 1 hour. • May cause false positive reading of Clinitest; false negative reading of Clinistix or Tes-Tape. • For symptoms and treatment of anaphylaxis, see p. 1114.
Antacids (including $NaHCO_3$) and laxatives containing aluminum, calcium, and magnesium; food, milk, or other dairy products: decreased antibiotic absorption. Give antibiotic 1 hour before or 2 hours after any of the above. *Ferrous sulfate and other iron products, zinc:* decreased antibiotic absorption. Give demeclocycline 3 hours after or 2 hours before iron administration. *Methoxyflurane:* may cause nephrotoxicity with tetracyclines. Monitor carefully.	• Use with extreme caution in impaired renal or hepatic function. • Obtain cultures before starting therapy. • Check expiration date. Outdated or deteriorated demeclocycline may cause nephrotoxicity. • Do not expose these drugs to light or heat; store in tight container. • Watch for overgrowth of nonsensitive organisms. Check patient's tongue for monilia organisms. Stress good oral hygiene. If superinfection occurs, drug should be discontinued. • Observe patient for diarrhea. • Use of these drugs during last half of pregnancy and in children younger than age 8 may cause permanent discoloration of teeth, enamel defects, and retardation of bone growth. • May cause false positive reading of Clinitest; false negative reading of Clinistix or Tes-Tape. • Warn patient to avoid direct sunlight and ultraviolet light. Photosensitivity persists for some time after discontinuation of drug. • Effectiveness is reduced when taken with milk or dairy products, food, antacids, or iron products. Explain this to patient. Tell patient to take each dose with a full glass of water on an empty stomach, at least 1 hour before meals or 2 hours afterward. Give at least 1 hour before bedtime to prevent esophagitis. • Instruct patient to take medication for as long as prescribed, exactly as prescribed, even after he feels better. Treat streptococcal infections for at least 10 days. • Has been used to treat the syndrome of inappropriate ADH secretion. • For symptoms and treatment of anaphylaxis, see p. 1114.

NAME	INDICATIONS & DOSAGE	SIDE EFFECTS
doxycycline hyclate Doxychel, Vibramycin◆	*Infections caused by sensitive gram-negative and gram-positive organisms, trachoma, amebiasis (with amebecide)—* **Adults:** 100 mg P.O. q 12 hours on first day, then 100 mg P.O. daily; or 200 mg I.V. on first day in 1 or 2 infusions, then 100 to 200 mg I.V. daily. **Children over 8 years (under 45 Kg):** 4.4 mg/Kg P.O. or I.V. daily, divided q 12 hours first day, then 2.2 to 4.4 mg/Kg daily. Over 45 Kg, same as adults. Give I.V. infusion slowly (minimum time 1 hour). Infusion must be completed within 12 hours (within 6 hours in lactated Ringer's solution or 5% dextrose in lactated Ringer's. *Gonorrhea in patients allergic to penicillin—* **Adults:** 200 mg P.O. initially, followed by 100 mg P.O. at bedtime, and 100 mg P.O. b.i.d. for 3 days; or 300 mg P.O. initially and repeat dose in 1 hour. *Primary or secondary syphilis in patients allergic to penicillin—* **Adults:** 300 mg P.O. daily in divided doses for 10 days. Do not inject intramuscularly or subcutaneously. Avoid extravasation.	*Blood:* hemolytic anemia, thrombocytopenia, neutropenia, eosinophilia. *CNS:* benign intracranial hypertension (adults). *CV:* pericarditis. *EENT:* sore throat, glossitis, dysphagia. *GI:* anorexia, epigastric distress, nausea, vomiting, diarrhea, enterocolitis, inflammatory lesions in anogenital region. *Skin:* maculopapular and erythematous rashes, photosensitivity, increased pigmentation, urticaria. *Other:* anaphylaxis, anaphylactoid purpura, exacerbation of systemic lupus erythematosus, angioneurotic edema.
methacycline hydrochloride Rondomycin	*Infections caused by sensitive gram-negative and gram-positive organisms, trachoma, amebiasis (with amebecide)—* **Adults:** 150 mg P.O. q 6 hours or 300 mg q 12 hours. **Children over 8 years:** 6 to 12 mg/Kg P.O. daily, divided q 6 hours to q 12 hours. *Gonorrhea in patients sensitive to penicillin—* **Adults:** 900 mg P.O. initially, then 300 mg P.O. q.i.d. for total of 5.4 g. *Syphilis in patients sensitive to penicillin—* **Adults:** total dose of 18 to 24 g in equally divided doses over 10 to 15 days.	*Blood:* hemolytic anemia, thrombocytopenia, neutropenia, eosinophilia. *CV:* pericarditis. *EENT:* dysphagia, glossitis. *GI:* anorexia, epigastric distress, nausea, vomiting, diarrhea, enterocolitis. *GU:* inflammatory lesions in anogenital region. *Metabolic:* increased BUN. *Skin:* maculopapular and erythematous rashes, photosensitivity, urticaria. *Other:* anaphylaxis, anaphylactoid purpura, exacerbation of systemic lupus erythematosus, angioneurotic edema.

INTERACTIONS	NURSING CONSIDERATIONS
Antacids (including $NaHCO_3$) and laxatives containing aluminum, magnesium, or calcium: decreased antibiotic absorption. Give antibiotic 1 hour before or 2 hours after any of the above. *Ferrous sulfate and other iron products, zinc:* decreased antibiotic absorption. Give doxycycline 3 hours after or 2 hours before iron administration. *Phenobarbital, carbamazepine, alcohol:* decreased antibiotic effect. Avoid if possible.	• Patient may develop thrombophlebitis with I.V. administration. • Use of these drugs during last half of pregnancy and in children younger than age 8 may cause permanent discoloration of teeth, enamel defects, and retardation of bone growth. • Obtain cultures before starting therapy. • Check expiration date. • Don't expose to light or heat. Protect from sunlight during infusion. • Watch for overgrowth of nonsensitive organisms. Check patient's tongue for monilia organisms. Stress good oral hygiene. If superinfection occurs, drug should be discontinued. • Observe patient for diarrhea. • May be taken with milk or food if GI side effects develop. • Do not give with antacids. • Tell patient to take medication exactly as prescribed, even after he feels better. Treat streptococcal infections for at least 10 days. • Reconstitute powder for injection with sterile water for injection. Use 10 ml for 100-mg vial and 20 ml in 200-mg vial. Dilute solution to 100 to 1,000 ml before giving. Do not infuse solutions more concentrated than 1 mg per ml. • Reconstituted solution is stable for 72 hours refrigerated. • Doxycycline may be used in patients with renal impairment; does not accumulate in or cause a significant rise in BUN. • May cause false positive reading of Clinitest; false negative reading of Clinistix or Tes-Tape. • Should not be taken within 1 hour of bedtime. • For symptoms and treatment of anaphylaxis, see p. 1114.
Antacids (including $NaHCO_3$) and laxatives containing aluminum, magnesium, or calcium; food, milk, or other dairy products: decreased antibiotic absorption. Give antibiotic 1 hour before or 2 hours after any of the above. *Ferrous sulfate and other iron products, zinc:* decreased antibiotic absorption. Give tetracyclines 3 hours after or 2 hours before iron administration.	• Use with extreme caution in impaired renal or hepatic function. Use during last half of pregnancy and in children younger than age 8 may cause permanent discoloration of teeth, enamel defects, and retardation of bone growth. • Obtain cultures before starting therapy. • Check expiration date. Outdated or deteriorated methacycline may cause nephrotoxicity. • Do not expose these drugs to light or heat. • Watch for overgrowth of nonsensitive organisms. Check patient's tongue for monilia organisms. Stress good oral hygiene. If superinfection occurs, drug should be discontinued. • Observe patient for diarrhea. • Warn patient to avoid direct sunlight and ultraviolet light. Photosensitivity persists for considerable time after discontinuation of drug. • Effectiveness is reduced when taken with milk or dairy products, food, antacids, or iron products. Explain this to patient. Tell patient to take each dose with a full glass of water on an empty stomach, at least 1 hour before meals or 2 hours afterward. Dose should be given at least 1 hour before bedtime to prevent esophagitis. • Instruct patient to take medication exactly as prescribed, even after he feels better. Treat streptococcal infections for at least 10 days. • May cause false positive reading of Clinitest; false negative reading of Clinistix or Tes-Tape. • For symptoms and treatment of anaphylaxis, see p. 1114.

NAME	INDICATIONS & DOSAGE	SIDE EFFECTS
minocycline hydrochloride Minocin◆, Ultramycin◆◆, Vectrin	*Infections caused by sensitive gram-negative and gram-positive organisms, trachoma, amebiasis (with amebicide)—* **Adults:** initially, 200 mg P.O., I.V.; then 100 mg q 12 hours or 50 mg P.O. q 6 hours. **Children over 8 years:** initially, 4 mg/Kg P.O., I.V.; then 4 mg/Kg P.O. daily, divided q 12 hours. Give I.V. in 500 to 1,000 ml solution which does not contain calcium over 6 hours. *Gonorrhea in patients sensitive to penicillin—* **Adults:** initially, 200 mg, then 100 mg q 12 hours for 4 days. *Syphilis in patients sensitive to penicillin—* **Adults:** initially, 200 mg, then 100 mg q 12 hours for 10 to 15 days. *Meningococcal carrier state—* 100 mg P.O. q 12 hours for 5 days.	*Blood:* hemolytic anemia, thrombocytopenia, neutropenia, eosinophilia. *CNS:* light-headedness, dizziness. *CV:* pericarditis. *EENT:* dysphagia, glossitis, black hairy tongue, hoarseness. *GI:* anorexia, epigastric distress, nausea, vomiting, diarrhea, enterocolitis, inflammatory lesions in anogenital region. *Metabolic:* increased BUN. *Skin:* maculopapular and erythematous rashes, photosensitivity, increased pigmentation, urticaria. *Other:* anaphylaxis, anaphylactoid purpura, exacerbation of systemic lupus erythematosus, angioneurotic edema.
oxytetracycline hydrochloride Dalimycin, Oxlopar, Oxy-Kesso-Tetra, Oxy-Tetrachel, Oxytetrachlor, Terramycin◆, Uri-tet	*Infections caused by sensitive gram-negative and gram-positive organisms, trachoma, amebiasis (with amebicide)—* **Adults:** 250 mg P.O. q 6 hours; 100 mg I.M. q 8 to 12 hours; 250 mg I.M. q 12 hours; or 250 to 500 mg I.V. q 6 to 12 hours. **Children over 8 years:** 25 to 50 mg/Kg P.O. daily, divided q 6 hours; 15 to 25 mg/Kg I.M. daily, divided q 8 to 12 hours; or 10 to 20 mg/Kg I.V. daily, divided q 12 hours. *Brucellosis—* **Adults:** 500 mg P.O. q.i.d. for 3 weeks with streptomycin 1 g I.M. q 12 hours first week, once daily second week. *Syphilis in patients sensitive to penicillin—* **Adults:** 30 to 40 g total dose P.O., divided equally over 10 to 15 days. *Gonorrhea in patients sensitive to penicillin—* **Adults:** initially, 1.5 g P.O. followed by 0.5 g q.i.d. for a total of 9 g.	*Blood:* hemolytic anemia, thrombocytopenia, neutropenia, eosinophilia. *CNS:* benign intracranial hypertension (adults). *CV:* pericarditis. *EENT:* dysphagia, glossitis. *GI:* anórexia, nausea, vomiting, diarrhea, enterocolitis, inflammatory lesions in anogenital region. *Local:* irritation after I.M. injection. *Metabolic:* increased BUN. *Skin:* maculopapular and erythematous rashes, urticaria, photosensitivity, increased pigmentation. *Other:* anaphylaxis, purpura, exacerbation of systemic lupus erythematosus, angioneurotic edema.

INTERACTIONS	NURSING CONSIDERATIONS
Antacids (including $NaHCO_3$*,) or laxatives containing aluminum, magnesium, or calcium:* decreased antibiotic absorption. Give antibiotic 1 hour before or 2 hours after any of the above. *Ferrous sulfate or other iron products, zinc:* decreased antibiotic absorption. Tetracyclines should be given 3 hours after or 2 hours before iron administration. *Methoxyflurane:* may cause severe nephrotoxicity with tetracyclines. Monitor carefully.	• Use with extreme caution in impaired renal or hepatic function. Use during last half of pregnancy and in children younger than age 8 may cause permanent discoloration of teeth, enamel defects, and retardation of bone growth. • Patient may develop thrombophlebitis with I.V. administration of this drug. Avoid extravasation. • Obtain cultures before starting therapy. • Check expiration date. • Do not expose these drugs to light or heat. Keep cap tightly closed. • Watch for overgrowth of nonsensitive organisms. Check patient's tongue for monilia organisms. Stress good oral hygiene. If superinfection occurs, drug should be discontinued. • Observe patient for diarrhea. • Effectiveness is reduced when taken with antacids or iron products. Explain this to patient.Tell patient to take medication exactly as prescribed, even after he feels better.Treat streptococcal infections for at least 10 days, syphilis for 10 to 15 days, gonorrhea for at least 4 days, and meningococcal carriers for 5 days. • Reconstitute 100 mg powder with 5 ml sterile water for injection with further dilution of 500 to 1,000 ml for I.V. infusion. Stable for 24 hours at room temperature. • May cause false positive reading of Clinitest; false negative reading of Clinistix or Tes-Tape. • Vestibular toxicity resulting in dizziness can occur with this drug. • For symptoms and treatment of anaphylaxis, see p. 1114.
Antacids (including $NaHCO_3$*) and laxatives containing aluminum, magnesium, or calcium; food, milk, or other dairy products:* decreased antibiotic absorption. Give antibiotic 1 hour before or 2 hours after any of the above. *Ferrous sulfate and other iron products, zinc:* decreased antibiotic absorption. Give tetracyclines 3 hours after or 2 hours before iron administration. *Methoxyflurane:* may cause severe nephrotoxicity with tetracyclines. Monitor carefully.	• Use with extreme caution in impaired renal or hepatic function. Use during last half of pregnancy and in children younger than age 8 may cause permanent discoloration of teeth, enamel defects, and retardation of bone growth. • Patient may develop thrombophlebitis with I.V. administration. Avoid extravasation. • Obtain cultures before starting therapy. • Check expiration date. Outdated or deteriorated oxytetracycline may cause nephrotoxicity. • Do not expose these drugs to light or heat. • Inject I.M. dosage deeply. Warn that it may be painful. Rotate sites. I.M. preparations contain a local anesthetic; ask patient about hypersensitivity to local anesthetics. • Watch for overgrowth of nonsensitive organisms. Check patient's tongue for monilia organisms. Stress good oral hygiene. If superinfection occurs, drug should be discontinued. • Observe patient for diarrhea. • Effectiveness is reduced when taken with milk or dairy products, food, antacids, or iron products. Explain this to patient. Tell patient to take each dose with a full glass of water on an empty stomach, at least 1 hour before meals or 2 hours afterward. Give at least 1 hour before bedtime to prevent esophagitis. • Tell patient to take medication exactly as prescribed, even after he feels better. • For I.V. use, reconstitute 250 mg and 500 mg powder for injection with 10 ml sterile water for injection. • Dilute to at least 100 ml in 5% dextrose in water, normal saline, or Ringer's solution. Do not mix with any other drug. • Store reconstituted solutions in refrigerator. Stable for 48 hours. • May cause false positive reading of Clinitest; false negative reading of Clinistix or Tes-Tape. • For symptoms and treatment of anaphylaxis, see p. 1114.

NAME	INDICATIONS & DOSAGE	SIDE EFFECTS
tetracycline hydrochloride Achromycin♦, Amer-Tet, Amtet, Bicycline, Bio-Tetra♦♦, Bristacycline, Cefracycline♦♦, Centet-250, Cycline, Cyclopar, Desamycin, Duratet, G-Mycin, Maso-Cycline, Maytrex, Medicycline♦♦, Mericycline, Neo-Tetrine♦♦, Nor-Tet 500, Novotetra♦♦ Paltet 250, Panmycin, Partrex, Piracaps, Retet, Robitet, Sarocycline, Scotrex, SK-Tetracycline, Sumycin♦, T-125, T-250, Tet-Cy Tetra-C, Tetrachel, Tetraclor, Tetra-Co, Tetracrine♦♦, Tetracyn♦, Tetralan, Tetralean♦♦, Tetram, Tetram-S, Tetramax, Trexin, Triacycline♦♦ **tetracycline phosphate complex** Tetrex♦	*Infections caused by sensitive gram-negative and gram-positive organisms, trachoma, amebiasis (with amebicide)—* **Adults:** 250 to 500 mg P.O. q 6 hours; 250 mg I.M. daily or 150 mg I.M. q 12 hours; or 250 to 500 mg I.V. q 8 to 12 hours (I.M. and I.V. hydrochloride salt only). **Children over 8 years:** 25 to 50 mg/Kg P.O. daily, divided q 6 hours; 15 to 25 mg/Kg/day (maximum 250 mg) I.M. single dose or divided q 8 to 12 hours; or 10 to 20 mg/Kg I.V. daily, divided q 12 hours. *Brucellosis—* **Adults:** 500 mg P.O. q 6 hours for 3 weeks with streptomycin 1 g I.M. q 12 hours week 1 and daily week 2. *Gonorrhea in patients sensitive to penicillin—* **Adults:** initially, 1.5 g P.O., then 500 mg q 6 hours for total of 9 g. *Syphilis in patients sensitive to penicillin—* **Adults:** 30 to 40 g total in equally divided doses over 10 to 15 days. *Acne—* **Adults and adolescents:** initially, 250 mg P.O. q 6 hours, then 125 to 500 mg P.O. daily or every other day.	*Blood:* anemia, hemolytic anemia, thrombocytopenia, neutropenia, eosinophilia. *CNS:* dizziness, headache. *CV:* pericarditis. *EENT:* sore throat, glossitis, black hairy tongue, hoarseness, dysphagia. *GI:* anorexia, epigastric distress, nausea, vomiting, diarrhea, bulky loose stools, stomatitis, enterocolitis, inflammatory lesions in anogenital region. *Local:* irritation after I.M. injection. *Metabolic:* increased BUN. *Skin:* maculopapular and erythematous rashes, urticaria, photosensitivity, increased pigmentation. *Other:* anaphylaxis, anaphylactoid purpura, exacerbation of systemic lupus erythematosus, serum sickness-like reactions, angioneurotic edema.

INTERACTIONS	NURSING CONSIDERATIONS
Antacids (including $NaHCO_3$) and laxatives containing aluminum, magnesium, or calcium; food, milk, or other dairy products: decreased antibiotic absorption. Give antibiotic 1 hour before or 2 hours after any of the above. *Ferrous sulfate and other iron products, zinc:* decreased antibiotic absorption. Give tetracyclines 3 hours after or 2 hours before iron administration. *Methoxyflurane:* may cause severe nephrotoxicity with tetracyclines. Monitor carefully.	• Use with extreme caution in impaired renal or hepatic function. Use during last half of pregnancy and in children younger than age 8 may cause permanent discoloration of teeth, enamel defects, and retardation of bone growth. • Obtain cultures before starting therapy. • Effectiveness reduced when taken with milk or dairy products, food, antacids, or iron products. Explain this to patient. Tell patient to take each dose with a full glass of water on an empty stomach, at least 1 hour before meals or 2 hours afterward. Give at least 1 hour before bedtime to prevent esophagitis. • Patient may develop thrombophlebitis with I.V. administration. Avoid extravasation. • Check expiration date. Outdated or deteriorated tetracycline may cause nephrotoxicity. • Discard I.M. solutions after 24 hours because they deteriorate. Exception: discard Achromycin solution in 12 hours. • Do not expose these drugs to light or heat. • Inject I.M. dosage deeply. Warn patient that it may be painful. Rotate sites. I.M. preparations often contain a local anesthetic; ask patient about hypersensitivity to local anesthetics. • Watch for overgrowth of nonsensitive organisms. Check patient's tongue for monilia organisms. Stress good oral hygiene. If superinfection occurs, drug should be discontinued. • Observe patient for diarrhea. • Tell patient to take medication exactly as prescribed, even after he feels better. Treat streptococcal infections for at least 10 days. • For I.V. use, reconstitute 100 mg and 250 mg powder for injection with 5 ml sterile water; with 10 ml for 500 mg. Dilute in 100 to 1,000 ml volume of 5% dextrose in 0.9% saline. Refrigerate dilute solution for I.V. use and use within 24 hours. Exception: use Achromycin solution immediately. • Do not mix tetracycline solution with any other I.V. additive. • For I.M. use, reconstitute 100 mg powder for injection with 2 ml sterile water for injection. Concentration will be 50 mg/ml. Amount of diluent for 250 mg injection varies according to brand. Check with pharmacy or follow manufacturer's instructions. • May cause false positive readings of Clinitest; false negative reading of Clinistix or Tes-Tape. • For symptoms and treatment of anaphylaxis, see p. 1114.

14

Sulfonamides

co-trimoxazole
sulfachlorpyridazine
sulfacytine
sulfadiazine
sulfamerazine
sulfameter
sulfamethizole
sulfamethoxazole
sulfamethoxypyridazine
sulfapyridine
sulfasalazine
sulfisoxazole

This group of drugs is effective in treating susceptible gram-positive and gram-negative bacteria, including most *E. coli*, *H. influenza*, and *Nocardia*. They do not reliably prevent postinfection complications in patients with group A streptococcal infections. Recently, increased resistance of meningococci and gonococci to the sulfonamides has reduced their effectiveness.

Major uses

- To treat urinary tract infections.
- To treat *Pneumocystis* pneumonitis infections in seriously ill patients.
- As prophylaxis for rheumatic heart disease in patients allergic to penicillin.
- To provide pre- and postoperative suppression of bowel flora and in treatment of ulcerative colitis.
- Adjunctive treatment in toxoplasmosis.
- To treat dermatitis herpetiformis (sulfapyridine).

Mechanism of action

- These drugs interfere with the bacterial synthesis of folic acid from para-aminobenzoic acid (PABA) and thereby inhibit the growth and multiplication of susceptible bacteria (those that must synthesize their own folic acid).

Absorption, distribution, and excretion

- Except for those especially designed for local effects in the bowel, these drugs are rapidly and adequately absorbed in the gastrointestinal tract.
- All sulfonamides are readily distributed throughout the body.
- They are largely metabolized in the liver and excreted in the urine.
- Urinary solubility of these drugs is pH dependent.

Onset and duration

- Peak blood levels usually appear 2 to 8 hours after oral administration and within minutes of I.V. administration.

- Peak blood levels usually appear 4 to 6 hours after S.C. or I.M. injections.
- These drugs have a half-life in the blood of 5 to 40 hours.

Combination drugs

AZO GANTANOL: sulfamethoxazole 500 mg and phenazopyridine hydrochloride 100 mg.
AZO GANTRISIN: sulfisoxazole 500 mg and phenazopyridine hydrochloride 50 mg.
AZOTREX: sulfamethizole 250 mg, tetracycline phosphate complex 125 mg, and phenazopyridine hydrochloride 50 mg.
SULADYNE: sulfamethizole 125 mg, sulfadiazine 125 mg, and phenazopyridine hydrochloride 75 mg.
THIOSULFIL-A: sulfamethizole 250 mg and phenazopyridine hydrochloride 50 mg.
TRIPLE SULFA: sulfadiazine 167 mg, sulfamerazine 167 mg, and sulfamethazine 167 mg.
UROBIOTIC 250: sulfamethizole 250 mg, oxytetracycline hydrochloride 125 or 250 mg, and phenazopyridine hydrochloride 50 mg.

SCORING WITH FLUIDS

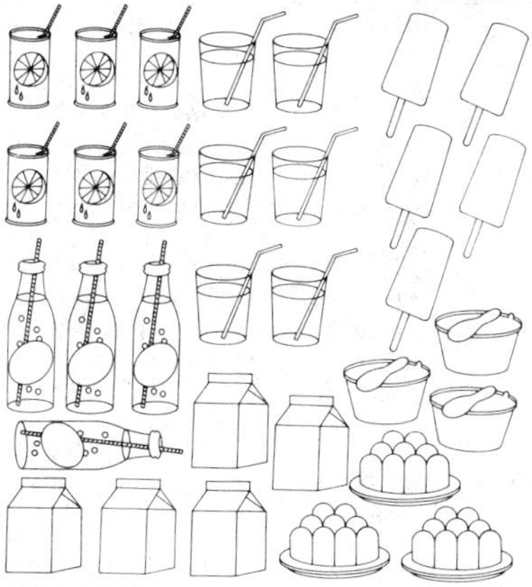

Patients who are taking sulfonamide preparations need to be well hydrated to help prevent crystalluria. To encourage children to take fluids, draw a scorecard using various symbols to represent fluids: soda bottles, popsicles, ice cream, jello, milk, and water. After the child takes the fluid, he colors the appropriate symbol on his scorecard.

Remember that sulfonamides may cause serious renal toxicity (crystalluria, hematuria, and obstruction). Monitor the patient's intake and output, encourage fluid intake, and visually examine the hospitalized patient's urine for crystals.

NAME	INDICATIONS & DOSAGE	SIDE EFFECTS
co-trimoxazole (sulfamethoxazole-trimethoprim) Bactrim◆, Bactrim DS◆, Septra◆, Septra DS◆	*Urinary tract infections and shigellosis*— **Adults:** 160 mg trimethoprim/800 mg sulfa q 12 hours for 10 to 14 days in urinary tract infections and 5 days in shigellosis. **Children:** 8 mg/Kg trimethoprim/ 40 mg/Kg sulfa per 24 hours, in 2 divided doses q 12 hours (10 days for urinary tract infections; 5 days in shigellosis). *Otitis media*— **Children:** 8 mg/Kg trimethoprim/ 40 mg/Kg sulfa per 24 hours, in 2 divided doses q 12 hours for 10 days. *Pneumocystis carinii pneumonitis*— **Adults:** 20 mg/Kg trimethoprim/ 100 mg/Kg sulfa per 24 hours, in equally divided doses q 6 hours for 14 days. **Children (36 Kg/80 lb):** 160 mg trimethoprim/800 mg sulfa q 6 hours for 14 days. Not recommended for infants less than 2 years old. Available as tablets or suspension only.	*Blood:* agranulocytosis, aplastic anemia, megaloblastic anemia, thrombocytopenia, leukopenia, hemolytic anemia, purpura, hypoprothrombinemia, methemoglobinemia. *CNS:* headache, peripheral neuritis, mental depression, convulsions, ataxia, hallucinations, tinnitus, vertigo, insomnia, apathy, fatigue, muscle weakness, nervousness. *CV:* allergic myocarditis, periarteritis nodosa. *EENT:* periorbital edema, conjunctival and scleral injection, tinnitus. *GI:* nausea, emesis, abdominal pain, diarrhea, anorexia, stomatitis. *GU:* toxic nephrosis with oliguria and anuria, crystalluria. *Skin:* erythema multiforme (Stevens-Johnson syndrome), generalized skin eruption, epidermal necrolysis, urticaria, pruritus, exfoliative dermatitis, photosensitization. *Other:* serum sickness, drug fever, chills, pancreatitis, hepatitis, L.E. phenomenon.
sulfachlorpyridazine Cosulid, Sonilyn, Vetisulid	*Urinary tract infections and some systemic infections*— **Adults:** 2 to 4 g P.O. initially, then 500 mg to 1 g P.O. q 6 hours. **Children over 2 months:** 75 mg/Kg P.O. initially, then 150 mg/Kg daily, divided into doses given q 6 hours. Maximum daily dose 6 g.	*Blood:* agranulocytosis, aplastic anemia, thrombocytopenia, leukopenia, hemolytic anemia, hypoprothrombinemia, methemoglobinemia, purpura. *CNS:* arthralgia, headache, peripheral neuritis, mental depression, convulsions, ataxia, hallucinations, vertigo, insomnia, restlessness, drowsiness. *CV:* allergic myocarditis, cyanosis, periarteritis nodosa. *EENT:* periorbital edema, conjunctival and scleral injection, tinnitus, pharyngitis, glossitis, sore throat. *GI:* nausea, emesis, abdominal pains, diarrhea, anorexia, stomatitis, gastroenteritis. *GU:* toxic nephrosis with oliguria and anuria, renal damage, crystalluria, hematuria. *Skin:* erythema multiforme (Stevens-Johnson syndrome), generalized skin eruption, epidermal necrolysis, urticaria, pruritus, exfoliative dermatitis, photosensitization, pallor. *Other:* serum sickness, drug fever, chills, anaphylaxis, cross-sensitization, weakness, L.E. phenomenon, pancreatitis, jaundice.

◆ Also available in Canada.
◆◆ Available in Canada only.
Unmarked trade names available in United States only.

INTERACTIONS	NURSING CONSIDERATIONS
Ammonium chloride, ascorbic acid, paraldehyde: doses sufficient to acidify urine may cause precipitation of sulfonamide and crystalluria. Don't use together. *PABA-containing local anesthetics and other PABA drugs:* inhibited antibacterial action. Don't use together.	• Contraindicated in porphyria. Use cautiously and in reduced dosages in impaired hepatic or renal function and in severe allergy or bronchial asthma, G-6-PD deficiency, blood dyscrasias. • Tell patient to drink a full glass of water with each dose and to drink plenty of water during the day to prevent crystalluria. Monitor fluid intake and urinary output. • This combination is often used in extremely ill immunosuppressed patients when prescribed for treatment of *Pneumocystis* pneumonia. • Oral suspension available for patients who cannot swallow large tablets. • Note that the "DS" product means "double strength." • Tell doctor if skin rash, sore throat, fever, or mouth sores occur. • Should be taken 1 hour before or 2 hours after meals for best absorption. • Used effectively for treatment of chronic bacterial prostatitis. • Used prophylactically for recurrent urinary tract infections in women. • Most side effects develop within 2 weeks of onset of therapy. • For treatment of anaphylaxis, see p. 1114.
Ammonium chloride, ascorbic acid, paraldehyde: doses sufficient to acidify urine may cause precipitation of sulfonamide and crystalluria. Don't use together. *PABA-containing local anesthetics and other PABA drugs:* inhibited antibacterial action. Don't use together.	• Contraindicated in porphyria. Use cautiously and in reduced dosages in impaired hepatic or renal function, asthma or blood dyscrasias, G-6-PD deficiency, history of multiple allergies. • Tell patient to drink a full glass of water with each dose and to drink plenty of water throughout the day to prevent crystalluria. Monitor fluid intake and urinary output. Intake should be sufficient to produce output of 1,500 ml daily. • To aid in prevention of crystalluria, sodium bicarbonate may be administered to alkalinize urine. • Tell patient to take medication for as long as prescribed, even after he feels better. • Monitor urinary cultures, CBC, and urinalysis before and during therapy. • Vitamin K_1 may reverse sulfonamide-induced hypoprothrombinemia. • Tell patient to report early signs of blood dyscrasias (sore throat, fever, pallor, or jaundice) immediately and to stop taking drug. Warn patient to avoid direct sunlight and ultraviolet light to prevent photosensitivity reaction. • For treatment of anaphylaxis, see p. 1114.

NAME	INDICATIONS & DOSAGE	SIDE EFFECTS
sulfacytine Renoquid	*Urinary tract infections—* **Adults:** initially, 500 mg P.O., then 250 mg P.O. q.i.d. for 10 days.	*Blood:* agranulocytosis, aplastic anemia, thrombocytopenia, leukopenia, hemolytic anemia, hypoprothrombinemia, methemoglobinemia, purpura. *CNS:* arthralgia, headache, peripheral neuritis, mental depression, convulsions, ataxia, hallucinations, vertigo, insomnia. *CV:* allergic myocarditis, periarteritis nodosa. *EENT:* periorbital edema, conjunctival and scleral injection, tinnitus. *GI:* nausea, emesis, abdominal pains, diarrhea, anorexia, stomatitis. *GU:* toxic nephrosis with oliguria and anuria, crystalluria. *Skin:* erythema multiforme (Stevens-Johnson syndrome), generalized skin eruption, epidermal necrolysis, urticaria, pruritus, exfoliative dermatitis, photosensitization. *Other:* serum sickness, drug fever, chills, anaphylaxis, L.E. phenomenon, jaundice, pancreatitis, hepatitis.
sulfadiazine Microsulfon, Neo-Quinette	*Urinary tract infection—* **Adults:** initially, 2 to 4 g P.O., then 500 mg to 1 g P.O. q 6 hours. **Children:** initially, 75 mg/Kg or 2 g/m² P.O., then 150 mg/Kg or 4 g/m² P.O. in 4 to 6 divided doses daily. Maximum daily dose 6 g. *Rheumatic fever prophylaxis, as an alternative to penicillin—* **Children over 30 Kg:** 1 g P.O. daily. **Children under 30 Kg:** 500 mg P.O. daily. *Adjunctive treatment in toxoplasmosis—* **Adults:** 4 g P.O. in divided doses q 6 hours for 3 to 4 weeks, discontinued for 1 week, then repeated; given with pyrimethamine 75 mg P.O. daily for 1 to 3 days, then 25 mg P.O. daily for 3 to 4 weeks, discontinued for 1 week, then repeated using 25 mg P.O. daily. **Children:** 100 mg/Kg P.O. in divided doses q 6 hours for 3 to 4 weeks, discontinued for 1 week, then repeated; given with pyrimethamine 1 mg/Kg P.O. daily for 1 to 3 days, then 0.5 mg/Kg P.O. daily for 3 to 4 weeks, discontinued for 1 week, then repeated using 0.5 mg/Kg P.O. daily.	*Blood:* agranulocytosis, aplastic anemia, thrombocytopenia, leukopenia, hemolytic anemia, hypoprothrombinemia, methemoglobinemia, purpura. *CNS:* arthralgia, headache, peripheral neuritis, mental depression, convulsions, ataxia, hallucinations, vertigo, insomnia, restlessness, drowsiness. *CV:* allergic myocarditis, periarteritis nodosa, cyanosis. *EENT:* periorbital edema, conjunctival and scleral injection, tinnitus, pharyngitis, glossitis, sore throat. *GI:* nausea, emesis, abdominal pains, diarrhea, anorexia, stomatitis, gastroenteritis. *GU:* toxic nephrosis with oliguria and anuria, renal damage, crystalluria, hematuria. *Skin:* erythema multiforme (Stevens-Johnson syndrome), generalized skin eruption, epidermal necrolysis, urticaria, pruritus, exfoliative dermatitis, photosensitization, pallor. *Other:* serum sickness, drug fever, chills, anaphylaxis, weakness, pancreatitis, jaundice, L.E. phenomenon.

INTERACTIONS	NURSING CONSIDERATIONS
Ammonium chloride, ascorbic acid, paraldehyde: doses sufficient to acidify urine may cause precipitation of sulfonamide and crystalluria. Don't use together. *PABA-containing local anesthetics and other PABA drugs:* inhibited antibacterial action. Don't use together.	• Contraindicated in porphyria. Use cautiously and in reduced dosages in impaired hepatic or renal function, bronchial asthma, history of multiple allergies, G-6-PD deficiency, blood dyscrasias. • Tell patient to drink a full glass of water with each dose and to drink plenty of water throughout the day to prevent crystalluria. Monitor fluid intake and urinary output. Intake should be sufficient to produce output of 1,500 ml daily. • To aid in prevention of crystalluria, sodium bicarbonate may be administered to alkalinize urine. • Tell patient to take medication for as long as prescribed, even after he feels better. Warn patient to avoid direct sunlight and ultraviolet light to prevent photosensitivity reaction. • Monitor urinary cultures, CBC, and urinalysis before and during therapy. • Tell patient to report early signs of blood dyscrasias (sore throat, fever, pallor, or jaundice) immediately and to stop taking drug. • Vitamin K_1 may reverse sulfonamide-induced hypoprothrombinemia. • For treatment of anaphylaxis, see p. 1114.
Ammonium chloride, ascorbic acid, paraldehyde: doses sufficient to acidify urine may cause precipitation of sulfonamide and crystalluria. Don't use together. *PABA-containing local anesthetics and other PABA drugs:* inhibited antibacterial action. Don't use together.	• Contraindicated in porphyria or in infants younger than 2 months (except in congenital toxoplasmosis). Use cautiously and in reduced dosages in impaired hepatic or renal function, bronchial asthma, history of multiple allergies, G-6-PD deficiency, blood dyscrasias. • Tell patient to drink a full glass of water with each dose and to drink plenty of water throughout the day to prevent crystalluria. Monitor fluid intake and urinary output. Intake should be sufficient to produce output of 1,500 ml daily. To aid in prevention of crystalluria, sodium bicarbonate may be administered to alkalinize urine. • Tell patient to take medication for as long as prescribed, even if he feels better. Warn patient to avoid direct sunlight and ultraviolet light to prevent photosensitivity reaction. • Give drug on schedule to maintain constant blood level. • Watch for signs of blood dyscrasias (purpura, ecchymosis, sore throat, fever, pallor, or jaundice). Report them immediately. • When giving I.V., make sure drug is well diluted. Infuse I.V. dosages slowly. If extravasation occurs, stop infusion and notify the doctor. • Monitor urinary cultures, CBC, and urinalysis before and during therapy. • Mix with dextrose 5% in normal saline or Ringer's solution for I.V. infusion; any acidic solution (especially with pH below 9) causes precipitation. Use diluent cautiously. Discard solution if precipitation occurs. • Sulfadiazine with pyrimethamine for treatment of toxoplasmosis may be continued for life. Therapy controls but does not cure toxoplasmosis. • Folic or folinic acid may be used during rest periods in toxoplasmosis therapy to reverse hematopoietic depression and/or anemia associated with pyrimethamine and sulfadiazine. • Vitamin K_1 may reverse sulfonamide-induced hypoprothrombinemia. • Protect drug from light. • For treatment of anaphylaxis, see p. 1114.

NAME	INDICATIONS & DOSAGE	SIDE EFFECTS
sulfamerazine	*Antibacterial (rarely used alone)*— **Adults:** initially, 2 to 4 g P.O., then 500 mg to 1 g P.O. q 6 hours. **Children over 2 months:** initially, 75 mg/Kg or 2 g/m², then 150 mg/Kg or 4 g/m² P.O. daily in 4 to 6 equally divided doses. Maximum daily dose 6 g.	*Blood:* agranulocytosis, aplastic anemia, thrombocytopenia, leukopenia, hemolytic anemia, hypoprothrombinemia, methemoglobinemia, purpura. *CNS:* arthralgia, headache, peripheral neuritis, mental depression, convulsions, ataxia, hallucinations, vertigo, insomnia, restlessness, drowsiness. *CV:* allergic myocarditis, periarteritis nodosa, cyanosis. *EENT:* periorbital edema, conjunctival and scleral injection, tinnitus, pharyngitis, glossitis, sore throat. *GI:* nausea, emesis, abdominal pains, diarrhea, anorexia, stomatitis, gastroenteritis. *GU:* toxic nephrosis with oliguria and anuria, renal damage, crystalluria, hematuria. *Skin:* erythema multiforme (Stevens-Johnson syndrome), generalized skin eruption, epidermal necrolysis, urticaria, pruritus, exfoliative dermatitis, photosensitization, pallor. *Other:* serum sickness, drug fever, chills, anaphylaxis, weakness, pancreatitis, jaundice, L.E. phenomenon.
sulfameter Sulla◆	*Urinary tract infections only*— **Adults, and children over 12:** initially, 1.5 g P.O., then 500 mg daily.	*Blood:* agranulocytosis, aplastic anemia, hemolytic anemia, thrombocytopenia, purpura, methemoglobinemia, hypoprothrombinemia. *CNS:* arthralgia, headache, peripheral neuritis, mental depression, ataxia, vertigo, insomnia, fatigue, psychosis. *CV:* periarteritis. *EENT:* tinnitus. *GI:* anorexia, nausea, vomiting, abdominal pain. *GU:* crystalluria, toxic nephrosis. *Skin:* maculopapular and bullous eruptions, exfoliative dermatitis, pruritus, urticaria, erythema nodosum, erythema multiforme (Stevens-Johnson syndrome), photosensitization. *Other:* L.E. phenomenon, serum sickness, hepatotoxicity, jaundice.

INTERACTIONS	NURSING CONSIDERATIONS
Ammonium chloride, ascorbic acid, paraldehyde: doses sufficient to acidify urine may cause precipitation of sulfonamide and crystalluria. Don't use together. *PABA-containing local anesthetics and other PABA drugs:* inhibited antibacterial action. Don't use together.	• Contraindicated in infants younger than 2 months (except in congenital toxoplasmosis); and in porphyria. Use cautiously in impaired hepatic or renal function, asthma, blood dyscrasias, G-6-PD deficiency, history of multiple allergies. • Although drug has low incidence of crystalluria, tell patient to drink a full glass of water with each dose and to drink plenty of water throughout the day to prevent crystalluria. Monitor fluid intake and urinary output. Intake should be sufficient to produce output of 1,500 ml daily. To aid in prevention of crystalluria, sodium bicarbonate may be administered to alkalinize urine. • Tell patient to take medication for as long as prescribed, even after he feels better. Warn patient to avoid direct sunlight and ultraviolet light to prevent photosensitivity reaction. Instruct patient to report early signs of blood dyscrasias (sore throat, fever, pallor, or jaundice) immediately and to stop taking drug. • Monitor urinary cultures, CBC, and urinalysis before and during therapy. • Used in combination sulfonamide preparations such as Triple Sulfa in conjunction with pyrimethamine to treat toxoplasmosis. • Watch for signs of GI superinfection during long-term therapy. • When given preop, the patient should receive a low-residue diet and a minimum of enemas and cathartics. • Vitamin K_1 may reverse sulfonamide-induced hypoprothrombinemia. • For treatment of anaphylaxis, see p. 1114.
Ammonium chloride, ascorbic acid, paraldehyde: doses sufficient to acidify urine may cause precipitation of sulfonamide and crystalluria. Don't use together. *PABA-containing local anesthetics and other PABA drugs:* inhibited antibacterial action. Don't use together.	• Contraindicated in patients weighing less than 45 Kg (100 pounds); porphyria. Use cautiously and in reduced dosages in impaired hepatic or renal function, those receiving oral hypoglycemic agents (sulfonylurea), in early pregnancy, blood dyscrasias, G-6-PD deficiency, asthma, and in patients with history of multiple allergies. • Tell patient to drink a full glass of water with each dose and to drink plenty of water throughout the day to prevent crystalluria. Monitor fluid intake and urinary output. Intake should be sufficient to produce output of 2,000 to 2,500 ml daily. To aid in prevention of crystalluria, sodium bicarbonate may be administered to alkalinize urine. • Tell patient to take medication for as long as prescribed, even after he feels better. Warn patient to avoid direct sunlight and ultraviolet light to prevent photosensitivity reaction. Instruct patient to report early signs of blood dyscrasias (sore throat, fever, pallor, or jaundice) immediately and to stop taking drug. • Check patient's urine pH frequently. If it's very acidic, the doctor may want to order sodium bicarbonate to alkalinize it. • Monitor urinary cultures, CBC, and urinalysis before and during therapy. • Long-acting sulfonamide; never use in place of short-acting sulfonamides to treat systemic infections. • Associated with increased incidence of severe and fatal adverse reactions. • Vitamin K_1 may reverse sulfonamide-induced hypoprothrombinemia. • For treatment of anaphylaxis, see p. 1114.

NAME	INDICATIONS & DOSAGE	SIDE EFFECTS
sulfamethizole Bursul, Microsul, Proklar-M, Sulfasol, Sulfstat, Sulfurine, Thiosulfil◆, Unisul, Uri-Pak, Urifon, Utrasul	*Urinary tract infections only—* **Adults:** 500 mg to 1 g P.O. t.i.d. to q.i.d. **Children over 2 months:** 30 to 45 mg/Kg P.O. daily, divided into doses given q 6 hours.	*Blood:* agranulocytosis, aplastic anemia, thrombocytopenia, leukopenia, hemolytic anemia, hypoprothrombinemia, methemoglobinemia, purpura. *CNS:* arthralgia, headache, peripheral neuritis, mental depression, convulsions, ataxia, hallucinations, vertigo, insomnia. *CV:* allergic myocarditis, periarteritis nodosa. *EENT:* periorbital edema, conjunctival and scleral injection, tinnitus. *GI:* nausea, emesis, abdominal pain, diarrhea, anorexia, stomatitis. *GU:* toxic nephrosis with oliguria and anuria, crystalluria. *Skin:* erythema multiforme (Stevens-Johnson syndrome), generalized skin eruption, epidermal necrolysis, urticaria, pruritus, exfoliative dermatitis, photosensitization. *Other:* serum sickness, drug fever, chills, anaphylaxis, L.E. phenomenon, pancreatitis, hepatitis.
sulfamethoxazole Gantanol◆	*Urinary tract and systemic infections—* **Adults:** initially, 2 g P.O., then 1 g P.O. b.i.d. up to t.i.d. for severe infections. **Children and infants over 2 months:** initially, 50 to 60 mg/Kg P.O., then 25 to 30 mg/Kg b.i.d. Maximum dose should not exceed 75 mg/Kg daily.	*Blood:* agranulocytosis, aplastic anemia, thrombocytopenia, leukopenia, hemolytic anemia, hypoprothrombinemia, methemoglobinemia, purpura. *CNS:* arthralgia, headache, peripheral neuritis, mental depression, convulsions, ataxia, hallucinations, vertigo, insomnia. *CV:* allergic myocarditis, periarteritis nodosa. *EENT:* periorbital edema, conjunctival and scleral injection, tinnitus. *GI:* nausea, emesis, abdominal pain, diarrhea, anorexia, stomatitis. *GU:* toxic nephrosis with oliguria and anuria, crystalluria. *Skin:* erythema multiforme (Stevens-Johnson syndrome), generalized skin eruption, epidermal necrolysis, urticaria, pruritus, exfoliative dermatitis, photosensitization. *Other:* serum sickness, drug fever, chills, pancreatitis, hepatitis, L.E. phenomenon.

INTERACTIONS	NURSING CONSIDERATIONS
Ammonium chloride, ascorbic acid, paraldehyde: doses sufficient to acidify urine may cause precipitation of sulfonamide and crystalluria. Don't use together. *PABA-containing local anesthetics and other PABA drugs:* inhibited antibacterial action. Don't use together. *Phenytoin:* inhibited metabolism of phenytoin. Use together cautiously.	• Contraindicated in porphyria. Use cautiously and in reduced dosages in impaired hepatic or renal function, blood dyscrasias, G-6-PD deficiency, asthma, history of multiple allergies. • Tell patient to drink a full glass of water with each dose and to drink plenty of water throughout the day to prevent crystalluria. Monitor fluid intake and urinary output. Intake should be sufficient to produce output of 1,500 ml daily. To aid in prevention of crystalluria, sodium bicarbonate may be administered to alkalinize urine. • Tell patient to take medication for as long as prescribed, even after he feels better. Warn patient to avoid direct sunlight and ultraviolet light to prevent photosensitivity reaction. Instruct patient to report early signs of blood dyscrasias (sore throat, fever, pallor, or jaundice) immediately and to stop taking drug. • Monitor urinary cultures, CBC, and urinalysis before and during therapy. • Vitamin K_1 may reverse sulfonamide-induced hypoprothrombinemia. • For treatment of anaphylaxis, see p. 1114.
Ammonium chloride, ascorbic acid, paraldehyde: doses sufficient to acidify urine may cause precipitation of sulfonamide and crystalluria. Don't use together. *PABA-containing local anesthetics and other PABA drugs:* inhibited antibacterial action. Don't use together.	• Contraindicated in porphyria or in infants younger than 2 months (except in congenital toxoplasmosis). Use cautiously and in reduced dosages in impaired hepatic or renal function and in those with severe allergy or bronchial asthma, G-6-PD deficiency, blood dyscrasias. • Tell patient to drink a full glass of water with each dose and to drink plenty of water during the day to prevent crystalluria. Monitor fluid intake and urinary output. Intake should be sufficient to produce output of 1,500 ml daily. To aid in prevention of crystalluria, sodium bicarbonate may be administered to alkalinize urine. • Tell patient to take medication for as long as prescribed, even after he feels better. Warn patient to avoid direct sunlight and ultraviolet light to prevent photosensitivity reaction. • Monitor urinary cultures, CBC, and urinalysis before and during therapy. • Sulfamethoxazole is also used in adjunctive therapy for treatment of toxoplasmosis following therapy with other first line agents. • Instruct patient to report early signs of blood dyscrasias (sore throat, fever, pallor, or jaundice) immediately and to stop taking drug. • Vitamin K_1 may reverse sulfonamide-induced hypoprothrombinemia. • For treatment of anaphylaxis, see p. 1114.

NAME	INDICATIONS & DOSAGE	SIDE EFFECTS
sulfamethoxy-pyridazine Midicel	*Urinary and systemic infections*— **Adults over 60 Kg:** initially, 1 g P.O. followed by 500 mg daily or 1 g every other day. For severe infection, initially, 2 g P.O. followed by 500 mg daily. **Adults under 60 Kg:** initially, 1 g P.O. followed by 250 mg P.O. daily. **Children over 2 months:** initially, 30 mg/Kg P.O. followed by 15 mg/Kg P.O. daily. Maximum initial dose 1 g, and 500 mg thereafter.	*Blood:* agranulocytosis, aplastic anemia, thrombocytopenia, leukopenia, hemolytic anemia, hypoprothrombinemia, methemoglobinemia, purpura. *CNS:* arthralgia, headache, peripheral neuritis, mental depression, convulsions, ataxia, hallucinations, vertigo, insomnia, restlessness, drowsiness. *CV:* allergic myocarditis, periarteritis nodosa. *EENT:* periorbital edema, conjunctival and scleral injection, tinnitus, pharyngitis, glossitis, sore throat. *GI:* nausea, emesis, abdominal pain, diarrhea, anorexia, stomatitis, gastroenteritis. *GU:* toxic nephrosis with oliguria and anuria, renal damage, crystalluria, hematuria. *Skin:* erythema multiforme (Stevens-Johnson syndrome), generalized skin eruption, epidermal necrolysis, urticaria, pruritus, exfoliative dermatitis, photosensitization, pallor. *Other:* serum sickness, drug fever, chills, anaphylaxis, cross-sensitization, weakness, pancreatitis, L.E. phenomenon, hepatitis.
sulfapyridine Dagenan◆◆	*Dermatitis herpetiformis*— **Adults:** 500 mg P.O. q.i.d. until improvement noted, then decrease dose by 500 mg every 3 days until minimum effective maintenance dose achieved.	*Blood:* agranulocytosis, aplastic anemia, thrombocytopenia, hemolytic anemia, hypoprothrombinemia, purpura, methemoglobinemia, leukopenia. *CNS:* arthralgia, headache, peripheral neuritis, mental depression, convulsions, ataxia, hallucinations, vertigo, insomnia, restlessness, drowsiness. *CV:* allergic myocarditis, periarteritis nodosa. *EENT:* periorbital edema, conjunctival and scleral injection, tinnitus, pharyngitis, glossitis, sore throat. *GI:* nausea, emesis, abdominal pain, diarrhea, anorexia, stomatitis, gastroenteritis. *GU:* toxic nephrosis with oliguria and anuria, renal damage, crystalluria, hematuria. *Skin:* erythema multiforme (Stevens-Johnson syndrome), generalized skin eruption, epidermal necrolysis, urticaria, pruritus, exfoliative dermatitis, photosensitization, pallor. *Other:* serum sickness, drug fever, chills, anaphylaxis, cross-sensitization, weakness, pancreatitis, L.E. phenomenon, hepatitis.

INTERACTIONS	NURSING CONSIDERATIONS
Ammonium chloride, ascorbic acid, paraldehyde: doses sufficient to acidify urine may cause precipitation of sulfonamide and crystalluria. Don't use together. *PABA-containing local anesthetics and other PABA drugs:* inhibited antibacterial action. Don't use together. *Oxacillin:* inhibited GI absorption of oxacillin. Don't use together.	• Contraindicated in porphyria. Use cautiously and in reduced dosages in impaired hepatic or renal function, asthma, blood dyscrasias, G-6-PD deficiency, history of multiple allergies. • Administer immediately after meals. • Watch for signs of Stevens-Johnson syndrome (high fever, rash, severe headache, stomatitis, conjunctivitis). Stop drug at once if these occur. • Tell patient to drink a full glass of water with each dose and to drink plenty of water during the day to prevent crystalluria. Monitor fluid intake and urinary output. Intake should be sufficient to produce output of 1,500 ml daily. To aid in prevention of crystalluria, sodium bicarbonate may be administered to alkalinize urine. • Tell patient to take medication for as long as prescribed, even after he feels better. Warn patient to avoid direct sunlight and ultraviolet light to prevent photosensitivity reaction. • Monitor urinary cultures, CBC, and urinalysis before and during therapy. • Sulfamethoxypyridazine is a long-acting sulfonamide and should never be used in place of short-acting sulfonamides to treat systemic infections. • Vitamin K_1 may reverse sulfonamide-induced hypoprothrombinemia. • For treatment of anaphylaxis, see p. 1114.
Ammonium chloride, ascorbic acid, paraldehyde: doses sufficient to acidify urine may cause precipitation of sulfonamide and crystalluria. Don't use together. *PABA-containing local anesthetics and other PABA drugs:* inhibited antibacterial action. Don't use together.	• Contraindicated in porphyria. Use cautiously and in reduced dosages in impaired hepatic or renal function, G-6-PD deficiency, history of multiple allergies, asthma, or blood dyscrasias. • Tell patient to drink a full glass of water with each dose and to drink plenty of water during the day to prevent crystalluria. Monitor fluid intake and urinary output. Intake should be sufficient to produce output of 1,500 ml daily. • Alkalinization of the urine may decrease the danger of crystalluria but may greatly increase renal tubular reabsorption of the drug, sustained blood levels, and risk of toxicity. • Tell patient to take medication for as long as prescribed, even after he feels better. Warn patient to avoid direct sunlight and ultraviolet light to prevent photosensitivity reaction. • Monitor urinary cultures, CBC, and urinalysis before and during therapy. • Sulfapyridine is an intermediate-acting sulfonamide with a high potential for toxicity; its use is restricted to treatment of dermatitis herpetiformis when sulfone therapy is contraindicated. • Tell patient to report any side effects at once and to stop drug. • Vitamin K_1 may reverse sulfonamide-induced hypoprothrombinemia. • For treatment of anaphylaxis, see p. 1114.

NAME	INDICATIONS & DOSAGE	SIDE EFFECTS
sulfasalazine Azulfidine, Azulfidine En-Tabs, SAS-500, Sulcolon	*Mild to moderate ulcerative colitis, adjunctive therapy in severe ulcerative colitis—* **Adults:** initially, 3 to 4 g P.O. daily in evenly divided doses; usual maintenance dose is 1.5 to 2 g P.O. daily in divided doses q 6 hours. May need to start with 1 to 2 g initially, with a gradual increase in dose to minimize side effects. **Children over 2 years:** initially, 40 to 60 mg/Kg P.O. daily, divided into 3 to 6 doses; then 30 mg/Kg daily in 4 doses. May need to start at lower dose if gastrointestinal intolerance occurs.	*Blood:* agranulocytosis, aplastic anemia, thrombocytopenia, leukopenia, hemolytic anemia, hypoprothrombinemia, purpura, eosinophilia, methemoglobinemia. *CNS:* arthralgia, headache, vertigo, peripheral neuropathy, ataxia, convulsions, insomnia, mental depression, drowsiness, hallucinations. *CV:* allergic myocarditis, periarteritis nodosa. *EENT:* tinnitus, hearing loss, periorbital edema, conjunctival and sclera injection. *GI:* anorexia, nausea, vomiting, diarrhea. *GU:* crystalluria, hematuria, proteinuria, nephrotic syndrome, toxic nephrosis with oliguria and anuria. *Skin:* generalized skin eruptions, erythema multiforme (Stevens-Johnson syndrome), parapsoriasis varioliformis acuta, exfoliative dermatitis, epidermal necrolysis, pruritus, urticaria, photosensitization. *Other:* alopecia, hepatitis, pancreatitis, L.E. phenomenon, cyanosis, decreased pulmonary function.
sulfisoxazole Barazole, Gantrisin♦, G-Sox, J-Sul, Lipo Gantrisin, Novosoxazole♦♦, Rosoxol, SK-Soxazole, Sosol, Soxa, Soxomide, Sulfagan, Sulfalar Sulfizin, Sulfizole♦♦, Urisoxin, Urizole, Velmatrol	*Urinary tract and systemic infections—* **Adults:** initially, 2 to 4 g P.O., then 1 to 2 g P.O. q.i.d.; extended-release suspension 4 to 5 g P.O. q 12 hours. **Children over 2 months:** initially, 75 mg/Kg P.O. daily or 2 g/m^2 P.O. daily in divided doses q 6 hours, then 150 mg/Kg or 4 g/m^2 P.O. daily in divided doses q 6 hours; extended-release suspension 60 to 70 mg/Kg P.O. q 12 hours. **Adults, and children over 2 months:** parenteral dosages (sulfisoxazole diolamine) initially, 50 mg/Kg or 1.125 g/m^2 by slow I.V. injection, then 100 mg/Kg daily or 2.25 g/m^2 daily in divided doses q 6 hours by slow I.V. injection.	*Blood:* agranulocytosis, aplastic anemia, thrombocytopenia, leukopenia, hemolytic anemia, hypoprothrombinemia, methemoglobinemia, purpura. *CNS:* arthralgia, headache, peripheral neuritis, mental depression, convulsions, ataxia, hallucinations, vertigo, insomnia. *CV:* allergic myocarditis, periarteritis nodosa. *EENT:* periorbital edema, conjunctival and scleral injection, tinnitus. *GI:* nausea, emesis, abdominal pain, diarrhea, anorexia, stomatitis. *GU:* toxic nephrosis with oliguria and anuria, crystalluria. *Skin:* erythema multiforme (Stevens-Johnson syndrome), generalized skin eruption, epidermal necrolysis, urticaria, pruritus, exfoliative dermatitis, photosensitization. *Other:* serum sickness, drug fever, chills, L.E. phenomenon, pancreatitis, hepatitis.

INTERACTIONS	NURSING CONSIDERATIONS
Ammonium chloride, ascorbic acid, paraldehyde: doses sufficient to acidify urine may cause precipitation of sulfonamide and crystalluria. Don't use together. *PABA-containing local anesthetics and other PABA drugs:* inhibited antibacterial action. Don't use together.	• Contraindicated in porphyria. Use cautiously and in reduced dosages in impaired hepatic or renal function and in those with severe allergy or bronchial asthma, G-6-PD deficiency. • Tell patient to drink a full glass of water with each dose and to drink plenty of water during the day to prevent crystalluria. Monitor fluid intake and urinary output. Intake should be sufficient to produce output of 1,500 ml daily. • Instruct patient to take medication for as long as prescribed, even after he feels better. Warn patient to avoid direct sunlight and ultraviolet light to prevent photosensitivity reaction. • Monitor urinary cultures, CBC, and urinalysis before and during therapy. • Colors urine orange-yellow. • Side effects are usually those affecting the GI tract. Minimize symptoms by spacing doses evenly. • For treatment of anaphylaxis, see p. 1114.
PABA-containing local anesthetics and other PABA drugs: inhibited antibacterial action. Don't use together. *Ammonium chloride, ascorbic acid, paraldehyde:* doses sufficient to acidify urine may cause crystalluria and precipitation of sulfonamide. Don't use together.	• Contraindicated in porphyria and in infants younger than 2 months (except in congenital toxoplasmosis). Use cautiously in impaired hepatic or renal function, severe allergy or bronchial asthma, G-6-PD deficiency. • Tell patient to drink a full glass of water with each dose and to drink plenty of water throughout the day to prevent crystalluria. Monitor fluid intake and urinary output. Intake should be sufficient to produce output of 1,500 ml daily. To aid in prevention of crystalluria, sodium bicarbonate may be administered to alkalinize urine. • Tell patient to take medication for as long as prescribed, even after he feels better. Warn patient to avoid direct sunlight and ultraviolet light to prevent photosensitivity reaction. • Monitor urinary cultures, CBC, and urinalysis before and during therapy. • Parenteral form can be given I.M. or S.C., but these routes are discouraged. Administration of this form with parenteral fluids is not recommended. • Diluents other than sterile distilled water may cause precipitation. • Gantrisin suspension and Lipo Gantrisin suspension cannot be interchanged, since the latter is an extended-release preparation. • Sulfisoxazole/pyrimethamine combination used to treat toxoplasmosis. • Tell patient to report early signs of blood dyscrasias (sore throat, fever, pallor, or jaundice) immediately and to stop taking drug. • Watch for signs of GI superinfection during long-term therapy. • When given preop, the patient should receive a low-residue diet and a minimum of enemas and cathartics. • Vitamin K_1 may reverse sulfonamide-induced hypoprothrombinemia. • For treatment of anaphylaxis, see p. 1114.

15

Urinary tract germicides

methenamine hippurate
methenamine mandelate
methenamine sulfosalicylate
methylene blue
nalidixic acid
nitrofurantoin
oxolinic acid

Urinary tract germicides are antibacterial drugs which are concentrated in the renal tubules, and other areas of the kidneys and bladder. These drugs do not reach effective serum levels for treating systemic infections. For these reasons, they can be thought of as locally acting antibacterial agents specifically for urinary tract infections.

Major uses

- Treatment of bacteriuria, pyelonephritis, pyelitis, and cystitis.
- Methylene blue is also used in treatment of idiopathic and drug-induced methemoglobinemia, and in treatment of cyanide poisoning.

Mechanism of action

- In acid urine, methenamines are hydrolyzed to form ammonia and the bacterial agent formaldehyde, which is responsible for antibacterial action against gram-positive and gram-negative organisms.
- Methylene blue is a dye with mild antiseptic action. In high concentrations it converts the ferrous iron of reduced hemoglobin to ferric iron to form methemoglobin. This action is the basis for its use as an antidote in cyanide poisoning. Low concentrations of methylene blue can hasten conversion of methemoglobin to hemoglobin.
- Nalidixic and oxolinic acids are bacteriostatic agents that inhibit protein synthesis in microorganisms.
- Nitrofurantoin is bacteriostatic in low concentration and may be bactericidal in higher concentration. It is presumed to interfere with bacterial enzyme systems.

Absorption, distribution, and excretion

- Methenamines are rapidly absorbed and are excreted in the urine (90% within 24 hours). They are inactive in the serum and are converted to ammonia and formaldehyde in the urine if its pH is 5.5 or less.
- Methylene blue is poorly absorbed orally, but once in the tissues it is rapidly reduced and slowly excreted into the bile and urine.
- Nalidixic acid is readily absorbed after oral administration. It is partially metabolized in the liver and is rapidly excreted through the kidneys.
- Nitrofurantoin is usually well absorbed from the GI tract in either the crystalline or macrocrystalline form. Bioequivalence differences may exist among various products. Rapidly metabolized, the drug reaches therapeutic concentration only in the urine, where it is rapidly excreted.

Onset and duration

- Onset of antibacterial activity occurs within 30 minutes with nitrofurantoin and methenamine hippurate; within 4 hours with nalidixic acid and oxolinic acid.
- Antibacterial levels are sustained with twice-a-day dosing with methenamine hippurate and oxolinic acid. All others require more frequent dosing.

Combination products

AZO-CYST: methenamine 120 mg, phenazopyridine HC1 50 mg, calcium mandelate 120 mg, sodium biphosphate 120 mg, hyoscyamine HBr 0.1037 mg, scopolamine HBr 0.0065 mg, and atropine sulfate 0.0194 mg.
AZO GANTANOL: sulfamethoxazole 500 mg and phenazopyridine HC1 100 mg.
AZO GANTRISIN: sulfisoxazole 500 mg and phenazopyridine HC1 50 mg.
AZOLATE: methenamine mandelate 500 mg and phenazopyridine HC1 50 mg.
AZO-MANDELAMINE: methenamine mandelate 500 mg and phenazopyridine HC1 50 mg.
AZO-SOXAZOLE: sulfisoxazole 500 mg and phenazopyridine HC1 50 mg.
AZOSUL: sulfisoxazole 500 mg and phenazopyridine HC1 50 mg.
AZO-SULFSTAT: sulfamethizole 500 mg and phenazopyridine HC1 50 mg.
AZOTREX: tetracycline phosphate complex equivalent to 125 mg tetracycline HC1 activity, sulfamethizole 250 mg, and phenazopyridine HC1 50 mg.
CYSTEX: methenamine 162 mg, salicylamine 65 mg, sodium salicylate 97 mg, and benzoic acid 32 mg.
CYSTISED (Improved): methenamine 40.8 mg, phenyl salicylate 18.1 mg, atropine sulfate 0.03 mg, hyoscyamine 0.03 mg, benzoic acid 4.5 mg, methylene blue 5.4 mg, and gelsemium 6.1 mg.
CYSTREA: methenamine 130 mg, phenyl salicylate 32 mg, atropine sulfate 0.0325 mg, hyoscyamine sulfate 0.0325 mg, and benzoic acid 6.5 mg, and methylene blue 13 mg.
HEXALOL: methenamine 40.8 mg, phenyl salicylate 18 mg, atropine sulfate 0.03 mg, hyoscyamine 0.03 mg, benzoic acid 4.5 mg, and methylene blue 5.4 mg.
METHENAMINE AND SODIUM BIPHOSPHATE: methenamine 325 mg and sodium biphosphate 325 mg.
PROSED: methylene blue 5.4 mg, methenamine 40.8 mg, phenyl salicylate 18.1 mg, atropine sulfate 0.03 mg, hyoscyamine 0.03 mg, and benzoic acid 4.5 mg.
RENAL: methenamine 130 mg, phenyl salicylate 32 mg, atropine sulfate 0.065 mg, hyoscyamine sulfate 0.0325 mg, benzoic acid 8 mg, and methylene blue 6.5 mg.
SULADYNE: sulfamethizole 125 mg, sulfadiazine 125 mg, and phenazopyridine HC1 75 mg.
THIOSULFIL-A: sulfamethizole 250 mg and phenazopyridine HC1 50 mg.
URO-PHOSPHATE: methenamine 300 mg and sodium acid phosphate 500 mg.
UROQID-ACID: methenamine mandelate 350 mg and sodium acid phosphate 200 mg.
UROQID-ACID NO. 2: methenamine mandelate 500 mg and sodium acid phosphate 500 mg.

NAME	INDICATIONS & DOSAGE	SIDE EFFECTS
methenamine hippurate Hiprex, Hip-Rex••, Urex	*Long-term prophylaxis or suppression of chronic urinary tract infections—* **Adults, and children over 12 years:** 1 g P.O. q 12 hours. **Children 6 to 12 years:** 500 mg to 1 g P.O. q 12 hours.	*GI:* nausea. *GU:* with high doses, urinary tract irritation, dysuria, frequency, albuminuria, hematuria. *Skin:* rashes.
methenamine mandelate Mandacon, Mandelamine•, Mandelets, Mandelurine••, Methandine••, Prov-U-Sep, Renelate, Sterine••	*Urinary tract infections, infected residual urine in patients with neurogenic bladder—* **Adults:** 1 g P.O. q.i.d. after meals. **Children 6 to 12 years:** 500 mg P.O. q.i.d. after meals. **Children under 6 years:** 50 mg/Kg divided in 4 doses after meals.	
methenamine sulfosalicylate Hexalet	*Long-term prophylaxis or suppression of chronic urinary tract infections—* **Adults, and children over 12:** 1 g P.O. q.i.d. after meals with ½ glass of water. **Children 6 to 12 years:** 500 mg P.O. q.i.d. after meals with ½ glass of water.	
methylene blue M-B Tabs, MG-Blue, Urolene Blue, Wright's Stain	*Cystitis, urethritis—* **Adults:** 65 mg P.O. b.i.d. or t.i.d. after meals with glass of water. *Methemoglobinemia and cyanide poisoning—* **Adults and children:** 1 to 2 mg/Kg of 1% sterile solution I.V. slowly.	*Blood:* anemia (long-term use). *GI:* nausea, vomiting, diarrhea. *GU:* dysuria, bladder irritation. *Other:* fever (large doses).
nalidixic acid NegGram•	*Acute and chronic urinary tract infections caused by susceptible gram-negative organisms (Proteus, Klebsiella, Enterobacter, and E. coli)—* **Adults:** 1 g P.O. q.i.d. for 7 to 14 days; 2 g daily for long-term use. **Children over 3 months:** 55 mg/Kg P.O. daily divided q.i.d. for 7 to 14 days; 33 mg/Kg/day for long-term use.	*Blood:* eosinophilia. *CNS:* drowsiness, weakness, headache, dizziness, vertigo, myalgia, convulsions in epileptics. *CV:* dyspnea. *EENT:* sensitivity to light, change in color perception, diplopia, blurred vision. *GI:* abdominal pain, nausea, vomiting, diarrhea. *Skin:* pruritus, photosensitivity, urticaria, rash. *Other:* angioedema, fever, chills, increased intracranial pressure and bulging fontanels in infants and children.

• Also available in Canada.
•• Available in Canada only.
Unmarked trade names available in United States only.

INTERACTIONS	NURSING CONSIDERATIONS
Alkalinizing agents: inhibited methenamine action. Don't use together. *Acetazolamide:* antagonized methenamine effect. Use together cautiously.	• Contraindicated in renal insufficiency, severe liver disease, or severe dehydration. • Ineffective against *Candida* infection. • Oral suspension contains vegetable oil. Administer cautiously to elderly or debilitated patients because aspiration could cause lipid pneumonia. • Monitor intake/output. Intake should be at least 1,500 to 2,000 ml/day. • Obtain clean voided urine specimen for culture and sensitivity before starting therapy and repeat p.r.n. • Limit intake of alkaline foods, such as vegetables, milk, peanuts, fruits, and fruit juices, except cranberry, plum, and prune juices. These juices or ascorbic acid may be used to acidify urine. • Warn patient not to take antacids, including Alka-Seltzer and sodium bicarbonate. • Maintain urine pH at 5.5 or less. Use Nitrazine paper to check pH. • *Proteus* and *Pseudomonas* tend to raise urine pH; urinary acidifiers are usually necessary when treating these infections. • Obtain liver function studies periodically during long-term therapy. • Administer after meals to lessen GI upset. • If rash appears, hold dose and contact doctor.
None significant.	• Contraindicated in patients with renal insufficiency. • Monitor intake/output carefully. Intake should be at least 2,000 ml/day. • Monitor hemoglobin; possibility of anemia from accelerated destruction of erythrocytes. • Turns urine and stool blue-green. • Seldom used as urinary antiseptic.
Nitrofurantoin: may antagonize nalidixic acid effect. Use together cautiously.	• Contraindicated in convulsive disorders. Use with caution in impaired hepatic or renal function, epilepsy, or severe cerebral arteriosclerosis. • Not effective against *Pseudomonas.* • Report visual disturbances; usually disappear with reduced dose. • Obtain clean voided urine specimen for culture and sensitivity before starting therapy and repeat p.r.n. • Obtain CBC, renal and liver function studies during long-term therapy. • Resistant bacteria may emerge within first 48 hours of therapy. • May cause a false positive Clinitest reaction. Use Clinistix or Tes-Tape to monitor urine glucose. Also gives false elevations in urinary vanilmandelic acid (VMA) and 17 ketosteroids. Repeat tests after therapy completed. • Avoid undue exposure to sunlight due to photosensitivity. Patient may continue to be photosensitive up to 3 months after drug is discontinued.

NAME	INDICATIONS & DOSAGE	SIDE EFFECTS
nitrofurantoin Cyantin, Furadantin, Furalan, Furatine◆◆, Furantoin, Ivadantin, J-Dantin, Nephronex◆◆, Nifuran◆◆, Nitrex, Novofuran◆◆, Parfuran, Sarodant **nitrofurantoin macrocrystals** Macrodantin◆	*Pyelonephritis, pyelitis, and cystitis due to susceptible E. coli, S. aureus, enterococci; certain strains of Klebsiella, Proteus, Pseudomonas, and Enterobacter—* **Adults, and children over 12:** 50 to 100 mg P.O. q.i.d. with meals. Or, 180 mg I.M. or I.V. b.i.d. in patients over 55 Kg; 5 to 7 mg/Kg daily I.M. or I.V. in patients under 55 Kg. **Children 1 month to 12 years:** 5 to 7 mg/Kg P.O. daily, divided q.i.d.	*Blood:* granulocytopenia, leukopenia, eosinophilia, megaloblastic anemia; hemolysis in patients with G-6-PD deficiency (reversed after stopping drug). *CNS:* peripheral neuropathy, headache, dizziness, drowsiness, ascending polyneuropathy with high doses or renal impairment. *EENT:* nystagmus. *GI:* anorexia, nausea, vomiting, abdominal pain, diarrhea. *GU:* crystalluria. *Skin:* maculopapular, erythematous, or eczematous eruption; pruritus; urticaria; angioedema; transient alopecia. *Other:* sensitivity reactions, asthmatic attacks in patients with history of asthma; anaphylaxis; drug fever; arthralgia; overgrowth of nonsusceptible organisms in the urinary tract; cholestatic jaundice; pulmonary sensitivity reactions (cough, chest pains, fever, chills, dyspnea).
oxolinic acid Utibid	*Cystitis, urethritis, pyelonephritis, pyelitis, caused by susceptible gram-negative organisms (Proteus, Klebsiella, E. coli, and Enterobacter)—* **Adults:** 1 tablet (750 mg) P.O. b.i.d. for 2 weeks.	*Blood:* transient leukopenia; transient increase in SGOT and alkaline phosphatase blood levels. *CNS:* insomnia, dizziness, nervousness, drowsiness, headache, impaired alertness, impaired physical coordination, weakness. *GI:* nausea, abdominal cramps, anorexia, vomiting, diarrhea, constipation.

INTERACTIONS	NURSING CONSIDERATIONS
None significant.	• Contraindicated in moderate to severe renal impairment, anuria, oliguria, creatinine clearance under 40 ml/min; in G-6-PD deficiency. • Obtain clean voided urine specimen for culture and sensitivity before starting therapy and repeat p.r.n. • Give with food or milk to minimize GI distress. • I.M. route painful and should not be used for more than 5 days. • Have patient rinse his mouth after taking liquid preparation to prevent staining tooth enamel. • Dilute I.V. nitrofurantoin to 500 ml of suitable I.V. solution before administering.Constitute in sterile water without preservatives. • Monitor intake/output carefully. May turn urine brown or darker. • Store in amber container. Keep away from metals other than stainless steel or aluminum to avoid precipitate formation. Warn patients not to use pillboxes made of these materials. • Continue treatment for 3 days after sterile urines obtained. • Monitor pulmonary status. • For symptoms and treatment of anaphylaxis, see p. 1114.
Nitrofurantoin: decreased response to oxolinic acid. Avoid if possible.	• Contraindicated in convulsive disorders. Use cautiously in impaired renal function; in older patients, as the drug may cause CNS stimulation. • Safe use when taken concurrently with other CNS stimulants not established. • Before and during therapy, monitor for development of resistant organisms by obtaining urine specimens for culture and sensitivity. • Warn patient that drug may cause dizziness. • Monitor intake/output.

16

Miscellaneous

amantadine hydrochloride
bacitracin
chloramphenicol palmitate
chloramphenicol sodium succinate
clindamycin hydrochloride
clindamycin palmitate hydrochloride
clindamycin phosphate
colistimethate sodium
erythromycin base
erythromycin estolate
erythromycin ethylsuccinate
erythromycin gluceptate
erythromycin lactobionate
erythromycin stearate
furazolidone
lincomycin hydrochloride
novobiocin calcium
novobiocin sodium
polymyxin B sulfate
spectinomycin dihydrochloride
troleandomycin phosphate
vancomycin hydrochloride
vidarabine monohydrate

These drugs have a lethal and/or inhibiting effect on a variety of infective agents, primarily bacterial and viral.

Major uses

- Treatment of various infections; often used as alternatives to other antibiotics, such as penicillin, in case of known hypersensitivity or resistance.

Mechanism of action

- These drugs are thought to exert their antimicrobial effect by interfering with protein synthesis, cell-wall synthesis, or enzyme systems of susceptible organisms.

Absorption, distribution, and excretion

- Amantadine HCl is well absorbed from the GI tract. Over 90% is excreted unchanged in the urine.
- Bacitracin is not absorbed orally but is absorbed quickly and completely after I.M. administration, widely distributed, and slowly excreted by glomerular filtration.
- Chloramphenicol is readily absorbed from the GI tract, rapidly diffuses with highest concentrations in the liver and kidneys. CSF levels reach about half of plasma level; 90% is metabolized in the liver and excreted by the kidneys, with the remainder excreted in the urine unchanged.
- Clindamycin is almost completely absorbed, whether in capsule or solution. Food may delay but not decrease absorption. It is widely distributed. The drug is metabolized by the

liver and excreted in the bile, with only 5% to 10% excreted unchanged in the urine.
• Colistimethate sodium is not absorbed orally and is excreted mainly in the urine.
• Erythromycin absorption varies greatly with the particular salt and form of dosage. Widely distributed, except in the brain and CSF. Partly metabolized in the liver; excreted via bile.
• Furazolidone is poorly absorbed orally and doesn't give therapeutic blood levels. About 5% is excreted in the urine.
• Lincomycin absorption is impaired by food; in the fasting state, about 30% is absorbed. Widely distributed, except in CSF. Partly metabolized by the liver and excreted primarily in the bile.
• Novobiocin is readily absorbed from GI tract. Diffuses well into pleural, joint, and ascitic fluids (but not spinal fluid, unless meninges inflamed); excreted in bile, urine, and feces.
• Polymyxin B sulfate is not absorbed from GI tract; blood levels are low, as the drug loses 50% of its activity in serum. Excreted slowly by the kidneys; tissue diffusion is poor.
• Troleandomycin is more readily absorbed orally than erythromycin; 18% to 24% is excreted in the urine, with large amounts in the bile.
• Vancomycin HCl is not absorbed orally but after I.V. administration is widely distributed, except in CSF. Excreted in urine, 80% to 90% unchanged.
• Vidarabine is poorly absorbed from the GI tract. It is widely distributed in all tissues, including the CSF; excreted over 24 hours by the kidneys.

Onset and duration
• Orally absorbed drugs (amantadine, chloramphenicol, clindamycin, erythromycin, lincomycin, novobiocin, troleandomycin) give peak blood levels usually within 2 hours.
• Drugs given I.M. (bacitracin, clindamycin, colistimethate, lincomycin, novobiocin, polymyxin B, spectinomycin) give peak blood levels usually within 1 hour.
• Drugs given I.V. (chloramphenicol, clindamycin, colistimethate, erythromycin, lincomycin, novobiocin, polymyxin B, vancomycin, vidarabine) give peak blood levels almost immediately and should be given by that route in acute, life-threatening situations.
• Duration of effect varies from 2 to 6 hours except for amantadine, which has an effect lasting up to 24 hours.

Combination products
None.

NAME	INDICATIONS & DOSAGE	SIDE EFFECTS
amantadine hydrochloride Symmetrel♦	*Prophylaxis or symptomatic treatment of influenza type A virus, respiratory tract illnesses—* **Adults, and children over 9 years:** 200 mg P.O. daily in a single dose or divided b.i.d. **Children 1 to 9 years:** 4.4 to 8.8 mg/Kg P.O. daily, divided b.i.d. or t.i.d. Don't exceed 150 mg daily. Symptomatic treatment should continue for 24 to 48 hours after symptoms disappear. Prophylaxis should start as soon as possible after initial exposure and continue for at least 10 days after exposure. May continue prophylactic treatment up to 90 days for repeated or suspected exposures if influenza vaccine unavailable. If used with influenza vaccine, continue dose for 2 to 3 weeks until protection from vaccine develops. To treat Parkinson's disease, see p. 1110.	*CNS:* depression, fatigue, confusion, dizziness, psychosis, hallucinations, anxiety, irritability, ataxia, insomnia, weakness, headache. *CV:* peripheral edema, orthostatic hypotension, congestive heart failure. *GI:* anorexia, nausea, constipation, vomiting, dry mouth. *GU:* urinary retention. *Skin:* livedo reticularis, particularly when used in parkinsonism.
bacitracin	*Pneumonia or empyema caused by susceptible staphylococci—* **Infants over 2.5 Kg:** 1,000 units/Kg I.M. daily, divided q 8 to 12 hours. **Infants under 2.5 Kg:** 900 units/Kg I.M. daily, divided q 8 to 12 hours. Although the F.D.A. approves the use of bacitracin in infants only, adults with susceptible staphylococcal infections may receive 10,000 to 25,000 units I.M. q 6 hours (maximum 25,000 units/dose, 100,000 units/day).	*Blood:* bone marrow toxicities, blood dyscrasias, eosinophilia. *GI:* nausea, vomiting, anorexia, diarrhea, rectal itching or burning. *GU:* nephrotoxicity (albuminuria, cylindruria, oliguria, anuria, increased BUN, tubular and glomerular necrosis). *Local:* pain at injection site. *Skin:* urticaria, rash. *Other:* superinfection, fever, anaphylaxis.
chloramphenicol palmitate, sodium succinate Amphicol, Chloromycetin♦, Mychel, Novochlorocap♦♦	*Hemophilus influenzae, meningitis, acute S. typhi infection, severe infections caused by sensitive Salmonella species, Rickettsia, lymphogranuloma, psittacosis, various sensitive gram-negative organisms causing meningitis, bacteremia, or other serious infections—* **Adults and children:** 50 to 100 mg/Kg P.O. or I.V. daily, divided q 6 hours. Maximum dose is 100 mg/Kg/day.	*Blood:* aplastic anemia, hypoplastic anemia, granulocytopenia, thrombocytopenia. *CNS:* headache, mild depression, confusion, delirium, peripheral neuropathy with prolonged therapy. *EENT:* optic neuritis (cystic fibrosis patients), glossitis, decreased visual acuity. *GI:* nausea, vomiting, stomatitis, diarrhea, enterocolitis. *Other:* infections by nonsusceptible organisms, hypersensitivity reaction

♦ Also available in Canada.
♦♦ Available in Canada only.
Unmarked trade names available in United States only.

INTERACTIONS	NURSING CONSIDERATIONS
None significant.	• Use cautiously in history of epilepsy, congestive heart failure, peripheral edema, hepatic disease, mental illness, eczematoid rash, renal impairment, orthostatic hypotension, cardiovascular disease, and in elderly patients. • For best absorption, drug should be taken after meals. • Instruct patient to report side effects to the doctor, especially dizziness, depression, anxiety, nausea, and urinary retention. • Monitor renal function, BUN, creatinine clearance, electrolyte balance, and urinary output. Frequently check SGOT levels and vital signs. • If orthostatic hypotension occurs, instruct patient not to stand or change positions too quickly. • If insomnia occurs, dose should be taken several hours before bedtime. • Prophylactic use recommended for patients who can't receive influenza virus vaccine.
None significant.	• Contraindicated in impaired renal function. Use cautiously in superinfections or neuromuscular disease. • Culture and sensitivity test should be done initially and p.r.n. • For I.M. administration only. Give deeply I.M.; injection may be painful; often diluted with procaine hydrochloride. Do not give if patient is sensitive to procaine or PABA derivatives. • Maintain adequate fluid intake and monitor urinary output closely. • Obtain baseline renal function studies before starting therapy. Monitor renal function (BUN, serum creatinine, creatinine clearance) daily during therapy. Notify doctor of any change. • Dilute in solution containing sodium chloride and 2% procaine hydrochloride. Concentration of bacitracin should be between 5,000 and 10,000 units/ml. Store in refrigerator. Drug is inactivated at room temperature. • Report side effects to the doctor immediately. • May be used with neomycin as a bowel prep, or in solution as a wound irrigant. • For treatment of anaphylaxis, see p. 1114.
Penicillins: antagonized antibacterial effect. Give penicillin at least 1 hour before.	• Use cautiously in impaired hepatic or renal function, with other drugs causing bone marrow depression or blood disorders. Don't use for infections susceptible to other agents or for trivial infections such as colds. • Culture and sensitivity test should be done initially and p.r.n. • Monitor CBC, platelets, serum iron, and reticulocytes before and every 2 days during therapy. Stop drug immediately if anemia, reticulocytopenia, leukopenia, or thrombocytopenia develops. • Give I.V. slowly over 1 minute. Check injection site daily for phlebitis and irritation. • Instruct patient to report side effects to the doctor, especially nausea, vomiting, diarrhea, fever, confusion, sore throat, or mouth sores. • Tell patient to take medication for as long as prescribed, exactly as directed, even if he feels better.

(continued on following page)

NAME	INDICATIONS & DOSAGE	SIDE EFFECTS
chloramphenicol palmitate, sodium succinate *(continued)*	**Prematures and neonates (2 weeks or younger):** 25 mg/Kg P.O. or I.V. daily, divided q 6 hours. I.V. route must be used to treat meningitis.	(fever, rash, urticaria, anaphylaxis), "gray baby syndrome" (abdominal distention, cyanosis, vasomotor collapse, death within a few hours of onset of symptoms).
clindamycin hydrochloride, palmitate, phosphate Cleocin, Dalcin C••	*Infections caused by sensitive Staphylococci, Streptococci, Pneumococci, Bacteroides, Fusobacterium, Clostridium perfringens, and other sensitive aerobic and anaerobic organisms—* **Adults:** 150 to 450 mg P.O. q 6 hours or 300 mg I.M. or I.V. q 6, 8, or 12 hours. Up to 2,700 mg I.M. or I.V. daily, divided q 6, 8, or 12 hours. May be used for severe infections. **Children over 1 month:** 8 to 25 mg/Kg P.O. daily, divided q 6 to 8 hours; or 15 to 40 mg/Kg I.M. or I.V. daily, divided q 6 hours.	*Blood:* transient leukopenia, eosinophilia, agranulocytosis, thrombocytopenia. *GI:* nausea, vomiting, abdominal pain, diarrhea, colitis, pseudomembranous colitis, esophagitis, flatulence, anorexia, bloody or tarry stools. *Local:* pain, induration, sterile abscess with I.M. injection; thrombophlebitis, erythema, and pain following I.V. administration. *Metabolic:* elevated SGOT, creatinine phosphokinase, alkaline phosphatase, bilirubin. *Skin:* maculopapular rash, urticaria. *Other:* unpleasant or bitter taste, anaphylaxis, jaundice.
colistimethate sodium Colistin Sulfate, Coly-Mycin M•, Coly-Mycin S Oral	*Enterocolitis caused by sensitive E. coli, sensitive Shigella, gastroenteritis—* **Infants and children:** 5 to 15 mg/Kg P.O. daily, divided q 6 to 8 hours. *Severe infections, especially of urinary tract caused by sensitive Pseudomonas, Enterobacteria, E. coli, and Klebsiella—* **Adults and children:** 2.5 to 5 mg/Kg I.M. or I.V. daily, divided q 6 to 12 hours. Maximum daily dose not to exceed 5 mg/Kg day in patients with normal renal function.	*CNS:* circumoral and lingual paresthesias; paresthesias of extremities; neuromuscular blockage with respiratory arrest, especially in patients with impaired renal function; dizziness; slurring of speech. *GI:* GI distress. *GU:* nephrotoxicity (decreased urine output, increased blood urea nitrogen, increased serum creatinine). *Local:* pain at I.M. site. *Skin:* pruritus, urticaria. *Other:* "drug fever," overgrowth of susceptible organisms.
erythromycin base E-Mycin•, Erythromid••, Ethril 500, Ilotycin•, Novorythro•• **erythromycin estolate** Ilosone•, Novorythro•• **erythromycin ethylsuccinate**	*Acute pelvic inflammatory disease caused by N. gonorrhoeae—* **Women:** 500 mg I.V. (erythromycin gluceptate, lactobionate) q 6 hours for 3 days, then 250 mg (erythromycin base, estolate, stearate) or 400 mg (erythromycin ethylsuccinate) P.O. q 6 hours for 7 days. *Endocarditis prophylaxis for dental procedures—* **Adults:** 500 mg (erythromycin base, estolate, stearate) P.O.	*GI:* abdominal pain and cramping, nausea, vomiting, diarrhea. *Local:* venous irritation, thrombophlebitis following I.V. injection. *Skin:* urticaria, rashes. *Other:* overgrowth of nonsusceptible bacteria or fungi; anaphylaxis, fever, cholestatic hepatitis (with erythromycin estolate).

INTERACTIONS	NURSING CONSIDERATIONS
	• Reconstitute 1 g vial of powder for injection with 10 ml sterile water for injection. Concentration will be 100 mg/ml. Stable for 30 days at room temperature but refrigeration recommended. Do not use cloudy solutions. • For treatment of anaphylaxis, see p. 1114.
Erythromycin: antagonist that may block access of clindamycin to its site of action; don't use together.	• Contraindicated in known hypersensitivity to antibiotic congener lincomycin; also in history of GI disease, especially colitis. Use cautiously in renal or hepatic disease, asthma, newborns, allergies. • Culture and sensitivity test should be performed initially and p.r.n. • Don't use in meningitis. Drug does not get into CSF. • Don't refrigerate reconstituted oral solution, as it will thicken. Drug is stable for 2 weeks at room temperature. • Instruct patient to report side effects to the doctor, especially diarrhea. Warn patient not to treat diarrhea himself. • Don't give diphenoxylate (Lomotil) to treat drug-induced diarrhea. May prolong and worsen diarrhea. • Give deep I.M. Rotate sites. Warn that I.M. injection may be painful. Doses greater than 600 mg per injection are not recommended. • When giving I.V., check site daily for phlebitis and irritation. For I.V. infusion, dilute each 300 mg in 50 ml solution, and give no faster than 30 mg/minute. • Monitor renal and hepatic function during prolonged therapy. • Superinfections likely to occur if therapy exceeds 10 days. • For treatment of anaphylaxis, see p. 1114.
None significant.	• Contraindicated in patients with known hypersensitivity to antibiotic congener polymyxin B. Use cautiously in renal impairment. • Give deep I.M. Rotate sites. Warn that I.M. injection may be painful. • When giving I.V., check site daily for phlebitis and irritation. For direct intermittent I.V. administration, inject ½ daily dose over 3 to 5 minutes at 12-hour intervals. • For continuous I.V. infusion, infuse ½ daily dose over 3 to 5 minutes; then infuse remainder 1 to 2 hours later at rate of 5 mg/hour. • Monitor renal function (BUN, creatinine clearance, urinary output). • Report side effects immediately, especially speech impairment or paresthesias. Watch for signs of superinfection. • Store reconstituted oral suspension at 2° to 15° C. (35.6° to 59° F.) and use within 7 days. • Use sterile water for injection to reconstitute. When mixing, swirl solution gently to avoid frothing. Always prepare I.V. infusion fresh. Use within 24 hours.
Clindamycin, lincomycin: may be antagonistic. Don't use together. *Penicillins:* antagonized antibacterial effect. Give penicillin at least 1 hour before.	• Erythromycin estolate contraindicated in hepatic disease. Use other erythromycin salts cautiously in impaired hepatic function. • Culture and sensitivity test should be performed initially and p.r.n. • For best absorption, instruct patient to take oral form of drug with a full glass of water 1 hour before or 2 hours after meals. If tablets are coated, they may be taken with meals. Don't drink fruit juice with medication. Chewable erythromycin tablets should not be swallowed whole. • May cause an overgrowth of nonsusceptible bacteria or fungi. Watch for signs and symptoms of superinfections. • Tell patient to take medication for as long as prescribed, exactly as directed, even if he feels better. Treat streptococcal infections for 10 days. • Report side effects, especially nausea, abdominal pain, or fever. • Erythromycin estolate may cause serious hepatotoxicity in adults

(continued on following page)

NAME	INDICATIONS & DOSAGE	SIDE EFFECTS
(continued) **erythromycin ethylsuccinate** E.E.S., Erythrocin◆, Pediamycin, Wyamycin Liquid **erythromycin gluceptate** Ilotycin◆ **erythromycin lactobionate** Erythrocin◆ **erythromycin stearate** Bristamycin, E-Biotic, Ethril, Erypar, Erythrocin◆, Novorythro◆◆, Pfizer E, Romycin, Wintrocin, Wyamycin	before procedure, followed by 250 mg P.O. q 6 hours for 4 doses afterward; or 800 mg (erythromycin ethylsuccinate) P.O. before procedure, followed by 400 mg P.O. q 6 hours for 4 doses afterward. **Children:** 30 to 50 mg/Kg (oral erythromycin salts) P.O. daily, divided q 6 hours. Give 1 dose before procedure and 4 doses afterward. *Intestinal amebiasis—* **Adults:** 250 mg (erythromycin base, estolate, stearate) P.O. q 6 hours for 10 to 14 days. **Children:** 30 to 50 mg/Kg (erythromycin base, estolate, stearate) P.O. daily, divided q 6 hours for 10 to 14 days. *Mild-to-moderately severe respiratory tract, skin and soft tissue infections caused by sensitive group A beta-hemolytic streptococci, Diplococci pneumoniae, Mycoplasma pneumoniae, Corynebacterium diphtheriae, Bordetella pertussis, Listeria monocytogenes—* **Adults:** 250 mg to 500 mg (erythromycin base, estolate, stearate) P.O. q 6 hours; or 400 to 800 mg (erythromycin ethylsuccinate) P.O. q 6 hours; or 15 to 20 mg/Kg I.V. daily, as continuous infusion or divided q 6 hours. **Children:** 30 mg/Kg to 50 mg/Kg (oral erythromycin salts) P.O. daily, divided q 6 hours; or 15 to 20 mg/Kg I.V. daily, divided q 4 to 6 hours. *Syphilis—* **Adults:** 500 mg (erythromycin base, estolate, stearate) P.O. q.i.d. for 15 days.	
furazolidone Furoxone	*Gastroenteritis, adjunctive therapy in cholera—* **Adults:** 100 mg P.O. q.i.d. **Children 5 to 12 years:** 25 to 50 mg P.O. q.i.d. **Children 1 to 4 years:** 17 to 25 mg P.O. q.i.d. **Infants (1 month to 1 year):** 8 to 17 mg P.O. q.i.d. Dosage based on 5 mg/Kg daily; maximum dose 8.8 mg/Kg daily.	*Blood:* hemolytic anemia in infants under 1 month and G-6-PD deficiency; hypoglycemia; agranulocytosis. *CNS:* headache, malaise. *GI:* nausea, vomiting, abdominal pain, diarrhea. *GU:* may turn urine brown. *Other:* hypersensitivity reaction (arthralgia, fever, hypotension, rash, urticaria, angioedema).

INTERACTIONS	NURSING CONSIDERATIONS
	(reversible cholestatic hepatitis). Monitor hepatic function (bilirubin, SGOT, SGPT, alkaline phosphatase). Other erythromycin salts cause hepatotoxicity to a lesser degree. • I.V. dose should be administered over 20 to 60 minutes. Dilute each 250 mg in at least 100 ml 5% dextrose in water or 0.9% normal saline solution. • Sterile water without preservatives should be used to reconstitute I.V. erythromycin to prevent precipitation. • Has been used successfully in the treatment of Legionnaire's disease. • For treatment of anaphylaxis, see p. 1114.
None significant.	• Tell patient to take medication exactly as directed, even if he feels better. • Report side effects to the doctor, especially fever, rash, abdominal pain. • Store medication in dark place at 2° to 15° C. (36.5° to 59° F.). • Warn patient not to use over-the-counter nasal sprays or cold and hay fever products. • Drug may turn urine brown. Flushing, nausea, sweating may occur following ethanol ingestion. • Tell patient not to drink alcohol or use alcohol-containing medication. • If patient is taking drug for more than 5 days, tell him not to eat broad beans, cheese, beer, wine, pickled herring, chicken livers, yeast extracts, or fermented products. • May cause false positive urine glucose with Benedict's Reagent.

NAME	INDICATIONS & DOSAGE	SIDE EFFECTS
lincomycin hydrochloride Lincocin◆	*Respiratory tract, skin and soft tissue, and urinary tract infections; osteomyelitis, septicemia, caused by sensitive group A beta-hemolytic streptococci, pneumococci, and staphylococci—* **Adults:** 500 mg P.O. q 6 to 8 hours (not to exceed 8 g daily); or 600 mg I.M. daily or q 12 hours; or 600 mg to 1 g I.V. q 8 to 12 hours (not to exceed 8 g daily). **Children over 1 month:** 30 to 60 mg/Kg P.O. daily, divided q 6 to 8 hours; or 10 mg/Kg I.M. daily or divided q 12 hours; or 10 to 20 mg/Kg I.V. daily, divided q 6 to 8 hours. For I.V. infusion, dilute to 100 ml and infuse over 1 hour to avoid hypotension.	*Blood:* neutropenia. leukopenia, agranulocytosis, thrombocytopenia, purpura. *CNS:* dizziness, angioedema, headache. *CV:* hypotension with rapid I.V. infusion. *EENT:* glossitis, tinnitus. *GI:* nausea, vomiting, persistent diarrhea, abdominal cramps, enterocolitis, stomatitis, pruritus ani. *GU:* vaginitis. *Local:* pain at injection site. *Skin:* rashes, urticaria. *Other:* hypersensitivity, cholestatic hepatitis.
novobiocin calcium, sodium Albamycin	*Serious infections from sensitive Staphylococcus aureus and Proteus when other antibiotics are contraindicated—* **Adults:** 250 to 500 mg P.O. q 6 hours or 500 mg to 1 g q 12 hours (not to exceed 2 g daily). **Children:** 15 to 45 mg/Kg P.O. daily, divided q 6 hours.	*Blood:* pancytopenia, leukopenia, agranulocytosis, anemia, thrombocytopenia, eosinophilia. *GI:* nausea, vomiting, anorexia, diarrhea, intestinal hemorrhage. *Local:* pain at injection site. *Skin:* urticaria, maculopapular dermatitis. *Other:* erythema multiforme, fever in hypersensitivity reactions, swollen joints, jaundice, overgrowth of nonsusceptible organisms.
polymyxin B sulfate Aerosporin◆	*Acute urinary tract infections or septicemia caused by sensitive P. aeruginosa, or when other antibiotics are ineffective or contraindicated; bacteremia caused by sensitive A. aerogenes and K. pneumoniae or acute urinary tract infections caused by E. coli—* **Adults and children:** 15,000 to 25,000 units/Kg/day I.V. infusion, divided q 12 hours; or 25,000 to 30,000 units/Kg/day, divided q 4 to 8 hours. I.M. advised due to severe pain at injection site. *Meningitis caused by sensitive P. aeruginosa or H. influenzae when other antibiotics ineffective or contraindicated—* **Adults, and children over 2 years:** 50,000 units intrathecally once daily for 3 to 4 days, then 50,000 units every other day for at least 2 weeks after cerebrospinal fluid tests are negative and cerebrospinal fluid sugar is normal.	*CNS:* irritability, drowsiness, weakness, ataxia, respiratory paralysis, headache and meningeal irritation with intrathecal administration, peripheral and perioral paresthesias, convulsions, coma. *CV:* facial flushing. *EENT:* blurred vision. *GU:* nephrotoxicity (albuminuria, cylindruria, hematuria, proteinuria, decreased urine output, increased BUN). *Local:* pain at I.M. injection site, thrombophlebitis with I.V. injection. *Skin:* urticaria. *Other:* hypersensitivity reactions with fever, anaphylaxis.

INTERACTIONS	NURSING CONSIDERATIONS
Antidiarrheal medication (kaolin, pectin, attapulgite): reduced oral absorption of lincomycin as much as 90%. Antidiarrheals should be avoided or given at least 2 hours before lincomycin.	• Contraindicated in known hypersensitivity to clindamycin. Use cautiously in history of GI disorders (especially colitis); asthma or other allergy; in hepatic or renal disease; and in endocrine or metabolic disorders. • Culture and sensitivity tests should be done initially and p.r.n. • For best absorption, instruct patient to take drug with a full glass of water 1 hour before or 2 hours after meals. • Tell patient to take medication exactly as directed, even if he feels better. • Tell patient to report side effects to doctor, especially diarrhea. Warn him not to treat diarrhea himself. Watch for signs of superinfection. • Never treat drug-induced diarrhea with diphenoxylate (Lomotil); may prolong or worsen diarrhea. • Monitor CBC and platelets. Stop drug immediately if neutropenia, leukopenia, or other blood disorders develop. • Give deep I.M. Rotate sites. Warn that I.M. injection may be painful. • When giving I.V., check site daily for phlebitis and irritation. • Monitor hepatic function (alkaline phosphatase, SGOT, SGPT, bilirubin).
None significant.	• Use cautiously in liver disease or blood disorders. Do not use in infants, as it may cause kernicterus. • Culture and sensitivity tests should be done initially and p.r.n. • For best absorption, instruct patient to take drug with a full glass of water 1 hour before or 2 hours after meals. • Tell patient to take medication for as long as prescribed exactly as directed, even if he feels better. • Report side effects, especially skin rash, fever, jaundice, or GI distress. • Stop drug immediately if blood dyscrasias develops. Notify doctor. • Monitor liver function (bilirubin, SGOT, SGPT, alkaline phosphatase). • Monitor CBC, platelet and reticulocyte counts before and during therapy.
None significant.	• Use cautiously in impaired renal function or myasthenia gravis. • Give only to hospitalized patients under constant medical supervision. • For meningitis, must give intrathecally to achieve adequate CSF levels. • Give deep I.M. Warn that injection may be painful. If patient isn't allergic to procaine, use 1% procaine as diluent to decrease pain. Rotate sites. • Don't give solution containing local anesthetics I.V. or intrathecally. • When giving I.V., check site daily for phlebitis and irritation. Dilute each 500,000 units in 300 to 500 ml 5% dextrose in water; infuse over 60 to 90 minutes. • Monitor renal function (BUN, serum creatinine, creatinine clearance, urinary output) before and during therapy. Intake should be sufficient to maintain output at 1,500 ml/day. • Notify doctor immediately if patient develops fever, CNS side effects, rash, or symptoms of nephrotoxicity. • For treatment of anaphylaxis, see p. 1114.

(continued on following page)

NAME	INDICATIONS & DOSAGE	SIDE EFFECTS
polymyxin B sulfate *(continued)*	**Children under 2 years:** 20,000 units intrathecally once daily for 3 to 4 days, then 25,000 units every other day for at least 2 weeks after cerebrospinal fluid tests are negative and cerebrospinal fluid sugar is normal.	
spectinomycin dihydrochloride Trobicin◆	*Gonorrhea—* **Adults:** 2 to 4 g I.M. single dose injected deeply into the upper outer quadrant of the buttock.	*CNS:* insomnia, dizziness. *GI:* nausea. *GU:* decreased urine output. *Local:* pain at injection site. *Skin:* urticaria. *Other:* fever, chills (may mask or delay symptoms of incubating syphilis).
troleandomycin phosphate Tao	*Sensitive pneumococcal pneumonia or group A beta-hemolytic streptococcal respiratory tract infection—* **Adults:** 250 to 500 mg P.O. q 6 hours. **Children:** 6.6 to 11 mg/Kg P.O. daily, q 6 hours.	*GI:* nausea, vomiting, diarrhea. *Skin:* urticaria and rashes in hypersensitivity reactions. *Other:* cholestatic hepatitis (abdominal pain), jaundice, anaphylaxis.
vancomycin hydrochloride Vancocin◆	*Severe staphylococcal infections when other antibiotics ineffective or contraindicated—* **Adults:** 500 mg I.V. q 6 hours or 1 g q 12 hours. **Children:** 44 mg/Kg I.V. daily, divided q 6 hours. **Neonates:** 10 mg/Kg I.V. daily, divided q 6 to 12 hours. *Staphylococcal enterocolitis—* **Adults:** 500 mg P.O. in 30 ml water q 6 hours. **Children:** 44 mg/Kg P.O. daily, divided q 6 hours with 30 ml water.	*Blood:* eosinophilia, transient eosinophilia. *EENT:* tinnitus, ototoxicity (deafness). *GI:* nausea. *GU:* nephrotoxicity (hyaline casts in urine, albuminuria, increased BUN). *Local:* pain or thrombophlebitis with I.V. administration. *Other:* chills, fever, anaphylaxis, overgrowth of nonsusceptible organisms.
vidarabine monohydrate Vira-A	*Herpes simplex virus encephalitis—* **Adults:** 15 mg/Kg/day for 10 days. Slowly infuse the total daily dose by I.V. infusion at a constant rate over 12 to 24 hour period. Avoid rapid or bolus injection.	*Blood:* anemia, neutropenia, thrombocytopenia. *CNS:* tremor, dizziness, hallucinations, confusion, psychosis, ataxia. *GI:* anorexia, nausea, vomiting, diarrhea. *Skin:* pruritus, rash. *Local:* pain at injection site. *Other:* elevated SGOT, bilirubin, weight loss.

INTERACTIONS	NURSING CONSIDERATIONS
None significant.	• Not effective in the treatment of syphilis. • Serologic test for syphilis should be done before treatment dose and 3 months after. • Use 20-gauge needle to administer drug. • Shake vial vigorously after reconstitution and before withdrawing dose. Store at room temperature after reconstitution and use within 24 hours. • Should be reserved for penicillin-resistant strains of gonorrhea.
None significant.	• Use cautiously in hepatic impairment. • Drug is not recommended for routine use. • For best absorption, instruct patient to take drug with a full glass of water 1 hour before or 2 hours after meals. • Tell patient to take medication for as long as prescribed, exactly as directed, even if he feels better. Treat streptococcal infections at least 10 days. • Monitor liver function (bilirubin, SGOT, SGPT, alkaline phosphatase). • Report side effects, especially abdominal pain, nausea, or jaundice. • For treatment of anaphylaxis see p. 1114.
None significant.	• Contraindicated in patients receiving other neurotoxic, nephrotoxic, or ototoxic drugs. Use cautiously in impaired liver, renal function; also in preexisting hearing loss; in patients over 60 years; and in patients with allergies to other antibiotics. • Tell patient to take medication exactly as directed, even if he feels better. Treat staphylococcal endocarditis for at least 3 weeks. • Patients should receive auditory function tests before and during therapy. • Tell patient to report side effects at once, especially dizziness, fullness or ringing in ears. Stop drug immediately. • Do not give drug I.M. • For I.V. infusion, dilute in 200 ml solution and infuse over 20 to 30 minutes. Check site daily for phlebitis and irritation. Report pain at infusion site. Avoid extravasation. Severe irritation and necrosis can result. • Monitor renal function (BUN, serum creatinine, urinalysis, creatinine clearance, urinary output) before and during therapy. Watch for signs of superinfection. • Refrigerate I.V. solution after reconstitution and use within 96 hours. • Oral preparation stable for 2 weeks if refrigerated. • Has been used recently to treat pseudomembranous colitis caused by clindamycin. • For treatment of anaphylaxis, see p. 1114.
None significant.	• Will reduce mortality caused by herpes simplex virus encephalitis from 70% to 28%. No evidence that vidarabine is effective in encephalitis due to other viruses. • Don't give I.M. or S.C. because of low solubility and poor absorption. • Monitor hematologic tests such as hemoglobin, hematocrit, WBC, and platelets during therapy. • Patient with impaired renal function may need dosage adjustment. • Once in solution, vidarabine is stable at room temperature for at least 2 weeks.

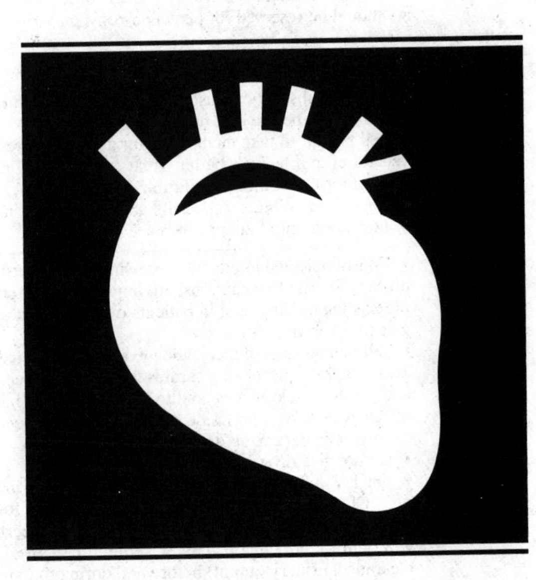

Cardiovascular System

17

Cardiotonic glycosides

deslanoside
digitalis leaf
digitoxin
digoxin
gitalin
lanatoside C
ouabain

Cardiotonic glycosides are used to treat congestive heart failure and atrial tachyarrhythmias. The range between toxic and therapeutic doses is extremely narrow. Toxic doses may vary with absorption rates, drug interactions, serum electrolytes, patient's age and condition, acid-base balance, and organ of excretion malfunction. Glycosides are obtained from plants (mainly digitalis).

Major uses

- Increase circulation impaired by congestive heart failure.
- Alleviation of atrial fibrillation and flutter, paroxysmal atrial tachycardia, and premature extrasystoles.

Mechanism of action

- Increase myocardial contractility (positive inotropic action) by a direct action on the myocardium.
- Increase calcium in myocardial cells to promote muscle protein binding and thus strengthen cardiac contraction.
- Inhibit activity of sodium- and potassium-activated adenosinetriphosphatase (ATPase), enzyme responsible for potassium loss and sodium gain in myocardial cells.
- Decrease impulse conduction through atrioventricular (AV) node to slow heart rate.
- Prolong effective refractory period of AV node through a direct effect and by a sympatholytic effect.

Absorption, distribution, and excretion

DESLANOSIDE
- I.V. or I.M. administration.
- Excreted in urine.

DIGITALIS LEAF
- 20% to 40% of oral dose absorbed.
- Metabolized in liver.
- Excreted in urine and bile.

DIGITOXIN
- 90% to 100% absorbed.
- Distributed through most body tissues.
- Metabolized in liver.

- Excreted in urine and bile.

DIGOXIN, LANATOSIDE C (converts to digoxin in stomach)

- 60% to 85% oral dose absorbed (wide variation between tablets of various manufacturers).
- Intramuscular injection poorly absorbed and is discouraged.
- Not distributed to fatty tissue.
- Excreted in urine.

GITALIN

- Well absorbed with oral administration.
- Excreted in urine primarily.

OUABAIN

- I.V. administration.
- Excreted in urine and via nonbiliary gastrointestinal route.

Onset and duration

Drug	Onset	Peak effect	Half-life	Duration of therapeutic effect
deslanoside	⅙ to ½ hour	1 to 2 hours	36 hours	2 to 5 days
digitalis leaf digitoxin	¼ to 2 hours	4 to 12 hours	5 to 7 days	2 to 3 weeks
digoxin lanatoside C	¼ to ½ hour	1½ to 5 hours	36 hours	2 to 3 days
gitalin	½ to 2 hours	12 to 20 hours	8 to 12 days	10 to 12 days
ouabain	5 to 10 minutes	½ to 2 hours	21 hours	1 to 2.5 days

Combination products

None.

NAME	INDICATIONS & DOSAGE	SIDE EFFECTS
deslanoside Cedilanid-D	*Congestive heart failure, paroxysmal atrial tachycardia, atrial fibrillation and flutter—* **Adults:** loading dose 1.2 to 1.6 mg I.M. or I.V. in 2 divided doses over 24 hours; for maintenance use another glycoside. Not recommended for children.	*Signs of toxicity:* *CNS:* headache, fatigue, malaise, drowsiness, generalized muscle weakness, dizziness, vertigo, syncope, insomnia, agitation, convulsions, opisthotonos, stupor, coma, severe pain, neuralgia, paresthesias, tremors, disorientation, depression, memory impairment, aphasia, delirium, hallucinations, personality changes. *CV:* increased severity of congestive heart failure, arrhythmias (most commonly conduction disturbances with or without AV block, premature ventricular contractions, and supraventricular arrhythmias), hypotension. Toxic effects on heart may be life-threatening and require immediate attention. *EENT:* yellow-green halos around visual images, blurred vision, light flashes, photophobia, diplopia, macropsia, micropsia, retrobulbar neuritis, amblyopia, scotoma. *GI:* anorexia, nausea, abdominal pain, vomiting, diarrhea, excessive salivation, abdominal distention.
digitalis leaf Digifortis, Pil-Digis	*Congestive heart failure, atrial fibrillation, paroxysmal atrial tachycardia, supraventricular tachyarrhythmias—* **Adults:** loading dose 1.2 to 1.8 g P.O. in divided doses over 24 hours; maintenance 100 mg P.O. daily. Not recommended for children.	*Signs of toxicity:* *CNS:* headache, fatigue, malaise, drowsiness, generalized muscle weakness, dizziness, vertigo, syncope, insomnia, agitation, convulsions, opisthotonos, stupor, coma, severe pain, neuralgia, paresthesias, tremors, disorientation, depression, memory impairment, aphasia, personality changes, delirium, hallucinations. *CV:* increased severity of congestive heart failure, arrhythmias (most commonly conduction disturbances with or without AV block, premature ventricular contractions, and supraventricular arrhythmias), hypotension. Toxic effects on heart may be life-threatening and require immediate attention. *EENT:* yellow-green halos around visual images, blurred vision, light flashes, photophobia, diplopia, macropsia, micropsia, retrobulbar neuritis, amblyopia, central scotoma. *GI:* anorexia, nausea, abdominal

INTERACTIONS	NURSING CONSIDERATIONS
Amphotericin B, carbenicillin, sodium polystyrene sulfonate, glucose and insulin infusions, glucagon, ticarcillin, corticosteroids, and diuretics, including chlorthalidone, ethacrynic acid, furosemide, metolazone, and thiazides: hypokalemia, predisposing patient to digitalis toxicity. Monitor serum potassium. *Parenteral calcium, thiazides:* hypercalcemia, predisposing patient to digitalis toxicity. Monitor serum calcium.	• Contraindicated in presence of any digitalis-induced toxicity; ventricular fibrillation; ventricular tachycardia unless caused by congestive heart failure. Administering calcium salts to digitalized patient is contraindicated. Calcium affects contractility and excitability of heart very much as glycosides do and may lead to serious arrhythmias in digitalized patient. Use with extreme caution with acute myocardial infarction, incomplete AV block, chronic constrictive pericarditis, idiopathic hypertrophic subaortic stenosis, renal insufficiency, severe pulmonary disease, hypothyroidism; and in the elderly. • Hypothyroid patients are very sensitive to glycosides; hyperthyroid patients may need larger doses. • Obtain baseline data (heart rate and rhythm, blood pressure, electrolytes, BUN, serum creatinine) before giving first dose. • Question patient about recent use of cardiotonic glycosides (within the previous 2 to 3 weeks) before administering a loading dose. Always divide loading dose over first 24 hours unless clinical situation indicates otherwise. • Use only for rapid digitalization, not maintenance. • Dose is adjusted to patient's clinical condition and is monitored by serum levels of cardiotonic glycoside, calcium, potassium, magnesium, and by EKG. • Take apical-radial pulse for a full minute. Record and report to doctor any significant changes (sudden increase or decrease in rate, pulse deficit, irregular beats, and particularly regularization of a previously irregular rhythm). Check blood pressure and obtain 12-lead EKG with these changes. • Observe eating pattern. Ask patient about nausea, vomiting, anorexia, visual disturbances, and other symptoms of toxicity. • I.M. injection is painful; give I.V. if possible. • Monitor serum potassium carefully. Take corrective action *before* hypokalemia occurs. • For symptoms and treatment of toxicity, see p. 1116.
Aminosalicylic acid, antacids, cholestyramine, kaolin-pectin, neomycin, colestipol: decreased absorption of digitoxin, the main active component of the leaf. Space doses as far as possible from administration of digitalis leaf. *Amphotericin B, carbenicillin, sodium polystyrene sulfonate, glucose and insulin infusions, glucagon, ticarcillin, corticosteroids, and diuretics, including chlorthalidone, ethacrynic acid, furosemide, metolazone, and thiazides:* hypokalemia, predisposing patient to digitalis toxicity. Mon-	• Contraindicated in presence of any digitalis-induced toxicity; ventricular fibrillation; ventricular tachycardia unless caused by congestive heart failure. Administering calcium salts to digitalized patient is contraindicated. Calcium affects contractility and excitability of heart very much as glycosides do and may lead to serious arrhythmias in digitalized patient. Use with extreme caution in acute myocardial infarction, incomplete AV block, chronic constrictive pericarditis, idiopathic hypertrophic subaortic stenosis, renal insufficiency, severe pulmonary disease, hypothyroidism; and in the elderly. • Hypothyroid patients are very sensitive to glycosides; hyperthyroid patients may need larger doses. • Obtain baseline data (heart rate and rhythm, blood pressure, electrolytes, BUN, serum creatinine) before giving first dose. • Question patient about recent use of cardiotonic glycosides (within the previous 2 to 3 weeks) before administering a loading dose. Always divide loading dose over first 24 hours unless clinical situation indicates otherwise. • Dose is adjusted to patient's clinical condition and is monitored by serum levels of cardiotonic glycoside, calcium, potassium, magnesium, and by EKG. • Take apical-radial pulse for a full minute. Record and report to doctor any significant changes (sudden increase or decrease in rate, pulse deficit, irregular beats, and particularly regularization of a previously irregular rhythm). Check blood pressure and obtain 12-lead EKG with these changes. • Observe eating pattern. Ask patient about nausea, vomiting, anorexia,

(continued on following page)

NAME	INDICATIONS & DOSAGE	SIDE EFFECTS
digitalis leaf *(continued)*		pain, vomiting, diarrhea, excessive salivation, abdominal distention.
digitoxin Crystodigin, De-Tone, Purodigin◆	*Congestive heart failure, atrial fibrillation and flutter, paroxysmal atrial tachycardia—* **Adults:** loading dose 1.2 to 1.6 mg I.V. or P.O. in divided doses over 24 hours; maintenance 0.1 mg daily. **Children 2 to 12 years:** loading dose 0.03 mg/Kg or 0.75 mg/m² I.M., I.V., or P.O. in divided doses over 24 hours; maintenance 1/10 loading dose or 0.003 mg/Kg or 0.075 mg/m² daily. Monitor closely for toxicity. **Children 1 to 2 years:** loading dose 0.04 mg/Kg over 24 hours in divided doses; maintenance 0.004 mg/Kg daily. Monitor closely for toxicity. **Children 2 weeks to 1 year:** loading dose 0.045 mg/Kg I.M., I.V., or P.O. in divided doses over 24 hours; maintenance 0.0045 mg/Kg daily. Monitor closely for toxicity. **Premature infants, neonates, severely ill older infants:** loading dose 0.022 mg/Kg I.M., I.V., or P.O. in divided doses over 24 hours; maintenance 0.0022 mg/Kg daily. Monitor closely for toxicity.	*Signs of toxicity:* *CNS:* headache, fatigue, malaise, drowsiness, generalized muscle weakness, dizziness, vertigo, syncope, insomnia, agitation, convulsions, stupor, severe pain, neuralgia, paresthesias, tremors, disorientation, depression, memory impairment, aphasia, delirium, hallucinations. *CV:* increased severity of congestive heart failure, arrhythmias (most commonly conduction disturbances with or without AV block, premature ventricular contractions, and supraventricular arrhythmias), hypotension. Toxic effects on heart may be life-threatening and require immediate attention. *EENT:* yellow-green halos around visual images, blurred vision, light flashes, photophobia, diplopia, macropsia, micropsia, retrobulbar neuritis, amblyopia, central scotoma. *GI:* anorexia, nausea, abdominal pain, vomiting, diarrhea, excessive salivation, abdominal distention.

INTERACTIONS	NURSING CONSIDERATIONS
itor serum potassium. *Parenteral calcium, thiazides:* hypercalcemia, predisposing patient to digitalis toxicity. Monitor serum calcium. *Phenylbutazone, phenobarbital, phenytoin, rifampin:* faster metabolism and shorter duration of action of digitoxin. Observe for underdigitalization.	visual disturbances, and other symptoms of toxicity. • Monitor serum potassium carefully. Take corrective action *before* hypokalemia occurs. • Digitalis leaf is a long-acting drug; watch for cumulative effects. • Withhold for 1 to 2 days before elective electrocardioversion. Adjust dosage after cardioversion. • Instruct patient and responsible family member about drug action, dosage regimen, how to take pulse, reportable signs, and follow-up plans. • Therapeutic blood levels of serum digitoxin (the active agent in the leaf) range from 25 to 35 ng/ml. • For symptoms and treatment of toxicity, see p. 1116.
Aminosalicylic acid, antacids, cholestyramine, colestipol, kaolin-pectin, neomycin: decreased absorption of oral digitoxin. Space dose times as far as possible from oral digitoxin administration. *Amphotericin B, carbenicillin, ticarcillin, sodium polystyrene sulfonate, glucagon, glucose and insulin infusions, corticosteroids, and diuretics, including chlorthalidone, ethacrynic acid, furosemide, metolazone, and thiazides:* hypokalemia, predisposing patient to digitalis toxicity. Monitor serum potassium. *Parenteral calcium, thiazides:* hypercalcemia, predisposing patient to digitalis toxicity. Monitor serum calcium. *Phenylbutazone, phenobarbital, phenytoin, rifampin:* faster metabolism and shorter duration of digitoxin. Observe for underdigitalization.	• Contraindicated in presence of any digitalis-induced toxicity; ventricular fibrillation; ventricular tachycardia unless caused by congestive heart failure. Administering calcium salts to digitalized patient is contraindicated. Calcium affects contractility and excitability of heart very much as glycosides do and may lead to serious arrhythmias in digitalized patient. Use with extreme caution in acute myocardial infarction, incomplete AV block, chronic constrictive pericarditis, idiopathic hypertrophic subaortic stenosis, renal insufficiency, severe pulmonary disease, hypothyroidism; and in the elderly. • Hypothyroid patients are very sensitive to glycosides; hyperthyroid patients may need larger doses. • Obtain baseline data (heart rate and rhythm, blood pressure, electrolytes, BUN, serum creatinine) before giving first dose. • Question patient about recent use of cardiotonic glycosides (within the previous 2 to 3 weeks) before administering a loading dose. Always divide loading dose over first 24 hours unless clinical situation indicates otherwise. • Dose is adjusted to patient's clinical condition and is monitored by serum levels of cardiotonic glycoside, calcium, potassium, magnesium, and by EKG. • Take apical-radial pulse for a full minute. Record and report to doctor any significant changes (sudden increase or decrease in rate, pulse deficit, irregular beats, and particularly regularization of a previously irregular rhythm). Check blood pressure and obtain 12-lead EKG with these changes. • Observe eating pattern. Ask patient about nausea, vomiting, anorexia, visual disturbances, and other symptoms of toxicity. • Watch closely for signs of toxicity, especially in children and the elderly. • Monitor serum potassium carefully. Take corrective action *before* hypokalemia occurs. • I.M. injection is painful; give I.V. if parenteral route is necessary. • Digitoxin is a long-acting drug; watch for cumulative effects. • Withhold for 1 to 2 days before elective electrocardioversion. Adjust dose after cardioversion. • Protect solution from light. • Instruct patient and responsible family member about drug action, dosage regimen, how to take pulse, reportable signs, and follow-up plans. • Do not substitute one brand for another. • Therapeutic blood levels of digitoxin range from 25 to 35 ng/ml. • For symptoms and treatment of toxicity, see p. 1116.

NAME	INDICATIONS & DOSAGE	SIDE EFFECTS
digoxin Lanoxin◆, Masoxin, Rougoxin◆◆, SK-Digoxin	*Congestive heart failure, atrial fibrillation and flutter, paroxysmal atrial tachycardia—* **Adults:** loading dose 0.5 to 1 mg I.V. or P.O. in divided doses over 24 hours; maintenance 0.125 to 0.5 mg I.V. or P.O. daily (average 0.25 mg). Larger doses are often needed for treatment of arrhythmias, depending on patient response. **Children over 2 years:** loading dose 0.06 mg/Kg P.O. divided q 8 hours over 24 hours; maintenance 0.02 mg/Kg P.O. daily divided q 12 hours. **Children 1 month to 2 years:** loading dose 0.06 to 0.075 mg/Kg P.O. divided into three doses over 24 hours; maintenance 0.02 to 0.025 mg/Kg P.O. daily divided q 12 hours. **Neonates under 1 month:** loading dose 0.05 mg/Kg P.O. divided q 8 hours over 24 hours; maintenance 0.0167 mg/Kg P.O. daily divided q 12 hours. **Premature infants:** loading dose 0.04 mg/Kg I.V. divided into 3 doses over 24 hours; maintenance 0.0133 mg/Kg I.V. daily divided q 12 hours.	*Signs of toxicity:* *CNS:* headache, fatigue, malaise, drowsiness, generalized muscle weakness, dizziness, vertigo, syncope, insomnia, agitation, convulsions, opisthotonos, stupor, coma, severe pain, neuralgia, paresthesias, tremors, disorientation, confusion, depression, memory impairment, aphasia, personality changes, delirium, hallucinations. *CV:* increased severity of congestive heart failure, arrhythmias (most commonly conduction disturbances with or without AV block, supraventricular arrhythmias, and premature ventricular contractions), hypotension. Toxic effects on heart may be life-threatening and require immediate attention. *EENT:* yellow-green halos around visual images, blurred vision, light flashes, photophobia, diplopia, macropsia, micropsia, retrobulbar neuritis, amblyopia, central scotoma. *GI:* anorexia, nausea, vomiting, abdominal distention and pain.
gitalin Gitaligin	*Congestive heart failure, atrial fibrillation and flutter, paroxysmal atrial tachycardia—* **Adults:** loading dose 2.5 mg P.O. initially, then 0.75 mg q 6 hours until therapeutic effect is attained (not to exceed 6 mg total in 24 hours); maintenance 0.25 to 1.25 mg daily. Not recommended for children.	*Signs of toxicity:* *CNS:* headache, fatigue, malaise, drowsiness, generalized muscle weakness, dizziness, vertigo, syncope, insomnia, agitation, convulsions, stupor, severe pain, neuralgia, paresthesias, tremors, disorientation, depression, memory impairment, aphasia, delirium, hallucinations. *CV:* increased severity of congestive heart failure, arrhythmias (most commonly conduction disturbances with or without AV block, supraventricular arrhythmias, and premature ventricular contractions), hypotension. Toxic effects on heart may be life-threatening and require immediate attention. *EENT:* yellow-green halos around

INTERACTIONS	NURSING CONSIDERATIONS
Aminosalicylic acid, antacids, cholestyramine, colestipol, kaolin-pectin, neomycin: decreased absorption of oral digoxin. Space dose times as far as possible from oral digoxin administration. *Amphotericin B, carbenicillin, ticarcillin, sodium polystyrene sulfonate, glucagon, glucose and insulin infusions, corticosteroids, and diuretics, including chlorthalidone, ethacrynic acid, furosemide, metolazone, and thiazides:* hypokalemia, predisposing patient to digitalis toxicity. Monitor serum potassium. *Parenteral calcium, thiazides:* hypercalcemia, predisposing patient to digitalis toxicity. Monitor serum calcium.	• Contraindicated in presence of any digitalis-induced toxicity; ventricular fibrillation; ventricular tachycardia unless caused by congestive heart failure. Administering calcium salts to digitalized patient is contraindicated. Calcium affects contractility and excitability of heart very much as glycosides do and may lead to serious arrhythmias in digitalized patient. Use with extreme caution in acute myocardial infarction, incomplete AV block, chronic constrictive pericarditis, idiopathic hypertrophic subaortic stenosis, renal insufficiency, severe pulmonary disease, hypothyroidism; and in the elderly. Dose must be reduced in renal impairment. • Hypothyroid patients are very sensitive to glycosides; hyperthyroid patients may need larger doses. • Obtain baseline data (heart rate and rhythm, blood pressure, electrolytes, BUN, serum creatinine) before giving first dose. • Question patient about recent use of cardiotonic glycosides (within the previous 2 to 3 weeks) before administering a loading dose. Always divide loading dose over first 24 hours unless clinical situation indicates otherwise. • Dose is adjusted to patient's clinical condition and is monitored by serum levels of cardiotonic glycoside, calcium, potassium, magnesium, and by EKG. • Take apical-radial pulse for a full minute. Record and report to doctor any significant changes (sudden increase or decrease in rate, pulse deficit, irregular beats, and particularly regularization of a previously irregular rhythm). Check blood pressure and obtain 12-lead EKG with these changes. • Observe eating pattern. Ask patient about nausea, vomiting, anorexia, visual disturbances, and other symptoms of toxicity. • I.M. injection is poorly and unpredictably absorbed, and is very painful. Give I.V. if parenteral route is necessary. • Monitor serum potassium carefully. Take corrective action *before* hypokalemia occurs. • Withhold for 1 to 2 days before elective electrocardioversion. Adjust dose after cardioversion. • Instruct patient and responsible family member about drug action, dosage regimen, how to take pulse, reportable signs, and follow-up plans. • Don't substitute one brand for another. • Therapeutic blood levels of digoxin range from 0.5 to 2.5 ng/ml. • For symptoms and treatment of toxicity, see p. 1116.
Aminosalicylic acid, antacids, cholestyramine, colestipol, kaolin-pectin, neomycin: decreased absorption of oral gitalin. Space dose times as far as possible from oral gitalin administration. *Amphotericin B, carbenicillin, ticarcillin, sodium polystyrene sulfonate, glucagon, glucose and insulin infusions, corticosteroids, and diuretics, including chlorthalidone,*	• Contraindicated in presence of any digitalis-induced toxicity; ventricular fibrillation; ventricular tachycardia unless caused by congestive heart failure. Administering calcium salts to digitalized patient is contraindicated. Calcium affects contractility and excitability of heart very much as glycosides do and may lead to serious arrhythmias in digitalized patient. Use with extreme caution in acute myocardial infarction, incomplete AV block, chronic constrictive pericarditis, idiopathic hypertrophic subaortic stenosis, renal insufficiency, severe pulmonary disease, hypothyroidism; and in the elderly. • Hypothyroid patients are very sensitive to glycosides; hyperthyroid patients may need larger doses. • Obtain baseline data (heart rate and rhythm, blood pressure, electrolytes, BUN, serum creatinine) before giving first dose. • Question patient about recent use of cardiotonic glycosides (within the previous 2 to 3 weeks) before administering a loading dose. Always divide loading dose over first 24 hours unless clinical situation indicates otherwise. • Dose is adjusted to patient's clinical condition and is monitored by serum levels of cardiotonic glycoside, calcium, potassium, magnesium, and by EKG.

(continued on following page)

NAME	INDICATIONS & DOSAGE	SIDE EFFECTS
gitalin *(continued)*		visual images, blurred vision, light flashes, photophobia, diplopia, macropsia, micropsia, retrobulbar neuritis, amblyopia, central scotoma. *GI:* anorexia, nausea, abdominal distention and pain, vomiting.
lanatoside C Cedilanid◆	*Congestive heart failure, atrial fibrillation and flutter, paroxysmal atrial tachycardia—* **Adults:** average total dose for digitalization is 10 mg P.O. given as follows: loading dose. First day, 3.5 mg; second day, 2.5 mg; third day, 2 mg; thereafter 1.5 mg per day until digitalization obtained; maintenance 0.5 to 1.5 mg daily. Not recommended for children.	*Signs of toxicity:* *CNS:* headache, fatigue, malaise, drowsiness, generalized muscle weakness, dizziness, vertigo, syncope, insomnia, agitation, convulsions, stupor, coma, severe pain, neuralgia, paresthesias, tremors, disorientation, confusion, depression, memory impairment, aphasia, personality changes, delirium, hallucinations. *CV:* increased severity of congestive heart failure, arrhythmias (most commonly conduction disturbances with or without AV block, supraventricular arrhythmias, and premature ventricular contractions), hypotension. Toxic effects on heart may be life-threatening and require immediate attention. *EENT:* yellow-green halos around visual images, blurred vision, light flashes, photophobia, diplopia, macropsia, micropsia, retrobulbar neuritis, amblyopia, central scotoma. *GI:* anorexia, nausea, abdominal distention and pain, vomiting, diarrhea, excessive salivation.

INTERACTIONS	NURSING CONSIDERATIONS
ethacrynic acid, furosemide, metolazone, and thiazides: hypokalemia, predisposing patient to digitalis toxicity. Monitor serum potassium. *Parenteral calcium, thiazides:* hypercalcemia, predisposing patient to digitalis toxicity. Monitor serum calcium.	• Take apical-radial pulse for a full minute. Record and report to doctor any significant changes (sudden increase or decrease in rate, pulse deficit, irregular beats, and particularly regularization of a previously irregular rhythm). Check blood pressure and obtain 12-lead EKG with these changes. • Observe eating pattern. Ask patient about nausea, vomiting, anorexia, visual disturbances, and other symptoms of toxicity. • Monitor serum potassium carefully. Take corrective action *before* hypokalemia occurs. • Gitalin is a long-acting drug; watch for cumulative effects. • Withhold for 1 to 2 days before elective electrocardioversion. Adjust dose after cardioversion. • Instruct patient and responsible family member about drug action, dosage regimen, how to take pulse, reportable signs, and follow-up plans. • For symptoms and treatment of toxicity, see p. 1116.
Aminosalicylic acid, antacids, cholestyramine, kaolin-pectin, neomycin, colestipol: decreased absorption of digoxin formed in stomach from lanatoside C. Space dose times as far as possible from lanatoside C administration. *Amphotericin B, carbenicillin, ticarcillin, sodium polystyrene sulfonate, glucagon, glucose and insulin infusions, corticosteroids, and diuretics, including chlorthalidone, ethacrynic acid, furosemide, metolazone, and thiazides:* hypokalemia, predisposing patient to digitalis toxicity. Monitor serum potassium. *Parenteral calcium, thiazides:* hypercalcemia, predisposing patient to digitalis toxicity. Monitor serum calcium.	• Contraindicated in presence of any digitalis-induced toxicity; ventricular fibrillation; ventricular tachycardia unless caused by congestive heart failure. Administering calcium salts to digitalized patient is contraindicated. Calcium affects contractility and excitability of heart very much as glycosides do and may lead to serious arrhythmias in digitalized patient. Use with extreme caution in acute myocardial infarction, incomplete AV block, chronic constrictive pericarditis, idiopathic hypertrophic subaortic stenosis, renal insufficiency, severe pulmonary disease, hypothyroidism; and in the elderly. Dose should be reduced in renal impairment. • Hypothyroid patients are very sensitive to glycosides; hyperthyroid patients may need larger doses. • Obtain baseline data (heart rate and rhythm, blood pressure, electrolytes, BUN, serum creatinine) before giving first dose. • Question patient about recent use of cardiotonic glycosides (within the previous 2 to 3 weeks) before administering a loading dose. Always divide loading dose over first 24 hours unless clinical situation indicates otherwise. • Dose is adjusted to patient's clinical condition and is monitored by serum levels of cardiotonic glycoside, calcium, potassium, magnesium, and by EKG. • Take apical-radial pulse for a full minute. Record and report to doctor any significant changes (sudden increase or decrease in rate, pulse deficit, irregular beats, and particularly regularization of a previously irregular rhythm). Check blood pressure and obtain 12-lead EKG with these changes. • Observe eating pattern. Ask patient about nausea, vomiting, anorexia, visual disturbances, and other symptoms of toxicity. • Monitor serum potassium carefully. Take corrective action *before* hypokalemia occurs. • Withhold for 1 to 2 days before elective electrocardioversion. Adjust dose after cardioversion. • Instruct patient and responsible family member about drug action, dosage regimen, how to take pulse, reportable signs, and follow-up plans. • For symptoms and treatment of toxicity, see p. 1116.

NAME	INDICATIONS & DOSAGE	SIDE EFFECTS
ouabain	*Congestive heart failure, atrial fibrillation and flutter, paroxysmal atrial tachycardia*— **Adults:** loading dose 0.25 to 0.5 mg by slow I.V. injection divided over 24 hours; for maintenance use another glycoside. Not recommended for children.	*Signs of toxicity:* *CNS:* headache, fatigue, malaise, drowsiness, generalized muscle weakness, dizziness, vertigo, syncope, insomnia, agitation, convulsions, stupor, coma, severe pain, neuralgia, paresthesias, tremors, disorientation, confusion, depression, memory impairment, aphasia, personality changes, delirium, hallucinations. *CV:* increased severity of congestive heart failure, arrhythmias (most commonly conduction disturbances with or without AV block, supraventricular arrhythmias, and premature ventricular contractions), hypotension. Toxic effects on heart may be life-threatening and require immediate attention. *EENT:* yellow-green halos around visual images, blurred vision, light flashes, photophobia, diplopia, macropsia, micropsia, retrobulbar neuritis, amblyopia, central scotoma. *GI:* anorexia, nausea, abdominal distention and pain, vomiting, diarrhea, excessive salivation.

INTERACTIONS	NURSING CONSIDERATIONS
Amphotericin B, carbenicillin, ticarcillin, sodium polystyrene sulfonate, glucagon, glucose and insulin infusions, corticosteroids, and diuretics, including chlorthalidone, ethacrynic acid, furosemide, metolazone, and thiazides: hypokalemia, predisposing patient to toxicity. Monitor serum potassium. *Parenteral calcium, thiazide:* hypercalcemia, predisposing patient to toxicity. Monitor serum calcium.	• Contraindicated in presence of any digitalis-induced toxicity; ventricular fibrillation; ventricular tachycardia unless caused by congestive heart failure. Administering calcium salts to digitalized patient is contraindicated. Calcium affects contractility and excitability of heart very much as glycosides do and may lead to serious arrhythmias in digitalized patient. Use with extreme caution in acute myocardial infarction, incomplete AV block, chronic constrictive pericarditis, idiopathic hypertrophic subaortic stenosis, renal insufficiency, severe pulmonary disease, hypothyroidism; and in the elderly. Dose should be reduced in renal impairment. • Hypothyroid patients are very sensitive to glycosides; hyperthyroid patients may need larger doses. • Obtain baseline data (heart rate and rhythm, blood pressure, electrolytes, BUN, serum creatinine) before giving first dose. • Question patient about recent use of cardiotonic glycosides (within the previous 2 to 3 weeks) before administering a loading dose. Always divide loading dose over first 24 hours unless clinical situation indicates otherwise. • Use only for rapid digitalization, not maintenance. • Dose is adjusted to patient's clinical condition and is monitored by serum levels of cardiotonic glycoside, calcium, potassium, magnesium, and by EKG. • Take apical-radial pulse for a full minute. Record and report to doctor any significant changes (sudden increase or decrease in rate, pulse deficit, irregular beats, and particularly regularization of a previously irregular rhythm). Check blood pressure and obtain 12-lead EKG with these changes. • Observe eating pattern. Ask patient about nausea, vomiting, anorexia, visual disturbances, and other symptoms of toxicity. • I.M. route is painful; absorption is unpredictable. Not recommended. • Monitor serum potassium carefully. Take corrective action *before* hypokalemia occurs. • Not a digitalis glycoside; derived from seeds of *strophanthus gratus* plant. • For symptoms and treatment of toxicity, see p. 1116.

18

Antiarrhythmics

atropine sulfate
bretylium tosylate
disopyramide
disopyramide phosphate
isoproterenol hydrochloride
lidocaine hydrochloride
phenytoin
phenytoin sodium
procainamide hydrochloride
propranolol hydrochloride
quinidine bisulfate
quinidine gluconate
quinidine polygalacturonate
quinidine sulfate

Antiarrhythmics are used to treat atrial and ventricular arrhythmias of various causes, including those secondary to myocardial infarction or cardiac glycoside toxicity. As a group, they have low toxic-therapeutic ratio, and their toxic effects are usually serious. Monitoring therapy is imperative. Before antiarrhythmic treatment is undertaken, underlying causes (if known) should be corrected when possible, as in electrolyte imbalances or hypoxia. Two alternative antiarrhythmic treatments are effective and may be used if drug therapy fails: electrocardioversion and electrical pacemakers.

Major uses

- Treatment of atrial and ventricular arrhythmias of various causes.
- Treatment and prophylaxis of arrhythmias after myocardial infarction.

Mechanism of action

- Disopyramide, quinidine, and procainamide decrease cardiac automaticity, increase the cardiac refractory period, reduce conduction impulses through the A-V conduction system, and decrease transport of sodium through cardiac membranes.
- Phenytoin and lidocaine decrease cardiac automaticity, increase conduction of impulses

through the A-V conduction system, and increase transport of potassium through cardiac membranes.

- Propranolol decreases conduction of impulses through the A-V conduction system, increases the refractory period, and decreases transport of sodium and potassium through cardiac membranes.
- Bretylium acts as an antiadrenergic, with no significant membrane effect. Its antiarrhythmic action may be mediated by the sympathetic nervous system. Early effects may be due to sympathetic stimulation resulting from the inhibition or re-uptake and resultant accumulation of norepinephrine at the nerve terminal; later effects may be due to effective adrenergic blockade resulting from depletion of releasable norepinephrine stores.
- Atropine blocks the vagal effects on the S-A node pacemaker, relieving severe nodal or sinus bradycardia, or A-V block. Increased conduction through the A-V node speeds the heart rate.
- Isoproterenol, a potent beta-adrenergic-cardiac stimulator, increases ventricular automaticity and conduction through the A-V node.

Absorption, distribution, and excretion

- Most are readily absorbed orally, except bretylium.
- Bretylium is poorly absorbed from the gastrointestinal tract so therapeutic blood levels cannot be maintained; given parenterally.
- Lidocaine is absorbed orally, but is metabolized so rapidly that therapeutic blood levels can't be maintained; given parenterally.
- Phenytoin is usually given orally or intravenously.
- All are widely distributed through body tissues and metabolize in the liver. Metabolites are excreted in urine.

Onset and duration

Drug	Onset	Peak effects	Duration of therapeutic effects
atropine	I.V.: immediate	within minutes	4 to 6 hours
bretylium	I.V.: within minutes I.M.: up to 2 hours	within 20 minutes 6 to 9 hours	up to 10 hours
disopyramide	P.O.: 30 minutes	2 hours	6 to 8 hours
isoproterenol	I.V.: immediate	within minutes	brief
lidocaine	I.V.: immediate I.M.: 5 to 15 minutes	immediate (after I.V. bolus)	I.V.: 10 to 20 minutes I.M.: 60 to 90 minutes
phenytoin	I.V.: immediate P.O.: 2 hours	I.V.: immediate P.O.: 6 hours	up to 24 hours
procainamide	I.V.: immediate P.O.: 30 minutes	I.V.: 25 to 60 minutes P.O.: 60 minutes	3 to 4 hours
propranolol	I.V.: immediate P.O.: 30 minutes	I.V.: 2 to 4 hours P.O.: 60 to 90 minutes	3 to 6 hours
quinidine (base)	P.O., I.V., I.M.: 30 minutes	P.O.: 1 to 3 hours I.V.: immediate I.M.: 30 to 90 minutes	6 to 8 hours

Combination products
None.

COMMON ARRHYTHMIAS

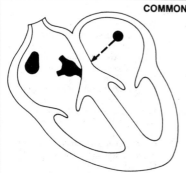

PACs

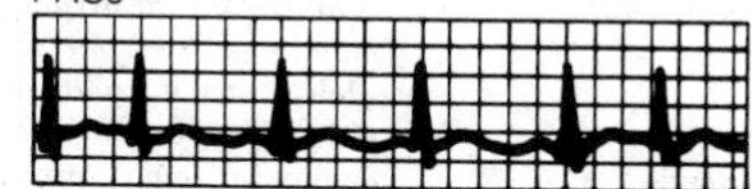

Treatment: Often none; possibly quinidine or procainamide.

PAT

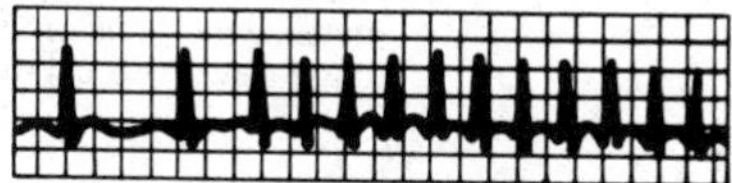

Treatment: Carotid sinus pressure or propranolol.

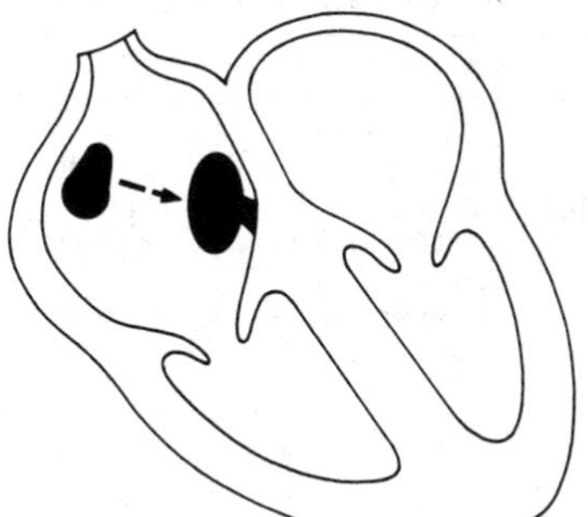

A-V BLOCK — SECOND DEGREE

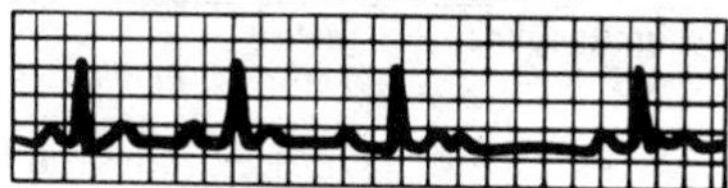

Treatment: Atropine, isoproterenol, or pacemaker.

A-V BLOCK — THIRD DEGREE

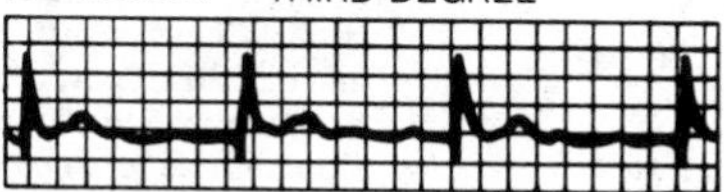

Treatment: Atropine, isoproterenol, or pacemaker.

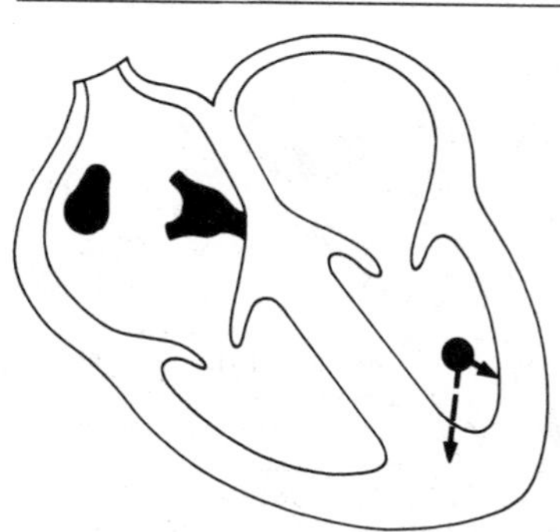

PVCs

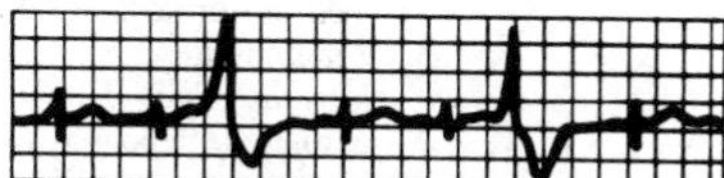

Treatment: Lidocaine, quinidine, or procainamide.

VENTRICULAR TACHYCARDIA

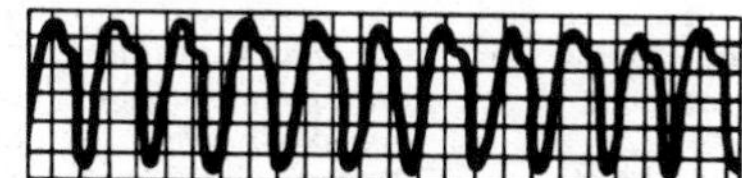

Treatment: Cardioversion (except for patients on digitalis) or lidocaine.

NAME	INDICATIONS & DOSAGE	SIDE EFFECTS
atropine sulfate	*Bradycardia, bradyarrhythmia (junctional or escape rhythm)*— **Adults:** usually 0.5 to 1 mg I.V. push; repeat q 5 minutes, to maximum 2 mg. Lower doses (less than 0.5 mg) can cause bradycardia. **Children:** 0.01 mg/Kg dose up to maximum 0.4 mg; or 0.3 mg/M^2 dose; may repeat q 4 to 6 hours.	*Blood:* leukocytosis. *CNS:* with doses greater than 5 mg—headache, restlessness, speech difficulty, ataxia, excitement, disorientation, hallucinations, delirium, coma. *CV:* 1 to 2 mg—tachycardia, palpitations; greater than 2 mg—extreme tachycardia. *EENT:* 1 mg—slight mydriasis, photophobia; 2 mg—blurred vision, mydriasis. *GI:* dry mouth (common even at low doses), thirst, constipation. *GU:* urinary retention. *Skin:* 2 mg—flushed, dry skin; 5 mg or more—hot, dry, reddened skin.
bretylium tosylate Bretylol	**Adults:** *Ventricular fibrillation*—5 mg/Kg by rapid I.V. injection. If necessary, increase dose to 10 mg/Kg and repeat q 15 to 30 minutes until 30 mg/Kg has been given. *Other ventricular arrhythmias*—initially, 500 mg diluted to 50 ml with 5% dextrose or normal saline and infused I.V. over more than 8 minutes at 5 to 10 mg/Kg. Dose may be repeated in 1 to 2 hours. Thereafter, dose q 6 to 8 hours. *I.V. maintenance*—infused in diluted solution of 500 ml 5% dextrose or normal saline at 1 to 2 mg/minute. *I.M. injection*—5 to 10 mg/Kg undiluted. Repeat in 1 to 2 hours. Not recommended for children.	*CNS:* vertigo, dizziness, lightheadedness, syncope (usually secondary to hypotension). *CV:* severe hypotension, transient hypertension, increased frequency of arrhythmias, bradycardia, anginal pain. *GI:* severe nausea, vomiting (with rapid infusion).
disopyramide Rythmodan◆ **disopyramide phosphate** Norpace◆	*Premature ventricular contractions (unifocal, multifocal, or coupled); ventricular tachycardia not severe enough to require electric cardioversion*— **Adults:** Usual maintenance dose 150 to 200 mg P.O. q 6 hours; for lightweight patients or those with renal, hepatic, or cardiac impairment—100 mg P.O. q 6 hours. Recommended doses in advanced renal insufficency: Creatinine clearance 15 to 40 ml/minute: 100 mg q 10 hours; creatinine clearance 5 to 15 ml/minute: 100	*CNS:* dizziness, fatigue, muscle weakness, syncope. *CV:* hypotension, edema, weight gain, shortness of breath. *EENT:* blurred vision. *GI:* nausea, vomiting, anorexia, bloating, abdominal pain, constipation, dry mouth. *GU:* urinary retention and hesitancy. *Skin:* rash in 1% to 3% of patients.

◆ Also available in Canada.
◆◆ Available in Canada only.
Unmarked trade names available in United States only.

INTERACTIONS	NURSING CONSIDERATIONS
Methotrimeprazine: may produce extra-pyramidal symptoms. Monitor patient carefully.	• Side effects vary considerably with dose. Most common are dry mouth, which can be treated with pilocarpine syrup, and thirst. Recommend sucking sour hard candy. • Watch for tachycardia in cardiac patients; report to doctor. • Antidote for atropine overdose is physostigmine salicylate. • Other anticholinergic drugs may increase vagal blockage. • For symptoms and treatment of toxicity, see p. 1115.
All antihypertensives: may potentiate hypotension. Monitor blood pressure.	• Contraindicated in digitalis-induced arrhythmias. Use cautiously in fixed cardiac output to avoid severe and sudden drop in blood pressure. • Monitor blood pressure, heart rate, and rhythm frequently. Notify doctor immediately of any change. If supine systolic blood pressure falls below 75 mm Hg, notify doctor, who may order norepinephrine or dopamine, or volume expansion to raise blood pressure. • Keep patient supine until tolerance to hypotension develops. • Follow dosage directions carefully to avoid nausea and vomiting. • Give I.V. injections for ventricular fibrillation as rapidly as possible. Do not dilute. • Rotate I.M. injection sites, and don't exceed 5 ml volume. Do not dilute. Do not inject into or near major nerve sites. • To be used with other cardioresuscitative measures. • Avoid subtherapeutic doses (less than 5 mg/Kg), since such doses may cause hypotension. • Ventricular tachycardia and other ventricular arrhythmias respond less rapidly to treatment than does ventricular fibrillation. • Dosage should be decreased in renal impairment. • Monitor carefully if pressor amines (sympathomimetics) are given to correct hypotension, as bretylium potentiates pressor amines. • Not first-line therapy; used for refractory arrhythmias only. Ineffective treatment for atrial arrhythmias. • Observe for increased anginal pain in susceptible patients. • Observe patient for side effects and notify doctor.
None significant.	• Contraindicated in cardiogenic shock or second- or third-degree heart block with no pacemaker. Use cautiously in congestive heart failure, underlying conduction abnormalities, urinary tract diseases (especially prostatic hypertrophy), hepatic or renal impairment, myasthenia gravis, glaucoma. Adjust dosage in renal insufficiency. • Discontinue if heart block develops, if QRS complex widens by more than 25%, or if QT interval lengthens by more than 25% above baseline. • Correct any underlying electrolyte abnormalities before use. • Watch for recurrence of arrhythmias; check for side effects; notify doctor. • Check apical pulse before administering drug. Notify doctor if pulse is less than 60 beats per minute or greater than 120 beats per minute. • Teach patient the importance of taking drug on time, exactly as prescribed. To do this, he may have to use an alarm clock for night dosages. • Relieve discomfort of dry mouth with chewing gum or hard candy. • Manage constipation with proper diet or bulk laxatives. • Use of disopyramide with other antiarrhythmics may cause further myocardial depression.

NAME	INDICATIONS & DOSAGE	SIDE EFFECTS
isoproterenol hydrochloride Isuprel◆	*Bradyarrhythmia—* **Adults:** constant infusion or drip of 2 mg in 500 ml 5% dextrose in water at 0.1 to 0.2 mg/minute, ranging from 0.5 to 0.3 mg/minute. Infusion should be adjusted to maintain a ventricular rate of 60 to 70/minute. **Children:** titrate drip to child's response using 1 mg/100 ml 5% dextrose in water I.V.	*CNS:* headache, nervousness, tremors. *CV:* hypotension or hypertension, tachycardia, palpitations, ventricular tachycardia, ventricular fibrillation. *Skin:* flushing of face, sweating.
lidocaine hydrochloride Lido Pen Auto-Injector, Xylocaine◆	*Ventricular arrhythmias from myocardial infarction or cardiac glycosides, ventricular tachycardia—* **Adults:** 50 to 100 mg (1 mg/Kg) I.V. bolus at 25 to 50 mg/minute. Give half this amount to elderly or lightweight patients, and to those with congestive heart failure or hepatic disease. Repeat bolus q 3 to 5 minutes until arrhythmias subside or side effects develop. Don't exceed 300 mg total bolus. Simultaneously, begin constant infusion: 1 to 4 mg/minute. Use lower dose in those with congestive heart failure or hepatic disease, or in elderly or lightweight patients. If single bolus has been given, repeat smaller bolus 15 to 20 minutes after start of infusion to maintain therapeutic serum level. After 24 hours continuous infusion, decrease rate by half. *I.M. administration:* 200 to 300 mg in deltoid muscle only. Recommended only in emergencies when I.V. therapy isn't possible and the benefits of using this route outweigh risks.	*CNS:* confusion, lethargy, stupor, restlessness, slurred speech, euphoria, depression, light-headedness, muscle twitches, convulsions, coma. *CV:* hypotension, bradycardia, further arrhythmias. *EENT:* tinnitus, blurred or double vision. *Other:* anaphylaxis.
phenytoin Dilantin Infatab◆, Dilantin Pediatric **phenytoin sodium** Dantoin◆◆, Dihycon, Dilantin◆, Di-Phen, Diphenylan Sodium, EKKO, Toin Unicelles	*Ventricular arrhythmias unresponsive to lidocaine or procainamide; supraventricular and ventricular arrhythmias induced by cardiac glycosides—* **Adults:** loading dose 1 g P.O. divided over first 24 hours, followed by 500 mg daily for 2 days, then maintenance dose 300 mg P.O. daily; 250 mg I.V. over 5	*Blood:* thrombocytopenia, leukopenia, agranulocytosis, pancytopenia, lymphadenopathy, megaloblastic anemia. *CNS:* ataxia, slurred speech, insomnia, headache, muscle twitching, lethargy. *CV:* severe hypotension, vascular collapse (with rapid I.V. infusions greater than 50 mg/minute), vasodila-

INTERACTIONS	NURSING CONSIDERATIONS
Propranolol: may inhibit the beta adrenergic effects of isoproterenol. Use together cautiously.	• Contraindicated in tachycardia caused by cardiac glycoside intoxication as a result of I.V. push. Use with caution in coronary insufficiency, diabetes, hyperthyroidism, cardiac failure with limited cardiac reserve, sensitivity to sympathomimetic amines. • Adjust speed of infusion to heart rate, ideally 90 to 100 beats per minute. If heart rate exceeds 110 beats per minute, decrease infusion. Heart rate in excess of 130 beats per minute may induce ventricular arrhythmias. • Never leave patient receiving an isoproterenol infusion unattended. He should be on a cardiac monitor the entire time. Time infusion and monitor to heart rate desired. Use an infusion pump or microdropper for accurate and safe dosing, especially for infusions lasting longer than crisis therapy. • Infusions can usually be stopped when stable supraventricular rhythm (sinus rhythm or atrial fibrillation) is obtained. Closely monitor vital signs. • Isoproterenol is usually used only after atropine has failed. • Side effects vary greatly according to dose and are short-lived. A decrease in dose usually terminates side effects.
Barbiturates: may decrease patient's response to lidocaine. Adjust dose. *Phenytoin;* additive cardiac depressant effects. Monitor carefully. *Procainamide:* may increase neurologic side effects. Monitor carefully.	• Contraindicated in complete or second-degree heart block. Use of lidocaine with epinephrine (for local anesthesia) to treat arrhythmias contraindicated. Use with caution in congestive heart failure, renal or hepatic disease, or in elderly or lightweight patients. Such patients will need a reduced dose. • If toxic signs (dizziness) occur, stop drug at once and tell doctor. Continued infusion could lead to convulsions and coma. Give O_2 via nasal cannula, if not contraindicated. Keep O_2 and CPR equipment handy. • Patients receiving infusions must be *attended at all times.* Use an infusion pump or a microdropper and timer for monitoring infusion precisely. Never exceed an infusion rate of 4 mg/minute, if possible. A faster rate greatly increases the risk of toxicity. • Monitor patient's response, especially blood pressure, serum electrolytes, BUN, and creatinine. Notify doctor promptly if abnormalities develop. • A bolus dose not followed by infusion will have a short-lived effect. • A patient who has received lidocaine I.M. will show a 7-fold increase in serum CPK level. Such CPK originates in the skeletal muscle, not the heart. Test isoenzymes if using I.M. route. • For treatment of anaphylaxis, see p. 1114.
Alcohol, barbiturates, folic acid, Loxitane: monitor for decreased phenytoin activity. *Oral anticoagulants, antihistamines, chloramphenicol, diazepam, diazoxide, disulfiram, INH, phenylbutazone,*	• Contraindicated in heart block, sinus bradycardia, Stokes-Adams attacks. Use cautiously in congestive heart failure, hepatic or renal dysfunction, elderly or debilitated patients, hypotension, myocardial insufficiency, respiratory depression. Cardiac patients on thyroid replacement therapy should be given I.V. phenytoin cautiously to prevent supraventricular tachycardia. • Don't stop abruptly in epileptic patients; this may precipitate seizures. • Administer drug slow I.V. push, not to exceed 50 mg/minute in adults. • Monitor blood pressure and EKG. Notify doctor if side effects occur. • Don't mix with 5% dextrose I.V. fluids, as crystallization will occur.

(continued on following page)

NAME	INDICATIONS & DOSAGE	SIDE EFFECTS
phenytoin *(continued)*	minutes until arrhythmias subside, side effects develop, or 1 g has been given. Infusion rate should never exceed 50 mg/minute (slow I.V. push). *Alternate method:* 100 mg I.V. q 15 minutes until side effects develop, arrhythmias are controlled, or 1 g has been given. I.M. dose not recommended because of pain and erratic absorption. **Children:** 3 to 8 mg/Kg P.O. or slow I.V. daily or 250 mg/M² daily given as single dose or divided in 2 doses.	tion, asystole, ventricular fibrillation, A-V block. *EENT:* nystagmus, diplopia, blurred vision. *GI:* gingival hyperplasia, nausea, vomiting, constipation. *Skin:* rash (morbilliform most common), dermatitis (bullous, exfoliative, purpuric), lupus erythematosus, Stevens-Johnson syndrome. *Other:* dysarthria, toxic hepatitis, hypoglycemia.
procainamide hydrochloride Pronestyl◆, Sub-Quin	**Adults:** *Premature ventricular contractions, ventricular tachycardia, atrial arrhythmias unresponsive to quinidine, paroxymal atrial tachycardia*—100 mg q 5 minutes slow I.V. push, no faster than 25 to 50 mg/minute until arrhythmias disappear, side effects develop, or 1 g has been given. Once arrhythmias disappear, give continuous infusion of 2 to 6 minute. Usual effective dose 500 to 600 mg. If arrhythmias recur, repeat bolus as above and increase infusion rate; 0.5 to 1 g I.M. q 4 to 8 hours until oral therapy begins. *Loading dose for atrial fibrillation or paroxysmal atrial tachycardia*—1 to 1.25 g P.O. If arrhythmias persist after 1 hour, give additional 750 mg. If no change occurs, give 500 mg to 1 g q 2 hours until arrhythmias disappear or side effects occur. Maintenance 0.5 to 1 g q 4 to 6 hours. *Loading dose for ventricular tachycardia*—1 g P.O. Maintenance 50 mg/Kg daily given at 3-hour intervals; average 250 to 500 mg q 3 hours.	*Blood:* thrombocytopenia, agranulocytosis, hemolytic anemia, increased ANA titer. *CNS:* psychosis, hallucinations, confusion, convulsions, hyperactivity, depression. *CV:* severe hypotension, bradycardia, A-V block, ventricular fibrillation (after parenteral use). *GI:* nausea, vomiting, anorexia, diarrhea, bitter taste. *Skin:* rash. *Other:* fever, lupus erythematosus syndrome (especially if drug is administered over long periods), myalgia, hepatitis.

INTERACTIONS	NURSING CONSIDERATIONS
phenyramidol, salicylates, sulfamethizole, valproate: monitor for increased phenytoin activity.	Flush I.V. line with saline before and after administration. • Watch patients on phenytoin and other antiarrhythmics (disopyramide, quinidine, procainamide, propranolol) closely for signs of additive cardiac depression. • Phenytoin can be diluted in normal saline and infused without precipitation. Such infusions should not take longer than 1 hour. • Shake oral suspensions well to make dosage uniform. After giving suspension by nasogastric tube, flush tube with water to facilitate passage to stomach. • Give drug with food or large glass of water to minimize gastric irritation. • Avoid I.M. route of administration. • Teach patient importance of taking drug on time, exactly as prescribed. • Dose should be decreased in hepatic dysfunction. • Serum levels greater than 20 mcg/ml may be toxic. The difference between therapeutic and toxic levels of phenytoin in the blood is very slight. If toxic symptoms occur, draw blood for serum level determination. • Stress need for good oral hygiene, to minimize gingival hyperplasia. • Uremic patients may require dose adjustment for stabilization. • Patients concurrently on phenytoin and barbiturates, prednisone, or isoniazid should have serum phenytoin levels checked frequently. Observe for phenytoin toxicity and for failure to respond adequately to phenytoin. • Patients concurrently on digitoxin and phenytoin may need larger doses. • Warn patient not to drink alcohol as he may lose control of previously stable antiarrhythmic effects.
None significant.	• Contraindicated in hypersensitivity to procaine and related drugs; in those with complete, second-, or third-degree heart block unassisted by electric pacemaker, or with myasthenia gravis. Use with caution in congestive heart failure or other conduction disturbances, such as bundle branch block or cardiac glycoside intoxication, or with hepatic or renal insufficiency. • Patients receiving infusions must be *attended at all times.* Use an infusion pump or a microdropper and timer to monitor the infusion precisely. • Monitor blood pressure and EKG continuously during I.V. administration. Watch for prolonged Q-T and Q-R intervals, heart block, or increased arrhythmias. If these occur, withhold drug, obtain rhythm strip, and notify doctor immediately. • Keep patient in supine position for I.V. administration. • Watch closely for side effects and notify doctor if they occur. Instruct patient to report fever, rash, muscle pain, diarrhea, or pleuritic chest pain. • Decrease dose in hepatic and renal dysfunction, and give over 6 hours. Half-life of procainamide is increased as much as threefold in these states. • Patient with congestive heart failure has a lower volume of distribution and can be treated with lower doses. • Positive antinuclear antibody titer common in about 60% of patients who don't have symptoms of lupus erythematosus syndrome. This response seems related to prolonged use, not dosage. • After long-standing atrial fibrillation, restoration of normal rhythm may result in thromboembolism, due to dislodgement of thrombi from atrial wall. Anticoagulation usually advised, before restoration of normal sinus rhythm. • Stress importance of taking drug exactly as prescribed. Patient may have to set an alarm clock for night dosage.

NAME	INDICATIONS & DOSAGE	SIDE EFFECTS
propranolol hydrochloride Inderal◆	*Supraventricular, ventricular, and atrial arrhythmias; tachyarrhythmias due to excessive catecholamine action during anesthesia, hyperthyroidism, and pheochromocytoma; hypertension and angina—* **Adults:** 1 to 3 mg I.V. diluted in 50 ml 5% dextrose in water or normal saline infused slowly, not to exceed 1 mg/minute. After 3 mg have been infused, another dose may be given in 2 minutes; subsequent doses no sooner than q 4 hours. Maintenance 10 to 80 mg P.O. t.i.d. or q.i.d. Value and safety of doses greater than 320 mg/daily has not been established.	*Blood:* eosinophilia, thrombocytopenia, agranulocytosis. *CNS:* giddiness, depression, hallucinations, light-headedness, insomnia, weakness, fatigue, short-term memory loss, disorientation to time and place, emotional liability, clouded sensorium. *CV:* severe hypotension, bradycardia, congestive heart failure, angina, myocardial infarction, syncope, shock. *EENT:* visual disturbances. *GI:* nausea, vomiting, abdominal cramps, diarrhea, constipation. *Metabolic:* hypoglycemia without symptoms. *Skin:* rash, reversible alopecia. *Other:* bronchospasm, wheezing, asthma, fever, laryngospasm.
quinidine bisulfate (66% quinidine base) Biquin Durules◆◆ **quinidine gluconate** (62% quinidine base) Quinaglute Dura-Tabs◆, Quinate◆◆ **quinidine polygalacturonate** (60.5% quinidine base) Cardioquin◆ **quinidine sulfate** (83% quinidine base) CinQuin, Quinidex Extentabs◆, Quinora	*Atrial flutter or fibrillation—* **Adults:** 200 mg P.O. q 2 to 3 hours for 5 to 8 doses with subsequent daily increases until sinus rhythm is restored or toxic effects develop. Administer quinidine only after digitalization to avoid increasing A-V block. Maximum 3 to 4 g daily. *Congestive heart failure, hepatic disease—* **Adults:** quinidine sulfate or equivalent base 200 mg P.O. q 6 hours. *Paroxysmal supraventricular tachycardia—* **Adults:** 400 to 600 mg I.M. q 2 to 3 hours until toxic side effects develop or arrhythmia subsides. *Premature atrial and ventricular contractions; paroxysmal atrioventricular junctional rhythm; paroxysmal atrial tachycardia, fibrillation, and flutter; paroxysmal ventricular tachycardia; maintenance after cardioversion of atrial fibrillation or flutter—*	*Blood:* hemolytic anemia, thrombocytopenia, agranulocytosis. *CNS:* vertigo, headache, confusion, restlessness, cold sweat, pallor, fainting. *CV:* premature ventricular contractions; severe hypotension; SA and A-V block; ventricular fibrillation, tachycardia; aggravated congestive heart failure; EKG changes (particularly widening of QRS complex, notched P waves, widened QT interval, ST segment depression); cardiac arrest. *EENT:* tinnitus, excessive salivation, visual disturbances. *GI:* diarrhea, nausea, vomiting. *Skin:* rash, petechial hemorrhage of buccal mucosa. *Other:* angioedema, acute asthmatic attack, respiratory arrest, fever, cinchonism, nausea, vomiting, diarrhea, light-headedness, headache, vertigo, neurologic changes, emotional reactions, blurred vision, optic and auditory nerve damage.

INTERACTIONS	NURSING CONSIDERATIONS
Insulin, hypoglycemic drugs (oral): can alter requirements for these drugs in previously stabilized diabetics. Monitor for hypoglycemia. *Cardiac glycosides:* caused excessive bradycardia and increased depressant effect on myocardium. Use together cautiously. *Aminophylline:* antagonized beta blocking effects of propranolol. Use together cautiously. *Isoproterenol, glucagon:* antagonized propranolol effect. May be used therapeutically and in emergencies. *Indomethacin:* possible decreased antihypertensive response. Monitor B.P.	• Contraindicated in diabetes mellitus, asthma, or allergic rhinitis; during ethyl ether anesthesia; in sinus bradycardia and in heart block greater than first degree; in cardiogenic shock; in right ventricular failure secondary to pulmonary hypertension. Use with caution in congestive heart failure or respiratory disease. • Always withdraw drug slowly. Abrupt withdrawal might precipitate myocardial infarction or aggravate angina, thyrotoxicosis, or pheochromocytoma. Abrupt withdrawal in thyrotoxicosis may exacerbate hyperthyroidism or precipitate thyroid storm. In thyrotoxicosis, propranolol may mask clinical signs of hyperthyroidism. • *Don't discontinue* before surgery for pheochromocytoma. Before any surgical procedure, notify anesthesiologist that patient is on propranolol. • Double-check dose and route. I.V. doses much smaller than P.O. • Check apical pulse rate and blood pressure before giving drug. If extremes in pulse rate, withhold drug and notify doctor at once. Severe bradycardia may be treated with atropine 0.25 to 1 mg I.V. • After long-standing atrial fibrillation, restoration of normal sinus rhythm may result in thromboembolism due to dislodgement of thrombi from atrial wall. Anticoagulation often advised before restoration of normal atrial rhythm. • Monitor blood pressure, EKG, heart rate, and rhythm frequently, especially during I.V. administration. When propranolol is used with other antihypertensives, monitor blood pressure while patient's sitting and standing. • Auscultate patient's lungs for rales and his heart for gallop rhythm or for third or fourth heart sounds. If these develop, notify doctor at once.
Acetazolamide, antacids, sodium bicarbonate: may increase quinidine blood levels due to alkaline urine. Monitor for increased effect. *Barbiturates, phenytoin:* may antagonize quinidine activity. Monitor for decreased quinidine effect.	• Contraindicated in cardiac glycoside toxicity when A-V conduction is grossly impaired; complete A-V block with A-V nodal or idioventricular pacemaker. Use with caution in myasthenia gravis. Anticholinergic drug doses may have to be increased. • Dosage varies—some patients may require drug q 4 hours, others q 6 hours. Titrate dose by both clinical response and blood levels. • When changing route of administration, alter dosage to compensate for variations in quinidine base content. • Check apical pulse rate and blood pressure before starting therapy. For extremes in pulse rate, withhold drug and notify doctor at once. • Lidocaine may be effective in treating quinidine-induced arrhythmias, since it increases A-V conduction. • GI side effects, especially diarrhea, are signs of toxicity. Notify doctor. Check quinidine blood levels, which are toxic when greater than 0.08 mg/ml. Decrease GI symptoms by giving with meals or antacids. Monitor drug response carefully. Doctor may order amphogel, since it doesn't affect quinidine absorption. • After long-standing atrial fibrillation, restoration of normal sinus rhythm may result in thromboembolism due to dislodgement of thrombi from atrial wall. Anticoagulation often advised before restoration of normal atrial rhythm. • Never use discolored (brownish) quinidine solution.

(continued on following page)

NAME	INDICATIONS & DOSAGE	SIDE EFFECTS
quinidine *(continued)*	**Adults:** test dose 50 to 200 mg P.O., then monitor vital signs before beginning therapy. Quinidine sulfate or equivalent base 200 to 400 mg P.O. q 4 to 6 hours; or initially, quinidine gluconate 600 mg I.M., then up to 400 mg q 2 hours, p.r.n.; or quinidine gluconate 800 mg I.V. diluted in 40 ml of 5% dextrose in water, infused at 1 mg/minute. **Children:** test dose 2 mg/Kg; 3 to 6 mg/Kg q 2 to 3 hours for 5 doses P.O. daily.	

INTERACTIONS	NURSING CONSIDERATIONS

19

Antihypertensives

alkavervir
alseroxylon
clonidine hydrochloride
cryptenamine
deserpidine
diazoxide
guanethidine sulfate
hydralazine hydrochloride
mecamylamine hydrochloride
methyldopa
metoprolol tartrate
nitroprusside sodium
pargyline hydrochloride
phenoxybenzamine hydrochloride
phentolamine
prazosin hydrochloride
propranolol hydrochloride
rauwolfia serpentina
rescinnamine
reserpine
trimethaphan camsylate

Doctors estimate that 15% of the adult population is hypertensive. Only about half these people realize they are ill because they remain asymptomatic until complications occur. If hypertension is left untreated, it can lead to stroke, heart disease, and renal disease. Compliance with prescribed drug regimens is one of the biggest problems in the treatment of this disorder, because, to the patient, the side effects from the drugs may seem worse than the disease.

Major uses

• Antihypertensive drugs are used primarily to treat mild to severe essential hypertension. Most parenteral drugs of this type are reserved for treatment of hypertensive emergencies, such as hypertensive encephalopathy and malignant hypertension.
• Two antihypertensives—phenoxybenzamine and phentolamine—are used to diagnose and manage pheochromocytoma.

Drug	Mechanism of action	Characteristic onset	Duration
methyldopa	Alpha-adrenergic stimulator; alters central sympathetic outflow	P.O. 12 to 24 hours I.V. 4 to 6 hours	24 to 48 hours
clonidine	Alters central sympathetic outflow	P.O. 30 to 60 minutes	8 hours
reserpine	Depletes norepinephrine stores	I.V. 4 min to 1 hour I.M. 2 hours P.O. days, weeks	6 to 8 hours 10 to 12 hours
propranolol *metoprolol*	Beta-adrenergic blocking agent; inhibits renin	I.M. 1 hour P.O. days, weeks	up to 12 hours

Drug	Mechanism of action	Characteristic onset	Duration
hydralazine	Relaxes arteriolar smooth muscle; vasodilator	I.V. 5 to 20 minutes	2 to 6 hours
		I.M. 10 to 30 minutes	2 to 6 hours
		P.O. 20 to 30 minutes	2 to 4 hours
prazosin	Relaxes venous and arteriolar smooth muscles; vasodilator	P.O. 2 hours	less than 24 hours
nitroprusside	Vasodilator	I.V. immediate	effect dissipates rapidly in 1 to 10 minutes
diazoxide	Vasodilator	I.V. 5 minutes	3 to 12 hours
trimethaphan	Ganglionic blocking agent	I.V. immediate	effect dissipates in 1 to 10 minutes
guanethidine	Direct inhibition of norepinephrine release	P.O. 1 to 3 weeks	1 to 3 weeks

Absorption, distribution, and excretion

• P.O. antihypertensives are absorbed rapidly from the GI tract with the exception of methyldopa and alkavervir, which are erratically absorbed. All are widely distributed in the body tissues. All mostly excreted through the kidneys, with the exception of prazosin (excreted through bile-feces).

Combination products

ALDOCLOR-150: chlorothiazide 150 mg and methyldopa 250 mg.
ALDOCLOR-250: chlorothiazide 250 mg and methyldopa 250 mg.
ALDORIL-15♦: hydrochlorothiazide 15 mg and methyldopa 250 mg.
ALDORIL-25♦: hydrochlorothiazide 25 mg and methyldopa 250 mg.
ALDORIL D30: hydrochlorothiazide 30 mg and methyldopa 500 mg.
ALDORIL D50: hydrochlorothiazide 50 mg and methyldopa 500 mg.
APRESAZIDE 25/25: hydrochlorothiazide 25 mg and hydralazine HCl 25 mg.
APRESAZIDE 50/50: hydrochlorothiazide 50 mg and hydralazine HCl 50 mg.
APRESAZIDE 100/50: hydrochlorothiazide 50 mg and hydralazine HCl 100 mg.
APRESOLINE-ESIDRIX: hydrochlorothiazide 15 mg and hydralazine HCl 25 mg.
COMBIPRES 0.1 MG♦: chlorthalidone 15 mg and clonidine HCl 0.1 mg.
COMBIPRES 0.2 MG: chlorthalidone 15 mg and clonidine HCl 0.2 mg.
DEMI-REGROTON: chlorthalidone 25 mg and reserpine 0.125 mg.

DIUPRES-250◆: chlorothiazide 250 mg and reserpine 0.125 mg.
DIUPRES-500: chlorothiazide 500 mg and reserpine 0.125 mg.
DIUTENSEN◆: methyclothiazide 2.5 mg and cryptenamine 2 mg.
DIUTENSEN-R◆: methyclothiazide 2.5 mg and reserpine 0.1 mg.
ENDURONYL: methyclothiazide 5 mg and deserpidine 0.25 mg.
ENDURONYL-FORTE: methyclothiazide 5 mg and deserpidine 0.5 mg.
ESIMIL: hydrochlorothiazide 25 mg and guanethidine monosulfate 10 mg.
EUTRON: methyclothiazide 5 mg and pargyline HCl 25 mg.
EXNA-R TABLETS: benzthiazide 50 mg and reserpine 0.125 mg.
HYDROMOX-R: quinethazone 50 mg and reserpine 0.125 mg.
HYDROPRES-25◆: hydrochlorothiazide 25 mg and reserpine 0.125 mg.
HYDROPRES-50◆: hydrochlorothiazide 50 mg and reserpine 0.125 mg.
HYDROSERP: hydrochlorothiazide 50 mg and reserpine 0.1 mg.
HYDROTENSIN-25 TABLETS: hydrochlorothiazide 25 mg and reserpine 0.125 mg.
HYDROTENSIN-50: hydrochlorothiazide 50 mg and resperine 0.125 mg.
HYSTOL TABLETS: hydrochlorothiazide 15 mg and hydralazine 25 mg.
INDERIDE 40/25: propranolol 40 mg and hydrochlorothiazide 25 mg.
INDERIDE 80/25: propranolol 80 mg and hydrochlorothiazide 25 mg.
METATENSIN TABLETS: trichlormethiazide 2 or 4 mg and resperine 0.1 mg.
NAQUIVAL: trichlormethiazide 4 mg and reserpine 0.1 mg.
NATURETIN W/K 2.5 MG◆: bendroflumetniazide 2.5 mg and potassium chloride 500 mg.
NATURETIN W/K 5 MG◆: bendroflumetniazide 5 mg and potassium chloride 500 mg.
ORETICYL FORTE: hydrochlorothiazide 25 mg and deserpidin.
ORETICYL FORTE: hydrochlorothiazide 25 mg and deserpidine 0.25 mg.
ORETICYL 25: hydrochlorothiazide 25 mg and deserpidine 0.125 mg.
ORETICYL 50: hydrochlorothiazide 50 mg and deserpidine 0.125 mg.
RAUTRAX: flumethiazide 400 mg, whole root rauwolfia 50 mg, and potassium chloride 400 mg.
RAUTRAX-N: bendroflumethiazide 4 mg, whole root rauwolfia 50 mg, and potassium chloride 400 mg.
RAUTRAX-N MODIFIED: bendroflumethiazide 5 mg, whole root rauwolfia 50 mg, and potassium chloride 400 mg.
RAUZIDE: bendroflumethiazide 4 mg and rauwolfia serpentina 50 mg.
REGROTON: chlorthalidone 50 mg and reserpine 0.25 mg.
RENESE-R: polythiazide 2 mg and reserpine 0.25 mg.
SALUTENSIN◆: hydroflumethiazide 50 mg and resperine 0.125 mg.
SALUTENSIN DEMI: hydroflumethiazide 25 mg and reserpine 0.125 mg.
SER-AP-ES◆: hydrochlorothiazide 15 mg, resperine 0.1 mg, and hydralazine HC1 25 mg.
SERPASIL-APRESOLINE #1: reserpine 0.1 mg and hydralazine HCl 25 mg.
SERPASIL-APRESOLINE #2◆: reserpine 0.2 mg and hydralazine HCl 50 mg.
SERPASIL-ESIDRIX #1◆: hydrochlorothiazide 25 mg and reserpine 0.1 mg.
SERPASIL-ESIDRIX #2◆: hydrochlorothiazide 50 mg and reserpine 0.1 mg.
THIA-SERP-25: hydrochlorothiazide 25 mg and reserpine 0.125 mg.
THIA-SERP-50: hydrochlorothiazide 50 mg and reserpine 0.125 mg.
THIA-ZINE TABLETS: hydrochlorothiazide 15 mg and hydralazine HCl 25 mg.
UNIPRES: hydrochlorothiazide 15 mg, reserpine 0.1 mg, and hydralazine HCl 25 mg.

PATIENT TEACHING AID — METHYLDOPA

Dear Patient:
Here's what you should know about the drug your doctor has prescribed for you. Methyldopa is used to treat high blood pressure. It will bring your blood pressure into a normal range and help keep it there.

To make sure you get the most from your therapy, follow these instructions carefully:

1. Take methyldopa only as prescribed. Never skip a dose or increase, decrease, or change your dose in any way without an order from your doctor.
2. Stay on the diet your doctor has given you. Don't drink alcohol without asking him first.
3. Tell every doctor who treats you that you are taking methyldopa.
4. Because methyldopa can cause drowsiness, be careful if you have to drive or perform other tasks that require mental alertness. This drowsiness usually disappears in time.
5. Avoid sudden rising or prolonged standing. If you have been lying down or sitting for a long period of time, stand up slowly to avoid dizziness.

Call the doctor *immediately* if you notice any of the following: depression, dizziness, fainting, mouth dryness, extreme drowsiness, nasal congestion, fatigue, headache, numbness, constipation, fever, rash, joint pains, impotence, nightmares, confusion, dark urine, excessive bruising, or changes in skin color.

PATIENT TEACHING AID — RESERPINE

Dear Patient:
Here's what you should know about the drug your doctor has prescribed for you. Reserpine is used to treat high blood pressure. It will bring your blood pressure into a normal range and help keep it there.

To make sure you get the most from your therapy, follow these instructions carefully:

1. Take this drug only as prescribed. Never skip a dose, increase it, or decrease it without asking your doctor.
2. Stay on the diet your doctor has given you.
3. Tell every doctor who treats you that you are taking this drug, especially if he plans surgery and you will be given an anesthetic.
4. This drug can cause drowsiness (which will disappear in time). Be careful if you have to drive or perform other tasks that require mental alertness.
5. Avoid sudden rising or prolonged standing. Stand up slowly to avoid dizziness.
6. *Notify your doctor if you become pregnant.*

Call the doctor *immediately* if you notice any of the following: depression, dizziness, fainting, diarrhea, stomach distress, black stools, weight gain greater than 2 lbs in 1 day or 7 lbs in 1 week, chest pains, heart palpitations, impotence, nightmares, rash, nasal congestion, or hives.

NAME	INDICATIONS & DOSAGE	SIDE EFFECTS
alkavervir Veriloid	*Essential, renal or malignant hypertension; toxemia of pregnancy*— **Adults:** 3 to 5 mg P.O. daily, given in 3 to 4 divided doses not less than 4 hours apart. Give after meals. Initial recommended dose is 8 to 9 mg. No dosing recommendations for children.	*CNS:* mental confusion. *CV:* orthostatic hypotension, cardiac arrhythmias, bradycardia. *EENT:* blurred vision, excessive salivation, unpleasant taste. *GI:* nausea, vomiting, epigastric burning, hiccups. *Other:* respiratory depression, bronchial constriction, sweating.
alseroxylon Raudolfin, Rautensin, Rauwiloid, Vio-Serpine	*Mild, labile hypertension*— **Adults:** initially, 4 mg P.O. daily as a single dose or divided in 2 doses for 1 to 3 weeks. Maintenance dose: 2 mg or less daily. No dosing recommendations for children.	*CNS:* mental confusion, depression, drowsiness, nervousness, anxiety, insomnia, nightmares, sedation, Parkinsonism. *CV:* orthostatic hypotension, fatigue. *EENT:* mouth dryness, nasal stuffiness, glaucoma. *GI:* hypersecretion of gastric acid, nausea, vomiting, gastrointestinal bleeding, biliary colic. *Skin:* pruritus, rash. *Other:* impotence, edema, weight gain.
clonidine hydrochloride Catapres♦	*Essential, renal, and malignant hypertension*— **Adults:** initially, 0.1 mg P.O. b.i.d. Then increase by 0.1 to 0.2 mg daily on a weekly basis. Usual dose range: 0.2 to 0.8 mg daily in divided doses. Infrequently, doses as high as 2.4 mg daily. No dosing recommendations for children.	*CNS:* drowsiness, dizziness, fatigue, sedation, behavioral changes, nightmares, nervousness, headache. *CV:* orthostatic hypotension, bradycardia, CHF. *EENT:* mouth dryness. *GI:* constipation. *GU:* urinary retention. *Other:* impotence.

♦ Also available in Canada.
♦♦ Available in Canada only.
Unmarked trade names available in United States only.

INTERACTIONS	NURSING CONSIDERATIONS
None significant.	• Contraindicated in patients with pheochromocytoma. Use cautiously in patients with angina, cerebrovascular disease, bronchial asthma, or those receiving other antihypertensive drugs. • Rarely used to treat hypertension because of unsatisfactory response and high incidence of side effects. • The range between therapeutic and toxic doses of this drug is narrow. Call the doctor immediately if patient develops side effects. • Monitor blood pressure and pulse rate closely. Keep phenylephrine or ephedrine handy in case severe hypotension develops. If patient develops bradycardia, he may require atropine. • Teach patient about his disease and therapy. Explain why it's important to take this drug exactly as prescribed, even when he's feeling well. Tell patient not to stop this drug suddenly, but to call the doctor if unpleasant side effects develop. • Tell patient to avoid alcohol and follow prescribed diet. • Inform patient that orthostatic hypotension can be minimized by rising slowly and avoiding sudden position changes. Unpleasant taste can be relieved with chewing gum, hard sour candy, or ice chips; nausea and vomiting by not eating for at least 4 hours after each dose. • In very hot weather, patient may require smaller doses. • Give this drug after meals.
MAO inhibitors: may cause excitability and hypertension. Avoid if possible. *Methotrimeprazine:* may increase hypotension. Observe patient carefully.	• Use cautiously in patients with severe cardiac or cerebrovascular disease, peptic ulcer, ulcerative colitis, renal disease, gallstones, mental depressive disorders, or those undergoing surgery. • Use cautiously in patients taking other antihypertensive drugs. • Monitor patient's blood pressure and pulse rate frequently. • Teach patient about his disease and therapy. Explain why it's important to take this drug exactly as prescribed, even when he's feeling well. Tell patient not to discontinue this drug suddenly, but to call the doctor if unpleasant side effects, such as mental depression, nightmares or insomnia, develop. Watch patient closely for signs of mental depression. • Warn patient that this drug can cause drowsiness. • Warn female patient to notify doctor if she becomes pregnant. • Tell patient to avoid alcohol and to follow prescribed diet. • Inform patient that orthostatic hypotension can be minimized by rising slowly and avoiding sudden position changes. Mouth dryness can be relieved with chewing gum, hard sour candy, or ice chips. • Tell patient to contact doctor if relief is needed for nasal stuffiness. • Give this drug with meals. • Patient should weigh himself daily and notify doctor of any weight gain.
Tricyclic antidepressants: may decrease antihypertensive effect. Use together cautiously. *Metoprolol, propranolol:* if clonidine is withdrawn, monitor for hypertensive response.	• Use cautiously in patients with severe coronary insufficiency, myocardial infarction, cerebral vascular disease, chronic renal failure, history of depression, or those taking other antihypertensives. • Monitor blood pressure and pulse rate frequently. Dosage is usually adjusted to patient's blood pressure and tolerance. • Reduce dose gradually over 2 to 4 days. If discontinued abruptly, this drug may cause severe hypertension. • Monitor liver function studies and blood glucose. • Teach patient about his disease and therapy. Explain why it's important to take this drug exactly as prescribed, even when he's feeling well. Tell patient not to discontinue this drug suddenly, but to call the doctor if unpleasant side effects develop. Warn that this drug can cause drowsiness. • Tell patient to avoid alcohol and to follow prescribed diet. • Inform patient that orthostatic hypotension can be minimized by rising slowly and avoiding sudden position changes. Mouth dryness can be relieved with chewing gum, hard sour candy, or ice chips. • Last dose should be taken immediately before retiring. • Has been used to decrease the subjective symptoms of opiate withdrawal.

NAME	INDICATIONS & DOSAGE	SIDE EFFECTS
cryptenamine acetate Unitensen Aqueous **cryptenamine tannate** Unitensen, Unitensyl••	*Mild to moderate hypertension, toxemia—* **Adults:** initially, 2 mg P.O. b.i.d., increased at weekly intervals, depending on response. Total daily dose not to exceed 12 mg daily. I.V. (for hypertensive crises and convulsive toxemia)—0.5 ml (130 CSR units) diluted to 20 ml with 5% dextrose in water. Administer at infusion rate of 1 ml/min. When giving this drug I.V., record blood pressure every minute. Stop injection immediately after first 20 mm.-drop in systolic blood pressure or 10 mm.-drop in diastolic blood pressure. If no further drop occurs in 5 minutes, continue to administer diluted drug at rate of 1 ml/min., stopping when blood pressure is at desired level. After first blood pressure drop, record blood pressure every 5 minutes. Give ½ previously effective dose when blood pressure exceeds desired level. When interval between I.V. doses exceeds 1 hour, give drug I.M. I.M. (for impending hypertensive crises and nonconvulsive toxemia)—0.5 ml (130 CSR units) deep injection. When giving this drug I.M., record heart rate and blood pressure every 15 minutes. If no hypotensive response in 1 hour, dosage may be increased in increments of 0.1 ml. When hypotensive response occurs, repeat injections as often as necessary. Oral therapy may begin when blood pressure is controlled.	*CNS:* mental confusion. *CV:* orthostatic hypotension, cardiac arrhythmias, bradycardia. *EENT:* blurred vision, excessive salivation, unpleasant taste. *GI:* nausea, vomiting, epigastric burning, hiccups. *Other:* respiratory depression, bronchial constriction.
deserpidine Harmonyl	*Mild essential hypertension—* **Adults:** 0.25 mg P.O. t.i.d. to q.i.d. for up to 2 weeks, then maintenance dose of 0.25 mg or less daily. No dosing recommendations for children.	*CNS:* mental confusion, depression, drowsiness, nervousness, anxiety, nightmares, sedation, Parkinsonism. *CV:* bradycardia. *EENT:* mouth dryness, nasal stuffiness, glaucoma. *GI:* hypersecretion of gastric acid, nausea, vomiting, gastrointestinal bleeding, biliary colic. *Skin:* pruritus, rash. *Other:* impotence, edema, weight gain.

INTERACTIONS	NURSING CONSIDERATIONS
None significant.	• Contraindicated in patients with pheochromocytoma. Use cautiously in patients with angina, cerebrovascular disease, bronchial asthma, renal insufficiency, or those taking other antihypertensives. • Monitor blood pressure and pulse rate closely. If severe hypotension develops, stop infusion and notify doctor, as he may use phenylephrine or ephedrine to counteract effect. Hypotension should dissipate in 60 to 90 minutes. If patient develops bradycardia, he may require atropine. Notify doctor promptly. • The range between therapeutic and toxic doses of this drug is narrow. Call doctor immediately if patient develops side effects. • Teach patient about his disease and therapy. Explain why it's important to take this drug exactly as prescribed, even when he's feeling well. Tell patient not to discontinue this drug suddenly, but to call the doctor if unpleasant side effects develop. Warn that this drug can cause drowsiness. • Tell patient to avoid alcohol and follow prescribed diet. • Inform patient that orthostatic hypotension can be minimized by rising slowly and avoiding sudden position changes. Unpleasant taste can be relieved with chewing gum, sour hard candy, or ice chips.
Methotrimeprazine: may increase hypotension. Don't use together. *MAO inhibitors:* may cause excitability and hypertension. Avoid if possible.	• Contraindicated in patients with mental depression. Use cautiously in patients with severe cardiac or cerebrovascular disease, peptic ulcer, ulcerative colitis, gallstones, or mental depressive disorders; patients undergoing surgery; and in patients taking other antihypertensives or anticonvulsants. • Monitor patient's blood pressure and pulse rate frequently. • Teach patient about his disease and therapy. Explain why it's important to take this drug exactly as prescribed, even when he's feeling well. Tell patient not to discontinue this drug suddenly, but to call the doctor if unpleasant side effects, such as mental depression, insomnia, or loss of appetite, develop. Warn that drug can cause drowsiness. • Warn female patient to notify doctor if she becomes pregnant.

(continued on following page)

NAME	INDICATIONS & DOSAGE	SIDE EFFECTS
deserpidine *(continued)*		
diazoxide Hyperstat◆ (I.V. only), Proglem, Proglycem	*Hypertensive crisis—* **Adults:** 300 mg I.V. bolus push, administered in 30 seconds or less into peripheral vein. Repeat at intervals of 4 to 24 hours, p.r.n. Switch to therapy with oral antihypertensives as soon as possible. **Children:** 5 mg/Kg I.V. rapid bolus push.	*Blood:* leukopenia. *CNS:* sweating, flushing, warmth, dizziness, light-headedness, euphoria. *CV:* sodium and water retention, angina, hypotension, myocardial ischemia, arrhythmias, EKG changes. *GI:* nausea, vomiting, abdominal discomfort. *GU:* decreased urinary output. *Local:* inflammation and pain from extravasation. *Metabolic:* hyperglycemia, hyperosmolar coma. *Skin:* rash. *Other:* dyspnea, cough, choking sensation, fever.
guanethidine sulfate Ismelin◆	*For moderate to severe hypertension; usually used in combination with other antihypertensives—* **Adults:** initially, 10 mg P.O. daily. Increase by 10 mg at weekly to monthly intervals, p.r.n. Usual dose is 25 to 50 mg daily. **Children:** initially, 200 mcg/Kg P.O. daily. Increase gradually every 1 to 3 weeks to maximum of 8 times initial dose.	*CNS:* dizziness, weakness, syncope. *CV:* orthostatic hypotension, bradycardia, congestive heart failure, arrhythmias. *EENT:* nasal stuffiness, mouth dryness. *Other:* edema, weight gain. *GI:* diarrhea. *GU:* inhibition of ejaculation.
hydralazine hydrochloride Apresoline◆, Dralzine, Hydralyn, Nor-Pres 25, Rolazine	*Essential hypertension—(oral, alone or in combination with other antihypertensives); to reduce afterload in severe congestive heart failure (with nitrates); and, severe essential hypertension (parenteral to lower blood pressure quickly).* **Adults:** initially, 10 mg P.O. q.i.d.; gradually increased to 50 mg q.i.d. Maximum recommended dosage is 200 mg daily. I.V.—20 to 40 mg given slowly and repeated as necessary, generally	*Blood:* leukopenia, thrombocytopenia, eosinophilia. *CNS:* peripheral neuritis, headache, dizziness. *CV:* orthostatic hypotension, tachycardia, arrhythmias, angina, palpitations, sodium retention. *GI:* nausea, vomiting, diarrhea, anorexia. *Skin:* rash. *Other:* lupus erythematosus, weight gain.

INTERACTIONS	NURSING CONSIDERATIONS
	• Watch patient closely for signs of mental depression. Warn him to notify doctor promptly if he starts having nightmares. • Tell patient to avoid alcohol and to follow prescribed diet. • Mouth dryness can be relieved with chewing gum, sour hard candy, or ice chips. Tell patient to contact doctor if relief is needed for nasal stuffiness. • Give this drug with meals to increase absorption. • Patient should weigh himself daily and notify doctor of any weight gain.
Hydralazine: may cause severe hypotension. Use together cautiously. *Thiazide diuretics:* may increase the effects of diazoxide. Use together cautiously.	• Use cautiously in patients with impaired cerebral or cardiac function, diabetes, uremia, or those taking other antihypertensives. • Monitor blood pressure frequently. Notify doctor immediately if severe hypotension develops. Keep levarterenol available. • Monitor patient's intake and output carefully. If fluid or sodium retention develops, doctor may want to order furosemide. • Take care to avoid extravasation. • Weigh patients daily. Notify doctor of any weight increase. • Watch diabetics closely for signs of severe hyperglycemia or hyperosmolar nonketotic coma. Insulin may be needed. • Check patient's blood sugar, uric acid levels, and white blood cell count frequently. Report abnormalities to doctor. • Inform patient that orthostatic hypotension can be minimized by rising slowly and avoiding sudden position changes. • This drug may alter requirements for insulin, diet, or oral hypoglycemic drugs in previously controlled diabetics. Monitor blood glucose daily.
Levodopa, alcohol, methotrimeprazine: may increase hypotensive effect of guanethidine. Use together cautiously. *MAO inhibitors, ephedrine, levarterenol, methylphenidate, amphetamines, tricyclic antidepressants, phenothiazines:* may inhibit the antihypertensive effect of guanethidine. Adjust dose accordingly.	• Contraindicated in patients with pheochromocytoma. Use cautiously in patients with severe cardiac disease, recent MI, cerebrovascular disease, peptic ulcer, impaired renal function, bronchial asthma, or those taking other antihypertensives. • Discontinue drug 2 to 3 weeks before elective surgery. • Teach patient about his disease and therapy. Explain why it's important to take this drug exactly as prescribed, even when he's feeling well. Tell patient not to discontinue this drug suddenly, but to call the doctor if unpleasant side effects develop. Warn that this drug can cause drowsiness. • Tell patient to avoid alcohol, follow prescribed diet, and avoid strenuous exercise. • Inform patient that orthostatic hypotension can be minimized by rising slowly and avoiding sudden position changes. Mouth dryness can be relieved with chewing gum, hard sour candy, or ice chips. • Give this drug with meals to increase absorption. • If patient develops diarrhea, doctor may prescribe atropine or paregoric.
Diazoxide: may cause severe hypotension. Use together cautiously.	• Use cautiously in patients with cardiac disease or those taking other antihypertensives. • Monitor patient's blood pressure and pulse rate frequently. • Watch patient closely for sore throat, fever, muscle and joint aches, skin rash. Call doctor immediately if any of these develop. • Monitor blood studies (complete blood count, Coombs') before and periodically during therapy. • Teach patient about his disease and therapy. Explain why it's important to take this drug exactly as prescribed, even when he's feeling well. Tell patient not to discontinue this drug suddenly, but to call the doctor if unpleasant side effects develop. • Tell patient to avoid alcohol and to follow prescribed diet. • Inform patient that orthostatic hypotension can be minimized by rising slowly and avoiding sudden position changes.

(continued on following page)

NAME	INDICATIONS & DOSAGE	SIDE EFFECTS
hydralazine hydrochloride *(continued)*	q 4 to 6 hours. Switch to oral antihypertensives as soon as possible. I.M.—20 to 40 mg repeated as necessary, generally q 4 to 6 hours. Switch to oral antihypertensives as soon as possible. **Children:** initially, 0.75 mg/Kg P.O. daily in 4 divided doses (25 mg/M^2 daily). May increase gradually to 10 times this dose, if necessary. I.V.—give slowly 1.7 to 3.5 mg/Kg daily or 50 to 100 mg/M^2 daily in 4 to 6 divided doses. I.M.—1.7 to 3.5 mg/Kg daily or 50 to 100 mg/M^2 daily in 4 to 6 divided doses.	
mecamylamine hydrochloride Inversine	*For moderate to severe essential hypertension and uncomplicated malignant hypertension*— **Adults:** initially, 2.5 mg P.O. b.i.d. Increase by 2.5 mg daily every 2 days. Average daily dose 25 mg given in 3 divided doses. No dosing recommendations for children. To change patient from another ganglionic blocking agent to mecamylamine, proceed as follows: Reduce daily dose of previous drug by 25% and replace with 25% of estimated daily dose of mecamylamine. Repeat this process at weekly intervals until complete conversion is accomplished. This should take 3 to 4 weeks.	*CNS:* dilated pupils, blurred vision, paresthesias, sedation, fatigue, tremor, choreiform movements, convulsions, psychic changes, dizziness, weakness. *CV:* orthostatic hypotension. *EENT:* mouth dryness, glossitis. *GI:* anorexia, nausea, vomiting, constipation, adynamic ileus, diarrhea. *GU:* urinary retention, impotence. *Other:* decreased libido.
methyldopa Aldomet♦, Dopamet♦♦, Medimet-250♦♦, Novomedopa♦♦	*For sustained mild-to-severe hypertension; should not be used for acute treatment of hypertensive emergencies*— **Adults:** initially, 250 mg P.O. b.i.d. to t.i.d. in first 48 hours. Then increase as needed every 2 days. Dosages may need adjustment if other antihypertensive drugs are added or deleted from therapy. Maintenance dosages—500 mg to 2 g daily in 2 to 4 divided doses. Maximum recommended daily dose is 3 g. I.V.—500 mg to 1 g q 6 hours, diluted in 5% dextrose in water,	*Blood:* hemolytic anemia, reversible granulocytopenia, thrombocytopenia. *CNS:* sedation, headache, asthenia, weakness, dizziness, decreased mental acuity, involuntary choreoathetotic movements, psychic disturbances, depression. *CV:* bradycardia, orthostatic hypotension, aggravated angina, myocarditis. *EENT:* nasal stuffiness. *GI:* dry mouth, distress, diarrhea, hepatic necrosis. *GU:* impotence. *Other:* gynecomastia, lactation, skin rash, drug-induced fever, anemia.

INTERACTIONS	NURSING CONSIDERATIONS
	• Give this drug with meals to increase absorption. • Compliance may be improved by administering this drug b.i.d. Check with doctor.
Sodium bicarbonate: may increase effect of mecamylamine. Use together cautiously. Watch for increased hypotensive effects.	• Contraindicated in patients with recent MI, uremia, chronic pylonephritis. Use cautiously in patients with lower urinary tract pathology, renal insufficiency, glaucoma, pyloric stenosis, coronary insufficiency, cerebral vascular insufficiency, or those taking other antihypertensives. • Effects of this drug are increased by high environmental temperature, fever, stress, or severe illness. • Don't withdraw this drug suddenly; rebound hypertension may occur. Tell patient to call the doctor if unpleasant side effects develop. • Monitor patient's blood pressure frequently while he's standing. • Give with meals for better absorption. Don't restrict sodium intake. • If patient develops constipation from this drug, the doctor may want him to take milk of magnesia. Instruct patient to avoid bulk laxatives. • Teach patient about his disease and therapy. Explain why it's important to take this drug exactly as prescribed, even when he's feeling well. Warn that this drug can cause drowsiness. • Tell patient to avoid alcohol and to follow prescribed diet. • Instruct patient that orthostatic hypotension can be minimized by rising slowly and avoiding sudden position changes. Mouth dryness can be relieved with chewing gum, sour hard candy, or ice chips.
Methotrimeprazine: increased hypotensive effects. Monitor carefully. *Norepinephrine, propranolol:* possible hypertensive effects. Monitor carefully.	• Use cautiously in patients receiving other antihypertensives or MAO inhibitors. Monitor blood pressure and pulse rate frequently. • Observe patient for side effects, particularly unexplained fever. Report side effects to doctor. • If patient requires blood transfusion, make sure he gets direct and indirect Coombs' tests to avoid cross-matching problems. • If patient has been on this drug for several months, positive reaction to direct Coombs' tests indicate hemolytic anemia. • Weigh patient daily. Notify doctor of any weight increase. Salt and water retention may occur but can be relieved with diuretics. • Tell patient that urine may turn dark in toilet bowls treated with bleach. • Monitor blood studies (complete blood count) before and during therapy. • Teach patient about his disease and therapy. Explain why it's important to take this drug exactly as prescribed, even when he's feeling well. Tell patient not to stop this drug suddenly, but to call the doctor if unpleasant side effects develop. Warn that this drug can cause drowsiness. Once-

(continued on following page)

NAME	INDICATIONS & DOSAGE	SIDE EFFECTS
methyldopa *(continued)*	and administered over 30 to 60 minutes. Switch to oral antihypertensives as soon as possible. **Children:** initially, 10 mg/Kg/day P.O. in 2 to 3 divided doses; or 20 to 40 mg/Kg/day I.V. in 4 divided doses. Increase dose daily until desired response. Maximum daily dose 65 mg/Kg.	
metoprolol tartrate Betaloc◆◆, Lopresor◆◆, Lopressor	*For hypertension; may be used alone or in combination with other antihypertensives—* **Adults:** P.O. for hypertension: 200 to 400 mg daily in 2 to 3 divided doses. No dosage recommendations for children.	*Blood:* eosinophilia, thrombocytopenia, agranulocytosis. *CNS:* giddiness, depression, hallucinations, visual disturbances, drowsiness. *CV:* bradycardia, congestive heart failure, angina, myocardial infarction, hypotension, syncope, shock *Metabolic:* hypoglycemia without symptoms. *Skin:* rash. *Other:* bronchospasm, wheezing, asthma.
nitroprusside sodium Nipride◆	*To lower blood pressure quickly in hypertensive emergencies; to control hypotension during anesthesia; to reduce pre-load and after-load in cardiac pump failure or cardiogenic shock; may be used with or without dopamine—* **Adults:** 50-mg vial diluted with 2 to 3 ml of dextrose 5% in water I.V. and then added to 500 to 1,000 ml dextrose 5% in water. Infuse at 0.5 to 10 mcg/Kg/min. Average dose: 3 mcg/Kg/min. Maximum infusion rate: 10 mcg/Kg/min. Patients taking other antihypertensive drugs along with nitroprusside are very sensitive to this drug. Adjust dosage accordingly.	*CNS:* headache, dizziness, ataxia, loss of consciousness, coma, weak pulse, absent reflexes, widely dilated pupils, restlessness. *CV:* distant heart sounds, hypotension, dyspnea, palpitations, shallow breathing. *GI:* vomiting, nausea. *Local:* tissue sloughing and necrosis with extravasation. *Metabolic:* acidosis. *Skin:* pink color.

INTERACTIONS	NURSING CONSIDERATIONS
	daily dosage given at bedtime will minimize drowsiness during daytime. Check with doctor. • Tell patient to avoid alcohol and to follow prescribed diet. • Inform patient that orthostatic hypotension can be minimized by rising slowly and avoiding position changes. Mouth dryness can be relieved with chewing gum, hard sour candy, or ice chips.
Insulin, hypoglycemic drugs (oral): can alter requirements for these drugs in previously stabilized diabetics. Observe patient carefully. *Cardiac glycosides:* excessive bradycardia and increased depressant effect on myocardium. Use together cautiously. *Indomethacin:* possible decreased antihypertensive response. Monitor carefully.	• Use cautiously in patients with heart block, congestive heart failure, diabetes, respiratory disease, or those taking other antihypertensives. Always check patient's apical pulse rate before giving this drug. If it's less than 60 beats/minute, hold drug and call doctor immediately. Treat excessive bradycardia with atropine. • Monitor blood pressure frequently. If patient develops severe hypotension, administer a vasopressor. • Don't discontinue abruptly; abrupt discontinuation can exacerbate angina and MI. • Teach patient about his disease and therapy. Explain why it's important to take this drug, even when he's feeling well. Tell patient not to discontinue this drug suddenly, but to call the doctor if unpleasant side effects develop. Warn that this drug can cause drowsiness. • Tell patient to avoid alcohol and to stay on diet prescribed by doctor. • Inform patient that orthostatic hypotension can be minimized by rising slowly and avoiding sudden position changes. • Food may increase the absorption of metoprolol. Give consistently with meals.
None significant.	• Use cautiously in patients with hypothyroidism, hepatic or renal disease, or those receiving other antihypertensives. • Due to light sensitivity, wrap I.V. solution and tubing in foil or black tape. Fresh solution should have faint brownish tint. Discard after 4 hours. • Obtain baseline vital signs before giving this drug and find out what parameters the doctor wants to achieve. • Check blood pressure every 5 minutes at start of infusion and every 15 minutes thereafter. If severe hypotension occurs, turn off I.V. Nipride—effects of drug quickly reversed. Notify doctor. If possible, an arterial pressure line should be started. Regulate drug flow to specified level. • Don't use bacteriostatic water for injection, or sterile saline for reconstitution. • Infuse with motorized infusion pump. • This drug is best run piggyback through a peripheral line with no other medication. Don't regulate rate of main I.V. line while this drug is running. Even small bolus of nitroprusside can cause severe hypotension. • This drug can cause cyanide toxicity, so check serum thiocyanate levels every 72 hours. Watch for signs of thiocyanate toxicity: profound hypotension, metabolic acidosis, dyspnea, headache, loss of consciousness, ataxia, vomiting. If these occur, discontinue drug immediately and notify doctor. • Tissue irritation can occur with extravasation.

NAME	INDICATIONS & DOSAGE	SIDE EFFECTS
pargyline hydrochloride Eutonyl	*For moderate-to-severe hypertension, usually given in combination with other drugs*— **Adults:** initially, 25 to 50 mg P.O. once daily, if not receiving any other antihypertensive drugs. Then increase dosage by 10 mg daily at weekly intervals. Maximum daily dosage 200 mg. Usual daily dose for patients over age 65 or those who've had sympathectomy: 10 to 25 mg. When used in combination with other drugs, total daily dose pargyline should not exceed 25 mg. No dosage recommendations for children.	*CNS:* tremors, convulsions, choreiform movements, psychic changes, nightmares, hyperexcitability, sweating, dizziness, fainting, drowsiness. *CV:* palpitations, orthostatic hypotension. *EENT:* mouth dryness, optic damage. *GI:* nausea, vomiting, increased appetite. *GU:* impotence. *Other:* fluid retention, hypoglycemia.
phenoxybenzamine hydrochloride Dibenzyline	*To control hypertension and sweating secondary to pheochromocytoma; may be used in combination with propranolol to control excessive tachycardia*— **Adults:** initially, 10 mg P.O. daily. Increase by 10 mg daily every 4 days. Maintenance dose: 20 to 60 mg daily. **Children:** initially, 0.2 mg/Kg or 6 mg/M² P.O. daily in a single dose. Maintenance dose: 12 to 36 mg/M² daily as a single dose or in divided doses.	*CNS:* lethargy, drowsiness. *CV:* orthostatic hypotension, tachycardia, shock. *EENT:* nasal stuffiness, miosis. *GI:* vomiting, abdominal distress. *GU:* impotence.
phentolamine hydrochloride Rogitine **phentolamine methanesulfonate** Regitene, Rogitine♦♦	*To aid in diagnosis of pheochromocytoma; to control or prevent hypertension before or during pheochromocytomectomy*— **Adults:** P.O. therapeutic dose: 50 mg q.i.d. I.V. diagnostic dose: 5 mg, with close monitoring of blood pressure.	*CNS:* dizziness, weakness, flushing. *CV:* hypotension, shock, arrhythmias, palpitations, tachycardia, angina pectoris, myocardial infarction. *GI:* diarrhea, abdominal pain, nausea, hyperperistalsis. *Other:* nasal stuffiness, hypoglycemia.

INTERACTIONS	NURSING CONSIDERATIONS
Amphetamines, ephedrine, levodopa, metaraminol, methotrimeprazine, methylphenidate, phenylephrine, phenylpropanolamine, pseudophedrine: enhanced pressor effects. Use together cautiously. *Alcohol, barbiturates, and other sedatives; tranquilizers; narcotics; dextromethorphan; tricyclic antidepressants:* unpredictable interactions. Should be used with caution and in reduced dosage.	• Contraindicated in patients with advanced renal failure, pheochromocytoma, hyperthyroidism, or Parkinson's disease; in patients who are hyperactive and hyperexcitable. Use cautiously in patients receiving other antihypertensives, or who have liver disease. • Discontinue this drug at least 2 weeks before elective surgery. • Hypotensive effects of this drug are increased by high temperatures, fever, stress, or severe illness. If patient develops severe hypotension, counteract with ephedrine or phenylephrine. • Monitor blood pressure and pulse rate frequently. Take blood pressure while patient is standing. • Patient should have periodic ophthalmic evaluations during therapy. • If patient is scheduled for surgery and has been taking this drug, be sure narcotic dosages are reduced. • This drug may require up to several weeks to reach optimal effect. • Warn patient not to take any other medications, including over-the-counter cold remedies, without first asking doctor. • This drug is an MAO inhibitor. Tell patient not to eat foods with high tyramine content, for example, aged cheese, chianti wine, sour cream, canned figs, raisins, chicken livers, yeast extract, chocolate, pickled herring, caffeine, cyclamates, cola drinks. • Teach patient about his disease and therapy. Explain why it's important to take this drug exactly as prescribed, even when he's feeling well. Tell patient not to discontinue this drug suddenly, but to call the doctor if unpleasant side effects develop. Warn that this drug can cause drowsiness. • Tell patient to avoid alcohol and to follow prescribed diet. • Inform patient that orthostatic hypotension can be minimized by rising slowly and avoiding sudden position changes. Mouth dryness can be relieved with chewing gum, sour hard candy, or ice chips.
None significant.	• Use cautiously in patients with cerebrovascular or coronary insufficiency, advanced renal disease, respiratory disease. • Watch patient closely for side effects, and call doctor promptly if they occur. If severe hypotension develops, patient may require levarterenol to counteract effect. • Patient with tachycardia may require concurrent propranolol therapy. • Monitor patient's heart rate and blood pressure frequently. • This drug may take several weeks to achieve optimal effect. • Monitor respiratory status carefully. This drug may aggravate symptoms of pneumonia and asthma. • Teach patient about his disease and therapy. Explain why it's important to take this drug exactly as prescribed, even when he's feeling well. Tell patient not to discontinue this drug suddenly, but to call the doctor if unpleasant side effects develop. Warn that this drug can cause drowsiness. • Tell patient to avoid alcohol and to follow prescribed diet. • Inform patient that orthostatic hypotension can be minimized by rising slowly and avoiding sudden position changes. Mouth dryness can be relieved with chewing gum, sour hard candy, or ice chips.
None significant.	• Contraindicated in angina, coronary artery disease, and history of MI. Use cautiously in patients with gastritis or peptic ulcer and in those receiving other antihypertensives. • When this drug is given for diagnostic test, check patient's blood pressure first. Make frequent blood pressure checks during administration. • Diagnosis positive for pheochromocytoma if severe hypotension results from I.V. test dose. • Administer levarterenol to counteract severe hypotensive effect of this

(continued on following page)

NAME	INDICATIONS & DOSAGE	SIDE EFFECTS
phentolamine *(continued)*	Prior to surgical removal of tumor give 2 to 5 mg I.M. or I.V. During surgery, patient may need small I.V. doses (1 mg) or small I.M. doses (3 mg). **Children:** P.O. therapeutic dose: 5 mg/Kg daily or 150 mg/M^2 daily in 4 to 6 divided doses. I.V. diagnostic dose: 0.1 mg/Kg or 3 mg/M^2 as single dose, with close monitoring of blood pressure. Prior to surgical removal of tumor give 1 mg I.V. or 3 mg I.M. During surgery, patient may need small I.V. doses (1 mg).	
prazosin hydrochloride Minipress◆	*For mild-to-moderate hypertension; used alone or in combination with a diuretic or other antihypertensive drugs; also used to decrease afterload in severe chronic congestive heart failure—* **Adults:** P.O. test dose: 1 mg given before bedtime to prevent "first-dose syncope." Initial dose: 1 mg t.i.d. Increase dosage slowly. Maximum daily dose 20 mg. Maintenance dose: 3 to 20 mg daily in 3 divided doses. A few patients have required dosages larger than this (up to 40 mg daily). If other antihypertensive drugs or diuretics are given along with this drug, decrease prazosin dosage to 1 to 2 mg t.i.d.	*CNS:* dizziness, headache, drowsiness, weakness, "first-dose syncope," depression. *CV:* orthostatic hypotension, palpitations. *EENT:* blurred vision. *GI:* vomiting, diarrhea, abdominal cramps, dry mouth, constipation.
propranolol hydrochloride Inderal◆	*Hypertension (usually used with thiazide diuretics)—* **Adults:** initial treatment of hypertension: 80 mg P.O. daily in 4 divided doses. Increase at 3- to 7-day intervals to maximum daily dose of 640 mg. Usual maintenance dose for hypertension: 160 to 480 mg daily. No dosing recommendations for children. For use as an antiarrhythmic, see Chapter 18.	*Blood:* eosinophilia, thrombocytopenia, agranulocytosis. *CNS:* giddiness, depression, hallucinations, visual disturbances. *CV:* bradycardia, congestive heart failure, angina, myocardial infarction, hypotension, syncope, shock. *GI:* nausea, vomiting, epigastric distress, diarrhea. *Metabolic:* hypoglycemia without symptoms. *Skin:* rash. *Other:* bronchospasm, wheezing, asthma.

INTERACTIONS	NURSING CONSIDERATIONS
	drug. Don't administer epinephrine to raise blood pressure, as this may cause further drop. • Don't give sedatives or narcotics 24 hours prior to diagnostic test.
None significant.	• Use cautiously in patients receiving other antihypertensive drugs. • Monitor patient's blood pressure and pulse rate frequently. • If initial dose is greater than 1 mg, patient may develop severe syncope with loss of consciousness (first-dose syncope). Increase dosage slowly. Instruct patient to sit or lie down if he experiences dizziness. • Teach patient about his disease and therapy. Explain why it's important to take this drug exactly as prescribed, even when he's feeling well. Tell patient not to discontinue this drug suddenly, but to call the doctor if unpleasant side effects develop. Warn that this drug can cause drowsiness. • Tell patient to avoid alcohol and to follow prescribed diet. • Inform patient that orthostatic hypotension can be minimized by rising slowly and avoiding sudden position changes. Mouth dryness can be relieved with chewing gum, sour hard candy, or ice chips. • Compliance may be improved by giving this drug on a once-daily basis. Check with doctor.
Insulin, hypoglycemic drugs (oral): can alter requirements for these drugs in previously stabilized diabetics. Monitor for hypoglycemia. *Cardiac glycosides:* excessive bradycardia and increased depressant effect on myocardium. Use together cautiously. *Aminophylline:* antagonized beta blocking effects of propranolol. Use	• Contraindicated in diabetes mellitus, asthma, allergic rhinitis; during ethyl ether anesthesia; in sinus bradycardia and heart block greater than first degree; in cardiogenic shock; in right ventricular failure secondary to pulmonary hypertension. Use with caution in congestive heart failure, respiratory disease, and patients taking other antihypertensive drugs. • Always check patient's apical pulse rate before giving this drug. If extremes in pulse rates, hold medication and call the doctor immediately. Treat excessive bradycardia with atropine. • Monitor blood pressure frequently. If patient develops severe hypotension, notify doctor, as he may prescribe a vasopressor. • Don't discontinue abruptly; abrupt discontinuation can exacerbate angina and MI. • Teach patient about his disease and therapy. Explain why it's important to take this drug exactly as prescribed, even when he's feeling well. Tell patient not to discontinue this drug suddenly, but to call the doctor if unpleasant side effects develop. • Tell patient to avoid alcohol and to stay on diet prescribed by doctor.

(continued on following page)

NAME	INDICATIONS & DOSAGE	SIDE EFFECTS
propranolol hydrochloride *(continued)*		
rauwolfia serpentina HBP, Hiwolfia, Hyper-Rauw, Hywolfia, Rau, Raudixin◆, Rauja, Raumason, Rauneed, Raupoid, Rauserpa, Rauserpin, Rausertina, Rauval, Rauwoldin, Rawfola, Ru-Hy-T, Serfia, Serfolia, T-Rau, Wolfina	*Mild-to-moderate hypertension*— **Adults:** initially and for 1 to 3 weeks thereafter, 200 mg P.O. daily as a single dose or in 2 divided doses. Maintenance dose: 150 mg or less daily. No dosing recommendations for children.	*CNS:* mental confusion, depression, drowsiness, nervousness, anxiety, nightmares, sedation, parkinsonism, headache. *CV:* orthostatic hypotension, bradycardia. *EENT:* mouth dryness, nasal stuffiness, glaucoma. *GI:* hypersecretion, nausea, vomiting, gastrointestinal bleeding, biliary colic. *Skin:* pruritus, rash. *Other:* impotence, edema, weight gain.
rescinnamine Anaprel, Cinnasil, Moderil	*For mild-to-moderate hypertension; may be used alone or in combination with other antihypertensives*— **Adults:** initially, 500 mcg P.O. once daily or in 2 divided doses for up to 2 weeks. Maintenance dose: 250 mcg or less daily. No dosing recommendations for children.	*CNS:* mental confusion, depression, drowsiness, nervousness, anxiety, nightmares, sedation, parkinsonism. *CV:* orthostatic hypotension. *EENT:* mouth dryness, nasal stuffiness, glaucoma. *GI:* hypersecretion, nausea, vomiting, gastrointestinal bleeding, biliary colic. *Skin:* pruritus, rash. *Other:* impotence, edema, weight gain.

INTERACTIONS	NURSING CONSIDERATIONS
together cautiously. *Isoproterenol, glucagon:* antagonized propranolol effect. May be used therapeutically and in emergencies. *Indomethacin:* possible decreased antihypertensive response.	• Inform patient that orthostatic hypotension can be minimized by rising slowly and avoiding sudden position changes. Mouth dryness can be relieved with chewing gum, sour hard candy, or ice chips. • This drug masks common signs of shock and hypoglycemia. • Food may increase the absorption of proprandol. Give consistently with meals. • Compliance may be improved by administering this drug on a twice-daily basis. Check with doctor.
MAO inhibitors: may cause excitability and hypertension. Use together cautiously. *Methotrimeprazine:* may increase hypotension. Monitor carefully.	• Contraindicated in patients with depression. Use cautiously in patients with severe cardiac or cardiovascular disease, impaired renal function, peptic ulcer, ulcerative colitis, gallstones; those undergoing surgery; or taking other antihypertensives or tricyclic antidepressants. • Monitor patient's blood pressure and pulse rate frequently. • Teach patient about his disease and therapy. Explain why it's important to take this drug exactly as prescribed, even when he's feeling well. Tell patient not to discontinue this drug suddenly, but to call the doctor if unpleasant side effects develop. Warn that this drug can cause drowsiness. • Warn female patient to notify the doctor if she becomes pregnant. • Watch patient closely for signs of mental depression. Warn him to notify doctor promptly if he starts having nightmares. • Tell patient to avoid alcohol and to follow prescribed diet. • Inform patient that orthostatic hypotension can be minimized by rising slowly and avoiding sudden position changes. Mouth dryness can be relieved with chewing gum, sour hard candy, or ice chips. Tell patient to contact doctor if relief is needed for nasal stuffiness. • Give this drug with meals. • Patient should weigh himself daily and notify doctor of any weight gain. • Effects of this drug may last for 10 days after it's been discontinued.
Methotrimeprazine: may increase hypotension. Use together cautiously. *MAO inhibitors:* may cause excitability and hypertension. Use together cautiously.	• Contraindicated in patients with depression. Use cautiously in patients with severe cardiac or cardiovascular disease, peptic ulcer, ulcerative colitis, gallstones, or those undergoing surgery. Also use cautiously in patients taking other antihypertensives. • Monitor patient's blood pressure and pulse rate frequently. • Teach patient about his disease and therapy. Explain why it's important to take this drug exactly as prescribed, even when he's feeling well. Tell patient not to discontinue this drug suddenly, but to call the doctor if unpleasant side effects develop. Warn that this drug can cause drowsiness. • Warn female patient to notify doctor if she becomes pregnant. • Watch patient closely for signs of mental depression. Warn him to notify doctor promptly if he starts having nightmares. • Tell patient to avoid alcohol and to follow prescribed diet. • Inform patient that orthostatic hypotension can be minimized by rising slowly and avoiding sudden position changes. Mouth dryness can be relieved with chewing gum, sour hard candy, or ice chips. Tell patient to contact doctor if relief is needed for nasal stuffiness. • Give this drug with meals. • Patient should weigh himself daily and notify doctor of any weight gain. • Effects of this drug may last for 10 days after it's been discontinued.

NAME	INDICATIONS & DOSAGE	SIDE EFFECTS
reserpine Alkarau, Arcum R-S, Bonapene, Broserpine, De Serpa, Elserpine, Geneserp #2, Hiserpia, Hyperine, Maso-Serpine, Neo-Serp••, Rauloydin, Raurine, Rau-Sed, Rauserpin, Releserp-5, Reserjen, Reserfia••, Reserpanca••, Reserpaneed, Reserpoid, Rolserp, Sandril, Serp, Serpalan, Serpena, Serpanray, Serpasil•, Serpate, Sertabs, Sertina, Tensin, T-Serp, Tri-Serp, Vio-Serpine, Zepine	*Mild-to-moderate essential hypertension (oral); hypertensive emergencies (parenteral)*— **Adults:** initially, 0.5 mg P.O. daily for 1 to 2 weeks. Maintenance dose: 0.1 to 0.5 mg daily. I.M—initially, 0.5 to 1 mg, followed by doses of 2 to 4 mg at 2-hour intervals. Maximum recommended dose 4 mg. **Children:** 0.07 mg/Kg or 2 mg/M^2 with hydralazine I.M. every 12 to 24 hours.	*CNS:* mental confusion, depression, drowsiness, nervousness, anxiety, nightmares, sedation, parkinsonism. *CV:* orthostatic hypotension. *EENT:* mouth dryness, nasal stuffiness, glaucoma. *GI:* hyperacidity, nausea, vomiting, gastrointestinal bleeding, biliary colic. *Skin:* pruritus, rash. *Other:* impotence, edema, weight gain.
trimethaphan camsylate Arfonad•	*To lower blood pressure quickly in hypertensive emergencies; for controlled hypotension during surgery*— **Adults:** 500 mg (10 ml) diluted in 500 ml dextrose 5% in water to yield concentration of 1 mg/ml I.V. Start I.V. drip at 1 to 2 mg/min and titrate to achieve desired hypotensive response. Range: 0.3 mg to 6 mg/min.	*CNS:* dilated pupils. *CV:* severe hypotension, tachycardia. *GI:* anorexia, nausea, vomiting, dry mouth. *GU:* urinary retention. *Other:* respiratory depression.

INTERACTIONS	NURSING CONSIDERATIONS
MAO inhibitors: may cause excitability and hypertension. Use together cautiously. *Methotrimeprazine:* may increase hypotension. Use together cautiously.	• Contraindicated in patients with depression. Use cautiously in patients with severe cardiac or cerebrovascular disease, peptic ulcer, ulcerative colitis, gallstones, mental depressive disorders; those undergoing surgery; and those taking other antihypertensive drugs. • Monitor patient's blood pressure and pulse rate frequently. • Teach patient about his disease and therapy. Explain why it's important to take this drug exactly as prescribed, even when he's feeling well. Tell patient not to discontinue this drug suddenly, but to call doctor if unpleasant side effects develop. Warn that this drug can cause drowsiness. • Warn female patient to notify doctor if she becomes pregnant. • Watch patient closely for signs of mental depression. Warn him to notify doctor promptly if he starts having nightmares. • Tell patient to avoid alcohol and to stay on diet prescribed by doctor. • Inform patient that orthostatic hypotension can be minimized by rising slowly and avoiding sudden position changes. Mouth dryness can be relieved with chewing gum, sour hard candy, or ice chips. Tell patient to contact doctor if relief is needed for nasal stuffiness. • Give this drug with meals. • Patient should weigh himself daily and notify doctor of any weight gain. • Effects of this drug may last for 10 days after it's been discontinued. • Parenteral form erratically absorbed; largely replaced by other antihypertensives for hypertensive emergencies.
None significant.	• Contraindicated in patients with anemia, respiratory insufficiency. Use cautiously in patients with arteriosclerosis; cardiac, hepatic, or renal disease; degenerative CNS disorders; Addison's disease; diabetes; those receiving glucocorticoids; or those receiving other antihypertensives. • Monitor patient's blood pressure and vital signs frequently. • If extreme hypotension occurs, discontinue drug and call doctor. Use phenylephrine or mephentermine to counteract hypotension. • Watch closely for respiratory distress, especially if large doses are used. • Use infusion pump to administer this drug slowly. • Discontinue drug before wound closure in surgery. • Position patient to avoid cerebral anoxia. • Patient should receive oxygen therapy during use of this agent.

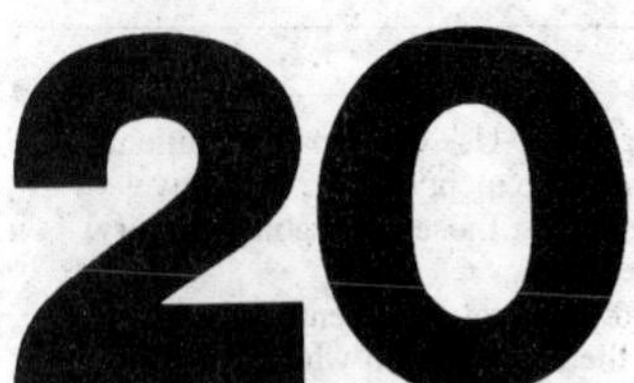

Vasodilators

amyl nitrite
cyclandelate
dioxyline phosphate
dipyridamole
erythrityl tetranitrate
ethaverine hydrochloride
isosorbide dinitrate
isoxsuprine hydrochloride
mannitol hexanitrate
nicotinyl alcohol
nitroglycerin
nylidrin hydrochloride
papaverine hydrochloride
pentaerythritol tetranitrate
tolazoline hydrochloride

Vasodilator drugs can be grouped into two therapeutic categories. Group I—drugs used to treat peripheral vascular diseases—includes cyclandelate, dioxyline phosphate, ethaverine hydrochloride, isoxsuprine hydrochloride, nicotinyl alcohol, nylidrin hydrochloride, papaverine hydrochloride, and tolazoline hydrochloride. Group II—loosely categorized as the coronary vasodilators—includes the nitrates, the nitrites, and dipyridamole.

Major uses

- Treatment of vasospastic and peripheral vascular diseases.
- Treatment and prophylaxis of acute and chronic angina pectoris.
- Adjunctive therapy in treatment of chronic congestive heart failure.
- Antiplatelet activity, in combination with warfarin, to decrease thrombus formation (dipyridamole).
- Antiplatelet activity, in combination with aspirin, to decrease risk of platelet thrombus (dipyridamole).

Mechanism of action

- Relaxation of smooth muscles, especially of blood vessels, resulting in vasodilation.
- Preferential redistribution of blood flow (Group I).
- Pooling of blood in peripheral circulation by venodilation, thus reducing heart's workload (decrease preload) and oxygen consumption (Group II).
- Dilation of arteries, decreasing resistance to ventricular ejection (decreased afterload) and oxygen consumption (Group II).

Absorption, distribution, and excretion

- Varies, depending on drug used, form selected, and route of administration.
- Usually rapidly absorbed.
- Usually rapidly excreted.

Onset and duration

- Varies, depending on drug used, form selected, and route of administration.
- Onset may vary from instantaneous (amyl nitrite) to 60 minutes.
- Peak and duration may also vary: duration of amyl nitrite is 4 to 8 minutes; of mannitol hexanitrate, 4 to 6 hours. (See table.)

Drug	Onset	Duration
amyl nitrite	instantaneous	4 to 8 min.
erythrityl tetranitrate		
sublingual	5 to 10 minutes	3 to 4 hours
oral	30 minutes	3 to 4 hours
isosorbide dinitrate		
sublingual	2 minutes	1 to 2 hours
oral	30 minutes	4 hours
mannitol hexanitrate	15 to 30 minutes	4 to 6 hours
nitroglycerin		
sublingual	1 to 2 minutes	30 minutes
oral (extended release)	60 minutes	4 to 6 hours
topical	15 to 30 minutes	4 to 6 hours
pentaerythritol tetranitrate	1 hour	4 to 5 hours

Combination products

ANTIME FORTE CAPSULES: pentaerythritol tetranitrate 30 mg and secobarbital 50 mg.
ANTORA-B: TD CAPSULES: pentaerythritol tetranitrate 30 mg and secobarbital 50 mg.
CARDILATE-P: erythrityl tetranitrate 10 mg and phenobarbital 15 mg.
CARTRAX-10: pentaerythritol tetranitrate 10 mg and hydroxyzine HCl 10 mg.
CARTRAX-20: pentaerythritol tetranitrate 20 mg and hydroxyzine HCl 10 mg.
COROVAS TYMCAPS: pentaerythritol tetranitrate 30 mg and secobarbital 50 mg.
EQUINITRATE 10♦: pentaerythritol tetranitrate 10 mg and meprobamate 200 mg.
EQUINITRATE 20: pentaerythritol tetranitrate 20 mg and meprobamate 200 mg.
HYDERGINE: dihydroergocornine mesylate 0.167 mg, dihydroergocristine mesylate 0.167 mg, and dihydroergocryptine mesylate 0.167 mg.
ISORDIL WITH PHENOBARBITAL: isosorbide dinitrate 10 mg and phenobarbital 15 mg.
MILTRATE: pentaerythritol tetranitrate 10 or 20 mg and meprobamate 200 mg.
PAPAVATRAL L.A. CAPSULES: pentaerythritol tetranitrate 50 mg and ethavarine HCl 30 mg.
PAVATRAL 10: pentaerythritol tetranitrate 10 mg and ethaverine HCl 30 mg.
PAVATRAL 20: pentaerythritol tetranitrate 20 mg and ethaverine HCl 30 mg.
PENNPHENO TABLETS: pentaerythritol tetranitrate 10 mg and phenobarbital 15 mg.
PENNPHENO DOUBLE STRENGTH TABLETS: pentaerythritol tetranitrate 20 mg and phenobarbital 15 mg.
PERITRATE WITH NITROGLYCERIN: pentaerythritol tetranitrate 10 mg and nitroglycerin 0.3 mg.
PERITRATE WITH PHENOBARBITAL♦: pentaerythritol tetranitrate 10 mg and phenobarbital 15 mg.
ROBAM-PETN 10 TABLETS: pentaerythritol tetranitrate 10 mg and meprobamate 200 mg.
ROBAM-PETN 20 TABLETS: pentaerythritol tetranitrate 20 mg and meprobamate 20 mg.

PATIENT TEACHING AID — NITROGLYCERIN

Dear Patient:
Here's what you should know about the drug your doctor has prescribed for you. Nitroglycerin relieves anginal pain by temporarily dilating (widening) veins and arteries. This brings more blood and oxygen to the heart when it needs it most, and your heart doesn't have to work so hard.

To make sure you get the most from your therapy, follow these instructions carefully:

1. When you get anginal pain, stop what you are doing, lie down, and put a pill under your tongue. Let it dissolve completely and hold the saliva in your mouth for 1 to 2 minutes before swallowing. Always sit or lie down when you take your pill or you may get dizzy. If you feel headachy or your face flushes after taking your pill, don't worry. These effects are only temporary.

2. Take up to 3 pills — 1 every 10 minutes — for pain. Record each dosage. *If the pain doesn't go away after 30 minutes or is unusually severe, call the doctor at once or go to the hospital emergency ward.*

3. Don't drink alcohol without asking your doctor first.

4. Never stop taking your pills altogether without your doctor's permission. However, don't worry about taking them as needed, because they are not habit-forming.

5. Keep your pills in their original container with the cotton removed. They will lose their strength if they're exposed to light, moisture, or heat — or if they're more than 3 months old. Get fresh ones after 3 months. Fresh pills produce a slight burning sensation under your tongue.

Call the doctor immediately if you notice any of the following: unusually severe or prolonged pain, fainting, or dizziness.

NAME	INDICATIONS & DOSAGE	SIDE EFFECTS
amyl nitrite	*Antidote for cyanide poisoning—* 0.2 or 0.3 ml by inhalation for 30 to 60 seconds q 5 minutes until conscious; 10 ml of 3% injection I.V. at rate of 2.5 to 5 ml/minute, then 50 ml of 25% sodium thiosulfate injection I.V. *Relief of angina pectoris, bronchospasm, biliary spasm—* **Adults and children:** 0.2 to 0.3 ml by inhalation (1 glass ampule inhaler), p.r.n.	*Blood:* methemoglobinemia. *CNS:* headache, sometimes with throbbing; dizziness; weakness. *CV:* orthostatic hypotension, tachycardia, flushing, palpitations, fainting. *GI:* nausea, vomiting. *Skin:* cutaneous vasodilation. *Other:* hypersensitivity reactions.
cyclandelate Cyclanfor, Cyclospasmol♦	*Adjunct in intermittent claudication, arteriosclerosis obliterans, vasospasm and muscular ischemia associated with thrombophlebitis, nocturnal leg cramps, Raynaud's phenomenon, selected cases of ischemic cerebral vascular disease—* **Adults:** initially, 200 mg P.O. q.i.d. (before meals and h.s.); maximum 400 mg P.O. q.i.d. When clinical response is noted, decrease dosage gradually until maintenance dosage is reached. Maintenance dose 400 to 800 mg daily in divided doses.	*CNS:* headache, tingling, dizziness. *CV:* mild flushing, tachycardia. *GI:* pyrosis, pain, eructation, nausea, heartburn. *Other:* sweating.
dioxyline phosphate Paveril♦ phosphate	*Treatment of angina pectoris and conditions in which there is reflex spasm of blood vessels in arms, legs, or lungs; smooth-muscle spasm—* **Adults:** 100 to 400 mg 3 to 4 times daily, as required.	*CNS:* dizziness, sedation. *CV:* sweating, flushing. *GI:* nausea, abdominal cramps.
dipyridamole Persantine♦	*Long-term therapy of chronic angina pectoris, prevention of recurrent transient ischemic attack—* **Adults:** 50 mg P.O. t.i.d. at least 1 hour before meals, to maximum of 400 mg daily. *Inhibition of platelet adhesion in patients with prosthetic heart valves, in combination with warfarin—* **Adults:** 100 to 400 mg P.O. daily. *Transient ischemic attack—* **Adults:** 100 mg P.O. daily as a single dose.	*CNS:* headache, dizziness. *CV:* flushing, fainting, hypotension. *GI:* intolerance, nausea, vomiting, diarrhea. *Skin:* rash. *Other:* weakness.

♦ Also available in Canada.
♦♦ Available in Canada only.
Unmarked trade names available in United States only.

INTERACTIONS	NURSING CONSIDERATIONS
None significant.	• Contraindicated in hypersensitivity to nitrites. Use with caution in cerebral hemorrhage, hypotension, head injury, and glaucoma. • Watch for orthostatic hypotension. Have patient sit down and avoid rapid position changes while inhaling drug. • Extinguish all cigarettes before using or ampule may ignite. • Wrap ampule in cloth and crush. Hold near patient's nose and mouth so vapor is inhaled. • Effective within 30 seconds but has a short duration (4 to 8 minutes). • Head-low position, deep breathing, and movement of extremities may help relieve dizziness, syncope, or weakness from postural hypotension. • Drug is often abused. Claimed to have aphrodisiac benefits. Sometimes called "Amy."
None significant.	• Use with extreme caution in severe obliterative coronary artery or cerebral vascular disease, since circulation to these diseased areas may be compromised by vasodilatory effects of the drug elsewhere (coronary steal syndrome). Use with caution in glaucoma, hypotension. • Give with food or antacids to lessen GI distress. • Use in conjunction with, not as a substitute for appropriate medical or surgical therapy of peripheral or cerebral vascular disease. • Short-term therapy of little benefit. Instruct patient to expect long-term treatment and to continue to take medication. • Side effects usually disappear after several weeks of therapy.
None significant.	• Alert patient to possible side effects.
None significant.	• Use with caution in hypotension, anticoagulant therapy. • Observe for side effects, especially with large doses. Monitor blood pressure. • Administer 1 hour before meals. • Watch for signs of bleeding, prolonged bleeding time (large doses, long-term). • Clinical response to antianginal therapy may not be evident before second or third month. Tell patient to continue drug despite lack of observable response.

NAME	INDICATIONS & DOSAGE	SIDE EFFECTS
erythrityl tetranitrate Anginar, Cardilate◆	*Prophylaxis and long-term management of frequent or recurrent anginal pain, reduced exercise tolerance associated with angina pectoris*— **Adults:** 5 mg sublingually or bucally t.i.d. or 10 mg P.O., a.c. chewed t.i.d., increasing in 2 to 3 days if needed.	*CNS:* headache, sometimes with throbbing; dizziness; weakness. *CV:* orthostatic hypotension, tachycardia, flushing, palpitations, fainting. *GI:* nausea, vomiting. *Local:* sublingual burning. *Skin:* cutaneous vasodilation. *Other:* hypersensitivity reactions.
ethaverine hydrochloride Cebral, Circubid, Etalent, Ethaquin, Ethatab, Ethavex, Isovex, Laverin, Myoquin, Neopavrin, Pavaspan, Roldiol, Spasodil	*Long-term treatment of peripheral and cerebrovascular insufficiency associated with arterial spasm; spastic conditions of gastrointestinal and genitourinary tracts*— **Adults:** 100 to 200 mg P.O. t.i.d. or 150 mg of sustained-release preparation P.O. q 12 hours.	*CNS:* headache, drowsiness. *CV:* hypotension, flushing, sweating, vertigo, cardiac depression, arrhythmias. *GI:* nausea; anorexia; abdominal distress; dryness of throat; constipation; diarrhea; hepatic hypersensitivity manifested by GI symptoms, eosinophilia, jaundice, altered hepatic function tests. *Skin:* rash. *Other:* respiratory depression, malaise, lassitude.
isosorbide dinitrate Angidil, Coronex◆◆, Iso-Bid, Iso-D, Isosorb, Isordil◆, Isotrate, Neo-Corovas-80, Onset, Sorate, Sorbide, Sorbitrate, Sorquad, Vasotrate	*Treatment of acute anginal attacks (sublingual and chewable only); prophylaxis in situations likely to cause attacks; treatment of chronic ischemic heart disease (by preload reduction); adjunct with other vasodilators, such as hydralazine and prazosin in treatment of severe chronic congestive heart failure*— **Adults:** *Sublingual form*—2.5 to 10 mg under the tongue for prompt relief of anginal pain, repeated q 2 to	*CNS:* headache, sometimes with throbbing; dizziness; weakness. *CV:* orthostatic hypotension, tachycardia, palpitations, fainting. *GI:* nausea, vomiting. *Local:* sublingual burning. *Skin:* cutaneous vasodilation, flushing. *Other:* hypersensitivity reactions.

INTERACTIONS	NURSING CONSIDERATIONS
None significant.	• Contraindicated in hypersensitivity to nitrites, idiosyncrasy, head trauma, cerebral hemorrhage, severe anemia. Use with caution in hypotension. • Monitor blood pressure, and intensity and duration of response to drug. • May cause headaches, especially at first. Treat headache with aspirin or acetaminophen. Dosage may need to be reduced temporarily, but tolerance usually develops. • Tell patient to take medication regularly, even long-term, if ordered, and to keep it easily accessible at all times. Physiologically necessary but not habit-forming. • Additional dose may be taken before anticipated stress or at bedtime if angina is nocturnal. • Advise patient to avoid alcoholic beverages; they may produce unpleasant antabuse-like side effects. • May cause orthostatic hypotension. Patient should get out of bed, go up and down stairs, and change position slowly, and should lie down at first sign of dizziness. • Teach patient to take sublingual tablet at first sign of attack. He should wet the tablet with saliva, place it under the tongue until completely absorbed, and sit down and rest. Burning sensation indicates potency. Dose may be repeated every 10 to 15 minutes for a maximum of 3 doses. If no relief, patient should call doctor or go to hospital emergency room. If patient complains of tingling, he may try holding tablet in buccal pouch. • Teach patient to take oral tablet on empty stomach, either ½ hour before or 1 to 2 hours after meals; to swallow oral tablets whole; and, chew chewable tablets thoroughly before swallowing. • Store medication in cool place, in tightly closed container, away from light. To assure freshness, replace supply every 3 months. Remove cotton from container, since it absorbs drug.
None significant.	• Contraindicated in complete A-V dissociation and in severe hepatic disease. Use with caution in women who are pregnant or of childbearing age; and in glaucoma or pulmonary embolus; may precipitate arrhythmias. • Hold dose and call doctor if signs of hepatic hypersensitivity develop. • Monitor and record vital signs during therapy.
None significant.	• Contraindicated in hypersensitivity to nitrites, idiosyncrasy, head trauma, cerebral hemorrhage, severe anemia. Use with caution in hypotension. • Monitor blood pressure, and intensity and duration of response to drug. • May cause headaches, especially at first. Treat headache with aspirin or acetaminophen. Dosage may need to be reduced temporarily, but tolerance usually develops. • Tell patient to take medication regularly, even long-term, if ordered, and to keep it easily accessible at all times. Physiologically necessary but not habit-forming. • Additional dose may be taken before anticipated stress or at bedtime if angina is nocturnal. • Advise patient to avoid alcoholic beverages; they may produce unpleasant antabuse-like side effects. • May cause orthostatic hypotension. Patient should get out of bed, go up

(continued on following page)

NAME	INDICATIONS & DOSAGE	SIDE EFFECTS
isosorbide dinitrate *(continued)*	3 hours during acute phase, or q 4 to 6 hours for prophylaxis. *Chewable form*—5 to 10 mg, p.r.n., for acute attack or q 2 to 3 hours for prophylaxis but only after initial test dose of 5 mg to determine risk of severe hypotension. *Oral form*—5 to 30 mg P.O. q.i.d. for prophylaxis only (use smallest effective dose); sustained-release forms 40 mg P.O. q 6 to 12 hours.	
isoxsuprine hydrochloride Rolisox, Vasodilan♦, Vasoprine	*Adjunct for relief of symptoms associated with cerebral vascular insufficiency, peripheral vascular diseases (such as arteriosclerosis obliterans, thromboangitis obliterans, Raynaud's disease); inhibition of uterine contractions in premature labor, threatened abortion, dysmenorrhea*— **Adults:** 10 to 20 mg P.O. t.i.d. or q.i.d.; initially, 5 to 10 mg I.M. b.i.d. or t.i.d. in severe or acute conditions, to maximum of 10 mg. Intramuscular doses greater than 10 mg may be associated with hypotension and tachycardia and are not recommended.	*CNS:* dizziness, nervousness, weakness, trembling. *CV:* hypotension, tachycardia, transient palpitations. *GI:* vomiting, abdominal distress, intestinal distention. *Skin:* severe rash.
mannitol hexanitrate Mannex, Vascunitol	*Chronic prophylaxis against attacks of angina pectoris*— **Adults:** 15 to 60 mg P.O. q 4 to 6 hours.	*Blood:* methemoglobinemia. *CNS:* headache, sometimes with throbbing; dizziness; weakness. *CV:* orthostatic hypotension, tachycardia, flushing, palpitations, fainting. *GI:* nausea, vomiting. *Local:* sublingual burning. *Skin:* cutaneous vasodilation. *Other:* hypersensitivity, rise in intraocular tension, increased intracranial pressure.

INTERACTIONS	NURSING CONSIDERATIONS
	and down stairs, and change position slowly, and should lie down at first sign of dizziness. • Teach patient to take sublingual tablet at first sign of attack. He should wet the tablet with saliva, place it under the tongue until completely absorbed, and sit down and rest. Burning sensation indicates potency. Dose may be repeated every 10 to 15 minutes for a maximum of 3 doses. If no relief, patient should call doctor or go to hospital emergency room. If patient complains of tingling, he may try holding tablet in buccal pouch. • Warn patient not to confuse sublingual with oral form. • Teach patient to take oral tablet on empty stomach, either ½ hour before or 1 to 2 hours after meals; to swallow oral tablets whole; and, chew chewable tablets thoroughly before swallowing. • Withdraw gradually, over 4 to 6 weeks. • Store in cool place, in tightly closed container, away from light.
None significant.	• Contraindicated in immediate postpartum period, arterial bleeding; I.M. contraindicated in hypotension or tachycardia. • Safe use in pregnancy and lactation not established, although drug has been used to inhibit contractions in premature labor. • Do not give intravenously. • Observe for hypotension with parenteral use. • Discontinue if rash develops.
None significant.	• Contraindicated in idiosyncrasy, head trauma, cerebral hemorrhage, severe anemia. Use with caution in hypotension. • Monitor blood pressure, and intensity and duration of response to drug. • Medication may cause headaches, especially at first. Treat headache with aspirin or acetaminophen. Dosage may need to be reduced temporarily, but tolerance usually develops. • Tell patient to take medication regularly, even long-term, if ordered. Physiologically necessary but not habit-forming. • Additional doses may be taken before anticipated stress or at bedtime if angina is nocturnal. • Alcoholic beverages should be avoided, since they may produce unpleasant antabuse-like side effects. • Medication may cause orthostatic hypotension. Patient should get out of bed, go up and down stairs, or change position slowly, and should lie down at first sign of dizziness. • Store medication in cool dark place in tightly covered container. • Effective within 15 to 30 minutes; duration 4 to 6 hours.

NAME	INDICATIONS & DOSAGE	SIDE EFFECTS
nicotinyl alcohol Roniacol♦	*Treatment of conditions of deficient circulation such as peripheral vascular disease, vascular spasm, varicose ulcers, decubital ulcers, Meniere's syndrome, vertigo—* **Adults:** 50 to 100 mg regular tablets P.O. b.i.d. or t.i.d. (may increase to 150 to 200 mg P.O. t.i.d. or q.i.d.); 150 to 300 mg sustained-release tablets P.O. b.i.d.; 5 to 10 ml of elixir P.O. t.i.d.	*CNS:* paresthesias. *CV:* transient flushing. *GI:* gastric disturbances. *Skin:* minor rashes. *Other:* allergic reactions.
nitroglycerin Ang-O-Span, Cardabid, Corobid, Glyceryl Trinitrate, Gly-Trate, Nitrine, Nitrobid, Nitrocap, Nitrocels, Nitro-Dial, Nitroglyn, Nitrol♦, Nitro-Lyn, Nitrong♦, Nitrospan, Nitrostabilin♦♦, Nitrostat♦, Nitrotym, Nitro-TD, Nitrozem, Nyglycon, Trates, Vasoglyn	*Prophylaxis against chronic anginal attacks—* **Adults:** 1 sustained-release capsule q 8 to 12 hours; or 2% ointment: Start with ½ inch ointment, increasing with ½-inch increments until headache occurs, then decreasing to previous dose. Range of dosage with ointment 2 to 5 inches. Usual dose 1 to 2 inches. *Relief of acute angina pectoris, prophylaxis to prevent or minimize anginal attacks when taken immediately prior to stressful events—* **Adults:** 1 sublingual tablet (gr. 1/400, 1/200, 1/150, 1/100) dissolved under the tongue or in the buccal pouch immediately upon indication of anginal attack. May repeat q 5 minutes for 15 minutes. Maximum of 3 0.4-mg tablets.	*CNS:* headache, sometimes with throbbing; dizziness; weakness; syncope. *CV:* orthostatic hypotension, tachycardia, flushing, palpitations, fainting. *GI:* nausea, vomiting. *Local:* sublingual burning. *Skin:* cutaneous vasodilation. *Other:* hypersensitivity reactions.
nylidrin hydrochloride Arlidin♦, Pervadil♦♦, Rolidrin	*To increase blood supply in vasospastic disorders (arteriosclerosis obliterans, thromboangitis obliterans, diabetic vascular disease, night leg cramps, Raynaud's phenomenon and disease, ischemic ulcer, frostbite, acrocyanosis, acroparasthesia, sequelae of thrombophlebitis); and in circulatory disturbances of the middle ear (primary cochlear ischemia, cochlear striae, vascular*	*CNS:* trembling, nervousness, weakness, dizziness. *CV:* palpitations, hypotension, flushing. *GI:* nausea, vomiting.

INTERACTIONS	NURSING CONSIDERATIONS
Clonidine: may inhibit vasodilation. Observe for lack of response.	• Contraindicated in active peptic ulcer or gastritis. • Tolerance to side effects develops with continued therapy.
None significant.	• Contraindicated in hypersensitivity to nitrites, idiosyncrasy, head trauma, cerebral hemorrhage, severe anemia. Use with caution in hypotension. • Monitor blood pressure, and intensity and duration of response to drug. • May cause headaches, especially at first. Treat headache with aspirin or acetaminophen. Dosage may need to be reduced temporarily, but tolerance usually develops. • Tell patient to take medication regularly, even long-term, if ordered, and to keep it easily accessible at all times. Physiologically necessary but not habit-forming. • Additional dose may be taken before anticipated stress or at bedtime if angina is nocturnal. • Advise patient to avoid alcoholic beverages; they may produce unpleasant antabuse-like side effects. • May cause orthostatic hypotension. Patient should get out of bed, go up and down stairs, and change position slowly, and should lie down at first sign of dizziness. • Teach patient to take sublingual tablet at first sign of attack. He should wet the tablet with saliva; place it under the tongue until completely absorbed and sit down and rest. Burning sensation indicates potency. Dose may be repeated every 10 to 15 minutes for a maximum of 3 doses. If no relief, patient should call doctor or go to hospital emergency room. If patient complains of tingling, he may try holding tablet in buccal pouch. • Teach patient to take oral tablet on empty stomach, either ½ hour before or 1 to 2 hours after meals; to swallow oral tablets whole; and chew chewable tablets thoroughly before swallowing. • Store in cool dark place, in tightly closed container. To assure freshness, replace supply every 3 months. Remove cotton from container, since it absorbs drug. • To apply ointment, spread in uniform thin layer on any nonhairy area. Do not rub in. Cover with plastic film to aid absorption and to protect clothing.
None significant.	• Contraindicated in acute myocardial infarction, paroxysmal tachycardia, angina pectoris, thyrotoxicosis. Use with caution in uncompensated heart disease or peptic ulcer.

(continued on following page)

NAME	INDICATIONS & DOSAGE	SIDE EFFECTS
nylidrin hydrochloride *(continued)*	*ischemia, macular or ampullar ischemia), other disturbances due to labyrinth artery spasm or obstruction—* **Adults:** 3 to 12 mg P.O. t.i.d. or q.i.d.	
papaverine hydrochloride Blupav, BP-Papaverine, Cerebid, Cerespan, Cirbed, Delapav, Dylate-SR, J-Pav, Kavrin, Lapay, Lem-Pav-Ty-Med, Myobid, Papacon, Papalease, Papital T.R., Pap-Kaps-150 Meta-Kaps, P-A-V, Pava-2, Pavabid, Pavacap, Pavacen, Pavaclor, Pavacron, Pavadel, Pavadur, Pavadyl, Pavakey S.A., Pavalyn, Pava-Par, Pava-Rx, Pavasule, Pavatime, Pavatran T.D., Pava-Wol, Paverolan, Pavex, PT-300, Ro-Papav, S.M.R.-Kaps, Sustaverine, Vasal, Vasocap, Vasospan, Vazosan	*Relief of cerebral and peripheral ischemia associated with arterial spasm and myocardial ischemia; treatment of smooth-muscle spasm (coronary occlusion, angina pectoris, sequelae of peripheral and pulmonary embolism, certain cerebral angiospastic states); and visceral spasms (biliary, ureteral, or gastrointestinal colic)—* **Adults:** 100 to 300 mg P.O. 3 to 5 times daily, or 150 to 300 mg sustained-release preparations q 8 to 12 hours; 30 to 120 mg I.M. or I.V. q 3 hours, as indicated.	*CNS:* headache. *CV:* increased heart rate, increased blood pressure (with parenteral use), depressed AV and intraventricular conduction, arrhythmias. *GI:* constipation. *Other:* sweating, flushing, malaise, increased depth of respiration.
pentaerythritol tetranitrate Angijen Green, Angitrate, Antora, Arcotrate Nos. 1 & 2, Baritrate, Blaintrate, Desatrate 30, Desatrate 50, Dilar, Dinate, Duotrate, El-PETN, Kaytrate, Maso-Trol, Naptrate, Nitrin, Penta-Cap-No. 1, Penta-E., Penta-E. S.A., Pentaforte-T, Penta-Tal No. 1 & 2, Pentestan-80, Pentetra, Pentrate T.D., Pentritol, Pent-T-80, Pentylan, Peritrate♦, PETN, Petro-20 mg, P-T♦♦, P-T-T, Quintrate, Rate, Reithritol, Vasitol, Vasolate, Vasolate-80	*Prophylaxis against angina pectoris—* **Adults:** 10 to 20 mg P.O. q.i.d.; may be titrated upward to 40 mg P.O. q.i.d. ½ hour before or 1 hour after meals and h.s.; 80 mg sustained-release preparations P.O. b.i.d.	*CNS:* headache, sometimes with throbbing; dizziness; weakness. *CV:* orthostatic hypotension, tachycardia, flushing, palpitations, fainting. *GI:* nausea, vomiting. *Skin:* cutaneous vasodilation. *Other:* hypersensitivity reactions.

INTERACTIONS	NURSING CONSIDERATIONS
None significant.	• Contraindicated for I.V. use in complete A-V block. Use with caution in glaucoma. • Monitor blood pressure, heart rate and rhythm, especially in cardiac disease. Hold dose and notify doctor immediately if changes occur. • Not often used parenterally, except when immediate effect is desired. • Give I.V. slowly (over 1 to 2 minutes) to avoid side effects. • Most effective when given early in the course of a disorder. • Tell patient to take medication regularly; long-term therapy is required. • Do not add to lactated Ringer's injection; will precipitate.
None significant.	• Contraindicated in idiosyncrasy, head trauma, cerebral hemorrhage, severe anemia. Use with caution in hypotension and glaucoma. • Monitor blood pressure, and intensity and duration of response to drug. • Medication may cause headaches, especially at first. Treat with aspirin or acetaminophen. Dosage may need to be reduced temporarily, but tolerance usually develops. • Medication should be taken regularly, even long-term, if ordered. Physiologically necessary but not habit-forming. • Additional doses may be taken before anticipated stress or at bedtime for nocturnal angina. • Alcoholic beverages should be avoided, since they may produce unpleasant antabuse-like side effects. • Medication may cause orthostatic hypotension. Patient should get out of bed, go up and down stairs, or change position slowly, and should lie down at first sign of dizziness. • Store medication in cool place in tightly covered, light-resistant container.

NAME	INDICATIONS & DOSAGE	SIDE EFFECTS
tolazoline hydrochloride Priscoline•, Tazol, Toloxan, Tolzol	*Spastic peripheral vascular disorders associated with acrocyanosis, acroparasthesia, arteriosclerosis obliterans, Buerger's disease, causalgia, diabetic arteriosclerosis, gangrene, endarteritis, sequelae of frostbite, post-thrombotic conditions, Raynaud's disease, scleroderma—* **Adults:** *Oral*—25 mg 4 to 6 times daily, gradually increasing to maximum of 50 mg 6 times daily; 80 mg sustained-release tablet P.O. q 12 hours. *Parenteral*—10 to 50 mg S.C., I.V., or I.M. q.i.d. Start with low dose, increasing gradually until optimal response (as determined by appearance of flushing) is reached. *Intra-arterial*—50 to 75 mg/ injection, depending on response; 1 or 2 injections may be required initially, then dose of 2 or 3 injections weekly to maintain circulation, possibly coupled with oral tolazoline between injections.	*CV:* arrhythmias, anginal pain, hypertension, hypotension, tachycardia, flushing, burning sensation (following intra-arterial injection), transient postural vertigo, palpitations. *GI:* nausea, vomiting, diarrhea, epigastric discomfort, exacerbation of peptic ulcer. *Other:* weakness, paradoxical response in seriously damaged limbs, increased pilomotor activity, tingling, chilliness, apprehension.

INTERACTIONS	NURSING CONSIDERATIONS
Ethyl alcohol: possible antabuse reaction from accumulation of acetaldehyde. Use together cautiously.	• Contraindicated in coronary artery disease, active peptic ulcer, or following cerebrovascular accident. Use with caution in history of peptic ulcer disease, gastritis, or known or suspected mitral stenosis. • Keep patient warm during parenteral administration to increase response. • Appearance of flushing usually indicates maximum tolerable dose. • Monitor vital signs. Watch especially for blood pressure changes, arrhythmias. • Instruct patient to avoid alcohol. • Due to risks, technique, and precautions, intra-arterial injection should be done only by experienced personnel, in selected cases, and only after maximum benefit has been achieved with oral and parenteral therapy. • Warn against exposure to cold, which can aggravate tissue damage. • Often used to distinguish between functional (vasospastic) and organic (obstructive) forms of peripheral insular disease.

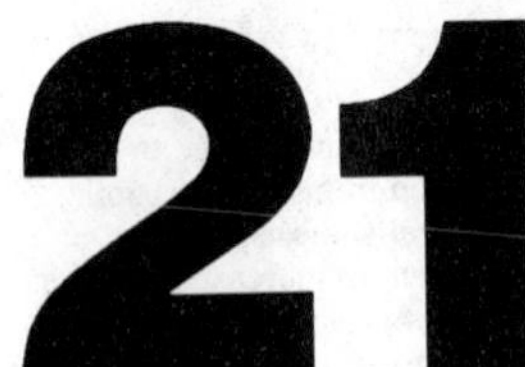

Antilipemics

cholestyramine
clofibrate
colestipol hydrochloride
dextrothyroxine sodium
niacin
probucol
sitosterols

In current practice, antilipemic agents are used primarily to manage primary hyperlipoproteinemias. Their effectiveness in primary and secondary coronary heart disease remains uncertain. They may prove of value in programs designed to reduce multiple risk factors, such as obesity and hypertension.

Hyperlipoproteinemias may be primary or secondary to underlying diseases, such as hypothyroidism, obstructive jaundice, nephrotic syndrome, or poorly controlled diabetes mellitus. In such cases, control of the underlying disease will correct the lipid disorder. Antilipemic agents should be prescribed only when dietary measures fail.

Major uses

• Treatment of hyperlipoproteinemias.

Mechanism of action

• All antilipemics lower the amount of serum lipids in the bloodstream, though their precise mechanism of action may differ.
• Cholestyramine combines with bile acid to form an insoluble compound which is then excreted. Cholestyramine lowers cholesterol; it raises or may have no effect on triglycerides.
• Clofibrate increases clearance of triglyceride and cholesterol; it lowers cholesterol and triglycerides.
• Colestipol hydrochloride combines with bile acid to form an insoluble compound which is then excreted. It lowers cholesterol; it raises or may have no effect on triglycerides.
• Dextrothyroxine sodium increases rate of catabolism of cholesterol in the liver and increases bile secretion. It lowers cholesterol and triglycerides.
• Niacin decreases synthesis of low-density lipoproteins and inhibits lipolysis in adipose tissue. It lowers cholesterol and triglycerides.
• Probucol inhibits transport of cholesterol from intestine and may also affect cholesterol synthesis. It lowers cholesterol but has a variable effect on triglycerides.
• Sitosterols interfere with intestinal absorption of cholesterol; they lower cholesterol but have a variable effect on triglycerides.

Absorption, distribution, and excretion

• Cholestyramine, sitosterols, and colestipol are not appreciably absorbed from the GI tract and are excreted in the feces.

• Probucol is absorbed only in small amounts and then secreted by the biliary tract into the GI tract. It takes 1 to 2 months to reach maximum effect of probucol and clofibrate.
• Response to antilipemic agents varies with adherence to drug and dietary regimens. For maximum benefit, plasma cholesterol and triglyceride should be tested several times during the first few months of antilipemic therapy and periodically thereafter.

Onset and duration
• None established.

Combination products
None.

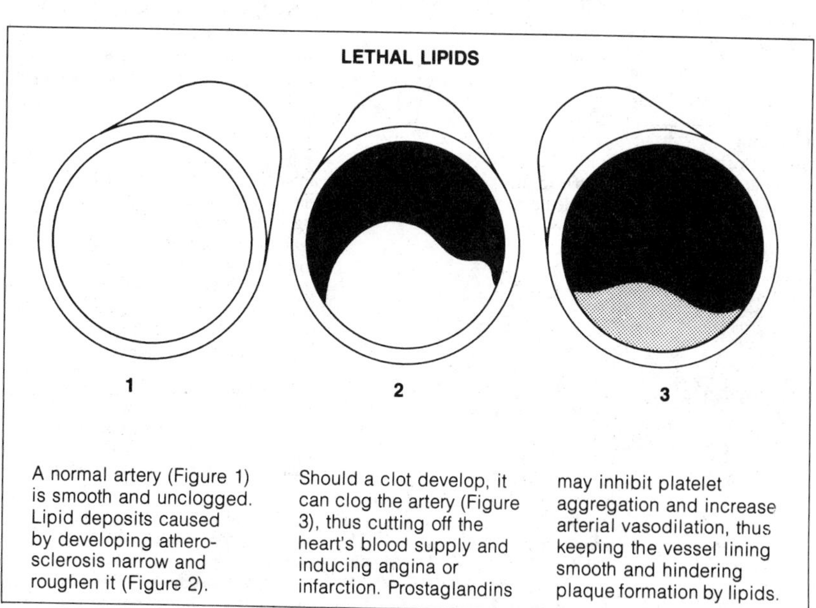

A normal artery (Figure 1) is smooth and unclogged. Lipid deposits caused by developing athero-sclerosis narrow and roughen it (Figure 2). Should a clot develop, it can clog the artery (Figure 3), thus cutting off the heart's blood supply and inducing angina or infarction. Prostaglandins may inhibit platelet aggregation and increase arterial vasodilation, thus keeping the vessel lining smooth and hindering plaque formation by lipids.

NAME	INDICATIONS & DOSAGE	SIDE EFFECTS
cholestyramine Questran◆	*Primary hyperlipidemia, pruritus, and diarrhea due to excess bile acid—* **Adults:** 4 g before meals and h.s., not to exceed 32 g daily. Each scoop or packet of Questran contains 4 g cholestyramine. **Children:** 240 mg/Kg/day P.O. in 3 divided doses with beverage or food. Safe dosage not established for children under 6.	*GI:* constipation (common, may require decreasing the dosage), fecal impaction, hemorrhoids, abdominal discomfort, flatulence, nausea, vomiting, steatorrhea. *Skin:* rashes, irritation of skin, tongue, and perianal area. *Other:* vitamin deficiency A, D, and K from decreased absorption; hyperchloremic acidosis with long-term use or very high dosage.
clofibrate Atromid-S◆	*Hyperlipidemia and xanthoma tuberosum—* **Adults:** 2 g P.O. daily in divided doses. Some patients may respond to lower doses as assessed by serum lipid monitoring.	*Blood:* leukopenia, anemia. *CNS:* fatigue, weakness, drowsiness, dizziness, headache. *CV:* angina, arrhythmias, swelling, phlebitis at xanthoma sites. *GI:* nausea, diarrhea, hepatomegaly, transient and reversible elevations of hepatic function tests, gallstones, vomiting, stomatitis, gastroenteritis, dyspepsia. *GU:* decreased libido. *Skin:* allergic rashes, urticaria, pruritus, dry skin and hair. *Other:* myalgias and arthralgias, resembling a flu-like syndrome, weight gain, polyphagia.
colestipol hydrochloride Colestid	*Primary hypercholesterolemia and xanthomas—* **Adults:** 15 to 30 g P.O. daily in 2 to 4 divided doses.	*GI:* constipation (common, may require decreasing the dosage), fecal impaction, hemorrhoids, abdominal discomfort, flatulence, nausea, vomiting, steatorrhea. *Skin:* rashes, irritation of skin, tongue, and perianal area. *Other:* vitamin deficiency A, D, and K from decreased absorption; hyperchloremic acidosis with long-term use or very high dosage.
dextrothyroxine sodium Choloxin◆	*Hyperlipidemia in euthyroid patients, especially when cholesterol and triglyceride levels are elevated—* **Adults:** initial dose 1 to 2 mg daily, increased by 1 to 2 mg daily at monthly intervals to a total of 4 to 8 mg daily. **Children:** initial dose 0.05 mg/Kg daily, increased by 0.05 mg/Kg daily at monthly intervals to a total of 4 mg daily.	*CV:* palpitations, angina pectoris, arrhythmias, ischemic myocardial changes on EKG, increased heart size, myocardial infarction. *EENT:* visual disturbances, ptosis, tinnitus. *GI:* dyspepsia, nausea, vomiting, diarrhea, constipation, decreased appetite. *Metabolic:* insomnia, weight loss, sweating, flushing, hyperthermia, hair loss, menstrual irregularities. *Other:* rarely, hoarseness, tinnitus, libido changes, "bitter taste," dizziness, psychic changes, paresthesias, muscle pain.

◆ Also available in Canada.
◆◆ Available in Canada only.
Unmarked trade names available in United States only.

INTERACTIONS	NURSING CONSIDERATIONS
None significant.	• To mix, sprinkle powder on surface of preferred beverage or wet food. Let stand a few minutes, then stir to obtain uniform suspension. • Mixing with carbonated beverages may result in excess foaming. To avoid, use large glass, mix slowly. • Administer all other medications at least 1 hour before or 4 to 6 hours after cholestyramine to avoid blocking their absorption. • Observe bowel habits; treat constipation as needed. If severe constipation develops, decrease dosage or discontinue drug. • Monitor cardiac glycoside levels for patients receiving both medications concurrently. Should cholestyramine therapy be discontinued, cardiac glycoside toxicity may result unless dosage is adjusted. • Watch for deficiencies of vitamins A, D, and K.
Oral contraceptives: may antagonize clofibrate's lipid-lowering effect. Monitor serum lipid level.	• Contraindicated in patients with severe renal or hepatic disease. • Warn patient to report flu-like symptoms to doctor immediately. • Monitor renal and hepatic function, blood counts, serum electrolyte, and blood sugar levels. If hepatic function tests show steady rise, clofibrate should be discontinued. • Should not be used indiscriminately. May pose increased risk of gallstones and cancer.
Oral hypoglycemics: may antagonize response to colestipol. Monitor serum lipid level.	• Administer all other medications at least 1 hour before or 4 to 6 hours after colestipol to avoid blocking their absorption. • Monitor cardiac glycoside levels for patients receiving both medications concurrently. Should colestipol therapy be discontinued, cardiac glycoside toxicity may result unless dosage is adjusted. • Watch for vitamin A, D, and K deficiency.
None significant.	• Contraindicated for pregnant women, lactating mothers, patients with hepatic or renal disease, or iodism. Patients with history of heart disease, including arrhythmias, hypertension, or angina pectoris should receive very small doses. • May increase need for insulin, diet therapy, or oral hypoglycemics in diabetics. • Discontinue drug 2 weeks before surgery. • Observe patient for signs of hyperthyroidism, such as nervousness, insomnia, weight loss. If these occur, dosage should be decreased or drug discontinued.

NAME	INDICATIONS & DOSAGE	SIDE EFFECTS
niacin Diacin, Efacin, Niac, Niacalex, Niacels, NICL, Nicobid, Nicocap, Nico-400, Nicolar, NiCord XL, nico-Span, Nicotinex, Ni-Span, Tega-Span, Tinic, Wampocap	*Adjunctive treatment of hyperlipidemias, especially associated with hypercholesterolemia—* **Adults:** 1.5 to 3.0 g daily in 3 divided doses with or after meals, increased at intervals to 6 g daily.	*Blood:* elevates serum uric acid, which may precipitate gout. *CV:* flushing, which usually subsides in a few weeks. *GI:* nausea, dyspepsia, vomiting, diarrhea, anorexia, flatulence, epigastric pain. *Metabolic:* glucose intolerance resulting in hyperglycemia in previously well-controlled diabetics. *Skin:* urticaria, dry skin.
probucol Lorelco◆	*Primary hypercholesterolemia—* **Adults:** 2 tablets (500 mg total) P.O. b.i.d. with morning and evening meals.	*GI:* diarrhea (in approximately 10% of patients), flatulence, abdominal pain, nausea, vomiting. *Other:* hyperhidrosis, fetid sweat, angioneurotic edema, dizziness, syncope, chest pain.
sitosterols Cytellin	*Adjunctive therapy for hypercholesterolemia or hyperbetalipoproteinemia—* **Adults:** 15 ml (3 g) P.O. before meals to a total of 45 ml (9 g) daily. May increase to 30 ml before large or high-fat meals; give fraction of usual dose before snacks.	*GI:* anorexia, diarrhea, abdominal cramps, bulky, light-colored stools.

INTERACTIONS	NURSING CONSIDERATIONS
None significant.	• Use cautiously in asthma, gout, tuberculosis, diabetes, gallbladder or hepatic disease, peptic ulcer, bronchial disease, or those patients receiving ganglionic blocking agents. • Advise patient that pruritus and flushing noted in first few weeks of therapy usually lessen with continued use. • Begin therapy with small doses; then increase gradually. • Give with meals to minimize GI irritation. Cold water eases swallowing.
None significant.	• Drug's effect is enhanced when taken with food.
None significant.	• Administer other medications 1 hour before or 4 hours after sitosterols. • Give sitosterols immediately before meals or snacks. • Mix with milk, tea, coffee, or fruit juice for palatability. • Maximum therapeutic effect during second and third month of therapy.

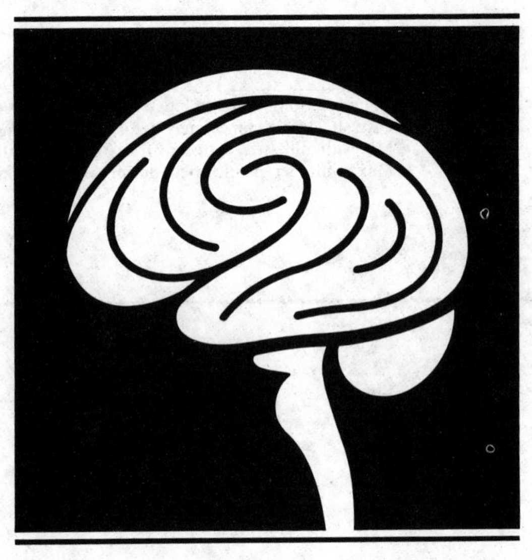

Central Nervous System

22
Nonnarcotic analgesics and antipyretics

acetaminophen
aspirin
butorphanol tartrate
calcium carbaspirin
choline salicylate
ethoheptazine citrate
ethoxazene hydrochloride
fenoprofen calcium
ibuprofen
indomethacin
magnesium salicylate
mefenamic acid
methotrimeprazine
nalbuphine hydrochloride
naproxen
oxyphenbutazone
pentazocine
phenacetin
phenazopyridine hydrochloride
phenylbutazone
propoxyphene hydrochloride
propoxyphene napsylate
salicylamide
salsalate
sodium salicylate
sodium thiosalicylate
sulindac
tolmetin sodium

Nonnarcotic analgesics and antipyretics are widely used. Many are available without a doctor's prescription, often combined with other analgesics to increase their therapeutic effect.

Major uses

- Relief of mild to moderate pain and fever.
- Reduction of inflammation associated with rheumatoid arthritis, gout, osteoarthritis, and other inflammatory conditions.

Mechanism of action

- Depress peripheral chemoreceptors to block pain impulses.
- Directly affect hypothalamus to lower body temperature.
- Decrease capillary permeability and may inhibit prostaglandins to reduce inflammation.
- Ethoxazene and phenazopyridine produce local, topical analgesia or anesthesia of urinary tract mucosa.

Absorption, distribution, and excretion

- Absorbed well from gastrointestinal tract after oral administration.
- Distributed throughout most body tissues.
- Metabolized in liver.

• Excreted in urine.

Onset and duration
• Begin acting within 60 minutes after oral administration and 30 minutes after parenteral administration.
• Peak within 2 hours.
• Duration—4 to 6 hours.

Combination products
ANACIN: aspirin 400 mg and caffeine 32 mg.
A.P.C.: aspirin 227 mg, phenacetin 162 mg and caffeine 32 mg.
A.S.A. COMPOUND: aspirin 227 mg, phenacetin 160 mg, and caffeine 32.5 mg.
BUTAZOLIDIN ALKA: phenylbutazone 100 mg, dried aluminum hydroxide gel 100 mg, and magnesium trisilicate 150 mg.
DARVOCET-N 50: acetaminophen 325 mg and propoxyphene napsylate 50 mg.
DARVON COMPOUND-65: aspirin 227 mg, phenacetin 162 mg, caffeine 32 mg, and propoxyphene HC1 65 mg.
DOLENE AP-65: acetaminophen 650 mg and propoxyphene HC1 65 mg.
DOLENE COMPOUND-65: aspirin 227 mg, phenacetin 162 mg, propoxyphene HC1 65 mg, and caffeine 32 mg.
EMPIRIN: aspirin 227 mg, phenacetin 162 mg, and caffeine 32 mg.
EQUAGESIC: aspirin 250 mg, ethoheptazine 75 mg, and meprobamate 150 mg.
EXCEDRIN: aspirin 195 mg, acetaminophen 97 mg, caffeine 65 mg, and salicylamide 130 mg.
FEMCAPS: aspirin 162 mg, phenacetin 65 mg, caffeine 32 mg, ephedrine 8 mg, and atropine 0.0325 mg.
FIORINAL: butalbital 50 mg, aspirin 200 mg, phenacetin 13 mg, caffeine 40 mg.
SYNALGOS: promethazine 6.25 mg, aspirin 194.4 mg, phenacetin 162 mg, caffeine 30 mg.
TALWIN COMPOUND: aspirin 325 mg and pentazocine 12.5 mg.
TRILISATE: choline salicylate 293 mg and magnesium salicylate 362 mg.
VANQUISH: aspirin 227 mg, acetaminophen 194 mg, caffeine 32 mg, dried aluminum hydroxide gel 25 mg, and magnesium hydroxide 50 mg.
ZACTIRIN: aspirin 325 mg and ethoheptazine 75 mg.

NAME	INDICATIONS & DOSAGE	SIDE EFFECTS
acetaminophen Acephen, Atasol◆◆, Campain◆◆, Datril, Dolanex, Liquiprin, Paralgin◆◆, Phendex, Robigesic◆◆, Rounox◆◆, SKA-pap, Tapar, Tempra◆, Tenlap, Tivrin◆◆, Tylenol◆, Valadol	*Mild pain or fever—* **Adults, and children over 10 years:** 325 to 650 mg P.O. or rectally q 4 hours, p.r.n. Maximum 2.6 g daily. **Children under 1 year:** 15 to 60 mg/dose **1 year:** 60 mg/dose **2 years:** 120 mg/dose **3 years:** 180 mg/dose **4 years:** 240 mg/dose **5 to 10 years:** 325 mg/dose May give P.O. or rectally q 4 to 6 hours. Maximum 1.2 q daily.	*Skin:* rash, urticaria. *Other:* hypersensitivity (laryngeal edema, anaphylaxis), thrombocytopenic purpura.
aspirin Acetal◆◆, Acetophen◆◆, Acetyl-Sal◆◆, Ancasal◆◆, A.S.A., Aspergum, Aspirjen Jr., Aspirin◆◆, Bayer Timed-Release, Buffinol, Decaprin, Ecotrin◆, Empirin, Entrophen◆◆, Measurin, Neopirine No. 25◆◆, Nova-Phase◆◆, Novasen◆◆, Rhonal◆◆, Sal-Adult◆◆, Sal-Infant◆◆, Supasa◆◆, Triaphen-10◆◆	**Adults:** *Arthritis*—2.6 to 5.2 g P.O. daily in divided doses. *Mild pain or fever—* 325 to 650 mg P.O. or rectally q 4 hours, p.r.n. *Thromboembolic disorders*—325 to 650 mg P.O. daily or b.i.d. **Children:** *Arthritis*—90 to 130 mg/Kg P.O. daily divided q 4 to 6 hours. *Fever*—40 to 80 mg/Kg P.O. or rectally daily divided q 6 hours, p.r.n. *Mild pain*—65 to 100 mg/Kg P.O. or rectally daily divided q 4 to 6 hours, p.r.n.	*Blood:* hemolysis in G-6-PD deficiency, prolonged bleeding time. *GI:* occult blood loss, nausea, vomiting, gastritis, ulcer, bleeding. *Other:* hypersensitivity reactions (range from urticaria to anaphylaxis), salicylism.
butorphanol tartrate Stadol	*Moderate to severe pain—* **Adults:** 1 to 4 mg I.M. q 3 to 4 hours, p.r.n.; or 0.5 to 2 mg I.V. q 3 to 4 hours, p.r.n.	*CNS:* sedation, headache, vertigo, floating sensation, lethargy, confusion, nervousness, unusual dreams, agitation, euphoria, hallucinations, flushing, warm and cold sensations. *CV:* palpitations, hypertension or hypotension. *EENT:* diplopia, blurred vision. *GI:* nausea, vomiting, dry mouth. *Skin:* rash, hives, clamminess, excessive sweating. *Other:* respiratory depression.
calcium carbaspirin Calurin	*Arthritis—* **Adults:** up to 1.75 g daily in divided doses. *Mild pain or fever—* **Adults:** 1 to 2 tablets P.O. q 4 hours, p.r.n. **Children 3 to 6 years:** ½ tablet q 4 hours, p.r.n. Each 382 mg tablet equals 300 mg aspirin.	*Blood:* hemolysis in G-6-PD deficiency, prolonged bleeding time. *GI:* occult blood loss, nausea, vomiting, gastritis, ulcer, bleeding. *Other:* hypersensitivity reactions (range from urticaria to anaphylaxis), salicylism.

◆ Also available in Canada.
◆◆ Available in Canada only.
Unmarked trade names available in United States only.

INTERACTIONS	NURSING CONSIDERATIONS
None significant.	• Has no anti-inflammatory effect. • Warn patient that high doses or unsupervised chronic use can cause hepatic damage. • Has little or no effect on prothrombin time. • For symptoms and treatment of acute toxicity, see p. 1114.
Ammonium chloride (and other urine acidifiers): increased blood levels of aspirin products. Monitor for aspirin toxicity. *Antacids (and other urine alkalinizers):* decreased levels of aspirin products. Monitor for decreased aspirin effect. *Oral anticoagulants:* increased risk of bleeding. Avoid using together if possible.	• Contraindicated in G-6-PD deficiency, GI ulcer, GI bleeding, aspirin hypersensitivity, and newborns. Use cautiously in hypoprothrombinemia, vitamin K deficiency, bleeding disorders, asthmatics with nasal polyps (may cause severe bronchospasm), and Hodgkin's disease (may cause profound hypothermia). • Febrile, dehydrated children can develop toxicity rapidly. • Give with food, milk, antacid, or large glass of water to reduce GI side effects. • Enteric-coated or timed-release preparations are absorbed erratically and are not good for chronic therapy. • Warn patients to check with doctor or pharmacist before taking over-the-counter combinations containing aspirin. • Therapeutic serum salicylate level in arthritis is 20 to 30 mg/100 ml. • Alcohol may increase gastrointestinal blood loss. • For symptoms and treatment of acute toxicity, see p. 1122.
None significant.	• Contraindicated in narcotic addiction. Use cautiously in head injury, increased intracranial pressure, acute MI, ventricular dysfunction, coronary insufficiency, respiratory diseases or depression, renal or hepatic dysfunction. • Unlikely to cause dependence.
Ammonium chloride (and other urine acidifiers): increased blood levels of aspirin products. Monitor for aspirin toxicity. *Antacids (and other urine alkalinizers):* decreased levels	• Contraindicated in G-6-PD deficiency, GI ulcer, GI bleeding, aspirin hypersensitivity, and newborns. Use cautiously in hypoprothrombinemia, vitamin K deficiency, bleeding disorders, asthmatics with nasal polyps (may cause severe bronchospasm), and Hodgkin's disease (may cause profound hypothermia). • Febrile, dehydrated children can develop toxicity rapidly. • Warn patient to check with doctor before taking over-the-counter drugs containing aspirin. • Therapeutic serum salicylate level in arthritis is 20 to 30 mg/100 ml.

(continued on following page)

NAME	INDICATIONS & DOSAGE	SIDE EFFECTS
calcium carbaspirin *(continued)*		
choline salicylate Arthropan♦	*Arthritis—* **Adults:** 5 to 10 ml P.O. q.i.d. *Minor pain or fever—* **Adults:** 870 mg (5 ml) P.O. q 3 to 4 hours, p.r.n. **Children 3 to 6 years:** 105 to 210 mg P.O. q 4 hours, p.r.n. Each 870 mg (5 ml) equals 650 mg aspirin.	*Blood:* hemolysis in G-6-PD deficiency, prolonged bleeding time. *GI:* occult blood loss, nausea, vomiting, gastritis, ulcer, bleeding. *Other:* hypersensitivity reactions (range from urticaria to anaphylaxis), salicylism.
ethoheptazine citrate Zactane	*Mild pain—* **Adults:** 75 to 150 mg P.O. t.i.d. or q.i.d.	*CNS:* dizziness, headache, syncope, nervousness. *EENT:* visual disturbances. *GI:* nausea, vomiting. *Skin:* pruritus.
ethoxazene hydrochloride Serenium	*Pain with urinary tract irritation or infection—* **Adults:** 100 mg a.c. P.O. t.i.d.	*GI:* nausea, vomiting.
fenoprofen calcium Nalfon♦	*Rheumatoid and osteoarthritis—* **Adults:** 300 to 600 mg P.O. q.i.d. Maximum 3.2 g daily.	*Blood:* prolonged bleeding time. *CNS:* headache, drowsiness, dizziness, fatigue, nervousness, tremor, confusion, insomnia, depression. *CV:* palpitations, peripheral edema. *EENT:* tinnitus, hearing loss, blurred vision. *GI:* anorexia, nausea, vomiting, constipation, diarrhea, flatus, hemorrhage, occult blood loss, peptic ulcer, indigestion. *Skin:* pruritus, rash, urticaria, sweating. *Other:* increased BUN, increased liver enzymes.
ibuprofen Motrin♦	*Arthritis, primary dysmenorrhea, post extraction dental pain—* **Adults:** 300 to 400 mg P.O. q.i.d. Maximum 2.4 g daily.	*CNS:* headache, dizziness, nervousness, insomnia, depression. *CV:* edema, hypertension. *EENT:* tinnitus, blurred vision. *GI:* anorexia, nausea, vomiting, constipation, diarrhea, flatus, hemorrhage, melena, peptic ulcer, heartburn. *Skin:* pruritus, rash, urticaria.

INTERACTIONS	NURSING CONSIDERATIONS
of aspirin products. Monitor for decreased aspirin effect. *Oral anticoagulants:* increased risk of bleeding. Avoid using together if possible.	• Alcohol may increase gastrointestinal blood loss. • For symptoms and treatment of acute toxicity, see p. 1122.
Ammonium chloride (and other urine acidifiers): increased blood levels of aspirin products. Monitor for aspirin toxicity. *Antacids (and other urine alkalinizers):* decreased levels of aspirin products. Monitor for decreased aspirin effect. *Oral anticoagulants:* increased risk of bleeding. Avoid using together if possible.	• Contraindicated in G-6-PD deficiency, GI ulcer, GI bleeding, aspirin hypersensitivity, and newborns. Use cautiously in hypoprothrombinemia, vitamin K deficiency, bleeding disorders, asthmatics with nasal polyps (may cause severe bronchospasm), and Hodgkin's disease (may cause profound hypothermia). • May cause less GI distress than aspirin. If antacid needed, give 2 hours after meals and give choline salicylate before meals. • May mix drug with water, fruit juice, or carbonated drinks. • Febrile, dehydrated children can develop toxicity rapidly. • Warn patient to check with doctor before taking over-the-counter combinations containing aspirin. • Therapeutic serum salicylate level in arthritis is 20 to 30 mg/100 ml. • Alcohol may increase gastrointestinal blood loss. • For symptoms and treatment of acute toxicity, see p. 1122.
None significant.	• May use with aspirin for arthritic pain. • Doesn't lower fever; may use alone when fever is valuable for diagnosis. • Side effects other than GI distress and pruritus usually occur only when recommended dosage exceeded.
None significant.	• Contraindicated in hepatic and renal disease. Use cautiously in GI disorders. • Colors urine reddish-orange. May stain fabrics. • Use only as analgesic. Use with antibiotic to treat urinary tract infection.
None significant.	• Contraindicated in renal disease and in asthmatics with nasal polyps. Use cautiously in GI disorders or allergy to other noncorticosteroid anti-inflammatory drugs, cardiac disease. • Tell patient therapeutic effect may be delayed for 2 to 3 weeks. • Check renal, hepatic and auditory function periodically in long-term therapy. Stop drug if abnormalities occur. • Give dose 30 minutes before or 2 hours after meals. If GI side effects occur, give with milk or meals.
None significant.	• Contraindicated in asthmatics with nasal polyps. Use cautiously in GI disorders, allergy to other noncorticosteroid anti-inflammatory drugs, hepatic or renal disease, cardiac decompensation. • Tell patient therapeutic effect may be delayed for 2 to 3 weeks. • Check renal and hepatic function periodically in long-term therapy. Stop drug if abnormalities occur. • Tell patient to report to doctor immediately any GI symptoms or signs of bleeding, visual disturbances, skin rashes, weight gain, or edema. • Give with meals or milk to reduce GI side effects.

NAME	INDICATIONS & DOSAGE	SIDE EFFECTS
indomethacin Indocid◆◆, Indocin	*Moderate to severe arthritis*— **Adults:** 25 mg P.O. b.i.d. or t.i.d. with food or antacids; may increase dose by 25 mg daily q 7 days up to 200 mg daily. *Acute gouty arthritis*—50 mg t.i.d. Reduce dose as soon as possible, then stop.	*Blood:* hemolytic anemia, aplastic anemia, agranulocytosis, leukopenia, thrombocytopenic purpura, iron deficiency anemia. *CNS:* headache, dizziness, depression, drowsiness, confusion, peripheral neuropathy, coma, convulsions, psychic disturbances, syncope. *CV:* hypertension, edema. *EENT:* blurred vision, corneal and retinal damage, hearing loss, tinnitus. *GI:* nausea, vomiting, anorexia, diarrhea, ulcer. *GU:* hematuria, acute renal failure. *Skin:* pruritus, urticaria, angioedema. *Other:* hypersensitivity (shock-like symptoms, rash, respiratory distress).
magnesium salicylate Analate, Arthrin, Lorisal, Magan, Mobidin, MSG-600, Triact	**Adults:** *Arthritis*—up to 9.6 g daily in divided doses. *Mild pain or fever*—600 mg P.O. t.i.d. or q.i.d.	*Blood:* hemolysis in G-6-PD deficiency, prolonged bleeding time. *GI:* occult blood loss, nausea, vomiting, gastritis, ulcer. *Other:* hypersensitivity reactions (range from urticaria to anaphylaxis), salicylism.
mefenamic acid Ponstan◆◆, Ponstel	*Mild to moderate pain*— **Adults, and children over 14 years:** 500 mg P.O. initially, then 250 mg q 4 hours, p.r.n. Maximum therapy 1 week.	*Blood:* hemolytic anemia, leukopenia, thrombocytopenia, agranulocytosis, aplastic anemia. *CNS:* drowsiness, dizziness, nervousness, headache, insomnia. *EENT:* blurred vision, eye irritation, ear pain. *GI:* nausea, vomiting, diarrhea, hemorrhage. *GU:* dysuria, hematuria, nephrotoxicity. *Skin:* rash, urticaria. *Other:* hepatotoxicity.
methotrimeprazine Levoprome, Nozinan◆◆	*Moderate to severe pain in nonambulatory patients*— **Adults:** 10 to 20 mg deep I.M. into large muscle mass, q 4 to 6 hours, p.r.n. Maximum dose 40 mg.	*CNS:* confusion, dizziness, sedation, weakness. *CV:* orthostatic hypotension. *EENT:* nasal congestion. *GI:* dry mouth, nausea, vomiting. *GU:* difficult urination. *Local:* pain, inflammation at injection site. *Other:* chills, slurred speech.

INTERACTIONS	NURSING CONSIDERATIONS
Probenecid: decreased indomethacin excretion; watch for increased incidence of indomethacin side effects. *Furosemide:* impaired response to both drugs. Avoid if possible.	• Contraindicated in aspirin allergy, GI disorders. Use cautiously in epilepsy, parkinsonism, hepatic or renal disease, infection, history of mental illness, and in elderly patients. • Severe headache may occur within 1 hour. Stop drug if headache persists. • Tell patient to notify doctor immediately if any visual changes occur. Patients taking drug long-term should have regular eye examinations. • Very irritating to GI tract. Give with meals. • Monitor for bleeding in patients receiving anticoagulants.
Ammonium chloride (and other urine acidifiers): increased blood levels of aspirin products. Monitor for aspirin toxicity. *Antacids (and other urine alkalinizers):* decreased levels of aspirin products. Monitor for decreased aspirin effect. *Oral anticoagulants:* increased risk of bleeding. Avoid using together if possible.	• Contraindicated in severe chronic renal insufficiency because of risk of magnesium toxicity; in G-6-PD deficiency, GI ulcer, GI bleeding, aspirin hypersensitivity, and newborns. Use cautiously in hypoprothrombinemia, vitamin K deficiency, bleeding disorders, and Hodgkin's disease (may cause profound hypothermia). • Febrile, dehydrated children can develop toxicity rapidly. • Give with food, milk, antacid, or large glass of water to reduce GI side effects. • Warn patient to check with doctor before taking over-the-counter combinations containing aspirin. • Therapeutic serum salicylate level in arthritis is 20 to 30 mg/100 ml. • Alcohol may increase gastrointestinal blood loss. • For symptoms and treatment of acute toxicity, see p. 1122.
None significant.	• Contraindicated in GI ulceration or inflammation. Use cautiously in hepatic or renal disease, blood dyscrasias, diabetes mellitus, asthmatics with nasal polyps. • Warn patient not to drive car or operate dangerous machinery until response to drug is determined. • Severe hemolytic anemia may occur with prolonged use. • Stop drug if rash or diarrhea develops. • Should not be administered for more than 1 week at a time. • Administer with food to minimize GI side effects. • Can be used to treat menstrual pain.
All antihypertensive agents: increased orthostatic hypotension. Select another analgesic.	• Contraindicated in phenothiazine hypersensitivity; cardiac, renal or hepatic disease; hypotension; coma; convulsive disorders. Use with extreme caution in elderly or debilitated patients with heart disease or any patients who may suffer severe consequences from a sudden drop in blood pressure. • Used mainly in nonambulatory patients because of hypotension. Keep patient in bed or assist when out of bed for at least 6 hours after initial dose. Tolerance to this effect usually develops, but watch patient closely after each dose. • May mix with atropine or scopolamine. Do not mix with other drugs.

NAME	INDICATIONS & DOSAGE	SIDE EFFECTS
nalbuphine hydrochloride Nubain	*Moderate to severe pain*— S.Q., I.M., or I.V. **Adults:** 10 to 20 mg q 3 to 6 hours p.r.n. Maximum daily dose of 160 mg.	*CNS:* sedation, nervousness, depression, restlessness, crying, euphoria, hostility, unusual dreams, confusion, hallucinations, delusions. *CV:* hypotension, bradycardia, tachycardia. *EENT:* blurred vision. *GI:* cramps, dyspepsia, bitter taste. *GU:* urinary urgency. *Skin:* itching, burning, urticaria. *Other:* respiratory depression, physical and psychological dependence, speech difficulty, difficulty, flushing and warmth.
naproxen Naprosyn◆	*Arthritis*— **Adults:** 250 mg P.O. b.i.d. Maximum 750 mg daily.	*Blood:* prolonged bleeding time. *CNS:* headache, drowsiness, dizziness, depression, inability to concentrate. *CV:* edema, palpitations, dyspnea. *EENT:* tinnitus, hearing loss, blurred vision. *GI:* nausea, vomiting, constipation, diarrhea, melena, hemorrhage, peptic ulcer, heartburn, stomatitis. *Skin:* pruritus, rash, urticaria, sweating. *Other:* increased BUN, dyspnea.
oxyphenbutazone Oxalid, Tandearil	*Pain, inflammation in arthritis, bursitus, superficial venous thrombosis*— **Adults:** 100 to 200 mg P.O. with food or milk t.i.d. or q.i.d.	*Blood:* bone marrow depression (fatal aplastic anemia, agranulocytosis, leukopenia, thrombocytopenia), hemolytic anemia. *CNS:* restlessness, confusion, lethargy. *CV:* hypertension, pericarditis, myocarditis, cardiac decompensation. *EENT:* optic neuritis, blurred vision, retinal hemorrhage or detachment, hearing loss. *GI:* nausea, vomiting, diarrhea, ulcer, bleeding, occult blood loss. *Metabolic:* toxic and nontoxic goiter, edema, respiratory alkalosis and metabolic acidosis. *Renal:* proteinuria, hematuria, glomerulonephritis, nephrotic syndrome, renal failure, ureteral obstruction. *Skin:* petechiae, pruritus, purpura, various dermatoses from rash to toxic necrotizing epidermolysis. *Other:* hepatitis (may be fatal).

INTERACTIONS	NURSING CONSIDERATIONS
None significant.	• Contraindicated in emotional instability, drug abuse, head injury, increased intracranial pressure. • Use cautiously in hepatic and renal disease. These patients may overreact to customary doses. • Causes respiratory depression which at 10 mg is equal to the respiratory depression produced by 10 mg of morphine. • Psychological and physiological dependence may occur, but it is less than that of pentazocine (Talwin). • Respiratory depression can be reversed with naloxone. • Also acts as a narcotic antagonist. • Warn patient not to drive a car or operate dangerous machinery until response to drug is determined.
None significant.	• Use cautiously in renal disease, GI disorders, allergy to noncorticosteroid anti-inflammatory agents, and asthmatics with nasal polyps. • Tell patient therapeutic effect may be delayed 2 to 3 weeks. • Check renal and hepatic function periodically in long-term therapy. Stop drug if abnormalities occur. • Dose can be given once daily very effectively. May increase patient compliance.
Methandrostenolone: may increase oxyphenbutazone levels. Give together cautiously.	• Contraindicated in senile patients; GI ulcer; blood dyscrasias; renal, hepatic, cardiac, and thyroid disease; polymyalgia rheumatica and temporal arteritis. • Tell patient to stop drug and notify doctor immediately if fever, sore throat, mouth ulcers, GI discomfort, black or tarry stools, bleeding, bruising, rash, or weight gain occur. • Warn patient to remain under close medical supervision and to keep all doctor and lab appointments. • Record patient's weight, intake, and output daily. • Response should be seen in 2 or 3 days. Drug should be stopped if no response seen within 1 week. • Monitor CBC every 2 weeks, or weekly in elderly patients. Report any abnormality to doctor immediately. • Patient over 60 years should not receive drug for longer than 1 week.

NAME	INDICATIONS & DOSAGE	SIDE EFFECTS
pentazocine Controlled substance Schedule IV Talwin◆	*Moderate to severe pain—* **Adults:** 50 to 100 mg P.O. q 3 to 4 hours, p.r.n. Maximum 600 mg daily or 30 mg I.M., I.V., or S.C. q 3 to 4 hours, p.r.n. Maximum 360 mg daily. Doses above 30 mg I.V. or 60 mg I.M. or S.C. not recommended.	*CNS:* visual disturbances, hallucinations, drowsiness, dizziness, lightheadedness, confusion, euphoria, headache. *CV:* hypertension, tachycardia, palpitations. *GI:* nausea, vomiting, dry mouth. *GU:* urinary retention. *Local:* induration, nodules, sloughing, and sclerosis of injection site. *Other:* respiratory depression, sweating, flushing, allergic reactions.
phenacetin	*Mild pain or fever—* **Adults:** 300 mg P.O. q 3 to 4 hours, p.r.n. Maximum 2.4 g daily.	*Blood:* methemoglobinemia in toxic doses, hemolytic anemia in G-6-PD deficiency. *GI:* nausea, vomiting. *GU:* papillary necrosis and chronic interstitial nephritis with long-term high doses. *Skin:* rash.
phenazopyridine hydrochloride Azodine, Azogesic, Azo-Pyridon, Azo-Standard, Azo-Sulfizin, Baridium, Di-Azo, Diridone, Phenazo◆◆, Phen-Azo, Phenazodine, Phenyl-Idium, Pyridiate, Pyridium◆, Urodine	*Pain with urinary tract irritation or infection—* **Adults:** 100 to 200 mg P.O. t.i.d.	*GI:* nausea.
phenylbutazone Algoverine◆◆, Anevral◆◆, Azolid, Butagesic◆◆, Butazolidin◆, Intrabutazone◆◆, Malgesic◆◆, Nadozone◆◆, Neo-Zoline◆◆, Phen-butazone◆◆, Phenylbetazone◆◆	*Pain, inflammation in arthritis, bursitis, acute superficial thrombophlebitis—* **Adults:** initially, 100 to 200 mg P.O. t.i.d. or q.i.d. Maximum dose 600 mg per day. When improvement is obtained, decrease dose to 100 mg t.i.d. or q.i.d.	*Blood:* bone marrow depression (fatal aplastic anemia, agranulocytosis, leukopenia, thrombocytopenia), hemolytic anemia. *CNS:* agitation, confusion, lethargy. *CV:* hypertension, pericarditis, myocarditis, cardiac decompensation. *EENT:* optic neuritis, blurred vision, retinal hemorrhage or detachment, hearing loss. *GI:* nausea, vomiting, diarrhea, ulcer, bleeding, occult blood loss. *Metabolic:* hyperglycemia, toxic and nontoxic goiter, edema, respiratory alkalosis, and metabolic acidosis. *Renal:* proteinuria, hematuria, glomerulonephritis, nephrotic syndrome, renal failure, ureteral obstruction. *Skin:* petechiae, pruritus, purpura, various dermatoses from rash to toxic necrotizing epidermolysis. *Other:* hepatitis (may be fatal).

INTERACTIONS	NURSING CONSIDERATIONS
None significant.	• Contraindicated in emotional instability, drug abuse, head injury, increased intracranial pressure. Use cautiously in hepatic or renal disease, myocardial infarction with nausea, respiratory depression. • Tablets not well absorbed. • Psychological and physiological dependence may occur. • Respiratory depression can be reversed with naloxone. • Do not mix in same syringe with soluble barbiturates. • Warn patient not to drive a car or operate dangerous machinery.
None significant.	• Repeated use contraindicated in anemia; cardiac, pulmonary, hepatic, or renal disease. • Contained in many analgesic combinations. Warn patient to check ingredients of combination over-the-counter products.
None significant.	• Contraindicated in renal and hepatic insufficiency. • Colors urine red or orange. May stain fabrics. • Use only as analgesic. Use with antibiotic to treat urinary tract infection. • Drug may be stopped in 3 days if pain relieved. • May alter Clinistix or Tes-Tape results. Use Clinitest for accurate urinary glucose test results. • Stop drug if skin or sclera becomes yellow tinged. May indicate accumulation due to impaired renal excretion.
Barbiturates, antidepressants: may impair phenylbutazone effect. Use together cautiously. *Cholestyramine:* may alter phenylbutazone absorption. Give 1 hour before cholestyramine.	• Contraindicated in senility; GI ulcer; blood dyscrasias; renal, hepatic, cardiac, and thyroid disease; polymyalgia rheumatica; temporal arteritis; and hypertension. • Warn patient to stop drug and notify doctor immediately if fever, sore throat, mouth ulcers, GI discomfort, black or tarry stools, bleeding, bruising, rash, or weight gain occur. • He should remain under close medical supervision and keep all doctor and lab appointments. • Record patient's weight, intake, and output daily. • Monitor CBC every 2 weeks or weekly in elderly patients. Report any abnormalities to doctor right away. • Response should be seen in 3 to 4 days. Stop drug if no response within 1 week. • Patients over 60 years should not receive drug for longer than 1 week.

NAME	INDICATIONS & DOSAGE	SIDE EFFECTS
propoxyphene hydrochloride Darvon, Depronal♦♦, Dolene, Doraphen, Harmar, Myospaz, Pargesic 65, Pro-65♦♦, Pro-Pox 65, Proxagesic, Ropoxy, Scrip-Dyne, SK-65, S-Pain-65, 642♦♦	*Mild to moderate pain*— **Adults:** 65 mg P.O. q 4 hours, p.r.n.	*CNS:* dizziness, headache, sedation, paradoxical excitement, insomnia. *GI:* nausea, vomiting, constipation. *Other:* euphoria, decreased 17-hydroxy and ketosteroid tolerance, psychological and physical dependence.
propoxyphene napsylate Darvocet-N, Darvon-N♦	*Mild to moderate pain*— **Adults:** 100 mg P.O. q 4 hours, p.r.n.	
salicylamide Amid-Sal, Doldram, Salamide	*Mild pain or fever*— **Adults:** 650 mg P.O. q.i.d., p.r.n.	*Blood:* hemolysis in G-6-PD deficiency, prolonged bleeding time. *GI:* occult blood loss, nausea, vomiting, gastritis, ulcer, bleeding. *Other:* hypersensitivity reactions (range from urticaria to anaphylaxis), salicylism.
salsalate Disalcid	*Minor pain or fever, arthritis*— **Adults:** 1 g P.O. t.i.d. or q.i.d., p.r.n.	*Blood:* hemolysis in G-6-PD deficiency, prolonged bleeding time. *GI:* occult blood loss, nausea, vomiting, gastritis, ulcer, bleeding. *Other:* hypersensitivity reactions (range from urticaria to anaphylaxis), salicylism.
sodium salicylate Uracel	*Minor pain or fever*— **Adults:** 325 to 650 mg P.O. q 4 to 6 hours, p.r.n., or 500 mg slow I.V. infusion over 4 to 8 hours. Maximum dose 1 g daily. **Children:** 40 to 100 mg/Kg P.O. q	*Blood:* hemolysis in G-6-PD deficiency, prolonged bleeding time. *GI:* occult blood loss, distress, gastritis, ulcer, bleeding. *Local:* thrombophlebitis or tissue slough if drug extravasates.

INTERACTIONS	NURSING CONSIDERATIONS
None significant.	• Use cautiously in narcotic addicts. • Warn patient not to drive car or operate dangerous machinery until response to drug has been established. • Warn patient not to exceed recommended dosage. • Do not use caffeine or amphetamines to treat overdose; may cause fatal convulsions. Use narcotic antagonist instead. • May cause false decreases in urinary steroid excretion tests. • 65 mg propoxyphene HCl equals 100 mg propoxyphene napsylate. • Can be considered a mild narcotic analgesic. • For symptoms and treatment of acute toxicity, see p. 1121.
Ammonium chloride (and other urine acidifiers): increased blood levels of aspirin products. Monitor for aspirin toxicity. *Antacids (and other urine alkalinizers):* decreased levels of aspirin products. Monitor for decreased aspirin effect. *Oral anticoagulants:* increased risk of bleeding. Avoid using together if possible.	• Contraindicated in G-6-PD deficiency, GI ulcer, GI bleeding, aspirin hypersensitivity, and newborns. Use cautiously in hypoprothrombinemia, vitamin K deficiency, bleeding disorders, and Hodgkin's disease (may cause profound hypothermia). • Give with food, milk, antacid, or large glass of water to reduce GI side effects. • Warn patient to check with doctor before taking over-the-counter combinations containing aspirin. • Alcohol may increase gastrointestinal blood loss. • For symptoms and treatment of acute toxicity, see p. 1122.
Ammonium chloride (and other urine acidifiers): increased blood levels of aspirin products. Monitor for aspirin toxicity. *Antacids (and other urine alkalinizers):* decreased levels of aspirin products. Monitor for decreased aspirin effect. *Oral anticoagulants:* increased risk of bleeding. Avoid using together if possible.	• Contraindicated in G-6-PD deficiency, GI ulcer, GI bleeding, aspirin hypersensitivity, and newborns. Use cautiously in hypoprothrombinemia, vitamin K deficiency, bleeding disorders, and Hodgkin's disease (may cause profound hypothermia). • Give with food, milk, antacid, or large glass of water to reduce GI side effects. • Warn patient to check with doctor before taking over-the-counter combinations containing aspirin. • Therapeutic serum salicylate level in arthritis is 20 to 30 mg/100 ml. • Alcohol may increase gastrointestinal blood loss. • For symptoms and treatment of acute toxicity, see p. 1122.
Ammonium chloride (and other urine acidifiers): increased blood levels of aspirin products. Monitor for aspirin toxicity.	• Contraindicated in G-6-PD deficiency, GI ulcer, GI bleeding, aspirin hypersensitivity, and newborns. Use cautiously in hypoprothrombinemia, vitamin K deficiency, bleeding disorders, asthmatics with nasal polyps (may cause severe bronchospasm), and Hodgkin's disease (may cause profound hypothermia). • Febrile, dehydrated children can develop toxicity rapidly.

(continued on following page)

NAME	INDICATIONS & DOSAGE	SIDE EFFECTS
sodium salicylate *(continued)*	4 to 6 hours, p.r.n.	*Other:* hypersensitivity reactions (range from urticaria to anaphylaxis).
sodium thiosalicylate Arthrolate, Nalate, Osteolate, Thiodyne, Thiolate, Thiosal, TH Sal	**Adults:** *mild pain*—50 to 100 mg I.M. daily or every other day. *Arthritis*—100 mg I.M. daily. *Rheumatic fever*—100 to 150 mg I.M. b.i.d. until asymptomatic. *Acute gout*—100 mg I.M. q 3 to 4 hours for 2 days, then 100 mg I.M. daily until asymptomatic.	*Blood:* hemolysis in G-6-PD deficiency, prolonged bleeding time. *GI:* occult blood loss, distress, gastritis, ulcer, bleeding. *Other:* hypersensitivity reactions (range from urticaria to anaphylaxis).
sulindac Clinoril	*Osteoarthritis, rheumatoid arthritis, ankylosing spondylitis*— **Adults:** 150 mg P.O. b.i.d. initially; may increase to 200 mg P.O. b.i.d. *Acute subacromial bursitis or supraspinatus tendinitis, acute gouty arthritis*— **Adults:** 200 mg P.O. b.i.d. for 7 to 14 days. Dose may be reduced as symptoms subside.	*Blood:* inhibits platelet aggregation; increased bleeding. *CNS:* dizziness, headache, nervousness. *EENT:* tinnitus. *GI:* pain, dyspepsia, nausea, vomiting, diarrhea, constipation, flatus, anorexia, cramps, ulceration and bleeding, gastritis, gastroenteritis, stomatitis. *Skin:* rash, pruritus, dry mucous membranes. *Other:* edema, hypersensitivity, hepatitis.
tolmetin sodium Tolectin♦	*Rheumatoid arthritis and juvenile rheumatoid arthritis*— **Adults:** 400 mg P.O. t.i.d. or q.i.d. Maximum 2 g daily. **Children: (2 yrs or older):** 15 to 30 mg/Kg/day in divided doses.	*Blood:* prolonged bleeding time. *CNS:* headache, dizziness, nervousness, drowsiness. *CV:* peripheral edema. *GI:* nausea, vomiting, constipation, heartburn, ulcer, bleeding. *Skin:* rash, urticaria, pruritus. *Other:* sodium retention.

INTERACTIONS	NURSING CONSIDERATIONS
Antacids (and other urine alkalinizers): decreased levels of aspirin products. Monitor for decreased aspirin effect. *Oral anticoagulants:* increased risk of bleeding. Avoid using together if possible.	• Give with food, milk, antacid, or large glass of water to reduce GI side effects. • Enteric-coated or timed-release preparations are absorbed erratically and are not good for chronic therapy. • Warn patient to check with doctor before taking over-the-counter combinations containing aspirin. • Therapeutic serum salicylate level in arthritis is 20 to 30 mg/ml. • Tinnitus, headache, dizziness, confusion, fever, sweating, thirst, drowsiness, dim vision, hyperventilation, and increased pulse rate are signs of mild toxicity. • Alcohol may increase gastrointestinal blood loss. • For symptoms and treatment of acute toxicity, see p. 1122.
Ammonium chloride (and other urine acidifiers): increased blood levels of aspirin products. Monitor for aspirin toxicity. *Antacids (and other urine alkalinizers):* decreased levels of aspirin products. Monitor for decreased aspirin effect. *Oral anticoagulants:* increased risk of bleeding. Avoid using together if possible.	• Contraindicated in G-6-PD deficiency, GI ulcer, GI bleeding, aspirin hypersensitivity, and newborns. Use cautiously in hypoprothrombinemia, vitamin K deficiency, bleeding disorders, asthmatics with nasal polyps (may cause severe bronchospasm), and Hodgkin's disease (may cause profound hypothermia). • Give with food, milk, antacid, or large glass of water to reduce GI side effects. • Tinnitus, headache, dizziness, confusion, fever, sweating, thirst, drowsiness, dim vision, hyperventilation, and increased pulse rate are signs of mild toxicity. • Alcohol may increase gastrointestinal blood loss. • For symptoms and treatment of acute toxicity, see p. 1122.
None significant.	• Contraindicated in acute asthmatics whose condition is precipitated by aspirin or other nonsteroidal anti-inflammatory agents; in active ulcers and GI bleeding. Use cautiously in history of ulcers and GI bleeding, renal dysfunction, compromised cardiac function, hypertension. • To reduce GI side effects, give with food, milk, or antacids. • Patient should notify doctor and have complete visual exam if any visual disturbances occur. • Tell patient to notify doctor immediately if prolonged bleeding occurs. • If hepatic function test abnormalities occur, drug should be stopped.
None significant.	• Contraindicated in asthmatics with nasal polyps. Use cautiously in cardiac and GI renal disease, and bleeding disorders. • Give with food, milk, or antacids (except sodium bicarbonate) to reduce GI side effects. • Tell patient therapeutic effect should begin within 1 week.

23

Narcotic analgesics

alphaprodine hydrochloride
anileridine hydrochloride
Brompton's cocktail
codeine phosphate
codeine sulfate
fentanyl citrate
hydromorphone hydrochloride
hydromorphone sulfate
levorphanol tartrate
meperidine hydrochloride
methadone hydrochloride
morphine sulfate
oxycodone hydrochloride
oxymorphone hydrochloride

Narcotic analgesics effectively relieve pain without producing loss of consciousness but may cause physical and sometimes psychologic dependence. These drugs are all controlled substances as defined in the Comprehensive Drug Abuse Prevention and Control Act of 1970.

Major uses

- Relief of moderate to severe pain.
- Preoperative sedation, alone or in combination with tranquilizers (such as chlorpromazine, diazepam, or hydroxyzine) or sedatives (such as pentobarbital).

Mechanism of action

- May act on the sensory cortex of the brain to produce analgesia, but precise mechanism of action is not known.
- May interfere with pain conduction or central nervous system response to pain; may alter patient's emotional response to pain.

Absorption, distribution, and excretion

- Parenteral administration is generally more effective than oral administration.
- Distributed in skeletal muscle, kidneys, liver, intestinal tract, lungs, spleen, and brain.
- Cross placenta.
- Excreted primarily in urine.

Onset and duration (based on I.M. or S.C. injection)

Drug	Onset	Duration of analgesia
alphaprodine hydrochloride	5 to 10 minutes	1 to 2 hours
anileridine hydrochloride	within 15 minutes	2 to 3 hours
Brompton's cocktail	10 to 15 minutes	3 to 8 hours
codeine phosphate	15 to 30 minutes	4 to 6 hours
codeine sulfate	15 to 30 minutes	4 to 6 hours

Drug	Onset	Duration of analgesia
fentanyl citrate	5 to 15 minutes	1 to 2 hours
hydromorphone hydrochloride	15 to 30 minutes	4 to 5 hours
hydromorphone sulfate	15 to 30 minutes	4 to 5 hours
levorphanol tartrate	within 60 minutes	4 to 5 hours
meperidine hydrochloride	10 to 15 minutes	2 to 4 hours
methadone hydrochloride	10 to 15 minutes	4 to 6 hours
morphine sulfate	within 30 minutes	4 to 5 hours
oxycodone hydrochloride (P.O.)	10 to 15 minutes	4 to 5 hours
oxymorphone hydrochloride	5 to 10 minutes	4 to 5 hours

Combination products

B & O SUPPRETTES #15A: powdered opium 30 mg and powdered belladonna extract 15 mg.
B & O SUPPRETTES #16A: powdered opium 60 mg and powdered belladonna extract 15 mg.
EMPIRIN COMPOUND #2: aspirin 325 mg and codeine phosphate 15 mg.
EMPIRIN COMPOUND #3: aspirin 325 mg and codeine phosphate 30 mg.
EMPIRIN COMPOUND #4: aspirin 325 mg and codeine phosphate 60 mg.
FIORINAL WITH CODEINE #1: butalbital 50 mg, caffeine 40 mg, aspirin 200 mg, phenacetin 130 mg, codeine 7.5 mg.
FIORINAL WITH CODEINE #2♦: butalbital 50 mg, caffeine 40 mg, aspirin 200 mg, phenacetin 130 mg, codeine 15 mg.
FIORINAL WITH CODEINE #3♦: butalbital 50 mg, caffeine 40 mg, aspirin 200 mg, phenacetin 130 mg, codeine 30 mg.
INNOVAR (INJECTION)♦: fentanyl citrate 0.05 mg, droperidol 2.5 mg, and lactic acid to adjust pH.
PANTOPON♦: hydrochlorides of opium alkaloids 20 mg.
PERCOCET-5♦: acetaminophen 325 mg and oxycodone hydrochloride 5 mg.
PERCODAN♦: oxycodone hydrochloride 4.5 mg, oxycodone terephthalate 0.38 mg, aspirin 224 mg, phenacetin 160 mg, and caffeine 32 mg.
PERCODAN-DEMI♦: oxycodone hydrochloride 2.25 mg, oxycodone terephthalate 0.19 mg, aspirin 224 mg, phenacetin 160 mg, and caffeine 32 mg.
TYLENOL WITH CODEINE #1♦: acetaminophen 300 mg and codeine phosphate 7.5 mg.
TYLENOL WITH CODEINE #2♦: acetaminophen 300 mg and codeine phosphate 15 mg.
TYLENOL WITH CODEINE #3♦: acetaminophen 300 mg and codeine phosphate 30 mg.
TYLENOL WITH CODEINE #4♦: acetaminophen 300 mg and codeine phosphate 60 mg.
TYLOX: acetaminophen 500 mg, oxycodone hydrochloride 4.5 mg, and oxycodone terephthalate 0.38 mg.

NAME	INDICATIONS & DOSAGE	SIDE EFFECTS
alphaprodine hydrochloride Controlled substance Schedule II Nisentil♦	*Moderate to severe pain—* **Adults:** 0.4 to 0.6 mg/Kg I.V. or 0.4 to 1.2 mg/Kg, S.C. q 2 hours, p.r.n. Maximum 240 mg daily. Don't give I.M.	*CNS:* dizziness, drowsiness, syncope. *Other:* sweating, urticaria, respiratory depression.
anileridine hydrochloride Controlled substance Schedule II Leritine♦	*Adjunct to anesthesia—* **Adults:** 50 to 100 mg added to 500 ml 5% dextrose in water for slow I.V. infusion; initially, 5 to 10 mg followed by slow infusion of 0.6 mg/min. Maximum dose 200 mg daily. *Moderate to severe pain—* **Adults:** 25 to 50 mg P.O., I.M., or S.C. q 4 to 6 hours, p.r.n. *Preop—* **Adults:** 50 to 75 mg I.M. or S.C.	*CNS:* dizziness, restlessness, euphoria, light-headedness, excitement. *CV:* bradycardia, hypotension. *GI:* nausea, vomiting. *Local:* pain at injection site, local tissue irritation, and induration after S.C. injection; phlebitis after I.V. injection. *Skin:* pruritus. *Other:* tolerance, physical and psychological dependence, sweating.
Brompton's cocktail (Mixture containing varying amounts of the following ingredients): morphine or methadone, cocaine or amphetamine, syrup or honey, alcohol (90% to 98%) or gin, chloroform water Controlled substance Schedule II	*Severe chronic pain of terminal cancer—* **Adults:** 10 to 20 ml of (standard pharmacy-prepared mixture) q 3 to 4 hours (if morphine is used) or q 6 to 8 hours (if methadone is used). Must be given around-the-clock. Dosage titrations can be made at 48- to 72-hour intervals. Maximum dose totally dependent on patient response.	*CNS:* excess sedation, euphoria. *CV:* hypotension. *GI:* nausea. *Other:* respiratory depression, physical and psychological dependence.

♦ Also available in Canada.
♦♦ Available in Canada only.
Unmarked trade names available in United States only.

INTERACTIONS	NURSING CONSIDERATIONS
None significant.	• Use with extreme caution in head injury, increased intracranial pressure, shock, elderly or debilitated patients, increased cerebrospinal fluid pressure, CNS depression, asthma, COPD, respiratory depression, seizures, hepatic or renal disease, hypothyroidism, Addison's disease, alcoholism. • Keep narcotic antagonist (naloxone) available when giving drug I.V. • Monitor respirations of newborns exposed to drug during labor. • Rapid but short-lived effect makes drug useful in minor surgery or in urologic procedures; not useful for relief of chronic pain. • Monitor respiratory and circulatory status carefully. • Related to meperidine. • If used with other narcotic analgesics, general anesthetics, tranquilizers, sedatives, hypnotics, alcohol, tricyclic antidepressants, or MAO inhibitors, depressant effect is increased. Reduce narcotic dose. Use together with extreme caution. • For symptoms and treatment of toxicity, see p. 1119.
None significant.	• Use with extreme caution in increased intracranial pressure, increased cerebrospinal fluid pressure, CNS depression, head injury, asthma, COPD, respiratory depression, seizures, hepatic or renal disease, hypothyroidism, Addison's disease, elderly or debilitated patients, alcoholism, shock. • Keep narcotic antagonist (naloxone) available when giving drug I.V. • Warn ambulatory patient to avoid activities that require alertness. • Monitor respirations of newborns exposed to drug during labor. • S.C. injection more likely to cause tissue irritation than I.M. route. • Stopping drug after long-term use may initiate withdrawal symptoms. • Related to meperidine. • Carefully aspirate before S.C. or I.M. injection. Sudden I.V. injection of more than 10 mg can cause cardiac arrest. • Monitor respiratory and circulatory status carefully. • If used with other narcotic analgesics, general anesthetics, tranquilizers, sedatives, hypnotics, alcohol, tricyclic antidepressants, or MAO inhibitors, depressant effect is increased. Reduce narcotic dose. Use together with extreme caution. • For symptoms and treatment of toxicity, see p. 1119.
None significant.	• Originated in Brompton Hospital in England to keep cancer patients in constant pain-free and euphoric state. • Not commercially prepared—must be prepared by pharmacy. • Has frequently proven to be effective when narcotic analgesics alone have failed to provide pain relief. • Around-the-clock administration reduces patient's anticipation of pain and is major reason for effectiveness. • If cocaine is ingredient in mixture—advise patient to swish mixture in mouth to aid absorption as cocaine is only absorbed through oral mucosa. • Phenothiazines are occasionally added to increase analgesic effect and prevent nausea. • Most formulations are stable for up to 4 weeks at room temperature; storage in refrigerator may increase stability to 8 weeks.

NAME	INDICATIONS & DOSAGE	SIDE EFFECTS
codeine phosphate **codeine sulfate** Controlled substance Schedule II	*Mild to moderate pain—* **Adults:** 15 to 60 mg P.O. or 15 to 60 mg (phosphate) S.C. q 4 hours, p.r.n. Don't give I.M. or I.V. **Children:** 3 mg/Kg daily P.O. divided q 4 hours, p.r.n. See antitussive dosage, p. 468.	*CNS:* drowsiness. *CV:* orthostatic hypotension. *GI:* nausea, vomiting, constipation. *Skin:* pruritus. *Other:* sweating, flushing, tolerance, physical and psychological dependence, respiratory depression, suppression of cough reflex.
fentanyl citrate Controlled substance Schedule II Sublimaze♦	*Adjunct to general anesthesia—* **Adults:** 0.05 to 0.1 mg I.V. repeated q 2 to 3 minutes p.r.n. Dose should be reduced in elderly and poor-risk patients. *Postop—* **Adults:** 0.05 to 0.1 mg I.M. q 1 to 2 hours, p.r.n. **Children 2 to 12 years:** 0.02 mg/9 Kg/dose. *Preop—* **Adults:** 0.05 to 0.1 mg I.M. 30 to 60 minutes prior to surgery.	*CNS:* dizziness, light-headedness, euphoria. *CV:* bradycardia, hypotension. *EENT:* blurred vision, miosis. *GI:* nausea, vomiting. *Skin:* pruritus. *Other:* tolerance, physical and psychological dependence, sweating, muscle rigidity, respiratory depression, apnea, laryngospasm.
hydromorphone hydrochloride **hydromorphone sulfate** Controlled substance Schedule II Dilaudid♦	*Moderate to severe pain—* **Adults:** 2 to 4 mg P.O. (hydrochloride) q 4 to 6 hours, p.r.n.; or 2 to 4 mg I.M., S.C., or I.V. (sulfate or hydrochloride) q 4 to 6 hours, p.r.n. I.V. dose should be given over 3 to 5 minutes; or 3 mg rectal suppository (hydrochloride) at bedtime, p.r.n. See antitussive dosage, p. 470.	*CNS:* dizziness, somnolence. *CV:* hypotension. *GI:* nausea, vomiting, anorexia, constipation. *Local:* induration with repeated S.C. injection. *Other:* respiratory depression, tolerance, physical and psychological dependence.

INTERACTIONS	NURSING CONSIDERATIONS
None significant.	• Use with extreme caution in head injury, increased intracranial pressure, increased cerebrospinal fluid pressure, hepatic or renal disease, hypothyroidism, Addison's disease, acute alcoholism, seizures, severe CNS depression, bronchial asthma, COPD, respiratory depression, shock, elderly or debilitated patients. • Warn ambulatory patient to avoid activities that require alertness. • Monitor respiratory and circulatory status, pupil size, bowel function. • For full analgesic effect, give before patient has intense pain. • Codeine and aspirin have additive effect. Give together for maximum pain relief. • Do not administer discolored injection solution. • If used with general anesthetics, other narcotic analgesics, tranquilizers, sedatives, hypnotics, alcohol, tricyclic antidepressants, or MAO inhibitors, CNS depression is increased. Use together with extreme caution. Monitor patient's response. • For symptoms and treatment of toxicity, see p. 1119.
None significant.	• Contraindicated in patients who have received MAO inhibitors within 14 days and with myasthenia gravis. Use cautiously in head injury, increased cerebrospinal fluid pressure, asthma, COPD, respiratory depression, seizures, hepatic or renal disease, hypothyroidism, Addison's disease, alcoholism, increased intracranial pressure, CNS depression, shock, elderly or debilitated patients. • Keep narcotic antagonist (naloxone) and resuscitative equipment available when giving drug I.V. • Monitor respirations of newborns exposed to drug during labor. • As postop analgesic, use only in recovery room. Make sure another analgesic is ordered for later use. • Often used with droperidol (as Innovar) to produce neuroleptanalgesia. • Monitor circulatory and respiratory status carefully. • If used with other narcotic analgesics, general anesthetics, tranquilizers, alcohol, sedatives, hypnotics, tricyclic antidepressants, or MAO inhibitors, respiratory depression, hypotension, profound sedation, and coma may result. Fentanyl citrate dose should be reduced by ¼ to ⅓. Also give above drugs in reduced dosages. • For symptoms and treatment of toxicity, see p. 1119.
None significant.	• Contraindicated in increased intracranial pressure, status asthmaticus. Use with extreme caution in increased cerebrospinal fluid pressure, respiratory depression, hepatic or renal disease, hypothyroidism, shock, elderly or debilitated patients, Addison's disease, acute alcoholism, seizures, head injury, severe CNS depression, brain tumor, bronchial asthma, COPD. • Warn ambulatory patient to avoid activities that require alertness. • Monitor respiratory and circulatory status, pupil size, and bowel function. • For full analgesic effect, give before patient has intense pain. • Keep narcotic antagonist (naloxone) available. • Respiratory depression and hypotension can occur with I.V. administration. Give very slowly and monitor constantly. • Rotate injection sites to avoid induration with S.C. injection. • Commonly abused narcotic. • If used with general anesthetics, other narcotic analgesics, tranquilizers, sedatives, hypnotics, alcohol, tricyclic antidepressants, or MAO inhibitors, CNS depression is increased. Hydromorphone dose should be reduced. Use together with extreme caution. Monitor patient's response. • For symptoms and treatment of toxicity, see p. 1119.

NAME	INDICATIONS & DOSAGE	SIDE EFFECTS
levorphanol tartrate Controlled substance Schedule II Levo-Dromoran◆	*Moderate to severe pain*— **Adults:** 2 to 3 mg P.O. or S.C. q 6 to 8 hours, p.r.n.	*CNS:* drowsiness, sedation, dizziness.. *CV:* orthostatic hypotension, arrhythmias. *GI:* nausea, vomiting. *GU:* urinary retention. *Skin:* urticaria. *Other:* tolerance, physical and psychological dependence, respiratory depression.
meperidine hydrochloride Controlled substance Schedule II Demer-Idine◆◆, Demerol◆, Pethidine HCl B.P.◆◆	*Moderate to severe pain*— **Adults:** 50 to 150 mg P.O., I.M., or S.C. q 3 to 4 hours, p.r.n. **Children:** 1 mg/Kg P.O., I.M., or S.C. q 4 to 6 hours. Maximum—100 mg q 4 hours, p.r.n. *Preop*— **Adults:** 50 to 100 mg I.M. or S.C. 30 to 90 minutes before surgery. **Children:** 1 to 2.2 mg/Kg I.M. or S.C. 30 to 90 minutes before surgery.	*CNS:* dizziness, euphoria, lightheadedness, restlessness, transient hallucinations and disorientation, sedation, convulsions with high doses. *CV:* tachycardia, bradycardia, palpitations, hypotension, shock. *GI:* nausea, vomiting, dry mouth, constipation, biliary tract spasm. *GU:* urinary retention. *Local:* pain at injection site, local tissue irritation and induration after S.C. injection; phlebitis after I.V. injection. *Skin:* pruritus, rash, urticaria. *Other:* tolerance, physical and psychological dependence, sweating, respiratory depression, weakness.
methadone hydrochloride Controlled substance Schedule II Dolophine, Westadone	*Severe pain*— **Adults:** 2.5 to 10 mg P.O., I.M., or S.C. q 3 to 4 hours, p.r.n. *Narcotic abstinence syndrome*— **Adults:** 15 to 40 mg P.O. daily (highly individualized). **Maintenance:** 20 to 120 mg P.O. daily. Adjust dose as needed. Daily doses greater than 120 mg require special state and federal approval.	*CNS:* light-headedness, dizziness, euphoria, headache, insomnia, disorientation, suppression of cough reflex, drowsiness, sedation; in large doses: convulsions, excitation. *CV:* orthostatic hypotension, bradycardia, palpitations. *EENT:* miosis, red eyes. *GI:* nausea, vomiting, dry mouth, constipation, biliary tract spasm. *GU:* urinary urgency and retention, impotence. *Local:* pain at injection site, tissue

INTERACTIONS	NURSING CONSIDERATIONS
None significant.	• Contraindicated in acute alcoholism, bronchial asthma, increased intracranial pressure, respiratory depression, and anoxia. Use with extreme caution in hepatic or renal disease, hypothyroidism, Addison's disease, seizures, head injury, severe CNS depression, brain tumor, COPD, shock, elderly or debilitated patients. • Warn ambulatory patient to avoid activities that require alertness. • Monitor circulatory and respiratory status, pupil size, bowel function. • For full analgesic effect, give before patient has intense pain. More potent than morphine. • Warn patient drug has bitter taste. • Protect from light. • Keep narcotic antagonist (naloxone) available. • If used with general anesthetics, other narcotic analgesics, tranquilizers, sedatives, hypnotics, alcohol, tricyclic antidepressants, or MAO inhibitors, CNS depression is increased. Reduce levorphanol dose. Use together with extreme caution. Monitor patient's response. • For symptoms and treatment of toxicity, see p. 1119.
MAO inhibitors, isoniazid: increased CNS excitation or depression can be severe or fatal. Don't use together.	• Contraindicated if patient has used MAO inhibitors within 14 days. Use with extreme caution in increased intracranial pressure, increased cerebrospinal fluid pressure, shock, children under 12, CNS depression, head injury, asthma, COPD, respiratory depression, supraventricular tachycardias, seizures, acute abdominal conditions, hepatic or renal disease, hypothyroidism, Addison's disease, urethral stricture, prostatic hypertrophy, alcoholism, elderly or debilitated patients. • Meperidine may be given slowly I.V., preferably as a diluted solution. S.C. injection very painful. • Keep narcotic antagonist (naloxone) available when giving drug I.V. • Warn ambulatory patient to avoid activities that require alertness. • Monitor respirations of newborns exposed to drug during labor. Have resuscitation equipment available. • P.O. dose less than half as effective as parenteral dose. Give I.M. if possible. When changing from parenteral to P.O., dose should be increased. • Syrup has local anesthetic effect. Give with full glass of water. • Chemically incompatible with barbiturates. Don't mix. • Monitor respiratory and cardiovascular status carefully. Don't give if respirations below 12/min. or if change in pupils. • Watch for withdrawal symptoms if stopped abruptly after long-term use. • If used with other narcotic analgesics, general anesthetics, phenothiazines, sedatives, hypnotics, tricyclic antidepressants, or alcohol, respiratory depression, hypotension, profound sedation, or coma may occur. Reduce meperidine dose. Use together with extreme caution. • For symptoms and treatment of toxicity, see p. 1119.
Pentazocine, rifampin, butorphanol: withdrawal symptoms; reduced blood levels of methadone. Use together cautiously. *Ammonium chloride, phenytoin:* may reduce methadone effect. Monitor for decreased pain control.	• Contraindicated in obstetric analgesia. Give with extreme caution in acute abdominal conditions, elderly or debilitated patients, severe hepatic or renal impairment, hypothyroidism, Addison's disease, prostatic hypertrophy, urethral stricture, head injury, increased intracranial pressure, asthma, COPD, respiratory depression, CNS depression. • Safe use in adolescents as maintenance drug not established. • Oral dose is half as potent as injected dose. • Rotate injection sites. • Has cumulative effect; marked sedation can occur after repeated doses. • Monitor circulatory and respiratory status, pupil size, bowel function. • Warn ambulatory patient to avoid activities that require alertness. • One daily dose adequate for maintenance. No advantage to divide doses. • Oral form legally required in maintenance programs.

(continued on following page)

NAME	INDICATIONS & DOSAGE	SIDE EFFECTS
methadone hydrochloride *(continued)*		irritation, induration following S.C. injections. *Skin:* pruritus, urticaria, edema. *Other:* sweating, bone and muscle pain, tolerance, physical and psychological dependence.
morphine sulfate◆ Controlled substance Schedule II	*Severe pain—* **Adults:** 5 to 15 mg S.C., I.M. q 4 hours, p.r.n. or injected slow I.V. (over 4 to 5 minutes) diluted in 4 to 5 ml water for injection. P.O. route not recommended. **Children:** 0.1 to 0.2 mg/Kg dose S.C. Maximum 15 mg.	*CNS:* suppression of cough reflex, drowsiness, sedation, mood changes, euphoria, restlessness; in large doses: convulsions, excitation. *CV:* bradycardia, orthostatic hypotension. *EENT:* miosis, red eyes. *GI:* nausea, vomiting, constipation, dry mouth, biliary colic. *GU:* urinary urgency, retention, impotence. *Skin:* pruritus, urticaria. *Other:* sweating, flushing, tolerance, physical and psychological dependence, respiratory depression.
oxycodone hydrochloride Controlled substance Schedule II Supeudol◆◆ Combinations: Percocet◆, Percocet-Demi◆◆, Percodan◆, Percodan-Demi◆◆, Tylox	*Moderate pain—* **Adults:** available only in U.S. in combination with other drugs, such as aspirin, phenacetin, and caffeine (Percodan, Percodan-Demi), or acetaminophen (Percocet, Percocet-Demi, Tylox). 1 to 2 tablets P.O. q 6 hours, p.r.n. **Adults:** (Supeudol) 1 to 3 suppositories rectally/day, p.r.n. **Children:** (Percodan-Demi) ¼ to ½ tablet P.O. q 6 hours, p.r.n.	*CNS:* light-headedness, dizziness, sedation, euphoria, dysphoria. *GI:* nausea, vomiting, constipation. *Skin:* pruritus. *Other:* respiratory depression, tolerance, physical and psychological dependence.

INTERACTIONS	NURSING CONSIDERATIONS
	• Give maintenance doses as oral liquid. Completely dissolve tablets in 120 ml of orange juice or powdered citrus drink. • Constipation often severe with maintenance. Make sure stool softener or other laxative is ordered. • Patient treated for narcotic abstinence syndrome will usually require an additional analgesic if pain control necessary. • If used with general anesthetics, tranquilizers, sedatives, hypnotics, alcohol, tricyclic antidepressants or MAO inhibitors, respiratory depression, hypotension, profound sedation, or coma may occur. Use together with extreme caution. Monitor patient's response. • For symptoms and treatment of toxicity, see p. 1119.
None significant.	• Use with extreme caution in head injury, increased intracranial pressure, seizures, asthma, COPD, alcoholism, prostatic hypertrophy, severe hepatic or renal disease, acute abdominal conditions, hypothyroidism, Addison's disease, increased cerebrospinal fluid pressure, urethral stricture, cardiac arrhythmias, reduced blood volume, toxic psychosis, elderly or debilitated patients. • Warn ambulatory patient to avoid activities that require alertness. • Monitor circulatory and respiratory status, pupil size, bowel function. Don't give if respirations below 12/min. • For full analgesic effect, give before patient has intense pain. • Drug of choice in relieving pain of myocardial infarction. May cause transient decrease in blood pressure. • Keep narcotic antagonist (naloxone) and resuscitative equipment available. • When used postop, encourage turning, coughing, and deep breathing to avoid atelectasis. • If used with general anesthetics, tranquilizers, sedatives, hypnotics, alcohol, tricyclic antidepressants, or MAO inhibitors, respiratory depression, hypotension, profound sedation, or coma may occur. Reduce morphine dose. Use together with extreme caution. Monitor patient's response. • For symptoms and treatment of toxicity, see p. 1119.
Anticoagulants: oxycodone hydrochloride products containing aspirin may increase anticoagulant effect. Monitor clotting times. Use together cautiously.	• Use with extreme caution in head injury, increased intracranial pressure, increased cerebrospinal fluid pressure, seizures, asthma, COPD, alcoholism, prostatic hypertrophy, severe hepatic or renal disease, acute abdominal conditions, urethral stricture, hypothyroidism, Addison's disease, cardiac arrhythmias, reduced blood volume, toxic psychosis, elderly or debilitated patients. • Don't give to children, except for Percodan-Demi and Percocet-Demi. • Warn ambulatory patient to avoid activities that require alertness. • Monitor circulatory and respiratory status, pupil size, bowel function. Do not give if respirations below 12/min. • For full analgesic effect, give before patient has intense pain. • High level of analgesia when given P.O. but poor choice due to high risk of addiction and presence of phenacetin in some combinations. • Give after meals or with milk. • If used with general anesthetics, other narcotic analgesics, tranquilizers, sedatives, hypnotics, alcohol, tricyclic antidepressants, or MAO inhibitors, CNS depression is increased. Reduce oxycodone dose. Use together with extreme caution. Monitor patient's response. • For symptoms and treatment of toxicity, see p. 1119.

NAME	INDICATIONS & DOSAGE	SIDE EFFECTS
oxymorphone hydrochloride Controlled substance Schedule II Numorphan◆	*Moderate to severe pain—* **Adults:** 1 to 1.5 mg I.M. or S.C. q 4 to 6 hours, p.r.n. or 0.5 mg I.V. q 4 to 6 hours, p.r.n., or 2.5 to 5 mg rectally q 4 to 6 hours, p.r.n.	*CNS:* light-headedness, headache, drowsiness, sedation, euphoria, restlessness, fainting; in large doses: convulsions, excitation. *CV:* bradycardia, orthostatic hypotension. *EENT:* miosis, red eyes. *GI:* nausea, vomiting, dry mouth. *GU:* urinary urgency, retention, impotence. *Skin:* pruritus, urticaria. *Other:* sweating, flushing, tolerance, physical and psychological dependence, respiratory depression.

INTERACTIONS	NURSING CONSIDERATIONS
None significant.	• Use with extreme caution in head injury, increased intracranial pressure, seizures, asthma, COPD, alcoholism, increased cerebrospinal fluid pressure, acute abdominal conditions, prostatic hypertrophy, severe hepatic or renal disease, urethral stricture, CNS depression, respiratory depression, hypothyroidism, Addison's disease, cardiac arrhythmias, reduced blood volume, toxic psychosis, elderly or debilitated patients. • Warn ambulatory patient to avoid activities that require alertness. • Monitor cardiovascular and respiratory status. Don't give if respirations below 12/minute. • For full analgesic effect, give before patient has intense pain. • Well absorbed rectally. Alternative to narcotics with more limited dosage forms. • Narcotic antagonists (naloxone) should be available. • If used with general anesthetics, tranquilizers, sedatives, hypnotics, alcohol, tricyclic antidepressants, or MAO inhibitors, CNS depression is increased. Reduce oxymorphone dose. Use together with extreme caution. Monitor patient response. • For symptoms and treatment of toxicity, see p. 1119.

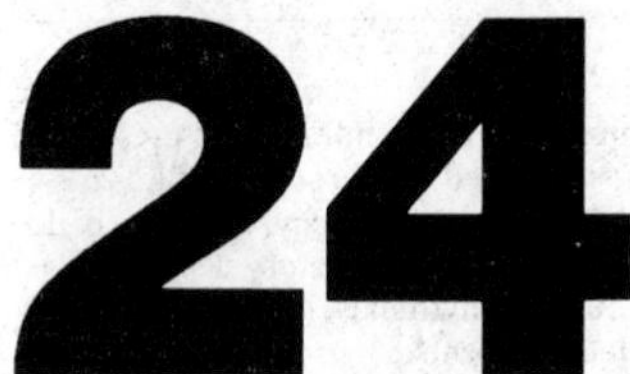

Narcotic antagonists

levallorphan tartrate
naloxone

Narcotic antagonists are very similar chemically to narcotics. However, they're much more potent: a narcotic antagonist can reverse respiratory depression caused by a narcotic dose 10 to 100 times as great. It also reverses a narcotic's analgesic, cardiovascular, and gastrointestinal effects.

Except for naloxone, narcotic antagonists are ineffective against barbiturate or anesthetic-induced respiratory depression. Indeed, levallorphan can produce respiratory depression and will worsen such depression caused by nonnarcotic drugs. Naloxone does not worsen nonnarcotic respiratory depression and is the antagonist of choice for respiratory depression of unknown cause. Naloxone can reverse respiratory depression caused by pentazocine and propoxyphene.

Narcotic antagonists are mainly used as antidotes for narcotic overdoses.

Major uses
- Antidote for narcotic-induced respiratory depression including asphyxia neonatorum.
- Diagnosis of suspected acute opiate overdosage (naloxone).

Mechanism of action
- Compete with narcotics for receptor sites (competitive antagonism).
- Also possess some agonistic activity (levallorphan tartrate).
- Naloxone is essentially a pure antagonist, with little or no agonistic activity.
- The precise mechanism of narcotic antagonism is unknown.

Absorption, distribution, and excretion
- Well absorbed after parenteral administration.
- Rapidly metabolized in liver.
- Excreted in the urine.
- Crosses placenta.

Onset and duration
- Onset within 1 to 2 minutes after I.V. administration; 5 to 20 minutes after I.M. or S.C. administration.
- Duration of action 1 to 4 hours.

Combination products
None.

CLEAR THE AIRWAY

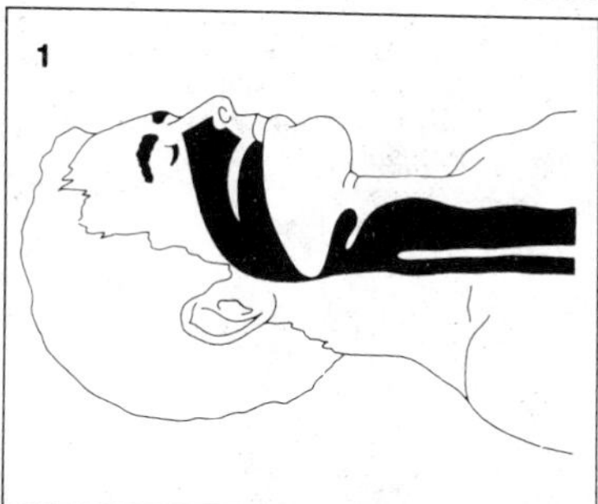

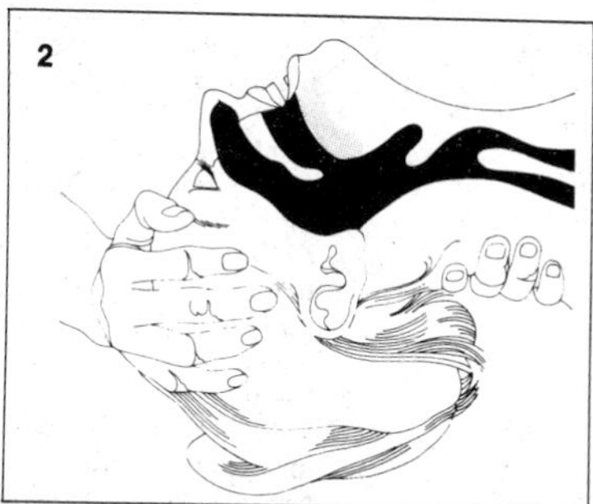

When an unconscious patient lies in a supine position, his relaxed muscles allow his lower jaw to drop backward and permit the back of his tongue to block his airway (see Figure 1).

To relieve this obstruction easily and quickly, use the head-tilt maneuver shown in Figure 2. This raises the tongue away from the back of the throat, and in some cases may be enough to start the patient breathing.

If the head tilt does not open the patient's airway, try the jaw thrust. Place your fingers behind the angles of the patient's jaw and push it forward. Exert enough pressure to maintain the head tilt.

Caution: Whenever you suspect neck injury, avoid using the head tilt and try to open the airway with a modified jaw thrust. Push the jaw forward, but don't hyperextend the neck or move the head to either side.

If you still need to ventilate the patient, use mouth-to-mouth or mouth-to-nose technique. Maintain his head tilt position with your hands, and pinch his nostrils with your thumb and index finger. Take a deep breath; open your mouth wide and make a tight seal with your mouth over the patient's open mouth. Blow air into his mouth; remove your mouth from his so he can exhale. Try to the start the breathing now by delivering four or five quick, full breaths with no time between for full lung deflation.

If his chest still doesn't rise, quickly check for a foreign substance obstructing the airway. Turn the patient's head to one side and forcibly open his mouth using your thumb and index finger and try to remove the blockage.

Another alternative method is mouth-to-nose. Use this method when the patient has a mouth injury or you're unable to form a tight seal over his mouth because he has no teeth.

If the patient has a stoma from a temporary tracheotomy, ventilate him by pinching his nostrils shut and sealing his lips with your hand to prevent leakage. Then put your mouth over his stoma and blow in air. Remove mouth, so he can exhale.

NAME	INDICATIONS & DOSAGE	SIDE EFFECTS
levallorphan tartrate Lorfan	*Severe narcotic-induced respiratory depression—* **Adults:** 1 mg I.V., then 1 to 2 doses of 0.5 mg at 10- to 15-minute intervals, p.r.n. Maximum total dose 3 mg. **Children:** 0.02 mg/Kg I.V. May give 0.01 to 0.02 mg/Kg in 10 to 15 minutes. **Neonates** (asphyxia neonatorum): 0.05 to 0.1 mg I.V. into umbilical vein immediately after delivery. May repeat in 5 to 10 minutes.	*CNS:* lethargy, dizziness, drowsiness, restlessness, sense of heaviness in limbs; with high doses: psychic disturbances (hallucinations, disorientation, weird dreams); in neonates: irritability, increased crying. *CV:* pallor. *EENT:* miosis, pseudoptosis. *GI:* nausea. *Other:* sweating, respiratory depression.
naloxone Narcan♦	*Pentazocine, propoxyphene, and narcotic-induced respiratory depression—* **Adults:** 0.4 mg I.V., S.C., or I.M. May repeat q 2 to 3 minutes, p.r.n., for 3 doses. *Postop narcotic depression*—0.1 to 0.2 mg I.V. q 2 to 3 minutes, p.r.n. Adult concentration is 0.4 mg/ml. **Children:** 0.01 mg/Kg dose I.M., I.V., S.C. May repeat q 2 to 3 minutes for 3 doses. **Neonates** (asphyxia neonatorum): 0.01 mg/Kg I.V. into umbilical vein. May repeat q 2 to 3 minutes for 3 doses. Neonatal concentration (for children also) is 0.02 mg/ml.	*With higher-than-recommended doses:* nausea, vomiting. *In narcotic addicts:* withdrawal symptoms.

♦ Also available in Canada.
♦♦ Available in Canada only.
Unmarked trade names available in United States only.

INTERACTIONS	NURSING CONSIDERATIONS
None significant.	• Contraindicated in mild respiratory depression and in narcotic addiction (violent withdrawal symptoms may occur). • Monitor respiratory depth and rate. Be prepared to give O_2, ventilation, and other resuscitative measures. • May increase mild respiratory depression or that caused by nonnarcotic agents. Repeated doses may produce tolerance and increased respiratory depression.
None significant.	• Use cautiously in cardiac irritability and narcotic addiction. • Safest drug to use when cause of respiratory depression uncertain. • Monitor respiratory depth and rate. Be prepared to give O_2, ventilation, and other resuscitative measures. • Ineffective in respiratory depression caused by nonnarcotics except pentazocine and propoxyphene. • May dilute adult concentration (0.4 mg) by mixing 0.5 ml with 9.5 ml sterile water or saline for injection to make neonatal concentration (0.02 mg/ml).

25

Sedatives and hypnotics

amobarbital
amobarbital sodium
aprobarbital
barbital
butabarbital
butabarbital sodium
chloral hydrate
ethchlorvynol
ethinamate
flurazepam hydrochloride
glutethimide
hexobarbital
mephobarbital
methaqualone
methaqualone hydrochloride
methotrimeprazine hydrochloride
methyprylon
paraldehyde
pentobarbital
pentobarbital sodium
phenobarbital
phenobarbital sodium
propiomazine hydrochloride
secobarbital
secobarbital sodium
talbutal
triclofos sodium

Sedatives and hypnotics are used primarily to treat insomnia and to provide preoperative sedation and relief of anxiety. They may also be used to ease alcohol withdrawal or as anticonvulsants. Most are barbiturates or have similar effects, including the risk of toxicity, drug dependence, and severe withdrawal symptoms.

Major uses

- Treatment of insomnia or induction of sleep before an operative or test procedure.
- Sedation and relief of anxiety.
- Alleviation of alcohol withdrawal syndrome.
- Control of status epilepticus, acute convulsive episodes, or acute psychotic agitation.
- Treatment of hyperbilirubinemia or chronic cholestasis.
- Prevention of nausea and vomiting.
- Some are used as basal or general anesthetics.

Mechanism of action

All depress the central nervous system, and most can produce effects ranging from mild sedation to hypnosis, deep coma, and death, depending on dosage; route of administration, absorption, distribution, metabolism, and excretion of the individual drug; and patient susceptibility. Some may relax skeletal muscles, alter temperature regulation, produce amnesia, cause local anesthesia, moderate convulsions, or have an antiemetic effect.

Absorption, distribution, and excretion

barbiturates:

- Absorbed well from all administration routes.
- Sodium salts absorbed more rapidly than acids.
- Absorption rate increased by alcohol, by ingestion of sodium salt as a dilute solution, or on an empty stomach.
- Absorption from I.V. route is almost immediate.
- Distributed to all tissues and fluids, with high concentrations in brain and liver. Appears in breast milk at lower levels than in plasma.
- Readily cross the placenta to fetal tissues and fluids.
- Metabolized slowly in the liver.
- Excreted unchanged in urine.
- Trace amounts are excreted in feces and sweat.

chloral hydrate:

- Absorbed from gastrointestinal tract after oral or rectal administration.
- Rapidly reduced and distributed through all tissues; drug and/or active metabolites detected in cerebrospinal fluid, umbilical cord blood, fetal blood, and amniotic fluid.
- Metabolized by liver and erythrocytes.
- Appears in breast milk and passes the placental barrier.
- Excreted primarily in urine, bile, and partially in feces.

ethchlorvynol:

- Absorbed rapidly from gastrointestinal tract after oral administration.
- Extensively localized in adipose tissues.
- Drug and/or metabolites detected in liver, kidneys, spleen, brain, bile, and cerebrospinal fluid.
- Metabolism is primarily in the liver and is influenced by the kidneys.

ethinamate:

- Absorbed well from gastrointestinal tract.
- Tissue distribution unknown; rapidly destroyed in the tissues.
- Liver is not significantly involved in the metabolism.
- Small amount is excreted in urine.

flurazepam hydrochloride:
- Absorbed from gastrointestinal tract after oral administration.
- Distributed to all tissues.
- Metabolized in liver.
- Excreted primarily in urine, partially in feces.

glutethimide:
- Absorbed irregularly from gastrointestinal tract after oral administration.
- Extensively concentrated in adipose tissues.
- Drug and/or metabolites detected in liver, kidneys, brain, and bile.
- Crosses placenta.
- Small quantities appear in breast milk.
- Metabolized in liver.
- Excreted in urine and feces.

mephobarbital:
- Approximately 50% is absorbed in gastrointestinal tract.
- Primary route of mephobarbital metabolism is by the liver to form phenobarbital.
- Excreted in the urine unchanged.

methaqualone, methaqualone hydrochloride:
- Absorbed rapidly from gastrointestinal tract after oral administration.
- Extensive localization in adipose tissues.
- Drug and/or metabolites detected in liver, kidneys, heart, brain, spleen, cerebrospinal fluid, and skeletal muscles.
- Metabolized in liver.
- Excreted in urine, bile, and feces.

methotrimeprazine hydrochloride:
- Absorbed rapidly after intramuscular injection.
- Crosses placenta and enters cerebrospinal fluid.
- Metabolized in liver.
- Excreted slowly in urine and feces.

methyprylon:
- Absorption and distribution not well known.
- Metabolized in liver.
- Metabolites secreted in bile and reabsorbed.
- Excreted in urine.

paraldehyde:
- Absorbed rapidly from gastrointestinal tract or intramuscular injection sites.
- Tissue distribution not well known, but drug concentration in cerebrospinal fluid is lower than in blood.
- Diffuses across placenta and appears in fetal circulation.
- Metabolized in liver.
- Excreted in urine and through lungs. Significant quantities exhaled unchanged with characteristic odor.

propiomazine hydrochloride:
- Absorbed well from parenteral sites.
- Distributed throughout the body.
- Metabolized in the liver.
- Excreted in urine and bile.

triclofos sodium:
- Rapidly absorbed from gastrointestinal tract.
- Tissue distribution not well known, but metabolite enters the cerebrospinal fluid and crosses the placenta.
- Metabolized primarily in the liver and the kidneys.
- Slowly excreted in urine and feces, and sometimes in the bile.

Onset and duration	**P.O./I.M.**	**I.V.**
Ultra short-acting: few minutes onset; short-term duration	hexobarbital	amobarbital ethchlorvynol pentobarbital phenobarbital
Short-acting: 10 to 15 minutes onset; 3 hours or less duration	paraldehyde pentobarbital secobarbital	
Intermediate-acting: 10 to 30 minutes onset; 3 to 6 hours duration	amobarbital aprobarbital butabarbital chloral hydrate ethchlorvynol ethinamate methotrimeprazine propiomazine talbutal tricloflos	
Long-acting: 30 to 60 minutes onset; 6 or more hours duration	barbital flurazepam glutethimide mephobarbital methaqualone methyprylon phenobarbital	

Combinations products—barbiturates

BUTATRAX CAPSULES: amobarbital 20 mg and butabarbital 30 mg.

ETHOBRAL CAPSULE: phenobarbital sodium 50 mg, butabarbital sodium 30 mg, and secobarbital sodium 50 mg.

HYPTRAN TABLET: secobarbital 60 mg and phenyltoloxamine citrate 25 mg in outer layer, phenyltoloxamine citrate 75 mg in core (delayed release).

NIDAR TABLET: phenobarbital 7.5 mg, butabarbital sodium 7.5 mg, and secobarbital sodium 25 mg, and pentobarbital 25 mg.

RUCK-SED KAPLETS: mephobarbital sodium 20 mg and butabarbital sodium 40 mg.

RUCK-SED LIQUID: amobarbital sodium 10 mg and butabarbital sodium 20 mg.

SECANAP TABLETS: phenobarbital 30 mg, secobarbital sodium 30 mg, and secobarbital sodium 50 mg.

TRI-BARBS CAPSULE: phenobarbital 32 mg, butabarbital sodium 32 mg, and secobarbital sodium 32 mg.

TRIPLE-BARB TABLET: phenobarbital sodium 16 mg, pentobarbital sodium 16 mg, and butabarbital sodium 16 mg.

TRIPLE-BARB TABLET: phenobarbital sodium 48 mg, pentobarbital sodium 48 mg, and butabarbital sodium 48 mg.

TRIPLE-BARB TABLET: phenobarbital sodium 97 mg, pentobarbital sodium 97 mg, and butabarbital sodium 97 mg.

TUINAL 50 MG: amobarbital sodium 25 mg and secobarbital sodium 25 mg Pulvules.

TUINAL 100 MG♦: amobarbital sodium 50 mg and secobarbital sodium 50 mg Pulvules.

TUINAL 200 MG♦: amobarbital sodium 100 mg and secobarbital sodium 100 mg.

Combination products—chloral hydrate

CARBRITAL KAPSEALS: pentobarbital sodium 48.7 mg and carbromal 260 mg.

CARBRITAL KAPSEALS: pentobarbital sodium 97.5 mg and carbromal 260 mg.

LORYL: chloral hydrate 337.5 mg and phenyltoloxamine citrate 37.5 mg.

PROMOTING GOOD SLEEP

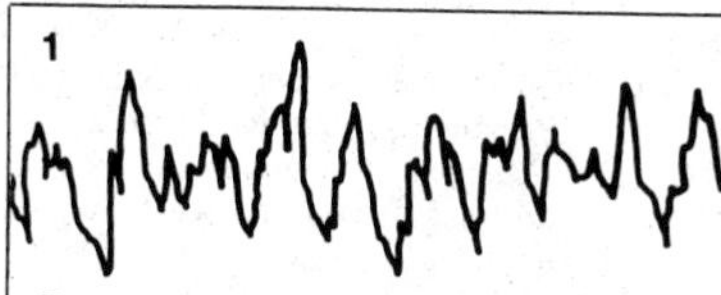

Delta waves which are very slow and high mark the start of stage four sleep.

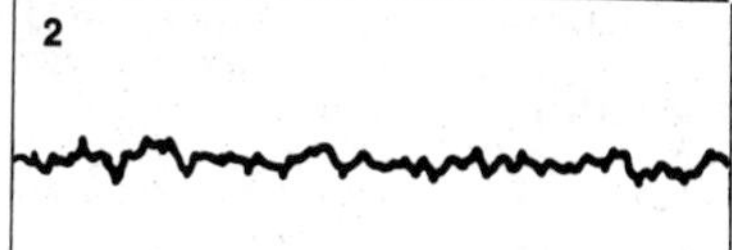

R.E.M., final sleep cycle, waves show an active EEG.

Each nursing shift can help promote good sleep without resorting to hypnotics and sedatives by following these suggestions.

DAY STAFF:

- Encourage naps in the morning rather than the afternoon. Morning naps are mostly a continuation of R.E.M. sleep — and because it is a light sleep, it usually leaves the patient feeling refreshed. Also, if your patient naps in the morning, he will more likely feel tired enough by evening to fall asleep again.
- If your patient's condition permits it, try to keep him as busy as possible during the day.
- Check your patient's history for unresolved anxiety — situations at home that may be worrying him in the hospital, i.e., financial problems, invalid spouse at home. Help end the worry by getting your patient in touch with a hospital social worker.

EVENING STAFF:

- Find out what your patient's sleep routine was at home and, whenever possible, try to let him follow it. Certain rituals, i.e., a bedtime snack or a favorite pillow, can aid sleep.
- Offer backrubs.
- Straighten out linens.
- Pull curtain closed to block out light from the unit.
- If advisable, close the door to patient's room.
- If your patient requires pain medication, try to give it early so he'll be relaxed by bedtime.

NIGHT STAFF:

- Find out who isn't sleeping and why.
- Be sure unit lights are dim and unnecessary lights are out.
- When checking on your patient, be as quiet as possible.
- Turn off nurses' station radio or make sure the patients can't hear it.
- After establishing a successful sleep plan for a specific patient, write it down so that it can be followed again.

NAME	INDICATIONS & DOSAGE	SIDE EFFECTS
amobarbital Amytal◆, Isobec◆◆ **amobarbital sodium** Controlled substance Schedule II Amytal Sodium◆	*Sedation—* **Adults:** usually 30 to 50 mg P.O. b.i.d. or t.i.d. but may range from 15 to 120 mg b.i.d. to q.i.d. **Children:** 3 to 6 mg/Kg/day P.O. divided into 4 equal doses. *Insomnia—* **Adults:** 65 to 200 mg P.O. or deep I.M. at bedtime; I.M. injection not to exceed 5 ml in any one site. Maximum dose 500 mg. **Children:** 3 to 5 mg/Kg deep I.M. at bedtime; I.M. injection not to exceed 5 ml in any one site. *Preanesthetic sedation—* **Adults and children:** 200 mg P.O. or I.M. 1 to 2 hours before surgery. *Manic reactions; anticonvulsant—* **Adults, and children over 6 years:** 65 to 500 mg slow I.V.; rate not to exceed 100 mg/minute. Maximum dose 1 g. **Children under 6 years:** 3 to 5 mg/Kg slow I.V. or I.M.	*CNS:* drowsiness, vertigo, headache, depression, residual sedation after hypnotic dose, paradoxical excitement. *GI:* nausea, vomiting, diarrhea. *Local:* pain at injection site. *Skin:* hypersensitivity reactions; jaundice. *Other:* respiratory depression, apnea, hypotension with I.V. administration; discontinuance of hypnotic doses may induce nightmares or insomnia.
aprobarbital Controlled substance Schedule III Alurate, Alurate Verdum	*Sedation—* **Adults:** 15 to 40 mg P.O. t.i.d. or q.i.d.; usual dose 40 mg t.i.d. *Insomnia—* **Adults:** 40 to 160 mg P.O. at bedtime.	*CNS:* drowsiness, vertigo, headache, depression, residual sedation after hypnotic dose, paradoxical excitement. *GI:* nausea, vomiting, diarrhea. *Skin:* hypersensitivity reactions, jaundice. *Other:* respiratory depression, apnea, hypotension; discontinuance of hypnotic doses may induce nightmares or insomnia.
barbital Controlled substance Schedule IV Barbital sodium	*Insomnia—* **Adults:** 300 to 600 mg P.O. or I.M. 1 to 2 hours before bedtime. *Sedative—* **Adults:** 65 to 130 mg P.O. or I.M. b.i.d. or t.i.d.	*CNS:* drowsiness, vertigo, headache, depression, residual sedation after hypnotic dose, paradoxical excitement. *GI:* nausea, vomiting, diarrhea. *Local:* pain, swelling, thrombophlebitis, necrosis, nerve injury. *Skin:* hypersensitivity reactions, jaundice. *Other:* respiratory depression, hiccuping; discontinuance of hypnotic doses may induce nightmares or insomnia.

◆ Also available in Canada.
◆◆ Available in Canada only.
Unmarked trade names available in United States only.

INTERACTIONS	NURSING CONSIDERATIONS
Alcohol or other CNS depressants, including other narcotic analgesics: excessive CNS and respiratory depression. Don't use together. *MAO inhibitors:* inhibited metabolism of barbiturates; may cause prolonged CNS depression. Reduce barbiturate dosage. *Rifampin:* may decrease barbiturate levels. Monitor for decreased effect.	• Contraindicated in uncontrolled severe pain, respiratory disease with dyspnea or obstruction, hypersensitivity to barbiturates, previous addiction to sedatives, porphyria. Use with caution in hepatic or renal impairment. • Use injection solution within 30 minutes after opening container to minimize deterioration. Don't use cloudy or precipitated solution. • Reserve I.V. injection for emergency treatment. Give under close supervision. Be prepared to give artificial respiration. Administer slowly I.V.; not to exceed 100 mg/minute. • Administer I.M. injection deeply. Superficial injection may cause pain, sterile abscess, and slough. • Because barbiturates potentiate narcotics, reduce dose when giving during labor. Excessive dose may cause respiratory depression in neonate. • Remove cigarettes if patient receives hypnotic dose. • Supervise walking; raise bed rails, especially for elderly patients. • Long-term high dosage may cause drug dependence and severe withdrawal symptoms. Withdraw barbiturates gradually. • Prevent hoarding or self-overdosing by patients who are depressed, suicidal, or drug-dependent, or who have a history of drug abuse. Warn patient about increased alcohol effects and against hazardous activity requiring alertness or skill. • Watch for signs of barbiturate toxicity: coma, pupillary constriction, cyanosis, clammy skin, hypotension. Overdose can be fatal. • Monitor prothrombin times carefully when patient on amobarbital starts or ends anticoagulant therapy. Anticoagulant dose may need to be adjusted. • For treatment of toxicity, see p. 1115.
Alcohol or other CNS depressants, including narcotic analgesics: excessive CNS and respiratory depression. Don't use together. *MAO inhibitors:* inhibited metabolism of barbiturates; may cause prolonged CNS depression. Reduce barbiturate dosage. *Rifampin:* may decrease barbiturate levels. Monitor for decreased effect.	• Contraindicated in uncontrolled severe pain, respiratory disease with dyspnea or obstruction, hypersensitivity to barbiturates, previous addiction to sedatives, porphyria. Use with caution in hepatic or renal impairment. • Remove cigarettes if patient receives hypnotic dose. • Supervise walking; raise bed rails, especially for elderly patients. • Long-term high dosage may cause drug dependence and severe withdrawal symptoms. Withdraw barbiturates gradually. • Prevent hoarding or self-overdosing by patients who are depressed, suicidal, or drug-dependent, or who have a history of drug abuse. Warn patient about increased alcohol effects and against hazardous activity requiring alertness or skill. • Available as elixir only, with alcohol 20%. • Monitor prothrombin times carefully when patient on aprobarbital starts or ends anticoagulant therapy. Anticoagulant dose may need to be adjusted. • Watch for signs of barbiturate toxicity: coma, pupillary constriction, cyanosis, clammy skin, hypotension. Overdose can be fatal. • For treatment of toxicity, see p. 1115.
Alcohol or other CNS depressants, including narcotic analgesics: excessive CNS and respiratory depression. Don't use together. *MAO inhibitors:* inhibited metabolism of barbiturates; may cause prolonged CNS depression.	• Contraindicated in uncontrolled severe pain, respiratory disease with dyspnea or obstruction, hypersensitivity to barbiturates, previous addiction to sedatives and porphyria. Use with caution in hepatic, renal, cardiac, or respiratory impairment; hyperthyroidism; diabetes mellitus; anemia; elderly or debilitated patients. • Use injection solution within 30 minutes after opening container to minimize deterioration. Don't use cloudy solution. • Administer I.M. injection deeply. Superficial injection may cause pain, sterile abscess, and slough. • Because barbiturates potentiate narcotics, reduce dose when giving during labor. Excessive dose may cause respiratory depression in neonate. • Remove cigarettes if patient receives hypnotic dose.

(continued on following page)

NAME	INDICATIONS & DOSAGE	SIDE EFFECTS
barbital *(continued)*		
butabarbital Buta-Barb◆◆, Butisol, Day-Barb◆◆, Medarsed, Neo-Barb◆◆ **butabarbital sodium** Controlled substance Schedule III BBS, Butal, Buta-zem, Buticaps, Butisol Sodium◆, Sarisol No. 1, Soduben	*Sedation—* **Adults:** 15 to 30 mg P.O. t.i.d. or q.i.d. **Children:** 6 mg/Kg P.O. divided t.i.d. Dosage range 7.5 to 30 mg P.O. t.i.d. *Preop—* **Adults:** 50 to 100 mg P.O. 60 to 90 minutes before surgery. *Insomnia—* **Adults:** 50 to 100 mg P.O. at bedtime.	*CNS:* drowsiness, vertigo, headache, depression, residual sedation after hypnotic dose, paradoxical excitement. *GI:* nausea, vomiting, diarrhea. *Skin:* hypersensitivity reactions (fever, serum sickness, urticaria, rash, edema, erythema), jaundice. *Other:* respiratory depression, paradoxical excitement and confusion in the elderly and children; discontinuance of hypnotic doses may induce nightmares or insomnia.
chloral hydrate Controlled substance Schedule IV Aquachloral Supprettes, Chloral-van◆◆, Cohidrate, Noctec◆, Novo-chlorhydrate◆◆, Oradrate	*Sedation—* **Adults:** 250 mg P.O. or rectally t.i.d. after meals. **Children:** 8 mg/Kg P.O. t.i.d. Maximum 500 mg t.i.d. *Insomnia—* **Adults:** 500 mg to 1 g P.O. or rectally 15 to 30 minutes before bedtime. **Children:** 50 mg/Kg single dose. Maximum dose 1 g. *Premedication for EEG—* **Children:** 25 mg/Kg single dose.	*CNS:* residual headache, drowsiness, nightmares, dizziness, hangover, ataxia. *GI:* nausea, vomiting, diarrhea, flatulence. *GU:* renal dysfunction. *Skin:* hypersensitivity reactions. *Other:* fever.

INTERACTIONS	NURSING CONSIDERATIONS
Reduce barbiturate dosage. *Rifampin:* may decrease barbiturate levels. Monitor for decreased effect.	• Supervise walking; raise bed rails, especially for elderly patients. • Long-term high dosage may cause drug dependence and severe withdrawal symptoms. Withdraw barbiturates gradually. • Prevent hoarding or self-overdosing by patients who are depressed, suicidal, or drug-dependent, or who have a history of drug abuse. Warn about increased alcohol effects and against hazardous activity requiring alertness or skill. • No analgesic action. May cause restlessness or delirium in presence of pain. • Monitor prothrombin times carefully when patient on barbital starts or ends anticoagulant therapy. Anticoagulant dose may need to be adjusted. • Watch for signs of barbiturate toxicity: coma, pupillary constriction, cyanosis, clammy skin, hypotension. Overdose can be fatal. • For treatment of toxicity, see p. 1115.
Alcohol or other CNS depressants, including narcotic analgesics: excessive CNS and respiratory depression. Don't use together. *MAO inhibitors:* inhibit the metabolism of barbiturates; may cause prolonged CNS depression. Reduce barbiturate dosage. *Rifampin:* may decrease barbiturate levels. Monitor for decreased effect.	• Contraindicated in uncontrolled severe pain, respiratory disease with dyspnea or obstruction, hypersensitivity to barbiturates, previous addiction to sedatives, porphyria. Use with caution in hepatic or renal impairment. • Remove cigarettes if patient receives hypnotic dose. • Supervise walking; raise bed rails, especially for elderly patients. • Long-term high dosage may cause drug dependence and severe withdrawal symptoms. Withdraw barbiturates gradually. • Prevent hoarding or self-overdosing by patients who are depressed, suicidal, or drug-dependent, or who have a history of drug abuse. Warn patient about increased alcohol effects and against hazardous activity requiring alertness or skill. • Butisol sodium elixir is sugar-free. • Monitor prothrombin times carefully when patient on butabarbital starts or ends anticoagulant therapy. Anticoagulant dose may need to be adjusted. • Watch for signs of barbiturate toxicity: coma, pupillary constriction, cyanosis, clammy skin, hypotension. Overdose can be fatal. • For treatment of toxicity, see p. 1115.
Alcohol or other CNS depressants, including narcotic analgesics: excessive CNS depression or vasodilation reaction. Use together cautiously. *Furosemide, I.V.:* sweating, flushes, variable blood pressure, uneasiness. Use together cautiously. Use a different hypnotic drug.	• Contraindicated in hepatic or renal impairment, hypersensitivity to chloral hydrate or triclofos. Oral administration contraindicated in gastric disorders. Use with caution in severe heart disease, mental depression, suicidal tendencies; also, in pregnancy, lactation, drug dependency. • Dilute or administer with liquid to minimize unpleasant taste and stomach irritation. Administer after meals. • Prevent hoarding by patients who are depressed, suicidal, or drug-dependent, or who have a history of drug abuse. Warn about increased alcohol effects and against hazardous activity requiring alertness or skill. • Remove cigarettes if patient receives hypnotic dose. • Supervise walking; raise bed rails, especially for elderly patients. • Large dosage may raise BUN level. • May cause false positives in glycosuria tests using cupric sulfate as Benedict's solution. Use Clinitest, Clinistix, or Tes-Tape. • May interfere with fluorometric tests for urine catecholamines and Reddy, Jenkins, Thorn test for urinary 17-hydroxycorticosteroids. Do not administer drug for 48 hours before fluorometric test. • Aqueous solutions incompatible with alkaline substances. • Store in dark container. Store suppositories in refrigerator. • If patient is given anticoagulant, monitor for increased prothrombin times during the first several days of therapy. Anticoagulant dose may need to be adjusted.

NAME	INDICATIONS & DOSAGE	SIDE EFFECTS
ethchlorvynol Controlled substance Schedule IV Placidyl◆	*Sedation—* **Adults:** 100 to 200 mg P.O. b.i.d. or t.i.d. *Insomnia—* **Adults:** 500 mg to 1 g P.O. at bedtime. May repeat 100 to 200 mg if awakened in early a.m.	*Blood:* thrombocytopenia. *CNS:* facial numbness, drowsiness, fatigue, nightmares, dizziness, residual sedation, prolonged hypnosis, muscular weakness, syncope, ataxia. *CV:* hypotension. *EENT:* unpleasant aftertaste, blurred vision. *GI:* distress, nausea, vomiting. *Skin:* rashes, urticaria, cholestatic jaundice. *Other:* mild hangover, unpleasant aftertaste.
ethinamate Controlled substance Schedule IV Valmid	*Insomnia—* **Adults:** 500 mg to 1 g P.O. 20 minutes before bedtime. Starting dose may be 250 mg for elderly or debilitated patients. *Preanesthetic—* **Adults:** 500 mg to 1 g P.O. 2½ hours preoperatively.	*Blood:* thrombocytopenia. *GI:* mild upset. *Skin:* rashes, purpura. *Other:* fever (allergic reaction).
flurazepam hydrochloride Controlled substance Schedule IV Dalmane◆	*Insomnia—* **Adults:** 15 to 30 mg P.O. at bedtime.	*Blood:* leukopenia, granulocytopenia. *CNS:* residual sedation, dizziness, drowsiness, disturbed coordination, lethargy, confusion, headache, coma, anxiety, talkativeness, irritability, euphoria, mental depression, restlessness, hallucinations, nightmares, faintness, weakness, slurred speech. *CV:* palpitations, hypotension. *EENT:* bitter taste, swollen tongue, dry mouth, excessive salivation, burning eyes, visual disturbances. *GI:* heartburn, nausea, vomiting, diarrhea, constipation, anorexia, pain.

INTERACTIONS	NURSING CONSIDERATIONS
Alcohol or other CNS depressants, including narcotic analgesics: excessive CNS depression. Use together cautiously.	• Contraindicated in uncontrolled pain and porphyria. Use cautiously in hepatic or renal impairment; in elderly or debilitated patients; in mental depression with suicidal tendencies; if patient has previously overreacted to barbiturates or alcohol. • Give with milk or food to minimize transient dizziness or ataxia caused by rapid absorption. • Avoid prolonged use; may cause dependence and severe withdrawal symptoms. • Prevent hoarding or self-overdosing by patients who are depressed, suicidal, or drug-dependent, or who have a history of drug abuse. Overdosage very difficult to treat and has a high mortality rate. Warn about increased alcohol effects and against hazardous activity requiring alertness or skill. • Watch for toxicity signs, such as poor muscle coordination, confusion, hypothermia, speech or vision disturbances, tremors, or weakness. • Remove cigarettes if patient receives hypnotic dose. • Supervise walking; raise bed rails, especially for elderly patients. • Slight darkening of liquid from exposure to air and light doesn't affect safety or potency, but store in tight, light-resistant container to avoid possible deterioration. • Monitor prothrombin times carefully when patient on ethchlorvynol starts or ends anticoagulant therapy. Anticoagulant dose may need to be adjusted. • Drug is effective for short-term use only.
None significant.	• Contraindicated for uncontrolled pain. Use cautiously in mental depression, suicidal tendencies, or history of drug abuse. • Not usually given for daytime sedation due to short duration of effect. • Long-term use may cause dependence and severe withdrawal symptoms. • Prevent hoarding or self-overdosing by patients who are depressed, suicidal, or drug-dependent, or who have a history of drug abuse. Warn about increased alcohol effects and against hazardous activity requiring alertness or skill. • Abrupt withdrawal may cause blood pressure and pulse rate changes, sweating, and hallucinations. • Remove patient's cigarettes after giving dose. • Supervise walking; raise bed rails, especially for elderly patients. • In overdosage, treat CNS and respiratory depression same as barbiturate intoxication; ethinamate is dialyzable. • May cause falsely elevated urinary 17-ketosteroid (modified Zimmerman reaction) and 17-hydroxycorticosteroid levels (Porter-Silber test). • Prolonged therapy not recommended; drug is not effective for more than 7 days.
None significant.	• Use cautiously in impaired hepatic or renal function, mental depression, suicidal tendencies, or history of drug abuse. Use caution and low end of dose range for elderly or debilitated patients. • Prevent hoarding or self-overdosing by patients who are depressed, suicidal, or drug-dependent, or who have a history of drug abuse. Warn about increased alcohol effects and against hazardous activity requiring alertness or skill. • Remove patient's cigarettes after giving dose. • Supervise walking; raise bed rails, especially for elderly patients. • Not for prolonged use; but if unavoidable, monitor blood, and hepatic and renal function periodically.

(continued on following page)

NAME	INDICATIONS & DOSAGE	SIDE EFFECTS
flurazepam hydrochloride *(continued)*		*Skin:* sweating, flushes, pruritus, rash. *Other:* hangover, shortness of breath, chest and joint pains. The above side effects are usually mild and disappear when the drug is discontinued. Prolonged therapy may cause hepatic or renal impairment.
glutethimide Controlled substance Schedule III Doriden♦, Rolathimide	*Insomnia—* **Adults:** 250 to 500 mg P.O. at bedtime. May be repeated, but not less than 4 hours before intended awakening. Total daily dose should not exceed 1 g. *Preop—* **Adults:** 500 mg night before surgery; 500 mg to 1 g 1 hour before anesthesia. *First stage of labor—* 500 mg at onset of labor; repeat once if necessary. *Sedative—* **Adults:** 125 to 250 mg t.i.d. after meals.	*CNS:* residual sedation, paradoxical excitation, headache, vertigo. *EENT:* dry mouth, blurred vision. *GI:* irritation, nausea, diarrhea. *Skin:* rashes, urticaria. *Other:* hiccups, residual hangover.
hexobarbital Controlled substance Schedule III Sombulex	*Sedation—* **Adults:** 250 mg P.O., repeated as needed, q 2 to 3 hours. *Insomnia—* **Adults:** 250 to 500 mg P.O. at bedtime.	*CNS:* drowsiness, vertigo, headache, depression, residual sedation after hypnotic dose, paradoxical excitement. *GI:* nausea, vomiting, diarrhea. *Skin:* hypersensitivity reactions, jaundice. *Other:* respiratory depression, apnea; discontinuance of hypnotic doses may induce nightmares or insomnia.
mephobarbital Controlled substance Schedule IV Mebaral♦.	*Sedation—* **Adults:** 32 to 100 mg P.O. t.i.d. to q.i.d. **Children:** 16 to 32 mg P.O. t.i.d. to q.i.d. *Incipient or active delirium tremens—* 200 mg P.O. t.i.d.	*CNS:* drowsiness, vertigo, headache, depression, residual sedation after hypnotic dose, paradoxical excitement. *GI:* nausea, vomiting, diarrhea. *Skin:* hypersensitivity reactions, jaundice. *Other:* respiratory depression, apnea; discontinuance of hypnotic doses may induce nightmares or insomnia.

INTERACTIONS	NURSING CONSIDERATIONS
Alcohol or other CNS depressants, including narcotic analgesics: excessive CNS depression. Use together cautiously.	• Contraindicated in uncontrolled pain, severe renal impairment, porphyria. Use cautiously in mental depression, suicidal tendencies, history of drug abuse, prostatic hypertrophy, stenosing peptic ulcer, pyloroduodenal or bladder neck obstruction, narrow-angle glaucoma, cardiac arrhythmias. • Drug is effective for short-term use only. • Remove patient's cigarettes after giving dose. • Supervise walking; raise bed rails, especially for elderly patients. • Prevent hoarding or self-overdosing by patients who are depressed, suicidal, or drug-dependent, or who have a history of drug abuse. Warn about increased alcohol effects and against hazardous activity requiring alertness or skill for 7 to 8 hours after receiving this drug. • Abrupt withdrawal may produce nausea, vomiting, nervousness, tremors, chills, fever, nightmares, insomnia, tachycardia, delirium, numbness of extremities, hallucinations, dysphagia, convulsions. Withdraw gradually. • Monitor prothrombin times carefully when patient on glutethimide starts or ends anticoagulant therapy. Anticoagulant dose may need to be adjusted.
Alcohol or other CNS depressants, including narcotic analgesics: excessive CNS and respiratory depression. Do not use together. *MAO inhibitors:* inhibited metabolism of barbiturates; may cause prolonged CNS depression. Reduce barbiturate dosage. *Rifampin:* may decrease barbiturate levels. Monitor for decreased effect.	• Contraindicated in uncontrolled severe pain, respiratory disease with dyspnea or obstruction, hypersensitivity to barbiturates, previous addiction to sedatives, porphyria. Use with caution in hepatic or renal impairment. • May be used preop with atropine when morphine contraindicated. • Because barbiturates potentiate narcotics, reduce dose when giving during labor. Excessive dose may cause respiratory depression in neonate. • Remove patient's cigarettes if he receives hypnotic dose. • Supervise walking; raise bed rails, especially for elderly patients. • Long-term high dosage may cause drug dependence and severe withdrawal symptoms. Withdraw barbiturates gradually. • Prevent hoarding or self-overdosing by patients who are depressed, suicidal, or drug-dependent, or who have a history of drug abuse. Warn about increased alcohol effects and against hazardous activity requiring alertness or skill. • Monitor prothrombin times carefully when patient on hexobarbital starts or ends anticoagulant therapy. Barbiturate dose may need to be adjusted. • Watch for signs of toxicity: coma, pupillary constriction (pupillary dilation with severe poisoning), clammy skin, hypotension. Overdose can be fatal. • For treatment of toxicity, see p. 1115.
Alcohol or other CNS depressants, including narcotic analgesics: excessive CNS and respiratory depression. Do not use together. *MAO inhibitors:* inhibited metabolism of barbiturates;	• Contraindicated in uncontrolled severe pain, respiratory disease with dyspnea or obstruction, hypersensitivity to barbiturates, previous addiction to sedatives, porphyria. Use with caution in hepatic or renal impairment, or impaired cardiac or respiratory function. • Remove cigarettes if patient receives hypnotic dose. • Supervise walking; raise bed rails, especially for elderly patients. • Long-term high dosage may cause drug dependence and severe withdrawal symptoms. Withdraw barbiturates gradually. • Prevent hoarding or self-overdosing by patients who are depressed, suicidal, or drug-dependent, or who have a history of drug abuse. Warn about

(continued on following page)

NAME	INDICATIONS & DOSAGE	SIDE EFFECTS
mephobarbital *(continued)*		
methaqualone Mequin, Quaalude, Sopor **methaqualone hydrochloride** Controlled substance Schedule II Parest, Parest 400, Rouqualone♦♦, Sedalone♦♦, Somnafac, Somnafac Forte, Triador♦♦, Tualone♦♦, Vitalone♦♦	*Sedation (methaqualone)*— **Adults:** 75 mg P.O. t.i.d. or q.i.d. *Insomnia (methaqualone)*— **Adults:** 150 to 300 P.O. at bedtime. *Insomnia (methaqualone hydrochloride)*— **Adults:** 200 to 400 mg P.O. at bedtime.	*CNS:* headache, dizziness, torpor, fatigue, residual sedation, transient paresthesias of extremities, restlessness, anxiety. *EENT:* dry mouth, cracking at corners of mouth, nosebleed. *GI:* anorexia, nausea, vomiting, epigastric discomfort, diarrhea, constipation. *GU:* menstrual disturbances. *Skin:* rashes, urticaria. *Other:* foul-smelling perspiration.
methotrimeprazine hydrochloride Levoprome, Nozinan♦♦	*Postop analgesia*— **Adults, and children over 12 years:** initially, 2.5 to 7.5 mg I.M. q 4 to 6 hours, then adjust dose. *Preanesthetic medication*— **Adults, and children over 12 years:** 2 to 20 mg I.M. 45 minutes to 3 hours prior to surgery. *Sedation, analgesia*— **Adults, and children over 12 years:** 10 to 20 mg deep I.M. q 4 to 6 hours as required. **Elderly:** 5 to 10 mg I.M. q 4 to 6 hours.	*Blood:* agranulocytosis and other dyscrasias after long-term high dosage. *CNS:* orthostatic hypotension, fainting, weakness, dizziness, drowsiness, excessive sedation, amnesia, disorientation, euphoria, headache, slurred speech. *CV:* drop in blood pressure, palpitations, tachycardia, bradycardia. *EENT:* dry mouth, nasal congestion. *GI:* nausea, vomiting, abdominal discomfort. *GU:* difficulty urinating. *Local:* pain, inflammation, swelling at injection site. *Other:* chills, respiratory depression, jaundice.
methyprylon Controlled substance Schedule III Noludar♦	*Insomnia*— **Adults:** 200 to 400 mg P.O. 15 minutes before bedtime. **Children over 3 months:** 50 mg P.O. at bedtime, increased to 200 mg, if necessary. Maximum 400 mg/day. *Sedation*— **Adults:** 150 to 400 mg t.i.d. or q.i.d. **Children:** 150 to 200 mg t.i.d. or q.i.d.	*CNS:* morning drowsiness, dizziness, headache, paradoxical excitation. *GI:* nausea, vomiting, diarrhea, esophagitis. *Skin:* rash.

INTERACTIONS	NURSING CONSIDERATIONS
may cause prolonged CNS depression. Reduce barbiturate dosage. *Rifampin:* may decrease barbiturate levels. Monitor for decreased effect.	increased alcohol effects and against hazardous activity requiring alertness or skill. • Mephobarbital is metabolized to phenobarbital, the active agent. • Monitor prothrombin times carefully when patient on mephobarbital starts or ends anticoagulant therapy. Barbiturate dose may need adjustment. • Watch for signs of toxicity. • For treatment of toxicity, see p. 1115.
Alcohol or other CNS depressants, including narcotic analgesics: excessive CNS depression. Use together cautiously.	• Contraindicated in hypersensitivity to barbiturates or history of drug abuse. Use cautiously in hepatic impairment, history of porphyria, mental depression, suicidal tendencies. • Remove cigarettes if patient receives hypnotic dose. • Supervise walking; raise bed rails, especially for elderly patients. • Warn about increased alcohol effects and against hazardous activity requiring alertness or skill. • Switching from another hypnotic to methaqualone requires 5 to 7 consecutive nights of therapy to obtain satisfactory hypnotic effect. • One of major drugs of abuse "on the street." Because of high abuse potential, methaqualone is rarely clinically indicated. • For symptoms and treatment of toxicity, see p. 1115.
All antihypertensive agents: increased orthostatic hypotension. Don't use together.	• Contraindicated in concurrent antihypertensive drug therapy, including MAO inhibitors; also, in history of convulsive disorders; hypersensitivity to phenothiazines; severe cardiac, hepatic, or renal disease; previous overdose of CNS depressant; coma. Use with extreme caution in elderly or debilitated patient with heart disease or in any patient who may suffer serious consequences from a sudden drop in blood pressure. • Use low initial dose in susceptible patient; increase gradually while frequently checking pulse, blood pressure, and circulation. • Expect drop in blood pressure 10 to 20 minutes after I.M. injection. • Keep patient in bed or closely supervised for 6 to 12 hours after initial doses because of orthostatic hypotension. If hypotension is severe, combat it with phenylephrine, methoxamine, or levarterenol. Don't use epinephrine. • Don't use for longer than 30 days except in terminal illness or when narcotics are contraindicated. • In prolonged use, monitor hepatic function and blood studies periodically. • Inject I.M. into large muscle masses. Rotate sites. Do not administer S.C., as local irritation results. I.V. injection not recommended. • May be mixed in same syringe with reduced dose of atropine and scopolamine. Do not mix with other drugs. Protect solution from light.
None significant.	• Contraindicated in intermittent porphyria. Use cautiously in renal or hepatic impairment. • Periodic blood counts are advisable during repeated or long-term use. • Long-term high dosage may cause drug dependence and severe life-threatening withdrawal symptoms. Withdrawal should be gradual and closely monitored. • Prevent hoarding or self-overdosing by patients who are depressed, suicidal, or drug-dependent, or who have a history of drug abuse. Warn about increased alcohol effect and against hazardous activity requiring alertness or skill. • Remove patient's cigarettes after giving dose. • Supervise walking; raise bed rails, especially for elderly patients.

(continued on following page)

NAME	INDICATIONS & DOSAGE	SIDE EFFECTS
methyprylon *(continued)*		
paraldehyde Controlled substance Schedule IV Paral	*Sedation—* **Adults:** 4 to 10 ml P.O. or 5 ml deep I.M. in upper outer quadrant of buttock. 3 to 5 ml I.V. (in emergency only). **Children:** 0.15 ml/Kg P.O. or deep I.M. *Insomnia—* **Adults:** 10 to 30 ml P.O.; 10 ml I.M. or I.V. **Children:** 0.3 ml/Kg P.O. or deep I.M. *Alcohol withdrawal syndrome—* **Adults:** 5 to 10 ml P.O. or 5 ml deep I.M. q 4 to 6 hours for the first 24 hours, not to exceed a total of 60 ml P.O. or 30 ml I.M.; then q 6 hours on following days, not to exceed 40 ml P.O. or 20 ml I.M. per 24 hours. *Status epilepticus—* **Adults:** 5 to 10 ml I.M. or 0.2 to 0.4 ml/Kg I.V. in 0.9% sodium chloride injection. **Children:** 0.15 ml/Kg I.M. q 4 to 6 hours or 0.1 to 0.15 ml/Kg I.V. in 0.9% sodium chloride injection. *Tetanus—* **Adults:** 4 to 5 ml I.V. (well diluted) or 12 ml (diluted 1:10) via gastric tube q 4 hours, p.r.n.; 5 to 10 ml I.M., p.r.n. to control seizures.	*CV:* I.V. administration may cause pulmonary edema or hemorrhage, dilation of right side of heart, circulatory collapse, respiratory distress. *GI:* irritation. *GU:* nephrosis with prolonged use. *Local:* pain, sterile abscesses, sloughing of skin, fat necrosis, muscular irritation, nerve damage at I.M. injection site (if injection is near nerve trunk). *Skin:* erythematous rash. *Other:* toxic hepatitis with prolonged use; oral or rectal administration of decomposed paraldehyde may cause severe corrosion of stomach or rectum, metabolic acidosis, or death.
pentobarbital Controlled substance Schedule III Nebralin **pentobarbital sodium** Maso-Pent, Nembutal Sodium♦, Nova-Rectal♦♦, Penital, Pentogen♦♦	*Sedation—* **Adults:** 20 to 40 mg P.O. b.i.d., t.i.d., or q.i.d. **Children:** 2 to 3 mg P.O. or rectally q 8 hours, p.r.n. *Insomnia—* **Adults:** 100 to 200 mg P.O. at bedtime or 150 to 200 mg deep I.M.; 120 to 200 mg rectally. **Children:** 3 to 5 mg/Kg I.M. Maximum dose: 100 mg. Rectal dosages: 2 months to 1 year, 30 mg; 1 to 4 years, 30 to 60 mg; 5 to 12 years, 60 mg; 12 to 14 years, 60 to 120 mg. *Preanesthetic medication—* **Adults:** 150 to 200 mg I.M. or P.O. in 2 divided doses.	*CNS:* drowsiness, vertigo, headache, depression, residual sedation after hypnotic dose, paradoxical excitement. *GI:* nausea, vomiting, diarrhea. *Skin:* hypersensitivity reactions, jaundice. *Other:* respiratory depression, apnea, laryngospasm, bronchospasm, or hypotension with I.V. administration; discontinuance of hypnotic doses may induce nightmares or insomnia.

INTERACTIONS	NURSING CONSIDERATIONS
	• Value of this drug as a sedative has not been established. • Overdosage symptoms include somnolence, confusion, constricted pupils, respiratory depression, hypotension, coma. Hemodialysis is useful in severe intoxication. • For treatment of toxicity, see p. 1119.
Alcohol: excessive CNS depression. Use with caution. *Disulfiram (antabuse):* increase in paraldehyde and acetaldehyde blood levels. Use together cautiously. May produce toxic disulfiram reaction.	• Contraindicated in bronchopulmonary disease or gastroenteritis with ulceration. Use cautiously in hepatic impairment. • Don't use for obstetric anesthesia because drug crosses placenta and appears in fetal bloodstream. • Give rectal dose in olive oil as retention enema: 1 part paraldehyde, 2 parts oil, and 200 ml 0.9% sodium chloride solution. • Dilute oral dose with iced juice or milk to mask taste and odor and to reduce GI distress. • Use fresh supply; discard bottles opened more than 24 hours. Don't use if liquid has a brownish color, vinegary odor, or contains a precipitate. • Drug reacts with plastic. Use glass syringe for parenteral dose, and don't put liquid in Styrofoam cup. • Give I.M. injection deeply, away from nerve trunks, and massage injection site. Do not give more than 5 ml per injection site. • Watch closely for respiratory depression, especially with repeated doses. • Long-term high dosage may cause drug dependence and severe withdrawal symptoms. Withdraw gradually, with close monitoring. • Remove cigarettes if patient receives hypnotic dose. • Supervise walking; raise bed rails, especially for elderly patients. • Ventilate patient's room well to remove exhaled paraldehyde. • No analgesic effect. May produce excitement or delirium in presence of pain.
Alcohol or other CNS depressants, including narcotic analgesics: excessive CNS and respiratory depression. Do not use together. *MAO inhibitors:* inhibited metabolism of barbiturates; may cause prolonged CNS depression. Reduce barbiturate dosage. *Rifampin:* may decrease barbiturate levels. Monitor for decreased effect.	• Contraindicated in uncontrolled severe pain, respiratory disease with dyspnea or obstruction, hypersensitivity to barbiturates, previous addiction to sedatives, porphyria. Use with caution in hepatic or renal impairment. • Use injection solution within 30 minutes after opening container to minimize deterioration. Don't use cloudy solution. • Parenteral solution alkaline. Avoid extravasation; may cause tissue necrosis. • I.V. injection should be reserved for emergency treatment and should be given under close supervision. Be prepared to give artificial respiration. • Administer I.M. injection deeply. Superficial injection may cause pain, sterile abscess, and slough. • Do not mix with any other medication. • Because barbiturates potentiate narcotics, reduce dose when giving during labor. Excessive dose may cause respiratory depression in neonate. • Remove cigarettes if patient receives hypnotic dose. • Supervise walking; raise bed rails, especially for elderly patients. • Long-term high dosage may cause drug dependence and severe withdrawal symptoms. Withdraw barbiturates gradually. • Prevent hoarding or self-overdosing by patients who are depressed, suici-

(continued on following page)

NAME	INDICATIONS & DOSAGE	SIDE EFFECTS
pentobarbital sodium *(continued)*		
phenobarbital Barbipil, Barbita, Eskabarb◆, Gardenal◆, Henomint, Luminal◆, Orprine, PBR 12, Pheno-Squar, Solfoton, Solu-barb, Stental **phenobarbital sodium** Controlled substance Schedule IV Luminal Sodium◆	*Sedation—* **Adults:** 30 to 120 mg P.O. daily in 2 or 3 divided doses. **Children:** 6 mg/Kg P.O. divided t.i.d. *Insomnia—* **Adults:** 100 to 320 mg P.O. or I.M. **Children:** 3 to 6 mg/Kg. *Preop sedation—* **Adults:** 100 to 200 mg I.M. 60 to 90 minutes before surgery. **Children:** 16 to 100 mg I.M. 60 to 90 minutes before surgery. *Hyperbilirubinemia—* **Neonates:** 7 mg/Kg/day P.O. from first to fifth day of life, or 5 mg/Kg/day I.M. on first day, repeated P.O. on second to seventh days. *Chronic cholestasis—* **Adults:** 90 to 180 mg P.O. daily in 2 or 3 divided doses. **Children under 12 years:** 3 to 12 mg/Kg/day P.O. in 2 or 3 divided doses.	*CNS:* drowsiness, vertigo, headache, depression, residual sedation after hypnotic dose, paradoxical excitement. *GI:* nausea, vomiting, diarrhea. *Local:* pain, swelling, thrombophlebitis, necrosis, nerve injury. *Skin:* hypersensitivity reactions, jaundice. *Other:* respiratory depression, hiccups, laryngospasm, embolism with I.V. use; discontinuance of hypnotic doses may induce nightmares or insomnia.
propiomazine hydrochloride Largon	*Sedation—* **Adults:** 20 to 40 mg I.M. or I.V. *Preop—* **Adults:** 10 to 20 mg I.M. or I.V. *During surgery; in conjunction with local, nerve block, or spinal anesthetic—* **Adults:** 20 to 40 mg I.M. or I.V. during early stages of labor, repeated q 3 hours, if necessary. *Sedation the night before surgery as a preanesthetic, or postop—* **Children under 27 Kg:** 0.55 to 1.1 mg/Kg I.M. or I.V. **Children 6 to 12 years:** 25 mg I.M. or I.V. in a single dose. **Children 4 to 6 years:** 15 mg I.M. or I.V. in a single dose.	*CNS:* dizziness, confusion, amnesia (primarily in the elderly), restlessness. *CV:* tachycardia, rise in blood pressure, transient hypotension with rapid I.V. infusion. *EENT:* dry mouth. *GI:* distress. *Skin:* rashes. *Other:* respiratory depression, changes in breathing pattern, vein irritation and thrombophlebitis following I.V. injection.

INTERACTIONS	NURSING CONSIDERATIONS
	dal, or drug-dependent, or who have a history of drug abuse. Warn about increased alcohol effects and against hazardous activity requiring alertness or skill. • No analgesic effect. May cause restlessness or delirium in presence of pain. • Monitor prothrombin times carefully when patient on pentobarbital starts or ends anticoagulant therapy. Anticoagulant dose may need to be adjusted. • Watch for signs of barbiturate toxicity: coma, pupillary constriction, cyanosis, clammy skin, hypotension. Overdose can be fatal. • For treatment of toxicity, see p. 1115.
Alcohol or other CNS depressants, including narcotic analgesics: excessive CNS and respiratory depression. Do not use together. *MAO inhibitors:* inhibited metabolism of barbiturates; may cause prolonged CNS depression. Reduce barbiturate dosage. *Rifampin:* may decrease barbiturate levels. Monitor for decreased effect. *Primidone:* monitor for excessive phenobarbital blood levels.	• Contraindicated in uncontrolled severe pain, respiratory disease with dyspnea or obstruction, hypersensitivity to barbiturates, previous addiction to sedatives, porphyria. Use with caution in impaired hepatic, renal, cardiac, or respiratory function; hyperthyroidism; diabetes mellitus; anemia; elderly or debilitated patients. • Use injection solution within 30 minutes after opening container to minimize deterioration. Don't use cloudy solution. • I.V. injection should be reserved for emergency treatment and should be given under close supervision. Be prepared to give artificial respiration. • When given I.V., do not give more than 60 mg/minute. • Give I.M. injection deeply. Superficial injection may cause pain, sterile abscess, and slough. • Because barbiturates potentiate narcotics, reduce dose when giving during labor. Excessive dose may cause respiratory depression in neonate. • Remove cigarettes if patient receives hypnotic dose. • Supervise walking; raise bed rails, especially for elderly patients. • Long-term high dosage may cause drug dependence and severe withdrawal symptoms. Withdraw barbiturates gradually. • Prevent hoarding or self-overdosing by patients who are depressed, suicidal, or drug-dependent, or who have a history of drug abuse. Warn about increased alcohol effects and against hazardous activity requiring alertness or skill. • No analgesic action. May cause restlessness or delirium in presence of pain. • Monitor prothrombin times carefully when patient on phenobarbital starts or ends anticoagulant therapy. Anticoagulant dose may need to be adjusted. • Watch for signs of barbiturate toxicity: coma, pupillary constriction, cyanosis, clammy skin, hypotension. Overdose can be fatal. • For treatment of toxicity, see p. 1115.
None significant.	• Contraindicated if patients have received large doses of other CNS depressants or are comatose. Use extreme caution with patients in hypertensive crisis. • Give I.V. injection slowly to avoid transient fall in blood pressure. • Inject in large, undamaged vein to minimize irritation. Avoid extravasation. Don't inject into artery; irritation may cause severe arteriospasm, impaired circulation, and gangrene. • Do not give subcutaneously. • Do not use solution for injection if it is cloudy or contains a precipitate. • Antiemetic effect may mask signs of drug overdose or other disorders. • Warn about increased effects of alcohol, tranquilizers, antihistamines, and other CNS depressants and against hazardous activity requiring alertness or skill. • Supervise walking; raise bed rails, especially in elderly patients.

NAME	INDICATIONS & DOSAGE	SIDE EFFECTS
secobarbital Seconal **secobarbital sodium** Controlled substance Schedule III Seco-8, Secogen Sodium◆◆, Seconal Sodium◆, Seral◆◆	*Sedation, preop—* **Adults:** 200 to 300 mg P.O. 1 to 2 hours before surgery. **Children:** 50 to 100 mg P.O. or 4 to 5 mg/Kg rectally 1 to 2 hours before surgery. *Insomnia—* **Adults:** 100 to 200 mg P.O. or I.M. **Children:** 3 to 5 mg/Kg I.M., not to exceed 100 mg, with no more than 5 ml injected in any one site. 4 to 5 mg/Kg rectally. *Acute tetanus convulsion—* **Adults and children:** 5.5 mg/Kg I.M. or slow I.V., repeated q 3 to 4 hours, if needed; I.V. injection rate not to exceed 50 mg per 15 seconds. *Acute psychotic agitation—* **Adults:** 50 mg/minute I.V. up to 250 mg I.V. initially, additional doses given cautiously after 5 minutes if desired response is not obtained. Not to exceed 500 mg total. *Status epilepticus—* **Adults and children:** 250 to 350 mg I.M. or I.V.	*CNS:* drowsiness, vertigo, headache, depression, residual sedation after hypnotic dose, paradoxical excitement. *GI:* nausea, vomiting, diarrhea. *Skin:* hypersensitivity reactions, jaundice. *Other:* respiratory depression, apnea, laryngospasm, hypotension if given rapidly I.V.; discontinuance of hypnotic doses may induce nightmares or insomnia.
talbutal Controlled substance Schedule III Lotusate	*Sedation—* **Adults:** 30 to 60 mg P.O. b.i.d. or t.i.d. *Insomnia—* **Adults:** 120 mg P.O. at bedtime.	*CNS:* drowsiness, vertigo, headache, depression, residual sedation after hypnotic dose, paradoxical excitement. *GI:* nausea, vomiting, diarrhea. *Skin:* hypersensitivity reactions, jaundice. *Other:* respiratory depression, apnea, hypotension with I.V. administration; discontinuance of hypnotic doses may induce nightmares or insomnia.

INTERACTIONS	NURSING CONSIDERATIONS
Alcohol or other CNS depressants, including narcotic analgesics: excessive CNS and respiratory depression. Do not use together. *MAO inhibitors:* inhibited metabolism of barbiturates; may cause prolonged CNS depression. Reduce barbiturate dosage. *Rifampin:* may decrease barbiturate levels. Monitor for decreased effect.	• Contraindicated in uncontrolled severe pain, respiratory disease with dyspnea or obstruction, hypersensitivity to barbiturates, previous addiction to sedatives, porphyria. Use with caution in hepatic or renal impairment; also, in pregnant women with toxemia; or history of bleeding. • Use injection solution within 30 minutes after opening container to minimize deterioration. Don't use cloudy solution. • I.V. injection should be reserved for emergency treatment and should be given under close supervision. Be prepared to give artificial respiration. • Give I.M. injection deeply. Superficial injection may cause pain, sterile abscess, and slough. • Because barbiturates potentiate narcotics, reduce dose when giving during labor. Excessive dose may cause respiratory depression in neonate. • Remove cigarettes if patient receives hypnotic dose. • Supervise walking; raise bed rails, especially for elderly patients. • Long-term high dosage may cause drug dependence and severe withdrawal symptoms. Withdraw barbiturates gradually. • Prevent hoarding or self-overdosing by patients who are depressed, suicidal, or drug-dependent, or who have a history of drug abuse. Warn about increased alcohol effects and against hazardous activity requiring alertness or skill. • If patient has renal insufficiency, use sterile drug reconstituted with sterile water for injection. Avoid commercial solution containing polyethylene glycol; may irritate kidneys. • Secobarbital in polyethylene glycol must be refrigerated. • Secobarbital sodium injection not compatible with lactated Ringer's solution. • Sterile secobarbital sodium compatible with bacteriostatic water and Ringer's injection. • To reconstitute, rotate ampule. Do not shake. • Monitor prothrombin times carefully when patient on secobarbital starts or ends anticoagulant therapy. Anticoagulant dose may need to be adjusted. • Watch for signs of barbiturate toxicity: coma, pupillary construction, cyanosis, clammy skin, hypotension. Overdose can be fatal. • For treatment of toxicity, see p. 1115.
Alcohol or other CNS depressants, including narcotic analgesics: excessive CNS and respiratory depression. Don't use together. *MAO inhibitors:* inhibited the metabolism of barbiturates; may cause prolonged CNS depression. Reduce barbiturate dosage. *Rifampin:* may decrease barbiturate levels. Monitor for decreased effect.	• Contraindicated in uncontrolled severe pain, respiratory disease with dyspnea obstruction, hypersensitivity to barbiturates, previous addiction to sedatives, porphyria. Use with caution in hepatic or renal impairment. • Remove cigarettes if patient receives hypnotic dose. • Supervise walking; raise bed rails, especially for elderly patients. • Long-term high dosage may cause drug dependence and severe withdrawal symptoms. Withdraw barbiturates gradually. • Prevent hoarding or self-overdosing by patients who are depressed, suicidal, or drug-dependent, or who have a history of drug abuse. Warn about increased alcohol effects and against hazardous activity requiring alertness or skill. • Monitor prothrombin times carefully when patient on talbutal starts or ends anticoagulant therapy. Anticoagulant dose may need to be adjusted. • Watch for signs of barbiturate toxicity: coma, pupillary constriction, cyanosis, clammy skin, hypotension. Overdose can be fatal. • For treatment of toxicity, see p. 1115.

NAME	INDICATIONS & DOSAGE	SIDE EFFECTS
triclofos sodium Triclos	*Insomnia—* **Adults:** 1.5 g P.O. 15 to 20 minutes before bedtime. *To induce sleep in EEG—* **Children under 12 years:** 22 mg/Kg P.O.	*CNS:* light-headedness, dizziness, drowsiness, headache, ataxia, vertigo. *GI:* nausea, vomiting, flatulence, bad taste in mouth. *GU:* ketonuria. *Skin:* urticaria. *Other:* hangover, nightmares, malaise.

INTERACTIONS	NURSING CONSIDERATIONS
Alcohol or other CNS depressants, including narcotic analgesics: excessive CNS depression or vasodilation. Use together cautiously. *Furosemide I.V.:* possible sweating, flushes, variable blood pressure, uneasiness. Use together cautiously.	• Contraindicated in hepatic or renal impairment, hypersensitivity to triclofos sodium or chloral hydrate, women in labor. Use with caution in cardiac arrhythmias, severe cardiac disease, mental depression, suicidal tendencies, or drug dependency. • In prolonged use, monitor blood and hepatic function periodically. • Withdraw slowly after prolonged use to avoid delirium, tremors, hallucinations. • Prevent hoarding or self-overdosing by patients who are depressed, suicidal, or drug-dependent, or who have a history of drug abuse. Warn about increased alcohol effects and against hazardous activity requiring alertness or skill. • Supervise walking; raise bed rails, especially for elderly patients. • May cause false positives in glycosuria tests using cupric sulfate as Benedict's or Fehling's solution. Use Clinitest, Clinistix, or Tes-Tape. • May interfere with fluorometric tests for urine catecholamines and Reddy, Jenkins, Thorn test for urinary 17-hydroxycorticosteroids. Don't administer drug for 48 hours before fluorometric test. • Monitor prothrombin times carefully when patient on triclofos starts or ends anticoagulant therapy. Anticoagulant dose may need to be adjusted.

26

Anticonvulsants

acetazolamide
bromides
carbamazepine
clonazepam
diazepam
ethosuximide
ethotoin
magnesium sulfate
mephenytoin
mephobarbital
metharbital
methsuximide
paraldehyde
paramethadione
phenacemide
phenobarbital
phensuximide
phenytoin
primidone
trimethadione
valproic acid

Anticonvulsant drugs are used to treat, prevent, or reduce the frequency or severity of seizures caused by epilepsy, drugs, hypoglycemia, hypomagnesemia, eclampsia, meningitis, encephalitis, alcohol withdrawal, or head trauma. Each drug has indications for specific seizure disorders, and frequently, these drugs are used in combination to treat complex or mixed seizure disorders. In nonepileptic seizures, therapy is often aimed at the underlying cause as well.

Major uses

- Treatment, prevention, or reduction in number or severity of epileptic or nonepileptic (e.g., eclampsia, head trauma, encephalitis) seizures.
- Treatment of status epilepticus.

Mechanism of action

- Acetazolamide may inhibit carbonic anhydrase in CNS and decrease abnormal paroxysmal, or excessive neuronal discharge.
- Bromides depress all nerve tissue, but exact mechanism of CNS depression is unknown.
- Succinimide derivatives (ethosuximide, methsuximide, phensuximide) and oxazolidinedione derivatives (paramethadione, trimethadione) raise the seizure threshold in motor cortex and basal ganglia and decrease synaptic response to repeated low-frequency stimulation.
- Hydantoin derivatives (ethotoin, mephenytoin, phenacemide, phenytoin) may raise seizure threshold in motor cortex and limit spread of seizure activity. They may also stabilize nerve cell membrane against hyperexcitability and reduce post-tetanic potentiation at synapses.
- Magnesium sulfate may decrease amount of acetylcholine released by nerve impulse, but its anticonvulsant mechanism remains unknown.

• Barbiturate derivatives (mephobarbital, metharbital, phenobarbital) are CNS depressants; they reduce monosynaptic and polysynaptic impluse transmission, thus decreasing excitability in the entire nerve cell. They also prevent the spread of seizure activity and raise the seizure threshold in motor cortex.
• Primidone may have similar action to barbiturates.
• Valproic acid may increase brain levels of gamma-aminobutyric acid (which transmits inhibitory nerve impulses in CNS).
• Mechanism of action of carbamazepine, clonazepam, diazepam, and paraldehyde are unknown.

Absorption, distribution, and excretion
• Rate and degree of absorption from GI tract unknown. Most are well absorbed, but some more slowly than others.
• Most are distributed throughout the body, including CNS.
• Metabolized in liver.
• Excreted in varying amounts by kidneys. Paraldehyde is excreted in small amounts (7%) by lungs.
• Phenytoin is excreted in small amounts in saliva. Salivary phenytoin levels may be obtained to monitor serum levels.

Onset and duration
• Onset and duration are highly variable.
• Most anticonvulsants require several days to achieve adequate therapeutic serum levels.
• Anticonvulsants used in acute situations (status epilepticus and eclampsia) have an immediate onset.
• Treatment with phenytoin often begins with a loading dose (the amount necessary to achieve therapeutic serum levels within 24 hours) to produce anticonvulsant effect rapidly. Duration of effect is often long enough to permit once daily dosing, but side effects (GI and CNS) may be more noticeable with the larger dose needed for such use.

Combination products
DILANTIN WITH PHENOBARBITAL♦: phenytoin sodium 100 mg and phenobarbital 16 mg.
DILANTIN WITH PHENOBARBITAL♦: phenytoin sodium 100 mg and phenobarbital 32 mg.
PHELANTIN♦: phenytoin 100 mg, phenobarbital 30 mg, and methamphetamine hydrochloride 2.5 mg.

NAME	INDICATIONS & DOSAGE	SIDE EFFECTS
acetazolamide Acetazolam••, Diamox•, Hydrazol, Roxolamide	*Myoclonic seizures, refractory grand mal or petite mal, mixed seizures—* **Adults:** 375 mg P.O., I.M., or I.V. daily up to 250 mg q.i.d. Initial dose when used with other anticonvulsants usually 250 mg daily. **Children:** 8 to 30 mg/Kg daily, divided t.i.d. or q.i.d. Maximum dose 1.5 g daily, or 300 to 900 mg/m² daily.	*Blood:* bone marrow depression, agranulocytosis, thrombocytopenia, thrombocytopenic purpura, hemolytic anemia, leukopenia, pancytopenia. *CNS:* paresthesias, drowsiness, disorientation, flaccid paralysis, convulsions, weakness, nervousness. *EENT:* transient myopia, tinnitus. *GI:* anorexia, melena, hepatic insufficiency, constipation. *GU:* polyuria, glycosuria, hematuria, crystalluria, nephrolithiasis. *Local:* pain at injection site, sterile abscesses. *Skin:* rash, urticaria. *Other:* fever, hyperchloremic acidosis.
bromides Bromide, Lanabrom, Neurosine, Peacocks Bromides, Potassium Bromide, Sodium Bromide	*Major motor and myoclonic seizures—* **Adults:** 1 to 2 g t.i.d. **Children:** 50 to 100 mg/Kg daily, divided equally t.i.d. Or, 1.5 to 3 g/m² daily in divided doses t.i.d.	*CNS:* drowsiness, mental dullness, toxic psychosis. *Skin:* rashes (acneform, morbilliform, granulomatous), Stevens-Johnson syndrome.
carbamazepine Tegretol•	*Psychomotor, temporal lobe, grand mal, mixed seizure patterns—* **Adults, and children over 12 years:** 200 mg P.O. b.i.d. on day 1. May increase by 200 mg P.O. per day, in divided doses at 6- to 8-hour intervals. Adjust to minimum effective level when control achieved. Usual maintenance 800 to 1,200 mg daily. Don't exceed 1 g total daily dose in 12- to 15-year-olds and 1,200 mg P.O. daily in patients over 15 years. **Children under 12 years:** 10 to 20 mg/Kg P.O daily in 2 to 4 divided doses. *Trigeminal neuralgia—* **Adults:** 100 mg P.O. b.i.d. with meals on day 1. Increase by 100 mg q 12 hours until pain	*Blood:* aplastic anemia, leukopenia, agranulocytosis, eosinophilia, leukocytosis, thrombocytopenia, purpura. *CNS:* dizziness, vertigo, drowsiness, fatigue, ataxia, poor coordination, confusion, agitated depression, headache, visual hallucinations, talkativeness, tinnitus, hyperacusis, oculomotor and speech disturbances, abnormal involuntary movement, paresthesias, peripheral neuritis. *CV:* congestive heart failure, hypertension, hypotension, syncope and collapse, edema, thrombophlebitis, aggravation of coronary artery disease. *EENT:* conjunctivitis, dry mouth and pharynx, blurred vision, diplopia, nystagmus. *GI:* nausea, vomiting, abdominal pain, diarrhea, constipation, anorexia, stomatitis, glossitis.

• Also available in Canada.
•• Available in Canada only.
Unmarked trade names available in United States only.

INTERACTIONS	NURSING CONSIDERATIONS
Methenamine: antagonized methenamine effect. If used together, urine must be kept at pH 5.5 or lower.	• Contraindicated in sulfonamide sensitivity, chronic pulmonary disease, renal or hepatic dysfunction, Addison's disease (adrenocortical insufficiency), hyponatremia, hypokalemia, hyperchloremic acidosis, pregnancy (especially first trimester), chronic noncongestive angle-closure glaucoma. Use cautiously in hypercalcinuria, diabetes mellitus, gout, and respiratory acidosis. • Obtain CBC and serum electrolytes every 3 months; serum calcium every 6 months. • Don't withdraw drug suddenly. Call doctor if side effects develop. • Warn patient to avoid activities that require alertness and good psychomotor coordination until response to drug has been determined. • This drug is also a diuretic. Use diuretic precautions. • Chronic use results in tolerance to drug. • Reconstitute 500 mg vial with 5 ml sterile water for injection. Provides 100 mg/ml. Refrigerate reconstituted solution. Discard after 24 hours. • Oral liquid: soften 1 tablet in 2 teaspoonsful of very warm water and add to 2 teaspoonsful honey or syrup (chocolate, cherry). Don't use fruit juice. • May cause hyperglycemia in prediabetics or diabetics on insulin or oral drugs. Monitor these patients carefully. • Observe and report signs of hypokalemia or metabolic acidosis. • May worsen anticonvulsant-induced osteomalacia.
None significant.	• Contraindicated in cerebral arteriosclerosis, organic brain damage, impaired renal function, pregnancy, lactation, debilitated or dehydrated patients, alcoholics, severe depression, neurologic or psychologic disorders, tuberculosis or skin disorders (acne, dermatitis, herpetiformis). Especially in adults, use may lead to chronic toxicity (mental, psychic, GI, and neurologic disturbances; skin eruptions). May be mistaken for acute alcohol intoxication, tabes dorsalis, cerebral tumor, uremia, or multiple sclerosis. • Watch closely for toxicity In adults, serum levels above 5 mEq/liter may cause toxicity. • Therapeutic serum level in children is usually 20 to 25 mEq/liter (200 mg/100 ml), but range is 10 to 35 mEq/liter. • Effect may not be seen for 2 to 3 weeks. • Notify doctor if side effects develop.
Troleandomycin, erythromycin: may increase carbamazepine blood levels. Use cautiously. *Propoxyphene:* may raise carbamazepine levels. Use another analgesic.	• Contraindicated in bone marrow depression, lactation, hypersensitivity to carbamazepine or tricyclic antidepressants. Use cautiously in cardiac, renal, or hepatic damage, or increased intraocular pressure. • Warn patient to avoid activities that require alertness and good psychomotor coordination until response to drug has been determined. • Never stop suddenly. Notify doctor immediately if side effects occur. • Obtain CBC, platelet and reticulocyte counts, and serum iron weekly for first 3 months, then monthly. If bone marrow depression develops, stop drug. Obtain urinalysis, BUN, and hepatic function tests every 3 months. Periodic eye examinations recommended. • Tell patient to notify doctor immediately if fever, sore throat, mouth ulcers, or easy bruising occur. • Therapeutic anticonvulsant serum level is 3 to 9 mcg/ml. • When used for trigeminal neuralgia, an attempt should be made every 3 months to decrease dose or stop drug.

(continued on following page)

NAME	INDICATIONS & DOSAGE	SIDE EFFECTS
carbamazepine *(continued)*	relieved. Don't exceed 1.2 g daily. Maintenance dose 200 to 400 mg P.O. b.i.d.	*GU:* urinary frequency or retention, oliguria with elevated blood pressure, impotence, albuminuria, glycosuria, elevated blood urea nitrogen levels, microscopic deposits in urine. *Skin:* rash, urticaria, photosensitivity, abnormal pigmentation, exfoliative dermatitis, erythema multiforme, erythema nodosum, aggravation of systemic lupus erythematosus, alopecia. *Other:* diaphoresis, fever, chills, adenopathy, aching joints and muscles, leg cramps, abnormal hepatic function, cholestatic and hepatocellular jaundice.
clonazepam Controlled substance Schedule IV, Clonopin, Rivotril◆	*Petit mal and petit mal variant (Lennox Gastaut syndrome); akinetic and myoclonic seizures—* **Adults:** initial dose should not exceed 1.5 mg P.O. per day, divided into 3 doses. May be increased by 0.5 to 1 mg q 3 days until seizures controlled. Maximum recommended daily dose is 20 mg. **Children up to 10 years or 30 Kg:** 0.01 to 0.03 mg/Kg P.O. daily (not to exceed 0.05 mg/Kg daily), divided q 8 hours. Increase dosage by 0.25 to 0.5 mg q third day to a maximum maintenance dose of 0.1 mg to 0.2 mg/Kg daily.	*Blood:* anemia, leukopenia, thrombocytopenia, eosinophilia. *CNS:* drowsiness, coma, ataxia, or hypotonia, behavioral disturbances (especially in children), aphonia, choreiform movements, dysarthria, dysdiadochokinesia, glassy-eyed appearance, headache, hemiparesis, slurred speech, respiratory depression, tremor, dizziness, confusion, depression, forgetfulness, hallucinations, hysteria, insomnia, psychosis, suicidal tendencies. *CV:* palpitations. *EENT:* increased salivation, coated tongue, dry mouth, diplopia, nystagmus, abnormal eye movements, rhinorrhea. *GI:* constipation, diarrhea, encopresis, gastritis, change in appetite, weight change, nausea, abnormal thirst, sore gums. *GU:* dysuria, enuresis, nocturia, urinary retention, increased libido. *Skin:* hair loss, hirsutism, rash. *Other:* ankle and facial edema; dehydration; fever; lymphadenopathy; chest congestion; shortness of breath; hepatomegaly; increased SGOT, SGPT, and alkaline phosphatase; muscle weakness and pain.
diazepam Controlled substance Schedule IV Valium◆	*Status epilepticus—* **Adults:** 5 to 10 mg slow I.V. push 1 mg/min; may repeat q 10 minutes up to maximum total dose of 30 mg. Use 2 to 5 mg in elderly or debilitated patients. May repeat therapy in 2 to 4 hours with caution if seizures recur. **Children:** 0.1 to 0.3 mg/Kg slow I.V. push (1 mg/minute). May	*Blood:* neutropenia. *CNS:* fatigue, drowsiness, ataxia, dizziness, headache, dysarthria, slurred speech, tremor, depression, changes in EEG patterns, confusion, hypoactivity, syncope, hyperexcitability, sleep disturbances, insomnia, anxiety, hostility, hallucinations, rage. *CV:* hypotension, bradycardia, cardiovascular collapse.

INTERACTIONS	NURSING CONSIDERATIONS
None significant.	• Contraindicated in hepatic disease; chlordiazepoxide, diazepam, or other benzodiazepine sensitivity; acute narrow-angle glaucoma; or lactation. Use with caution in chronic respiratory disease, impaired renal function, open-angle glaucoma. • Warn patient to avoid activities that require alertness and good psychomotor coordination until response to drug has been determined. • Never withdraw suddenly. Call doctor at once if side effects develop. • Obtain periodic CBC and hepatic function tests. • Monitor patient for oversedation.
None significant.	• Contraindicated in shock, psychosis, coma, acute alcohol intoxication with depression of vital signs, acute narrow-angle glaucoma. Use cautiously in elderly or debilitated patients, those with limited pulmonary reserve, and those in whom blood pressure drop might cause cardiovascular complications; also in history of anxiety states with suicidal tendencies, blood dyscrasias, hepatic or renal damage, open-angle glaucoma, or alcoholism. • Monitor respirations every 5 to 15 minutes and before each I.V. repeated dose. Have emergency resuscitative equipment and oxygen at bedside. • Do not mix with other drugs or I.V. fluids. • Do not use small veins such as those on dorsum of hand or wrist.

(continued on following page)

NAME	INDICATIONS & DOSAGE	SIDE EFFECTS
diazepam *(continued)*	repeat q 15 minutes for 2 doses. Maximum single dose: children under 5 years—5 mg; children over 5 years—10 mg. *Adjunctive use in convulsive disorders—* **Adults and children:** 2 to 10 mg P.O. b.i.d., t.i.d., or q.i.d.	*EENT:* diplopia, blurred vision, nystagmus. *GI:* nausea, constipation, change in salivation. *GU:* incontinence, urinary retention. *Local:* pain, thrombosis, and phlebitis at injection site. *Skin:* rash, urticaria. *Other:* jaundice, hiccups.
ethosuximide Zarontin•	*Petit mal—* **Adults, and children over 6 years:** initially, 250 mg P.O. b.i.d. May increase by 250 mg q 4 to 7 days up to 1.5 g daily. **Children 3 to 6 years:** 250 mg P.O. daily or 125 mg P.O. b.i.d. May increase by 250 mg q 4 to 7 days up to 1.5 daily.	*Blood:* leukopenia, eosinophilia, agranulocytosis, pancytopenia, aplastic anemia. *CNS:* drowsiness, headache, fatigue, dizziness, ataxia, irritability, hiccups, euphoria, lethargy, hyperactivity. *EENT:* myopia. *GI:* nausea, vomiting, diarrhea, gum hypertrophy, weight loss, cramps, tongue swelling, anorexia, epigastric and abdominal pain. *GU:* vaginal bleeding. *Skin:* urticaria, pruritic and erythematous rashes, Stevens-Johnson syndrome, hirsutism. *Systemic:* systemic lupus erythematosus.
ethotoin Peganone	*Grand mal or psychomotor seizures—* **Adults:** initially, 250 mg P.O. q.i.d. after meals. May increase slowly over several days to 3 g daily divided q.i.d. **Children:** initially, 250 mg P.O. b.i.d. May increase up to 250 mg P.O. q.i.d.	*Blood:* thrombocytopenia, leukopenia, agranulocytosis, agranulocytopenia, pancytopenia, megaloblastic anemia. *CNS:* fatigue, insomnia, dizziness, headache, numbness. *CV:* chest pain. *EENT:* diplopia, nystagmus. *GI:* nausea, vomiting, diarrhea, gingival hyperplasia (rare). *Skin:* rash. *Other:* fever, lymphadenopathy, hepatotoxicity, reversible lupus erythematosus.
magnesium sulfate	*Hypomagnesemic seizures—* **Adults:** 1 to 2 g (as 10% solution) I.V. over 15 minutes, then 1 g I.M. q 4 to 6 hours, based on patient's response and serum magnesium levels. **Children:** seizures secondary to hypomagnesemia in acute nephritis—0.2 ml/Kg of 50% solution I.M. q 4 to 6 hours, p.r.n. or 100 mg/Kg of 10% solution I.V. very slowly. Titrate dosage according to serum magnesium levels and seizure response.	*CNS:* sweating, drowsiness, depressed reflexes, flaccid paralysis, hypothermia, hypocalcemic tetany. *CV:* hypotension, flushing, circulatory collapse, depressed cardiac function, heart block. *Other:* respiratory paralysis, hypocalcemia.

INTERACTIONS	NURSING CONSIDERATIONS
	• Do not infuse through plastic tubing. Do not store in plastic syringe. • Drug should not be withdrawn abruptly. • Avoid heavy use of alcohol or other CNS depressants. • For symptoms and treatment of toxicity, see p. 1123.
None significant.	• Contraindicated in hypersensitivity to succinimide derivatives. Use cautiously in hepatic or renal disease. • Never withdraw drug suddenly. Abrupt withdrawal may precipitate petit mal seizures. Call doctor immediately if side effects develop. • Warn patient to avoid activities that require alertness and good psychomotor coordination until response to drug has been determined. • Obtain CBC every 3 months; urinalysis and hepatic function tests every 6 months. • Therapeutic serum levels 40 to 80 mg/ml. • May increase frequency of grand mal seizures when used alone in mixed epilepsy. • May cause positive direct Coombs' test.
Alcohol, folic acid, Loxitane: monitor for decreased ethotoin activity. *Oral anticoagulants, antihistamines, chloramphenicol, diazepam, diazoxide, disulfiram, isoniazid, phenylbutazone, phenyramidol, salicylates, sulfamethizole, valproate:* monitor for increased ethotoin activity and toxicity.	• Contraindicated in hydantoin hypersensitivity and in hepatic or hematologic disorders. Use cautiously in patients receiving other hydantoin derivatives. • Never withdraw suddenly. Call doctor at once if side effects develop. • Warn patient to avoid activities that require alertness and good psychomotor coordination until response to drug has been determined. • Obtain CBC and urinalysis when therapy starts and monthly thereafter. • Give after meals. Schedule doses as evenly as possible over 24 hours. • Stop at once if lymphadenopathy or lupus-like syndrome develops. • Heavy use of alcohol may diminish benefits of drug. • Hydantoin derivative of choice in young adults who are prone to gingival hyperplasia caused by phenytoin.
Neuromuscular blocking agents: may cause increased neuromuscular blockade. Use cautiously.	• Contraindicated in impaired renal function, myocardial damage, heart block, women in labor. • Keep I.V. calcium gluconate available to reverse magnesium intoxication; however, don't use in digitalized patient due to danger of arrhythmias. • Monitor vital signs every 15 minutes when giving drug I.V. • Watch for respiratory depression and signs of heart block. Respirations should be approximately 16 per minute before each dose given. • Monitor intake and output. Urinary output should be 100 ml or more in 4-hour period before each dose. • Check serum magnesium levels after repeated doses. Disappearance of knee jerk and patellar reflexes are signs of pending magnesium toxicity. • Maximum infusion rate is 150 mg per minute. Rapid drip will induce uncomfortable feeling of heat. • Call doctor if side effects develop.

(continued on following page)

NAME	INDICATIONS & DOSAGE	SIDE EFFECTS
magnesium sulfate *(continued)*	*Prevention or control of seizures in pre-eclampsia or eclampsia*— **Women:** initially, 4 g I.V. in 250 ml 5% dextrose in water and 4 g deep I.M. each buttock; then 4 g deep I.M. into alternate buttock q 4 hours, p.r.n. Subsequent doses based on serum magnesium levels and urinary magnesium excretion. Do not exceed 40 g daily.	
mephenytoin Mesantoin◆	*Refractory grand mal, focal, or psychomotor seizures*— **Adults:** 50 to 100 mg P.O. daily. May increase by 50 to 100 mg at weekly intervals up to 200 mg P.O. t.i.d. **Children:** initial dose 50 to 100 mg P.O. daily or 100 to 450 mg/m² P.O. daily in 3 divided doses. May increase slowly by 50 to 100 mg at weekly intervals up to 200 mg P.O. t.i.d., divided q 8 hours. Dosage must be adjusted individually.	*Blood:* leukopenia, neutropenia, agranulocytosis, thrombocytopenia, pancytopenia, eosinophilia, leukocytosis, monocytosis. *CNS:* ataxia, drowsiness, fatigue, irritability, choreiform movements, depression, tremor, sleeplessness, dizziness (usually transient). *EENT:* photophobia, conjunctivitis, diplopia, nystagmus. *GI:* gingival hyperplasia, weight gain, nausea and vomiting (with prolonged use), gum hyperplasia. *Skin:* rashes, exfoliative dermatitis, erythema multiforme, toxic epidermal necrolysis, alopecia. *Systemic:* systemic lupus erythematosus. *Other:* hypertrichosis, edema, dysarthria, lymphadenopathy, polyarthropathy, pulmonary fibrosis.
mephobarbital Controlled substance Schedule IV Mebaral◆, Mentabal, Mephoral	*Grand or petit mal*— **Adults:** 400 to 600 mg P.O. daily or in divided doses. **Children:** 6 to 12 mg/Kg P.O. daily, divided q 6 to 8 hours (smaller doses are given initially and increased over 4 to 5 days as needed).	*Blood:* megaloblastic anemia, agranulocytosis, thrombocytopenia. *CNS:* dizziness, headache, hangover, confusion, paradoxical excitation, exacerbation of existing pain, drowsiness. *CV:* hypotension. *GI:* nausea, vomiting, epigastric pain. *Skin:* urticaria, morbilliform rash, blisters, purpura, erythema multiforme. *Other:* allergic reactions (facial edema).
metharbital Controlled substance Schedule III Gemonil	*Grand or petit mal; myoclonic or mixed seizures*— **Adults:** initially, 100 mg P.O. daily to t.i.d. May increase to 800 mg daily in divided doses, p.r.n. **Children:** 5 to 15 mg/Kg P.O.	*Blood:* megaloblastic anemia, agranulocytosis, thrombocytopenia. *CNS:* dizziness, irritability, drowsiness, headache, confusion, excitation. *CV:* hypotension. *GI:* distress.

INTERACTIONS	NURSING CONSIDERATIONS
	• Especially when given I.V. to toxemic mothers within 24 hours before delivery, observe newborn for signs of magnesium toxicity, including neuromuscular or respiratory depression.
Alcohol, folic acid, Loxitane: monitor for decreased mephenytoin activity. *Oral anticoagulants, antihistamines, chloramphenicol, diazepam, diazoxide, disulfiram, isoniazid, phenylbutazone, phenyramidol, salicylates, sulfamethizole, valproate:* monitor for increased mephenytoin activity and toxicity.	• Contraindicated in hydantoin hypersensitivity. Use cautiously in patients receiving other hydantoin derivatives. • Tell patient to notify doctor if fever, sore throat, bleeding, or rash occurs. • Check CBC and platelet count initially and every 2 weeks thereafter, up to 2 weeks after full dose attained; then monthly for first year and every 3 months thereafter. Stop drug if neutrophils less than 1,600/mm. • Never withdraw drug suddenly. Call doctor if side effects develop. • Warn patient to avoid activities that require alertness and good psychomotor coordination until response to drug has been determined. • Therapeutic serum level is 5 to 20 mcg/ml. • Heavy use of alcohol may diminish benefit of drug.
Alcohol and other CNS depressants, including narcotic analgesics: excessive CNS depression. Use cautiously. *MAO inhibitors:* potentiated barbiturate effect. Monitor patient for increased CNS and respiratory depression. *Rifampin:* may decrease barbiturate levels. Monitor for decreased effect.	• Contraindicated in barbiturate hypersensitivity, porphyria, and respiratory disease with dyspnea or obstruction. Use cautiously in hepatic, renal, cardiac, or respiratory function impairment, and in myasthenia gravis and myxedema. • Never withdraw suddenly. Call doctor at once if side effects develop. • Warn patient to avoid activities that require alertness and good psychomotor coordination until response to drug has been determined. • Store in light-resistant container. • In adults, give total or largest dose at night if seizures occur then. • Three quarters of drug metabolized to phenobarbital; therapeutic serum levels as phenobarbital are 15 to 40 mcg/ml. • Monitor prothrombin times carefully when patient on mephobarbital starts or ends anticoagulant therapy. Anticoagulant dose may need to be adjusted. • For symptoms and treatment of toxicity, see p. 1115.
Alcohol and other CNS depressants, including narcotic analgesics: excessive CNS depression. Use cautiously.	• Contraindicated in barbiturate hypersensitivity, in manifest or latent porphyria, and in respiratory disease with dyspnea or obstruction. Use cautiously in hepatic, cardiac, or renal impairment. • Don't stop drug abruptly. • Warn patient to avoid activities that require alertness and good psychomotor coordination until response to drug is determined.

(continued on following page)

NAME	INDICATIONS & DOSAGE	SIDE EFFECTS
metharbital *(continued)*	daily, divided t.i.d. May increase to 50 to 100 mg P.O. daily, b.i.d., or t.i.d.	*Skin:* rash, urticaria, purpura, erythema multiforme.
methsuximide Celontin♦	*Refractory petit mal—* **Adults and children:** initially, 300 mg P.O. daily. May increase by 300 mg weekly. Maximum daily dosage of 1.2 g.	*Blood:* eosinophilia, leukopenia, monocytosis, pancytopenia. *CNS:* drowsiness, ataxia, dizziness, irritability, nervousness, headache, hiccups, insomnia, confusion, depression, aggressiveness, hypochondriacal behavior, instability. *EENT:* blurred vision, photophobia, periorbital edema. *GI:* nausea, vomiting, anorexia, diarrhea, weight loss, abdominal or epigastric pain, constipation. *Skin:* Stevens-Johnson syndrome, urticaria, pruritic and erythematous rashes. *Systemic:* systemic lupus erythematosus. *Other:* hyperemia.
paraldehyde Controlled substance Schedule IV Paral	*Refractory grand mal seizures—* **Adults:** 5 to 10 ml I.M. (divide 10 ml dose into 2 injections); 0.2 to 0.4 ml/Kg in 0.9% saline injection I.V. **Children:** 0.15 ml/Kg dose deep I.M. q 4 to 6 hours, p.r.n.; or 0.3 ml/Kg rectally in olive oil q 4 to 6 hours; or 1 ml per year of age not to exceed 5 ml, repeated in 1 hour, p.r.n.; or dilute 5 ml in 95 ml 0.9% saline injection for I.V. infusion and titrate dose beginning at 5 ml/hour.	*CV:* I.V. administration may cause pulmonary edema or hemorrhage, dilatation of right side of heart, circulatory collapse, respiratory distress. *Local:* pain, sterile abscesses, sloughing of skin, fat necrosis, muscular irritation, nerve damage (if injection is near nerve trunk) at I.M. injection site. *Skin:* erythematous rash. *Other:* rectal administration of decomposed paraldehyde may cause severe corrosion of stomach or rectum, metabolic acidosis, and death.
paramethadione Paradione♦	*Refractory petit mal—* **Adults:** initially, 300 mg P.O. t.i.d. May increase by 300 mg weekly, up to 600 mg q.i.d., if needed. **Children over 6 years:** 0.9 g P.O. daily in divided doses t.i.d. or q.i.d. **Children 2 to 6 years:** 0.6 g P.O. daily in divided doses t.i.d. or q.i.d. **Children under 2 years:** 0.3 g P.O. daily in divided doses b.i.d.	*Blood:* neutropenia, leukopenia, eosinophilia, thrombocytopenia, pancytopenia, agranulocytosis, hypoplastic and aplastic anemia. *CNS:* drowsiness, fatigue, insomnia, vertigo, headache, paresthesias, grand mal, irritability, personality changes, hiccups. *CV:* hypertension, hypotension. *EENT:* hemeralopia, photo phobia, diplopia, epistaxis, retinal hemorrhage.

INTERACTIONS	NURSING CONSIDERATIONS
MAO inhibitors: potentiated barbiturate effect. Monitor patient for increased CNS and respiratory depression. *Rifampin:* may decrease barbiturate levels. Monitor for decreased effect.	• Monitor prothrombin times carefully when patient on metharbital starts or ends anticoagulant therapy. Anticoagulant dose may need to be adjusted. • For symptoms and treatment of toxicity, see p. 1115.
None significant.	• Contraindicated in hypersensitivity to succinimide derivatives. Use cautiously in hepatic or renal dysfunction. • Never change or withdraw drug suddenly. Abrupt withdrawal may precipitate petit mal seizures. Call doctor immediately if side effects develop. • Warn patient to avoid activities that require alertness and good psychomotor coordination until response to drug has been determined. • Obtain CBC every 3 months; urinalysis and hepatic function tests every 6 months. • May color urine pink or brown. • Therapeutic serum levels 40 to 100 mcg/ml. • May increase incidence of grand mal seizures when used alone in mixed epilepsy.
Alcohol: increased CNS depression. Use with caution. *Disulfiram:* increased paraldehyde and acetaldehyde blood levels; possible toxic disulfiram reaction. Use together cautiously.	• Contraindicated in gastroenteritis with ulceration. Use cautiously in impaired hepatic function, or in asthma or other pulmonary disease. • Use fresh supply. Don't expose to air. Don't use if liquid is brown, has a vinegary odor, or if container has been opened longer than 24 hours. • Watch closely for respiratory depression, especially in repeated doses. • Drug reacts with plastic. Use glass syringe and bottle for parenteral dose. Prepare fresh I.V. solution every 4 hours. I.V. administration very hazardous. • Give I.M. dose deeply, away from nerve trunks; massage injection site. • Dilute paraldehyde in olive oil or cottonseed oil 1:2 for rectal administration. Give as retention enema. • Keep patient's room well ventilated to remove exhaled paraldehyde. • Long-term high dosage may cause drug dependence and severe withdrawal symptoms.
None significant.	• Contraindicated in renal and hepatic dysfunction, severe blood dyscrasias. Use cautiously in retinal or optic nerve diseases. • Not recommended in trimester preceding planned pregnancy. • Never withdraw suddenly. Call doctor at once if side effects develop. • Therapeutic serum levels 6 to 71 mcg/ml. • Stop drug if scotomata or signs of hepatitis, SLE, lymphadenopathy, skin rash, nephrosis, hair loss, or grand mal seizures appear. • Tell patient to report sore throat, fever, malaise, bruises, petechiae, or epistaxis to doctor immediately. Advise patient to wear dark glasses if photophobia occurs. Warn him not to drive car or operate machinery. • Obtain hepatic function studies and urinalysis before therapy; then monthly.

(continued on following page)

NAME	INDICATIONS & DOSAGE	SIDE EFFECTS
paramethadione *(continued)*		*GI:* nausea, vomiting, abdominal pain, weight loss, bleeding gums. *GU:* albuminuria, vaginal bleeding. *Skin:* acneiform or morbilliform rash, exfoliative dermatitis, erythema multiforme, petechiae, alopecia. *Other:* lymphadenopathy, lupus erythematosus.
phenacemide Phenurone	*Refractory, mixed psychomotor, grand mal, petit mal and petit mal variant seizures—* **Adults:** 500 mg P.O. t.i.d. May increase by 500 mg t.i.d. weekly up to 5 g daily, p.r.n. **Children 5 to 10 years:** 250 mg P.O. q.i.d. May increase by 250 mg weekly, up to 1.5 g daily, p.r.n.	*Blood:* aplastic anemia, agranulocytosis, leukopenia. *CNS:* acute psychotic states, drowsiness, dizziness, insomnia, headaches, parethesias, depression, suicidal tendencies, aggressiveness. *GI:* anorexia, weight loss. *GU:* nephritis with marked albuminuria. *Skin:* rashes. *Other:* hepatitis, jaundice.
phenobarbital Bar, Barbipil, Barbita, Eskabarb◆, Floramine, Gardenal◆◆, Henomint, Luminal◆, Nova-Pheno◆◆, Orprine, PB, PBR, Pheno-Squar, Solfoton, Solu-Barb, Stental **phenobarbital sodium** Controlled substance Schedule IV Luminal Sodium◆	*All forms of epilepsy, febrile seizures in children—* **Adults:** 100 to 200 mg P.O. daily, divided t.i.d. or given as single dose at bedtime. **Children:** 4 to 6 mg/Kg P.O. daily, divided q 12 hours. *Status epilepticus—* **Adults:** 90 to 120 mg I.V., followed by 30 to 60 mg q 10 to 15 minutes, as needed, up to 500 mg total. **Children:** 5 to 10 mg/Kg I.V. May repeat q 10 to 15 minutes up to total of 20 mg/Kg. I.V. injection rate should not exceed 60 mg/min.	*CNS:* drowsiness, dizziness, headache, depression, residual sedation, paradoxical excitement, hangover, confusion. *CV:* hypotension. *GI:* nausea, vomiting. *Skin:* mild maculopapular, morbilliform or scarletiniform rashes. *Other:* respiratory depression, impotence.
phensuximide Milontin◆	*Petit mal—* **Adults and children:** 500 mg to 1 g P.O. b.i.d. to t.i.d.	*Blood:* agranulocytopenia, transient leukopenia, pancytopenia. *CNS:* muscular weakness, drowsiness, dizziness, ataxia, headache. *GI:* nausea, vomiting, anorexia. *GU:* urinary frequency, renal damage, hematuria. *Skin:* pruritus, eruptions, erythema, erythema multiforme, alopecia. *Other:* hyperemia.

INTERACTIONS	NURSING CONSIDERATIONS
	• Dilute oral solution with water before giving. • Monitor CBC. Discontinue if neutrophil count falls below 2,500/mm³.
None significant.	• Contraindicated in preexisting personality disturbances. Use with caution in hepatic dysfunction, history of allergy, and when hydantoin is used concomitantly. • Obtain hepatic function tests, CBC, and urinalysis before and at monthly intervals during therapy. • Tell patient to report sore throat or fever to doctor immediately. Warn him to avoid activities that require alertness or good psychomotor coordination until response to drug determined. • Never withdraw suddenly. Call doctor at once if side effects develop. • Tell patient's family to watch for personality or psychological changes and report them to doctor immediately. • Extremely toxic. Use only when other anticonvulsants are ineffective. • Notify doctor if patient develops personality changes, jaundice or other signs of hepatitis, abnormal urinary findings, or WBC below 4,000/mm³.
Alcohol and other CNS depressants, including narcotic analgesics: excessive CNS depression. Use cautiously. *MAO inhibitors:* potentiated barbiturate effect. Monitor for increased CNS and respiratory depression. *Rifampin:* may decrease barbiturate levels. Monitor for decreased effect. *Primidone:* monitor for excessive phenobarbital blood levels.	• Contraindicated in barbiturate hypersensitivity, porphyria, hepatic dysfunction, respiratory disease with dyspnea or obstruction, lactation, nephritis. Use cautiously in hyperthyroidism, diabetes mellitus, anemia, and in elderly or debilitated patients. • I.V. injection should be reserved for emergency treatment and should be given slowly under close supervision. Monitor respirations closely. • Watch for barbiturate toxicity signs, such as coma, asthmatic breathing, cyanosis, clammy skin, hypotension. Overdose can be fatal. • Warn patient to avoid activities that require alertness and good psychomotor coordination until response to drug is determined. • Don't stop drug abruptly. Call doctor immediately if side effects develop. • Full therapeutic effects not seen for 2 to 3 weeks. • Do not use injection solution if it contains a precipitate. • Therapeutic serum levels are 15 to 40 mg/ml. • Monitor prothrombin times carefully when patient on phenobarbital starts or ends anticoagulant therapy. Anticoagulant dose may need to be adjusted. • For symptoms and treatment of toxicity, see p. 1115.
None significant.	• Contraindicated in hypersensitivity to succinimide derivatives. Use cautiously in hepatic or renal disease. • Never withdraw suddenly. Abrupt withdrawal may precipitate petit mal seizures. Call doctor immediately if side effects develop. • Obtain CBC every 3 months; urinalysis and hepatic function tests every 6 months. • May color urine pink or red to reddish brown. • Therapeutic serum level 40 to 80 mcg/ml. • May increase incidence of grand mal seizures if used alone to treat mixed epilepsy.

NAME	INDICATIONS & DOSAGE	SIDE EFFECTS
phenytoin (formerly diphenylhydantoin) Dilantin Infatab◆, Dilantin Pediatric **phenytoin sodium** Dantoin◆◆, Dihycon, Dilantin Sodium, Di-Phen, Diphenylan Sodium, EKKO Jr. & Sr.	*Grand mal and psychomotor seizures, nonepileptic seizures (post head trauma, Reye's syndrome)—* **Adults:** loading dose 900 mg to 1.5 g I.V. at 50 mg/min or P.O. divided t.i.d., then start maintenance dose of 300 mg P.O. daily or divided t.i.d. **Children:** loading dose 15 mg/Kg I.V. at 50 mg/min or P.O. divided q 8 to 12 hours, then start maintenance dose of 5 to 7 mg/Kg P.O. or I.V. daily, divided q 12 hours. • *A loading dose is given if patient has not taken phenytoin in the past or has no detectible status epilepticus. If patient has not received phenytoin previously or has no detectible serum level, use loading dose—* **Adults:** 900 mg to 1.5 g I.V. divided into t.i.d. at 50 mg/min. Do not exceed 500 mg each dose. **Children:** 15 mg/Kg I.V. at 50 mg/min. *If patient has been receiving phenytoin but has missed one or more doses and has subtherapeutic levels—* **Adults:** 100 to 300 mg I.V. at 50 mg/min. **Children:** 5 to 7 mg/Kg I.V. at 50 mg/min. May repeat lower dose in 30 minutes if needed. *Neuritic pain (migraine, trigeminal neuralgia, Bell's palsy)—* **Adults:** 200 to 400 mg P.O. daily.	*Blood:* thrombocytopenia, leukopenia, agranulocytopenia, agranulocytosis, pancytopenia, macrocytosis, megaloblastic anemia. *CNS:* ataxia, slurred speech, confusion, dizziness, insomnia, nervousness, twitching, headache. *CV:* hypotension, ventricular fibrillation. *EENT:* nystagmus, diplopia, blurred vision. *GI:* nausea, vomiting, constipation, gingival hyperplasia. *Local:* pain, necrosis, and inflammation at injection site. *Skin:* scarletiniform or morbilliform rash; bullous, exfoliative or purpuric dermatitis; Stevens-Johnson syndrome; lupus erythematosus; hirsutism, toxic epidermal necrolysis. *Other:* toxic hepatitis, hepatic damage, periarteritis nodosa, lymphadenopathy, hyperglycemia, osteomalacia.
primidone Mysoline◆, Sertan◆◆	*Grand mal, psychomotor, and focal seizures—* **Adults, and children over 8 years:** 250 mg P.O. daily. Increase by 250 mg weekly, up to maximum 2 g daily, divided q.i.d. **Children under 8 years:** 125 mg P.O. daily. Increase by 125 mg weekly, up to maximum 1 g daily, divided q.i.d.	*Blood:* leukopenia, eosinophilia. *CNS:* drowsiness, ataxia, emotional disturbances, vertigo, hyperirritability, fatigue. *EENT:* diplopia, nystagmus, edema of the eyelids. *GI:* anorexia, nausea, vomiting. *GU:* impotence, polyuria. *Skin:* morbilliform rash, alopecia. *Other:* edema, thirst.
trimethadione Tridione, Trimedone◆◆	*Refractory, petit mal—* **Adults:** initially, 300 mg P.O. t.i.d. May increase by 300 mg weekly up to 600 mg P.O. q.i.d. **Children:** 20 to 50 mg/Kg P.O. daily, divided q 6 to 8 hours. May	*Blood:* neutropenia, leukopenia, eosinophilia, thrombocytopenia, pancytopenia, agranulocytosis, hypoplastic and aplastic anemia. *CNS:* drowsiness, fatigue, malaise, insomnia, dizziness, headache,

INTERACTIONS	NURSING CONSIDERATIONS
Alcohol, folic acid, loxipine: monitor for decreased phenytoin activity. *Oral anticoagulants, antihistamines, chloramphenicol, diazepam, diazoxide, disulfiram, isoniazid, phenylbutazone, phenyramidol, salicylates, sulfamethizole, valproate:* monitor for increased phenytoin activity and toxicity.	• Contraindicated in phenacemide or hydantoin hypersensitivity, bradycardia, S-A and A-V block, Stokes-Adams syndrome. Use cautiously in hepatic or renal dysfunction, elderly or debilitated patients, hypotension, myocardial insufficiency, respiratory depression, in patients receiving other hydantoin derivatives. • Don't withdraw suddenly. Call doctor at once if side effects develop. • Warn patient to avoid activities that require alertness and good psychomotor coordination until response to drug is determined. • Don't mix drug with 5% dextrose in water because it will precipitate. Clear I.V. tubing first with normal saline solution. Never use cloudy solution. May mix with 50 to 100 ml normal saline and give over 30 minutes. • Do not give I.M. unless dosage adjustments are made. Drug may precipitate at injection site, cause pain, and give erratic blood levels. • Obtain CBC and serum calcium every 6 months. Doctor may order folic acid and vitamin B_{12} if megaloblastic anemia is evident. • Drug may color urine pink or red to reddish brown. • Tell patient to carry identification stating that he's taking phenytoin. • Stress importance of good oral hygiene and regular dental exams. • Drug should be stopped if rash appears. If rash is scarlet or measles-like, drug may be resumed after rash clears. If rash reappears, therapy should be stopped. If rash is exfoliative, purpuric, or bullous, don't resume drug. • Use only clear solution for injection. Slight yellow color acceptable. Don't refrigerate. • Divided doses given with or after meals may decrease GI side effects. • Available as suspension. Shake well before each dose. Use solid form (chewable tablets or capsules) if possible. • Therapeutic serum level is 10 to 20 mcg/ml. • Heavy use of alcohol may diminish benefits of drug. • Phenytoin levels may be decreased in mononucleosis. Monitor for increased seizure activity.
Phenytoin: stimulated conversion of primidone to phenobarbital. Observe for increased phenobarbital effect.	• Contraindicated in phenobarbital hypersensitivity, porphyria. • Don't withdraw suddenly. Call doctor at once if side effects develop. • Warn patient to avoid activities that require alertness and good psychomotor coordination until response to drug determined. • Therapeutic serum levels of primidone 7 to 15 mg/ml. Therapeutic serum levels of phenobarbital 15 to 40 mcg/ml. • CBC and routine blood chemistry should be done every 6 months. • Metabolically converted to phenobarbital; use cautiously with phenobarbital. • For symptoms and treatment of toxicity, see p. 1115.
None significant.	• Contraindicated in paramethadione and trimethadione hypersensitivity, severe blood dyscrasias, severe hepatic dysfunction. Use with extreme caution in retinal and optic nerve diseases. • Do not use in trimester preceding planned pregnancy. • Don't withdraw drug suddenly. Abrupt withdrawal may precipitate petit mal seizures. Call doctor immediately if side effects develop.

(continued on following page)

NAME	INDICATIONS & DOSAGE	SIDE EFFECTS
trimethadione *(continued)*	increase by 150 to 300 mg. Usual maintenance 40 mg/Kg or 1 g/m² P.O. daily in divided doses t.i.d. or q.i.d.	parasthesias, grand mal seizures, irritability, personality changes, myasthenia gravis-like syndrome. *CV:* hypertension, hypotension. *EENT:* hemeralopia, diplopia, photophobia, epistaxis, retinal hemorrhage. *GI:* nausea, vomiting, anorexia, weight loss, abdominal pain, bleeding gums. *GU:* nephrosis, albuminuria, vaginal bleeding. *Skin:* acneiform and morbilliform rash, exfoliative dermatitis, erythema multiforme, petechiae, alopecia, lupus erythematosis. *Other:* lymphadenopathy.
valproic acid Depakene	*Simple and complex absence seizures (including petit mal), mixed seizure types (including absence seizures)—* **Adults and children:** initially, 15 mg/Kg P.O. daily divided b.i.d. or t.i.d.; then may increase by 5 to 10 mg/Kg daily at weekly intervals up to maximum of 30 mg/Kg daily, divided b.i.d. or t.i.d.	Because drug usually used in combination with other anticonvulsants, side effects reported may not be caused by valproic acid alone. *Blood:* inhibited platelet aggregation, increased bleeding time, leukopenia. *CNS:* sedation, emotional upset, depression, psychosis, aggression, hyperactivity, behavioral deterioration, muscle weakness, tremors. *GI:* nausea, vomiting, indigestion, diarrhea, abdominal cramps, constipation, increased appetite and weight gain, anorexia and weight loss. *Skin:* transient hair loss. *Other:* increased alkaline phosphatase and SGOT, dysarthria.

INTERACTIONS	NURSING CONSIDERATIONS
	• Check CBC, hepatic function, and urinalysis before starting therapy and monthly thereafter. Drug should be stopped if neutrophil count falls below 2,500/mm³. • Watch for impending toxicity; may precipitate grand mal seizure. • Warn patient to report skin rash, alopecia, sore throat, fever, bruises, or espistaxis to doctor immediately. • Warn patient to avoid activities that require alertness and good psychomotor coordination. • Suggest sunglasses if vision blurs in bright light. Notify doctor. • If scotomata or rash occurs, drug should be stopped. • Therapeutic serum levels 20 to 40 mcg/ml. • May increase incidence of grand mal seizures if used alone to treat mixed epilepsy.
None significant.	• Use cautiously in hepatic dysfunction. • Don't withdraw suddenly. Call doctor at once if side effects develop. • Obtain hepatic function studies, platelet counts, and prothrombin time before starting drug and every 2 months thereafter. • Warn patient to avoid activities that require alertness and good psychomotor coordination until response to drug is determined. • May give drug with food or milk to reduce GI side effects. Advise against chewing capsules; causes irritation of mouth and throat. • Tremors may indicate the need for dosage reduction.

27 Antidepressants

amitriptyline hydrochloride
desipramine hydrochloride
doxepin hydrochloride
imipramine hydrochloride
isocarboxazid
nortriptyline hydrochloride
phenelzine sulfate
protriptyline hydrochloride
tranylcypromine sulfate
trimipramine maleate

Depression is one of the most common psychiatric disorders and involves many body systems. Change in affect (mood) is a primary symptom, but sleep disturbances, decreased activity, appetite change, and morbid preoccupation also occur.

Amphetamines and other psychomotor stimulants, the original antidepressants, have recently been replaced by tricyclic antidepressants (TCA) and monoamine oxidase inhibitors (MAO inhibitors or MAOIs). Because the TCAs are less toxic, they are the drugs of first choice, and at least two TCAs are usually tried before MAO inhibitor therapy.

Major uses

- Treatment of psychotic and neurotic endogenous depressions; TCAs are less effective for reactive or mild depressions.
- Prevention of recurrent depression as in unipolar manic-depressive illness (TCAs).
- Treatment of enuresis in children and adolescents (imipramine, other TCAs).
- Treatment of symptoms of severe reactive or endogenous depression in closely supervised patients who are unresponsive to other antidepressant therapy (MAOIs).

Mechanism of action

- Precise mechanism unknown.
- Tricyclic antidepressants block re-uptake of certain central nervous system neurotransmitters, including norepinephrine and serotonin, allowing more build-up in terminals.
- Monoamine oxidase inhibitors block naturally occurring enzyme monoamine oxidase (which helps metabolize neurotransmitters at synapse), causing build-up of certain neurotransmitters and probably resulting in antidepressant action.

Absorption, distribution, and excretion

- Both TCAs and MAOIs have rapid but highly variable oral absorption.
- TCAs are widely distributed to liver, kidneys, stomach, lung, and brain tissues, but levels are low.
- TCAs are rapidly excreted in urine: 40% within 24 hours, 70% within 72 hours; the remainder is excreted in feces. They are metabolized in the liver.
- MAOIs are probably rapidly excreted, but enzyme inactivation is long.

Onset and duration

- TCAs produce sedative effects within a few hours after oral administration, with lessened sleep disturbances after a few days; anticholinergic effects soon after therapy begins; and antidepressant effects after 7 to 14 days due to slow effect on brain's neurotransmitter metabolism.

• TCAs' long therapeutic half-life permits dosing once daily, although divided doses are usually used in older patients. Their plasma levels vary widely.

• MAOIs produce some stimulation early in therapy but possible latent period of few days to several weeks.

Combination products

ETRAFON (2-10)♦: perphenazine 2 mg and amitriptyline 10 mg.
ETRAFON (2-25)♦: perphenazine 2 mg and amitriptyline 25 mg.
ETRAFON-A (4-10)♦: perphenazine 4 mg and amitriptyline 10 mg.
ETRAFON FORTE (4-25): perphenazine 4 mg and amitriptyline 25 mg.
LIMBITROL 10-25: chlordiazepoxide 10 mg and amitriptyline 25 mg.
LIMBITROL 5-12.5: chlordiazepoxide 5 mg and amitriptyline 12.5 mg.
TRIAVIL 2-10, Triavil 4-10, Triavil 2-25, Triavil 4-25 are products identical to the Etrafon products listed above. Triavil is also available as Triavil 4-50 (perphenazine 4 mg and amitriptyline 50 mg).

PATIENT TEACHING AID — FOODS TO AVOID

Dear Patient:
When you are taking MAO inhibitors, avoid foods with a high tyramine content (pictured below).

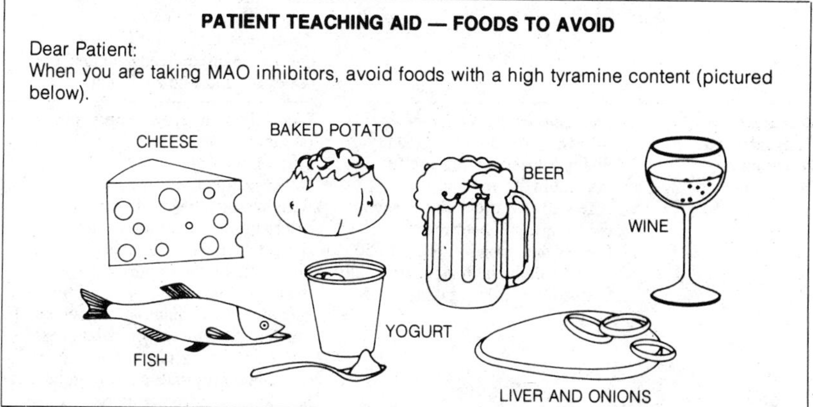

NAME	INDICATIONS & DOSAGE	SIDE EFFECTS
amitriptyline hydrochloride Amiline◆◆, Amitril, Deprex◆◆, Elavil◆, Endep, Levate◆◆, Meravil◆◆, Novotriptyn◆◆, Rolavil	*Endogenous depression—* **Adults:** 50 to 100 mg P.O., h.s. increasing to 200 mg daily; maximum 300 mg daily if needed; or 20 to 30 mg I.M. q.i.d. Alternatively, the entire dosage can be given at bedtime. **Elderly and adolescents:** 30 mg P.O. daily in divided doses.	*Blood:* bone marrow depression (agranulocytosis, thrombocytopenia, eosinophilia, purpura). *CNS:* sedation, dizziness, fatigue, weakness, confusion, headache, disorientation, disturbed concentration, delusions, hallucinations, anxiety, restlessness, excitement, insomnia, nightmares, ataxia, tremors, seizures, incoordination, numbness, tingling, paresthesias of extremities, altered EEG, extrapyramidal symptoms, inappropriate ADH (antidiuretic hormone) syndrome, increased psychotic symptoms. *CV:* hypotension or hypertension, tachycardia, palpitations, myocardial infarction, arrhythmias, heart block, stroke, EKG changes. *EENT:* blurred vision, tinnitus, increased intraocular pressure, mydriasis. *GI:* nausea, vomiting, dry mouth, epigastric distress, anorexia, stomatitis, peculiar taste, diarrhea or constipation, paralytic ileus, black tongue. *GU:* urinary retention or frequency, dilation of urinary tract, testicular swelling, changed libido. *Skin:* rash, urticaria, pruritus. *Other:* increased sweating, edema of face and tongue, changed blood sugar level, photosensitivity, angioedema, alopecia, weight changes, parotid swelling and gynecomastia in males, breast enlargement and galactorrhea in females. *Abrupt cessation after long-term therapy:* nausea, headache, malaise. (Does not indicate addiction.)
desipramine hydrochloride Norpramin◆, Pertofrane◆	*Endogenous depression—* **Adults:** 75 to 150 mg P.O. daily in divided doses, increasing to maximum 200 mg daily. Alternatively, the entire dosage can be given at bedtime. **Elderly and adolescents:** 25 to 50 mg P.O. daily, increasing gradually to maximum 100 mg daily.	*Blood:* bone marrow depression (agranulocytosis, thrombocytopenia, eosinophilia, purpura). *CNS:* sedation, dizziness, fatigue, weakness, confusion, headache, disorientation, disturbed concentration, delusions, hallucinations, anxiety, restlessness, excitement, insomnia, nightmares, ataxia, tremors, seizures, incoordination, numbness, tingling, paresthesias of extremities, altered EEG, extrapyramidal symptoms, inappropriate ADH (antidiuretic hormone) syndrome, increased psychotic symptoms. *CV:* orthostatic hypotension, hyper-

◆ Also available in Canada.
◆◆ Available in Canada only.
Unmarked trade names available in United States only.

INTERACTIONS	NURSING CONSIDERATIONS
MAO inhibitors: may cause severe excitation, hyperpyrexia, convulsions, usually with high dose. Use together cautiously. *Epinephrine, levarterenol:* increased hypertensive effect. Use with caution. *Barbiturates:* decreased TCA blood levels. Monitor for decreased antidepressant effect. *Methylphenidate:* increased TCA blood levels. Monitor for enhanced antidepressant effect.	• Contraindicated in acute recovery phase of myocardial infarction, and in prostatic hypertrophy. Use with caution in history of seizures, urinary retention, angle-closure glaucoma, increased intraocular pressure, cardiovascular disease, impaired hepatic function, hyperthyroidism, patients receiving thyroid medications, suicide risk, electroshock therapy, before elective surgery. • Reduce dose in elderly or debilitated persons and adolescents. • Do not withdraw abruptly. • If psychotic signs increase, reduce dose. Chart mood changes. Watch for suicidal tendencies. Allow minimum supply of tablets to lessen suicide risk. • Check for urinary retention and constipation. Increase fluids to lessen constipation. Suggest stool softener, if needed. • Warn patient to avoid activities that require alertness and good psychomotor coordination until response to drug is determined. Drowsiness and dizziness usually subside after first few weeks. • Photosensitivity reactions can be avoided by use of sunscreening agents and protective clothing. • Has strong anticholinergic effects; one of the most sedating tricyclic antidepressants. Avoid combining with alcohol or other depressants. • Expect time lag of up to 30 days before noticeable effect. • Dry mouth may be relieved with sugarless hard candy or gum. • Notify doctor and hold dose in symptoms of blood dyscrasias (sore throat, fever, infection, cellulitis, weakness).
MAO inhibitors: may cause severe excitation, hyperpyrexia, convulsions, usually with high dose. Use together cautiously. *Epinephrine, levarterenol:* increased hypertensive effect. Use with caution. *Barbiturates:* decreased TCA blood levels. Monitor for decreased antidepressant effect. *Methylphenidate:*	• Contraindicated in acute recovery phase of myocardial infarction and in prostatic hypertrophy. Use with caution in cardiovascular disease, urinary retention, glaucoma, thyroid disease or medication, seizure disorders, electroshock therapy, blood dyscrasias, suicide risk, before elective surgery, impaired hepatic function. • Reduce dose in elderly or debilitated persons, and adolescents. • Do not withdraw abruptly. • Notify doctor and hold dose in symptoms of blood dyscrasias (fever, sore throat, infection, cellulitis, weakness). • If psychotic signs increase, reduce dose. Chart mood changes. Watch for suicidal tendencies. Allow minimum supply of tablets to lessen suicide risk. • Check for urinary retention and constipation. Increase fluids to lessen constipation. Suggest stool softener if needed. • Warn patient to avoid activities that require alertness and good psychomotor coordination until response to drug is determined. Drowsiness and dizziness usually subside after a few weeks.

(continued on following page)

NAME	INDICATIONS & DOSAGE	SIDE EFFECTS
desipramine hydrochloride *(continued)*		tension, tachycardia, palpitations, myocardial infarction, arrhythmia, heart block, stroke. *EENT:* blurred vision, tinnitus, increased intraocular pressure, mydriasis. *GI:* nausea, vomiting, dry mouth, epigastric distress, anorexia, stomatitis, peculiar taste, diarrhea, constipation, paralytic ileus, black tongue. *GU:* urinary retention or frequency, nocturia, dilation of urinary tract, delayed micturition, testicular swelling and changed libido. *Skin:* rash, urticaria, petechial pruritus. *Other:* jaundice, altered hepatic function, increased sweating, flushing, edema of face and tongue, changed blood sugar level, photosensitivity, angioedema, alopecia, weight changes, parotid swelling and gynecomastia in males, breast enlargement and galactorrhea in females. *Abrupt cessation after long-term therapy:* nausea, headache, malaise. (Does not indicate addiction.)
doxepin hydrochloride Adapin, Sinequan◆	*Depression, anxiety—* **Adults:** initially, 30 to 75 mg P.O. daily in divided doses, to maximum 300 mg daily. Alternatively, entire dosage may be given at bedtime.	*Blood:* eosinophilia. *CNS:* sedation, dizziness, fatigue, weakness, confusion, headache, disorientation, hallucinations, ataxia, seizures, numbness, tingling, paresthesias, extrapyramidal symptoms. *CV:* hypotension, tachycardia. *EENT:* blurred vision, tinnitus. *GI:* dry mouth, nausea, vomiting, indigestion, anorexia, stomatitis, peculiar taste, diarrhea or constipation. *GU:* testicular swelling and changed libido. *Skin:* rash, pruritus. *Other:* sweating, edema, changed blood sugar level, photosensitivity, alopecia, chills, flushing, weight gain, jaundice, gynecomastia in males, breast enlargement and galactorrhea in females.
imipramine hydrochloride Antipress, Imavate, Impril◆◆, Janimine, Novopramine◆◆, Praminil◆◆, Presamine, Ropramine, SK-Pramine, Tofranil◆, W.D.D.	*Endogenous and other depression—* **Adults:** 75 to 100 mg P.O. or I.M. daily in divided doses, with 25 to 50 mg increments up to 200 mg. Maximum 300 mg daily. Alternatively, the entire dosage may be given at bedtime. (I.M. route rarely used.)	*Blood:* bone marrow depression (agranulocytosis, thrombocytopenia, eosinophilia, purpura). *CNS:* sedation, dizziness, fatigue, weakness, mania, confusion, headache, delusions, hallucinations, anxiety, restlessness, agitation, ataxia, tremors, seizures, incoordination, numbness, tingling, paresthesias

INTERACTIONS	NURSING CONSIDERATIONS
increased TCA blood levels. Monitor for enhanced antidepressant effect.	• Photosensitivity reactions can be avoided by use of sunscreening agents and protective clothing. • Dry mouth may be relieved with sugarless hard candy or gum. • Drug has anticholinergic effect, is a metabolite or imipramine, and produces less sedation than amitriptyline or doxepin. Alcohol may antagonize effects of desipramine.
MAO inhibitors: may cause severe excitation, hyperpyrexia, convulsions, usually with high dose. Use together cautiously. *Barbiturates:* decreased TCA blood levels. Monitor for decreased antidepressant effect. *Methylphenidate:* increased TCA blood levels. Monitor for enhanced antidepressant effect.	• Contraindicated in urinary retention, glaucoma, and prostatic hypertrophy. Use with caution in suicide risk. • Reduce dose in elderly or debilitated persons, adolescents, and those receiving other medications (especially anticholinergics). • Dilute oral concentrate with 120 ml water, milk, or juice (orange, grapefruit, tomato, prune, or pineapple). Avoid carbonated beverages. • Have patient take most of daily dose at bedtime. • If psychotic symptoms increase, reduce dose. Chart mood changes. Watch for suicidal tendencies. • Check for urinary retention and constipation. Increase fluids to lessen constipation. Suggest stool softener, if needed. • Warn patient to avoid activities that require alertness and good psychomotor coordination until response to drug is determined. Drowsiness and dizziness usually subside after a few weeks. • Expect time lag of 10 to 14 days before noticeable effect. • Dry mouth may be relieved with sugarless hard candy or gum. • Has strong anticholinergic effects; one of the most sedating tricyclic antidepressants. Avoid combining with alcohol or other depressants.
MAO inhibitors: may cause severe excitation, hyperpyrexia, convulsions, usually with high dose. Use together cautiously. *Epinephrine, levarterenol:* increased hypertensive effect.	• Contraindicated in acute recovery phase of myocardial infarction. Use with extreme caution in cardiovascular disease, urinary retention, narrow-angle glaucoma or increased intraocular pressure, thyroid disease or medication, seizure disorders, electroshock therapy, blood dyscrasias, suicide risk, before elective surgery, impaired hepatic function. • Reduce dose in elderly or debilitated persons, adolescents, and patients with aggravated psychotic symptoms. • Do not withdraw abruptly. • Notify doctor and hold dose in symptoms of blood dyscrasias (fever, sore

(continued on following page)

NAME	INDICATIONS & DOSAGE	SIDE EFFECTS
imipramine hydrochloride *(continued)*		of extremities, altered EEG, peripheral neuropathy, extrapyrimidal symptoms, increased psychotic symptoms. *CV:* hypotension or hypertension, tachycardia, palpitations, myocardial infarction, arrhythmias, heart block, stroke. *EENT:* blurred vision, tinnitus, increased intraocular pressure, mydriasis. *GI:* dry mouth, nausea, vomiting, epigastric distress, anorexia, stomatitis, peculiar taste, diarrhea or constipation, paralytic ileus, abdominal cramps, black tongue. *GU:* urinary retention or frequency, dilation of urinary tract, delayed micturition, testicular swelling and changed libido. *Skin:* rash, urticaria, pruritis. *Other:* increased sweating, jaundice, altered hepatic function, flushing, edema (general or of face and tongue), changed blood sugar level, photosensitivity, angioedema, alopecia, drug fever, weight changes, parotid swelling, gynecomastia in males, breast enlargement and galactorrhea in females. *Abrupt cessation after long-term therapy:* nausea, headache, malaise. (Does not indicate addiction.)
isocarboxazid Marplan♦	*Depression—* **Adults:** 30 mg P.O. daily in divided doses. Reduce to 10 to 20 mg daily when condition improves. Not recommended for children under 16 years.	*CNS:* dizziness, vertigo, weakness, headache, overactivity, hyperreflexia, tremors, muscle twitching, mania, insomnia, confusion, memory impairment, fatigue. *CV:* orthostatic hypotension, arrhythmias, paradoxical hypertension. *EENT:* blurred vision. *GI:* dry mouth, anorexia, nausea, diarrhea, constipation. *GU:* changed libido. *Skin:* rash. *Other:* peripheral edema, sweating, weight changes.

INTERACTIONS	NURSING CONSIDERATIONS
Use with caution. *Barbiturates:* decreased tricyclic blood levels. Monitor for decreased effect. *Methylphenidate:* increased TCA blood levels. Monitor for enhanced antidepressant effect.	throat, infection, cellulitis, weakness). • Watch for increased psychotic signs; reduce dose if they occur. Chart mood changes. Watch for suicidal tendencies. Allow only minimum supply of tablets to lessen suicide risk. • Check urinary retention and constipation. Increase fluids to lessen constipation. Suggest stool softener, if necessary. • Warn patient to avoid activities that require alertness and good psychomotor coordination until response to drug has been determined. Drowsiness and dizziness usually subside after a few weeks. • Don't combine with alcohol or other depressants. • Photosensitivity reactions can be avoided by using sunscreening agents and protective clothing. • Expect time lag of 10 to 14 days before noticeable effect. • Dry mouth may be relieved with sugarless hard candy or gum. • Not as effective as other tricyclics in severely depressed patients.
Amphetamines, ephedrine, levodopa, meperidine, metaraminol, methotrimeprazine, methylphenidate, phenylephrine, phenylpropanolamine: pressor effects of these drugs are enhanced by isocarboxazid. Use together cautiously. *Alcohol, barbiturates, and other sedatives; tranquilizers; narcotics; dextromethorphan; tricyclic antidepressants:* unpredictable interaction. Use with caution and in reduced dosage.	• Contraindicated in severe hepatic or renal impairment; congestive heart failure; pheochromocytoma; foods containing tryptophan or tyramine; excess caffeine; elderly or debilitated persons; hypertensive, cardiovascular, or cerebrovascular disease; severe or frequent headaches; therapy with other MAO inhibitor (including pargyline HCl, phenelzine sulfate, tranylcypromine sulfate) or within 10 days of such therapy; within 10 days of elective surgery requiring general anesthetic, cocaine, or local anesthetic containing sympathomimetic vasoconstrictors. Use cautiously with other psychotropic drugs or with spinal anesthetic; in hyperactive, agitated, or schizophrenic patients; in suicide risk, diabetes, epilepsy. • Recommended only when TCA or electroshock therapy is ineffective or contraindicated. • Hold dose and notify doctor if patient develops symptoms of overdosage: palpitations or frequent headaches, jaundice or other hepatic symptoms, or severe orthostatic hypotension. • Watch for suicidal tendencies. • Dose is usually reduced to maintenance level as soon as possible. • Do not withdraw drug abruptly. • Weigh patient biweekly; check for edema and urinary retention. • Warn patient to avoid foods high in tyramine or tryptophan; large amounts of caffeine; and self-medication with over-the-counter cold, hay fever, or reducing preparations. • Incidence of orthostatic hypotension is high. Supervise walking. Tell

(continued on following page)

NAME	INDICATIONS & DOSAGE	SIDE EFFECTS
isocarboxazid *(continued)*		
nortriptyline hydrochloride Aventyl◆, Pamelor	*Endogenous depression—* **Adults:** 25 mg P.O. t.i.d. or q.i.d., gradually increasing to maximum 100 mg daily. Alternatively, entire dose may be given at bedtime.	*Blood:* bone marrow depression (agranulocytosis, thrombocytopenia, eosinophilia, purpura). *CNS:* sedation, dizziness, fatigue, weakness, confusion, headache, delusions, hallucinations, anxiety, restlessness, agitation, insomnia, panic, nightmares, ataxia, tremors, seizures, incoordination, numbness, tingling, paresthesias of extremities, peripheral neuropathy, altered *EEG,* extrapyramidal symptoms, increased psychotic symptoms. *CV:* hypotension, hypertension, tachycardia, palpitations, myocardial infarction, arrhythmias, heart block, stroke. *EENT:* blurred vision, tinnitus, increased intraocular pressure, mydriasis. *GI:* dry mouth, nausea, vomiting, epigastric distress, anorexia, stomatitis, peculiar taste, diarrhea or constipation, paralytic ileus, abdominal cramps, black tongue. *GU:* urinary retention or frequency, dilation of urinary tract, delayed micturition, nocturia, testicular swelling and changed libido. *Skin:* rash, urticaria, pruritus, petechiae. *Other:* jaundice, altered hepatic function, increased sweating, flushing, edema (general or of face and tongue), changed blood sugar level, photosensitivity, alopecia, drug fever, weight changes, parotid swelling, gynecomastia in males, breast enlargement and galactorrhea in females. *Abrupt cessation after long-term therapy:* nausea, headache, malaise. (Does not indicate addiction.)
phenelzine sulfate Nardil◆	*Atypical, nonendogenous, neurotic depression—* **Adults:** 45 mg P.O. daily in divided doses, increasing rapidly to 60 mg daily. Maximum 90 mg daily. Not recommended for children under 16 years.	*CNS:* dizziness, vertigo, headache, overactivity, hyperreflexia, tremors, muscle twitching, mania, jitteriness, insomnia, confusion, memory impairment, drowsiness, weakness, fatigue. *CV:* paradoxical hypertension, orthostatic hypotension, arrhythmias. *GI:* dry mouth, anorexia, nausea, constipation.

INTERACTIONS	NURSING CONSIDERATIONS
	patient to get out of bed slowly, sitting up first for 1 minute. • Continue precautions 10 days after stopping drug; long-lasting effects. • Expect time lag of 1 to 4 weeks before noticeable effect. • Drug is MAO inhibitor and is generally less effective than tricyclic antidepressant. Avoid combining with alcohol or other depressant.
MAO inhibitors: may cause severe excitation, hyperpyrexia, convulsions, usually with high dose. Use together cautiously. *Epinephrine, levarterenol:* increased hypertensive effect. Use with caution. *Barbiturates:* decreased TCA blood levels. Monitor for decreased antidepressant effect. *Methylphenidate:* increased TCA blood levels. Monitor for enhanced antidepressant effect.	• Contraindicated in acute recovery phase of myocardial infarction and in prostatic hypertrophy. Use with caution in cardiovascular disease, urinary retention, glaucoma, thyroid disease or medication, seizure disorders, electroshock therapy, blood dyscrasias, suicide risk, before elective surgery. • Reduce dose in elderly or debilitated persons, and adolescents. • Do not withdraw abruptly. • Notify doctor and hold dose in symptoms of blood dyscrasias (fever, sore throat, infection, cellulitis, weakness). • If psychotic signs increase, reduce dose. Chart mood changes. Watch for suicidal tendencies. Allow minimum supply of tablets to lessen suicide risk. • Check for urinary retention and constipation. Increase fluids to lessen constipation. Suggest stool softener, if needed. • Warn patient to avoid activities that require alertness and good psychomotor coordination until response to drug is determined. Drowsiness and dizziness usually subside after a few weeks. • Photosensitivity reactions can be avoided by use of sunscreening agents and protective clothing. • Expect time lag of 10 to 14 days before noticeable effects. • Dry mouth may be relieved by sugarless hard candy or gum. • Drug is tricyclic antidepressant, similar in anticholinergic effects to other tricyclics. Avoid combining with alcohol or other depressants.
Amphetamines, ephedrine, levodopa, meperidine, metaraminol, methotrimeprazine, methylphenidate, phenylephrine, phenylpropanolamine: enhanced pressor ef-	• Contraindicated in hepatic impairment; congestive heart failure; pheochromocytoma; foods containing tryptophan (broad beans) or tyramine; excess caffeine or chocolate; elderly or debilitated persons; hypertension, cardiovascular, or cerebrovascular disease; severe or frequent headaches; therapy with other MAO inhibitor, including pargyline HCl, isocarboxazid, tranylcypromine sulfate, or within 10 days of such therapy; within 10 days of elective surgery requiring general anesthetic, cocaine, or local anesthetic containing sympathomimetic vasoconstrictors; hyperactive, agitated, or schizophrenic patients. Use cautiously with antihypertensive drugs

(continued on following page)

NAME	INDICATIONS & DOSAGE	SIDE EFFECTS
phenelzine sulfate *(continued)*		*Other:* peripheral edema, sweating, weight changes.
protriptyline hydrochloride Triptil••, Vivactil	*Depression—* **Adults:** 15 to 40 mg P.O. daily in divided doses, increasing gradually to maximum 60 mg daily.	*Blood:* bone marrow depression (agranulocytosis, thrombocytopenia, eosinophilia, purpura). *CNS:* sedation, dizziness, fatigue, weakness, mania, confusion, headache, delusions, hallucinations, anxiety, restlessness, agitation, insomnia, panic, nightmares, ataxia, tremors, seizures, incoordination, numbness, tingling, paresthesias of extremities, altered EEG, peripheral neuropathy, extrapyramidal symptoms, increased psychotic symptoms. *CV:* orthostatic hypotension, hypertension, tachycardia, palpitations, myocardial infarction, arrhythmias, heart block, stroke. *EENT:* blurred vision, tinnitus, increased intraocular pressure, mydriasis. *GI:* dry mouth, nausea, vomiting, epigastric distress, anorexia, stomatitis, peculiar taste, diarrhea or constipation, paralytic ileus, abdominal cramps, black tongue. *GU:* urinary retention or frequency, dilation of urinary tract, delayed micturition, nocturia, testicular swelling, changed libido. *Skin:* rash, urticaria, pruritus, petechiae. *Other:* jaundice, altered hepatic function, sweating, flushing, edema (general or of face and tongue), changed blood sugar level, photosensitivity, alopecia, drug fever, weight changes, parotid swelling, gynecomastia in males, breast enlargement and galactorrhea

INTERACTIONS	NURSING CONSIDERATIONS
fects. Use together cautiously. *Alcohol, barbiturates, and other sedatives; tranquilizers; narcotics; dextromethorphan; tricyclic antidepressants:* unpredictable interaction. Use with caution and in reduced dosage.	containing thiazide diuretics or with spinal anesthetic; in suicide risk, diabetes, epilepsy. • Use only when TCA or electroshock therapy are ineffective or contraindicated. • Hold dose and notify doctor if patient develops symptoms of overdose: jaundice or other hepatic symptoms, severe hypotension, palpitations or frequent headaches. • Watch for suicidal tendencies. • Dose is usually reduced to maintenance level as soon as possible. • Store drug in tight container, away from heat and light. • Have phentolamine (Regitine) available to counteract severe hypertension. • Warn patient to avoid foods high in tyramine or tryptophan; large amounts of caffeine; and self-medication with over-the-counter cold, hay fever, or reducing preparations. • Incidence of orthostatic hypotension is high. Supervise walking. Tell patient to get out of bed slowly, sitting up first for 1 minute. • Continue precautions 10 days after stopping drug; long-lasting effects. • Expect time lag of 1 to 4 weeks before noticeble effect. • Drug is MAO inhibitor and is generally less effective than tricyclic antidepressant. Avoid combining with alcohol or other depressants.
MAO inhibitors: may cause severe excitation, hyperpyrexia, convulsions, and death, usually with high dose. Use together cautiously. *Epinephrine, levarterenol:* increased hypertensive effect. Use with caution. *Barbiturates:* decreased TCA blood levels. Monitor for decreased antidepressant effect. *Methylphenidate:* increased TCA blood levels. Monitor for enhanced antidepressant effect.	• Contraindicated in acute recovery phase of myocardial infarction and in prostatic hypertrophy. Use with caution in cardiovascular disease, urinary retention, increased intraocular tension, elderly, thyroid disease or medication, seizure disorders, electroshock therapy, blood dyscrasias, suicide risk, before elective surgery. • Reduce dose in elderly or debilitated persons, and adolescents. • Do not withdraw abruptly. • Notify doctor and hold dose in symptoms of blood dyscrasias (fever, sore throat, infection, cellulitis, weakness). • Watch for increased psychotic signs, anxiety, agitation, or cardiovascular reactions; reduce dose if they occur. Chart mood changes. Watch for suicidal tendencies. Allow minimum supply of tablets to lessen suicide risk. • Check urinary retention and constipation. Increase fluids to lessen constipation. Suggest stool softener, if needed. • Warn patient to avoid activities that require alertness and good psychomotor coordination until response to drug is determined. Drowsiness and dizziness usually subside after a few weeks. • Photosensitivity reactions can be avoided by use of sunscreening agents and protective clothing. • Dry mouth may be relieved with sugarless hard candy or gum. • Expect time lag of 7 to 14 days before noticeable effect. • Drug is possibly the most rapid-acting but least sedating tricyclic antidepressant. Avoid combining with alcohol or other depressants. • Do not give entire dose at bedtime as patient may develop insomnia.

(continued on following page)

NAME	INDICATIONS & DOSAGE	SIDE EFFECTS
protriptyline hydrochloride *(continued)*		in females. *Abrupt cessation after long-term therapy:* nausea, headache, malaise. (Does not indicate addiction.)
tranylcypromine sulfate Parnate◆	*Severe reactive or endogenous depression—* **Adults:** 10 mg P.O. b.i.d. Increase to maximum 30 mg daily, if necessary, after 2 weeks. Not recommended for children under 16 years.	*CNS:* dizziness, vertigo, headache, overactivity, hyperreflexia, tremors, muscle twitching, mania, jitteriness, confusion, memory impairment, fatigue. *CV:* orthostatic hypotension, arrhythmias, paradoxical hypertension. *EENT:* blurred vision. *GI:* dry mouth, anorexia, nausea, diarrhea, constipation, abdominal pain. *GU:* changed libido, impotence. *Skin:* rash. *Other:* peripheral edema, sweating, weight changes, chills.
trimipramine maleate Surmontil	*Endogenous and other depression—* **Adults:** 75 mg daily in divided doses, increased to 200 mg per day. Dosages over 300 mg per day not recommended. *Enuresis—* **Children over 6:** initial dose 25 mg P.O. 1 hour before bedtime; if no response, increase dose to 50 mg in children under 12, and to 75 mg in children over 12.	*Blood:* bone marrow depression (agranulocytosis, thrombocytopenia, eosinophilia, purpura). *CNS:* sedation, dizziness, fatigue, weakness, mania, confusion, headache, delusions, hallucinations, anxiety, restlessness, agitation, ataxia, tremors, seizures, incoordination, numbness, tingling, paresthesias of extremities, altered EEG, peripheral neuropathy, extrapyramidal symptoms, increased psychotic symptoms. *CV:* hypotension or hypertension, tachycardia, palpitations, myocardial infarction, arrhythmias, heart block,

INTERACTIONS	NURSING CONSIDERATIONS
Amphetamines, ephedrine, levodopa, meperidine, metaraminol, methotrimeprazine, methylphenidate, phenylephrine, phenylpropanolamine: pressor effects of these drugs are enhanced by tranylcypromine. Use together cautiously. *Alcohol, barbiturates, and other sedatives; tranquilizers; narcotics; dextromethorphan; tricyclic antidepressants:* use with caution and in reduced dosage.	• Contraindicated in severe hepatic or renal impairment; congestive heart failure; pheochromocytoma; antihypertensive drugs; diuretics; patients for whom close supervision is not possible; foods containing tryptophan or tyramine; excess caffeine; elderly or debilitated persons; hypertension, cardiovascular, or cerebrovascular disease; severe or frequent headaches; therapy with other MAO inhibitor (including pargyline HCl, phenelzine sulfate, isocarboxazid) or within 7 days of such therapy; within 7 days of elective surgery requiring general anesthetic, cocaine, or local anesthetic containing sympathomimetic vasoconstrictors; hyperactive, agitated, or schizophrenic patients. Use cautiously with anti-Parkinson drugs, spinal anesthetic, renal disease, suicide risk, diabetes, epilepsy, and hyperthyroidism. • Use only when TCA or electroshock therapy are ineffective or contraindicated. • Hold dose and notify doctor if patient develops symptoms of overdose: palpitations, frequent headaches, jaundice or other hepatic symptoms, severe orthostatic hypotension. • Watch for suicidal tendencies. • Dose is usually reduced to maintenance level as soon as possible. • Do not withdraw drug abruptly. • Have phentolamine (Regitine) available to counteract severe hypertension. • Warn patient to avoid foods high in tyramine or trytophan; large amounts of caffeine; and self-medication with over-the-counter cold, hay fever, or reducing preparations. • Tell patient to get out of bed slowly, sitting up for 1 minute. • Continue precautions for 7 days after stopping drug; effects last that long. • Expect time lag of 1 to 3 weeks before noticeable effect. • More rapid onset of action than isocarboxazid or phenelzine sulfate. • MAO inhibitor most likely to cause hypertensive crisis in presence of high-tyramine ingestion. Generally less effective than an tricyclic antidepressant. Avoid combining with alcohol or other depressants.
MAO inhibitors: may cause severe excitation, hyperpyrexia, convulsions, usually with high dose. Use together cautiously. *Epinephrine, levarterenol:* increased hypertensive effect. Use with caution. *Barbiturates:* decreased TCA blood levels. Monitor for decreased antidepressant effect.	• Contraindicated in acute recovery phase of myocardial infarction; in prostatic hypertrophy. Use with extreme caution in cardiovascular disease, urinary retention, narrow-angle glaucoma or increased intraocular pressure, thyroid disease or medication, seizure disorders, electroshock therapy, blood dyscrasias, suicide risk, before elective surgery, impaired hepatic function. • Reduce dose in elderly or debilitated persons, and adolescents. • Do not withdraw abruptly. • Notify doctor and hold dose in symptoms of blood dyscrasias (fever, sore throat, infection, cellulitis, weakness). • If psychotic signs increase, reduce dose. Chart mood changes. Watch for suicidal tendencies. Allow minimum supply of tablets to lessen suicide risk. • Check for urinary retention and constipation. Increase fluids to lessen constipation. Suggest stool softener, if needed. • Warn patient to avoid activities that require alertness and good psycho-

(continued on following page)

NAME	INDICATIONS & DOSAGE	SIDE EFFECTS
trimipramine maleate *(continued)*		stroke. *EENT:* blurred vision, tinnitus, increased intraocular pressure, mydriasis. *GI:* dry mouth, nausea, vomiting, epigastric distress, anorexia, stomatitis, peculiar taste, diarrhea or constipation, paralytic ileus, abdominal cramps, black tongue. *GU:* urinary retention or frequency, dilation of urinary tract, delayed micturition, testicular swelling and changed libido. *Skin:* rash, urticaria, pruritus. *Other:* increased sweating, jaundice, altered hepatic function, flushing, edema (general or of face and tongue), changed blood sugar level, photosensitivity, angioedema, alopecia, drug fever, weight changes, parotid swelling, gynecomastia in males, breast enlargement and galactorrhea in females. *Abrupt cessation after long-term therapy:* nausea, headache, malaise. (Does not indicate addiction.)

INTERACTIONS	NURSING CONSIDERATIONS
Methylphenidate: increased TCA blood levels. Monitor for enhanced antidepressant effect.	motor coordination until response to drug is determined. Drowsiness and dizziness usually subside after a few weeks. • Photosensitivity reactions can be avoided by use of sunscreening agents and protective clothing. • Expect time lag of 10 to 14 days before noticeable effect. • Dry mouth may be relieved with sugarless hard candy or gum. • Most common tricyclic used for enuresis, but effectiveness may decrease over time. Similar in anticholinergic effects to other tricyclics. Avoid combining with alcohol or other depressants.

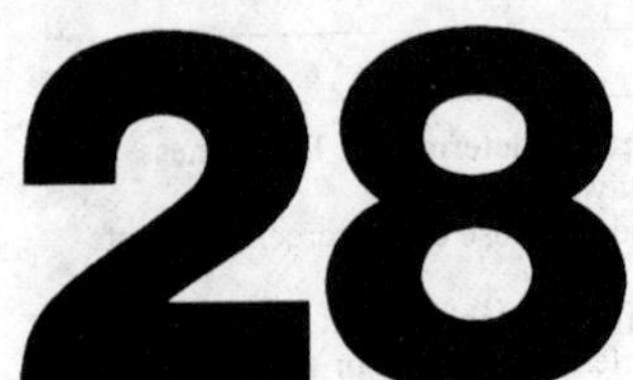

Tranquilizers

chlordiazepoxide hydrochloride
chlormezanone
clorazepate dipotassium
chlorazepate monopotassium
diazepam
hydroxyzine hydrochloride
hydroxyzine pamoate
lorazepam
meprobamate
oxazepam
prazepam
tybamate

Tranquilizers reduce anxiety without inducing sleep. They are indicated for patients suffering from various neuroses or mild depression. Most have muscle relaxant and anticonvulsive properties. They produce a dose-dependent, nonspecific central nervous system depression and closely resemble sedative-hypnotic drugs (barbiturates) in pharmacological properties.

There are three chemical groups of tranquilizers: the benzodiazepines (including chlordiazepoxide, diazepam, and others), the propanediols and thiazanones (meprobamate, tybamate, and chlormezanone), and sedating antihistamines, such as hydroxyzine. The barbiturates are an older class of drugs that have been used as antianxiety agents in doses lower than those used for sleep induction. See also Chapter 25.

Major uses

- Treatment of anxiety.
- Treatment and prevention of alcohol withdrawal symptoms.
- Premedication for anesthesia or intravenous general anesthesia for short procedures (especially diazepam).
- Prevention of convulsions and treatment of status epilepticus (especially intravenous diazepam).
- Relaxation of skeletal muscle (limited effectiveness).

Mechanism of action

- Most agents appear to depress the central nervous system at the limbic and subcortical levels of the brain, leading to sedative, skeletal muscle relaxant, and anticonvulsant effects.

Absorption, distribution, and excretion

- Oral absorption quite good and very rapid, but chlordiazepoxide absorbed more slowly.
- Intramuscular absorption of two benzodiazepines (diazepam and chlordiazepoxide) is slower, variable, unpredictable, and painful.
- Most benzodiazepines are metabolized to active products, resulting in long therapeutic

half-lives and permitting once-daily dosing when steady state levels are reached.
- Detoxified in liver, with metabolites excreted through feces and urine.

Onset and duration

- Meprobamate begins effect in 1 hour, peaks in 2 to 3 hours, has a half-life of approximately 10 hours, and is very well absorbed from the gastrointestinal tract. Tybamate is similar but has a much shorter half-life (3 hours).
- Oral diazepam has rapid onset of action, in 1 hour, and has a long half-life.
- Chlordiazepoxide is slowly absorbed and probably takes several hours to peak.
- Oxazepam and lorazepam probably have the shortest half-lives and therefore the shortest duration of all benzodiazepines.
- Chlormezanone acts within 15 to 30 minutes and lasts 6 hours.

Combination products

BAMADEX: meprobamate 300 mg and *d*-amphetamine sulfate 15 mg.
DEPROL: meprobamate 400 mg and benactyzine 1 mg.
EQUAGESIC: meprobamate 150 mg, ethoheprazine citrate 75 mg, and aspirin 250 mg.
EQUANITRATE♦: meprobamate 200 mg and pentaerythritol tetranitrate 10 mg or 20 mg.
LIBRAX♦: chlordiazepoxide hydrochloride 5 mg, and clidinium bromide 2.5 mg.
LIMBITROL 5-12.5: chlordiazepoxide 5 mg and amitriptyline 12.5 mg.
LIMBITROL 10-25: chlordiazepoxide 10 mg and amitriptyline 25 mg.
MENRIUM♦ 5-2: chlordiazepoxide 5 mg and conjugated estrogens 0.2 mg.
MENRIUM♦ 5-4: chlordiazepoxide 5 mg and conjugated estrogens 0.4 mg.
MENRIUM♦ 10-4: chlordiazepoxide 10 mg and conjugated estrogens 0.4 mg.
MILPATH 200: meprobamate 200 mg and tridihexethyl chloride 25 mg.
MILPATH 400: meprobamate 400 mg and tridihexethyl chloride 25 mg.
MILPREM: meprobamate 200 or 400 mg and conjugated estrogens 0.45 mg.
MILTRATE: meprobamate 200 mg and pentaerythritol tetranitrate 10 mg.
PATHIBAMATE-200 AND PATHIBAMATE-400♦ are identical to above Milpath products.
PMB 200: meprobamate 200 mg and conjugated estrogens 0.45 mg.
PMB 400: meprobamate 400 mg and conjugated estrogens 0.45 mg.
ROBAM-PETN-10: meprobamate 200 mg and pentaerythritol tetranitrate 10 mg.

NAME	INDICATIONS & DOSAGE	SIDE EFFECTS
chlordiazepoxide hydrochloride Controlled substance Schedule IV A-poxide, Chlordiazachel, Corax♦♦, C-Tran♦♦, J-Liberty, Libritabs, Librium♦, Medilium♦♦, Nack♦♦, Novopoxide♦♦, Protensin♦♦, Relaxil♦♦, Sereen, SK-Lygen, Solium♦♦, Tenax, Trilium♦♦, Zetran	*Mild to moderate anxiety and tension*— **Adults:** 5 to 10 mg t.i.d. or q.i.d. **Children over 6 years:** 5 mg P.O. b.i.d. to q.i.d. Maximum 10 mg P.O. b.i.d. to t.i.d. *Severe anxiety and tension*— **Adults:** 20 to 25 mg t.i.d. or q.i.d. *Withdrawal symptoms of acute alcoholism*— **Adults:** 50 to 100 mg P.O., I.M., or I.V. Maximum 300 mg daily. *Preop apprehension and anxiety*— **Adults:** 5 to 10 mg P.O. t.i.d. or q.i.d. on days preceding surgery or 50 to 100 mg I.M. 1 hour prior to surgery.	*Blood:* agranulocytosis. *CNS:* drowsiness, lethargy, fainting, vertigo, headache, weakness, muscle tenderness and spasm, slurred speech, EEG changes, mental confusion, ataxia. *CV:* hypotension, tachycardia, edema. *EENT:* blurred vision, tinnitus. *GI:* nausea, constipation. *GU:* minor menstrual irregularities, changed libido, failure to ejaculate, urinary frequency, acute hepatic necrosis or dysfunction. *Local:* pain at injection site. *Skin:* rash. *Other:* edema depressed thyroid ^{131}I uptake, photosensitivity, jaundice.
chlormezanone Fenarol, Trancopal♦	*Mild anxiety and tension, muscle relaxation*— **Adults:** 100 to 200 mg P.O. t.i.d. or q.i.d. **Children 5 to 12 years:** 50 to 100 mg P.O. t.i.d. or q.i.d.	*CNS:* drowsiness, mental depression, headache, dizziness, ataxia, lethargy, muscular weakness. *CV:* edema, flushing. *GI:* nausea, anorexia, dry mouth. *GU:* urinary retention. *Skin:* rash. *Other:* cholestatic jaundice.
chlorazepate dipotassium Controlled substance Schedule IV Tranxene♦	*Acute alcohol withdrawal*— **Adults:** Day 1—30 mg P.O. initially, followed by 30 to 60 mg P.O. in divided doses; Day 2—45 to 90 mg P.O. in divided doses; Day 3—22.5 to 45 mg P.O. in divided doses; Day 4—15 to 30 mg P.O. in divided doses; gradually reducing daily dose to 7.5 to 15 mg. *Anxiety*— **Adults:** 15 to 60 mg P.O. daily.	*Blood:* decreased hematocrit. *CNS:* drowsiness, fatigue, mental depression and confusion, dizziness, nervousness, headache, insomnia, ataxia. *CV:* decreased systolic blood pressure. *EENT:* blurred vision, diplopia. *GI:* dry mouth. *Skin:* transient rash.
chlorazepate monopotassium Controlled substance Schedule IV Azene	*Acute alcohol withdrawal*—in elderly or debilitated patients: 6.5 to 13 mg P.O. in divided doses. **Adults:** Day 1—26 mg P.O. initially, followed by 26 to 52 mg P.O. in divided doses; Day 2—39 to 78 mg P.O. in divided doses; Day 3—19.5 to 39 mg P.O. in divided doses; Day 4—13 to 26 mg P.O. in divided doses; gradually	

♦ Also available in Canada.
♦♦ Available in Canada only.
Unmarked trade names available in United States only.

INTERACTIONS	NURSING CONSIDERATIONS
None significant.	• Contraindicated in oral form for children under 6 years; in parenteral form for children under 12 years. Use with caution in mental depression, blood dyscrasias, hepatic or renal disease, or anticoagulant therapy. • Dosage should be reduced in elderly or debilitated patients. • Do not withdraw drug abruptly. • Possibility of abuse, addiction. Withdrawal symptoms similar to those of barbiturates. • Warn patient to avoid activities that require alertness and good psychomotor coordination until response to drug is determined. • Warn patient not to combine drug with alcohol or other depressants. • Although package recommends I.M. use only, drug may be given I.V. • Injectable form (as hydrochloride) comes as two ampules—the diluent and the powdered drug. For I.M., add 2 ml of diluent to powder and agitate gently until clear. Use immediately. I.M. form may be erratically absorbed. Do not give packaged diluent I.V. • For I.V., use 5 ml of saline injection or sterile water for injection as diluent; give slowly over 1 minute. Do not give such solution I.M. • Keep powder away from light; mix just before use; discard remainder. • Do not mix injectable form with any other parenteral drug. • Tell patient to use sun-screening agents and to avoid prolonged exposure to sunlight while taking drug. • For symptoms and treatment of toxicity, see p. 1123.
None significant.	• Use with caution in hepatic or renal disease. • Dosage should be reduced in elderly or debilitated patients. • Do not withdraw drug abruptly. • Possibility of abuse, addiction exists. • Warn patient to avoid activities that require alertness and good psychomotor coordination until response to drug is determined. • Warn patient not to combine drug with alcohol or other depressants. • Rapid onset of action (15 to 30 minutes), with effects lasting 4 to 6 hours. • Chemically unrelated to other antianxiety agents. • Suggest chewing gum or hard candy to relieve dry mouth.
None significant.	• Contraindicated in acute narrow-angle glaucoma, lactation, depressive neuroses, psychotic reactions, children under 18 years. Use with caution in hepatic or renal damage. • Dosage should be reduced in elderly or debilitated patients. • Do not withdraw drug abruptly. • Possibility of abuse, addiction exists. Withdrawal symptoms similar to those of barbiturates. • Warn patient to avoid activities that require alertness and good psychomotor coordination. • Warn patient not to combine drug with alcohol or other depressants. • Benzodiazepine derivative. • Suggest chewing gum or hard candy to relieve dry mouth. • May affect hepatic and renal function tests, producing abnormal results.

(continued on following page)

NAME	INDICATIONS & DOSAGE	SIDE EFFECTS
chlorazepate monopotassium *(continued)*	reduce to 6.5 to 13 mg P.O. and stop when patient stable. *Anxiety—* **Adults:** 13 to 52 mg P.O. in divided doses. Maximum—78 mg daily.	
diazepam Controlled substance Schedule IV D-Tran••, E-Pam••, Erital••, Meval••, NeoCalme••, Novodipam••, Paxel••, Serenack••, Stress-Pam••, Valium•, Vivol••	*Tension, anxiety, adjunct in convulsive disorders or skeletal muscle spasm—* **Adults:** 2 to 10 mg P.O. t.i.d. or q.i.d. **Children over 6 months:** 1 to 2.5 mg P.O. t.i.d. or q.i.d. *Tension, anxiety, muscle spasm, endoscopic procedures, convulsive seizures—* **Adults:** 5 to 10 mg I.V. initially, up to 30 mg in 1 hour or possibly more for cardioversion or status epilepticus, depending on response. **Children 5 years and over:** 1 mg I.V. or I.M. slowly q 2 to 5 minutes to maximum 10 mg. Repeat q 2 to 4 hours. **Children 30 days to 5 years:** 0.2 to 0.5 mg I.V. or I.M. slowly q 2 to 5 minutes to maximum 5 mg. Repeat q 2 to 4 hours. *Tetanic muscle spasms—* **Children over 5 years:** 5 to 10 mg I.M. or I.V. q 3 to 4 hours, p.r.n. **Infants over 30 days:** 1 to 2 mg I.M. or I.V. q 3 to 4 hours, p.r.n.	*Blood:* neutropenia. *CNS:* fatigue, drowsiness, ataxia, dizziness, headache, vertigo, weakness, fainting, slurred speech, depression, changed EEG pattern, increased muscle spasticity, sleep disturbances, anxiety, hostility, hallucinations. *CV:* hypotension. *EENT:* tinnitus, diplopia. *GI:* nausea, vomiting, epigastric distress, constipation. *GU:* urinary frequency, retention, decreased flow; changed libido. *Local:* desquamation, pain, phlebitis at injection site. *Skin:* maculopapular/rubelliform/morbilliform rash, pruritus, urticaria. *Other:* hyperpyrexia, hypothermia, weight gain, jaundice, brief period of apnea.
hydroxyzine hydrochloride Atarax•, Vistaril (parenteral) **hydroxyzine pamoate** Vistaril (oral)	*Anxiety and tension—* **Adults:** 25 to 100 mg P.O. t.i.d. or q.i.d. *Anxiety, tension, hyperkinesis—* **Children over 6 years:** 50 to 100 mg P.O. daily in divided doses. **Children under 6 years:** 50 mg P.O. daily in divided doses. *Preop and postop adjunctive therapy—* **Adults:** 25 to 100 mg I.M. q 4 to 6 hours. **Children:** 1.1 mg/Kg I.M. q 4 to 6 hours.	*CNS:* drowsiness, involuntary motor activity. *GI:* dry mouth. *Local:* marked discomfort at site of I.M. injection.

INTERACTIONS	NURSING CONSIDERATIONS
None significant.	• Contraindicated in shock, coma, acute alcohol intoxication, acute narrow-angle glaucoma, psychosis; in oral form for children under 6 months. Use with caution in blood dyscrasias, hepatic or renal damage, depression, open-angle glaucoma, elderly and debilitated patients, those with limited pulmonary reserve, and those in whom blood pressure drop might cause cardiovascular complications. • Dosage should be reduced in elderly or debilitated patients. • Do not withdraw drug abruptly. • Keep resuscitation equipment available. • Possibility of abuse, addiction exists. Withdrawal symptoms similar to those of barbiturates. • Warn patient to avoid activities that require alertness and good psychomotor coordination until response to drug is determined. • Warn patient not to combine drug with alcohol or other depressants. • Do not dilute with solutions or mix with other drugs: incompatible. • Avoid extravasation. Do not inject into small veins. • Watch for phlebitis at injection site. • Give I.V. slowly, at rate not exceeding 5 mg per minute. • I.V. route more reliable; I.M. absorption variable, to be discouraged. • Drug of choice (I.V. form) for status epilepticus. • Benzodiazepine derivative. • For symptoms and treatment of toxicity, see p. 1123.
None significant.	• Dosage should be reduced in elderly or debilitated patients. • Do not withdraw drug abruptly. • Possibility of abuse, addiction exists. • Warn patient to avoid activities that require alertness and good psychomotor coordination until response to drug is determined. • Warn patient not to combine drug with alcohol or other depressants. • Observe for excessive sedation due to potentiation with other CNS drugs. • Used as an antiemetic and antianxiety drug. • Used in psychogenically-induced allergic conditions, such as chronic urticaria and pruritus. • Parenteral form (hydroxyzine HCl) for I.M. use only; never I.V. • Aspirate injection carefully to prevent inadvertent intravascular injection.

NAME	INDICATIONS & DOSAGE	SIDE EFFECTS
lorazepam Controlled substance Schedule IV Ativan◆	*Anxiety, tension, agitation, irritability, especially in anxiety neuroses or organic (especially GI or CV) disorders—* **Adults:** 2 to 6 mg P.O. daily in divided doses. Maximum 10 mg daily. *Insomnia—* **Adults:** 2 to 4 mg h.s.	*CNS:* drowsiness, dizziness, weakness, lethargy, disorientation, ataxia, depression, psychomotor agitation, sleep disturbance, headache. *EENT:* blurred vision, diplopia. *GI:* nausea, change in appetite and weight, vomiting. *Skin:* rash.
meprobamate Controlled substance Schedule IV Arcoban, Bamate, Bamo-400, Equanil, Kalmm, Lan-Dol◆◆, Maso-Bamate, Meditran, Mep-E, Meprocon, Meprotabs, Meribam, Miltown◆, Neo-Tran◆◆, Novomepro◆◆, Pax-400, Quietal◆◆, Saronil, Sedabamate, SK-Bamate, Tranmep	*Sedation—* **Adults:** 1.2 to 1.6 g P.O. in 3 or 4 equally divided doses. Maximum 2.4 g daily. **Children 6 to 12 years:** 100 to 200 mg P.O. b.i.d. or t.i.d. Not recommended for children under 6 years.	*Blood:* thrombocytopenia, leukopenia, eosinophilia. *CNS:* drowsiness, ataxia, dizziness, slurred speech, headache, vertigo, weakness, paresthesia, euphoria, fast EEG activity. *CV:* palpitation, tachycardia, arrhythmias, fainting, hypotensive crisis. *EENT:* impaired vision. *GI:* anorexia, nausea, vomiting, diarrhea, stomatitis. *Skin:* pruritus, urticaria, erythematous maculopapular rash, petechiae, ecchymosis, exfoliative dermatitis, Stevens-Johnson syndrome, bullous dermatitis.
oxazepam Controlled substance Schedule IV Serax◆	*Alcohol withdrawal—* **Adults:** 15 to 30 mg P.O. t.i.d. or q.i.d. *Severe anxiety—* **Adults:** 15 to 30 mg P.O. t.i.d. or q.i.d. *Tension, mild to moderate anxiety—* **Adults:** 10 to 15 mg P.O. t.i.d. or q.i.d.	*Blood:* leukopenia. *CNS:* drowsiness, dizziness, vertigo, headache, sleep disturbances, excitement, fatigue, slurred speech, lethargy, tremor, ataxia. *CV:* palpitation, hypotension. *GI:* nausea, abdominal pain, hepatic dysfunction. *GU:* libido changes. *Skin:* rash, jaundice. *Other:* edema, hyperventilation, stomatitis.
prazepam Controlled substance Schedule IV Verstran	*Anxiety—* **Adults:** 30 mg P.O. in divided doses. Range 20 to 60 mg daily. May be administered as single daily dose at bedtime. Start with 20 mg.	*CNS:* fatigue, dizziness, weakness, drowsiness, light-headedness, ataxia, headache, confusion, tremor, vivid dreams, slurred speech, blurred vision, fainting. *CV:* palpitation, slight decrease in blood pressure, swelling of feet. *GI:* dry mouth, weight gain. *Skin:* pruritus, rash. *Other:* diaphoresis, joint pains.

INTERACTIONS	NURSING CONSIDERATIONS
None significant.	• Contraindicated in myasthenia gravis, acute narrow-angle glaucoma, psychosis, mental depression. Use with caution in organic brain syndrome, renal or hepatic impairment. • Dosage should be reduced in elderly or debilitated patients. • Do not withdraw drug abruptly. • Possibility of abuse, addiction exists. Withdrawal symptoms similar to those of barbiturates. • Warn patient not to drive or operate dangerous machinery until response to drug is determined. • Warn patient not to combine drug with alcohol or other depressants. • For symptoms and treatment of toxicity, see p. 1123.
None significant.	• Contraindicated in hypersensitivity to meprobamate, carisoprodol, mebutamate, tybamate, carbromal; renal insufficiency; porphyria. Use with caution in impaired hepatic or renal function, in lactation, and in patients with suicidal tendencies. • Dosage should be reduced in elderly or debilitated patients. • Withdraw drug gradually (over 2 weeks). • Possibility of abuse, addiction exists. • Warn patient to avoid activities that require alertness or good psychomotor coordination until response to drug is determined. • Warn patient not to combine drug with alcohol or other depressants. • Watch for respiratory failure, hypotension, EKG changes with doses over 800 mg. • Give I.M. deeply. • Give P.O. with meals to reduce gastric distress. • Therapeutic blood levels 0.5 to 2 mg/100 ml; levels above 20 mg/100 ml may cause coma and death.
None significant.	• Contraindicated in psychoses. Use cautiously in history of convulsive disorders, drug allergies, blood dyscrasias, hepatic or renal disease, depression. • Dose should be reduced in elderly or debilitated patients. • Do not withdraw drug abruptly. • Possibility of abuse, addiction exists. Withdrawal symptoms similar to those of barbiturates. • Warn patient to avoid activities that require alertness or good psychomotor coordination until response to drug is determined. • Warn patient not to combine drug with alcohol or other depressants. • Fewer cumulative effects due to short half-life. • For symptoms and treatment of toxicity, see p. 1123.
None significant.	• Contraindicated in acute narrow-angle glaucoma, psychosis, and psychiatric disorders not showing anxiety. Use with caution in renal or hepatic impairment. • Dosage should be reduced in elderly or debilitated patients. • Do not withdraw drug abruptly. • Possibility of abuse, addiction exists. Withdrawal symptoms similar to those of barbiturates. • Warn patient to avoid activities that require alertness and good psychomotor coordination until response to drug is determined. • Warn patient not to combine drug with alcohol or other depressants. • Benzodiazepine derivative. • May produce abnormal hepatic function tests. • For symptoms and treatment of toxicity, see p. 1123.

NAME	INDICATIONS & DOSAGE	SIDE EFFECTS
tybamate Controlled substance Schedule IV	*Anxiety and tension—* **Adults:** 750 mg to 2 g P.O. daily in divided doses; maximum 3 g daily. **Children 6 to 12 years:** 20 to 25 mg/Kg daily, divided into 3 or 4 doses.	*Blood:* dyscrasias. *CNS:* drowsiness, dizziness, fatigue, weakness, ataxia, depressive or panic reactions, paradoxical irritability, excitement, confusion, euphoria, insomnia, headache, paresthesia, petit and grand mal seizures (with large doses or when given with other psychotherapeutics). *CV:* flushing, light-headedness, hypotension, palpitation, tachycardia, fainting. *GI:* nausea, anorexia, dry mouth, glossitis. *Skin:* urticaria, pruritus, pruritus ani, rash.

INTERACTIONS	NURSING CONSIDERATIONS
None significant.	• Contraindicated in history of hypersensitivity to tybamate or related compounds, such as meprobamate, carisoprodol, or mebutamate; convulsive disorders; drug allergies; blood dyscrasias; lactation; porphyria. Use with caution in hepatic or renal dysfunction. • Dosage should be reduced in elderly or debilitated patients. • Do not withdraw drug abruptly. • Possibility of abuse, addiction exists. • Warn patient to avoid activities that require alertness and good psychomotor coordination until response to drug is determined. • Warn patient not to combine drug with alcohol or other depressants. • Shorter acting than meprobamate.

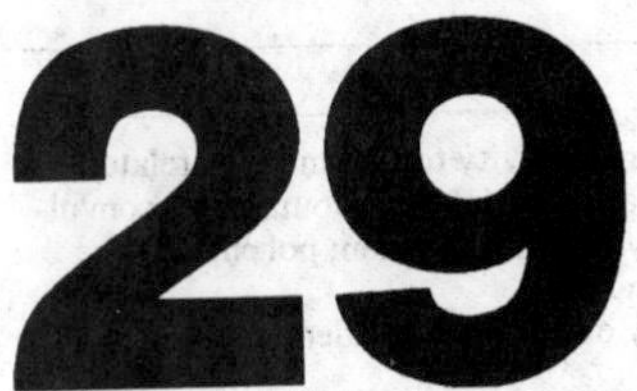

29 Antipsychotics

acetophanazine maleate
butaperazine maleate
carphenazine maleate
chlorpromazine hydrochloride
chlorprothixene
droperidol
fluphenazine
haloperidol
loxapine succinate
mesoridazine besylate
molindone hydrochloride
perphenazine
piperacetazine
prochlorperazine
promazine hydrochloride
thioridazine hydrochloride
thiothixene
trifluoperazine hydrochloride
triflupromazine hydrochloride

Antipsychotic (neuroleptic) drugs help control symptoms of acute and chronic schizophrenia but do not correct basic psychotic processes. They also treat organic psychoses and control acute mania in manic depression. These agents modify thought disorder, blunted affect, and psychomotor retardation, and lessen paranoid symptoms, agitation, hallucinations, delusions, and autistic behavior. Some are also used as antiemetics, antihistamines, or antipruritics. Since their advent in the early 1950s, these drugs have tremendously reduced the number of persons requiring institutionalization.

Five distinct chemical classes of drugs are used to treat schizophrenia: the phenothiazines, thiothixenes, butyrophenones, dibenzoxazepines, and the dihydroindoles. Many clinicians believe the phenothiazines should be treated as three distinct drug classes because of their differences in side effects (sedative properties, cardiovascular effects, and the potential for inducing neuromuscular or extrapyramidal syndromes). These three classes include the aliphatics (large potential to cause sedation and anticholinergic effects), the piperidines (large potential to cause sedation), and the piperazines (large potential to cause extrapyramidal reactions).

Because antipsychotics have many side effects, they should be reserved for major psychiatric illnesses. For lesser ailments, antianxiety drugs (chlordiazepoxide, meprobamate) or barbiturates (phenobarbital) are safer and probably more efficient.

Chlorpromazine was the first drug to be used as an antipsychotic, and 100 mg of chlorpromazine is the reference compound for all other drugs in this class.

Major uses

- Symptomatic treatment of acute and chronic psychoses, especially with increased psychomotor activity (including manic phase of manic-depressive illness, and schizophrenia).
- Control of nausea and vomiting.
- Control of agitation in organic brain syndromes.
- Management of acute agitation in alcohol withdrawal or alcoholic hallucinosis.

Mechanism of action

- Precise mechanism unknown.
- May block effects of dopamine, a neurotransmitter in brain. This blockage may also cause extrapyramidal side effects, which are common with many of these drugs.

Absorption, distribution, and excretion

- Oral absorption is good but highly variable from one patient to another. Oral absorption is best with the liquid concentrate forms.
- Intramuscular absorption is generally more complete. Approximately half of oral dose may be used parenterally for equal effect.
- Distributed to most body tissues.
- Highest concentrations of unchanged drug occur in the brain. Metabolites of the drugs predominate in lungs, liver, kidneys, and spleen.
- All antipsychotics metabolized in the liver.
- Phenothiazine metabolites are excreted in urine, bile, and feces; may be detected up to 6 months after stopping drug.

Onset and duration

- Peak plasma levels are reached in 2 to 6 hours for most agents.
- Some diminution of symptoms may occur with the first few doses, but maximum effects may not be seen for weeks to several months.
- Long half-lives permit once-daily dosing (usually bedtime).
- Divided dosages are sometimes necessary for drugs causing significant hypotension.
- Serum levels are variable, with tenfold differences possible between patients receiving identical doses.

Combination products

COMBID: prochlorperazine maleate 10 mg and isopropamide 5 mg.
ESKATROL: prochlorperazine maleate 7.5 mg and dextroamphetamine sulfate 15 mg.
ETRAFON (2-10): perphenazine 2 mg and amitriptyline 10 mg.
ETRAFON-A (4-10): perphenazine 2 mg and amitriptyline 25 mg.
ETRAFON-FORTE (4-25): perphenazine 4 mg and amitriptyline 25 mg.
LIMBITROL 10-25: chlordiazepoxide 10 mg and amitriptyline 25 mg.
LIMBITROL 5-12.5: chlordiazepoxide 5 mg and amitriptyline 12.5 mg.
TRIAVIL 2-10, TRIAVIL 4-10, TRIAVIL 2-25, TRIAVIL 4-25 are identical to Etrafon products listed above; TRIAVIL 4-50: perphenazine 4 mg and amitriptyline 50 mg.

NAME	INDICATIONS & DOSAGE	SIDE EFFECTS
acetophenazine maleate Tindal	*Psychosis, anxiety, tension, agitation, hyperexcitability in ambulatory patients—* **Adults:** initially, 20 mg P.O. t.i.d. or q.i.d. Daily dosage ranges from 40 to 80 mg in outpatients, or 80 to 120 mg in hospitalized patients, but in severe psychotic states up to 600 mg daily has been safely administered. Smallest effective dose should be used at all times.	The phenothiazines are related structurally and therefore have the potential to cause all the side effects listed; however, all may not have been reported with each drug. *Blood:* agranulocytosis and other dyscrasias. *CNS:* drowsiness, high incidence of extrapyramidal reactions (akathisia, acute dystonias, parkinsonism, tardive dyskinesias), EEG changes, headache, cerebral edema. *CV:* orthostatic hypotension (possible shock), hypertension, tachycardia, fainting, dizziness, bradycardia, pallor. *EENT:* visual impairment, nasal congestion. *GI:* anorexia, dyspepsia, constipation, diarrhea, cholestatic jaundice, paralytic ileus, excessive salivation, increased appetite, weight changes, "oral syndrome" (dry mouth; gum changes; stomatitis; cracked lips; white or black hairy tongue; bald, beefy, red tongue; pseudomembrane in mouth). *GU:* dark urine, difficult urination, incontinence, delayed ovulation, menstrual irregularities, changed libido, impotence, inhibited ejaculation, glycosuria. *Metabolic:* hyper- and hypoglycemia, hyper- and hypothermia. *Skin:* photosensitivity (yellowish-brown or grayish-purple pigment deposits after sun exposure), excessive sweating, dermatoses (erythematous and eczematous). *Other:* heat prostration, respiratory distress, asthma, edema (laryngeal, angioneurotic, peripheral), gynecomastia, lactation. *After abrupt withdrawal:* gastritis, nausea, vomiting, dizziness, tremors, feeling of warmth or cold, sweating, tachycardia, headache, insomnia.
butaperazine maleate Repoise	*Chronic schizophrenia—* **Adults:** initially, 5 to 10 mg P.O. t.i.d. Increase gradually to maximum 100 mg daily. Use lowest effective dose.	The phenothiazines are related structurally and therefore have the potential to cause all the side effects listed; however, all may not have been reported with each drug. *Blood:* agranulocytosis and other dyscrasias. *CNS:* drowsiness, high incidence of extrapyramidal reactions (akathisia,

• Also available in Canada.
•• Available in Canada only.
Unmarked trade names available in United States only.

INTERACTIONS	NURSING CONSIDERATIONS
Antacids: inhibited absorption of oral phenothiazines. Separate antacid and phenothiazine dosage by at least 2 hours. *Anticholinergics (including antidepressant and antiparkinson agents):* increased anticholinergic activity, aggravated parkinson-like symptoms. Use with caution. *Barbiturates:* may decrease phenothiazine effect. Observe patient.	• Contraindicated in history of coma; CNS depression; bone marrow depression; subcortical damage; use of spinal or epidural anesthesia, or adrenergic blocking agents. Use cautiously with other CNS depressants, anticholinergics; in hepatic disease, elderly or debilitated patients, arteriosclerosis or cardiovascular disease (may cause sudden drop in blood pressure), exposure to extreme heat or cold (including antipyretic therapy), respiratory disorders, hypocalcemia, convulsive disorders, severe reactions to insulin or electroshock therapy, suspected brain tumor or intestinal obstruction, glaucoma, or prostatic hypertrophy. • Hold dose and notify doctor if patient develops symptoms of blood dyscrasias (fever, sore throat, infection, cellulitis, weakness), persistent (longer than a few hours) extrapyramidal reactions, or any such reaction during pregnancy. • Dose of 20 mg is therapeutic equivalent of 100 mg chlorpromazine. • Monitor therapy by weekly bilirubin tests during first month; periodic blood tests (CBC, hepatic function, blood sugar) and ophthalmic tests (long-term use). • Check intake and output for urinary retention or constipation. • Tell patient to use sunscreening agents and protective clothing to avoid photosensitivity reactions. • Warn against activities that require alertness or good psychomotor coordination until response to drug is determined. • Watch for orthostatic hypotension. Advise patient to get up slowly. • Dry mouth may be relieved with gum, sour hard candy, or rinsing with mouthwash. • Avoid combining with alcohol or other depressants. • Do not withdraw abruptly unless required by severe side effects. • Patient on maintainence may take medication at bedtime to facilitate sleep and decrease sedation during daytime. • For symptoms and treatment of toxicity, see p. 1120.
Antacids: inhibited absorption of oral phenothiazines. Separate antacid and phenothiazine dosage by at least 2 hours. *Anticholinergics (including antidepressant and antiparkin-*	• Contraindicated in history of coma; CNS depression; bone marrow depression; subcortical damage; use of spinal or epidural anesthetic, or adrenergic blocking agents. Use cautiously with other CNS depressants, anticholinergics; in hepatic disease, elderly or debilitated patients, arteriosclerosis or cardiovascular disease (may cause sudden drop in blood pressure), exposure to extreme heat or cold (including antipyretic therapy), respiratory disorders, hypocalcemia, acutely ill or dehydrated children, convulsive disorders, severe reactions to insulin or electroshock therapy, suspected brain tumor or intestinal obstruction, glaucoma, or prostatic

(continued on following page)

NAME	INDICATIONS & DOSAGE	SIDE EFFECTS
butaperazine maleate *(continued)*		acute dystonias, parkinsonism, tardive dyskinesias), EEG changes, headache, cerebral edema. *CV:* orthostatic hypotension (possible shock), tachycardia, fainting, dizziness, bradycardia, pallor. *EENT:* visual impairment, nasal congestion. *GI:* anorexia, dyspepsia, constipation, diarrhea, cholestatic jaundice, paralytic ileus, excessive salivation, increased appetite, "oral syndrome" (dry mouth; gum changes; stomatitis; cracked lips; white or black hairy tongue; bald, beefy, red tongue). *GU:* dark urine, difficult urination, incontinence, delayed ovulation, menstrual irregularities, changed libido, impotence, inhibited ejaculation, glycosuria. *Metabolic:* hyper- and hypoglycemia, hyper- and hypothermia. *Skin:* photosensitivity (yellowish-brown or grayish-purple pigment deposits after sun exposure); excessive sweating; dermatoses (erythematous and eczematous). *Other:* heat prostration, respiratory distress, asthma, edema (laryngeal, angioneurotic, peripheral), gynecomastia, lactation. *After abrupt withdrawal:* gastritis, nausea, vomiting, dizziness, tremors, feeling of warmth or cold, sweating, tachycardia, headache, insomnia.
carphenazine maleate Proketazine	*Acute and chronic schizophrenia—* **Adults:** initially, 12.5 to 50 mg P.O., b.i.d. or t.i.d. Increase gradually to maximum 100 mg daily.	The phenothiazines are related structurally and therefore have the potential to cause all the side effects listed; however, all may not have been reported with each drug. *Blood:* agranulocytosis and other dyscrasias. *CNS:* headache, high incidence of extrapyramidal reactions (akathisia, acute dystonias, parkinsonism, tardive dyskinesias), moderate incidence of sedation, EEG changes, cerebral edema. *CV:* orthostatic hypotension (possible shock), tachycardia, fainting, dizziness, bradycardia, pallor. *EENT:* visual impairment, nasal congestion. *GI:* anorexia, dyspepsia, constipation, diarrhea, cholestatic jaundice, excessive salivation, paralytic ileus, in-

INTERACTIONS	NURSING CONSIDERATIONS
son agents): increased anticholinergic activity; aggravated parkinson-like symptoms. Use with caution. *Barbiturates:* may decrease phenothiazine effect. Observe patient.	hypertrophy. • Hold dose and notify doctor if patient develops symptoms of jaundice, blood dyscrasias (fever, sore throat, infection, cellulitis, weakness), persistent (longer than a few hours) extrapyramidal reactions, or any such reaction in children. • Patients on maintenance may take medication at bedtime to facilitate sleep and decrease sedation during the daytime. • Monitor therapy by weekly bilirubin tests during first month; periodic blood tests (CBC, hepatic function, blood sugar) and ophthalmic tests (long-term use). • Check intake and output for urinary retention or constipation. • Watch for possible addiction. • Tell patient to use sunscreening agents and protective clothing to avoid photosensitivity reactions. • Warn against activities that require alertness or good psychomotor coordination, until response to drug is determined. Drowsiness and dizziness usually subside after first few weeks. • Watch for orthostatic hypotension. Advise patient to get up slowly. • If dry mouth or nasal congestion occurs, symptoms may diminish in a week or two. Dry mouth may be relieved with gum, sour hard candy, or rinsing with mouthwash. • Do not withdraw abruptly unless required by severe side effects. • Avoid combining with alcohol or other depressants. • Dose of 10 mg is therapeutic equivalent of 100 mg chlorpromazine. • For symptoms and treatment of toxicity, see p. 1120.
Antacids: inhibited absorption of oral phenothiazines. Separate antacid and phenothiazine dosage by at least 2 hours. *Anticholinergics (including antidepressant and antiparkinson agents):* increased anticholinergic activity, aggravated parkinson-like symptoms. Use with caution. *Barbiturates:* may decrease phenothiazine effect. Observe patient.	• Contraindicated in history of coma; CNS depression; bone marrow depression; subcortical damage; use of spinal or epidural anesthesia, or adrenergic blocking agents. Use cautiously with other CNS depressants, anticholinergics; in hepatic disease, elderly or debilitated patients, arteriosclerosis or cardiovascular disease (may cause sudden drop in blood pressure), exposure to extreme heat or cold (including antipyretic therapy), respiratory disorders, hypocalcemia, acutely ill or dehydrated children, convulsive disorders, severe reactions to insulin or electroshock therapy, suspected brain tumor or intestinal obstruction, glaucoma, or prostatic hypertrophy. • Hold dose and notify doctor if patient develops symptoms of jaundice, blood dyscrasias (fever, sore throat, infection, cellulitis, weakness) or persistent (longer than a few hours) extrapyramidal reactions. • Monitor therapy by weekly bilirubin tests during first month; periodic blood tests (CBC, hepatic function, blood sugar) and ophthalmic tests (long-term use). • Check intake and output for urinary retention or constipation. • Tell patient to use sunscreening agents and protective clothing to avoid photosensitivity reactions. • Warn against activities that require alertness or good psychomotor coordination until response to drug is determined. Drowsiness and dizziness

(continued on following page)

NAME	INDICATIONS & DOSAGE	SIDE EFFECTS
carphenazine maleate *(continued)*		creased appetite, weight changes, "oral syndrome" (dry mouth; gum changes; stomatitis; cracked lips; white or black hairy tongue; bald, beefy, red tongue). *GU:* dark urine, difficult urination, incontinence, delayed ovulation, menstrual irregularities, changed libido, impotency, inhibited ejaculation, glycosuria. *Metabolic:* hyper- and hypoglycemia, hyper- and hypothermia. *Skin:* photosensitivity (yellowish-brown or grayish-purple pigment deposits after sun exposure), excessive sweating, dermatoses (erythematous and eczematous). *Other:* heat prostration, respiratory distress, asthma, edema (laryngeal, angioneurotic, peripheral), gynecomastia, lactation. *After abrupt withdrawal:* gastritis, nausea, vomiting, dizziness, tremors, feeling of warmth or cold, sweating, tachycardia, headache, insomnia.
chlorpromazine hydrochloride Chlorprom♦♦, Chlor-Promanyl♦♦, Chlorzine, Klorazine, Klomazine, Largactil♦♦, Omazine, Ormazine, Promachel, Promachlor, Promapar, Promaz, Sonazine, Terpium, Thoradex, Thorazine	*Intractable hiccups—* **Adults:** 25 to 50 mg P.O. or I.M. t.i.d. or q.i.d. *Mild alcohol withdrawal, acute intermittent porphyria, and tetanus—* **Adults:** 25 to 50 mg I.M. t.i.d. or q.i.d. *Nausea and vomiting—* **Adults:** 10 to 25 mg P.O. or I.M. q 4 to 6 hours, p.r.n.; or 50 to 100 mg rectally q 6 to 8 hours, p.r.n. **Children:** 0.25 mg/Kg P.O. q 4 to 6 hours; or 0.25 mg/Kg I.M. q 6 to 8 hours; or 0.5 mg/Kg rectally q 6 to 8 hours. *Psychosis—* **Adults:** 500 mg P.O. daily in divided doses, increasing gradually to 2 g; or 25 to 50 mg I.M. q 1 to 4 hours, p.r.n. **Children:** 0.25 mg/Kg P.O. q 4 to 6 hours; or 0.25 mg/Kg I.M. q 6 to 8 hours; or 0.5 mg/Kg rectally q 6 to 8 hours. Maximum dose is 40 mg in children under 5 years, and 75 mg in children 5 to 12 years.	The phenothiazines are related structurally and therefore have the potential to cause all the side effects listed; however, all may not have been reported with each drug. *Blood:* agranulocytosis and other dyscrasias. *CNS:* drowsiness, moderate incidence of extrapyramidal reactions (akathisia, acute dystonias, pseudoparkinsonism, tardive dyskinesias), headache, *EEG* changes, cerebral edema. *CV:* postural hypotension (possible shock), tachycardia, fainting, dizziness, arrhythmias, pallor. *EENT:* visual impairment, nasal congestion. *GI:* anorexia, dyspepsia, constipation, diarrhea, excessive salivation, cholestatic jaundice, paralytic ileus, increased appetite, weight gain, "oral syndrome" (dry mouth; gum changes; stomatitis; cracked lips; white or black hairy tongue; bald, beefy, red tongue; pseudomembrane in mouth). *GU:* dark or pinkish urine, difficult urination, incontinence, delayed ovulation, menstrual irregularities, changed libido, impotence, inhibited ejaculation, glycosuria. *Metabolic:* hyper- and hypoglycemia,

INTERACTIONS	NURSING CONSIDERATIONS
	usually subside after a few weeks. • Watch for orthostatic hypotension. Advise patient to get up slowly. • Avoid combining with alcohol or other depressants. • Do not withdraw abruptly unless required by severe side effects. • Dry mouth may be relieved by gum, sour hard candy, or rinsing with mouthwash. • Dose of 25 mg is therapeutic equivalent of 100 mg chlorpromazine. • For symptoms and treatment of toxicity, see p. 1120.
Antacids: inhibited absorption of oral phenothiazines. Separate antacid and phenothiazine dosage by at least 2 hours. *Anticholinergics (including antidepressant and antiparkinson agents):* increased anticholinergic activity, aggravated parkinson-like symptoms. Use with caution. *Barbiturates:* may decrease phenothiazine effect. Observe patient. *Lithium:* possible decreased response to chlorpromazine. Observe patient.	• Contraindicated in history of coma; CNS depression; bone marrow depression; subcortical damage; use of spinal or epidural anesthesia, or adrenergic blocking agents; Reye's syndrome. Use cautiously with other CNS depressants, anticholinergics; in hepatic disease, elderly or debilitated patients, arteriosclerosis or cardiovascular disease (may cause sudden drop in blood pressure), exposure to extreme heat or cold (including antipyretic therapy), respiratory disorders, hypocalcemia, acutely ill or dehydrated children, convulsive disorders, severe reactions to insulin or electroshock therapy, suspected brain tumor or intestinal obstruction, glaucoma, or prostatic hypertrophy. • Hold dose and notify doctor if patient develops jaundice, symptoms of blood dyscrasias (fever, sore throat, infection, cellulitis, weakness), persistent (longer than a few hours) extrapyramidal reactions, or any such reaction in pregnancy or in children. • Monitor therapy by weekly bilirubin tests during first month; periodic blood tests (CBC, hepatic function, blood sugar) and ophthalmic tests (long-term use). • Check intake and output for urinary retention or constipation. • Tell patient to use sunscreening agents and protective clothing to avoid photosensitivity reactions. • Warn against activities that require alertness or good psychomotor coordination until response to drug is determined. Drowsiness and dizziness usually subside after first few weeks. • Watch for orthostatic hypotension, especially with parenteral administration. Monitor blood pressure before and after I.M. administration. Keep patient supine for 1 hour afterward. Advise patient to get up slowly. • Avoid combining with alcohol or other depressants. • Give I.M. only in upper outer quadrant of buttocks. Massage slowly afterward to prevent sterile abscess. Injection may sting. • Prevent contact dermatitis by keeping drug off patient's skin and clothes. • Protect liquid concentrate from light. Dilute with fruit juice, milk, or

(continued on following page)

NAME	INDICATIONS & DOSAGE	SIDE EFFECTS
chlorpromazine hydrochloride *(continued)*		hyper- and hypothermia. *Skin:* photosensitivity (yellowish-brown or grayish-purple pigment deposits after sun exposure), excessive sweating, dermatoses (erythematous and eczematous). *Other:* heat prostration, respiratory distress, asthma, edema (laryngeal, angioneurotic, peripheral), gynecomastia, lactation. *After abrupt withdrawal:* gastritis, nausea, vomiting, dizziness, tremors, feeling of warmth or cold, sweating, tachycardia, headache, insomnia.
chlorprothixene Taractan, Tarasan◆◆	*Agitation of mild neurosis, depression, schizophrenia—* **Adults:** initially, 10 mg P.O. t.i.d. or q.i.d. Increase gradually to maximum 60 mg daily. **Children over 6 years:** 10 to 25 mg P.O. t.i.d. or q.i.d. *Agitation of severe neurosis, depression, schizophrenia—* **Adults:** 25 to 50 mg P.O. or I.M. t.i.d. or q.i.d. Increase as needed up to maximum 600 mg.	The thiothixenes are related structurally to the phenothiazines, and therefore have the potential to cause all the side effects listed; however, all may not have been reported with this drug. *Blood:* agranulocytosis and other dyscrasias. *CNS:* headache, low to moderate incidence of extrapyramidal reactions (akathisia, acute dystonias, parkinsonism, tardive dyskinesias), high incidence of sedation, EEG changes, cerebral edema. *CV:* orthostatic hypotension (possible shock), tachycardia, fainting, dizziness, bradycardia, pallor. *EENT:* visual impairment, nasal congestion. *GI:* anorexia, dyspepsia, constipation, diarrhea, excessive salivation, cholestatic jaundice, paralytic ileus, increased appetite, weight gain, "oral syndrome" (dry mouth; gum changes; stomatitis; cracked lips; white or black hairy tongue; bald, beefy, red tongue; pseudomembrane in mouth). *GU:* dark urine, difficult urination, anuria, bile and increased urinary acid in urine incontinence, delayed ovulation, menstrual irregularities, changed libido, impotence, inhibited ejaculation, glycosuria. *Metabolic:* hyper- and hypoglycemia, hyper- and hypothermia. *Skin:* photosensitivity (yellowish-brown or grayish-purple pigment deposits after sun exposure), excessive sweating, dermatoses (erythematous and eczematous). *Other:* heat prostration, respiratory distress, asthma, edema (laryngeal,

INTERACTIONS	NURSING CONSIDERATIONS
	semisolid food just before administration. • Slight yellowing of injection or concentrate is common; does not affect potency. Discard markedly discolored solutions. • Do not withdraw abruptly unless required by severe side effects. • Dry mouth may be relieved by gum, sour hard candy, or rinsing with mouthwash. • An aliphatic; has greater tendency to cause anticholinergic side effects. • For symptoms and treatment of toxicity, see p. 1120.
Anticholinergics (including antidepressant and antiparkinson agents): increased anticholinergic activity, aggravated parkinson-like symptoms. Use with caution.	• Contraindicated in coma, CNS depression, bone marrow depression, circulatory collapse, congestive failure, cardiac decompensation, coronary artery or cerebral vascular disorders, subcortical damage, use of spinal or epidural anesthesia or adrenergic blocking agents. Use cautiously with other CNS depressants, anticholinergics; in hepatic or renal disease, elderly or debilitated patients, arteriosclerosis or cardiovascular disease (may cause sudden drop in blood pressure), exposure to extreme heat or cold (including antipyretic therapy), respiratory disorders, hypocalcemia, acutely ill or dehydrated children, convulsive disorders, severe reactions to insulin or electroshock therapy, suspected brain tumor or intestinal obstruction, glaucoma, or prostatic hypertrophy. • Hold dose and notify doctor if patient develops symptoms of blood dyscrasias (fever, sore throat, infection, cellulitis, weakness), jaundice, persistent (longer than a few hours) extrapyramidal reactions, or any such reactions in children. • Monitor therapy by weekly bilirubin tests during first month; periodic blood tests (CBC, hepatic function, blood sugar) before and during therapy; and ophthalmic tests (long-term therapy). • Check intake and output for urinary retention or constipation. • Tell patient to use sunscreening agents and protective clothing to avoid photosensitivity reactions. • Warn against activities that require alertness or good psychomotor coordination until response to drug is determined. Drowsiness and dizziness usually subside after first few weeks. • Watch for orthostatic hypotension, especially with parenteral administration, since adrenergic blockage is high. Keep patient supine for 1 hour afterward. Advise patient to change positions slowly. • Avoid combining with alcohol or other depressants. • Give I.M. deeply only in upper outer quadrant of buttocks or midlateral thigh. Massage slowly afterward to prevent sterile abscess. Injection may sting. • Dilute liquid concentrate with fruit juice, milk, or semisolid food just before administration. • Protect medication from light. Slight yellowing of injection or concentrate is common; does not affect potency. Discard markedly discolored solutions. • Do not withdraw abruptly unless required by severe side effects. • Prevent contact dermatitis by keeping drug off patient's skin and clothes. • Dry mouth may be relieved by gum, sour hard candy, or rinsing with mouthwash. • Dose of 100 mg is therapeutic equivalent of 100 mg chlorpromazine.

(continued on following page)

NAME	INDICATIONS & DOSAGE	SIDE EFFECTS
chlorprothixene *(continued)*		angioneurotic, peripheral), gynecomastia, lactation. *After abrupt withdrawal:* gastritis, nausea, vomiting, dizziness, tremors, feeling of warmth or cold, sweating, tachycardia, headache, insomnia.
droperidol Inapsine♦	*Premedication—* **Adults:** 2.5 to 10 mg (1 to 4 ml) I.M. 30 to 60 minutes preop. **Children 2 to 12 years:** 1 to 1.5 mg (0.4 to 0.6 ml) I.M. per 20 to 25 lbs. of body weight. *As induction agent—* **Adults:** 2.5 mg (1 ml) per 20 to 25 lbs I.V. with analgesic and/or general anesthetic. **Children 2 to 12 years:** 1 to 1.5 mg (0.4 to 0.6 ml) per 20 to 25 lbs I.V. Dose should be titrated. **Elderly, debilitated:** initial dose should be decreased. *Maintenance dose in general anesthesia*—1.25 to 2.5 mg (0.5 to 1 ml) I.V.	*CNS:* extrapyramidal reactions (dystonia, akathisia), upward rotation of eyes and oculogyric crises, extended neck, flexed arms, fine tremor of limbs, dizziness, chills or shivering, facial sweating, restlessness. *CV:* hypotension, tachycardia.
fluphenazine decanoate Modecate Decanoate♦♦, Prolixin Decanoate **fluphenazine enanthate** Moditen♦, Prolixin Enanthate **fluphenazine hydrochloride** Moditen Hydrochloride♦♦, Permitil Hydrochloride, Prolixin Hydrochloride	*Psychomotor agitation in schizophrenia—* **Adults:** initially, 0.5 to 10 mg fluphenazine HCl P.O. daily in divided doses q 6 to 8 hours; may increase cautiously to 20 mg. Higher doses (50 to 100 mg) have been given. Maintenance: 1 to 5 mg P.O. daily. I.M. doses are ⅓ to ½ oral doses. Lower doses for geriatric patients (1 to 2.5 mg daily). **Children:** 0.25 to 3.5 mg fluphenazine HCl P.O. daily in divided doses q 4 to 6 hours; or ⅓ to ½ of oral dose I.M.; maximum 10 mg daily. **Adults, and children over 12 years:** 12.5 to 25 mg of long-acting esters (fluphenazine decanoate and enanthate) I.M. or S.C. q 1 to 6 weeks. Maintenance: 25 to 100 mg, p.r.n.	The phenothiazines are related structurally and therefore have the potential to cause all the side effects listed; however, all may not have been reported with each drug. *Blood:* agranulocytosis and other dyscrasias. *CNS:* headache, high incidence of extrapyramidal reactions (akathisia, acute dystonias, parkinsonism, tardive dyskinesias), low to moderate incidence of sedation, EEG changes, cerebral edema, mental depression. *CV:* orthostatic hypotension (possible shock), hypertension, blood pressure fluctuations, tachycardia, fainting, dizziness, pallor. *EENT:* visual impairment, nasal congestion. *GI:* anorexia, dyspepsia, nausea, constipation, diarrhea, excessive salivation, cholestatic jaundice, paralytic ileus, increased appetite, weight gain, "oral syndrome" (dry mouth; gum changes; stomatitis; cracked lips; white or black hairy tongue; bald, beefy red tongue; pseudomembrane in mouth). *GU:* dark urine, difficult urination,

INTERACTIONS	NURSING CONSIDERATIONS
None significant.	• Use cautiously in elderly or debilitated patients; hypotension or other cardiovascular disease; impaired hepatic or renal function; Parkinson's disease. • Watch for extrapyramidal reactions. Call doctor at once if any occur. • Approved by FDA *only* for use preop and during induction and maintenance of anesthesia. • A butyrophenone compound, related to haloperidol; has greater tendency to cause extrapyramidal reactions. • Keep intravenous fluids and vasopressors handy to manage hypotension. • If used with a narcotic analgesic such as fentamyl (Sublimaze), be familiar with the special properties of each drug, particularly the widely differing durations of action. Watch for respiratory depression, apnea, and muscular rigidity, which could lead to respiratory arrest if untreated. Have narcotic antagonist and CPR equipment on hand. • Monitor vital signs frequently; notify doctor of any changes immediately. • Give intravenous injections slowly. • Do not place patient in head-down position (i.e., shock), as severe hypotension and deeper anesthesia may result, causing respiratory arrest. • Has been used to prevent cis-platinum-associated nausea and vomiting.
Antacids: inhibited absorption of oral phenothiazines. Separate antacid and phenothiazine dosage by at least 2 hours. *Anticholinergics (including antidepressant and antiparkinson agents):* increased anticholinergic activity, aggravated parkinson-like symptoms. Use with caution. *Barbiturates:* may decrease phenothiazine effect. Observe patient.	• Contraindicated in coma, CNS depression, bone marrow depression or other blood dyscrasia, subcortical damage, use of spinal or epidural anesthesia or adrenergic blocking agents, hepatic damage, renal insufficiency. Use cautiously with other CNS depressants, anticholinergics; in hepatic disease, elderly or debilitated patients, pheochromocytoma, arteriosclerotic, cerebrovascular, or cardiovascular disease (may cause sudden drop in blood pressure), peptic ulcer, exposure to extreme heat or cold (including antipyretic therapy); respiratory disorders; hypocalcemia; acutely ill or dehydrated children; convulsive disorders; severe reactions to insulin or electroshock therapy; suspected brain tumor or intestinal obstruction; glaucoma; or prostatic hypertrophy. • Hold dose and notify doctor if patient develops symptoms of blood dyscrasias (fever, sore throat, infection, cellulitis, weakness), persistent (longer than a few hours) extrapyramidal reactions, or any such reactions in pregnancy or in children. • Monitor therapy by weekly bilirubin tests during first month; periodic blood tests (CBC, hepatic function, blood sugar); periodic renal function and ophthalmic tests (long-term use). • Check intake and output for urinary retention or constipation. • Tell patient to use sunscreening agents and protective clothing to avoid photosensitivity reactions. • Warn against activities that require alertness and good psychomotor coordination until response to drug is determined. Drowsiness and dizziness usually subside after first few weeks. • Avoid combining with alcohol or other depressants. • Watch for orthostatic hypotension, especially with parenteral administration. Monitor blood pressure before and after I.M. administration. Keep patient supine for 1 hour afterward. Advise him to change positions slowly. • Give I.M. deeply in upper outer quadrant of buttocks. Massage slowly afterward to prevent sterile abscess. Injection may sting.

(continued on following page)

NAME	INDICATIONS & DOSAGE	SIDE EFFECTS
fluphenazine *(continued)*		polyuria, incontinence, delayed ovulation, menstrual irregularities, changed libido, impotence, inhibited ejaculation, glycosuria. *Metabolic:* hyper- and hypoglycemia, hyper- and hypothermia. *Skin:* photosensitivity (yellowish-brown or grayish-purple pigment deposits after sun exposure), excessive sweating, dermatoses (erythematous and eczematous). *Other:* heat prostration, respiratory distress, fever, asthma, edema (laryngeal, angioneurotic, peripheral), gynecosmastia, lactation. *After abrupt withdrawal:* gastritis, nausea, vomiting, dizziness, tremors, feeling of warmth or cold, sweating, tachycardia, headache, insomnia.
haloperidol Haldol♦	*Agitation in schizophrenia, manic phase of manic-depressive psychosis, psychotic reactions in organic brain damage and mental retardation—* **Adults:** dosage varies for each patient. Initial range is 0.5 to 5 mg P.O. b.i.d. or t.i.d.; or 2 to 5 mg I.M. q 4 to 8 hours, increasing rapidly if necessary for prompt control. Maximum 100 mg P.O. daily. Doses over 100 mg have been used for severely resistant patients. *Control of tics, vocal utterances in Gilles de la Tourette's syndrome—* **Adults:** 0.5 to 5 mg P.O. b.i.d. or t.i.d., increasing p.r.n.	The butyrophenones are related structurally to the phenothiazines, and therefore have the potential to cause all the side effects listed; however, all may not have been reported with this drug. *Blood:* transient leukopenia and leukocytosis, decreased serum cholesterol and red blood cells. *CNS:* high incidence of severe extrapyramidal reactions (akathisia, acute dystonias, parkinsonism, tardive dyskinesias), oculogyric crisis, torticollis, opisthotonos, hyperreflexia, insomnia, restlessness, anxiety, euphoria, grand mal seizures, hallucinations, depression, confusion, headache, vertigo, low incidence of sedation. *CV:* low incidence of cardiovascular effects; peripheral edema, tachycardia, hypotension. *EENT:* blurred vision, ocular changes. *GI:* constipation, dry mouth, anorexia, diarrhea, nausea, vomiting, excessive salivation, dyspepsia, jaundice. *GU:* urinary retention, incontinence, impotence, mastalgia, menstrual irregularities, inhibited ejaculation, increased libido. *Metabolic:* hyper- and hypoglycemia. *Skin:* rash, sweating, cutaneous changes. *Other:* laryngospasm, bronchospasm, reduced depth of respiration, bronchopneumonia, breast engorgement

NAME	INDICATIONS & DOSAGE	SIDE EFFECTS
	• For long-acting forms (decanoate and enanthate), which are oil preparations, use a dry needle of at least 21 gauge. Allow 24 to 96 hours for onset of action. • Prevent contact dermatitis by keeping drug off patient's skin and clothes. • Dilute liquid concentrate with water, fruit juice, milk, or semisolid food just before administration. • Protect medication from light. Slight yellowing of injection or concentrate is common; does not affect potency. Discard markedly discolored solutions. • Dry mouth may be relieved by gum, sour hard candy, or rinsing with mouthwash. • Do not withdraw abruptly unless required by severe side effects. • Dose of 2 mg is therapeutic equivalent of 100 mg chlorpromazine. • For symptoms and treatment of toxicity, see p. 1120.	
Anticholinergics (including antidepressant and antiparkinson agents): increased anticholinergic activity; aggravated parkinson-like symptoms. Use with extreme caution. *Lithium:* lethargy and confusion with high doses. Observe patient. *Methyldopa:* possible symptoms of dementia. Observe patient.	• Contraindicated in seizures, parkinsonism, coma, severe depression, or CNS depression. Use with caution in severe cardiovascular disorders; allergies; elderly and debilitated patients; conjunction with anticonvulsant, anticoagulant, antiparkinson, or lithium medications; glaucoma; urinary retention. • Warn patient against activities that require alertness and good psychomotor coordination until response to drug is determined. Drowsiness and dizziness usually subside after a few weeks. • Avoid combining with alcohol or other depressants. • Monitor therapy by periodic blood tests (blood sugar, hepatic function, CBC). Monitor blood pressure before and after I.M. administration. Keep patient supine for 30 minutes afterward. • Give I.M. deeply. • Protect medication from light. Slight yellowing of injection or concentrate is common; does not affect potency. Discard markedly discolored solutions. • Prevent contact dermatitis by keeping drug off patient's skin and clothes. • Do not withdraw abruptly unless required by severe side effects. • Dry mouth may be relieved by gum, sour hard candy, and rinsing with mouthwash. • Dose of 2 mg is therapeutic equivalent of 100 mg chlorpromazine. • Only butyrophenone compound used as an antipsychotic in the U.S.	

(continued on following page)

NAME	INDICATIONS & DOSAGE	SIDE EFFECTS
haloperidol *(continued)*		and lactation, gynecomastia. *After abrupt withdrawal:* transient dyskinetic signs that are indistinguishable from tardive dyskinesias.
loxapine succinate Daxolin, Loxapac♦♦, Loxitane, Loxitane-C	*Disorientation, hallucinations, withdrawal, hostility of schizophrenia*— **Adults:** 10 mg P.O. b.i.d. to q.i.d., rapidly increasing to 60 to 100 mg P.O. daily for most patients; dose varies from patient to patient. Maximum 250 mg daily.	The dibenzoxazepines are related structurally to the phenothiazines, and therefore have the potential to cause all the side effects listed; however, all may not have been reported with this drug. *Blood:* dyscrasias. *CNS:* high incidence of extrapyramidal reactions (akathisia, acute dystonias, parkinsonism, tardive dyskinesias); high incidence of sedation, but tolerance usually develops with continued therapy; dizziness; lethargy; light-headedness; headache; ataxia; weakness; confusion; paresthesias; ptosis; dyspnea; hyperpyrexia; seizure. *CV:* hypotension, hypertension, tachycardia, fainting. *EENT:* blurred vision, retinopathy, tinnitus, nasal congestion. *GI:* constipation, nausea, dry mouth, vomiting, excessive salivation. *GU:* incontinence, impotence, inhibited ejaculation. *Skin:* dermatitis, pruritus, seborrhea, rashes, sweating. *Other:* polydipsia, flushed face, facial edema.
mesoridazine besylate Serentil♦	*Alcoholism*— **Adults, and children over 12 years:** 25 mg P.O. b.i.d. up to maximum 200 mg daily. *Behavioral problems associated with chronic brain syndrome*— **Adults, and children over 12 years:** 25 mg P.O. t.i.d. up to maximum of 300 mg daily. *Psychoneurotic manifestations (anxiety)*— **Adults, and children over 12 years:** 10 mg P.O. t.i.d. up to maximum 150 mg daily. *Schizophrenia*— **Adults, and children over 12 years:** initially, 50 mg P.O. t.i.d., increasing to maximum 400 mg daily, or 25 mg I.M. repeated in 30 to 60 minutes, p.r.n., up to 200 mg daily.	The phenothiazines are related structurally and therefore have the potential to cause all the side effects listed; however, all may not have been reported with each drug. *Blood:* agranulocytosis and other dyscrasias. *CNS:* high incidence of sedation, low incidence of extrapyramidal reactions (akathisia, acute dystonias, parkinsonism, tardive dyskinesias), headache, EEG changes, cerebral edema. *CV:* orthostatic hypotension (possible shock), tachycardia, fainting, dizziness, arrhythmias, pallor. *EENT:* visual impairment, nasal congestion. *GI:* anorexia, excessive salivation, dyspepsia, constipation, diarrhea, cholestatic jaundice, paralytic ileus, increased appetite, weight gain, "oral syndrome" (dry mouth; gum changes;

INTERACTIONS	NURSING CONSIDERATIONS
None significant.	• Contraindicated in convulsive disorders, coma, severe CNS depression, drug-induced depressed states. Use with caution in epilepsy, cardiovascular disorders, glaucoma, urinary retention, suspected intestinal obstruction or brain tumor, renal damage. • Warn against activities that require alertness and good psychomotor coordination until response to drug is determined. Drowsiness and dizziness usually subside after first few weeks. • Avoid combining with alcohol or other depressants. • Advise patient to get up slowly to avoid orthostatic hypotension. • Dilute liquid concentrate with orange or grapefruit juice just before giving. • Dry mouth may be relieved by gum, sour hard candy, or rinsing with mouthwash. • Monitor blood pressure. • Periodic ophthalmic tests recommended. • Tricyclic dibenzoxazepine; the only dibenzoxazepine derivative. • Dose of 10 mg is therapeutic equivalent of 100 mg chlorpromazine.
Antacids: inhibited absorption of oral phenothiazines. Separate antacid and phenothiazine dosage by at least 2 hours. *Anticholinergics (including antidepressant and antiparkinson agents):* increased anticholinergic activity, aggravated parkinson-like symptoms. Use with caution. *Barbiturates:* may decrease phenothiazine effect. Observe patient.	• Contraindicated in coma, CNS depression, bone marrow depression, subcortical damage, use of spinal or epidural anesthesia or adrenergic blocking agents. Use cautiously with other CNS depressants, anticholinergics; in hepatic disease, elderly or debilitated patients, arteriosclerosis or cardiovascular disease (may cause sudden drop in blood pressure), exposure to extreme heat or cold (including antipyretic therapy), respiratory disorders, hypocalcemia, acutely ill or dehydrated children, convulsive disorders, severe reactions to insulin or electroshock therapy, suspected brain tumor or intestinal obstruction, glaucoma, or prostatic hypertrophy. • Hold dose and notify doctor if patient develops jaundice, symptoms of blood dyscrasias (fever, sore throat, infection, cellulitis, weakness), persistent (longer than a few hours) extrapyramidal reactions, or any such reactions in pregnancy or in children over 12 years. • Monitor therapy by weekly bilirubin tests during first month; periodic blood tests (CBC, hepatic function, blood sugar) and ophthalmic tests (long-term use). • Check intake and output for urinary retention or constipation. • Tell patient to use sunscreening agents and protective clothing to avoid photosensitivity reactions. • Warn against activities that require alertness and good psychomotor coordination until response to drug is determined. Drowsiness and dizziness usually subside after a few weeks.

(continued on following page)

NAME	INDICATIONS & DOSAGE	SIDE EFFECTS
mesoridazine besylate *(continued)*		stomatitis; cracked lips; white or black hairy tongue; bald, beefy, red tongue; pseudomembrane in mouth). *GU:* glycosuria. *Metabolic:* hyper- and hypoglycemia, hyper- and hypothermia. *Other:* heat prostration, respiratory distress, asthma, edema (laryngeal, angioneurotic, peripheral). *After abrupt withdrawal:* gastritis, nausea, vomiting, dizziness, tremors, feeling of warmth or cold, sweating, tachycardia, headache, insomnia.
molindone hydrochloride Lidone, Moban	*Disorientation, hallucinations, withdrawal, tension of schizophrenia—* **Adults:** 50 to 75 mg P.O. daily, increasing to maximum 225 mg daily. Doses up to 400 mg may be required.	The dihydroindoles are related structurally to the phenothiazines, and therefore have the potential to cause all the side effects listed; however, all may not have been reported with this drug. *CNS:* moderate to high incidence of transient initial drowsiness, motor restlessness, moderate incidence of extrapyramidal reactions (akathisia, acute dystonias, parkinsonism, tardive dyskinesias), oculogyric crisis, spasticity, insomnia, headache, mental depression, suicidal tendencies, euphoria, dizziness, weakness. *CV:* orthostatic hypotension, tachycardia, nonspecific EKG changes. *EENT:* nasal congestion, tinnitus, visual impairment, pigmentary retinopathy. *GI:* dry mouth, excessive salivation, constipation, anorexia, nausea, weight changes. *GU:* menstrual irregularities, increased libido, incontinence, impotence, inhibited ejaculation, breast engorgement with lactation. *Skin:* rash, sweating.
perphenazine Phenazine♦♦, Trilafon♦	The lowest effective dosage should be employed at all times. *Hospitalized psychiatric patients—* **Adults:** initially, 8 to 16 mg P.O. b.i.d., t.i.d., or q.i.d., increasing to 64 mg daily. **Children over 12 years:** 6 to 12 mg P.O. daily in divided doses. *Mental disturbances, acute alcoholism, nausea, vomiting, hiccups—* **Adults, and children over 12 years:**	The phenothiazines are related structurally and therefore have the potential to cause all the side effects listed; however, all may not have been reported with each drug. *Blood:* agranulocytosis and other dyscrasias. *CNS:* low to moderate incidence of sedation, high incidence of extrapyramidal reactions (akathisia, acute dystonias, parkinsonism, tardive dyskinesias), EEG changes, headache, cerebral edema.

INTERACTIONS	NURSING CONSIDERATIONS
	• Avoid combining with alcohol or other depressants. • Watch for orthostatic hypotension, especially with parenteral administration. Advise patient to change positions slowly. • Give I.M. only in upper outer quadrant of buttocks. Massage slowly afterward to prevent sterile abscess. Injection may sting. • Protect medication from light. Slight yellowing of injection or concentrate is common; does not affect potency. Discard markedly discolored solutions. • Prevent contact dermatitis by keeping drug off patient's skin and clothes. • Dry mouth may be relieved with gum, sour hard candy, or rinsing with mouthwash. • Do not withdraw abruptly unless required by severe side effects. • Drug is a piperidine phenothiazine (a metabolite of thioridazine). • Dose of 50 mg is therapeutic equivalent of 100 mg chlorpromazine. • For symptoms and treatment of toxicity, see p. 1120.
None significant.	• Contraindicated in coma or severe CNS depression. Use with caution when increased physical activity would be harmful, as this agent increases activity; in seizures, suicide risk, suspected brain tumor, or intestinal obstruction. • Warn against activities that require alertness or good psychomotor coordination until response to drug is determined. Drowsiness and dizziness usually subside after first few weeks. • Avoid combining with alcohol or other depressants. • Dry mouth may be relieved with gum, sour hard candy, or rinsing with mouthwash. • Drug is the only dihydroindolone derivative. • Dose of 20 mg is therapeutic equivalent of 100 mg chlorpromazine.
Antacids: inhibited absorption of oral phenothiazines. Separate antacid and phenothiazine dosage by at least 2 hours. *Anticholinergics (including antidepressant and antiparkinson agents):* increased anticholinergic activity, aggravated parkinson-like symptoms.	• Contraindicated in coma, CNS depression, bone marrow depression, subcortical damage, use of spinal or epidural anesthesia or adrenergic blocking agents. Use cautiously with other CNS depressants, anticholinergics; in hepatic disease, elderly or debilitated patients, arteriosclerosis or cardiovascular disease (may cause sudden drop in blood pressure), exposure to extreme heat or cold (including antipyretic therapy), respiratory disorders, hypocalcemia, acutely ill or dehydrated children, convulsive disorders, severe reactions to insulin or electroshock therapy, suspected brain tumor or intestinal obstruction, glaucoma, or prostatic hypertrophy. • Hold dose and notify doctor if patient develops jaundice, symptoms of blood dyscrasias (fever, sore throat, infection, cellulitis, weakness), persistent (longer than a few hours) extrapyramidal reactions, or any such reactions in pregnancy or in children.

(continued on following page)

NAME	INDICATIONS & DOSAGE	SIDE EFFECTS
perphenazine *(continued)*	5 to 10 mg I.M., p.r.n. Maximum 15 mg daily in ambulatory, 30 mg daily in hospitalized patients. *Severe nausea and vomiting*— **Adults:** 5 mg I.M. Maximum dose is 30 mg daily.	*CV:* orthostatic hypotension (possible shock), tachycardia, fainting, dizziness, arrhythmias, pallor. *EENT:* visual impairment, nasal congestion. *GI:* anorexia, excessive salivation, dyspepsia, constipation, diarrhea, cholestatic jaundice, paralytic ileus, increased appetite, weight gain, "oral syndrome" (dry mouth, gum changes, white or black hairy tongue, bald and beefy, red tongue, pseudomembrane in mouth). *GU:* dark urine, difficult urination, incontinence, delayed ovulation, menstrual irregularities, changed libido, impotence, inhibited ejaculation, glycosuria. *Metabolic:* hyper- and hypoglycemia, hyper- and hypothermia. *Skin:* sweating, photosensitivity (yellow-brown or gray-purple pigment deposits after sun exposure), dermatoses (erythematous and eczematous). *Other:* heat prostration, respiratory distress, fever, asthma, edema (laryngeal, angioneurotic, peripheral), gynecomastia, lactation. *After abrupt withdrawal:* gastritis, nausea, vomiting, dizziness, tremors, feeling of warmth or cold, sweating, tachycardia, headache, insomnia.
piperacetazine Quide◆	*Hyperactivity, agitation, and anxiety in schizophrenia*— **Adults:** initially, 10 mg P.O. b.i.d. to q.i.d. Dosage may be gradually increased to 160 mg daily if necessary.	The phenothiazines are related structurally and therefore have the potential to cause all the side effects listed; however, all may not have been reported with each drug. *Blood:* agranulocytosis and other dyscrasias. *CNS:* moderate incidence of sedation, low to moderate incidence of extrapyramidal reactions (akathisia, acute dystonias, parkinsonism, tardive dyskinesias), EEG changes, cerebral edema, headache. *CV:* possible orthostatic hypotension (possible shock), tachycardia, fainting, dizziness, arrhythmias, pallor. *EENT:* visual impairment, nasal congestion. *GI:* anorexia, excessive salivation, dyspepsia, constipation, diarrhea, cholestatic jaundice, paralytic ileus, increased appetite, weight gain, "oral syndrome" (dry mouth, gum changes,

INTERACTIONS	NURSING CONSIDERATIONS
Use with caution. *Barbiturates:* may decrease phenothiazine effect. Observe patient.	• Monitor therapy by weekly bilirubin tests during first month; periodic blood tests (CBC, hepatic function, blood sugar) and ophthalmic tests (long-term use). • Check intake and output for urinary retention or constipation. • Tell patient to use sunscreening agents and protective clothing to avoid photosensitivity reactions. • Warn against activities that require alertness or good psychomotor coordination until response to drug is determined. Drowsiness and dizziness usually subside after a few weeks. • Avoid combining with alcohol or other depressants. • Watch for orthostatic hypotension, especially with parenteral administration. Keep patient supine for 1 hour afterward. Advise patient to change positions slowly. • Give I.M. deeply only in upper outer quadrant of buttocks. Massage slowly afterward to prevent sterile abscess. Injection may sting. • Do not withdraw abruptly unless required by severe side effects. • Protect from light. Slight yellowing of injection or concentrate is common; does not affect potency. Discard markedly discolored solutions. • Prevent contact dermatitis by keeping drug off patient's skin and clothes. • Dilute liquid concentrate with fruit juice, milk, carbonated beverage, or semisolid food just before giving. Exceptions: oral concentrate causes turbidity or precipitation in colas, black coffee, grape or apple juice, or tea. Do not mix with these liquids. • Dry mouth may be relieved with gum, sour hard candy, or rinsing with mouthwash. • Dose of 8 mg is therapeutic equivalent of 100 mg chlorpromazine. • For symptoms and treatment of toxicity, see p. 1120.
Antacids: inhibited absorption of oral phenothiazines. Separate antacid and phenothiazine dosage by at least 2 hours. *Anticholinergics (including antidepressant and antiparkinson agents):* increased anticholinergic activity, aggravated parkinson-like symptoms. Use with caution. *Barbiturates:* may decrease phenothiazine effect. Observe patient.	• Contraindicated in coma, CNS depression, bone marrow depression, thrombocytopenia and other blood dyscrasias, subcortical damage, use of spinal or epidural anesthesia or adrenergic blocking agents. Use cautiously with other CNS depressants, anticholinergics; in hepatic disease, elderly or debilitated patients, arteriosclerosis or cardiovascular disease (may cause sudden drop in blood pressure), exposure to extreme heat or cold (including antipyretic therapy), respiratory disorders, hypocalcemia, convulsive disorders, severe reactions to insulin or electroshock therapy, suspected brain tumor or intestinal obstruction, glaucoma, or prostatic hypertrophy. • Hold dose and notify doctor if patient develops jaundice, symptoms of blood dyscrasias (fever, sore throat, infection, cellulitis, weakness), persistent (longer than a few hours) extrapyramidal reactions, or any such reactions during pregnancy. • Monitor therapy by weekly bilirubin tests during first month; periodic blood tests (CBC, hepatic function, blood sugar) and ophthalmic tests (long-term use). • Check intake and output for urinary retention or constipation. • Tell patient to use sunscreening agents and protective clothing to avoid photosensitivity reactions. • Monitor blood pressure. • Warn against activities that require alertness or good psychomotor coordination until response to drug is determined. Drowsiness and dizziness usually subside after a few weeks.

(continued on following page)

NAME	INDICATIONS & DOSAGE	SIDE EFFECTS
piperacetazine *(continued)*		stomatitis, cracked lips, white or black hairy tongue, bald and beefy red tongue, pseudomembrane in mouth). *GU:* dark urine, difficult urination, incontinence, delayed ovulation, menstrual irregularities, changed libido, impotence, inhibited ejaculation, glycosuria. *Metabolic:* hyper- and hypoglycemia, hyper- and hypothermia. *Skin:* photosensitivity (yellowish-brown or grayish-purple pigment deposits after sun exposure), dermatoses (erythematous and eczematous). *Other:* heat prostration, respiratory distress, asthma, edema (laryngeal, angioneurotic, peripheral), gynecomastia, lactation. *After abrupt withdrawal:* gastritis, nausea, vomiting, dizziness, tremors, feeling of warmth or cold, sweating, tachycardia, headache, insomnia.
prochlorperazine edisylate **prochlorperazine maleate** Compazine, Stemetil♦♦	*Mild to moderate emotional disturbances—* **Adults:** 5 to 10 mg P.O. t.i.d. or q.i.d.; extended-release 15 mg P.O. in a.m. or 10 mg q 12 hours; 25 mg rectally b.i.d.; 5 to 10 mg I.M. q 3 to 4 hours. **Children weighing 18 to 38.5 Kg:** 5 mg P.O. or rectally b.i.d., to maximum of 15 mg daily. **Children weighing 13.5 to 17.5 Kg:** 2.5 mg P.O. or rectally b.i.d. or t.i.d., up to maximum 10 mg daily. **Children weighing 9 to 13 Kg:** 2.5 mg P.O. or rectally daily or b.i.d. to maximum 7.5 mg daily. I.M. dose 0.13 mg/Kg; repeat if necessary. Not recommended in children under 20 pounds. *Psychomotor agitation in schizophrenia; manic phase of manic-depressive psychosis; involutional toxic and senile psychoses—* **Adults:** initially, 10 mg P.O. t.i.d. to q.i.d., increasing up to 50 to 150 mg daily; or 10 to 20 mg I.M. q 1 to 4 hours, p.r.n., up to 100 mg daily, until symptoms are controlled. Prolonged I.M. dosage 10 to 20 mg q 4 to 6 hours.	The phenothiazines are related structurally and therefore have the potential to cause all the side effects listed; however, all may not have been reported with each drug. *Blood:* agranulocytosis and other dyscrasias. *CNS:* low to moderate incidence of sedation, high incidence of extrapyramidal reactions (akathisia, acute dystonias, parkinsonism, tardive dyskinesias), EEG changes, headache, cerebral edema. *CV:* orthostatic hypotension (possible shock), tachycardia, fainting, dizziness, arrhythmias, pallor. *EENT:* visual impairment, nasal congestion. *GI:* anorexia, excessive salivation, dyspepsia, constipation, diarrhea, cholestatic jaundice, paralytic ileus, increased appetite, weight gain, "oral syndrome" (dry mouth, gum changes, stomatitis, cracked lips, white or black hairy tongue, bald and beefy red tongue, pseudomembrane in mouth). *GU:* dark urine, difficult urination, incontinence, delayed ovulation, menstrual irregularities, changed libido, impotence, inhibited ejaculation, glycosuria. *Metabolic:* hyper- and hypoglycemia, hyper- and hypothermia. *Skin:* photosensitivity (yellowish-

INTERACTIONS	NURSING CONSIDERATIONS
	• Avoid combining with alcohol or other depressants. • Watch for orthostatic hypotension. • Protect tablets from light. • Do not withdraw abruptly unless required by severe side effects. • Dry mouth may be relieved with gum, sour hard candy, or rinsing with mouthwash. • Drug is a piperidine phenothiazine. • Dose of 10 mg is therapeutic equivalent of 100 mg chlorpromazine. • For symptoms and treatment of toxicity, see p. 1120.
Antacids: inhibited absorption of oral phenothiazines. Separate antacid and phenothiazine dosage by at least 2 hours. *Anticholinergics (including antidepressant and antiparkinson agents):* increased anticholinergic activity, aggravated parkinson-like symptoms. Use with caution. *Barbiturates:* may decrease phenothiazine effect. Observe patient.	• Contraindicated in coma, depression, CNS depression, bone marrow depression, subcortical damage, pediatric surgery, use of spinal or epidural anesthetic or adrenergic blocking agents, alcohol usage. Use cautiously with other CNS depressants, anticholinergics; in hepatic disease, elderly or debilitated patients, arteriosclerosis or cardiovascular disease (may cause sudden drop in blood pressure), exposure to extreme heat or cold (including antipyretic therapy), respiratory disorders, hypocalcemia, vomiting in children, acutely ill or dehydrated children, convulsive disorders or severe reactions to insulin or electroshock therapy, suspected brain tumor or intestinal obstruction, glaucoma, or prostatic hypertrophy. • Hold dose and notify doctor if patient develops jaundice, symptoms of blood dyscrasias (fever, sore throat, infection, cellulitis, weakness), persistent (longer than a few hours) extrapyramidal reactions, or any such reactions during pregnancy or in children. • Monitor therapy by weekly bilirubin tests during first month; periodic blood tests (CBC, hepatic function, blood sugar) and ophthalmic test (long-term therapy). • Check intake and output for urinary retention or constipation. • Monitor blood pressure and heart rate. • Tell patient to use sunscreening agents and protective clothing to avoid photosensitivity reactions. • Warn against activities that require alertness or good psychomotor coordination until response to drug is determined. Drowsiness and dizziness usually subside after a few weeks. • Avoid combining with alcohol or other depressants. • Watch for orthostatic hypotension, especially with parenteral administration. Advise patient to change positions slowly. • Give I.M. deeply only in upper outer quadrant of buttocks. Massage slowly afterward to prevent sterile abscess. Injection may sting. • Do not mix in same syringe with another drug. • Do not give S.C. • Protect from light. Slight yellowing of injection or concentrate is common; does not affect potency. Discard markedly discolored solutions. • Prevent contact dermatitis by keeping drug off patient's skin and clothes.

(continued on following page)

NAME	INDICATIONS & DOSAGE	SIDE EFFECTS
prochlorperazine *(continued)*		brown or grayish-purple pigment deposits after sun exposure), sweating, dermatoses (erythematous and eczematous). *Other:* heat prostration, respiratory distress, asthma, edema (laryngeal, angioneurotic, peripheral), gynecomastia, lactation. *After abrupt withdrawal:* gastritis, nausea, vomiting, dizziness, tremors, feeling of warmth or cold, sweating, tachycardia, headache, insomnia.
promazine hydrochloride Promabec◆◆, Promanyl◆◆, Promazettes◆◆, Sparine◆	*Psychosis—* **Adults:** 25 to 200 mg P.O. or I.M. q 4 to 6 hours, up to 1 g daily. I.V. dose in concentrations no greater than 25 mg/ml for acutely agitated patients. Initial dose 50 to 150 mg; repeat within 5 to 10 minutes if necessary. **Children over 12:** 10 to 25 mg P.O. or I.M. q 4 to 6 hours.	The phenothiazines are related structurally and therefore have the potential to cause all the side effects listed; however, all may not have been reported with each drug. *Blood:* agranulocytosis and other dyscrasias. *CNS:* moderate incidence of sedation, extrapyramidal reactions (akathisia, acute dystonias, parkinsonism, tardive dyskinesias), EEG changes, cerebral edema, headache. *CV:* moderate incidence of orthostatic hypotension (possible shock), tachycardia, fainting, dizziness, arrhythmias, pallor. *EENT:* visual impairment, nasal congestion. *GI:* anorexia, excessive salivation, dyspepsia, constipation, diarrhea, cholestatic jaundice, paralytic ileus, increased appetite, weight gain, "oral syndrome" (dry mouth, gum changes, stomatitis, cracked lips, white or black hairy tongue, bald and beefy red tongue, pseudomembrane in mouth). *GU:* dark urine, incontinence, difficult urination, delayed ovulation, menstrual irregularities, changed libido, impotence, inhibited ejaculation, glycosuria. *Metabolic:* hyper- and hypoglycemia, hyper- and hypothermia. *Skin:* photosensitivity (yellowish-brown or grayish-purple pigment deposits after sun exposure), dermatoses (erythematous and eczematous). *Other:* heat prostration, respiratory distress, asthma, edema (laryngeal, angioneurotic, peripheral), gynecomastia, lactation. *After abrupt withdrawal:* gastritis, nausea, vomiting, dizziness, tremors, feeling of warmth or cold, sweating, tachycardia, headache, insomnia.

INTERACTIONS	NURSING CONSIDERATIONS
	• Dilute liquid concentrate with fruit juice, milk, coffee, tea, carbonated beverages, or semisolid food just before giving. • Do not withdraw abruptly unless required by severe side effects. • Dry mouth may be relieved with gum, sour hard candy, or rinsing with mouthwash. • Piperidine phenothiazine; most commonly used as an antiemetic. • If more than 4 doses are needed in 24-hour period, notify doctor. • For symptoms and treatment of toxicity, see p. 1120.
Antacids: inhibited absorption of oral phenothiazines. Separate antacid and phenothiazine dosage by at least 2 hours. *Anticholinergics (including antidepressant and antiparkinson agents):* increased anticholinergic activity, aggravated parkinson-like symptoms. Use with caution. *Barbiturates:* may decrease phenothiazine effect. Observe patient.	• Contraindicated in coma, CNS depression, bone marrow depression, subcortical damage, use of spinal or epidural anesthesia or adrenergic blocking agents. Use cautiously with other CNS depressants, anticholinergics; in hepatic disease, elderly or debilitated patients, arteriosclerosis or cardiovascular disease (may cause sudden drop in blood pressure), exposure to extreme heat or cold (including antipyretic therapy), respiratory disorders, hypocalcemia, acutely ill or dehydrated children, convulsive disorders, severe reactions to insulin or electroshock therapy, suspected brain tumor or intestinal obstruction, glaucoma, or prostatic hypertrophy. • Hold dose and notify doctor if patient develops jaundice, symptoms of blood dyscrasias (fever, sore throat, infection, cellulitis, weakness), persistent (longer than a few hours) extrapyramidal reactions, or any such reactions during pregnancy or in children. • Monitor therapy by weekly bilirubin tests during first month; periodic blood tests (CBC, hepatic function, blood sugar) and ophthalmic tests (long-term use). • Check intake and output for urinary retention or constipation. • Tell patient to use sunscreening agents and protective clothing to avoid photosensitivity reactions. • Warn against activities that require alertness or good psychomotor coordination until response to drug is determined. Drowsiness and dizziness usually subside after a few weeks. • Avoid combining with alcohol or other depressants. • Monitor blood pressure lying and standing. • Watch for orthostatic hypotension, especially with parenteral administration. Keep patient supine for 1 hour afterward. Advise patient to change positions slowly. • Give I.M. only in upper outer quadrant of buttocks. Massage slowly afterward to prevent sterile abscess. Injection may sting. • Protect from light. Slight yellowing of injection or concentrate is common; does not affect potency. Discard markedly discolored solutions. • Prevent contact dermatitis by keeping drug off patient's skin and clothes. • Dilute liquid concentrate with fruit juice, milk, semisolid food, or chocolate-flavored drinks just before giving. For best taste, use at least 10 ml diluent per 25 mg drug. • Do not withdraw abruptly unless required by severe side effects. • Dry mouth may be relieved with gum, sour hard candy, or rinsing with mouthwash. • Drug is an aliphatic phenothiazine; rarely used for psychiatric treatment. • For symptoms and treatment of toxicity, see p. 1120.

NAME	INDICATIONS & DOSAGE	SIDE EFFECTS
thioridazine hydrochloride Mellaril◆, Novoridazine◆◆	*Psychosis—* **Adults:** initially, 50 to 100 mg P.O. t.i.d., with gradual increments up to 800 mg daily in divided doses, if needed. Dosage varies. Dose above 800 mg may be associated with ocular toxicity (pigmentary retinopathy). *Depressive neurosis, alcohol withdrawal, dementia in geriatrics—* **Adults:** initially, 25 mg P.O. t.i.d. Maintenance dose is 20 to 200 mg daily. **Children over 2 years:** 0.5 to 3 mg/Kg daily in divided doses.	The phenothiazines are related structurally and therefore have the potential to cause all the side effects listed; however, all may not have been reported with each drug. *Blood:* agranulocytosis, leukopenia, and other dyscrasias. *CNS:* extrapyramidal reactions (akathisia, acute dystonias, parkinsonism, high incidence of sedation, but less severe, tardive dyskinesias), headache, EEG changes, cerebral edema. *CV:* orthostatic hypotension (possible shock), tachycardia, fainting, dizziness, arrhythmias, pallor. *EENT:* visual impairment, pigmentary retinopathy, nasal congestion. *GI:* anorexia, dyspepsia, excessive salivation, constipation, diarrhea, cholestatic jaundice, paralytic ileus, increased appetite, weight gain, "oral syndrome" (dry mouth [very marked with this agent], gum changes, stomatitis, cracked lips, white or black hairy tongue, bald and beefy, red tongue, pseudomembrane in mouth). *GU:* dark urine, difficult urination, incontinence, delayed ovulation, menstrual irregularities, changed libido, impotence, inhibited ejaculation, glycosuria. *Metabolic:* hyper- and hypoglycemia, hyper- and hypothermia. *Skin:* photosensitivity (yellowish-brown or grayish-purple pigment deposits after sun exposure), sweating, dermatoses (erythematous and eczematous). *Other:* heat prostration, respiratory distress, asthma, edema (laryngeal, angioneurotic, peripheral), parotid gland swelling (reported infrequently), gynecomastia, lactation. *After abrupt withdrawal:* gastritis, nausea, vomiting, dizziness, tremors, feeling of warmth or cold, sweating, tachycardia, headache, insomnia.

INTERACTIONS	NURSING CONSIDERATIONS
Antacids: inhibited absorption of oral phenothiazines. Separate antacid and phenothiazine dosage by at least 2 hours. *Anticholinergics (including antidepressant and antiparkinson agents):* increased anticholinergic activity, aggravated parkinson-like symptoms. Use with caution. *Barbiturates:* may decrease phenothiazine effect. Observe patient.	• Contraindicated in coma, CNS depression, bone marrow depression, hypertensive or hypotensive cardiac disease, subcortical damage, use of spinal or epidural anesthesia or adrenergic blocking agents. Use cautiously with other CNS depressants, anticholinergics; in hepatic disease, elderly or debilitated patients, arteriosclerosis or cardiovascular disease (may cause sudden drop in blood pressure), exposure to extreme heat or cold (including antipyretic therapy), respiratory disorders, hypocalcemia, acutely ill or dehydrated children, convulsive disorders, severe reactions to insulin or electroshock therapy, suspected brain tumor or intestinal obstruction, glaucoma, or prostatic hypertrophy. • Hold dose and notify doctor if patient develops jaundice, symptoms of blood dyscrasias (fever, sore throat, infection, cellulitis, weakness), persistent (longer than a few hours) extrapyramidal reactions, or any such reactions during pregnancy or in children. • Monitor therapy by weekly bilirubin tests during first month; periodic blood tests (CBC, hepatic function, blood sugar) and ophthalmic tests (long-term therapy). • Check intake and output for urinary retention or constipation. • Watch for blurred vision, dry mouth; high incidence of anticholinergic effects. • Tell patient to use sunscreening agents and protective clothing to avoid photosensitivity reactions. • Monitor blood pressure. • Warn against activities that require alertness or good psychomotor coordination until response to drug is determined. Drowsiness and dizziness usually subside after a few weeks. • Avoid combining with alcohol or other depressants. • Watch for orthostatic hypotension especially with parenteral administration. Advise patient to change positions slowly. • Prevent contact dermatitis by keeping drug off patient's skin and clothes. • Dilute liquid concentrate with water or fruit juice just before giving. • Do not withdraw abruptly unless required by severe side effects. • Dry mouth may be relieved with gum, sour hard candy, or rinsing with mouthwash. • Piperidine phenothiazine; used to continue antipsychotic therapy when parkinsonian effects require withdrawal of other phenothiazines. • Dose of 100 mg is therapeutic equivalent of 100 mg chlorpromazine. • For symptoms and treatment of toxicity, see p. 1120.

NAME	INDICATIONS & DOSAGE	SIDE EFFECTS
thiothixene **thiothixene hydrochloride** Navane◆	*Acute agitation—* **Adults:** 4 mg I.M. b.i.d. to q.i.d. Maximum 30 mg daily I.M. Change to P.O. as soon as possible. *Mild to moderate psychosis—* **Adults:** initially, 2 mg P.O. t.i.d. May increase gradually to 15 mg daily. *Severe psychosis—* **Adults:** initially, 5 mg P.O. b.i.d. May increase gradually to 15 to 30 mg daily. Maximum recommended daily dose 60 mg. Not recommended in children under 12.	The thiothixenes are related structurally to the phenothiazines and therefore have the potential to cause all the side effects listed; however, all may not have been reported with this drug. *Blood:* agranulocytosis, transient leukopenia, leukocytosis. *CNS:* drowsiness, high incidence of extrapyramidal reactions (akathisia, acute dystonias, parkinsonism, low incidence of sedation, tardive dyskinesias), headache, EEG changes, cerebral edema. *CV:* orthostatic hypotension (possible shock), nonspecific ECG changes, tachycardia, fainting, dizziness, pallor. *EENT:* visual impairment, nasal congestion. *GI:* anorexia, excessive salivation, nausea, vomiting, dyspepsia, constipation, diarrhea, cholestatic jaundice, paralytic ileus, increased appetite, weight gain, "oral syndrome" (dry mouth, gum changes, stomatitis, cracked lips, white or black hairy tongue, bald and beefy red tongue). *GU:* dark urine, difficult urination, incontinence, delayed ovulation, menstrual irregularities, changed libido, impotence, inhibited or premature ejaculation, glycosuria. *Metabolic:* hyper- and hypoglycemia, hyper- and hypothermia. *Skin:* photosensitivity (yellowish-brown or grayish-purple pigment deposits after sun exposure), sweating, dermatoses (erythematous and eczematous), rash, pruritus, urticaria. *Other:* heat prostration, respiratory distress, asthma, edema (laryngeal, angioneurotic, peripheral), leg cramps, gynecomastia, lactation. *After abrupt withdrawal:* gastritis, nausea, vomiting, dizziness, tremors, feeling of warmth or cold, sweating, tachycardia, headache, insomnia.

INTERACTIONS	NURSING CONSIDERATIONS
Anticholinergics (including antidepressant and antiparkinson agents): increased anticholinergic activity, aggravated parkinson-like symptoms. Use with caution.	• Contraindicated in convulsive seizures, circulatory collapse, coma, CNS depression, blood dyscrasias, bone marrow depression, alcohol withdrawal, akathisia or restlessness, subcortical damage, use of spinal or epidural anesthesia or adrenergic blocking agents. Use cautiously with other CNS depressants, anticholinergics; in hepatic disease, elderly or debilitated patients, arteriosclerosis or cardiovascular disease (may cause sudden drop in blood pressure), exposure to extreme heat or cold (including antipyretic therapy), or undue sunlight, respiratory disorders, hypocalcemia, severe reactions to insulin or electroshock therapy, suspected brain tumor or intestinal obstruction, glaucoma, or prostatic hypertrophy. • Hold dose and notify doctor if patient develops jaundice, symptoms of blood dyscrasias (fever, sore throat, infection, cellulitis, weakness), persistent (longer than a few hours) extrapyramidal reactions, or any such reactions during pregnancy. • Monitor therapy by weekly bilirubin tests during first month; periodic blood tests (CBC, hepatic function, blood sugar) and ophthalmic test (long-term therapy). • Check intake and output for urinary retention or constipation. • Tell patient to use sunscreening agents and protective clothing to avoid photosensitivity reactions. • Warn against activities that require alertness or good psychomotor coordination until response to drug is determined. Drowsiness and dizziness usually subside after a few weeks. • Avoid combining with alcohol or other depressants. • Watch for orthostatic hypotension, especially with parenteral administration. Keep patient supine for 1 hour afterward. Advise patient to change positions slowly. • Give I.M. only in upper outer quadrant of buttocks or midlateral thigh. Massage slowly afterward to prevent sterile abscess. Injection may sting. • Slight yellowing of injection or concentrate is common; does not affect potency. Discard markedly discolored solutions. • Prevent contact dermatitis by keeping drug off patient's skin and clothes. • Dilute liquid concentrate with fruit juice, milk, or semisolid food just before giving. • Do not withdraw abruptly unless required by severe side effects. • Dry mouth may be relieved with gum, sour hard candy, or rinsing with mouthwash. • Drug is a thioxanthene derivative but produces responses similar to phenothiazine, butyrophenones, and chlorprothixene. • Dose of 4 mg is therapeutic equivalent of 100 mg chlorpromazine.

NAME	INDICATIONS & DOSAGE	SIDE EFFECTS
trifluoperazine hydrochloride Clinazine♦♦, Novoflurazine♦♦, Pentazine♦♦, Solazine♦♦, Stelazine♦, Terfluzine♦♦, Triflurin♦♦, Tripazine♦♦	*Anxiety states—* **Adults:** 1 to 2 mg P.O. b.i.d. *Schizophrenia and other psychotic disorders—* **Adults:** outpatients—1 to 2 mg P.O. b.i.d., up to 4 mg daily; hospitalized— 2 to 5 mg P.O. b.i.d.; may gradually increase to 40 mg daily. 1 to 2 mg I.M. q 4 to 6 hours, p.r.n. More than 6 mg daily is rarely needed. **Children 6 to 12 years (hospitalized or under close supervision):** 1 mg P.O. daily or b.i.d.; may increase gradually to 15 mg daily.	The phenothiazines are related structurally and therefore have the potential to cause all the side effects listed; however, all may not have been reported with each drug. *Blood:* agranulocytosis and other dyscrasias. *CNS:* low incidence of sedation, high incidence of extrapyramidal reactions (akathisia, acute dystonias, parkinsonism, tardive dyskinesias), headache, EEG changes, cerebral edema. *CV:* orthostatic hypotension (possible shock), tachycardia, fainting, dizziness, arrhythmias, pallor. *EENT:* visual impairment, nasal congestion. *GI:* anorexia, excessive salivation, dyspepsia, constipation, diarrhea, cholestatic jaundice, paralytic ileus, increased appetite, weight gain, "oral syndrome" (dry mouth, gum changes, stomatitis, cracked lips, white or black hairy tongue, bald and beefy red tongue, pseudomembrane in mouth). *GU:* dark urine, difficult urination, incontinence, delayed ovulation, menstrual irregularities, changed libido, impotence, inhibited ejaculation, glycosuria. *Metabolic:* hyper- and hypoglycemia, hyper- and hypothermia. *Skin:* photosensitivity (yellowish-brown or grayish-purple pigment deposits after sun exposure), sweating, dermatoses (erythematous and eczematous). *Other:* heat prostration, respiratory distress, asthma, edema (laryngeal, angioneurotic, peripheral), gynecomastia, lactation. *After abrupt withdrawal:* gastritis, nausea, vomiting, dizziness, tremors, feeling of warmth or cold, sweating, tachycardia, headache, insomnia.
triflupromazine hydrochloride Vesprin	*Acute, severely agitated—* **Adults:** 60 to 150 mg I.M. in 2 or 3 divided doses. **Children over 2½ years:** 0.2 to 0.25 mg/Kg in divided doses. Maximum dose 10 mg daily. *Nausea and vomiting—* **Adults:** 20 to 30 mg P.O. daily; or 1 to 3 mg I.V. daily; or 5 to 15 mg I.M. daily up to maximum	The phenothiazines are related structurally and therefore have the potential to cause all the side effects listed; however, all may not have been reported with each drug. *Blood:* agranulocytosis and other dyscrasias. *CNS:* low incidence of sedation, moderate incidence of extrapyramidal reactions (akathisia, acute dystonias,

INTERACTIONS	NURSING CONSIDERATIONS
Antacids: inhibited absorption of oral phenothiazines. Separate antacid and phenothiazine dosage by at least 2 hours. *Anticholinergics (including antidepressant and antiparkinson agents):* increased anticholinergic activity, aggravated parkinson-like symptoms. Use with caution. *Barbiturates:* may decrease phenothiazine effect. Observe patient.	• Contraindicated in coma, CNS depression, bone marrow depression, subcortical damage, use of spinal or epidural anesthesia or adrenergic blocking agents. Use cautiously with other CNS depressants, anticholinergics; in hepatic disease, elderly or debilitated patients, arteriosclerosis or cardiovascular disease (may cause drop in blood pressure), exposure to extreme heat or cold (including antipyretic therapy), respiratory disorders, hypocalcemia, acutely ill or dehydrated children, convulsive disorders, severe reactions to insulin or electroshock therapy, suspected brain tumor or intestinal obstruction, glaucoma, or prostatic hypertrophy. • Hold dose and notify doctor if patient develops jaundice, symptoms of blood dyscrasias (fever, sore throat, infection, cellulitis, weakness), persistent (longer than a few hours) extrapyramidal reactions, or any such reactions during pregnancy or in children. • Monitor therapy by weekly bilirubin tests during first month; periodic blood tests (CBC, hepatic function, blood sugar) and ophthalmic tests (long-term therapy). • Check intake and output for urinary retention or constipation. • Tell patient to use sunscreening agents and protective clothing to avoid photosensitivity reactions. • Warn against activities that require alertness or good psychomotor coordination until response to drug is determined. Drowsiness and dizziness usually subside after a few weeks. • Avoid combining with alcohol or other depressants. • Watch for orthostatic hypotension, especially with parenteral administration. Keep patient supine for 1 hour afterward. Advise patient to change positions slowly. • Give I.M. deeply only in upper outer quadrant of buttocks. Massage slowly afterward to prevent sterile abscess. Injection may sting. • Protect from light. Slight yellowing of injection or concentrate is common; does not affect potency. Discard markedly discolored solutions. • Prevent contact dermatitis by keeping drug off patient's skin and clothes. • Dilute liquid concentrate with 60 ml tomato or fruit juice, carbonated beverages, coffee, tea, milk, water, or semisolid food just before giving. • Do not withdraw abruptly unless required by severe side effects. • Dry mouth may be relieved with gum, sour hard candy, or rinsing with mouthwash. • Drug is a prototype piperazine phenothiazine. • Dose of 5 mg is therapeutic equivalent of 100 mg chlorpromazine. • For symptoms and treatment of toxicity, see p. 1120.
Antacids: inhibited absorption of oral phenothiazines. Separate antacid and phenothiazine dosage by at least 2 hours. *Anticholinergics (including antidepressant and antiparkinson agents):* increased	• Contraindicated in coma, CNS depression, blood dyscrasias, bone marrow depression, subcortical brain damage, use of spinal or epidural anesthesia or adrenergic blocking agents. Use cautiously with other CNS depressants, anticholinergics; in hepatic disease, elderly or debilitated patients, arteriosclerosis or cardiovascular disease (may cause sudden drop in blood pressure), exposure to extreme heat or cold (including antipyretic therapy), respiratory disorders, pheochromocytoma, hypocalcemia, acutely ill or dehydrated children, convulsive disorders, severe reactions to insulin or electroshock therapy, suspected brain tumor or intestinal obstruction, glaucoma, or prostatic hypertrophy.

(continued on following page)

NAME	INDICATIONS & DOSAGE	SIDE EFFECTS
triflupromazine hydrochloride *(continued)*	60 mg daily. **Children:** 0.2 mg/Kg P.O. or I.M. up to maximum 10 mg daily. *Psychotic disorders (mild to moderate symptoms)—* **Adults:** 10 to 25 mg P.O. b.i.d. **Children over 2½ years:** 10 mg P.O. t.i.d. **Elderly or debilitated:** 10 mg b.i.d. or t.i.d.; increase gradually to desired effect. *Severe symptoms—* **Adults:** 50 mg P.O. b.i.d. or t.i.d. **Children over 2½ years:** 2 mg/Kg P.O. in 3 divided doses; may increase gradually to 150 mg daily.	parkinsonism, tardive dyskinesias), headache, EEG changes, cerebral edema. *CV:* moderate incidence of orthostatic hypotension (possible shock), tachycardia, fainting, dizziness, arrhythmias, pallor. *EENT:* visual impairment, nasal congestion. *GI:* anorexia, excessive salivation, dyspepsia, constipation, diarrhea, cholestatic jaundice, paralytic ileus, increased appetite, weight gain, "oral syndrome" (dry mouth, gum changes, stomatitis, cracked lips, white or black hairy tongue, bald and beefy red tongue). *GU:* dark or pinkish urine, difficult urination, incontinence, delayed ovulation, menstrual irregularities, changed libido, impotence, inhibited ejaculation, glycosuria. *Metabolic:* hyper- and hypoglycemia, hyper- and hypothermia. *Skin:* photosensitivity (yellowish-brown or grayish-purple pigment deposits after sun exposure), sweating, dermatoses (erythematous and eczematous). *Other:* heat prostration, respiratory distress, fever, asthma, edema (laryngeal, angioneurotic, peripheral), gynecomastia, lactation. *After abrupt withdrawal:* gastritis, nausea, vomiting, dizziness, tremors, feeling of warmth or cold, sweating, tachycardia, headache, insomnia.

INTERACTIONS	NURSING CONSIDERATIONS
anticholinergic activity, aggravated parkinson-like symptoms. Use with caution. *Barbiturates:* may decrease phenothiazine effect. Observe patient.	• Hold dose and notify doctor if patient develops jaundice, symptoms of blood dyscrasias (fever, sore throat, infection, cellulitis, weakness), persistent (longer than a few hours) extrapyramidal reactions, or any such reactions during pregnancy or in children. • Monitor therapy by weekly bilirubin tests during first month; periodic blood tests (CBC, hepatic function, blood sugar) and ophthalmic tests (long-term therapy). • Check intake and output for urinary retention or constipation. • Watch for hypothermia reactions. • Tell patient to use sunscreening agents and protective clothing to avoid photosensitivity reactions. • Warn against activities that require alertness or good psychomotor coordination until response to drug is determined. Drowsiness and dizziness usually subside after a few weeks. • Avoid combining with alcohol or other depressants. • Watch for orthostatic hypotension, especially with parenteral administration. Keep patient supine for 1 hour afterward. Advise patient to change positions slowly. • Give I.M. only in upper outer quadrant of buttocks. Massage slowly afterward to prevent sterile abscess. Injection may sting. • Protect from light. Slight yellowing of injection or concentrate is common; does not affect potency. Discard markedly discolored solutions. • Keep liquid suspension tightly closed. • Prevent contact dermatitis by keeping drug off patient's skin and clothes. • Do not withdraw abruptly unless required by severe side effects. • Dry mouth may be relieved with gum, sour hard candy, or rinsing with mouthwash. • Drug is an aliphatic phenothiazine. • Dose of 25 mg is therapeutic equivalent of 10 mg chlorpromazine.

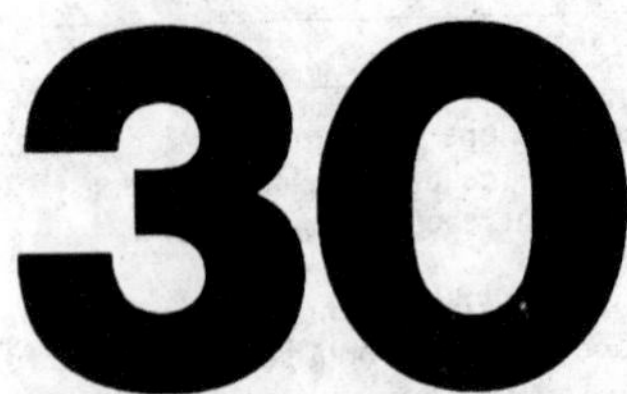

Miscellaneous psychotherapeutics

lithium carbonate
lithium citrate

Lithium carbonate has been used to treat manic-depressive psychosis: worldwide, for over twenty years; in the United States, only since 1970 because of many lithium-related deaths that occurred during the 1940s, when it was improperly used as a salt substitute.

Lithium does have several dangerous side effects. Moreover, the toxic level of the drug is very close to its therapeutic level. However, used with proper supervision, lithium carbonate can prevent and control the manic phase of manic-depressive illness.

Major uses

- Treatment of manic-depressive disorders during acute manic or hypomanic episodes.
- Prevention of recurring episodes of manic-depressive illness, sometimes during both mania and depression.

Mechanism of action

- Alters chemical transmitters in the central nervous system, possibly by interfering with ionic pump mechanisms in brain cells.
- Exact mechanism of action in mania is unknown.

Absorption, distribution, and excretion

- Readily absorbed orally.
- Widely distributed throughout body water; cross placenta.
- Almost entirely excreted through kidneys as unchanged lithium ions.

Onset and duration

- Plasma peak within 1 to 3 hours.
- Antimanic action delayed for 5 to 10 days.

Combination products

None.

HOW TO DETERMINE DAILY LITHIUM DOSAGE

Oral administration of lithium can effectively control recurrent and chronic mania. Lithium treatment does not impair intellectual activity, consciousness, or range or quality of emotional life. It does help patients to fully experience joy, grief, tenderness, sexual desire, and other normal affects.

When deciding daily dosage, remember to maintain the serum lithium concentration between 1 and 1.5 mEq per liter, which may be measured with a flame photometer. For long-term control, adjust the serum levels to remain between 0.6 and 1.5 mEq per liter, which usually requires an oral dose of 300 mg three times daily.

To determine the appropriate daily lithium dosage:

- Give a 600-mg priming dose of lithium.
- Measure lithium level in a sample collected 24 hours later. Now, refer to the chart to match the 24-hour serum level to the dosage required. (This chart minimizes serum fluctuation between 0.6 and 1.2 mEq per liter.)

DAILY LITHIUM DOSAGE

IF PATIENT'S 24-HOUR SERUM LEVEL AFTER SINGLE LOADING DOSE IS	LITHIUM DOSAGE REQUIRED IS
Less than 0.05	1,200 mg three times a day
0.05 to 0.09	900 mg three times a day
0.10 to 0.14	600 mg three times a day
0.15 to 0.19	300 mg four times a day
0.20 to 0.23	300 mg three times a day
0.24 to 0.30	300 mg twice a day
More than 0.30	300 mg twice a day*

Toxic symptoms may occur above serum levels of 1.5 mEq per liter. Signs to watch for include: nausea, abdominal cramps, vomiting, diarrhea, thirst, and polyuria. Reverse the toxic symptoms by promptly discontinuing the drug.

*Use extreme caution.

American Journal of Psychiatry (130:601-603, 1973). Copyright 1973. American Psychiatric Association. Adapted and reprinted with permission.

NAME	INDICATIONS & DOSAGE	SIDE EFFECTS
lithium carbonate Carbolith••, Eskalith, Lithane•, Lithizine••, Lithonate, Lithotabs **lithium citrate**	*Prevention or control of mania*— **Adults:** 300 to 600 mg P.O. up to 4 times daily, increasing on the basis of serum levels to achieve optimal dosage. Recommended therapeutic serum lithium levels: 1 to 1.5 mEq/liter for acute mania; 0.6 to 1.2 mEq/liter for maintenance therapy; and 2 mEq/liter as maximum. **Adults:** 0.5 ml lithium citrate (liquid) contains 8 mEq lithium equal to 300 mg lithium carbonate.	*Note:* Side effects seldom occur at serum levels below 1.5 mEq/l except for fine hand tremor, polyuria, mild thirst, and mild nausea. Symptoms listed below are signs of toxicity. *Blood:* leukocytosis of 14,000 to 18,000 (reversible). *CNS:* tremors, drowsiness, headache, confusion, restlessness, dizziness, psychomotor and mental retardation, stupor, lethargy, coma, "blackouts," epileptiform seizures, EEG changes, impaired speech, ataxia, muscle weakness, incoordination, hyperexcitability. *CV:* reversible EKG changes, arrhythmia, hypotension, peripheral circulatory failure and collapse, allergic vasculitis, ankle and wrist edema. *EENT:* tinnitus, impaired vision. *GI:* nausea, vomiting, anorexia, diarrhea, fecal incontinence, dry mouth, thirst, metallic taste. *GU:* polyuria, oliguria, albuminuria, glycosuria, incontinence. *Metabolic:* transient hyperglycemia, goiter, hypothyroidism (lowered T_3, T_4, and PBI, but elevated ^{131}I uptake), hyponatremia, diabetes insipidus. *Skin:* pruritus, rash, diminished or lost sensation, ulcers.

• Also available in Canada.
•• Available in Canada only.
Unmarked trade names available in United States only.

INTERACTIONS	NURSING CONSIDERATIONS
Diuretics: increased reabsorption of lithium by kidneys, with possible toxic effect. Use with extreme caution, and monitor lithium and electrolyte levels (especially sodium). *Haloperidol:* encephalopathic syndrome (lethargy, tremors, extrapyramidal symptoms). Watch for syndrome and stop drug if it occurs. *Aminophylline, sodium bicarbonate and sodium chloride:* ingestion of these salts increases lithium excretion. Avoid salt loads and monitor lithium levels.	• Contraindicated if therapy cannot be closely monitored; in renal or cardiovascular disease, brain damage, severe debilitation or dehydration, or sodium depletion; with diuretic usage; in first trimester of pregnancy and in lactation. Use with caution with haloperidol, other antipsychotics, neuromuscular blocking agents; in elderly or debilitated persons; thyroid disease and epilepsy. • Monitor baseline EKG, thyroid and renal studies, and electrolyte levels. Monitor serum lithium levels 8 to 12 hours after first dose, usually before a.m. dose, 2 to 3 times weekly first month, then weekly to monthly on maintenance. • Check fluid intake and output, especially when surgery is scheduled. • Warn patient and family to watch for signs of toxicity (diarrhea, vomiting, drowsiness, muscular weakness, ataxia) and to expect transient nausea, polyuria, thirst, and discomfort during first few days. He should withhold 1 dose and call doctor if toxic symptoms appear, but not stop drug abruptly. • Expect lag of 1 to 3 weeks before drug's beneficial effects are noticed. • Adjust fluid and salt ingestion to compensate if excessive loss occurs through protracted sweating or diarrhea. • Have outpatient follow-up of thyroid and renal functions every 6 to 12 months. Palpate thyroid to check for enlargement. • Carry identification/instruction card (available from pharmacy) with toxicity and emergency information. • Avoid activities that require alertness and good psychomotor coordination until response to drug is determined. • Check urine for specific gravity and report level below 1.015. • Has been used to treat syndrome of inappropriate ADH. • Tell patient not to switch brands of lithium without doctor's guidance. • For symptoms and treatment of toxicity, see p. 1118.

31
Cerebral stimulants

amphetamine
benzphetamine hydrochloride
caffeine
chlorphentermine hydrochloride
clortermine hydrochloride
deanol acetamidobenzoate
dextroamphetamine
diethylpropion hydrochloride
fenfluramine hydrochloride
mazindol
methamphetamine hydrochloride
methylphenidate hydrochloride
pemoline
phendimetrazine tartrate
phenmetrazine hydrochloride
phentermine

Amphetamines are the prototypes for this group of central nervous system stimulants. Amphetamine and its isomers stimulate the respiratory center of the brain and cause sympathomimetic activity. Historically, they are the first agents to be used as appetite suppressors or as anorexiants. They are not to be used to combat depressive states.

Major uses

- For appetite suppression and weight reduction in exogenous obesity. To be used as short-term adjunctive therapy to weight control and dieting.
- To treat narcolepsy.
- To treat minimal brain dysfunction in children (hyperkinesis), with other remedial measures.
- To treat nocturnal enuresis.

Mechanism of action

- Amphetamines stimulate the cerebral cortex and possibly the reticular-activating system. They probably promote nerve impulse transmission by releasing stored norepinephrine from brain nerve terminals.

Absorption, distribution, and excretion

- Most agents are readily absorbed from the gastrointestinal tract.
- Oral administration is most common, and distribution is to most body tissues, with high concentrations in the brain and cerebrospinal fluid.
- Excreted through the kidneys, largely unchanged, in about 3 hours.
- Amphetamines and fenfluramine hydrochloride are excreted more readily in acidic urine.
- Pemoline probably undergoes the greatest metabolic change.

Onset and duration

- Onset is usually within 1 to 4 hours.
- Duration of action is from 4 to 10 hours, with most agents requiring multiple doses for continued anorexiant effect. Some products are long-acting preparations (6 to 12 hours).

Combination products

AMPHAPLEX—10/Obetrol-10: dextroamphetamine saccharate 2.5 mg, amphetamine aspartate 2.5 mg, amphetamine sulfate 2.5 mg, dextroamphetamine sulfate 2.5 mg.
AMPHAPLEX—20/Obetrol-20: dextroamphetamine saccharate 5 mg, amphetamine aspartate 5 mg, amphetamine sulfate 5 mg, dextroamphetamine sulfate 5 mg.
BIPHETAMINE 7½: dextroamphetamine 3.75 mg and amphetamine 3.75 mg.
BIPHETAMINE 12½: dextroamphetamine 6.25 mg and amphetamine 6.25.
BIPHETAMINE 20: dextroamphetamine 10 mg and amphetamine 10 mg.
DEXAMYL♦: dextroamphetamine sulfate 5 mg and amobarbital 32 mg.
DEXAMYL #1: dextroamphetamine sulfate 10 mg and amobarbital 65 mg.
DEXAMYL #2: dextroamphetamine sulfate 15 mg and amobarbital 97 mg.
ESKATROL: dextroamphetamine sulfate 15 mg and prochlorperazine maleate 7.5 mg.

PREVENTING AND TREATING AMPHETAMINE ADDICTION

PREVENTION

- Educate the patient concerning the misuse of caffeine and amphetamines.
- Prevent medically induced amphetamine addiction by:

— teaching the obese patient on amphetamines to report such symptoms as nervousness, insomnia, and cardiac palpitations.

— observing the depressed patient who is being treated with amphetamines, for insomnia, loss of appetite, restlessness, and agitation.

— watching the patient on powerful central nervous system stimulants, such as dextroamphetamine, which is twice as potent as amphetamine. Dextroamphetamine, in large doses, is more likely to cause fatigue, mental depression, increased blood pressure, cyanosis, respiratory failure, disorientation, hallucinations, convulsions, and coma.

- Alert the doctor to drug-induced symptoms you've observed. He may want to stop medication.

TREATMENT

- Be aware of your own attitude toward drug addiction and abuse. Respect the amphetamine addict as a human being; his motivation will be increased. Be straightforward with him. Be firm in setting limits, but do not irritate or humiliate him unnecessarily when enforcing them.
- Make a special effort to establish a supportive relationship with the addicted patient during his withdrawal from amphetamines. This critical stage of rehabilitation can have a favorable effect on the patient's final recovery.

NAME	INDICATIONS & DOSAGE	SIDE EFFECTS
amphetamine hydrochloride **amphetamine phosphate** **amphetamine sulfate** Controlled substance Schedule II Benzedrine◆	*Minimal brain dysfunction—* **Children 6 years and older:** 5 mg P.O. daily, with 5 mg increments weekly, p.r.n. **Children 3 to 5 years:** 2.5 mg P.O. daily, with 2.5 mg increments weekly, p.r.n. *Narcolepsy—* **Adults:** 5 to 60 mg P.O. daily in divided doses. **Children over 12 years:** 10 mg P.O. daily, with 10 mg increments weekly, p.r.n. **Children 6 to 12 years:** 5 mg P.O. daily, with 5 mg increments weekly, p.r.n. *Short-term adjunct in exogenous obesity—* **Adults:** single 10 or 15 mg long-acting capsule daily, or 2 if needed, up to 30 mg daily; or 5 to 30 mg daily in divided doses 30 to 60 minutes before meals. Not recommended for children under 12 years old.	*CNS:* restlessness, tremor, hyperactivity, talkativeness, insomnia, irritability, dizziness, headache, chills, overstimulation, dysphoria. *CV:* tachycardia, palpitations, hypertension, hypotension. *GI:* nausea, vomiting, cramps, dry mouth, diarrhea, constipation, metallic taste, anorexia, weight loss. *Others:* urticaria, impotence, changes in libido.
benzphetamine hydrochloride Controlled substance Schedule III Didrex	*Short-term adjunct in exogenous obesity—* **Adults:** 25 to 50 mg P.O., daily, b.i.d., or t.i.d.	*CNS:* restlessness, tremor, hyperactivity, talkativeness, insomnia, irritability, dizziness, headache, chills, overstimulation, dysphoria. *CV:* tachycardia, palpitations, hypertension, hypotension. *GI:* nausea, vomiting, cramps, dry mouth, diarrhea, constipation, metallic taste, anorexia, weight loss. *Other:* urticaria, impotence, changes in libido.
caffeine Ban-Drowz, Kirkaffein, Nodoz, Stim 250, Stim-Tabs, Tirend, Vivarin **caffeine, citrated**	*Respiratory and central nervous system stimulant—* **Adults:** 100 to 200 mg anhydrous caffeine P.O.; 500 mg to 1 g I.M., caffeine sodium benzoate or I.V. in emergency only.	*CNS:* stimulation, insomnia, restlessness, nervousness, mild delirium, headache, excitement, agitation, muscle tremors, twitches. *CV:* tachycardia, arrhythmias, extrasystoles. *EENT:* scintillating scotoma, tinnitus. *GI:* pain, nausea, vomiting.

◆ Also available in Canada.
◆◆ Available in Canada only.
Unmarked trade names available in United States only.

INTERACTIONS	NURSING CONSIDERATIONS
MAO inhibitors: severe hypertension; possible hypertensive crisis. Don't use together. *Sodium bicarbonate, acetazolamide:* increased renal reabsorption. Monitor for enhanced effect. *Ammonium chloride, ascorbic acid:* observe for decreased amphetamine effect. *Phenothiazines, haloperidol:* observe for decreased amphetamine effect.	• Contraindicated in symptomatic cardiovascular diseases, hyperthyroidism, nephritis, diabetes mellitus, angina pectoris, moderate to severe hypertension, parkinsonism due to arteriosclerosis, certain types of glaucoma, advanced arteriosclerosis, agitated states, or history of drug abuse. Use with caution in elderly, debilitated, or hyperexcitable patients. • Psychic dependence or habituation may occur, especially in patients with history of drug addiction. Avoid prolonged administration. When used long-term, lower dosage gradually to prevent acute rebound depression. • When used for obesity, make sure patient is also on a weight reduction program. Give drug 30 to 60 minutes before meals. • Fatigue may result as drug effects wear off. Patient will need more rest. • Tell patient to avoid caffeine drinks, which increase the effects of amphetamines and related amines. • Check vital signs regularly. Observe for signs of excessive stimulation. • Urinary acidification enhances renal excretion; urinary alkalinization enhances renal reabsorption and recycling. • When tolerance to anorexic effect develops, dosage should not be increased, but drug discontinued. • Discourage use to combat fatigue. • Warn patient to avoid activities that require alertness or good psychomotor coordination until response to drug is determined. • May alter daily insulin needs. Monitor blood sugar and fractional urine. • Use as analeptic is usually discouraged, since CNS stimulation superimposed on CNS depression can lead to neuronal instability and seizures. • May reverse beneficial effect of antihypertensives. Monitor blood pressures.
MAO inhibitors: severe hypertension; possible hypertensive crisis. Don't use together. *Sodium bicarbonate, acetazolamide:* increased renal reabsorption. Monitor for enhanced effects. *Ammonium chloride, ascorbic acid:* observe for decreased benzphetamine effects. *Phenothiazines, haloperidol:* observe for decreased benzphetamine effects.	• Contraindicated in symptomatic cardiovascular diseases, hyperthyroidism, nephritis, diabetes mellitus, angina pectoris, moderate to severe hypertension, parkinsonism due to arteriosclerosis, certain types of glaucoma, advanced arteriosclerosis, agitated states, or history of drug abuse. Use with caution in elderly, debilitated, or hyperexcitable patients. • Psychic dependence or habituation may occur, especially in patients with history of drug addiction. Avoid prolonged administration. When used long-term, lower dosage gradually to prevent acute rebound depression. • Use in conjunction with weight reduction program. Give 30 to 60 minutes before meals. • Fatigue may result as drug effects wear off. Patient will need more rest. • Tell patient to avoid caffeine drinks, which increase the effects of amphetamines and related amines. • Check vital signs regularly. Observe for signs of excessive stimulation. • Urinary acidification enhances renal excretion; urinary alkalinization enhances renal reabsorption and recycling. • When tolerance to anorexic effect develops, dosage should not be increased, but drug discontinued. • Warn patient to avoid activities that require alertness or good psychomotor coordination until response to drug is determined. • May alter daily insulin needs. Monitor blood sugar and fractional urine.
None significant.	• Contraindicated for patients with gastric or duodenal ulcer. • Tolerance or psychological dependence may develop. • Be alert for signs of overdose: GI pain, mild delirium, insomnia, diuresis, dehydration, and fever. Treat with short-acting barbiturates, gastric emesis, or lavage. • Single dose should not exceed 1 g. • Caffeine content in cola beverages, 17 to 55 mg/180 ml; tea, 40 to 100 mg/180 ml; instant coffee, 60 to 180 mg/180 ml; brewed coffee, 100 to 150

(continued on following page)

NAME	INDICATIONS & DOSAGE	SIDE EFFECTS
caffeine *(continued)* **caffeine and sodium benzoate injection**		*GU:* diuresis. *Skin:* hyperesthesia.
chlorphentermine hydrochloride Controlled substance Schedule III Chlorophen, Pre-Sate♦	*Short-term adjunct in exogenous obesity—* **Adults:** 65 mg P.O. taken after breakfast.	*CNS:* insomnia, overstimulation, nervousness, dizziness, paradoxical sedation, headache. *CV:* tachycardia, palpitations, increased blood pressure. *GI:* nausea, dry mouth, constipation. *Skin:* urticaria.
clortermine hydrochloride Controlled substance Schedule III Voranil	*Short-term adjunct in exogenous obesity—* **Adults:** 50 mg P.O. taken at midmorning.	*CNS:* restlessness, dizziness, insomnia, euphoria, tremor, headache. *CV:* tachycardia, palpitations, arrhythmias, increased blood pressure. *GI:* dry mouth, diarrhea, constipation. *Skin:* urticaria. *Other:* impotence, libido changes.
deanol acetamidobenzoate Deaner, Deaner-100♦♦, Deaner-250	*Minimal brain dysfunction—* **Children over 6 years:** initially, 500 mg P.O. daily after breakfast; may reduce to maintenance 250 to 500 mg daily. Dose adjusted to patient's needs and response. *Dyskinesia, blepharospasm—* **Adults:** 600 mg to 1.6 g P.O. daily.	*CNS:* insomnia, mild overstimulation, irritability, dull occipital headache, muscle twitching, tenseness. *CV:* postural hypotension. *EENT:* increased nasal and oral secretions. *GI:* constipation. *Skin:* transient rash. *Other:* dyspnea.
dextroamphetamine hydrochloride Controlled substance Schedule II **dextroamphetamine phosphate** **dextroamphetamine sulfate**	*Narcolepsy—* **Adults:** 5 to 60 mg P.O. daily in divided doses. **Children over 12 years:** 10 mg P.O. daily, with 10 mg increments weekly, p.r.n. **Children 6 to 12 years:** 5 mg P.O. daily, with 5 mg increments weekly, p.r.n. *Short-term adjunct in exogenous obesity—*	*CNS:* restlessness, tremor, hyperactivity, talkativeness, insomnia, irritability, dizziness, headache, chills, overstimulation, dysphoria. *CV:* tachycardia, palpitations, hypertension, hypotension. *GI:* nausea, vomiting, cramps, dry mouth, diarrhea, constipation, metallic taste, anorexia, weight loss. *Other:* urticaria, impotence, changes in libido.

INTERACTIONS	NURSING CONSIDERATIONS
	mg/180 ml. • Caffeine does not reverse alcohol intoxication or depressant effects of alcohol. Overvigorous therapy with caffeine may aggravate depression in an already depressed patient. • Use as analeptic is discouraged.
MAO inhibitors: severe hypertension; possible hypertensive crisis. Don't use together. *Sodium bicarbonate, acetazolamide:* increased renal reabsorption. Monitor for enhanced effects. *Ammonium chloride, ascorbic acid:* observe for decreased chlorphentermine effects.	• Contraindicated in hyperexcitability states, hyperthyroidism, hypertension, angina pectoris, severe cardiovascular disease, glaucoma, or history of drug abuse. • Psychic dependence and habituation may occur. When tolerance to anorexic effect develops, dose should not be increased but stop drug. • May alter daily insulin needs. Monitor blood sugar and fractional urine. • Teach patient a good dietary plan and exercise program. • Withdraw drug gradually. • Fatigue may result as drug effects wear off. Patient will need more rest. • Tell patient to avoid caffeine drinks, which increase the effects of amphetamines and related amines. • Check vital signs regularly. Observe for signs of excessive stimulation. • Urinary acidification enhances renal excretion; urinary alkalinization enhances renal reabsorption and recycling.
MAO inhibitors: severe hypertension; possible hypertensive crisis. Don't use together. *Sodium bicarbonate, acetazolamide:* increased renal reabsorption. Monitor for enhanced effects. *Ammonium chloride, ascorbic acid:* observe for decreased clortermine effects.	• Contraindicated in hyperthyroidism, glaucoma, severe hypertension, cardiovascular diseases, agitated states, history of drug abuse. Use with caution in diabetes mellitus. Insulin requirements may be altered. Monitor blood sugar and fractional urine. • Warn patient to avoid activities that require alertness or good psychomotor coordination until response to drug is determined. • Be sure patient is following a sensible dietary regimen. • Drug should be discontinued when tolerance develops. • Fatigue may result as drug effects wear off. Patient will need more rest. • Tell patient to avoid caffeine drinks, which increase the effects of amphetamines and related amines. • Check vital signs regularly. Observe for signs of excessive stimulation. • Urinary acidification enhances renal excretion; urinary alkalinization enhances renal reabsorption and recycling.
None significant.	• Contraindicated for patients with grand mal epilepsy. • In long-term use, monitor child closely for signs of growth suppression. • Beneficial effects may not appear until after several weeks of therapy. • Used with some success in treatment of tardive dyskinesia.
MAO inhibitors: severe hypertension; possible hypertensive crisis. Don't use together. *Sodium bicarbonate, acetazolamide:* increased renal reabsorption. Monitor for enhanced amphetamine effects.	• Contraindicated in hyperthyroidism, nephritis, diabetes mellitus, severe hypertension, angina pectoris or other severe cardiovascular disease, some types of glaucoma, or history of drug abuse. Use with caution in elderly, debilitated, or hyperexcitable patients. • Psychic dependence or habituation may occur, especially in patients with history of drug addiction. Avoid prolonged administration. When used long-term, lower dosage gradually to prevent acute rebound depression. • When used for obesity, be sure patient is also on a weight reduction program. Give 30 to 60 minutes before meals. Avoid giving within 6 hours of bedtime. • Fatigue may result as drug effects wear off. Patient will need more rest.

(continued on following page)

NAME	INDICATIONS & DOSAGE	SIDE EFFECTS
dextroamphetamine sulfate *(continued)* Dexampex, Dexedrine♦, Ferndex, Robese, Spancap #1 and #4, Tidex	**Adults:** single 10 to 15 mg long-acting capsule up to 30 mg daily, or in divided doses, 5 to 10 mg 1/2 hour before meals. *Minimal brain dysfunction—* **Children 6 years and over:** 5 mg once daily or b.i.d., with 5 mg increments weekly, p.r.n. **Children 3 to 5 years:** 2.5 mg P.O. daily, with 2.5 mg increments weekly, p.r.n.	
diethylproprion hydrochloride Controlled substance Schedule IV Dietec♦♦, D.I.P.♦♦, Nobesine♦♦, Nu-Dispoz, o.b.c.t., Regibon♦♦, Ro-Diet, Tenuate♦, Tepanil	*Short-term adjunct in exogenous obesity—* **Adults:** 25 mg P.O. before meals, t.i.d., or 75 mg controlled-release tablet P.O. in midmorning.	*CNS:* headache, nervousness, dizziness. *CV:* tachycardia, palpitations, rise in blood pressure. *EENT:* blurred vision. *GI:* nausea, abdominal cramps, dry mouth, diarrhea, constipation. *Skin:* urticaria. *Other:* impotence, libido changes, menstrual upset.
fenfluramine hydrochloride Controlled substance Schedule IV Pondimin♦	*Short-term adjunct in exogenous obesity—* **Adults:** initially, 20 mg P.O. t.i.d. before meals. Maximum 40 mg t.i.d. Adjust dosage according to patient's response.	*CNS:* drowsiness, dizziness, confusion, incoordination, headache, euphoria or depression, anxiety, insomnia, weakness or fatigue, agitation, dysarthria, lethargy, vivid dreams, nightmares. *CV:* palpitations, hypotension, hypertension, chest pain. *EENT:* eye irritation, blurred vision. *GI:* diarrhea, dry mouth, nausea, vomiting, abdominal pain, constipation. *GU:* dysuria, increased urinary frequency, impotence, increased libido. *Skin:* rashes, urticaria, burning sensation. *Other:* fainting, sweating, chills, fever.
mazindol Controlled substance Schedule IV Sanorex♦	*Short-term adjunct in exogenous obesity—* **Adults:** 1 mg t.i.d. 1 hour before meals, or 2 mg daily 1 hour before lunch. Use lowest effective dose.	*CNS:* nervousness, restlessness, dizziness, insomnia, dysphoria, headache, depression, drowsiness, weakness, tremors. *CV:* palpitations, tachycardia. *GI:* dry mouth, nausea, constipation, diarrhea, unpleasant taste.

INTERACTIONS	NURSING CONSIDERATIONS
Ammonium chloride, ascorbic acid: observe for decreased amphetamine effects. *Phenothiazines, haloperidol:* observe for decreased amphetamine effects.	• Tell patient to avoid caffeine drinks, which increase the effects of amphetamines and related amines. • Check vital signs regularly. Observe for signs of excessive stimulation. • Urinary acidification enhances renal excretion; urinary alkalinization enhances renal reabsorption and recycling. • When tolerance to anorexic effect develops, dosage should not be increased, but drug discontinued. • Discourage use to combat fatigue. • Warn patient to avoid activities that require alertness or good psychomotor coordination until response to drug is determined. • May alter daily insulin needs. Monitor blood sugar and fractional urine. • Use as analeptic is usually discouraged, since CNS stimulation superimposed on CNS depression can lead to neuronal instability and seizures.
MAO inhibitors: hypertension; possible hypertensive crisis. Don't use together.	• Contraindicated in hyperthyroidism, hypertension, angina pectoris, severe cardiovascular disease, glaucoma, or history of drug abuse. Use with caution in epilepsy, diabetes mellitus, or hyperexcitability states. May alter insulin requirements. Monitor blood sugar and fractional urine. • When tolerance to anorexic effect develops, dosage should not be increased, but drug discontinued. • Habituation or psychic dependence may occur. • Be sure patient is also on a weight reduction program. • Can be used to stop nighttime eating. Rarely causes insomnia. • Fatigue may result as drug effects wear off. Patient will need more rest. • Tell patient to avoid caffeine drinks, which increase the effects of amphetamines and related amines. • Check vital signs regularly. Observe for signs of excessive stimulation. • Urinary acidification enhances renal excretion; urinary alkalinization enhances renal reabsorption and recycling. • Use as analeptic is usually discouraged, since CNS stimulation superimposed on CNS depression can lead to neuronal instability and seizures.
MAO inhibitors: severe hypertension; possible hypertensive crisis. Don't use together.	• Contraindicated in glaucoma, hypersensitivity to sympathomimetic amines, symptomatic cardiovascular disease, history of drug abuse, or alcoholism. Use with caution in hypertension, history of mental depression, diabetes mellitus. • Because of possible hypoglycemia, diabetics may have altered insulin or sulfonylureas requirements. Monitor blood sugar and fractional urine. • Check vital signs regularly. Observe patient for signs of excessive sedation, depression or excessive stimulation. Closely monitor blood pressure. • Be sure patient is on a weight reduction program. • Tolerance or dependence may occur. Avoid prolonged administration. • Fatigue may result as drug effects wear off. Patient will need more rest. • Tell patient to avoid caffeine drinks, which increase the effects of amphetamines and related amines.
MAO inhibitors: severe hypertension; possible hypertensive crisis. Don't use together.	• Contraindicated in glaucoma, cardiovascular disease including arrhythmias, agitated states, history of drug abuse. Use with caution in diabetes mellitus, hypertension, hyperexcitability states. • Warn patient to avoid activities that require alertness or good psychomotor coordination until response has been determined. • Fatigue may result as drug effects wear off. Patient will need more rest. • Tell patient to avoid caffeine drinks, which increase the effects of amphet-

(continued on following page)

NAME	INDICATIONS & DOSAGE	SIDE EFFECTS
mazindol *(continued)*		*GU:* difficulty initiating micturition, impotence, libido changes. *Skin:* rash, clamminess, pallor. *Other:* shivering, excessive sweating.
methamphetamine hydrochloride Controlled substance Schedule II Desoxyn, Methampex, Obedrin-LA	*Minimal brain dysfunction—* **Children 6 years and over:** 2.5 to 5 mg P.O. once daily or b.i.d., with 5 mg increments weekly, p.r.n. Usual effective dosage is 20 to 25 mg daily. *Short-term adjunct in exogenous obesity—* **Adults:** 2.5 to 5 mg P.O. once to t.i.d. daily 30 minutes before meals; or 1 long-acting 5 to 15 mg capsule daily before breakfast.	*CNS:* nervousness, insomnia, irritability, talkativeness, dizziness, headache, hyperexcitability, tremor. *CV:* hypertension or hypotension, tachycardia, palpitations, cardiac arrhythmias. *EENT:* blurred vision, mydriasis. *GI:* nausea, vomiting, abdominal cramps, diarrhea or constipation, dry mouth, anorexia, metallic taste. *GU:* impotence, libido changes. *Skin:* urticaria.
methylphenidate hydrochloride Controlled substance Schedule II Methidate◆◆, Ritalin◆	*Minimal brain dysfunction (hyperkinetic behavior disorders)—* **Children 6 years and over:** initial dose 5 to 10 mg P.O. daily before breakfast and lunch, with 5 to 10 mg increments weekly as needed, up to 60 mg daily. *Narcolepsy—* **Adults:** 10 mg P.O. b.i.d. or t.i.d., ½ hour before meals. Dosage varies with patient needs. Dosage range is 5 to 50 mg daily.	*CNS:* nervousness, insomnia, dizziness, headache, akathisia, dyskinesia, drowsiness. *CV:* palpitations, angina, cardiac arrhythmias, tachycardia, changes in blood pressure and pulse rate. *GI:* nausea, dry throat, abdominal pain, anorexia, weight loss. *EENT:* difficulty with accommodation and blurring of vision. *Skin:* rash, urticaria, exfoliative dermatitis, erythema multiforme.

INTERACTIONS	NURSING CONSIDERATIONS
	amines and related amines. • Check vital signs regularly. Observe for signs of excessive stimulation. • Tolerance or dependence may develop. Avoid prolonged use. • Be sure patient is also on a weight reduction program. • May alter insulin needs. Monitor blood sugar and fractional urine.
MAO inhibitors: severe hypertension; possible hypertensive crisis. Don't use together. *Sodium bicarbonate, acetazolamide:* increased renal reabsorption. Monitor for enhanced effects. *Ammonium chloride, ascorbic acid:* observe for decreased amphetamine effects. *Phenothiazines, haloperidol:* observe for decreased amphetamine effects.	• Contraindicated in hypertension, hyperthyroidism, nephritis, angina pectoris or other severe cardiovascular disease, diabetes, glaucoma, parkinsonism due to arteriosclerosis, agitated states, or history of drug abuse. Use with caution in patients who are elderly, debilitated, asthenic, psychopathic, or who have a history of suicidal or homicidal tendencies. • Warn that potential for abuse is high. Discourage use to combat fatigue. • May alter insulin needs. Monitor blood sugar and fractional urine. • When used for obesity, be sure patient is on a weight reduction program. • Tell patient to avoid caffeine drinks, which increase the effects of amphetamines and related amines. • Check vital signs regularly. Observe for signs of excessive stimulation. • Urinary acidification enhances renal excretion; urinary alkalinization enhances renal reabsorption and recycling. • When tolerance to anorexic effect develops, dosage should not be increased but drug discontinued. • Warn patient to avoid activities that require alertness or good psychomotor coordination until response to drug is determined.
MAO inhibitors: severe hypertension; possible hypertensive crisis. Don't use together.	• Contraindicated in symptomatic cardiac disease; hyperthyroidism; moderate to severe hypertension; angina pectoris; advanced arteriosclerosis; severe depression of either endogenous or exogenous forms; glaucoma; history of drug abuse or dependency; history of marked anxiety, tension, or agitation; parkinsonism. Use with caution in elderly, debilitated, or hyperexcitable patients and those with history of cardiovascular disease, diabetes, or seizures. • Closely monitor blood pressure. Observe for signs of excessive stimulation. • Discourage use to combat fatigue. • Observe for interactions, as treatment of other disease states may be affected. May alter daily insulin needs. Monitor blood sugar and fractional urine. May decrease seizure threshold in seizure disorder patients. • Drug of choice for minimal brain dysfunction. Usually stopped postpuberty. • Used in treatment for nocturnal enuresis in children. • Periodic CBC, differential, and platelet counts advised with long-term use. • Tolerance, psychic dependence or habituation may occur, especially in patients with history of drug addiction. High abuse potential. Avoid prolonged administration. When used long-term, lower dosage gradually to prevent acute rebound depression. • Fatigue may result as drug effects wear off. Patient will need more rest. • Tell patient to avoid caffeine drinks, which increase the effects of amphetamines and related amines. • May endanger patient's ability to safely operate machinery or vehicles. • Warn patient to avoid activities that require alertness or good psychomotor coordination until response to drug is determined.

NAME	INDICATIONS & DOSAGE	SIDE EFFECTS
pemoline Controlled substance Schedule IV Cylert	*Minimal brain dysfunction—* **Children 6 years and over:** initially, 37.5 mg P.O. given in the morning. Daily dose can be raised by 18.75 mg weekly. Effective dosage range 56.25 to 75 mg daily; maximum is 112.5 mg daily.	*Blood:* elevated serum levels of glutamic-oxaloacetic transaminase, glutamic-pyruvic transaminase, alkaline phosphatase. *CNS:* insomnia (most frequent side effect), malaise, irritability, fatigue, mild depression, dizziness, headache, drowsiness, hallucinations, nervousness (large doses), seizures. *CV:* tachycardia (large doses). *GI:* anorexia, abdominal pain, nausea, diarrhea. *Skin:* rash.
phendimetrazine tartrate Controlled substance Schedule IV Adphen, Anorex, Bacarate, Banobese, Bontril PDM, Delcozine, Di-Ap-Trol, Di-Metrex, Ex-Obese, Limit, Melfiat, Metra, Minus, Obalan, Obepar, Obeval, Obezine, Phenazine♦, Phenzine, Plegine, Ropledge, SPRX 1,2,3, Statobex, Trimstat, Trimtabs, Weightrol	*Short-term adjunct in exogenous obesity—* **Adults:** 35 mg P.O. 2 to 3 times daily 1 hour before meals. Maximum dosage is 70 mg t.i.d. Use lowest effective dosage. Adjust dose to individual response.	*CNS:* nervousness, dizziness, insomnia, tremor, headache. *CV:* tachycardia, palpitations, rise in blood pressure. *EENT:* blurred vision. *GI:* dry mouth, nausea, abdominal cramps, diarrhea or constipation. *GU:* dysuria.
phenmetrazine hydrochloride Controlled substance Schedule II Preludin	*Short-term adjunct in exogenous obesity—* **Adults:** 25 mg P.O. b.i.d. or t.i.d. 1 hour before meals, up to 75 mg daily; or single 50 to 75 mg extended-release tablet daily in midmorning.	*CNS:* nervousness, dizziness, insomnia, headache. *CV:* tachycardia, palpitations, increased blood pressure. *EENT:* blurred vision. *GI:* dry mouth, nausea, abdominal cramps, constipation. *GU:* libido changes, impotence. *Skin:* urticaria.

INTERACTIONS	NURSING CONSIDERATIONS
None significant.	• Use with caution in impaired renal function. Drug may accumulate. • Safety and efficacy for more than 2 years of administration has not been established. Closely monitor patients on long-term therapy for possible hepatic function abnormalities and for growth suppression. • Structurally dissimilar to amphetamines or methylphenidate. • Therapeutic effects may not be evident for 2 to 3 weeks.
MAO inhibitors: severe hypertension; possible hypertensive crisis. Don't use together. *Sodium bicarbonate, acetazolamide:* increased renal reabsorption. Monitor for enhanced effects. *Ammonium chloride, ascorbic acid:* observe for decreased phendimetrazine effects. *Phenothiazines, haloperidol:* observe for decreased effect.	• Contraindicated in hyperthyroidism, hypertension, angina pectoris or other severe cardiovascular disease, glaucoma. Use with caution in hyperexcitability states or history of addiction. • Warn patient to avoid activities that require alertness or good psychomotor coordination until response to drug has been determined. • Be sure patient is following weight reduction program. • Tolerance or dependence can develop. Not advised for prolonged use. • Fatigue may result as drug effects wear off. Patient will need more rest. • Tell patient to avoid caffeine drinks, which increase the effects of amphetamines and related amines. • Check vital signs regularly. Observe for signs of excessive stimulation. • Urinary acidification enhances renal excretion; urinary alkalinization enhances renal reabsorption and recycling. • May alter daily insulin needs. Monitor blood sugar and fractional urine.
MAO inhibitors: severe hypertension; possible hypertensive crisis. Don't use together. *Sodium bicarbonate, acetazolamide:* increased renal reabsorption. Monitor for enhanced effects. *Ammonium chloride, ascorbic acid:* observe for decreased phenmetrazine effects. *Phenothiazines, haloperidol:* observe for decreased effect.	• Contraindicated in hyperthyroidism, hypertension, angina pectoris or other cardiovascular disease, glaucoma, or history of drug abuse. Use with caution in hyperexcitability states. • Tolerance or dependence may develop. High abuse potential. Not advised for prolonged use. • Be sure patient is also following weight reduction program. • Administer 1 hour before meals. • Fatigue may result as drug effects wear off. Patient will need more rest. • Tell patient to avoid caffeine drinks, which increase the effects of amphetamine and related amines. • Check vital signs regularly. Observe for signs of excessive stimulation. • Urinary acidification enhances renal excretion; urinary alkalinization enhances renal reabsorption and recycling.

NAME	INDICATIONS & DOSAGE	SIDE EFFECTS
phentermine Controlled substance Schedule IV Adipex, Ambesa-LA, Anoxine, Fastin, Ionamin◆, Parmine, Phentrol, Rolaphent, Wilpo, Wilpowr	*Short-term adjunct in exogenous obesity—* **Adults:** 8 mg P.O. t.i.d. ½ hour before meals (hydrochloride salt); or 15 to 30 mg daily before breakfast (resin complex).	*CNS:* nervousness, dizziness, insomnia. *CV:* palpitations, tachycardia, increased blood pressure. *GI:* dry mouth, unpleasant taste, nausea, constipation, diarrhea. *GU:* libido changes, impotence. *Skin:* urticaria.

INTERACTIONS	NURSING CONSIDERATIONS
MAO inhibitors: severe hypertension; possible hypertensive crisis. Don't use together. *Sodium bicarbonate, acetazolamide:* increased renal reabsorption. Monitor for enhanced effects. *Ammonium chloride, ascorbic acid:* observe for decreased phentermine effects. *Phenothiazines, haloperidol:* observe for decreased effect.	• Contraindicated in hyperthyroidism, hypertension, angina pectoris or other severe cardiovascular disease, glaucoma. Use with caution in hyperexcitability states or history of drug addiction. • Tolerance or dependence may develop. Avoid prolonged administration. • Use with weight reduction program. Give 30 minutes before meals. • Fatigue may result as drug effects wear off. Patient will need more rest. • Tell patient to avoid caffeine drinks, which increase the effects of amphetamine and related amines. • Check vital signs regularly. Observe for signs of excessive stimulation. • Urinary acidification enhances renal excretion; urinary alkalinization enhances renal reabsorption and recycling.

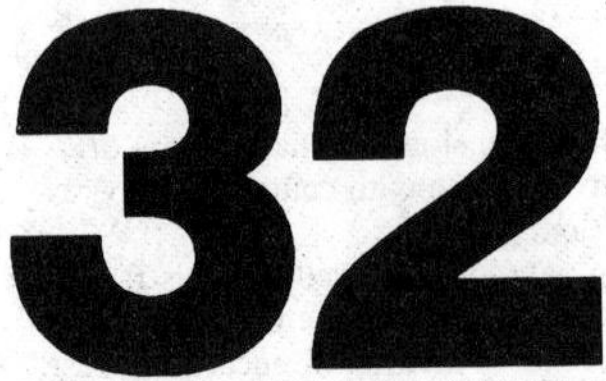

Respiratory stimulants

ammonia, aromatic spirits
doxapram hydrochloride
nikethamide
pentylenetetrazol

These agents have limited usefulness in treating respiratory depression in patients with postanesthetic apnea caused by drugs other than muscle relaxants. Doxapram is the most commonly used drug in this group. Pentylenetetrazol and nikethamide are seldom used today.

Major uses

- To combat effects of central nervous system depressants.
- To stimulate respiration through peripheral irritation (ammonia).
- To enhance physical and mental activity in elderly patients (pentylenetetrazol).

Mechanism of action

- These analeptics act directly on the central respiratory centers in the medulla or indirectly by stimulating the carotid chemoreceptors.

Absorption, distribution, and excretion

- Generally, these agents are quickly absorbed and well distributed.
- Nikethamide is partly metabolized to niacinamide, which is excreted in the urine as N-methylniacinamide.
- Pentylenetetrazol is readily absorbed following oral or intravenous administration; metabolized in the liver into at least 5 inactive metabolites, 75% of which are excreted in the urine. The excretory products have not been identified.

Onset and duration

- Onset is quick, usually within 1 minute.
- Duration is variable but short (usually 2 to 15 minutes).

Combination products

NICO-METRAZOL: pentylenetetrazol 100 mg, niacin 50 mg.

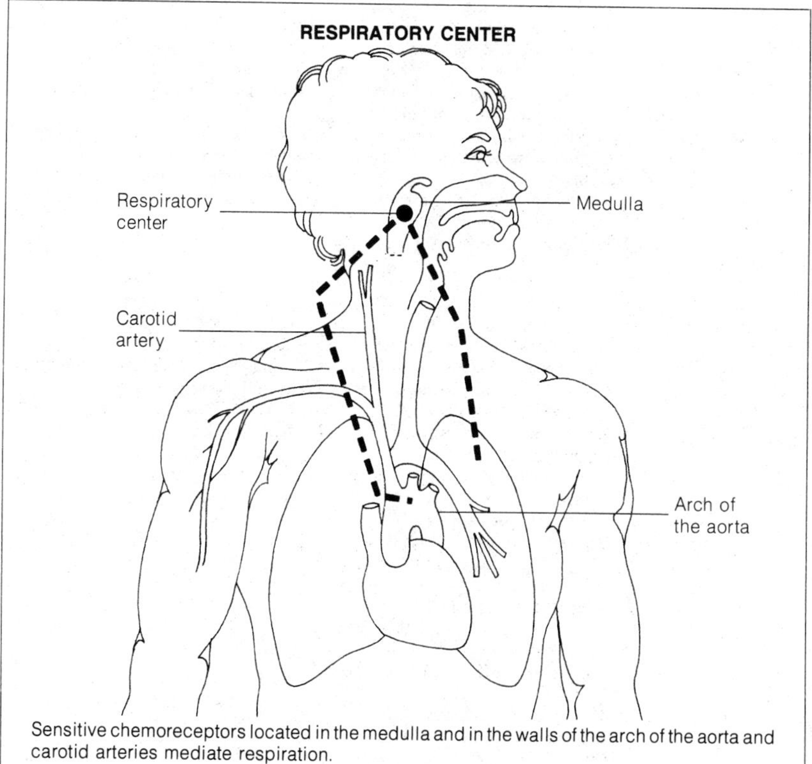

Sensitive chemoreceptors located in the medulla and in the walls of the arch of the aorta and carotid arteries mediate respiration.

NAME	INDICATIONS & DOSAGE	SIDE EFFECTS
ammonia, aromatic spirits	*Fainting—* **Adults and children:** inhale as needed.	None reported.
doxapram hydrochloride Dopram◆	*Postanesthesia respiratory stimulant, drug-induced central nervous system depression, and chronic pulmonary disease associated with acute hypercapnia—* **Adults:** 0.5 to 1 mg/Kg of body weight (up to 2 mg/Kg in CNS depression), I.V. injection or infusion. Maximum 4 mg/Kg up to 3 g in 1 day. Infusion rate 1 to 3 mg/min (initial: 5 mg/min for postanesthesia). *Chronic obstructive pulmonary disease—* **Adults:** infusion, 1 to 2 mg/min. Maximum 3 mg/min for a maximum duration of 2 hours.	*CNS:* headache, dizziness, apprehension, disorientation, pupillary dilation, bilateral Babinski signs, hyperpyrexia, flushing, sweating, pruritus, paresthesias. *CV:* lowered T-waves, hypotension, chest pain and tightness, variations in heart rate. *GI:* nausea, vomiting, diarrhea. *GU:* urinary retention, or stimulation of the urinary bladder with spontaneous voiding. *Other:* sneezing, coughing, laryngospasm, bronchospasm, hiccups, rebound hypoventilation, cerebral vasoconstriction, decreased cerebral circulation.
nikethamide Coramine◆, Kardonyl◆◆	**Adults:** *Acute alcoholism*—1.25 g to 5 g I.V.; repeat as necessary. *Carbon monoxide poisoning*—1.25 g to 2.5 g I.V. initially, then 1.25 g q 15 minutes for first hour, depending on response. *Cardiac arrest*—125 mg to 250 mg intracardially associated with anesthetic overdosage. *Combat respiratory paralysis*—3.75 g I.V.; repeat as required. *Overcome respiratory depression*—1.25 to 2.5 g I.V. *Shock*—2.5 g to 3.75 g I.V. or I.M. initially; repeat as indicated. *Shorten narcosis*—1 g I.V. or I.M. **Neonates:** *Adjunct in neonatal asphyxia*—3.75 mg injected into umbilical vein. Oral maintenance: **Adults and children:** 3 to 5 ml oral solution q 4 to 6 hours.	*CNS:* restlessness, muscle twitching or fasciculations. *CV:* increase in heart rate, respiratory rate, and blood pressure. *EENT:* unpleasant burning or itching at back of nose. *GI:* nausea, vomiting. *Other:* flushing, feeling of warmth, fear, sneezing, coughing, sweating.

◆ Also available in Canada.
◆◆ Available in Canada only.
Unmarked trade names available in United States only.

INTERACTIONS	NURSING CONSIDERATIONS
None significant.	• Stimulates mucous membranes of upper respiratory tract.
MAO inhibitors: potentiated adverse cardiovascular effects. Use together cautiously.	• Contraindicated in epilepsy, convulsive disorders, head injury, cardiovascular disorders, frank uncompensated heart failure, severe hypertension, cerebrovascular accidents, respiratory failure or incompetence secondary to neuromuscular disorders, muscle paresis, flail chest, obstructed airway, pulmonary embolism, pneumothorax, restrictive respiratory disease, acute bronchial asthma, extreme dyspnea, hypoxia not associated with hypercapnia. Use with caution in bronchial asthma, severe tachycardia or cardiac arrhythmias, cerebral edema or increased cerebrospinal fluid pressure, hyperthyroidism, pheochromocytoma, or profound metabolic disorders. • Establish adequate airway before administering drug. Prevent patient from aspirating vomitus. • Monitor blood pressure, heart rate, deep tendon reflexes, and arterial blood gases before giving drug and every 30 minutes afterward. • Be alert for signs of overdosage: hypertension, tachycardia, arrhythmias, skeletal muscle hyperactivity, dyspnea. Discontinue if patient shows signs of increased arterial carbon dioxide or oxygen tension, or if mechanical ventilation is started. May give I.V. injection of anticonvulsant for convulsions. • Use only in operating room or emergency room situations. • Do not combine with alkaline solutions.
None significant.	• Monitor patient's respiratory rate and volume. • Mechanical support of breathing is often preferred over nikethamide. • Don't inject intra-arterially; arterial spasm and thrombosis may result. • Watch for signs of overdosage: muscle tremors or spasm, retching, tachycardia, arrhythmias, hyperpyrexia, hyperpnea, convulsions, psychotic reactions, postictal depression. May give I.V. injection of diazepam or barbiturate such as thiopental sodium for convulsions. Induced emesis and gastric lavage aren't effective.

NAME	INDICATIONS & DOSAGE	SIDE EFFECTS
pentylenetetrazol Cenalene-M, Metrazol, Nelex-100, Nioric, Petrazole	*Overdose of CNS depressants*— **Adults:** 100 to 500 mg I.V. Repeat, if necessary, followed by 100 to 200 mg I.M., p.r.n. *In depression from barbiturates*— 5 ml of 10% solution I.V. within 3 to 5 seconds. If necessary, may be repeated until patient awakens. *To improve mental and physical activity in elderly patients*— **Adults:** 100 to 200 mg P.O. t.i.d.	Few side effects with oral administration; narrow margin of safety with parenteral administration. *Signs of overdose:* *CNS:* fasciculations, clonic convulsions. *CV:* slight increases in blood pressure, bradycardia. *GI:* nausea, vomiting. *Other:* hypersalivation, coughing, hyperthermia.

INTERACTIONS	NURSING CONSIDERATIONS
None significant.	• Use with caution in history of seizures or focal brain lesion. If dosage is high, use with caution in heart disease. • Analeptic use is not recommended. • False positive response to HCG pregnancy test.

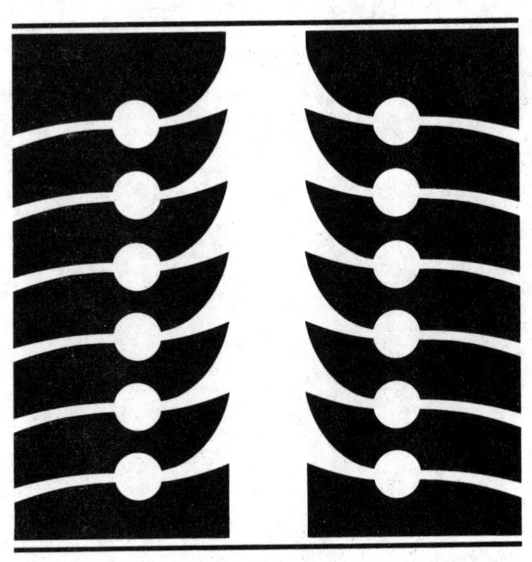

Autonomic System

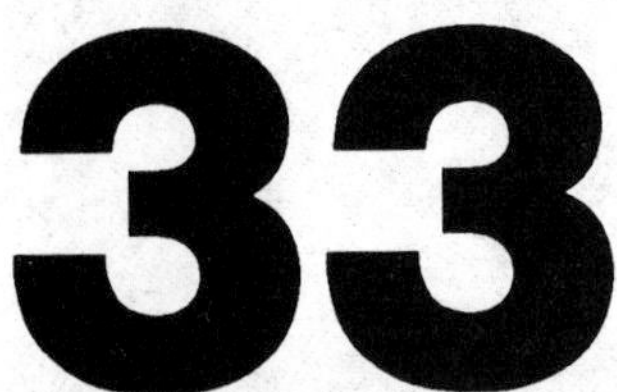

Cholinergics (parasympathomimetics)

bethanechol chloride
edrophonium chloride
neostigmine bromide
neostigmine methylsulfate
physostigmine salicylate
pyridostigmine bromide

The parasympathetic nervous system innervates a variety of body organs and systems; for example, eyes, sweat and salivary glands, heart, respiratory tract, stomach, liver, bladder, and intestines. Consequently drugs which stimulate the parasympathetic system (parasympathomimetics) have a variety of actions. These actions may be seen as a therapeutic response in one area of the body, as a side effect in another area.

Major uses

- To diagnose and treat myasthenia gravis.
- To prevent and treat postoperative abdominal distention and megacolon.
- To reverse the effect of neuromuscular blocking agents (muscle relaxants) used in surgical procedures.
- As antidote in anticholinergic (such as tricyclic drugs) poisoning (physostigmine salicylate).
- To treat postoperative urinary retention and neurogenic bladder.
- To treat paroxysmal atrial tachycardia (edrophonium chloride).

Mechanism of action

- Stimulate or increase the effect of acetylcholine, which serves as the neurotransmitter for impulses in the parasympathetic nervous system. In this way, parasympathomimetics mimic the effect of acetylcholine on the parasympathetic system.

Absorption, distribution, and excretion

- Absorption varies from fair to good, depending somewhat on how these drugs are administered.
- Widely distributed to organs innervated by the parasympathetic nervous system.
- Usually excreted by the kidneys as water-soluble metabolites.

Onset and duration

- Given orally, parasympathetic drugs start acting in 30 minutes and last from 2 to 6 hours.
- Given intramuscularly or subcutaneously, they start acting within 15 minutes and last from 2 to 6 hours.
- Given intravenously, they start acting immediately; their effects last from minutes for edrophonium to as long as 3 hours for neostigmine.

Combination products

None.

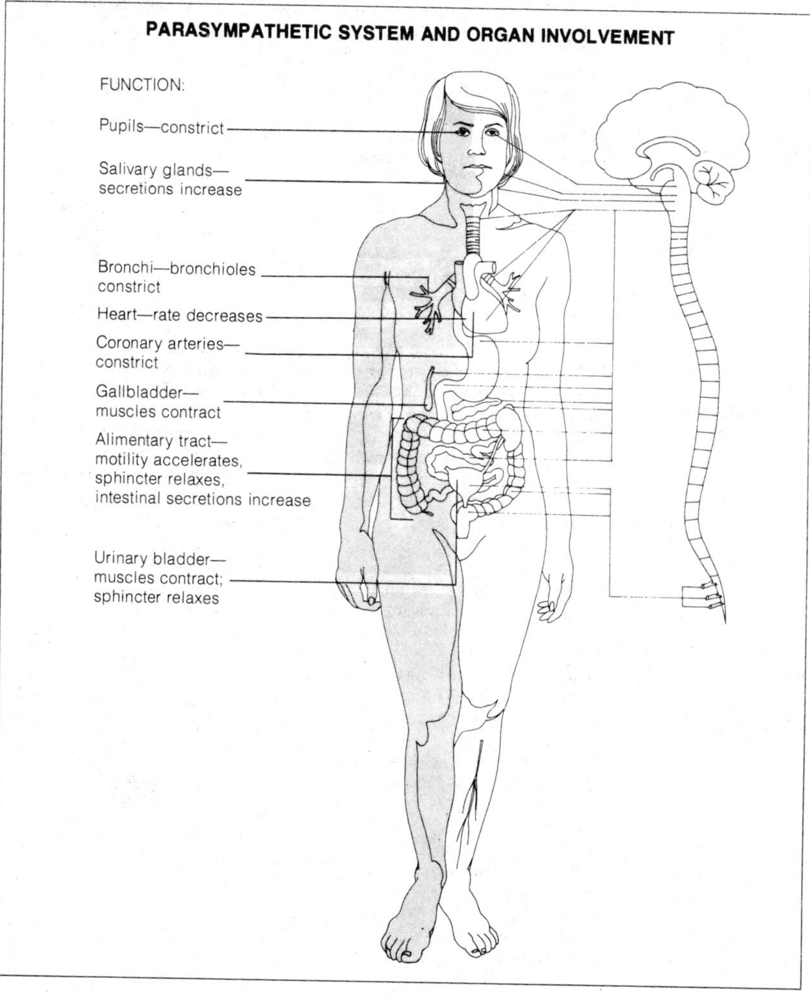
PARASYMPATHETIC SYSTEM AND ORGAN INVOLVEMENT
FUNCTION:
Pupils—constrict
Salivary glands—secretions increase
Bronchi—bronchioles constrict
Heart—rate decreases
Coronary arteries—constrict
Gallbladder—muscles contract
Alimentary tract—motility accelerates, sphincter relaxes, intestinal secretions increase
Urinary bladder—muscles contract; sphincter relaxes

NAME	INDICATIONS & DOSAGE	SIDE EFFECTS
bethanechol chloride Mictrol-10, Mictrol-25, Myotonachol, Urecholine◆, Urolax, Vesicholine	*Acute postop and postpartum nonobstructive (functional) urinary retention, neurogenic atony of urinary bladder with retention, abdominal distention, megacolon—* **Adults:** 10 to 30 mg P.O. t.i.d. to q.i.d. Never give I.M. or I.V. When used for urinary retention, some patients may require 50 to 100 mg P.O. per dose. Use such doses with extreme caution. Test dose: 2.5 mg S.C. repeated at 15- to 30-minute intervals to total of 4 doses to determine the minimal effective dose; then use minimal effective dose q 6 to 8 hours. All doses must be adjusted individually.	*Dose related:* *CNS:* headache, malaise. *CV:* bradycardia, hypotension, cardiac arrest, tachycardia. *EENT:* lacrimation, salivation, miosis. *GI:* abdominal cramps, diarrhea, nausea, vomiting, belching, borborygmi. *GU:* urinary urgency. *Skin:* flushing. *Other:* bronchoconstriction, sweating.
edrophonium chloride Tensilon◆	*As a curare antagonist (to reverse neuromuscular blocking action)—* **Adults:** 10 mg I.V. given over 30 to 45 seconds. Dose may be repeated as necessary to 40 mg maximum dose per patient. Larger doses may potentiate rather than antagonize effect of curare. *Diagnostic aid in myasthenia gravis—* **Adults:** 1 to 2 mg I.V. within 15 to 30 seconds, then 8 mg if no response (increase in muscle strength). **Children over 34 Kg.:** 2 mg I.V. If no response within 45 seconds, give 1 mg q 45 seconds to maximum of 10 mg. **Children up to 34 Kg.:** 1 mg I.V. If no response within 45 seconds, give 1 mg q 45 seconds to maximum of 5 mg. **Infants:** 0.5 mg I.V. *To differentiate myasthenic crisis from cholinergic crisis—* **Adults:** 1 mg I.V. If no response in 1 minute, repeat dose once. Increased muscular strength confirms myasthenic crisis; no increase or exaggerated weakness confirms cholinergic crisis.	*CNS:* weakness, respiratory paralysis. *CV:* hypotension, bradycardia. *EENT:* miosis. *GI:* nausea, vomiting, diarrhea, abdominal cramps, excessive salivation. *Other:* increased bronchial secretions, bronchospasm, muscle cramps, fasciculation, sweating.

◆ Also available in Canada.
◆◆ Available in Canada only.
Unmarked trade names available in United States only.

INTERACTIONS	NURSING CONSIDERATIONS
Procainamide, quinidine: may reverse cholinergic effects on muscle. Observe for lack of drug effect.	• Contraindicated in patients with uncertain strength or integrity of bladder wall; when increased muscular activity of GI or urinary tract is harmful; in mechanical obstructions of GI or urinary tract; in hyperthyroidism, peptic ulcer, latent or active bronchial asthma, cardiac or coronary artery disease, vagotonia, epilepsy, Parkinson's disease, bradycardia, chronic obstructive pulmonary disease, hypotension, hypertension, pregnancy, vasomotor instability, peritonitis, or other acute inflammatory conditions of GI tract. • Don't give I.M. or I.V.; could cause circulatory collapse, hypotension, severe abdominal cramping, bloody diarrhea, shock, cardiac arrest. • Should stop all other cholinergics before giving this drug. • Watch closely for side effects which may indicate drug toxicity, especially with S.C. administration. Call doctor promptly. • Monitor vital signs frequently, being especially careful to check respirations. Position patient to make breathing easier. Be prepared to give atropine 0.5 to 1 mg slow I.V. push, and provide respiratory support if needed. • If used to treat urinary retention, make sure bedpan is handy. Monitor intake/output. • When used to prevent abdominal distention and GI distress, the doctor may also order a rectal tube inserted to help passage of gas. • Poor and variable oral absorption requires larger oral doses. Oral and S.C. doses are *NOT* interchangeable. • Give on empty stomach; if taken after meals may cause nausea and vomiting. • For symptoms and treatment of toxicity, see p. 1117.
Procainamide, quinidine: may reverse cholinergic effects on muscle. Observe for lack of drug effect.	• Contraindicated in mechanical obstruction of intestine or urinary tract, bradycardia, hypotension. Use cautiously in hyperthyroidism, cardiac arrhythmias, peptic ulcer, bronchial asthma. • Should stop all other cholingerics before giving this drug. • Watch closely for side effects; may indicate toxicity. Call doctor promptly. • Monitor vital signs frequently, being especially careful to check respirations. Position patient to make breathing easier. Be prepared to give atropine 0.5 to 1 mg slow I.V. push, and provide respiratory support if needed. Have syringe available during test dose. • When giving drug to differentiate myasthenic crisis from cholinergic crisis, observe patient's muscle strength closely. • Edrophonium not effective against muscle relaxation induced by decamethonium bromide and succinylcholine chloride. • This cholinergic has the most rapid onset but shortest duration. • For easier parenteral administration, use a tuberculin syringe with an I.V. needle and leave in situ. • I.M. route may be used in children due to difficulty with the I.V. route: for children under 34 Kg, inject 2 mg I.M.; children over 34 Kg, 5 mg I.M. Expect same reactions as with I.V. test, but these appear after 2- to 10-minute delay. • When used as antidote for curariform drugs, record each dose given. • For symptoms and treatment of toxicity, see p. 1117.

NAME	INDICATIONS & DOSAGE	SIDE EFFECTS
neostigmine bromide Prostigmin Bromide♦ **neostigmine methylsulfate** Prostigmin♦	*Antidote for tubocurarine—* **Adults:** 0.5 to 2 mg I.V. slowly. Repeat p.r.n. Give 0.6 to 1.2 mg atropine sulfate I.V. before antidote dose. *Functional amenorrhea*—1 mg I.M. or S.C. daily for 3 days. *Postop abdominal distention and bladder atony—* **Adults:** 0.5 to 1 mg I.M. or S.C. q 4 to 6 hours. *Postop ileus—* **Adults:** 0.25 to 1 mg I.M. or S.C. q 4 to 6 hours. *Treatment of myasthenia gravis—* **Adults:** 15 to 30 mg t.i.d. (range 15 to 375 mg per day); or 0.5 to 2 mg I.M. or I.V. q 1 to 3 hours. Dose must be individualized, depending on response and tolerance of side effects. Therapy may be required day and night. **Children:** 7.5 to 15 mg P.O. t.i.d. to q.i.d. *Note:* 1:1,000 solution of injectable solution contains 1 mg/1 ml.	*CNS:* dizziness, muscle weakness, mental confusion, jitteriness, sweating, respiratory depression. *CV:* bradycardia, hypotension. *EENT:* miosis. *GI:* nausea, vomiting, diarrhea, abdominal cramps, excessive salivation. *Other:* bronchospasm, muscle cramps, bronchoconstriction.
physostigmine salicylate Antilirium♦	*Anticholinergic poisoning—* **Adults:** 0.5 to 4 mg I.M. or I.V. q 2 hours. *Tricyclic antidepressant poisoning—* **Adults:** 0.5 to 3 mg I.M. or I.V. (1 mg per minute I.V.) repeated as necessary if life-threatening signs recur (coma, convulsions, arrhythmias). For ophthalmic dose, see p. 822.	*CNS:* hallucinations, muscular twitching, muscle weakness, ataxia, restlessness, excitability, sweating. *CV:* irregular pulse, palpitations. *EENT:* miosis. *GI:* nausea, vomiting, epigastric pain, excessive salivation. *Other:* bronchospasm, bronchial constriction, dyspnea.

INTERACTIONS	NURSING CONSIDERATIONS
Procainamide, quinidine: may reverse cholinergic effect on muscle. Observe for lack of drug effect.	• Contraindicated in peritonitis, decreased GI motility, hypersensitivity to cholinergics or to bromide, mechanical obstruction of the intestine or urinary tract, bradycardia, hypotension. Use with extreme caution in bronchial asthma. Use cautiously in epilepsy, recent coronary occlusion, vagotonia, hyperthyroidism, cardiac arrhythmias, or peptic ulcer. • Should stop all other cholinergics before giving this drug. • Watch closely for side effects; may indicate toxicity. Call doctor promptly. • Monitor vital signs frequently, being especially careful to check respirations. Position patient to make breathing easier. Be prepared to give atropine 0.5 to 1 mg slow I.V. push, and provide respiratory support if needed. • Difficult to judge optimum dose. Help doctor by documenting patient's response after each dose. Show patient how to observe and record variations in muscle strength. • When using for myasthenia gravis, explain that this drug will relieve lid drooping, double vision, difficulty in chewing and swallowing, trunk and limb weakness. Stress importance of taking drug exactly as ordered. Explain that drug must be taken for life. Explain the drug's effect on myasthenic symptoms. • If patient has dysphagia, schedule dose 30 minutes before each meal. • When used to prevent abdominal distention and GI distress, the doctor may order a rectal tube inserted to help passage of gas. • Patients sometimes develop a resistance to neostigmine. • When used for functional amenorrhea, check for vaginal bleeding and instruct patient to report any vaginal bleeding. If no bleeding in 72 hours after third injection, the patient has nonfunctional amenorrhea. • If muscle weakness is severe, doctor determines if drug-induced toxicity or exacerbation of myasthenia gravis. Test dose of edrophonium I.V. will aggravate drug-induced weakness but will temporarily relieve weakness caused by disease. • Hospitalized patients with long-standing myasthenia may request bedside supply of tablets. Seek approval, if indicated, but continue to oversee medication regimen. • For symptoms and treatment of toxicity, see p. 1117.
Procainamide, quinidine: may reverse cholinergic effects on muscle. Observe for lack of drug effect.	• Contraindicated in mechanical obstruction of intestine or urogenital tract, bronchial asthma, gangrene, diabetes, cardiovascular disease, vagotonia, bradycardia, hypotension, epilepsy, or Parkinson's disease. Use cautiously in hyperthyroidism, peptic ulcer. • Should stop all other cholinergics before giving this drug. • Watch closely for side effects, particularly CNS disturbances. Use side rails if patient becomes restless or hallucinates. Side effects may indicate drug toxicity. Call doctor promptly. • Monitor vital signs frequently, being especially careful to check respirations. Position patient to make breathing easier. Be prepared to give atropine 0.5 to 1 mg slow I.V. push, and provide respiratory support if needed. • Use only clear solution. Darkening may indicate loss of potency. • Best administered in presence of doctor. • Give I.V. at controlled rate; use slow, direct injection at no more than 1 mg/min. • For symptoms and treatment of toxicity, see p. 1117.

NAME	INDICATIONS & DOSAGE	SIDE EFFECTS
pyridostigmine bromide Mestinon◆, Regonol◆	*Curariform antagonist—* **Adults:** 10 to 30 mg I.V. followed by atropine sulfate 0.6 to 1.2 mg I.V. *Myasthenia gravis—* **Adults:** 60 to 180 mg P.O. b.i.d. or q.i.d. Usual dose 600 mg daily but higher doses may be needed (up to 1,500 mg per day). Give 1/30th of oral dose I.M. or I.V. Dose must be adjusted for each patient, depending on response and tolerance of side effects.	*CNS:* headache (with high doses), weakness, sweating, convulsions. *CV:* bradycardia, hypotension, thrombophlebitis after I.V. administration. *EENT:* miosis. *GI:* abdominal cramps, nausea, vomiting, diarrhea, excessive salivation. *Skin:* rash. *Other:* bronchospasm, bronchoconstriction, increased bronchial secretions, muscle cramps, fasciculation.

INTERACTIONS	NURSING CONSIDERATIONS
Procainamide, quinidine: may reverse cholinergic effects on muscle. Observe for lack of drug effect.	• Contraindicated in mechanical obstruction of intestine or urinary tract, bradycardia, hypotension. Use with extreme caution in bronchial asthma. Use cautiously in epilepsy, recent coronary occlusion, vagotonia, hyperthyroidism, cardiac arrhythmias, peptic ulcer. Avoid large doses in decreased gastrointestinal motility or megacolon. • Difficult to judge optimum dosage. Help doctor by recording patient's response after each dose. • Should stop all other cholinergics before giving this drug. • Watch closely for side effects; may indicate toxicity. Call doctor promptly. • Monitor vital signs frequently, being especially careful to check respirations. Position patient to make breathing easier. Be prepared to give atropine 0.5 to 1 mg slow I.V. push, and provide respiratory support if needed. • If muscle weakness is severe, doctor determines if drug-induced toxicity or exacerbation of myasthenia gravis. Test dose of edrophonium I.V. will aggravate drug-induced weakness but will temporarily relieve weakness caused by disease. • When using for myasthenia gravis, stress importance of taking drug exactly as ordered, on time, in evenly spaced doses. If doctor has ordered extended-release tablets, explain how these work. Patient must take them at the same time each day, at least 6 hours apart. Explain that he must take this drug for life. Tell about the drug's effect on myasthenic symptoms. • Has longest duration of the cholinergics used for myasthenia gravis. • Available in 60 mg tablets, sustained-release (180 mg) tablets, injection, and syrup. • For symptoms and treatment of toxicity, see p. 1117.

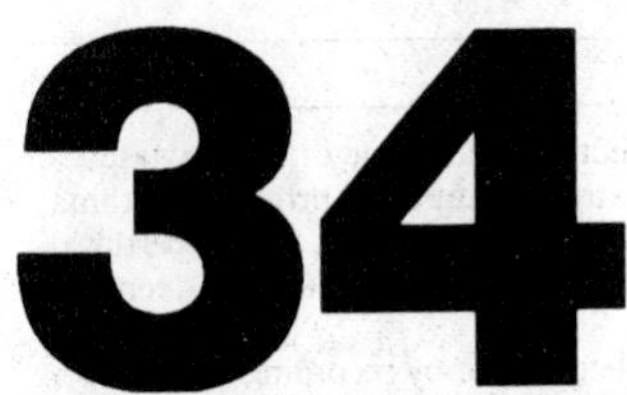

Cholinergic blockers (parasympatholytics)

atropine sulfate
benztropine mesylate
biperiden
chlorphenoxamine hydrochloride
cycrimine hydrochloride
ethopropazine hydrochloride
glycopyrrolate
methscopolamine bromide
procyclidine hydrochloride
scopolamine hydrobromide
trihexyphenidyl hydrochloride

The parasympathetic nervous system innervates a variety of body organs and systems; for example, eyes, sweat and salivary glands, heart, respiratory tract, stomach, liver, bladder, and intestines. Consequently, drugs which inhibit or block the actions of the parasympathetic system (parasympatholytics) have a variety of actions. In one area of the body, their action may be seen as a therapeutic response; in another, as a side effect. Major parasympathetic responses are triggered by the body's natural release of the neurotransmitter, acetylcholine. Nerve fibers transmitting these responses are largely cholinergic.

For cholinergic blockers used specifically for gastrointestinal disorders, see Chapter 46.

Major uses

• To reduce normal body secretions; for example, gastric acid, salivation, perspiration, and bronchial mucus.
• To reduce spasm or smooth-muscle contraction of the gastrointestinal tract, bladder, or respiratory tract.
• To treat parkinsonism, paralysis agitans, and drug-induced extrapyramidal disorders.

Mechanism of action

• Inhibit or block the effect of acetylcholine, which serves as the neurotransmitter for impulses in the parasympathetic nervous system. This inhibition or blocking takes place at the junction between the postganglionic nerve endings and the effector organs.

Absorption, distribution, and excretion

• Oral absorption of these drugs ranges from moderately poor to moderately good.
• After administration, these drugs are widely distributed to organs innervated by the parasympathetic nervous system. CNS penetration is more likely with atropine, benztropine, biperiden, scopolamine, and trihexyphenidyl.
• These drugs are excreted unchanged in the urine.

Onset and duration

• When given intravenously, onset is immediate; duration of effect, from 1 to 4 hours.

- When given intramuscularly or subcutaneously, onset is within 30 minutes; duration of effect, from 2 to 6 hours.
- When given orally, onset is from 30 to 60 minutes; duration of effect, from 4 to 6 hours.

Combination products
Cholinergic blocking agents are available in tablets and capsules in varying combinations including an anticholinergic and a sedative.

HOW CHOLINERGIC BLOCKERS WORK

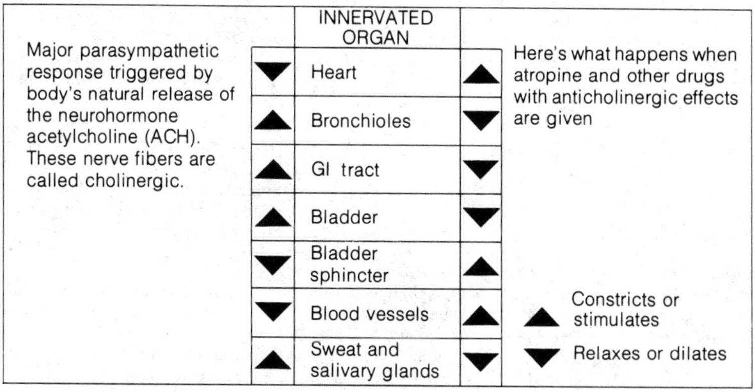

Major parasympathetic response triggered by body's natural release of the neurohormone acetylcholine (ACH). These nerve fibers are called cholinergic.

Here's what happens when atropine and other drugs with anticholinergic effects are given

	INNERVATED ORGAN	
▼	Heart	▲
▲	Bronchioles	▼
▲	GI tract	▼
▲	Bladder	▼
▼	Bladder sphincter	▲
▼	Blood vessels	▲
▲	Sweat and salivary glands	▼

▲ Constricts or stimulates

▼ Relaxes or dilates

Overstimulation of the parasympathetic system will decrease heart rate, leading to bradycardia. The anticholinergic drug atropine, which blocks the body's response to acetylcholine, turns this response around. It increases the heart rate, so the drug is useful as an antiarrhythmic.

NAME	INDICATIONS & DOSAGE	SIDE EFFECTS
atropine sulfate	*Antidote for anticholinesterase insecticide poisoning—* **Adults and children:** 2 mg I.M. or I.V. repeated at hourly intervals until muscarinic symptoms disappear. Severe cases may require up to 6 mg I.M. or I.V. q 1 hour. *Preop for diminishing secretions—* **Adults:** 0.4 to 0.6 mg I.M. 45 to 60 minutes before anesthesia. **Children:** 0.01 mg/Kg I.M. up to a maximum dose of 0.4 mg 45 to 60 minutes before anesthesia. For treatment of brady-arrhythmias, see Chapter 18.	*CNS:* disorientation, restlessness, irritability, incoherence, weakness, nervousness, drowsiness, dizziness, hallucinations, headache. *CV:* palpitations, tachycardia, paradoxical bradycardia with doses less than 0.4 mg. *EENT:* dilated pupils, blurred vision, photophobia, increased intraocular pressure, eye pain, dysphagia. *GI:* constipation, mouth dryness, nausea, vomiting, paralytic ileus, epigastric distress. *GU:* urinary hesitancy or retention. *Skin:* flushing, dryness, rash. *Other:* bronchial plugging, fever. Side effects above may be due to pending atropine toxicity and are dose-related. With usual doses of 0.4 to 0.6 mg, there are few side effects other than dry mouth. However, individual tolerance varies greatly.
benztropine mesylate Cogentin♦	*Acute dystonic reaction—* **Adults:** 2 mg I.V. or I.M. followed by 1 to 2 mg P.O. b.i.d. to prevent recurrence. *Parkinsonism—* **Adults:** 0.5 to 6 mg P.O. daily. Initial dose 0.5 to 1 mg. Increase 0.5 mg every 5 to 6 days. Adjust dosage to meet individual requirements.	*CNS:* disorientation, restlessness, irritability, incoherence, weakness, nervousness, drowsiness, dizziness, hallucinations, headache, sedation, depression, muscular weakness. *CV:* palpitations, tachycardia, paradoxical bradycardia. *EENT:* dilated pupils, blurred vision, photophobia, difficulty swallowing. *GI:* constipation, mouth dryness, nausea, vomiting, epigastric distress. *GU:* urinary hesitancy or retention. *Skin:* rash. Some side effects may be due to pending atropine-like toxicity and are dose-related.
biperiden hydrochloride or lactate Akineton♦	*Extrapyramidal disorders—* **Adults:** 2 to 6 mg P.O. daily, b.i.d., or t.i.d., depending on severity. Usual dose is 2 mg daily, or 2 mg I.M. or I.V. q ½ hour, not to exceed 4 doses or 8 mg total daily. *Parkinsonism—* **Adults:** 2 mg P.O. t.i.d. to q.i.d.	*CNS:* disorientation, euphoria, restlessness, irritability, incoherence, nervousness, drowsiness, dizziness, increased tremor. *CV:* transient postural hypotension. *EENT:* blurred vision. *GI:* constipation, mouth dryness, nausea, vomiting, epigastric distress. *GU:* urinary hesitancy or retention. Side effects are dose-related and may resemble atropine toxicity.

♦ Also available in Canada.
♦♦ Available in Canada only.
Unmarked trade names available in United States only.

INTERACTIONS	NURSING CONSIDERATIONS
Methotrimeprazine: extrapyramidal symptoms when used with anticholinergics. Use together with caution.	• Contraindicated in narrow-angle glaucoma, obstructive uropathy, obstructive disease of GI tract, asthma, myasthenia gravis, paralytic ileus, intestinal atony, unstable cardiovascular status in acute hemorrhage, and toxic megacolon. Use with caution in autonomic neuropathy, hyperthyroidism, coronary heart disease, cardiac arrhythmias, congestive heart failure, hypertension, hiatal hernia associated with reflux esophagitis, hepatic or renal disease, ulcerative colitis, in patients over 40 because of the increased incidence of glaucoma, and in children under 6 years. Use with caution in hot or humid environments. Drug-induced heat stroke possible. • Check all dosages carefully. Even slight overdose could lead to toxicity. • Monitor vital signs carefully. Watch closely for side effects, especially in elderly or debilitated patients. Call doctor promptly. • When given I.V., may cause paradoxical initial bradycardia. Usually disappears within 2 minutes. • Monitor intake/output. Drug causes urinary retention and hesitancy; have patient void before administering it. • For symptoms and treatment of toxicity, see p. 1115.
Amantadine: anticholinergic side effects, such as confusion and hallucinations. Reduce dosage before administering amantadine.	• Contraindicated in angle-closure glaucoma. Use cautiously in prostatic hypertrophy, tendency to tachycardia, and in elderly or debilitated patients; produces atropine-like side effects. • Monitor vital signs carefully. Watch closely for side effects, especially in elderly or debilitated patients. Call doctor promptly. • Never discontinue this drug abruptly. Dosages must be reduced gradually. • Warn patient to avoid activities that require alertness until response to drug is determined. If patient is to receive single daily dose, give at bedtime. • Explain that drug may take 2 to 3 days to exert full effect. • Monitor intake/output. • Watch for intermittent constipation, distention, abdominal pain; may be onset of paralytic ileus. • Relieve dry mouth with cool drinks, ice chips, sugarless gum, or hard candy. • To help prevent gastric irritation administer after meals. • For symptoms and treatment of toxicity, see p. 1115.
None significant.	• Use with caution in prostatism, cardiac arrhythmias, narrow-angle glaucoma. • Monitor vital signs carefully. Watch closely for side effects, especially in elderly or debilitated patients. Call doctor promptly. • Give oral doses with or after meals to decrease GI side effects. • When giving parenterally, keep patient supine. Parenteral administration may cause transient postural hypotension and coordination disturbances. • Because of possible dizziness, assist patient when he gets out of bed. • Tolerance may develop and may require increased dosage. • In severe parkinsonism, tremors may increase as spasticity is relieved. • Relieve dry mouth with cool drinks, ice chips, sugarless gum, or hard candy. • I.V. injections should be made very slowly. • For symptoms and treatment of toxicity, see p. 1115.

NAME	INDICATIONS & DOSAGE	SIDE EFFECTS
chlorphenoxamine hydrochloride Phenoxene◆	*Parkinsonism—* **Adults:** 50 mg P.O. t.i.d.; in severe cases, 300 to 400 mg daily, 100 mg t.i.d. to q.i.d.	*CNS:* drowsiness, sedation, increased tremors. *EENT:* blurred vision. *GI:* constipation, dry mouth, nausea, vomiting, epigastric distress.
cycrimine hydrochloride Pagitane Hydrochloride	*Idiopathic and arteriosclerotic parkinsonism—* **Adults:** initially, 1.25 to 2.5 mg P.O. t.i.d.; gradually increasing dosage to 5 mg q.i.d. *Postencephalitic parkinsonism—* **Adults:** 5 mg t.i.d. or up to 5 mg q 2 hours while awake.	*CNS:* disorientation, incoherence, weakness, drowsiness, dizziness. *EENT:* blurred vision. *GI:* epigastric distress, sore mouth and tongue, constipation, mouth dryness. Also transient nausea and anorexia 30 minutes to 1 hour after administration. *Skin:* flushing, dryness, rash. *Other:* fever.
ethopropazine hydrochloride Parsidol, Parsitan◆◆	*Parkinsonism—* **Adults:** initially, 10 mg P.O. q.i.d., then increase 10 mg per dose every 2 to 3 days until desired effect or tolerance is reached. Maintenance dose: 100 to 600 mg P.O. daily in divided doses.	*CNS:* drowsiness, dizziness, headache, confusion, paresthesia, ataxia, accentuation of parkinsonism. *EENT:* blurred vision. *GI:* mouth dryness, epigastric distress, constipation. *GU:* urinary retention.
glycopyrrolate Robinul, Robinul Forte◆	*To reverse neuromuscular blockade—* **Adults:** 0.2 mg for each 1 mg neostigmine or equivalent dose of pyridostigmine. May be given intravenously without dilution or may be added to dextrose injection and given by infusion.	*CNS:* disorientation, restlessness, irritability, incoherence, weakness, nervousness, drowsiness, dizziness, hallucinations, headache. *CV:* palpitations, tachycardia, paradoxical bradycardia. *EENT:* dilated pupils, blurred vision, photophobia, increased intraocular pressure, difficulty swallowing. *GI:* constipation, mouth dryness, nausea, vomiting, paralytic ileus, epigastric distress. *GU:* urinary hesitancy or retention. *Local:* burning at injection site. *Skin:* flushing, dryness, rash. *Other:* bronchial plugging, fever.

INTERACTIONS	NURSING CONSIDERATIONS
None significant.	• Use cautiously in narrow-angle glaucoma, tachycardia, or prostatic hypertrophy. • Monitor vital signs carefully. Watch closely for side effects, especially in elderly or debilitated patients. Call doctor promptly. • Warn patient to avoid activities that require alertness until reaction to drug is determined. • Administer doses with milk after meals to decrease GI side effects. • In severe parkinsonism, tremors may increase as spasticity is relieved. • Tolerance may develop and may require increased dosage. • Relieve dry mouth with cool drinks, ice chips, sugarless gum, or hard candy. • For symptoms and treatment of toxicity, see p. 1115.
None significant.	• Use with caution in narrow-angle glaucoma; in the elderly with arteriosclerotic changes; in tachycardia or any tendency toward urinary retention. • Monitor vital signs carefully. • Watch closely for side effects, especially vertigo, disorientation, and weakness. Call doctor promptly; he may want to stop or reduce dosage. • Explain that mild side effects, such as dry mouth, blurred vision, epigastric distress, disappear with continued administration. • Administer doses with milk or after meals to decrease GI side effects. • Relieve dry mouth with cool drinks, ice chips, sugarless gum, or hard candy. • For symptoms and treatment of toxicity, see p. 1115.
None significant.	• Contraindicated in hypersensitivity to phenothiazine, or in narrow-angle glaucoma. Use with caution in cardiac disease, prostatic hypertrophy, or pyloric obstruction. • Prolonged high dosage may result in restlessness, delirium, hallucinations, convulsions, overt hostility, paranoid psychosis. Call doctor promptly. • Monitor intake/output because of possible urinary retention. • Relieve dry mouth with cool drinks, ice chips, sugarless gum, or hard candy. • For symptoms and treatment of toxicity, see p. 1115.
None significant.	• Contraindicated in narrow-angle glaucoma, obstructive uropathy, obstructive disease of the GI tract, myasthenia gravis, paralytic ileus, intestinal atony, unstable cardiovascular status in acute hemorrhage, toxic megacolon. Use with caution in autonomic neuropathy, hyperthyroidism, coronary heart disease, cardiac arrhythmias, congestive heart failure, hypertension, hiatal hernia associated with reflux esophagitis, hepatic or renal disease, ulcerative colitis, and patients over 40 because of increased incidence of glaucoma. Use with caution in hot or humid environments. Drug-induced heat stroke possible. • Check all dosages carefully. Even slight overdose could lead to toxicity. • Don't mix with I.V. solution containing sodium chloride or bicarbonate. • When given parenterally, may retard gastric emptying. Have a nasogastric tube handy after 2 or more parenteral doses are administered. • Monitor vital signs carefully. Watch closely for side effects, especially in elderly or debilitated patients. Call doctor promptly. • Monitor intake/output. Causes urinary retention or hesitancy. • Side effects less likely than with other parasympatholytics, unless dosages are excessive. • For symptoms and treatment of toxicity, see p. 1115.

NAME	INDICATIONS & DOSAGE	SIDE EFFECTS
methscopolamine bromide Pamine◆, Scoline	*Adjunctive treatment of peptic ulcer and disorders associated with hypersecretion, hypermotility, or spasm—* **Adults:** 2.5 to 5 mg P.O. given 30 minutes before meals and h.s., or 0.25 to 1 mg I.M. or S.C. q 6 to 8 hours. **Children:** 0.2 mg/Kg P.O. daily or 6 mg/m² daily divided q.i.d.	*CNS:* disorientation, restlessness, irritability, incoherence, weakness, nervousness, drowsiness, dizziness, hallucinations, headache, decreased mental alertness. *CV:* palpitations, tachycardia, paradoxical bradycardia. *EENT:* dilated pupils, blurred vision, photophobia, increased intraocular pressure, difficulty swallowing. *GI:* constipation, mouth dryness, nausea, vomiting, paralytic ileus, epigastric distress, loss of taste. *GU:* urinary hesitancy or retention. *Skin:* flushing, dryness, rash. *Other:* bronchial plugging, fever. Side effects may be due to pending toxicity and are dose-related. Individual tolerance varies greatly.
procyclidine hydrochloride Kemadrin◆, Procyclid◆◆	*Parkinsonism, muscle rigidity—* **Adults:** initially, 2 to 2.5 mg P.O. t.i.d., after meals. Increase as needed to maximum 60 mg daily. Also used to relieve extrapyramidal dysfunction which accompanies treatment with phenothiazines and rauwolfia derivatives. Also controls sialorrhea from neuroleptic medications.	*CNS:* light-headedness, giddiness. *EENT:* blurred vision, mydriasis. *GI:* constipation, mouth dryness, nausea, vomiting, epigastric distress. *Skin:* rash.
scopolamine hydrobromide	*Postencephalitic parkinsonism and other spastic states—* **Adults:** 0.5 to 1 mg P.O. t.i.d. to q.i.d.; 0.3 to 0.6 mg S.C., I.M., or I.V. (with suitable dilution) t.i.d. to q.i.d. **Children:** 0.006 mg/Kg P.O. or S.C. t.i.d. to q.i.d.; or 0.20 mg/m².	*CNS:* disorientation, restlessness, irritability, incoherence, weakness, nervousness, drowsiness, dizziness, hallucinations, headache. *CV:* palpitations, tachycardia, paradoxical bradycardia. *EENT:* dilated pupils, blurred vision, photophobia, increased intraocular pressure, difficulty swallowing. *GI:* constipation, mouth dryness, nausea, vomiting, paralytic ileus, epigastric distress. *GU:* urinary hesitancy or retention. *Skin:* flushing, dryness, rash. *Other:* bronchial plugging, fever, depressed respirations. Side effects may be due to pending atropine-like toxicity and are dose-related. Individual tolerance varies greatly.

INTERACTIONS	NURSING CONSIDERATIONS
None significant.	• Contraindicated in acute or narrow-angle glaucoma; obstructive prostatic hypertrophy; paralytic ileus; pyloric, duodenal, or bladder neck obstruction; myasthenia gravis; tachycardia; ulcerative colitis. Use with caution in hepatic or renal disease, autonomic neuropathy, hyperthyroidism, coronary heart disease, cardiac arrhythmias, congestive heart failure, hypertension, or nonobstructive prostatic hypertrophy. • Heat prostration and fever possible with high environmental temperature. • Monitor vital signs carefully. Watch closely for side effects, especially in elderly or debilitated patients. Notify doctor. • Monitor intake/output. Causes urinary retention or hesitancy; have patient void before administering. • Warn patient to avoid activities that require alertness until response to drug is determined. • Relieve dry mouth with cool drinks, ice chips, sugarless gum, or hard candy. • For symptoms and treatment of toxicity, see p. 1115.
None significant.	• Contraindicated in angle-closure glaucoma. Use cautiously in tachycardia, hypotension, urinary retention, or prostatic hypertrophy. • Watch closely for mental confusion, disorientation, agitation, hallucinations, and psychotic symptoms, especially in elderly. Call doctor promptly. • In severe parkinsonism, tremors may increase as spasticity is relieved. • Give after meals. • Relieve dry mouth with cool drinks, ice chips, sugarless gum, or hard candy. • For symptoms and treatment of toxicity, see p. 1115.
Methotrimeprazine: extrapyramidal symptoms when used with anticholinergics. Use with caution.	• Contraindicated in narrow-angle glaucoma, obstructive uropathy, obstructive disease of the GI tract, asthma, chronic lung disease, myasthenia gravis, paralytic ileus, intestinal atony, unstable cardiovascular status in acute hemorrhage, or toxic megacolon. Use with caution in autonomic neuropathy, hyperthyroidism, coronary heart disease, cardiac arrhythmias, congestive heart failure, hypertension, hiatal hernia associated with reflux esophagitis, hepatic or renal disease, ulcerative colitis, in patients over 40 because of the increased incidence of glaucoma, and in children under 6 years. Use with caution in hot or humid environments. Drug-induced heat stroke possible. • Warn patient that he may experience transient amnesia after taking drug. • Some patients become temporarily excited or disoriented. Symptoms disappear when sedative effect is complete. Use bed rails as precaution. • Tolerance may develop when administered over a long period of time. • For symptoms and treatment of toxicity, see p. 1115.

NAME	INDICATIONS & DOSAGE	SIDE EFFECTS
trihexyphenidyl hydrochloride Aparkane♦♦, Artane♦, Hexaphen, Novohexidyl♦♦, T.H.P., Tremin, Trihexane, Trihexidyl, Trihexy♦♦, Trixyl♦♦	*Parkinsonism*— **Adults:** 1 mg P.O. 1st day, 2 mg 2nd day, then 2 mg every 3 to 5 days until total of 6 to 10 mg given daily. Usually given t.i.d. before meals and if need q.i.d. (last dose should be before bedtime). Postencephalitic parkinsonism may require 12 to 15 mg total daily dose.	*CNS:* nervousness, dizziness, headache, restlessness, agitation, confusion, delirium, hallucinations, euphoria, delusion, amnesia. *CV:* tachycardia. *EENT:* dry mouth, blurred vision, mydriasis, increased intraocular pressure. *GI:* nausea, vomiting, constipation. *GU:* urinary hesitancy or retention. Side effects are dose-related.

INTERACTIONS	NURSING CONSIDERATIONS
Amantadine: anticholinergic side effects, such as confusion and hallucinations. Reduce dosage before administering amantadine.	• Contraindicated in narrow-angle glaucoma. Use cautiously in cardiac, hepatic, or renal disorders; hypertension; obstructive disease of the GI and the genitourinary tracts; possible prostatic hypertrophy; patients over 60; and those with arteriosclerosis or history of drug hypersensitivities. • Warn patient to avoid activities that require alertness until response to drug is determined. • If giving before meals causes nausea, give after. • Relieve dry mouth with cool drinks, ice chips, sugarless gum, or hard candy. • Patient may develop a tolerance to this drug. • Gonioscopic evaluation and close monitoring of intraocular pressures advised. • For symptoms and treatment of toxicity, see p. 1115.

35

Adrenergics (sympathomimetics)

dobutamine hydrochloride
dopamine hydrochloride
ephedrine sulfate
epinephrine
epinephrine bitartrate
epinephrine hydrochloride
ethylnorepinephrine hydrochloride
isoproterenol hydrochloride
isoproterenol sulfate
levarterenol bitartrate (norepinephrine, noradrenaline)
mephentermine sulfate
metaproterenol sulfate
metaraminol bitartrate
methoxamine hydrochloride
methoxyphenamine hydrochloride
phenylephrine hydrochloride
protokylol hydrochloride
pseudoephedrine hydrochloride
terbutaline sulfate

The sympathetic nervous system regulates the body's expenditure of energy, especially in times of stress. In doing so, it innervates a variety of body organs and systems, for example, eyes, sweat and salivary glands, heart, respiratory tract, stomach, liver, bladder, and intestines. Because of this, drugs which stimulate the sympathetic nervous system (sympathomimetics) have a variety of actions. In one area of the body a drug's action may be seen as a therapeutic response, while in another area the same action may be a side effect.

Major sympathetic responses are triggered by the body's natural release of epinephrine (adrenaline) and norepinephrine. Nerve fibers transmitting these responses are largely adrenergic. In adrenergic nerves, two types of receptor cells exist that respond to stimulation: alpha and beta (B_1 and B_2) receptors. Stimulation of alpha receptors causes vasoconstriction, uterine muscle contraction, and sphincter contraction. $Beta_1$ stimulation increases heart rate, myocardial contraction, and atrioventricular conduction. $Beta_2$ stimulation causes bronchodilation, vasodilation, and uterine relaxation. The sympathomimetic amines may stimulate all or some of these receptors.

Dopamine exerts its own dopaminergic action on selected dopaminergic receptors and on alpha and beta receptors.

Major uses

• To improve blood pressure and cardiac output in severely decompensated states, such as cardiogenic shock and heart failure.
• To treat heart block, certain arrhythmias, paroxysmal atrial tachycardia (PAT), and cardiac arrest.
• To relieve bronchoconstriction.
• To treat anaphylaxis and other allergic reactions (common in asthmatic attacks), to relieve ophthalmic congestion, to control local hemorrhage, and to delay delivery in premature labor.

Mechanism of action

• Simulates or increases the effect of epinephrine and norepinephrine on alpha- and beta-adrenergic receptors within the sympathetic nervous system. Effects vary and include bronchodilation, release of glucose from liver, increased heart rate and contractility of ventricles, CNS excitation, dilation (beta effect) of blood vessels in skeletal muscles, and constriction (alpha effect) of blood vessels in cutaneous areas.

Absorption, distribution, and excretion

• The following drugs are absorbed well when given orally: ephedrine, metaproterenol, methoxyphenamine, protokylol, pseudoephedrine, and terbutaline.
• The following drugs are not effective when given orally but are rapidly absorbed when given intramuscularly or subcutaneously: epinephrine hydrochloride, isoproterenol hydrochloride, isoproterenol sulfate, metaraminol bitartrate, and methoxamine hydrochloride.
• All these drugs are widely distributed to organs innervated by the sympathetic nervous system. However, CNS penetration is more likely with ephedrine, isoproterenol, mephentermine, metaproterenol, methoxyphenamine, protokylol, pseudoephedrine, and terbutaline.
• Generally, these drugs are metabolized by the liver and are excreted unchanged or in metabolite form in the urine.

Onset and duration

- When given intravenously, the onset of these drugs is almost immediate; duration of action varies.
- When given intramuscularly, subcutaneously, or by inhalation, onset is within 15 minutes; duration varies.
- When given orally, onset is within 30 to 90 minutes; duration from 3 to 6 hours.

Combination products

Only a few of the many combinations are included here as examples of this group.

Inhalants

DUOHALER: isoproterenol hydrochloride 0.16 mg and phenylephrine bitartrate 0.24 mg per dose.
DUO-MEDIHALER: isoproterenol hydrochloride 0.16 mg and phenylephrine bitartrate 0.24 mg per dose.

Oral Bronchodilators

AMESEC◆: theophylline 130 mg, ephedrine 25 mg, and amobarbital 25 mg.
BRONCHOBID DURACAPS: theophylline 260 mg and pseudoephedrine HCl 50 mg.
MARAX◆: theophylline 130 mg, ephedrine 25 mg, and hydroxyzine HCl 10 mg.
QUADRINAL◆: theophylline calcium salicylate 130 mg, ephedrine hydrochloride 24 mg, potassium iodide 320 mg, and phenobarbital 24 mg.
QUIBRON PLUS: theophylline (anhydrous) 150 mg, ephedrine hydrochloride 25 mg, guaifenesin 100 mg, and butabarbital 20 mg.
TEDRAL-SA◆: theophylline 180 mg, ephedrine hydrochloride 48 mg, and phenobarbital 25 mg.
(OTC) ASMA-LIEF: theophylline 130 mg, ephedrine hydrochloride 24 mg, and phenobarbital 8 mg.
(OTC) TEDRAL◆: theophylline 130 mg, ephedrine hydrochloride 24 mg, and phenobarbital 8 mg.
(OTC) THALFED: theophylline (hydrous) 120 mg, ephedrine hydrochloride 25 mg, and phenobarbital 8 mg.

Decongestants

ACTIFED◆: pseudoephedrine hydrochloride 60 mg and triprolidine hydrochloride 2.5 mg.
CONGESPRIN: phenylephrine hydrochloride 1.25 mg and aspirin 8 mg.
DRISTAN: phenylephrine hydrochloride 5 mg, chlorpheniramine maleate 2 mg, aspirin 325 mg, and caffeine.
HISTASPAN PLUS◆: phenylephrine hydrochloride 20 mg and chlorpheniramine maleate 8 mg.
NALDECON: phenylpropanolamine hydrochloride 40 mg, phenylephrine hydrochloride 10 mg, chlorpheniramine 5 mg, and phenyltoloxamine citrate 15 mg.
ORNEX: phenylpropanolamine hydrochloride 18 mg and acetaminophen 325 mg.
PHENERGAN D: pseudoephedrine hydrochloride 60 mg and promethazine hydrochloride 6.25 mg.
SINUTAB II: phenylpropanolamine hydrochloride 25 mg and acetaminophen 325 mg.
TRIAMINIC: phenylpropanolamine hydrochloride 50 mg, pyrilamine maleate 25 mg, and pheniramine maleate 25 mg.

SYMPATHETIC SYSTEM AND ORGAN INVOLVEMENT

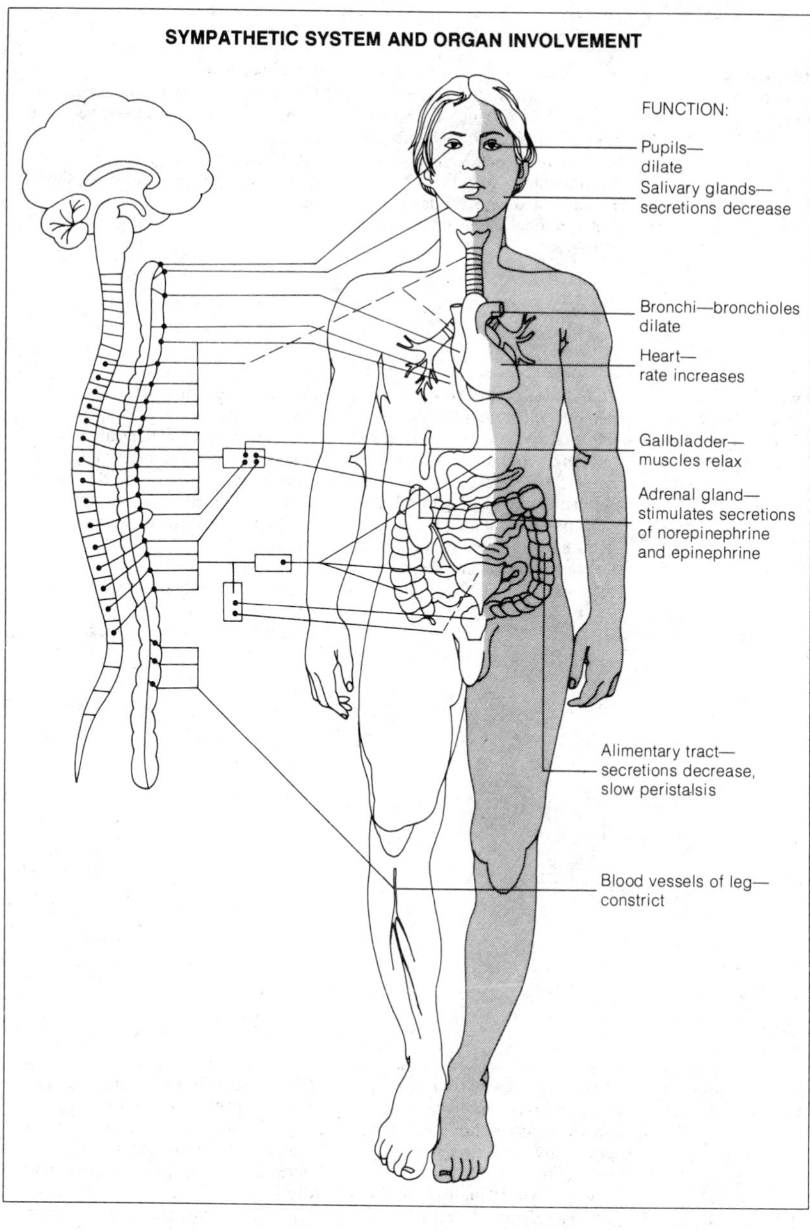

NAME	INDICATIONS & DOSAGE	SIDE EFFECTS
dobutamine hydrochloride Dobutrex	*Refractory heart failure and as adjunct in cardiac surgery—* **Adults:** 2.5 to 10 mcg/Kg/min as an I.V. infusion. Rarely, infusion rates up to 40 mcg/Kg/min have been required. May be reconstituted with 5% dextrose in water, normal saline, or lactated Ringer's.	*CNS:* headache. *CV:* increased heart rate, hypertension, premature ventricular beats, angina. *GI:* nausea, vomiting. *Other:* nonspecific chest pain, shortness of breath.
dopamine hydrochloride Intropin◆	*To treat shock and correct hemodynamic imbalances; to improve perfusion to vital organs, increase cardiac output; and to correct hypotension—* **Adults:** 2 to 5 mcg/Kg/min I.V. infusion up to 50 mcg/Kg/min. Titrate each patient to the desired hemodynamic and/or renal response.	*Blood:* azotemia. *CNS:* headache. *CV:* ectopic beats, tachycardia, anginal pain, palpitations, hypotension. Less frequently, bradycardia, widening of QRS intervals, hypertension, conduction disturbances, vasoconstriction. *GI:* nausea, vomiting. *Local:* necrosis and tissue sloughing with extravasation. *Other:* piloerection, dyspnea.
ephedrine sulfate Ectasule Minus III	*To correct hypotensive states; to support ventricular rate in Adams-Stokes syndrome; in myasthenia gravis to increase muscle strength—* **Adults:** 25 to 50 mg I.M. or S.C., or 10 to 25 mg I.V. p.r.n. to maximum 150 mg/24 hours.	*CNS:* insomnia, nervousness, dizziness, headache, muscle weakness, sweating, euphoria, confusion, delirium; in elderly patients, hallucinations, convulsions, CNS depression, death. *CV:* palpitations, tachycardia, hypertension, cardiac arrhythmias.

◆ Also available in Canada.
◆◆ Available in Canada only.
Unmarked trade names available in United States only.

INTERACTIONS	NURSING CONSIDERATIONS
Propranolol, metaprolol: these beta-blockers may make dobutamine ineffective. Do not use together.	• Contraindicated in idiopathic hypertrophic subaortic stenosis. • A unique agent. Increases contractility of failing heart without inducing marked tachycardia, except at high doses. • Dobutamine is a chemical modification of isoproterenol. • Often used with nitroprusside for additive effects. • EKG, blood pressure, pulmonary wedge pressure, and cardiac output should be monitored continuously. • Incompatible with alkaline solutions. Do not mix with sodium bicarbonate injection. • Infusions of up to 72 hours produce no more adverse effects than shorter infusions. • Oxidation of drug may slightly discolor admixtures containing dobutamine. This does not indicate a significant loss of potency. • Intravenous solutions remain stable for 24 hours.
Ergot alkaloids: extreme elevations in blood pressure. Don't use together.	• Contraindicated in uncorrected tachyarrhythmias, pheochromocytoma, ventricular fibrillation. Use cautiously in occlusive vascular disease, cold injuries, diabetic endarteritis, arterial embolism; also, in pregnant patients and those taking MAO inhibitors. • Not a substitute for blood or fluid volume deficits. If volume deficits exist, these should be replaced before vasopressors are administered. • Don't mix with alkaline solutions. Use 5% dextrose in water, normal saline or combination of 5% dextrose in water and saline. Mix just before use. • Dopamine solutions deteriorate after 24 hours. Discard at that time or earlier if solution is discolored. • Use large vein, as in antecubital fossa, to minimize risk of extravasation. Watch site carefully for signs of extravasation. If it occurs, stop infusion immediately and call doctor. He may want to counteract effect by infiltrating the area with 5 to 10 mg phentolamine and 10 to 15 ml normal saline. • Check blood pressure, pulse, urine output, and extremity color and temperature often during infusion. Titrate infusion rate according to findings, using doctor's guidelines. Use a microdrip or infusion pump to regulate flow rate. • Observe patient closely for side effects. If adverse effects develop, dosage may need to be adjusted or discontinued. • If a disproportionate rise in the diastolic pressure (a marked decrease in pulse pressure) is observed in patients receiving dopamine, decrease infusion rate and observe carefully for further evidence of predominant vasoconstrictor activity, unless such an effect is desired. • If doses exceed 50 mcg/Kg/min, check urine output often. If urine flow decreases without hypotension, consider reducing dose. • If drug is stopped, watch closely for sudden drop in blood pressure. • Do not mix other drugs in bottle containing dopamine. • Do not give alkaline drugs (sodium bicarbonate, phenytoin sodium) through I.V. line containing dopamine.
MAO inhibitors and tricyclic antidepressants: when given with sympathomimetics, may cause severe hypertension (hypertensive crisis). Don't use together.	• Contraindicated in porphyria, severe coronary artery disease, cardiac arrhythmias, patients on MAO inhibitor therapy, narrow-angle glaucoma, psychoneurosis. Use with caution in elderly patients, hypertension, hyperthyroidism, nervous or excitable states, cardiovascular disease, and prostatic hypertrophy. • Not a substitute for blood or fluid volume deficits. Volume deficit should be replaced before vasopressors are administered. • Give I.V. injection slowly.

(continued on following page)

NAME	INDICATIONS & DOSAGE	SIDE EFFECTS
ephedrine sulfate *(continued)*	**Children:** 3 mg/Kg S.C. or I.V. daily, divided into 4 to 6 doses. *Bronchodilator or nasal decongestant—* **Adults:** 12.5 to 50 mg P.O. b.i.d., t.i.d. or q.i.d. Maximum 400 mg/day in 6 to 8 divided doses. **Children:** 2 to 3 mg/Kg P.O. daily in 4 to 6 divided doses.	*EENT:* dryness of nose and throat. *GI:* nausea, vomiting, anorexia. *GU:* urinary retention, painful urination due to visceral sphincter spasm.
epinephrine Inhalants: Bronkaid Mist♦, Primatene Mist **epinephrine bitartrate** Inhalants: AsthmaHaler, Medihaler-Epi♦ **epinephrine hydrochloride** Adrenalin Chloride, Asmolin, Sus-Phrine♦	*Bronchospasm, hypersensitivity reactions, and anaphylaxis—* **Adults:** 0.1 to 0.5 ml of 1:1,000 S.C. or I.M. Repeat q 10 to 15 minutes p.r.n. or 0.1 to 0.25 ml 1:1,000 I.V. **Children:** 0.01 ml (10 mcg) of 1:1,000/Kg S.C. Repeat q 20 minutes to 4 hours p.r.n.; 0.005 ml/Kg of 1:200 (Sus-Phrine). Repeat 0.05 ml/Kg q 8 to 12 hours, p.r.n. *Hemostatic—* **Adults:** 1:50,000 to 1:1,000, applied topically. *Acute asthmatic attacks (inhalation)—* **Adults and children:** 1 or 2 inhalations of 1:100 or 2.25% racemic or inhaler p.r.n.; 0.2 mg/dose usual content. *To prolong anesthetic effect—* **Adults and children:** 0.2 to 0.4 ml of 1:1,000 intraspinal; 1:500,000 to 1:50,000 local. *To restore cardiac rhythm in cardiac arrest—* **Adults:** 0.5 to 1 mg I.V., or 0.1 to 0.2 mg intracardiac. **Children:** 10 mcg/Kg I.V., or 5 to 10 mcg (0.05 to 0.1 ml of 1:10,000)/Kg intracardiac.	*Blood:* hyperglycemia, glycosuria. *CNS:* pallor, nervousness, tremor, anxiety, coldness of extremities, vertigo, headache, sweating, cerebral hemorrhage, disorientation, agitation. In patients with Parkinson's disease, the drug increases rigidity and tremor. *CV:* palpitations; widened pulse pressure; hypertension; tachycardia; ventricular fibrillation; CVA; anginal pain; EKG changes, including a decrease in the T-wave amplitude. *EENT:* rebound nasal congestion and rhinitis with prolonged use of nasal products. *Other:* pulmonary edema, dyspnea.
ethylnorepinephrine hydrochloride Bronkephrine	*To relieve bronchospasm due to asthma—* **Adults:** 0.5 to 1 ml S.C. or I.M. **Children:** 0.1 to 0.5 ml S.C. or I.M.	*CV:* changes in blood pressure, elevation in pulse rate, palpitations. *Other:* headache, dizziness, nausea.

INTERACTIONS	NURSING CONSIDERATIONS
Methylodopa: may inhibit effect of ephedrine. Give together cautiously.	• Hypoxia, hypercapnia, and acidosis, which may reduce effectiveness or increase the incidence of adverse effects, must be identified and corrected before or during ephedrine administration. • Blood pressure should be elevated to slightly less than the patient's normal blood pressure. • Effectiveness decreases after 2 to 3 weeks. Then increased dosage may be needed. Tolerance develops, but not known to cause addiction. • To prevent insomnia, avoid giving within 2 hours of bedtime. • Warn patient not to take over-the-counter drugs that contain ephedrine without informing doctor.
Tricyclic antidepressants: when given with sympathomimetics, may cause severe hypertension (hypertensive crisis). Don't give together. *Propranolol:* vasoconstriction and reflex bradycardia. Monitor patient cautiously.	• Contraindicated in narrow-angle glaucoma, shock (other than anaphylactic shock), during general anesthesia with halogenated hydrocarbons or cyclopropane, organic brain damage, labor (may delay second stage), cardiac dilatation and coronary insufficiency, and patients with ventricular fibrillation. Use with extreme caution in patients with long-standing bronchial asthma and emphysema who have developed degenerative heart disease. Use with caution in elderly patients, hyperthyroidism, angina, hypertension, psychoneurosis, diabetes, pregnancy. • Don't mix with alkaline solutions. Use 5% dextrose in water, normal saline, or a combination of 5% dextrose in water and saline. Mix just before use. • Epinephrine is rapidly destroyed by oxidizing agents, such as iodine, chromates, nitrates, nitrites, oxygen, and salts of easily reducible metals such as iron. • Epinephrine solutions deteriorate after 24 hours. Discard after that time or before if solution is discolored or contains precipitate. Keep solution in light-resistant container and don't remove before use. • Massage site after injection to counteract possible vasoconstriction. Repeated local injection can cause necrosis at site due to vasoconstriction. • Avoid intramuscular administration of oil injection into buttocks. Gas gangrene may occur because epinephrine reduces oxygen tension of the tissues, encouraging the growth of contaminating organisms. • This drug may widen patient's pulse pressure. • In the event of a sharp blood pressure rise, rapid-acting vasodilators, such as the nitrites or alpha-adrenergic blocking agents, can be given to counteract the marked pressor effect of large doses of epinephrine. • Observe patient closely for side effects. If adverse effects develop, dosage may need to be adjusted or discontinued. • If patient has acute hypersensitivity reactions, it may be necessary to instruct him to self-inject epinephrine at home. • This drug may cause the following changes in lab test results: hyperglycemia, glycosuria, elevated BUN, decreased protein-bound iodine. • Drug of choice in emergency treatment of severe acute anaphylactic reactions, including anaphylactic shock.
None significant.	• Use with caution in cardiovascular disease or history of stroke. • Safer than epinephrine for use in hypertensive or severely ill patients in whom significant pressor effects are undesirable. • Valuable when used in children due to low incidence of adverse effects; may be useful in diabetic asthmatics due to low glycogenolytic activity. • Choose anatomical injection site carefully to avoid inadvertent intraneural or intravascular injection.

NAME	INDICATIONS & DOSAGE	SIDE EFFECTS
isoproterenol hydrochloride Isuprel◆, Proternol (tabs) Inhalants: Iprenol, Norisodrine, Vapo-Iso **isoproterenol sulfate** Iso-Autohaler, Luf-Iso Inhalation, Medihaler-Iso◆, Norisodrine	*Bronchial asthma and reversible bronchospasm—* **Adults:** 10 to 20 mg S.L. every 6 to 8 hours. **Children:** 5 to 10 mg S.L. q 6 to 8 hours. Not recommended for children under 6 years. *Bronchospasm—* **Adults and children:** acute dyspneic episodes: 1 inhalation initially. May repeat if needed after 2 to 5 minutes. Maintenance: 1 to 2 inhalations q.i.d. to 6 times daily. May repeat once more 10 minutes after second dose. Not more than 3 doses should be administered for each attack. *Cardiac standstill and cardiac arrhythmias—* **Adults:** initially, 0.02 to 0.06 mg I.V. Subsequent doses 0.01 to 0.2 mg I.V. or 5 mcg/min I.V.; or 0.2 mg I.M. initially, then 0.02 to 1 mg, p.r.n.; or 0.02 mg intracardiac in extreme cases. **Children:** may give ½ of initial adult dose. *Heart block and ventricular arrhythmias—* **Adults:** use I.V. therapy in acute heart block. Same dosage regimens as above. **Children:** same I.V. therapy as above in acute heart block. 5 to 10 mg dose S.L. q 6 to 8 hours, p.r.n. *Maintenance for Stokes-Adams disease or A-V block—* **Adults:** 30 to 180 mg timed-release tablets P.O. daily swallowed whole. *Shock—* **Adults and children:** 0.5 to 5 mcg/min by continuous I.V. infusion. Usual concentration: 1 mg (5 ml) in 500 ml 5% dextrose in water. Adjust rate according to heart rate, central venous pressure, blood pressure, and urine flow.	*CNS:* headache, mild tremor, dizziness, flushing of face, nervousness, insomnia. *CV:* cardiac arrhythmias, palpitations, tachycardia, anginal pain; blood pressure may be elevated and then fall. *GI:* nausea, vomiting. *Other:* weakness, sweating, bronchial edema and inflammation; with prolonged use, swelling of parotid glands.
levarterenol bitartrate (norepinephrine, noradrenaline) Levophed◆	*To restore blood pressure in acute hypotensive states and to treat cardiac arrest—* **Adults:** initially, 8 to 12 mcg/min I.V. infusion, then adjust to maintain normal blood pressure. Average maintenance dose 2 to 4 mcg/min.	*CNS:* headache, anxiety, weakness, dizziness, tremor, restlessness, insomnia. *CV:* bradycardia, severe hypertension, marked increase in peripheral resistance, decreased cardiac output, arrhythmias, ventricular tachycardia, bigeminal rhythm, atrioventricular dissociation and/or fibrillation, precordial pain.

INTERACTIONS	NURSING CONSIDERATIONS
Propranolol: blocked effect of isoproterenol and vice versa. Monitor patient carefully if used together.	• Contraindicated in tachycardia caused by digitalis intoxication and in patients with preexisting arrhythmias, especially tachycardia, because chronotropic effect on the heart may aggravate such disorders. Use cautiously in coronary insufficiency, diabetes, hyperthyroidism. • Not a substitute for blood or fluid volume deficits. If deficits exist, these should be replaced before vasopressors are administered. • If heart rate exceeds 110 beats/minute, it may be advisable to decrease infusion rate or temporarily stop infusion. Doses sufficient to increase the heart rate to more than 130 beats/minute may induce ventricular arrhythmias. • If precordial distress or anginal pain occurs, stop drug immediately. • When administering I.V. isoproterenol for shock, closely monitor blood pressure, CVP, EKG, arterial blood gas measurements, and urinary output. Carefully adjust infusion rate according to these measurements. • Oral and sublingual tablets are poorly and erratically absorbed. • Teach patient how to take sublingual tablet properly. Tell him to hold tablet under tongue until it dissolves and is absorbed and not to swallow saliva until that time. Prolonged use of sublingual tablets can cause tooth decay. Instruct patient to rinse mouth with water between doses. This will also help prevent dryness of oropharynx. • If possible, don't give at bedtime because it interrupts sleep patterns. • Oral tablets not for sublingual use must be swallowed whole, not broken. Store in cool, dry place in airtight, light-resistant container. Keep bottle tightly capped after opening. • This drug may cause a slight rise in systolic blood pressure and a slight to marked drop in diastolic blood pressure. • Use a microdrip or infusion pump to regulate infusion flow rate. • Observe patient closely for side effects. Dosage may need to be adjusted or discontinued. • Teach patient to use oral inhalation correctly. Give the following instructions for using a metered-dose nebulizer: —Clear nasal passages and throat. —Breathe out, expelling as much air from lungs as possible. —Place mouthpiece well into mouth as dose from nebulizer is released, and inhale deeply. —Hold breath for several seconds, remove mouthpiece, and exhale slowly. • Instructions for metered powder nebulizer are the same, except that deep inhalation is not necessary. • Patient may develop a tolerance to this drug. Warn against overuse. • Warn patient using oral inhalant that drug may turn sputum and saliva pink. • May cause these changes in test results: hyperglycemia, glycosuria, elevated BUN. • May aggravate ventilation perfusion abnormalities; even while ease of breathing is improved, arterial oxygen tension may fall paradoxically. • Discard inhalation solution if it is discolored or contains precipitate.
Tricyclic antidepressants: when given with sympathomimetics, may cause severe hypertension (hypertensive crisis). Don't give together.	• Contraindicated in mesenteric or peripheral vascular thrombosis, pregnancy, profound hypoxia, hypercarbia, hypotension from blood volume deficits, or during cyclopropane and halothane anesthesia. Use cautiously in hypertension, hyperthyroidism, severe heart disease. Use with extreme caution in patients receiving MAO inhibitors or tricyclic antidepressants. • Not a substitute for blood or fluid volume deficits. If deficits exist, these should be replaced before vasopressors are administered. • Levarterenol solutions deteriorate after 24 hours. Discard after that time. • Use large vein, as in antecubital fossa, to minimize risk of extravasation. Check site frequently for signs of extravasation. If it occurs, stop infusion

(continued on following page)

NAME	INDICATIONS & DOSAGE	SIDE EFFECTS
levarterenol bitartrate (norepinephrine, noradrenaline) *(continued)*		*GU:* decreased urine output. *Metabolic:* metabolic acidosis. *Other:* hyperglycemia, increased glycogenolysis, fever, respiratory difficulty.
mephentermine sulfate Wyamine♦	*Hypotension following spinal anesthesia—* **Adults:** 30 to 45 mg I.V. in a single injection, then 30 mg I.V. repeated, p.r.n. Maintenance of blood pressure: continuous I.V. infusion of 0.1% solution of mephentermine in 5% dextrose in water. *Hypotension following spinal anesthesia during obstetrical procedures—* **Adults:** initially, 15 mg I.V., p.r.n. *Prevention of hypotension during spinal anesthesia—* **Adults:** 30 to 40 mg I.M. 10 to 20 minutes prior to anesthesia. *Treatment of shock and hypotension—* **Adults:** 0.5 mg/Kg I.V. or I.M. **Children:** 0.4 mg/Kg I.V. or I.M.	*CNS:* euphoria, weeping, nervousness, anxiety, tremor, incoherence, drowsiness, convulsions. *CV:* arrhythmias, marked elevation of blood pressure (with large doses).
metaproterenol sulfate Alupent♦, Metaprel	*Acute episodes of bronchial asthma—* **Adults and children:** 2 to 3 inhalations. Should not repeat inhalations more often than q 3 to	*CNS:* nervousness, weakness, drowsiness, tremor. *CV:* tachycardia, hypertension, palpitations; with excessive use, cardiac arrest.

INTERACTIONS	NURSING CONSIDERATIONS
	immediately and call doctor. He may counteract effect by infiltrating area with 5 to 10 mg phentolamine and 10 to 15 ml normal saline. Also check for blanching along course of infused vein; may progress to superficial slough. During infusion, check blood pressure every 2 minutes until stabilized; then every 5 minutes. Also check pulse rates, urinary output, and color and temperature of extremities. Titrate infusion rate according to findings, using doctor's guidelines. In previously hypertensive patients, blood pressure should be raised no more than 40 mmHg below preexisting systolic pressure. • Never leave patient unattended. • Use a microdrip or infusion pump to regulate infusion flow rate. • Watch closely for side effects. If adverse effects develop, dosage may need to be adjusted or stopped. Have phentolamine handy to reverse effect. • For I.V. therapy, use bottle setup so I.V. can run if levarterenol is stopped. • Some doctors add phentolamine 5 to 10 mg to each liter of levarterenol to prevent tissue sloughing. • Report decreased urinary output to doctor immediately. • If prolonged I.V. therapy is necessary, change injection site frequently. • When stopping drug, slow infusion rate gradually. Monitor vital signs, even after stopping. Watch for possible severe drop in blood pressure. • Whole blood or plasma incompatible with levarterenol. Give separately. • Keep these emergency drugs on hand to reverse effects of levarterenol: atropine for reflex bradycardia and propranolol for arrhythmias. • Administer in dextrose and saline; saline alone is not recommended.
None significant.	• Contraindicated in concealed hemorrhage or hypotension from hemorrhage, except in emergencies; also in patients receiving phenothiazines, or who have received MAO inhibitors within 2 weeks. Use cautiously with arteriosclerosis, cardiovascular disease, hyperthyroidism, hypertension, and chronic illness. • Not a substitute for blood or fluid volume deficits. If deficits exist, these should be replaced before vasopressors are administered. • During infusion, check blood pressure every 5 minutes until stabilized; then every 15 minutes. • Observe patient closely for side effects. If adverse effects develop, dosage may need to be adjusted or discontinued. • Monitor blood pressure even after stopping drug. • I.M. route may be used since drug is not irritating to tissue. • I.V. drug is not irritating to tissue, and extravasation is not dangerous. To prepare 0.1% I.V. solution: add 20 ml mephentermine (30 mg/ml) to 500 ml 5% dextrose in water. • May increase uterine contractions during 3rd trimester of pregnancy. • Hypercapnia, hypoxia, and acidosis may reduce effectiveness or increase adverse effects. Identify and correct before and during administration.
None significant.	• Contraindicated in tachycardia and in arrhythmias associated with tachycardia. Use with caution in hypertension, coronary artery disease, hyperthyroidism, diabetes. • Safe use of inhalant in children under 12 not established. • Teach patient how to administer metered dose correctly. Instructions:

(continued on following page)

NAME	INDICATIONS & DOSAGE	SIDE EFFECTS
metaproterenol sulfate *(continued)*	4 hours. Should not exceed 12 inhalations daily. *Bronchial asthma and reversible bronchospasm—* **Adults:** 20 mg P.O. q 6 to 8 hours. **Children over 9 years or over 60 lbs.:** 20 mg P.O. q 6 to 8 hours. (0.4 mg to 0.9 mg/Kg/dose t.i.d.) **Children 6 to 9 years or less than 60 lbs.:** 10 mg P.O. q 6 to 8 hours. (0.4 mg to 0.9 mg/Kg/dose t.i.d.) Not recommended for children under 6 years.	*GI:* vomiting, nausea, bad taste. *Other:* paradoxical bronchiolar constriction with excessive use.
metaraminol bitartrate Aramine•	*Prevention of hypotension—* **Adults:** 2 to 10 mg I.M. or S.C. *Severe shock—* **Adults:** 0.5 to 5 mg direct I.V. followed by I.V. infusion. *Treatment of hypotension due to shock—* **Adults:** 15 to 100 mg in 500 ml normal saline or 5% dextrose in water I.V. infusion. Adjust rate to maintain blood pressure. *All indications—* **Children:** 0.01 mg/Kg as single I.V. injection; 1 mg/25 ml 5% dextrose in water as I.V. infusion. Adjust rate to maintain blood pressure in normal range. 0.1 mg/Kg I.M. as single dose, p.r.n. Allow at least 10 minutes to elapse before increasing the dose because the maximum effect is not immediately apparent.	*Blood:* plasma volume depletion, increased cholesterol levels, increased blood levels of fatty acids, hyperglycemia. *CNS:* apprehension, restlessness, dizziness, headache, tremor, weakness; with excess, convulsions. *CV:* hypertension; hypotension; precordial pain; palpitations; arrhythmias, including sinus or ventricular tachycardia; bradycardia; ventricular beats; nodal rhythm; supraventricular premature beats; atrioventricular dissociation. *GI:* nausea, vomiting. *GU:* decreased urinary output. *Skin:* flushing, pallor, sweating. *Other:* metabolic acidosis in hypovolemia, increased body temperature, respiratory distress.

INTERACTIONS	NURSING CONSIDERATIONS
	shake container; exhale through nose; administer aerosol while inhaling deeply on mouthpiece of inhaler; hold breath for a few seconds, then exhale slowly. Allow 2 minutes between inhalations. Store drug in light-resistant container. • Tell patient to notify doctor if no response to dosage. Warn against changing dose without calling doctor.
MAO inhibitors: may cause severe hypertension (hypertensive crisis). Don't use together.	• Contraindicated in peripheral or mesenteric thrombosis; pulmonary edema; cardiac arrest; untreated hypoxia; hypercarbia; and acidosis; during anesthesia with cyclopropane and halogenated hydrocarbon anesthetics. Use cautiously in hypertension, thyroid disease, diabetes, cirrhosis, or malaria, and in those receiving digitalis. • Not a substitute for blood or fluid volume deficits. Fluid deficit should be replaced before vasopressors are administered. • Keep solution in light-resistant container, away from heat. • Use large veins, as in antecubital fossa, to minimize risk of extravasation. Watch infusion site carefully for signs of extravasation. If it occurs, stop infusion immediately and call doctor. • During infusion check blood pressure every 5 minutes until stabilized; then every 15 minutes. Check pulse rates, urinary output, and color and temperature of extremities. Titrate infusion rate according to findings, using doctor's guidelines. • Use a microdrip or infusion pump to regulate infusion flow rate. • Observe patient closely for side effects. If adverse effects develop, dosage may need to be adjusted or discontinued. • For I.V. therapy, use 2-bottle setup so I.V. can run if this drug is stopped. • Blood pressure should be raised to slightly less than the patient's normal level. Be careful to avoid excessive blood pressure response. Rapidly induced hypertensive response can cause acute pulmonary edema, arrhythmias, and cardiac arrest. • Because of prolonged action, a cumulative effect is possible. With an excessive vasopressor response, elevated blood pressure may persist after stopping. • Urinary output may decrease initially, then increase as blood pressure reaches normal level. Report persistent decreased urine output. • When discontinuing therapy with this drug, slow infusion rate gradually. Continue monitoring vital signs, watching for possible severe drop in blood pressure. Keep equipment nearby to start drug again, if necessary. Pressor therapy should not be reinstated until the systolic blood pressure falls below 70 to 80 mm Hg. • Keep emergency drugs on hand to reverse effects of metaraminol: atropine for reflex bradycardia, phentolamine to decrease vasopressor effects, and propranolol for arrhythmias. • Closely monitor diabetics. Adjustment in insulin dose may be needed. • Metaraminol should not be mixed with other drugs.

NAME	INDICATIONS & DOSAGE	SIDE EFFECTS
methoxamine hydrochloride Vasoxyl♦	*Moderate fall in blood pressure—* **Adults:** 5 to 10 mg I.M. *Paroxysmal supraventricular tachycardia—* **Adults:** 5 to 15 mg I.V. injected slowly. 10 to 20 mg I.M. Allow 15 minutes before additional increased doses to evaluate effects of initial dose and prevent a cumulative effect. *Prevention of hypotension during spinal anesthesia—* **Adults:** 10 to 15 mg I.M. before or with spinal anesthesia. *Support and restoration of blood pressure during anesthesia (including cyclopropane); termination of paroxysmal supraventricular tachycardia; emergency situations; systolic falls below 60 mm Hg—* **Adults:** initially, 3 to 5 mg slow I.V. injection, followed by 10 to 15 mg I.M. to prolong effect. **Children:** direct I.V. dose is 80 mcg/Kg of body weight or 2.5 mg/m^2 of body surface area, injected slowly.	*Blood:* plasma volume depletion. *CNS:* paresthesias, chills, severe headache, restlessness, tremors, dizziness, anxiety, nervousness. *CV:* hypertension, bradycardia, cardiac depression, precordial pain, heart failure in diseased myocardium. *GI:* projectile vomiting. *GU:* urinary urgency, decreased urine output. *Skin:* gooseflesh, pallor. *Other:* respiratory distress, metabolic acidosis.
methoxyphenamine hydrochloride Orthoxine hydrochloride	*To treat allergies and bronchial asthma—* **Adults:** 100 mg P.O. q 4 to 6 hours. Maximum dose, 600 mg/day. **Children:** 25 to 50 mg P.O. q 4 to 6 hours.	*CNS:* insomnia, nervousness, dizziness, headache, sweating, anxiety, flushing. *CV:* palpitations, tachycardia, hypertension. *GI:* nausea, vomiting, dry mouth.
phenylephrine hydrochloride Neo-Synephrine♦	*Hypotensive emergencies during spinal anesthesia—* **Adults:** initially, 0.2 mg I.V., then subsequent doses of 0.1 to 0.2 mg. *Maintenance of blood pressure during spinal or inhalation anesthesia—* **Adults:** 2 to 3 mg S.C. or I.M. 3 or 4 minutes before anesthesia is administered. **Children:** 0.04 mg to 0.088 mg/Kg S.C. or I.M. *Mild to moderate hypotension—* **Adults:** 2 to 5 mg S.C. or I.M; 0.1 to 0.5 mg I.V. Not to be repeated more often than 10 to 15 minutes. *Paroxysmal supraventricular tachycardia—*	*Blood:* plasma volume depletion. *CNS:* trembling, sweating, pallor, sense of fullness in head, tingling in extremities, sleeplessness, dizziness, panesthesia in extremities from injection, light-headedness, weakness. *CV:* palpitations, tachycardia, extrasystoles, short paroxysms of ventricular tachycardia, hypertension, anginal pain. *EENT:* nasal burning, stinging, dryness, and sneezing; blurred vision; conjunctival allergy; stinging pain in eyes; rebound nasal congestion with high doses or prolonged use. *Skin:* gooseflesh, feeling of coolness. *Other:* tachyphylaxis may occur with continued use.

NAME	INDICATIONS & DOSAGE	SIDE EFFECTS
None significant.	• Contraindicated in severe heart disease or in those taking MAO inhibitors; in shock due to myocardial infarction, or peripheral or mesenteric vascular thrombosis; and in the elderly. Use cautiously in hyperthyroidism or hypertension; after use of ergot alkaloids; and in pregnancy. • Should not be used with local anesthetics to prolong their effect. • Not a substitute for blood volume or fluid volume deficits. If deficit exists, replace before vasopressors are given. Hypoxia and acidosis should also be corrected before or during therapy. • Methoxamine solutions deteriorate after 24 hours. Discard after that time or before if discolored or contains precipitate. • Has potent, prolonged pressor action. Does not increase cardiac rate or irritability of cyclopropane-sensitized heart. • Does not stimulate the CNS. • Monitor response by checking blood pressure. Adjust dose accordingly. Blood pressure should be raised to slightly less than normal level. In previously normotensive patients, systolic blood pressure should be maintained at 80 to 100 mm of mercury; in previously hypertensive patients, systolic blood pressure should be maintained at 30 to 40 mm of mercury below usual level. • Observe patient closely for side effects. Dosage may need to be adjusted or discontinued. • Keep these emergency drugs on hand to reverse effects of methoxamine: atropine for reflex bradycardia and propranolol for arrhythmias. • Monitor blood pressure and pulse rate even after stopping drug. Report sudden changes.	
None significant.	• Contraindicated in those who have used MAO inhibitors within past 2 weeks. Use cautiously in hypertension, hyperthyroidism, acute coronary disease, cardiac decompensation, and diabetes mellitus. • Only "possibly effective" in treating bronchial asthma, acute urticaria, allergic rhinitis, gastrointestinal allergy, and allergic headaches. • Effectiveness decreases after 2 to 3 weeks. Then increased dose may be needed. • Avoid giving this drug within 2 hours of bedtime. • Warn against using over-the-counter drugs containing sympathomimetics without informing doctor.	
MAO inhibitors: may cause severe hypertension (hypertensive crisis). Don't use together. *Tricyclic antidepressants:* increased pressor response. Observe patient carefully.	• Contraindicated in narrow-angle glaucoma; with MAO inhibitors, tricyclic antidepressants; hypotension; ventricular tachycardia; severe coronary disease or cardiovascular disease (including myocardial infarction). Use with extreme caution in heart disease, hyperthyroidism, diabetes, severe atherosclerosis, bradycardia, partial heart block, myocardial disease, and the elderly. • Longer acting than ephedrine and epinephrine. • Causes little or no CNS stimulation. • Monitor blood pressure frequently. Avoid excessive rise in blood pressure. Maintain blood pressure at slightly below the patient's normal level. In previously normotensive patients, maintain systolic blood pressure at 80 to 100 mm Hg; in previously hypertensive patients, maintain systolic blood pressure at 30 to 40 mm Hg below their usual level. • May reverse severe increase in blood pressure with phentolamine. • With I.V. infusions, avoid abrupt withdrawal. Monitor blood pressure throughout. Reverse therapy if blood pressure falls too rapidly.	

(continued on following page)

NAME	INDICATIONS & DOSAGE	SIDE EFFECTS
phenylephrine hydrochloride *(continued)*	**Adults:** initially, 0.5 mg rapid I.V.; subsequent doses should not exceed 1 mg. *Prolongation of spinal anesthesia—* **Adults:** 2 to 5 mg added to anesthetic solution. *Severe hypotension and shock (including drug induced)—* **Adults:** 10 mg in 500 ml 5% dextrose in water. Start 100 to 180 drops per minute I.V. infusion, then 40 to 60 drops per minute. Adjust to patient response. *Vasoconstrictor for regional anesthesia—* **Adults:** 1 mg phenylephrine added to 20 ml local anesthetic.	
protokylol hydrochloride Ventaire	*Bronchodilator—* **Adults:** 2 to 4 mg P.O. q.i.d. **Children:** 1 to 2 mg P.O. t.i.d. or q.i.d.	*CNS:* trembling, tenseness, insomnia, dizziness, weakness (all dose-related). *CV:* tachycardia, palpitations, angina, precordial distress (all dose-related). *GI:* nausea, gastric irritation. *GU:* difficulty in urination.
pseudoephedrine hydrochloride Besan, Cenafed, D-Feda, Eltor◆◆, Gyrocaps, Novafed, Robidrine◆◆, Ro-Fed-rin, Sudabid, Sudafed◆, Sudafed SA	*Nasal and eustachian tube decongestant—* **Adults:** 60 mg P.O. q 4 hours. **Children 6 to 12 years:** 30 mg P.O. q 4 hours. Maximum 120 mg/day. **Children 2 to 6 years:** 15 mg P.O. q 4 hours. Maximum, 60 mg/day. Extended-relief tablets: **Adults, and children over 12 years:** 60 to 120 mg P.O. of q 12 hours. This form contraindicated for children under 12.	*CNS:* anxiety, hallucinations, transient stimulation, tremors, dizziness, headache, insomnia, numbness of extremities, nervousness, hypersensitivity, drowsiness. *CV:* arrythmias, palpitations, tachycardia. *GI:* anorexia, nausea, vomiting, dry mouth. *GU:* difficulty in urination. *Skin:* pallor. *Other:* respiratory difficulties.
terbutaline sulfate Brethine, Bricanyl Tablets◆	*Bronchodilator—* **Adults:** 2.5 to 5 mg P.O. q 8 hours; or 0.25 to 0.5 mg S.C. If no improvement in 15 to 30 minutes, repeat dose. Do not exceed 0.5 mg in 4 hours. **Children 12 to 15 years:** 2.5 mg P.O. t.i.d. Not recommended for children under 12.	*CNS:* nervousness, tremors, headache, drowsiness, sweating. *CV:* palpitations, increased heart rate. *GI:* vomiting, nausea.

INTERACTIONS	NURSING CONSIDERATIONS
None significant.	• Contraindicated in cardiac arrhythmias, coronary insufficiency, and in patients receiving beta blocking drugs, such as propranolol hydrochloride. Use cautiously in cardiovascular disorders, diabetes mellitus, hyperthyroidism, prostatic hypertrophy, or glaucoma; and in patients receiving other sympathomimetic drugs. • Administer drug with meals to prevent gastrointestinal distress. • Stop drug and call doctor promptly if angina, precordial distress, or palpitations develop. • Store drug in dry place.
MAO inhibitors: may cause severe hypertension (hypertensive crisis). Don't use together.	• Contraindicated in severe hypertension or severe coronary artery disease; and in those receiving MAO inhibitors; nursing mothers. Use cautiously in hypertension, heart disease, glaucoma, hyperthyroidism, or prostatic hypertrophy. • Tell patient to stop drug if he becomes unusually restless and to notify doctor promptly. • Warn against using over-the-counter products containing ephedrine or other sympathomimetic amines. • Tell patient not to take drug within 2 hours of bedtime because it can cause insomnia. • Relieve dry mouth with gum or sour hard candy.
MAO inhibitors: when given with sympathomimetics may cause severe hypertension (hypertensive crisis). Don't use together. *Propranolol:* blocked effects of terbutaline. Monitor patient carefully if used together.	• Use cautiously in patients with diabetes, hypertension, hyperthyroidism, severe heart disease, or cardiac arrhythmias. • Protect injection from light. Do not use if discolored. • Make sure patient's family understands why patient is taking drug, so they can encourage continuation. • Give subcutaneous injections in lateral deltoid area. • Tolerance may develop with prolonged use.

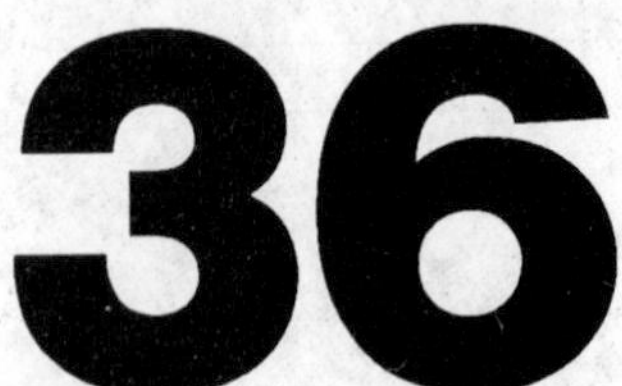

Adrenergic blockers (sympatholytics)

dihydroergotamine mesylate
ergotamine tartrate
methysergide maleate
phenoxybenzamine hydrochloride
phentolamine hydrochloride/mesylate
propranolol

Adrenergic blocking (sympatholytic) drugs inhibit or decrease the effects of epinephrine and norepinephrine released from sympathetic nerve endings, and of other sympathomimetic amines. Within the sympathetic nervous system are two types of receptors: alpha and beta. Alpha receptors are found in smooth muscle and cause smooth-muscle contraction, such as vasoconstriction, sphincter contraction, and uterine contraction. Beta receptors are classified as $beta_1$ and $beta_2$, according to their response to drugs. $Beta_1$ receptors—located mainly in the heart—increase heart rate, cardiac contraction, and atrioventricular conduction. $Beta_2$ receptors are responsible for smooth-muscle relaxation, such as vasodilation, bronchodilation, and uterine relaxation. Adrenergic blocking drugs have been synthesized for specific alpha or beta blocking effects.

Major uses

Alpha blocking agents

- Temporary treatment of hypertension caused by pheochromocytoma.
- Symptomatic treatment of spastic peripheral vascular diseases.
- Prophylaxis and treatment of vascular headaches.

Mechanism of action

- Block the effects of epinephrine and norepinephrine and of other sympathomimetic amines on smooth muscle and on exocrine glands, thereby preventing sympathetic stimulation.
- Methysergide specifically blocks serotonin (a neurotransmitter); other alpha-adrenergic blocking drugs may have some degree of antiserotonin effects.
- Propranolol prevents vasodilation of cerebral arteries due to its beta-adrenergic blocking action.

Absorption, distribution, and excretion

- Ergotamine, methysergide, and propranolol are well absorbed orally.
- Phenoxybenzamine is variably absorbed orally.
- Dihydroergotamine and ergotamine are well absorbed parenterally.
- Ergotamine is rapidly and well absorbed sublingually.

- After administration, these drugs are widely distributed to organs innervated by the sympathetic nervous system.
- Phenoxybenzamine HCl is excreted by the kidneys unchanged or as metabolites.
- Methysergide maleate is metabolized in the liver.
- Little is known about absorption, distribution, and excretion of phentolamine and ergotamine.

Onset and duration

- Onset after oral administration varies from 30 minutes for ergot alkaloids to several hours for phenoxybenzamine.
- Onset after parenteral administration (I.M., S.C.) is 15 to 30 minutes. Onset with intravenous administration is immediate and is recommended in acute situations.
- Duration varies from 3 to 4 hours for most drugs in this group to several hours for ergotamine and several days for phenoxybenzamine.

Combination products

ALLYLGESIC W/ERGOTAMINE: ergotamine tartrate 1 mg, allobarbital 15 mg, aspirin 150 mg, acetaminophen 100 mg and aluminum aspirin 100 mg.
CAFERGOT: ergotamine tartrate 1 mg, caffeine 100 mg.
CAFERGOT SUPPOSITORIES: ergotamine tartrate 2 mg and caffeine 100 mg.
CAFERGOT PB (SUPPOSITORIES): ergotamine tartrate 2 mg, caffeine 100 mg, pentobarbital sodium 30 mg, and belladonna alkaloids 0.125 mg.
DEAPRIL-ST: dihydroergocornine mesylate 0.167 mg, dihydroergocristine mesylate 0.167, and dihydroergokryptine mesylate 0.167 mg.
ERGOCAF: ergotamine tartrate 1 mg, and caffeine 100 mg.
MIGRAL: ergotamine tartrate 1 mg, caffeine 50 mg, and cyclizine 25 mg.
MIGRALAM: ergotamine 1 mg, caffeine 25 mg, pyrilamine 10 mg, salicylamide 150 mg, and phenacetin 150 mg.
WIGRAINE♦: ergotamine tartrate 1 mg, caffeine 100 mg, belladonna alkaloids 0.1 mg, and phenacetin 130 mg.
WIGRAINE SUPPOSITORIES: ergotamine tartrate 1 mg, caffeine 100 mg, belladonna alkaloids 0.1 mg, and phenacetin 130 mg.

NAME	INDICATIONS & DOSAGE	SIDE EFFECTS
dihydroergotamine mesylate D.H.E. 45	*Vascular or migraine headache*— **Adults:** 1 mg I.M. or I.V. May repeat q 1 to 2 hours, p.r.n., up to total of 3 mg. Maximum weekly dose is 6 mg.	*CV:* transient tachycardia or bradycardia, precordial distress and pain, increased arterial pressure. *GI:* nausea, vomiting. *Local:* numbness and tingling in fingers and toes, weakness in legs, muscle pains in extremities. *Skin:* itching. *Other:* localized edema.
ergotamine tartrate Ergomar•, Ergostat, Gynergen•, Medihaler-Ergotamine•	*Vascular or migraine headache*— **Adults:** initially, 2 mg P.O. S.L., then 1 to 2 mg P.O. q hour or S.L. q ½ hour, up to maximum 6 mg daily and 10 mg weekly; or initially, 0.25 mg I.M., S.C.; repeat in 40 minutes if needed. Maximum dose 0.5 mg/24 hours and 1 mg/week; or 1 inhalation initially, if not relieved in 5 minutes use another inhalation. May repeat inhalations at least 5 minutes apart up to maximum of 6/24 hours.	*CV:* transient tachycardia or bradycardia, precordial distress and pain, increased arterial pressure, angina pectoris. *GI:* nausea, vomiting, diarrhea, abdominal cramps. *Local:* numbness and tingling in fingers and toes, weakness in legs, muscle pains in extremities. *Skin:* itching. *Other:* localized edema.
methysergide maleate Sansert•	*Prevention of frequent, severe, uncontrollable, or disabling migraine or vascular headache*— **Adults:** 2 to 4 mg P.O. b.i.d. with meals.	*Blood:* neutropenia, eosinophilia. *CNS:* insomnia, drowsiness, euphoria, vertigo, ataxia, light-headedness, hyperesthesia, weakness, hallucinations or feelings of disassociation. *CV:* fibrotic thickening of cardiac valves and aorta, inferior vena cava, and common iliac branches; vasoconstriction, causing chest pain, abdominal pain, vascular insufficiency of lower limbs; cold, numb, painful extremities with or without paresthesias and diminished or absent pulses; postural hypotension; tachycardia; peripheral edema; murmurs; bruits. *EENT:* nasal stuffiness. *GI:* nausea, vomiting, diarrhea, constipation, epigastric pain. *Skin:* hair loss, dermatitis, sweating, flushing, rash. *Other:* retroperitoneal fibrosis, causing general malaise, fatigue, weight gain, backache, low grade fever, urinary obstruction; pulmonary fibrosis, causing dyspnea, tightness and pain in chest, pleural friction rubs and effusion, arthralgia, myalgia.

• Also available in Canada.
•• Available in Canada only.
Unmarked trade names available in United States only.

INTERACTIONS	NURSING CONSIDERATIONS
Propranolol: blocked natural pathway for vasodilation in patients receiving ergot alkaloids and thus could result in excessive vasoconstriction. Watch closely if drugs are used together.	• Contraindicated in peripheral and occlusive vascular disease, coronary heart disease, hypertension, hepatic or renal dysfunction, sepsis. • Avoid prolonged administration; don't exceed recommended dosage. • Tell patient to report any feeling of coldness in extremities or tingling of fingers and toes. These symptoms appear before onset of gangrene. • Most effective when used to prevent migraine or soon after onset. Provide a quiet, low-light environment to help patient relax. • Help patient evaluate underlying causes of stress. • Alpha-adrenergic blocker.
Propranolol: blocked natural pathway for vasodilation in patients receiving ergot alkaloids and thus could result in excessive vasoconstriction. Watch closely if drugs are used together.	• Contraindicated in peripheral and occlusive vascular diseases, coronary heart disease, hypertension, hepatic or renal dysfunction, sepsis. • Avoid prolonged administration, and don't exceed recommended dosage. • Most effective when used to prevent migraine or soon after onset. • Provide a quiet, low-light environment to help patient relax. • Help patient evaluate underlying causes of stress. • Instruct patient on long-term therapy to check for and report any feeling of coldness in extremities or tingling of fingers and toes. These symptoms appear before the onset of gangrene. • Alpha-adrenergic blocker. • Store drug in light-resistant container.
None significant.	• Contraindicated in severe hypertension, arteriosclerosis, peripheral vascular insufficiency, renal or hepatic disease, severe coronary artery diseases, thromboembolic disorders, phlebitis or cellulitis of lower limbs, fibrotic processes, valvular disease, debilitated patients. Use cautiously in peptic ulcers; in suspected coronary artery disease. EKG and cardiac status evaluation advisable before giving to patients over 40. • Stop drug every 6 months; then restart after at least 3 or 4 weeks. • Tell patient not to stop drug abruptly; may cause rebound headaches. Stop gradually over 2 to 3 weeks. • Patient should keep daily weight record and report unusually rapid weight gain. Teach him to check for peripheral edema. Explain and suggest low-salt diet if necessary. • Give drug for 3 weeks before evaluating effectiveness. Obtain renal function tests before starting therapy and every 4 to 6 months thereafter. • Tell patient to report to doctor promptly if he experiences cold, numb, or painful hands and feet; leg cramps when walking; girdle, chest, or flank pain. • Not for treatment of migraine or vascular headache in progress, or for treatment of tension (muscle contraction) headaches. • Indicated only for patients who are unresponsive to other drugs and who can be kept under close medical supervision.

NAME	INDICATIONS & DOSAGE	SIDE EFFECTS
phenoxybenzamine hydrochloride Dibenzyline	*To control or prevent hypertension and sweating associated with pheochromocytoma; Raynaud's syndrome, frostbite; acrocyanosis*— **Adults:** initially, 10 mg P.O., then increase by 10 mg q 4 days to a maximum of 60 mg daily.	*CNS:* sedation, fatigue, lassitude. *CV:* tachycardia, postural hypotension with dizziness. *EENT:* miosis, nasal congestion. *GI:* irritation. *GU:* inhibition of ejaculation.
phentolamine hydrochloride Regitine, Rogitine♦♦ **phentolamine mesylate**	*To control or prevent hypertension before or during pheochromocytomectomy*— **Adults:** 50 to 100 mg P.O. 4 to 6 times daily; or 5 mg I.M. or I.V. 1 to 2 hours preop. May repeat if needed. During surgery, 5 mg I.V. may be given as needed. **Children:** 25 mg P.O. daily, divided q 4 to 6 hours; or 1 mg I.M. or I.V. 1 to 2 hours preop. May repeat if needed. During surgery, 1 mg I.V. may be given as needed. *To prevent dermal necrosis and sloughing after extravasation of levarterenol I.V.*— add 10 mg phentolamine to each liter of levarterenol solution to prevent tissue damage. *To treat extravasation*— infiltrate area with 5 to 10 mg phentolamine in 10 ml 0.9% normal saline solution. Must be done within 12 hours.	*CV:* acute and prolonged hypotension, tachycardia, cardiac arrhythmia, angina, orthostatic hypotension, flushing. *EENT:* nasal congestion. *GI:* nausea, vomiting, diarrhea, exacerbation of peptic ulcer.
propranolol Inderal♦	*Prevention of frequent, severe, uncontrollable, or disabling migraine or vascular headache*— **Adults:** initially, 80 mg daily in divided doses. Usual maintenance	*Blood:* eosinophilia, thrombocytopenia, agranulocytosis. *CNS:* giddiness, depression, hallucinations, visual disturbances. *CV:* bradycardia, congestive heart

INTERACTIONS	NURSING CONSIDERATIONS
None significant.	• Contraindicated whenever a fall in blood pressure is undesirable. Use cautiously in cerebral or coronary arteriosclerosis, renal damage, or respiratory disease. • May aggravate symptoms of respiratory infections. • Safe use in pregnancy has not been established, but drug has been used during the third trimester to treat hypertension caused by pheochromocytoma without apparent harm to mother or fetus. • Reduce gastric irritation by giving with milk or in divided doses. • Place overdosed patient in Trendelenburg position; have I.V. solution ready. Treat hypotension with levarterenol (norepinephrine). • Full therapeutic effect may not be seen for several weeks. • Alpha-adrenergic blocking agent leaves beta-adrenergic receptors unopposed.
None significant.	• Contraindicated in angina, coronary artery disease, or in history of myocardial infarction. Use with caution in gastritis or peptic ulcer. • If cardiac arrhythmias occur, don't give digitalis glycosides until cardiac rhythm returns to normal. • Place overdosed patient in Trendelenburg position; have I.V. solution ready. Treat hypotension with levarterenol (norepinephrine). • Monitor blood pressure closely, especially after parenteral administration. • Alpha-adrenergic blocking agent and beta-adrenergic stimulator. • To reconstitute injection add 1 ml sterile water for injection to 5 mg vial of drug. Use immediately after reconstitution.
Insulin, hypoglycemic drugs (oral): can alter requirements for these drugs in previously stabilized	• Contraindicated in diabetes mellitus, asthma, or allergic rhinitis; during ethyl ether anesthesia; in sinus bradycardia and in heart block greater than first degree; in cardiogenic shock; in right ventricular failure secondary to pulmonary hypertension. Use with caution in congestive heart failure or respiratory disease.

(continued on following page)

NAME	INDICATIONS & DOSAGE	SIDE EFFECTS
propranolol *(continued)*	dose: 160 to 240 mg daily, divided t.i.d. or q.i.d.	failure, angina, myocardial infarction, hypotension, syncope, shock. *GI:* nausea, vomiting, epigastric distress, diarrhea. *Metabolic:* hypoglycemia without symptoms. *Skin:* rash. *Other:* bronchospasm, wheezing, asthma.

INTERACTIONS	NURSING CONSIDERATIONS
diabetics. Monitor for hypoglycemia. *Cardiac glycosides:* excessive bradycardia and increased depressant effect on myocardium. Monitor pulse. *Aminophylline:* antagonized beta blocking effects of propranolol. Use together cautiously. *Isoproterenol, glucagon:* antagonized propranolol effect. May be used therapeutically and in emergencies.	• Withdraw drug slowly. Abrupt withdrawal might precipitate myocardial infarction or aggravate angina, thyrotoxicosis, or pheochromoocytoma. Abrupt withdrawal in thyrotoxicosis may exacerbate hyperthroidism or precipitate thyroid storm. In thyrotoxicosis, propranolol may mask clinical signs of hyperthyroidism. • Don't stop before surgery for pheochromocytoma. Before any surgical procedure, notify anesthesiologist that patient is on propranolol. • Always check apical pulse rate before giving this drug. If less than 60 beats/minute, hold dose and call doctor promptly. Treat excessive bradycardia with atropine. • Monitor blood pressure frequently. If patient develops excessive hypotension, notify doctor, as he may order a vasopressor to counteract effect. Tell patient that orthostatic hypotension can be minimized by rising slowly and avoiding sudden position changes. • Relieve mouth dryness with gum, sour hard candy, or ice chips. • Remember, this drug masks common signs of shock and hypoglycemia.

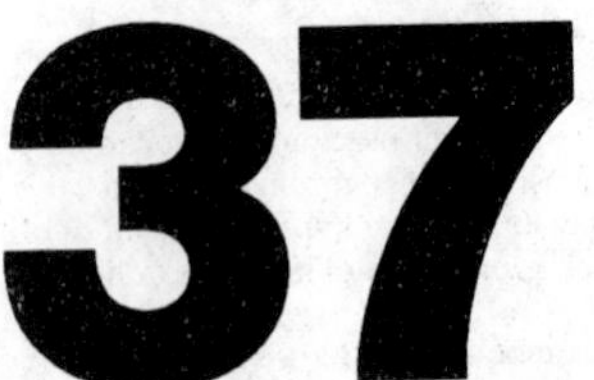

Skeletal muscle relaxants

baclofen
carisoprodol
chlorphenesin carbamate
chlorzoxazone
cyclobenzaprine
dantrolene sodium
metaxalone
methocarbamol
orphenadrine citrate

Skeletal muscle relaxants are of two distinct types: centrally acting agents, which are usually given orally; and neuromuscular blockers (Chapter 38), which must be given parenterally. Centrally acting agents are widely used for a variety of minor musculoskeletal disorders.

Major uses

- Relief of acute muscle spasm associated with trauma, inflammation, manipulations, or psychogenic disorders.
- Generally not useful for spasticity from multiple sclerosis or other CNS disorders (except baclofen and dantrolene sodium).

Mechanism of action

- Depresses transmission of nerve impulses from spinal cord to skeletal muscle.
- Directly inhibits skeletal muscle activation (dantrolene).

Absorption, distribution, and excretion

- Well absorbed orally and I.M.
- Widely distributed to body tissues, with high concentration in the brain.
- Metabolized in the liver, with renal excretion of unchanged drug and metabolites.

Onset and duration

- Onset within 1 hour.
- Peak effects at 2 to 3 hours.
- Duration 4 to 6 hours.

Combination products

NORGESIC: orphenadrine citrate 25 mg, aspirin 225 mg, phenacetin 160 mg, and caffeine 30 mg.
NORGESIC FORTE: orphenadrine citrate 50 mg, aspirin 450 mg, phenacetin 320 mg, and caffeine 60 mg.
PARAFON FORTE♦: chlorzoxazone 250 mg and acetaminophen 300 mg.
ROBAXISAL♦: methocarbamol 400 mg and aspirin 325 mg.
SOMA COMPOUND♦: carisoprodol 200 mg, phenacetin 160 mg, and caffeine 32 mg.
SOMA COMPOUND WITH CODEINE: carisoprodol 200 mg, phenacetin 160 mg, caffeine 32 mg, and codeine phosphate 16 mg.

PATIENT TEACHING AID — HOW TO RELIEVE MUSCLE SPASM

Dear Patient:

If you are taking muscle relaxants, remember these drugs are only a supplement, not a replacement for muscle spasm therapy. Your doctor will probably also recommend the simple measures of rest, cold and heat. If your pain is severe, stay in bed in a comfortable position; get up only to use the bathroom. Have someone apply cold or heat to the painful area for 20 to 30 minutes four times daily. Try cold first — it's more effective.

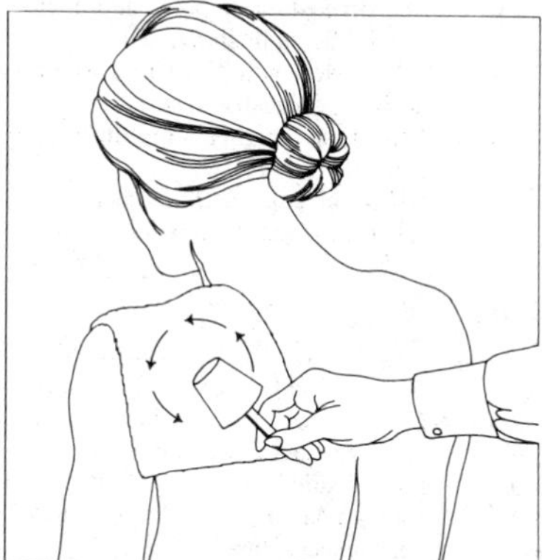

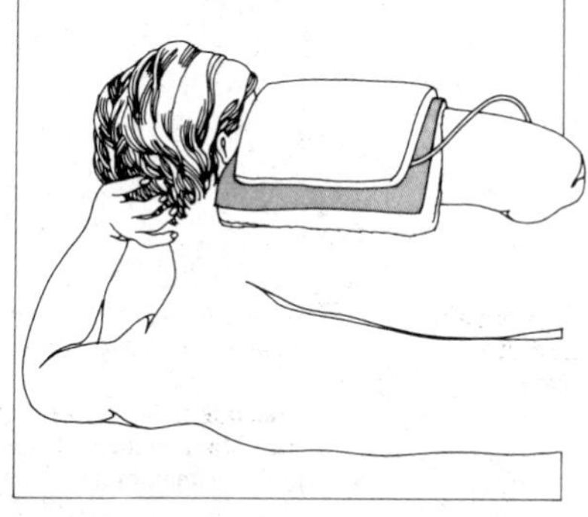

WHEN APPLYING COLD...

1. Place a tongue blade or popsicle stick in water in a paper cup; freeze; peel the paper off the ice. Or put crushed ice in a pillowcase or other type of cloth, not a plastic bag.
2. Place a cold cloth over the painful area to avoid frostbite and cold shock. Never apply ice directly to the skin.
3. Rub the ice back and forth over towel-covered skin.

Note: When applying cold to a joint that has begun to stiffen after an acute inflammatory attack, don't let the analgesic effect make you overconfident about using the joint.

The switch from cold to heat therapy can be made 24 to 72 hours after an injury or when cold no longer helps.

WHEN APPLYING HEAT...

1. Place a moist towel over the painful area. Moist heat is better because it's less drying to the skin; it's less likely to burn the skin; it doesn't result in sweating with excessive fluid and salt loss; and it penetrates more deeply.
2. Place plastic over the towel.
3. Put a heating pad — only use a pad that carries the Underwriter's seal — over the plastic. Set the heating pad at medium or low, never high. Also, never place the heating pad under the body.
4. Then cover the heating pad with a lightweight blanket.
5. Remove the heating pad and wet-pack after 20 to 30 minutes, never longer.

NAME	INDICATIONS & DOSAGE	SIDE EFFECTS
baclofen Lioresal	*Spasticity in multiple sclerosis, spinal cord injury—* **Adults:** initially, 5 mg t.i.d. for 3 days, 10 mg t.i.d. for 3 days, 15 mg t.i.d. for 3 days, 20 mg t.i.d. for 3 days. Increase according to response up to maximum 80 mg daily.	*CNS:* drowsiness, dizziness, headache, weakness, fatigue, confusion, insomnia. *CV:* hypotension. *EENT:* nasal congestion. *GI:* nausea, constipation. *GU:* urinary frequency. *Metabolic:* increased SGOT, alkaline phosphatase, blood sugar. *Skin:* rash, pruritus. *Other:* ankle edema, excessive perspiration, weight gain.
carisoprodol Rela•, Soma•	*As an adjunct in acute, painful musculoskeletal conditions—* **Adults, and children over 12:** 350 mg P.O. t.i.d. and at bedtime. Not recommended for children under 12.	*CNS:* drowsiness, dizziness, vertigo, ataxia, tremor, agitation, irritability, headache, depressive reactions, insomnia. *CV:* orthostatic hypotension, tachycardia, facial flushing. *GI:* nausea, vomiting, increased bowel activity, epigastric distress. *Skin:* rash, erythema multiforme, pruritus. *Other:* hiccups, asthmatic episodes, fever, angioneurotic edema, anaphylaxis.
chlorphenesin carbamate Maolate	*As an adjunct in short-term, acute, painful, musculoskeletal conditions—* **Adults:** initial dose 800 mg P.O. t.i.d. Maintenance 400 mg P.O. q.i.d. for maximum of 8 weeks.	*Blood:* blood dyscrasia. *CNS:* drowsiness, dizziness, confusion, headache, weakness. Dose-related side effects include paradoxical stimulation, agitation, insomnia, nervousness, headache. *GI:* nausea, epigastric distress. *Other:* anaphylaxis.
chlorzoxazone Paraflex	*As an adjunct in acute, painful, musculoskeletal conditions—* **Adults:** 250 to 750 mg t.i.d. or q.i.d. **Children:** 20 mg/Kg daily divided t.i.d. or q.i.d.	*CNS:* drowsiness, dizziness, lightheadedness, malaise, headache, overstimulation. *GI:* anorexia, nausea, vomiting, heartburn, abdominal distress, constipation, diarrhea. *GU:* urinary color change (orange or purple-red). *Skin:* urticaria, redness, itching, petechiae, bruising. *Other:* liver dysfunction.

• Also available in Canada.
•• Available in Canada only.
Unmarked trade names available in United States only.

INTERACTIONS	NURSING CONSIDERATIONS
None significant.	• Use cautiously in impaired renal function, stroke patients (minimal benefit, poor tolerance), epilepsy, spasticity used to sustain upright balance and locomotion or to obtain increased body function. • Give with meals or milk to prevent gastric distress. • Amount of relief determines if dosage (and drowsiness) can be reduced. • Watch for increased seizures in epileptics. • Watch for sensitivity reactions such as fever, skin eruptions, and respiratory distress. • Tell patient to avoid driving and other hazardous activities until response to drug is determined. Drowsiness usually transient. • Patient should follow doctor's orders regarding rest, physical therapy. • Do not withdraw abruptly unless required by severe side effects. May precipitate hallucinations or rebound spasticity. • Overdosage treatment supportive only; do not induce emesis or use respiratory stimulant in obtunded patients.
None significant.	• Contraindicated in hypersensitivity to related compounds (including meprobamate, tybamate); or intermittent porphyria. Use with caution in impaired hepatic or renal function. • Watch for idiosyncratic reactions after first to fourth dose (weakness, ataxia, visual and speech difficulties, fever, skin eruptions, mental changes) or severe reactions, including bronchospasm, hypotension, anaphylactic shock. Hold dose and notify doctor immediately of any unusual reactions. • Record amount of relief to determine whether dosage can be reduced. • Watch for signs of respiratory distress. • Withdrawal symptoms may occur if high doses are stopped abruptly. • Warn patient to avoid driving and other hazardous activities until response to drug is determined. Drowsiness is transient. • Avoid combining with alcohol or other depressants. • Patient should follow doctor's orders regarding rest, physical therapy. • For treatment of anaphylaxis, see p. 1114.
None significant.	• Use cautiously in hepatic disease or impaired renal function. • Safe use for periods exceeding 8 weeks not established. • Take with meals or milk to prevent gastric distress. • Amount of relief determines if dosage (and drowsiness) can be reduced. • Watch for sensitivity reactions such as fever, skin eruptions, and respiratory distress. Hold dose and notify doctor of any unusual reactions. • Monitor hepatic function tests and blood studies. • Watch for unusual bleeding and infectious problems which may indicate blood dyscrasia. • For treatment of anaphylaxis, see p. 1114.
None significant.	• Contraindicated in impaired hepatic function. Use cautiously in drug allergies. • Record amount of relief to determine whether dosage can be reduced. • Watch for signs of hepatic damage. Hold dose and notify doctor. • Warn patient to avoid driving and other hazardous activities until response to drug is determined. Drowsiness is transient. • Avoid combining with alcohol or other depressants. • Expect urine color to change. • Patient should follow doctor's orders regarding rest, physical therapy. • Give with meals or milk to prevent gastric distress.

NAME	INDICATIONS & DOSAGE	SIDE EFFECTS
cyclobenzaprine Flexeril◆	*Short-term treatment of muscle spasm—* **Adults:** 10 mg P.O. t.i.d. for 7 days. Maximum: 60 mg/day for 2 to 3 weeks.	*CNS:* drowsiness, euphoria, weakness, headache, insomnia, nightmares, paresthesias, dizziness. *CV:* tachycardia. *EENT:* blurred vision. *GI:* abdominal pain, dyspepsia, peculiar taste, constipation, dry mouth. *GU:* urinary retention. *Skin:* rash, urticaria, pruritus. *Other:* in high doses, watch for side effects like those of other tricyclic drugs (amitriptyline, imipramine).
dantrolene sodium Dantrium◆	*Spasticity and sequelae secondary to severe chronic disorders (multiple sclerosis, cerebral palsy, spinal cord injury, stroke)—* *Careful dose titration to lowest effective dose essential.* **Adults:** 25 mg P.O. daily. Increase gradually to 25 mg b.i.d. to q.i.d. to maximum of 800 mg/day for 4 to 7 days. **Children:** 1 mg/Kg/day P.O. Increase gradually as needed by 1 mg/Kg/day b.i.d. to q.i.d., to maximum of 100 mg q.i.d.	*CNS:* muscle weakness, drowsiness, dizziness, light-headedness, malaise, fatigue, headache, mental depression, confusion, increased nervousness, insomnia, speech disturbance. *CV:* tachycardia, blood pressure changes, phlebitis. *EENT:* excessive tearing, visual disturbances. *GI:* diarrhea, anorexia, constipation, cramping, dysphagia. *GU:* increased urinary frequency, incontinence, nocturia, dysuria, crystalluria, difficult erection. *Skin:* acneform rash, eczematoid eruption, pruritus, urticaria. *Other:* abnormal hair growth, drooling, peculiar taste, sweating, backache, myalgia, chills, fever, feeling of suffocation, photosensitivity, hepatotoxicity.
metaxalone Skelaxin◆	*As an adjunct in acute, painful musculoskeletal conditions—* **Adults, and children over 12 years:** 800 mg P.O. t.i.d. or q.i.d.	*Blood:* leukopenia, hemolytic anemia. *CNS:* drowsiness, dizziness, headache, nervousness, irritability, exacerbation of grand mal epilepsy. *GI:* nausea, vomiting, GI upset, jaundice. *Skin:* light rash with or without pruritus.

INTERACTIONS	NURSING CONSIDERATIONS
None significant.	• Contraindicated in patients who have received MAO inhibitors within 14 days; during acute recovery phase of myocardial infarction; and in heart block, arrhythmias, conduction disturbances, or congestive heart failure. Use cautiously in urinary retention, angle-closure glaucoma, increased intraocular pressure, cardiovascular disease, impaired hepatic function, elderly or debilitated patients, or seizures. • Withdrawal symptoms (nausea, headache, malaise) may occur if drug stopped abruptly after long-term therapy. • Watch for symptoms of overdose, including possible cardiotoxicity. Notify doctor immediately and have physostigmine available. • Check intake and output. Be alert for urinary retention. If constipation is a problem, increase fluid intake and get an order for a stool softener. • Warn patient to avoid driving and other hazardous activities until drug response is determined. Drowsiness and dizziness usually subside after 2 weeks. • Avoid combining alcohol or other depressants with cyclobenzaprine. • Expect a dry mouth. Relieve with sugarless candy or gum.
None significant.	• Contraindicated when spasticity is used to sustain upright balance and locomotion or to maintain increased body function; in spasms in rheumatic disorders, lactation. Use with caution in severely impaired cardiac or pulmonary function; preexisting hepatic disease; in females, and in patients over 35. • Safety and efficacy in long-term use not established; value may be determined by therapeutic trial. Do not give more than 45 days if no benefits observed. • Give with meals or milk to prevent gastric distress. • Prepare oral suspension for single dose by dissolving capsule contents in juice or other suitable liquid. For multiple dose, use acid vehicle, such as citric acid, in USP Syrup; refrigerate. Use in several days. • Test, initially and periodically, hepatic, renal, and hematopoietic functions. • Record amount of relief to determine whether dosage can be reduced. • Watch for hepatitis (fever, jaundice), severe diarrhea or weakness, or sensitivity reactions (fever, skin eruptions). Hold dose and notify doctor. • Watch for signs of respiratory distress. • Warn patient to avoid driving and other hazardous activities until response to drug is determined. Side effects should subside after 4 days. • Tell patient to avoid combining with alcohol or other depressants; to avoid photosensitivity reactions by using sunscreening agents and protective clothing; to report abdominal discomfort or GI problems immediately; and to follow doctor's orders regarding rest, physical therapy.
None significant.	• Contraindicated in impaired hepatic or renal function; history of drug-induced hemolytic or other anemias. • Test hepatic function periodically. May cause abnormalities in hepatic function studies; repeat tests after drug is discontinued. • Record amount of relief to determine if dosage can be reduced. • Watch for sensitivity reactions, such as rash with pruritus. • Warn patient to avoid combining with alcohol or other depressants. • Patient should follow doctor's orders regarding rest, physical therapy. • Give with meals or milk to prevent gastric distress. • False positive results in glucose tests if cupric sulfate is used. Use glucose oxidase instead.

NAME	INDICATIONS & DOSAGE	SIDE EFFECTS
methocarbamol Delaxin, Forbaxin, Metho-500, Robamol, Robaxin◆, Rometho-carb, Spenaxin	*As an adjunct in acute, painful, musculoskeletal conditions—* **Adults:** 1.5 g P.O. for 2 to 3 days, then 1 g P.O. q.i.d., or not more than 500 mg (5 ml) I.M. into each gluteal region. May repeat q 8 hours. I.V.: 1 to 3 g/day (10 to 30 ml) directly into vein at 3 ml/minute, or 10 ml may be added to no more than 250 ml of 5% dextrose in water or normal saline. Maximum dose 3 g/day. *Supportive therapy in tetanus management—* **Adults:** 1 to 2 g into tubing of running I.V. or 1 to 3 g in infusion bottle q 6 hours. **Children:** 15 mg/Kg I.V. q 6 hours.	*Blood:* hemolysis, increased hemoglobin (I.V. only). *CNS:* drowsiness, dizziness, lightheadedness, headache, vertigo, mild muscular incoordination (I.M. or I.V. only), convulsions (I.V. only). *CV:* hypotension, bradycardia (I.M. or I.V. only). *GI:* nausea, anorexia, GI upset. *GU:* red blood cells in urine (I.V. only). *Local:* thrombophlebitis, extravasation (I.V. only). *Skin:* urticaria, pruritus, rash. *Other:* fever, metallic taste, flushing, anaphylactic reactions (I.M. or I.V. only).
orphenadrine citrate Flexon, Myolin, Neocyten, Norflex◆, Ro-Orphena, Tega-Flex, X-Otag	*Adjunctive treatment in painful acute musculoskeletal conditions—* **Adults:** 100 mg P.O. b.i.d., or 60 mg I.V. or I.M. q 12 hours, p.r.n.	*CNS:* disorientation, restlessness, irritability, incoherence, weakness, drowsiness, headache, insomnia. *CV:* palpitations, tachycardia. *EENT:* dilated pupils, blurred vision, increased intraocular pressure, eye pain, difficulty swallowing. *GI:* constipation, dry mouth, nausea, vomiting, paralytic ileus, epigastric distress. *GU:* urinary hesitancy or retention. *Skin:* flushing, dryness, rash.

INTERACTIONS	NURSING CONSIDERATIONS
None significant.	• Contraindicated in impaired renal function (injection form), children under 12 years (except in tetanus), myasthenia gravis, patients receiving anticholinesterase agents, epilepsy (injection form). • I.V. irritates veins, may cause phlebitis, aggravates seizures, may cause fainting if injected rapidly. • In tetanus management, use methocarbamol with tetanus antitoxin, penicillin, tracheotomy, and aggressive supportive care. Long course of I.V. methocarbamol required. • Watch for sensitivity reactions such as fever, skin eruptions. • Warn patient to avoid driving and other hazardous activities until response to drug is determined. Drowsiness subsides. • Avoid combining with alcohol or other depressants. • Patient should follow doctor's orders regarding rest, physical therapy. • Tell patient urine may turn green, black, or brown. • Give with meals or milk to prevent gastric distress. • Watch for orthostatic hypotension, especially with parenteral administration. Keep patient supine for 15 minutes afterward, and supervise ambulation. Advise patient to get up slowly. • Give I.V. slowly. Maximum rate 300 mg (3 ml)/minute. Give I.M. deeply, only in upper outer quadrant of buttocks, with maximum of 5 ml in each buttock, and inject slowly. Do not give S.C. • Have epinephrine, antihistamines, corticosteroids available. • Prepare liquid by crushing tablets into water or saline solution. Give through nasogastric tube. • For treatment of anaphylaxis, see p. 1114.
None significant.	• Contraindicated in narrow-angle glaucoma; prostatic hypertrophy; pyloric, duodenal, or bladder neck obstruction; myasthenia gravis; tachycardia; severe hepatic or renal disease; ulcerative colitis; lactation. Use cautiously in elderly or debilitated patients with cardiac disease, and those exposed to high temperatures; arrhythmias. • Check all dosages carefully. Even a slight overdose can lead to toxicity. Early signs are excessive dry mouth, dilated pupils, blurred vision, skin flushing, fever. • Monitor vital signs carefully. Watch closely for side effects, particularly in elderly or debilitated patients. Call doctor promptly. • When given I.V., may cause paradoxical initial bradycardia. Usually disappears in 2 minutes. • Monitor intake and output. Causes urinary retention and hesitancy; have patient void before administering. • Relieve dry mouth with cool drinks, ice chips, sugarless gum, or hard candy. • Monitor blood, urine, and hepatic function periodically, especially with long-term use. • Patient may develop a tolerance to this drug.

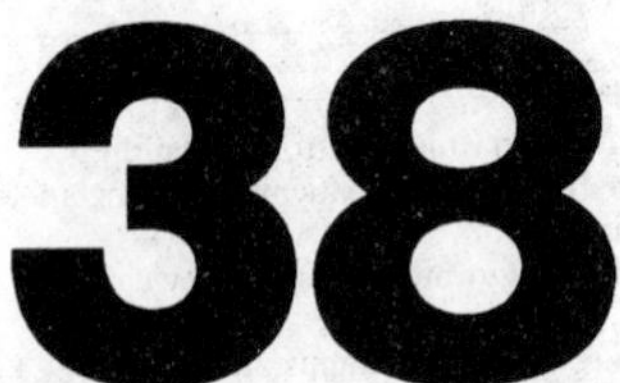

38 Neuromuscular blockers

decamethonium bromide
gallamine triethiodide
hexafluorenium bromide
metocurine iodide
pancuronium bromide
succinylcholine chloride
tubocurarine chloride

Neuromuscular blockers, the second of two types of skeletal muscle relaxants, are sometimes called peripherally acting skeletal muscle relaxants. Unlike the centrally acting agents (Chapter 37) which are usually used orally, neuromuscular blockers must be used parenterally. They are potent drugs with very specific uses and should only be administered by a doctor or under a doctor's direct supervision, with emergency respiratory support available. Because the effects of these drugs are frightening to conscious patients, they should be used only with adequate levels of general anesthesia.

Major uses

- Potentiation of surgical anesthesia, allowing use of lighter level of anesthesia.
- Facilitation of intubation, abdominal surgery, corrections of dislocations, and resetting of fractures.
- Control of respiration for patients on respirator.
- Diagnosis of myasthenia gravis (tubocurarine).
- Symptomatic control of muscle spasms in convulsive states (tetanus, status epilepticus, drug intoxication, black widow spider bites).
- Control of muscle contraction during electroconvulsive therapy.

Mechanism of action

- Blocks transmission of nerve impulses at the skeletal neuromuscular junction.

Absorption, distribution, and excretion

- Not effective orally (poorly absorbed from gastrointestinal tract); slowly and unpredictably absorbed from intramuscular sites.
- Rapidly distributed from intravenous sites.
- Poorly metabolized (except succinylcholine); remain effective in body until excreted via bile and urine as active unchanged drug.
- Succinylcholine is hydrolyzed by pseudocholinesterase in the plasma and liver.

Onset and duration

- Onset is immediate with I.V. use.

- Effects persist for 1½ to 2 hours.
- Effects accumulate with repeated doses.
- Succinylcholine is extremely short acting.

Combination products
None.

WHERE NEUROMUSCULAR BLOCKING AGENTS ACT

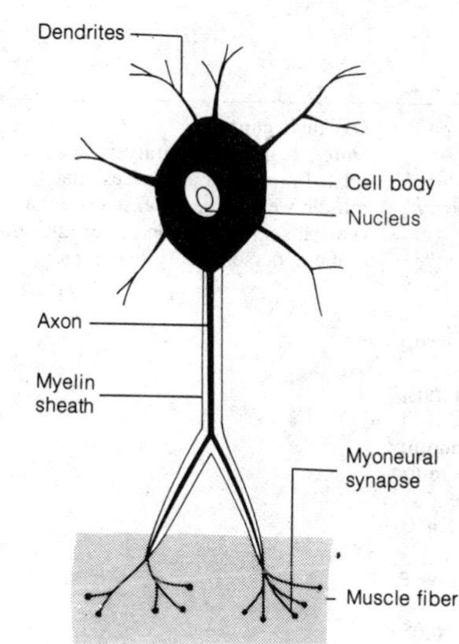

The basic unit of the nervous system is the nerve cell or neuron. Typically, it consists of a central cell body and a number of threadlike projections of cytoplasm known as nerve fibers. These are of two types: the axon, which conducts impulses away from the cell body, and the dendrite, which conducts impulses to the cell body. Most neurons have multiple dendrites and a single axon.

Axons are surrounded by a white fatty substance called myelin, which insulates and protects the delicate inner fiber.

Neurons receive and transmit impulses at junctions called synapses, where one structure almost touches another. When information flows, one of the structures releases a transmitting chemical which crosses the narrow cleft between them and activates the receiving cell.

Neuromuscular blocking agents block this chemical at the neuromuscular synapse.

NAME	INDICATIONS & DOSAGE	SIDE EFFECTS
decamethonium bromide Syncurine•	*Adjunct to anesthesia to induce skeletal muscle relaxation; facilitate intubation, lessen muscle contractions in pharmacologically or electrically induced convulsions; assist with mechanical ventilation—* Dose depends on anesthetic used, individual needs and response. Doses are representative and must be adjusted. **Adults:** initially, 0.5 to 3 mg I.V., at a rate of 0.5 mg to 1 mg per minute, then 0.5 to 1 mg q 10 to 30 minutes for sustained relaxation. **Children and infants:** initially, 0.05 to 0.08 mg/Kg I.V., then 0.02 to 0.03/Kg at intervals.	*CV:* bradycardia, tachycardia, cardiac arrest, hypo- and hypertension. *Other:* dose-related prolonged apnea, residual muscle weakness, increased oropharyngeal secretions, allergic or idiosyncratic hypersensitivity reactions, postoperative muscle pain.
gallamine triethiodide Flaxedil•	*Adjunct to anesthesia to induce skeletal muscle relaxation; facilitate intubation, reduction of fractures and dislocations; lessen muscle contractions in pharmacologically or electrically induced convulsions; assist with mechanical ventilation—* Dose depends on anesthetic used, individual needs and response. Doses are representative and must be adjusted. **Adults, and children over 1 month:** initially, 1 mg/Kg I.V. to maximum of 100 mg, regardless of patient's weight; then 0.5 mg to 1 mg/Kg q 30 to 40 minutes. **Children under 1 month but over 5 Kg (11 lbs.):** initially, 0.25 to 0.75 mg/Kg I.V., then 0.01 to 0.05 mg/Kg q 30 to 40 minutes.	*CV:* tachycardia. *Other:* respiratory paralysis, dose-related prolonged apnea, residual muscle weakness, increased oropharyngeal secretions, allergic or idiosyncratic hypersensitivity reactions.

• Also available in Canada.
•• Available in Canada only.
Unmarked trade names available in United States only.

INTERACTIONS	NURSING CONSIDERATIONS
Aminoglycoside antibiotics (including gentamicin, kanamycin, neomycin, streptomycin); polymyxin antibiotics (polymyxin B sulfate, colistin); clindamycin: potentiated neuromuscular blockade, leading to increased skeletal muscle relaxation and possible respiratory paralysis. Use cautiously during surgical and postop periods. *Narcotic analgesics:* potentiated neuromuscular blockade, leading to increased skeletal muscle relaxation and possible respiratory paralysis. Use with extreme caution.	• Contraindicated in hypersensitivity to bromides, impaired renal function, shock, myasthenia gravis, surgical procedures lasting longer than 20 minutes. Use cautiously in patients undergoing surgery in Trendelenburg or lithotomy positions; patients recently digitalized; elderly or debilitated patients; in hepatic or pulmonary impairment, respiratory depression; myasthenic syndrome of lung cancer, dehydration, thyroid disorders, collagen disease, porphyria; electrolyte disturbances; fractures; muscular spasms; and (in large doses) cesarean section. • Seldom used due to uncertain effects and lack of suitable antidote. • Multiple doses not often recommended; may cause reduced response, prolonged apnea. • Monitor baseline electrolyte determinations (electrolyte imbalance, especially K, Ca, and Mg, can potentiate neuromuscular effects) and vital signs, especially respiration. • Check intake and output (renal dysfunction prolongs duration of action, since drug is unchanged before excretion). • Maintain clear airway. Have emergency respiratory support (endotracheal equipment, respirator, oxygen, atropine, neostigmine, or edrophonium) on hand. • Reassure patient that postop stiffness is normal and will soon subside. • Determine whether patient has bromide allergy. • Use only fresh solutions. • Give I.V. slowly (not more than 1 mg/minute). • Do not give without direct supervision of doctor or experienced clinician.
Aminoglycoside antibiotics (gentamicin, kanamycin, neomycin, streptomycin); polymyxin antibiotics (polymyxin B sulfate, colistin); clindamycin: potentiated neuromuscular blockade, leading to increased skeletal muscle relaxation and possible respiratory paralysis. Use cautiously during surgical and postop periods. *Narcotic analgesics:* potentiated neuromuscular blockade, leading to increased skeletal muscle relaxation and possible respiratory paralysis. Use with extreme caution, and reduce dose of gallamine.	• Contraindicated in hypersensitivity to iodides; patients in whom tachycardia may be hazardous; impaired renal function, shock, myasthenia gravis. Use cautiously in cesarean section, hepatic or pulmonary impairment, respiratory depression, elderly or debilitated patients; myasthenic syndrome of lung cancer, dehydration, thyroid disorders, collagen diseases, porphyria; electrolyte disturbances; fractures; muscular spasm. • Monitor baseline electrolyte determinations (electrolyte imbalance can potentiate neuromuscular effects). • Watch respiration for early symptoms of paralysis, inability to keep eyelids open and eyes focused, difficulty in swallowing and speaking. Notify doctor immediately. • Take vital signs every 15 minutes, especially for developing tachycardia. Notify doctor immediately of changes. • Measure intake and output (renal dysfunction prolongs duration of action, since drug is unchanged before excretion). • Keep airway clear. Have emergency respiratory support (endotracheal equipment, respirator, oxygen, atropine, neostigmine) on hand. • Reassure patient that postop stiffness is normal and will soon subside. • Determine whether patient has iodide allergy. • Protect drug from light or excessive heat; use only fresh solutions. • Do not mix solution with meperidine HC1 or barbiturate solutions. • Give I.V. slowly (over 30 to 90 seconds). • Do not give without direct supervision of doctor.

NAME	INDICATIONS & DOSAGE	SIDE EFFECTS
hexafluorenium bromide Mylaxen	*Adjunct for use with succinylcholine to prolong neuromuscular blockade and reduce muscular fasciculations—* Dose depends on individual needs and response. Doses are representative and must be adjusted. **Adults and children:** use in ratio of 2 mg/1 mg succinylcholine. Maximum hexafluorenium bromide 10 to 36 mg; should not be administered more frequently than q 15 to 30 minutes.	*CNS:* prolonged neuromuscular blockade. *CV:* hypotension, hypertension, tachycardia, bradycardia, cardiac arrest. *EENT:* increased intraocular pressure. *Other:* increased bronchial tone, bronchospasm.
metocurine iodide Metubine	*Adjunct to anesthesia to induce skeletal muscle relaxation; facilitate intubation, reduction of fractures and dislocations—* Dose depends on anesthetic used, individual needs and response. Doses are representative and must be adjusted. Administer as sustained injection over 30 to 60 seconds. **Adults:** given cyclopropane: 2 to 4 mg I.V. (2.68 mg average). Given ether: 1.5 to 3 mg I.V. (2.1 mg average). Given nitrous oxide: 4 to 7 mg I.V. (4.79 mg average). Supplemental injections of 0.5 to 1 mg in 25 to 90 minutes, repeated p.r.n. *Lessen muscle contractions in pharmacologically or electrically induced convulsions—* **Adults:** 1.75 to 5.5 mg I.V.	*CV:* hypotension secondary to histamine release, ganglionic blockade in rapid dose or overdose. *Other:* dose-related prolonged apnea, residual muscle weakness, increased oropharyngeal secretions, allergic or idiosyncratic hypersensitivity reactions, bronchospasm.
pancuronium bromide Pavulon◆	*Adjunct to anesthesia to induce skeletal muscle relaxation; facilitate intubation, lessen muscle contractions in pharmacologically or electrically induced convulsions; assist with mechanical ventilation—* Dose depends on anesthetic used, individual needs and response. Doses are representative and must be adjusted.	*CV:* tachycardia, increased blood pressure. *Local:* burning sensation. *Skin:* transient rashes. *Other:* excessive sweating and salivation, prolonged dose-related apnea, residual muscle weakness, allergic or idiosyncratic hypersensitivity reactions.

INTERACTIONS	NURSING CONSIDERATIONS
None reported for this drug alone; always used with succinylcholine. See p. 446.	• Contraindicated in hypersensitivity to bromides, in bronchial asthma. Use cautiously in renal, hepatic, or pulmonary impairment, or respiratory depression; in elderly or debilitated patients; in myasthenia gravis; myasthenic syndrome of lung cancer, dehydration, thyroid disorders, collagen diseases, porphyria; electrolyte disturbances; (in large doses) cesarean section; glaucoma; or during ocular surgery. • Not used extensively in clinical practice. • Monitor baseline electrolyte determinations (electrolyte imbalance potentiates neuromuscular effects) and vital signs (watch respirations closely). • Keep airway clear. Have emergency respiratory support (endotracheal equipment, respirator, oxygen, atropine, neostigmine) on hand. • Reassure patient that postop stiffness is normal and will soon subside. • Determine whether patient has bromide allergy. • Use only fresh solutions; do not give without direct supervision of doctor.
Aminoglycoside antibiotics (including gentamicin, kanamycin, neomycin, streptomycin); polymyxin and polypeptide antibiotics (polymyxin B sulfate, colistin); clindamycin: potentiated neuromuscular blockade, leading to increased skeletal muscle relaxation and possible respiratory paralysis. Use cautiously during surgical and postop periods. *Narcotic analgesics:* potentiated neuromuscular blockade, leading to increased skeletal muscle relaxation and possible respiratory paralysis. Use with extreme caution, and reduce dose of metocurine iodide.	• Contraindicated in hypersensitivity to iodides: in patients in whom histamine release is a hazard (asthmatic or atopic patients). Use cautiously in myasthenia gravis; renal, hepatic, or pulmonary impairment; respiratory depression; elderly or debilitated patients; myasthenia gravis; myasthenic syndrome of lung cancer, dehydration, thyroid disorders, collagen diseases, porphyria; electrolyte disturbances; hyperthermia; (in large doses) cesarean section. • Neostigmine, edrophonium, and epinephrine may be used to reverse effects of metocurine because of their anticurare effects. • Doses of 1 mg therapeutic equivalent of 3 mg *d*-tubocurarine chloride. • Monitor baseline electrolyte determinations (electrolyte imbalance, especially K, Ca, and Mg, can potentiate neuromuscular effects) and vital signs, especially respiration. • Measure intake and output (renal dysfunction prolongs duration of action, since drug is mainly unchanged before excretion). • Keep airway clear. Have emergency respiratory support (endotracheal equipment, respirator, oxygen, atropine, edrophonium, epinephrine, and neostigmine) on hand. • Reassure patient that postop stiffness is normal and will soon subside. • Determine whether patient has iodide allergy. • Store solution away from heat, sunlight; do not mix with barbiturates, methohexital, or thiopental (precipitate will form). Use only fresh solutions. • Do not give without direct supervision of doctor.
Aminoglycoside antibiotics (including gentamicin, kanamycin, neomycin, streptomycin): polymyxin and polypeptide antibiotics (polymyxin B sulfate, colistin); clindamycin: potentiated neuromuscular	• Contraindicated in hypersensitivity to bromides; preexisting tachycardia; patients for whom even a minor increase in heart rate is undesirable. Use cautiously in renal, hepatic, or pulmonary impairment; respiratory depression; elderly or debilitated patients; myasthenia gravis; myasthenic syndrome of lung cancer, dehydration, thyroid disorders, collagen diseases, porphyria; electrolyte disturbances; hyperthermia; (in large doses) cesarean section; or in toxemic states. • Causes no histamine release or hypotension. • Dose of 1 mg approximates therapeutic equivalent of 5 mg *d*-tubocurarine chloride.

(continued on following page)

NAME	INDICATIONS & DOSAGE	SIDE EFFECTS
pancuronium bromide *(continued)*	**Adults:** initially, 0.04 to 0.1 mg/Kg I.V.; then 0.01 mg/Kg q 30 to 60 minutes. **Children over 10 years:** initially, 0.04 to 0.1 mg/Kg I.V., then 1/5 initial dose q 30 to 60 minutes.	
succinylcholine chloride Anectine◆, Anectine Flo-Pack Powder, Sucostrin, Sux-Cert	*Adjunct to anesthesia to induce skeletal muscle relaxation; facilitate intubation and assist with mechanical ventilation or orthopedic manipulations (drug of choice); lessen muscle contractions in pharmacologically or electrically induced convulsions*—Dose depends on anesthetic used, individual needs and response. Doses are representative and must be adjusted. **Adults:** 25 to 75 mg I.V., then 2.5 mg/minute, p.r.n. or 2.5 mg/Kg I.M. up to maximum 150 mg I.M. in deltoid muscle. **Children:** 1 to 2 mg/Kg I.M. or I.V. Maximum I.M. dose 150 mg. (Children may be less sensitive to succinylcholine than adults.) Test dose: 5 to 10 mg I.V.	*CV:* bradycardia, tachycardia, hyper- and hypotension, arrhythmias, cardiac arrest. *EENT:* increased intraocular pressure. *Other:* prolonged respiratory depression, apnea, malignant hyperthermia, muscle fasciculation, postoperative muscle pain, myoglobinemia, excessive salivation, allergic or idiosyncratic hypersensitivity reactions.

INTERACTIONS	NURSING CONSIDERATIONS
blockade, leading to increased skeletal muscle relaxation and possible respiratory paralysis. Use cautiously during surgical and postop periods. *Lithium, narcotic analgesics:* potentiated neuromuscular blockade, leading to increased skeletal muscle relaxation and possible respiratory paralysis. Use with extreme caution, and reduce dose of pancuronium.	• Monitor baseline electrolyte determinations (electrolyte imbalance can potentiate neuromuscular effects) and vital signs (watch respiration and heart rate closely). • Measure intake and output (renal dysfunction may prolong duration of action, since 25% of the drug is unchanged before excretion). • Have emergency respiratory support (endotracheal equipment, respirator, oxygen, atropine, neostigmine) on hand. • Allow succinylcholine effects to subside before giving pancuronium. • Store in refrigerator. Do not store in plastic containers or syringes, although plastic syringes may be used for administration. • Do not mix with barbiturate solutions; use only fresh solutions. • Do not give without direct supervision of doctor.
Aminoglycoside antibiotics (including gentamicin, kanamycin, neomycin, paromomycin, streptomycin); polymyxin and polypeptide antibiotics (polymyxin B sulfate, colistin): potentiated neuromuscular blockade, leading to increased skeletal muscle relaxation and possible respiratory paralysis. Use cautiously during surgical and postop periods. *Narcotic analgesics, lidocaine, procaine, methotrimeprazine:* potentiated neuromuscular blockade, leading to increased skeletal muscle relaxation and possible respiratory paralysis. Use with extreme caution. *MAO inhibitors,*	• Contraindicated in abnormally low plasma or pseudocholinesterase levels. Use with caution in severe burns or trauma, electrolyte imbalance, quinidine or digitalis therapy, hyperkalemia, paraplegia, spinal neuraxis injury, degenerative or dystrophic neuromuscular disease; patient with personal or family history of malignant hypertension or hyperthermia; hepatic, renal, or pulmonary impairment; respiratory depression; elderly or debilitated patients; myasthenia gravis; myasthenic syndrome of lung cancer, dehydration, thyroid disorders, collagen diseases, porphyria; fractures; muscular spasms; (in large doses) cesarean section; glaucoma; eye surgery or penetrating eye wounds; pheochromocytoma. • Drug of choice for short procedures (less than 3 minutes) and for orthopedic manipulations; use caution in fractures or dislocations. • Duration of action prolonged to 20 minutes by continuous I.V. infusion or single-dose administration, along with hexafluorenium bromide. • Repeated or continuous infusions of succinylcholine alone not advised; may cause reduced response or prolonged apnea. • Monitor baseline electrolyte determinations and vital signs (check respiration every 5 to 10 minutes during infusion). • Keep airway clear. Have emergency respiratory support (endotracheal equipment, respirator, oxygen, atropine, neostigmine) on hand. • Reassure patient that postop stiffness is normal and will soon subside. • Store injectable form in refrigerator. Store powder form at room temperature, tightly closed. Use immediately after reconstitution. Do not mix with alkaline solutions (thiopental, sodium bicarbonate, barbiturates). • Give test dose (10 mg I.M. or I.V.) after patient has been anesthetized. Normal response (no respiratory depression or transient depression lasting less than 5 minutes) indicates drug may be given. Do not give if patient develops respiratory paralysis sufficient to permit endotracheal intubation. (Recovery within 30 to 60 minutes.) • Do not give without direct supervision of doctor.

(continued on following page)

NAME	INDICATIONS & DOSAGE	SIDE EFFECTS
succinylcholine chloride *(continued)*		
tubocurarine chloride Tubarine◆◆	*Adjunct to anesthesia to induce skeletal muscle relaxation; facilitate intubation, orthopedic manipulations—* Dose depends on anesthetic used, individual needs and response. Doses listed are representative and must be adjusted. **Adults:** 1 unit/Kg or 0.15 mg/Kg I.V. slowly over 60 to 90 seconds. Average, initially, 40 to 60 units I.V. May give 20 to 30 units in 3 to 5 minutes. For longer procedures, give 20 units, p.r.n. **Children:** 1 unit/Kg or 0.15 mg/Kg. *Assist with mechanical ventilation—* **Adults and children:** initially, 0.0165 mg/Kg I.V. (average 1 mg or 7 units), then adjust subsequent doses to patient's response. *Diagnose myasthenia gravis—* **Adults and children:** 0.0041 to 0.033 mg/Kg I.V. or $^1/_{15}$ to $^1/_5$ normal adult dose for electroshock. Positive result: profound exaggeration of myasthenic symptoms. Dose may also be given I.M. when necessary. *Lessen muscle contractions in pharmacologically or electrically induced convulsions—* **Adults and children:** 1 unit/Kg or 0.15 mg/Kg slowly over 60 to 90 seconds. Initial dose 20 units (3 mg) less than calculated dose.	*CV:* hypotension, circulatory depression. *Other:* profound and prolonged muscle relaxation, respiratory depression to the point of apnea, hypersensitivity, idiosyncrasy, residual muscle weakness, bronchospasm.

INTERACTIONS	NURSING CONSIDERATIONS
lithium, echothiophate, cyclophosphamide: prolonged apnea. Use with caution. *Magnesium sulfate (parenterally):* potentiated neuromuscular blockade, increased skeletal muscle relaxation and possible respiratory paralysis. Use with caution, preferably with reduced doses. *Digitalis glycosides:* possible cardiac arrhythmias. Use together cautiously.	
Aminoglycoside antibiotics (including gentamicin, kanamycin, neomycin, paromomycin, streptomycin); polymyxin and polypeptide antibiotics (polymyxin B sulfate, colistin): potentiated neuromuscular blockade, leading to increased skeletal muscle relaxation and possible respiratory paralysis. Use cautiously during surgical and postop periods. *Quinidine:* prolonged neuromuscular blockade. Use together with caution. Monitor closely. *Thiazide diuretics, furosemide, ethacrynic acid, amphotericin B, propranolol, methotrimeprazine, narcotic analgesics:* potentiated neuromuscular blockade, leading to increased respiratory paralysis. Use with extreme caution during surgical and postop periods.	• Contraindicated in patients for whom histamine release is a hazard (asthmatics). Use cautiously in hepatic or pulmonary impairment; respiratory depression; elderly or debilitated patients; myasthenia gravis; myasthenic syndrome of lung cancer, dehydration, thyroid disorders, collagen diseases, porphyria; electrolyte disturbances; fractures; muscular spasms; and (in large doses) cesarean section. • Small margin of safety between therapeutic dose and dose causing respiratory paralysis. • Used to diagnose myasthenia gravis, but procedure is hazardous. • Allow succinylcholine effects to subside before giving tubocurarine. • Monitor baseline electrolyte determinations (electrolyte imbalance can potentiate neuromuscular effects). • Watch respiration closely for early symptoms of paralysis—inability to keep eyelids open and eyes focused or difficulty in swallowing and speaking; notify doctor immediately. • Check vital signs every 15 minutes. Notify doctor at once of changes. • Measure intake and output (renal dysfunction prolongs duration of action, since much of drug is unchanged before excretion). • Keep airway clear. Have emergency respiratory support (endotracheal equipment, respirator, oxygen, atropine, edrophonium, epinephrine, and neostigmine) on hand. • Reassure patient that postop stiffness is normal and will soon subside. • Decrease dose if inhalation anesthetics are used. • Do not mix with barbiturates. Use only fresh solutions; discard if discolored. • Give I.V. slowly (60 to 90 seconds); give I.M. deeply in deltoid muscle. • Do not give without direct supervision of doctor.

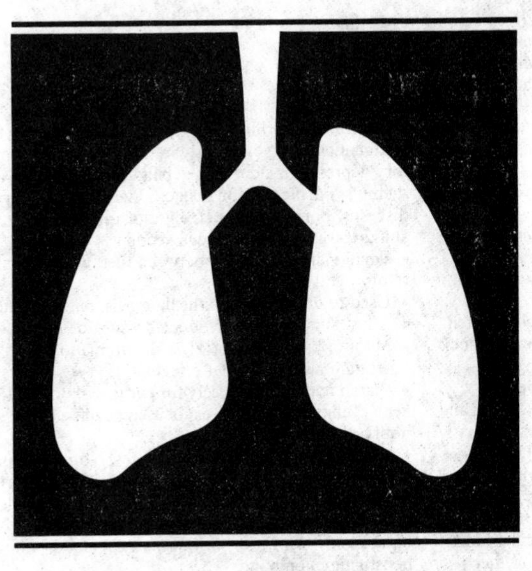

Respiratory Tract

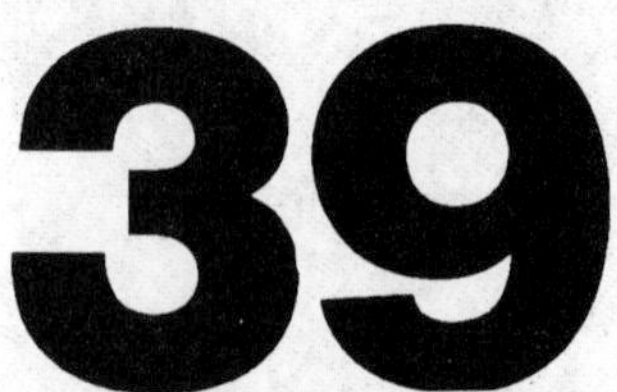

Antihistamines

azatadine maleate
brompheniramine maleate
carbinoxamine maleate
chlorpheniramine maleate
clemastine fumarate
cyproheptadine hydrochloride
dexbrompheniramine maleate
dexchlorpheniramine maleate
dimethindene maleate
dimethothiazine mesylate
diphenhydramine hydrochloride
diphenylpyraline hydrochloride
doxylamine succinate
methdilazine hydrochloride
promethazine hydrochloride
trimeprazine tartrate
tripelennamine hydrochloride
triprolidine hydrochloride

The antihistamines combat the effects of histamine, which causes the symptoms associated with allergic reactions. Several are related to phenothiazines and so are called phenothiazine antihistamines. These are dimethothiazine mesylate, methdilazine hydrochloride, promethazine hydrochloride, and trimeprazine tartrate.

Major uses

- Symptomatic relief of allergic rhinitis and conjunctivitis.
- Treatment of mild, uncomplicated urticaria or pruritus resulting from allergic dermatoses.
- Treatment of minor allergic reactions to drugs and blood or plasma.
- Adjunctive therapy in anaphylaxis.
- Sedation.
- Prevention of motion sickness.

Mechanism of action

- Occupy histamine receptor sites, thus preventing histamine action on the cell.
- Counter most of histamine's pharmacological actions.
- Cause CNS depression and, occasionally, CNS stimulation.
- Act on smooth muscle of bronchial tubes, GI tract, uterus, blood vessels, and capillaries.
- Exhibit anticholinergic effects.
- Cyproheptadine hydrochloride, azatadine maleate, and the phenothiazine antihistamines also block serotonin.
- Antiemetic effect may be related to central anticholinergic activity or to CNS depression.

Absorption, distribution, and excretion

- Rapidly absorbed following oral or parenteral administration.
- Metabolized in liver.
- Excreted in urine.

Onset and duration

- Begin to act in 15 to 30 minutes.
- Peak within 1 hour.
- Duration of 3 to 6 hours (sustained-release—8 to 10 hours).

Combination products

ALLEREST: phenylpropanolamine hydrochloride 18.7 mg and chlorpheniramine maleate 2 mg.
BENDECTIN: doxylamine succinate 10 mg and pyridoxine hydrochloride 10 mg.
CHLOR-TRIMETON DECONGESTANT: chlorpheniramine maleate 4 mg and *d*-isoephedrine sulfate 60 mg.
CODIMAL DH: hydrocodone bitartrate 1.66 mg, phenylephrine hydrochloride 5 mg, pyrilamine maleate 8.33 mg, potassium guaiacolsulfonate 83.3 mg, sodium citrate 216 mg, and citric acid 50 mg.
DIMETAPP EXTENTABS: brompheniramine maleate 12 mg, phenylephrine hydrochloride 15 mg, and phenylpropanolamine hydrochloride 15 mg.
DISOPHROL CHRONOTAB: dexbrompheniramine maleate 6 mg and *d*-isoephedrine sulfate 120 mg.
DRIXORAL•: dexbrompheniramine maleate 6 mg and *d*-isoephedrine sulfate 120 mg.
HISTASPAN-D: chlorpheniramine maleate 8 mg, phenylephrine hydrochloride 20 mg, and methscopolamine nitrate 2.5 mg.
NALDECON: phenylephrine hydrochloride 10 mg, phenylpropanolamine hydrochloride 40 mg, phenyltoloxamine citrate 15 mg, and chlorpheniramine maleate 5 mg.
NEOTEP: chlorpheniramine maleate 9 mg and phenylephrine hydrochloride 21 mg.
NOLAMINE: chlorpheniramine maleate 4 mg, phenindamine tartrate 24 mg, and phenylpropanolamine hydrochloride 50 mg.
NOVAFED A: pseudoephedrine hydrochloride 120 mg and chlorpheniramine maleate 8 mg.
NOVAHISTINE ELIXIR: phenylpropanolamine hydrochloride 18.75 mg, chlorpheniramine maleate 2 mg, and alcohol 5%/5 ml.
ORNADE: isopropamide iodide 2.5 mg, phenylpropanolamine hydrochloride 50 mg, and chlorpheniramine maleate 8 mg.
RHINEX D-LAY: acetaminophen 300 mg, salicylamide 300 mg, phenylpropanolamine hydrochloride 60 mg, and chlorpheniramine maleate 4 mg.
RONDEC T: carbinoxamine maleate 4 mg and pseudoephedrine hydrochloride 60 mg.
TRIAMINIC TIMED-RELEASE: phenylpropanolamine hydrochloride 50 mg, pheniramine maleate 25 mg, and pyrilamine maleate 25 mg.

NAME	INDICATIONS & DOSAGE	SIDE EFFECTS
azatadine maleate Optimine◆	*Rhinitis, allergy symptoms, chronic urticaria—* **Adults:** 1 to 2 mg P.O. b.i.d. Maximum 4 mg daily.	*Blood:* thrombocytopenia. *CNS:* drowsiness, dizziness, vertigo, disturbed coordination, sedation. *CV:* hypotension, palpitations. *GI:* anorexia, nausea, vomiting, dry mouth and throat. *GU:* urinary retention. *Skin:* urticaria, rash. *Other:* chills, thickening of bronchial secretions.
brompheniramine maleate Dimetane◆, Dimetane-Ten, Rolabromophen, Spentane, Veltane	*Rhinitis, allergy symptoms—* **Adults:** 4 to 8 mg P.O. t.i.d. or q.i.d.; or (timed-release) 8 to 12 mg P.O. b.i.d. or t.i.d.; or 5 to 20 mg q 6 to 12 hours I.M., I.V., or S.C. Maximum 40 mg daily. **Children over 6 years:** 4 mg t.i.d. or q.i.d.; or (timed-release) 8 to 12 mg q 12 hours; or 0.5 mg/Kg daily I.M., I.V., or S.C. divided t.i.d. or q.i.d. **Children under 6 years:** 0.5 mg/Kg daily P.O., I.M., I.V., or S.C. divided t.i.d. or q.i.d.	*Blood:* thrombocytopenia, agranulocytosis. *CNS:* dizziness, tremors, irritability, insomnia. *CV:* hypotension, palpitations. *GI:* anorexia, nausea, vomiting, dry mouth and throat. *GU:* urinary retention. *Skin:* urticaria, rash. *After parenteral administration:* local reaction, sweating, syncope may occur.
carbinoxamine maleate Clistin RA	*Rhinitis, allergy symptoms—* **Adults:** 4 to 8 mg P.O. t.i.d. to q.i.d., or (timed-release) 8 to 12 mg q 12 hours. **Children over 6 years:** 4 mg P.O. t.i.d. to q.i.d. **Children 3 to 6 years:** 2 to 4 mg P.O. t.i.d. to q.i.d. **Children 1 to 3 years:** 2 mg P.O. t.i.d. to q.i.d.	*CNS:* drowsiness, dizziness. *GI:* anorexia, nausea, vomiting, dry mouth.
chlorpheniramine maleate Allerbid, Allerid-O.D., AL-R, Antagonate, Chlor-100, Chloramate, Chlormene, Chlor-Pro, Chlortab, Chlor-Trimeton, Chlor-Tripolon◆◆, Ciramine, Histalon◆◆, Histaspan, Histex, Histrey, Novopheniram◆◆, Pyranistan, Ru-Hist, Teldrin	*Rhinitis, allergy symptoms—* **Adults:** 2 to 4 mg P.O. t.i.d. or q.i.d.; or (timed-release) 8 to 12 mg P.O. b.i.d. or t.i.d.; or 5 to 40 mg I.M., I.V., or S.C. Give I.V. injection over 1 minute. **Children 6 to 12 years:** 2 mg P.O. t.i.d. or q.i.d.; or (timed-release) 8 mg P.O. daily or b.i.d. **Children 2 to 6 years:** 1 mg P.O. t.i.d. or q.i.d.	*CNS:* sedation, drowsiness. *CV:* hypotension, palpitations. *GI:* epigastric distress, dry mouth. *GU:* urinary retention. *Other:* thickening of bronchial secretions. *After parenteral administration:* local stinging, burning sensation, pallor, weak pulse, transient hypotension may occur.

◆ Also available in Canada.
◆◆ Available in Canada only.
Unmarked trade names available in United States only.

INTERACTIONS	NURSING CONSIDERATIONS
None significant.	• Contraindicated in acute asthmatic attack, narrow-angle glaucoma, urinary retention, prostatic hypertrophy, bladder neck obstruction. Use cautiously in increased intraocular pressure, hyperthyroidism, elderly patients, cardiovascular or renal disease, hypertension, or bronchial asthma. • Warn patient against alcoholic beverages during therapy, and against driving or other hazardous activities until response to drug is determined. • Reduce GI distress by giving with food or milk. • Coffee or tea may reduce drowsiness. Gum, sour hard candy, or ice chips may relieve dry mouth. • Titrate each patient's dose; response to drug varies. • If tolerance develops, another antihistamine may be substituted. • Warn patient to stop taking drug the evening before allergy skin tests; otherwise, accuracy of tests may be affected.
None significant.	• Contraindicated in acute asthmatic attack, narrow-angle glaucoma, urinary retention, prostatic hypertrophy, bladder neck obstruction. Use cautiously in increased intraocular pressure, hyperthyroidism, elderly patients, cardiovascular or renal disease, hypertension, or bronchial asthma. • Warn patient against alcoholic beverages during therapy, and against driving or other hazardous activities until response to drug is determined. • Reduce GI distress by giving with food or milk. • Coffee or tea may reduce drowsiness. Gum, sour hard candy, or ice chips may relieve dry mouth. • Titrate each patient's dose; response to drug varies. • If tolerance develops, another antihistamine may be substituted. • Warn patient to stop taking drug the evening before allergy skin tests; otherwise, accuracy of tests may be affected. • Injectable form containing 10 mg per ml can be given diluted or undiluted very slowly I.V.
None significant.	• Contraindicated in acute asthmatic attack, narrow-angle glaucoma, urinary retention, prostatic hypertrophy, bladder neck obstruction. Use cautiously in increased intraocular pressure, hyperthyroidism, elderly patients, cardiovascular or renal disease, hypertension, or bronchial asthma. • Warn patient against alcoholic beverages during therapy, and against driving or other hazardous activities until response to drug is determined. • Reduce GI distress by giving with food or milk. • Coffee or tea may reduce drowsiness. Gum, sour hard candy, or ice chips may relieve dry mouth. • Titrate each patient's dose; response to drug varies. • If tolerance develops, another antihistamine may be substituted. • Warn patient to stop taking drug the evening before allergy skin tests; otherwise, accuracy of tests may be affected.
None significant.	• Contraindicated in acute asthmatic attack, narrow-angle glaucoma, urinary retention, prostatic hypertrophy, bladder neck obstruction. Use cautiously in increased intraocular pressure, hyperthyroidism, elderly patients, cardiovascular or renal disease, hypertension, or bronchial asthma. • Warn patient against alcoholic beverages and other CNS depressants during therapy, and against driving or other hazardous activities until response to drug is determined. • Coffee or tea may reduce drowsiness. • Titrate each patient's dose; response to drug varies. • If tolerance develops, another antihistamine may be substituted. • Warn patient to stop taking drug the evening before allergy skin tests; otherwise, accuracy of tests may be affected. • Only injectable forms *without* preservatives can be given I.V. Give *slowly.* • If symptoms occur after parenteral dose, stop drug. Notify doctor.

NAME	INDICATIONS & DOSAGE	SIDE EFFECTS
clemastine fumarate Tavist, Tavist-1	*Rhinitis, allergy symptoms—* **Adults:** 1.34 to 2.68 mg once daily. Maximum recommended daily dosage is 8.04 mg; or (timed-release) 1.34 mg (1 long-acting tablet) b.i.d., not to exceed 8.04 mg (6 long-acting tablets) per day. *Allergic skin manifestation of urticaria and angioedema—* **Adults:** 2.68 mg up to t.i.d. maximum.	*Blood:* hemolytic anemia, thrombocytopenia, agranulocytosis. *CNS:* sedation, drowsiness. *CV:* hypotension, palpitations, tachycardia. *GI:* epigastric distress, anorexia, nausea, vomiting, constipation, dry mouth. *GU:* urinary retention. *Skin:* rash, urticaria. *Other:* thickening of bronchial secretions.
cyproheptadine hydrochloride Periactin◆, Vimicon◆◆	*Allergy symptoms, pruritus—* **Adults:** 4 mg P.O. t.i.d. or q.i.d. Maximum 0.5 mg/Kg daily. **Children 7 to 14 years:** 4 mg P.O. b.i.d. or t.i.d. **Children 2 to 6 years:** 2 mg P.O. b.i.d. or t.i.d.	*CNS:* sedation, drowsiness, dizziness, headache, fatigue. *GI:* anorexia, nausea, vomiting, dry mouth. *Skin:* rash.
dexbrompheniramine maleate Disomer	*Rhinitis, allergy symptoms—* **Adults:** 2 to 4 mg P.O. t.i.d. or q.i.d. or (timed-release) 6 mg P.O. q 8 to 12 hours.	*Blood:* thrombocytopenia. *CNS:* sedation, dizziness, headache, drowsiness, irritability. *CV:* hypotension, palpitations, tachycardia, extrasystoles. *GI:* anorexia, nausea, vomiting, dry mouth. *Skin:* urticaria, rash.
dexchlorpheniramine maleate Polaramine◆	*Rhinitis, allergy symptoms, contact dermatitis, pruritus—* **Adults:** 2 to 4 mg P.O. t.i.d. or q.i.d.; or (timed-release) 4 to 6 mg b.i.d. or t.i.d. **Children 6 to 12 years:** 2 mg P.O. t.i.d. or q.i.d. **Children 2 to 6 years:** 1 to 2 mg P.O. t.i.d. or q.i.d. **Children under 2 years:** 0.5 mg P.O. t.i.d. or q.i.d. Do not use timed-release tablets for children.	*CNS:* drowsiness, dizziness. *GI:* nausea, dry mouth. *GU:* polyuria, dysuria.

INTERACTIONS	NURSING CONSIDERATIONS
None significant.	• Contraindicated in acute asthmatic attack, narrow-angle glaucoma, urinary retention, prostatic hypertrophy, bladder neck obstruction. Use cautiously in increased intraocular pressure, hyperthyroidism, elderly patients, cardiovascular or renal disease, hypertension, or bronchial asthma. • Warn patient against alcoholic beverages during therapy and against driving or other hazardous activities until response to drug is determined. • Coffee or tea may reduce drowsiness. Gum, sour hard candy, or ice chips may relieve dry mouth. • Titrate each patient's dose; response to drug varies. • If tolerance develops, another antihistamine may be substituted. • Warn patient to stop taking drug the evening before allergy skin tests; otherwise, accuracy of tests may be affected. • Tablets are available as 1.34 and 2.68 mg. Long-acting tablets are 1.34 mg.
None significant.	• Contraindicated in acute asthmatic attack, narrow-angle glaucoma, urinary retention, prostatic hypertrophy, bladder neck obstruction, and elderly patients. Use cautiously in increased intraocular pressure, hyperthyroidism, cardiovascular or renal disease, hypertension, or bronchial asthma. • Warn patient against alcoholic beverages during therapy and against driving or other hazardous activities until response to drug is determined. • Reduce GI distress by giving with food or milk. • Coffee or tea may reduce drowsiness. Gum, sour hard candy, or ice chips may relieve dry mouth. • Titrate each patient's dose; response to drug varies. • If tolerance develops, another antihistamine may be substituted. • Warn patient to stop taking drug the evening before allergy skin tests; otherwise, accuracy of tests may be affected. • Used experimentally to stimulate appetite and increase weight gain in children.
None significant.	• Contraindicated in acute asthmatic attack, narrow-angle glaucoma, urinary retention, prostatic hypertrophy, bladder neck obstruction. Use cautiously in increased intraocular pressure, hyperthyroidism, elderly patients, cardiovascular or renal disease, hypertension, or bronchial asthma. • Warn patient against alcoholic beverages during therapy and against driving or other hazardous activities until response to drug is determined. • Reduce GI distress by giving with food or milk. • Coffee or tea may reduce drowsiness. Gum, sour hard candy, or ice chips may relieve dry mouth. • Titrate each patient's dose; response to drug varies. • If tolerance develops, another antihistamine may be substituted. • Warn patient to stop taking drug the evening before allergy skin tests; otherwise, accuracy of tests may be affected.
None significant.	• Contraindicated in acute asthmatic attack, narrow-angle glaucoma, urinary retention, prostatic hypertrophy, bladder neck obstruction. Use cautiously in increased intraocular pressure, hyperthyroidism, elderly patients, cardiovascular or renal disease, hypertension, or bronchial asthma. • Warn patient against alcoholic beverages during therapy and against driving or other hazardous activities until response to drug is determined. • Coffee or tea may reduce drowsiness. • Titrate each patient's dose; response to drug varies. • If tolerance develops, another antihistamine may be substituted. • Warn patient to stop taking drug the evening before allergy skin tests; otherwise, accuracy of tests may be affected.

NAME	INDICATIONS & DOSAGE	SIDE EFFECTS
dimethindene maleate Triten	*Allergy symptoms—* **Adults, and children over 6 years:** 1 to 2 mg P.O. daily t.i.d.; or (timed-release) 2.5 mg P.O. daily b.i.d.	*CNS:* drowsiness, dizziness, insomnia, irritability, headache. *GI:* anorexia, nausea, vomiting, dry mouth, diarrhea. *GU:* urinary frequency.
dimethothiazine mesylate Promaquid♦♦	*Allergy symptoms, pruritus—* **Adults:** 20 mg P.O. b.i.d. or t.i.d. Maximum 120 mg daily. **Children 12 to 15 years:** 20 mg P.O. daily or b.i.d.	*CNS:* drowsiness, dizziness, fatigue, headache, restlessness, insomnia. *CV:* hypotension, palpitations, tachycardia, extrasystoles. *EENT:* blurred vision. *GI:* dry mouth. *Skin:* rash.
diphenhydramine hydrochloride Allerdryl, Baramine, Bax, Benachlor, Benadryl♦, Benahist, Ben-Allergin, Bendylate, Bentrac, Bonyl, Eldadryl, Fenylhist, Hyrexin, Nordryl, Notose, Phen-Amin 50, Phenamine, Rodryl, Rohydra, Span-Lanin, Valdrene, Wehdryl	*Rhinitis, allergy symptoms, motion sickness, antiparkinsonism—* **Adults:** 25 to 50 mg P.O. t.i.d. to q.i.d.; or 10 to 50 mg deep I.M. or I.V. Maximum 400 mg daily. **Children under 12 years:** 5 mg/Kg daily P.O., deep I.M., or I.V. divided q.i.d. Maximum 300 mg daily. *Sedation—* **Adults:** 25 to 50 mg P.O., deep I.M., p.r.n.	*CNS:* drowsiness, confusion, insomnia, headache, vertigo. *CV:* palpitations. *EENT:* photosensitivity, diplopia, nasal stuffiness. *GI:* nausea, vomiting, diarrhea, dry mouth, constipation. *GU:* dysuria. *Skin:* urticaria. *Other:* tightness of chest, wheezing.
diphenylpyraline hydrochloride Diafen, Hispril	*Rhinitis, allergy symptoms—* **Adults:** 2 mg P.O. q 4 hours, p.r.n.; or (timed-release) 5 mg P.O. q 12 hours. **Children over 6 years:** 2 mg P.O. q 6 hours, p.r.n.; or (timed-release) 5 mg P.O. daily. **Children 2 to 6 years:** 1 to 2 mg P.O. q 8 hours, p.r.n.	*CNS:* drowsiness, dizziness, headache. *EENT:* nasal congestion. *GI:* dry mouth and throat, epigastric distress. *Skin:* flushing.

INTERACTIONS	NURSING CONSIDERATIONS
None significant.	• Contraindicated in acute asthmatic attack, narrow-angle glaucoma, urinary retention, prostatic hypertrophy, bladder neck obstruction. Use cautiously in increased intraocular pressure, hyperthyroidism, elderly patients, cardiovascular or renal disease, hypertension, or bronchial asthma. • Warn patient against alcoholic beverages during therapy and against driving or other hazardous activities until response to drug is determined. • Reduce GI distress by giving with food or milk. • Coffee or tea may reduce drowsiness. Gum, sour hard candy, or ice chips may relieve dry mouth. • Titrate each patient's dose; response to drug varies. • If tolerance develops, another antihistamine may be substituted. • Warn patient to stop taking drug the evening before allergy skin tests; otherwise, accuracy of tests may be affected.
Other phenothiazines: increased effects. Use together cautiously.	• Contraindicated in narrow-angle glaucoma, peptic ulcer, intestinal obstruction, prostatic hypertrophy, bladder neck obstruction, epilepsy, bone marrow depression, coma, CNS depression, acutely ill or dehydrated children. Use cautiously in pulmonary, hepatic, or cardiovascular disease; asthma; hypertension; elderly or debilitated patients. • Warn patient against driving or other hazardous activities until response to drug is determined. • Coffee or tea may reduce drowsiness. • Titrate each patient's dose; response to drug varies. • If tolerance develops, another antihistamine may be substituted. • Warn patient to stop taking drug the evening before allergy skin tests; otherwise, accuracy of tests may be affected. • Blocks serotonin.
None significant.	• Contraindicated in acute asthmatic attack, narrow-angle glaucoma, prostatic hypertrophy, peptic ulcer, pyloroduodenal and bladder neck obstruction, and newborns. Use cautiously in pregnancy, lactation, and in asthmatic, hypertensive, or cardiac patients. • Alternate injection sites to prevent irritation. • Warn patient against alcoholic beverages during therapy and against driving or other hazardous activities until response to drug is determined. • Reduce GI distress by giving with food or milk. • Coffee or tea may reduce drowsiness. Gum, sour hard candy, or ice chips may relieve dry mouth. • Titrate each patient's dose; response to drug varies. • If tolerance develops, another antihistamine may be substituted. • Warn patient to stop taking drug the evening before allergy skin tests; otherwise, accuracy of tests may be affected. • Used with epinephrine in anaphylaxis. • One of most sedating antihistamines; often used as a nighttime sedative.
None significant.	• Contraindicated in acute asthmatic attack, narrow-angle glaucoma, urinary retention, prostatic hypertrophy, bladder neck obstruction. Use cautiously in increased intraocular pressure, hyperthyroidism, elderly patients, cardiovascular or renal disease, hypertension, diabetes mellitus, or bronchial asthma. • Warn patient against alcoholic beverages during therapy and against driving or other hazardous activities until response to drug is determined. • Reduce GI distress by giving with food or milk. • Coffee or tea may reduce drowsiness. Gum, sour hard candy, or ice chips may relieve dry mouth. • Titrate each patient's dose; response to drug varies. • If tolerance develops, another antihistamine may be substituted. • Warn patient to stop taking drug the evening before allergy skin tests; otherwise, accuracy of tests may be affected.

NAME	INDICATIONS & DOSAGE	SIDE EFFECTS
doxylamine succinate Decapryn	*Rhinitis, allergy symptoms—* **Adults:** 12.5 to 25 mg P.O. q 4 to 6 hours, p.r.n. **Children 6 to 12 years:** 6.25 to 12.5 mg P.O. q 4 to 6 hours, p.r.n.	*CNS:* drowsiness, dizziness, insomnia, disorientation, confusion, tremor, irritability, vertigo. *CV:* palpitations. *GI:* dry mouth and throat.
methdilazine hydrochloride Dilosyn♦♦, Tacaryl	*Pruritus—* **Adults:** 8 mg P.O. b.i.d. to q.i.d. or (chewable tablets) 7.2 mg P.O. b.i.d. to q.i.d. **Children over 3 years:** 4 mg P.O. b.i.d. to q.i.d. or (chewable tablets) 3.6 mg P.O. b.i.d. to q.i.d.	*CNS:* drowsiness, dizziness, headache. *GI:* nausea, dry mouth and throat, cholestatic jaundice. *Skin:* rash.
promethazine hydrochloride Fellozine, Ganphen, Histantil♦♦, K-Phen, Methazine, Pentazine♦, Phencen-50, Phenergan♦, Promethamead, Promethazine, Prorex, Provigan, Quadnite, Remsed, Rolamethazine, Sigazine, ZiPan	*Motion sickness—* **Adults:** 25 mg P.O. b.i.d. **Children:** 12.5 to 25 mg P.O., I.M., or rectally b.i.d. *Nausea—* **Adults:** 12.5 to 25 mg P.O., I.M., or rectally q 4 to 6 hours, p.r.n. **Children:** 0.25 to 0.5 mg/Kg I.M. or rectally q 4 to 6 hours, p.r.n. *Rhinitis, allergy symptoms—* **Adults:** 12.5 mg P.O. q.i.d.; or 25 mg P.O. at bedtime. **Children:** 6.25 to 12.5 mg P.O. t.i.d. or 25 mg P.O. at bedtime. *Sedation—* **Adults:** 25 to 50 mg P.O., I.M. at bedtime or p.r.n. **Children:** 12.5 to 25 mg P.O., I.M., or rectally at bedtime.	*CNS:* sedation, confusion, restlessness, tremors. *CV:* hypotension. *EENT:* transient myopia, nasal congestion. *GI:* anorexia, nausea, vomiting, diarrhea, constipation, dry mouth.

INTERACTIONS	NURSING CONSIDERATIONS
None significant.	• Contraindicated in acute asthmatic attack, narrow-angle glaucoma, urinary retention, prostatic hypertrophy, bladder neck obstruction. Use cautiously in increased intraocular pressure, hyperthyroidism, elderly patients, cardiovascular or renal disease, hypertension, or bronchial asthma. • Warn patient against alcoholic beverages during therapy and against driving or other hazardous activities until response to drug is determined. • Reduce GI distress by giving with food or milk. • Coffee or tea may reduce drowsiness. Gum, sour hard candy, or ice chips may relieve dry mouth. • Titrate each patient's dose; response to drug varies. • If tolerance develops, another antihistamine may be substituted. • Warn patient to stop taking drug the evening before allergy skin tests; otherwise, accuracy of tests may be affected.
Phenothiazines: increased effects. Don't use together.	• Contraindicated in acute asthmatic attack, narrow-angle glaucoma, peptic ulcer, prostatic hypertrophy, bladder neck obstruction, CNS depression, acutely ill or dehydrated children. Use cautiously in pulmonary, hepatic, or cardiovascular disease, asthma, hypertension, elderly or debilitated patients. • Warn patient against alcoholic beverages during therapy and against driving or other hazardous activities until response to drug is determined. • Reduce GI distress by giving with food or milk. • Coffee or tea may reduce drowsiness. Gum, sour hard candy, or ice chips may relieve dry mouth. • Titrate each patient's dose; response to drug varies. • If tolerance develops, another antihistamine may be substituted. • Available as chewable tablet for children. Instruct child to chew completely and swallow promptly; may cause local anesthetic effect in mouth. • Warn patient to stop taking drug the evening before allergy skin tests; otherwise, accuracy of tests may be affected.
Other phenothiazines: increased effects. Don't give together.	• Contraindicated in narrow-angle glaucoma, peptic ulcer, intestinal obstruction, prostatic hypertrophy, bladder neck obstruction, epilepsy, bone marrow depression, coma, CNS depression, pregnancy (except during labor), lactation, newborns, acutely ill or dehydrated children. Use cautiously in pulmonary, hepatic, or cardiovascular disease, asthma, hypertension, elderly or debilitated patients. • Warn patient against alcoholic beverages during therapy and against driving or other hazardous activities until response to drug is determined. • Reduce GI distress by giving with food or milk. • Coffee or tea may reduce drowsiness. Gum, sour hard candy, or ice chips may relieve dry mouth. • Titrate each patient's dose; response to drug varies. • If tolerance develops, another antihistamine may be substituted. • Warn patient to stop taking drug the evening before allergy skin tests; otherwise, accuracy of tests may be affected. • Pronounced sedative effect limits use in many ambulatory patients. • May cause false positive immunological urinary pregnancy test (Gravindex). Also may interfere with blood grouping in ABO system.

NAME	INDICATIONS & DOSAGE	SIDE EFFECTS
trimeprazine tartrate Panectyl◆◆, Temaril	*Pruritus—* **Adults:** 2.5 mg P.O. q.i.d.; or (timed-release) 5 mg P.O. b.i.d. **Children 3 to 12 years:** 2.5 mg P.O. t.i.d., p.r.n. **Children 6 months to 3 years:** 1.25 mg P.O. t.i.d., p.r.n.	*Blood:* agranulocytosis, leukopenia. *CNS:* drowsiness, dizziness, confusion, restlessness, tremors, irritability, insomnia. *CV:* hypotension, headache, palpitations, tachycardia. *GI:* anorexia, nausea, vomiting, dry mouth and throat. *GU:* urinary frequency or retention. *Skin:* urticaria, rash. *Other:* cholestatic jaundice, thickening of bronchial secretions.
tripelennamine hydrochloride PBZ-SR, Pyribenzamine◆, Ro-Hist	*Rhinitis, allergy symptoms—* **Adults:** 25 to 50 mg P.O. q 4 to 6 hours; or (timed-release) 100 mg b.i.d. to t.i.d. Maximum 600 mg daily. **Children over 5 years:** 50 mg P.O. q 8 to 12 hours (timed-release). **Children under 5 years:** 5 mg/Kg daily P.O. in 4 to 6 divided doses. Maximum 300 mg daily.	*CNS:* drowsiness, dizziness, confusion, restlessness, tremors, irritability, insomnia. *CV:* palpitations. *GI:* anorexia, diarrhea or constipation, nausea, vomiting, dry mouth. *GU:* urinary frequency or retention. *Skin:* urticaria, rash. *Other:* thickening of bronchial secretions.
triprolidine hydrochloride Actidil◆	*Colds and allergy symptoms—* **Adults:** 2.5 mg P.O. b.i.d. or t.i.d. **Children over 2 years:** 1.25 mg b.i.d. or t.i.d. **Children under 2 years:** 0.6 mg b.i.d. or t.i.d.	*CNS:* drowsiness, dizziness, confusion, restlessness, insomnia. *GI:* anorexia, diarrhea or constipation, nausea, vomiting, dry mouth. *GU:* urinary frequency or retention. *Skin:* urticaria, rash.

INTERACTIONS	NURSING CONSIDERATIONS
Other phenothiazines: increased effects. Don't use together.	• Contraindicated in acute asthmatic attack, narrow-angle glaucoma, peptic ulcer, intestinal obstruction, prostatic hypertrophy, bladder neck obstruction, epilepsy, bone marrow depression, coma, CNS depression, pregnancy (except during labor), lactation, acutely ill or dehydrated children. Use cautiously in pulmonary, hepatic, or cardiovascular disease, asthma, hypertension, elderly or debilitated patients. • Warn patient against alcoholic beverages during therapy and against driving or other hazardous activities until response to drug is determined. • Reduce GI distress by giving with food or milk. • Coffee or tea may reduce drowsiness. Gum, sour hard candy, or ice chips may relieve dry mouth. • Titrate each patient's dose; response to drug varies. • If tolerance develops, another antihistamine may be substituted. • Warn patient to stop taking drug the evening before allergy skin tests; otherwise, accuracy of tests may be affected.
None significant.	• Contraindicated in acute asthmatic attack, narrow-angle glaucoma, urinary retention, prostatic hypertrophy, bladder neck obstruction. Use cautiously in increased intraocular pressure, hyperthyroidism, elderly patients, cardiovascular or renal disease, hypertension, or bronchial asthma. • Warn patient against alcoholic beverages during therapy and against driving or other hazardous activities until response to drug is determined. • Reduce GI distress by giving with food or milk. • Coffee or tea may reduce drowsiness. Gum, sour hard candy, or ice chips may relieve dry mouth. • Titrate each patient's dose; response to drug varies. • If tolerance develops, another antihistamine may be substituted. • Warn patient to stop taking drug the evening before allergy skin tests; otherwise, accuracy of tests may be affected. • Used with epinephrine in anaphylaxis.
None significant.	• Contraindicated in acute asthma, narrow-angle glaucoma, urinary retention, prostatic hypertrophy, bladder neck obstruction. Use cautiously in increased intraocular pressure, hyperthyroidism, elderly patients, cardiovascular or renal disease, hypertension, diabetes mellitus, or bronchial asthma. • Warn patient against alcoholic beverages during therapy and against driving or other hazardous activities until response to drug is determined. • Reduce GI distress by giving with food or milk. • Coffee or tea may reduce drowsiness. Gum, sour hard candy, or ice chips may relieve dry mouth. • Titrate each patient's dose; response to drug varies. • Warn patient to stop taking drug the evening before allergy skin tests; otherwise, accuracy of tests may be affected.

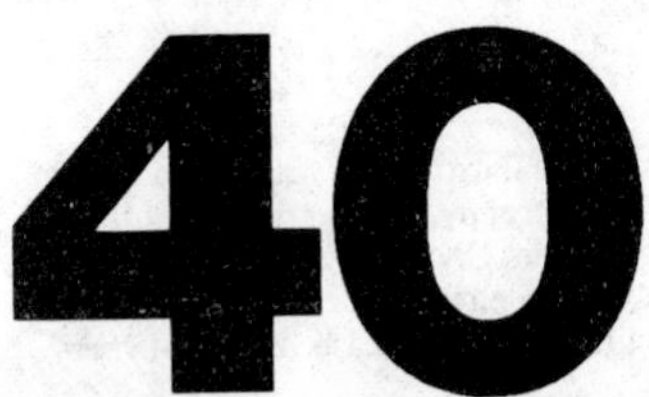

Expectorants and antitussives

acetylcysteine
ammonium chloride
benzonatate
calcium iodide
chlophedianol hydrochloride
codeine
codeine phosphate
codeine sulfate
dextromethorphan hydrobromide
diphenhydramine hydrochloride
guaifenesin
hydriodic acid
hydrocodone bitartrate
hydromorphone hydrochloride
iodinated glycerol
levopropoxyphene napsylate
noscapine hydrochloride
potassium iodide
terpin hydrate
tyloxapol

Expectorants loosen secretions in chronic pulmonary disorders and other similar conditions. Antitussives inhibit or suppress the cough reflex but are usually used only when a cough is nonproductive. In patients with chronic pulmonary disorders, cough preparations should be used only as part of a total rehabilitation plan. Expectorants, antitussives, and other cough preparations are available in many combinations.

Major uses

- Facilitate expectoration in pneumonia, bronchitis, tuberculosis, cystic fibrosis, emphysema, atelectasis, bronchial asthma.
- Suppress nonproductive coughs.

Mechanism of action

- Expectorants increase respiratory tract fluids to help liquify and reduce the viscosity of thick, tenacious sputum.
- Tyloxapol also lowers surface tension of sputum to facilitate expectoration.
- Antitussives inhibit or suppress the cough reflex by a direct effect on the cough center in the brain (codeine, hydrocodone bitartrate), by a local anesthetic effect (benzonatate), or by peripheral action on sensory nerve endings.

Absorption, distribution, and excretion

- All are well absorbed after oral administration.
- Benzonatate and tyloxapol are well absorbed after inhalation.
- Metabolized in liver.
- Excreted in urine. The iodides (calcium iodide, potassium iodide) are also excreted through the respiratory tract.

Onset and duration
- Begin to act within 30 minutes.
- Effect lasts from 4 to 6 hours, except benzonatate, which may act up to 8 hours.

Combination products
Preparations are available in the following combinations:
- antitussives with decongestants, antihistamines, or both.
- antitussives and expectorants.
- antitussives and expectorants with decongestants, antihistamines, or both.
- expectorants with decongestants, antihistamines, or both.

HOW TO FOSTER PRODUCTIVE COUGHING

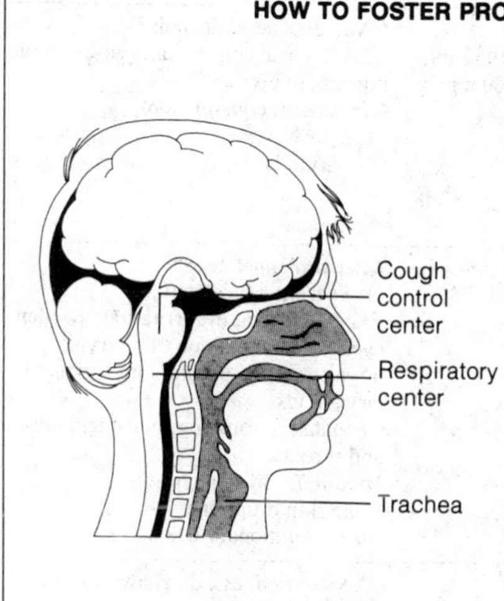

Coughing is an essential body defense mechanism which frees the respiratory tract of foreign matter. A productive cough raises sputum. Recognize a shallow nonproductive cough by its dry, hacking sound.

To encourage productive coughing:
— Instruct the patient in deep-breathing exercises.
— Perform postural drainage.
— Limit or ban the patient's smoking.
— Make sure the patient's fluid intake is adequate.

To monitor and control the patient's cough:
— Record the type of cough; its frequency; amount, color, and consistency of sputum; and odor.
— Instruct the patient to cough in several layers of tissues to be disposed of in a paper bag.
— Ask the patient to report any side effects of prescribed expectorants or antitussives.

NAME	INDICATIONS & DOSAGE	SIDE EFFECTS
acetylcysteine Airbron♦♦, Mucomyst♦, NAC♦♦	*Pneumonia, bronchitis, tuberculosis, cystic fibrosis, emphysema, atelectasis (adjunct), complications of thoracic surgery and CV surgery*— **Adults and children:** 1 to 2 ml 10% to 20% solution by direct instillation into trachea as often as every hour; or 3 to 5 ml 20% solution, or 6 to 10 ml 10% solution, by mouthpiece t.i.d. or q.i.d.	*EENT:* rhinorrhea, hemoptysis. *GI:* stomatitis, nausea. *Other:* bronchospasm (especially in asthmatics).
ammonium chloride	*As expectorant*— **Adults:** 250 to 500 mg P.O. q 2 to 4 hours.	*CNS:* headache, drowsiness, confusion, excitation alternating with coma, twitching, hyperreflexia, EEG abnormalities. *CV:* bradycardia. *GI:* anorexia, nausea, vomiting. *GU:* renal impairment, glycosuria. *Metabolic:* decreased potassium, hypocalcemic tetany, hyperglycemia. *Skin:* rash. *Other:* thirst.
benzonatate Tessalon♦	*Nonproductive cough*— **Adults, and children over 10 years:** 100 mg P.O. t.i.d.; up to 600 mg daily.	*CNS:* dizziness, drowsiness. *EENT:* nasal congestion, sensation of burning in eyes. *GI:* nausea, constipation. *Skin:* rash. *Other:* chills.
calcium iodide	*Asthma, bronchitis, emphysema (adjunct)*— **Adults:** 300 to 600 mg P.O. q 2 to 4 hours.	**After prolonged use:** *CNS:* frontal headache. *EENT:* coryza; eye irritation; swollen eyelids; inflammation of pharynx, larynx, tonsils, parotid and submaxillary glands. *GI:* nausea, vomiting, burning mouth and throat. *Metabolic:* hyperthyroidism. *Skin:* skin eruptions. *Other:* pulmonary edema.
chlophedianol hydrochloride Ulo, Ulone♦♦	*Nonproductive cough*— **Adults, and children over 12 years:** 25 mg P.O. t.i.d. or q.i.d. **Children 2 to 6 years:** 12.5 mg P.O. t.i.d. or q.i.d.	*CNS:* drowsiness, dizziness, excitation, irritability, nightmares, hallucinations. *GI:* nausea, vomiting.

♦ Also available in Canada.
♦♦ Available in Canada only.
Unmarked trade names available in United States only.

INTERACTIONS	NURSING CONSIDERATIONS
None significant.	• Use cautiously in asthma or severe respiratory insufficiency, in elderly or debilitated patients. • A mucolytic. • Use plastic, glass, stainless steel, or another nonreactive metal when administering by nebulization. Handbulb nebulizers not recommended because output too small and particle size too large. • After opening, store in refrigerator; use within 96 hours. • Incompatible with oxytetracycline, tetracycline, and erythromycin lactobionate. • Monitor cough type and frequency. • Discourage smoking. Offer hard candy. • Large doses are used P.O. to treat acetaminophen overdose. For dose in acetaminophen toxicity, see p. 1114.
Spironolactone: systemic acidosis. Use cautiously.	• Contraindicated in hepatic or renal impairment. Use cautiously in pulmonary insufficiency, congestive heart failure. • Give with full glass of water. • Monitor cough type and frequency. • Discourage smoking. Offer hard candy. • Encourage deep-breathing exercises. • Watch for potentiated diuresis when used with diuretics.
None significant.	• Patient should not chew tablets or leave in mouth to dissolve; local anesthesia will result. • A cough suppressant; don't use when cough is valuable as diagnostic sign or is beneficial (as after thoracic surgery). • Use with percussion and chest vibration. • Maintain fluid intake to help liquify sputum. • Discourage smoking. Offer hard candy. • Monitor cough type and frequency.
None significant.	• Contraindicated in hyperthyroidism, iodine hypersensitivity, acute inflammatory conditions of respiratory or GI mucosa. Not for long-term use. • Liquifies thick tenacious sputum; maintain fluid intake. • Monitor cough type and frequency. • Discourage smoking. Offer hard candy. • Encourage deep-breathing exercises.
None significant.	• An antitussive; don't use when cough is valuable as diagnostic sign or is beneficial (as after thoracic surgery). • Use with percussion and chest vibration. • CNS side effects disappear when drug is stopped. • Monitor cough type and frequency. • Discourage smoking. Offer hard candy.

NAME	INDICATIONS & DOSAGE	SIDE EFFECTS
codeine, codeine phosphate, codeine sulfate Controlled substance Schedule II Paveral	*Nonproductive cough—* **Adults:** 8 to 20 mg P.O. t.i.d. or q.i.d. **Children:** 1 to 1.5 mg/Kg P.O. daily in 6 divided doses.	*CNS:* dizziness, sedation. *CV:* palpitations. *GI:* nausea, vomiting; in repeated doses, constipation. *Skin:* pruritus. *Other:* tolerance and physical dependence.
dextromethorphan hydrobromide Balminil DM♦♦, Broncho-Grippol-DM♦♦, Contratuss♦♦, Pertussin 8-hour, Romilar Chewable Tablets for Children, St. Joseph's Cough Syrup for Children, Sedatuss♦♦. Silence Is Golden. More commonly available in combination products such as Benylin-DM, Coryban-D, Dimacol, Naldetuss, Novahistine DMX, Ornacol, Phenergan Expectorant with Dextromethorphan, Robitussin DM, Romilar CF, Rondec-DM, Triaminicol, Trind-DM, Tussi-Organidin-DM, 2G-DM	*Nonproductive cough—* **Adults:** 10 to 20 mg q 4 hours, or 30 mg q 6 to 8 hours. **Children 6 to 12 years**: 5 to 10 mg q 4 hours, or 15 mg q 6 to 8 hours. **Children 2 to 6 years**: 2.5 mg q 4 hours, or 7.5 mg q 6 to 8 hours.	*CNS:* drowsiness. *GI:* nausea.
diphenhydramine hydrochloride Allerdryl, Baramine, Bax, Benachlor, Benadryl♦, Benahist, Ben-Allergin, Bendylate, Bentrac, Benylin Cough Syrup♦♦, Eldadryl, Fenylhist, Hyrexin, Nordryl, Notose, Phen-Amin 50, Phenamine, Rodryl, Rohydra, Valdrene, Wehdryl	*Nonproductive cough—* **Adults:** 25 to 50 mg P.O. q 4 hours (not to exceed 300 mg/day). **Children 6 to 12 years**: 25 mg P.O. q 4 hours (not to exceed 150 mg/day). **Children 2 to 6 years:** 12.5 to 25 mg P.O. q 4 hours (not to exceed 100 mg/day). For rhinitis, allergy, and motion sickness, see p. 458.	*CNS:* sedation, confusion. restlessness, insomnia, headache. *CV:* palpitations. *EENT:* diplopia, blurred vision, nasal congestion. *GI:* dry mouth and throat, nausea, vomiting, diarrhea, constipation. *GU:* dysuria. *Skin:* urticaria. *Other:* photosensitivity, tightness of chest, wheezing.

INTERACTIONS	NURSING CONSIDERATIONS
None significant.	• Contraindicated in increased intracranial or CSF pressure. Use cautiously in asthma, emphysema, head injury, after thoracotomies or laporotomies, in debilitated patients, in dehydrated postop patients; history of drug abuse, hepatic or renal disease, hypothyroidism, Addison's disease, acute alcoholism, seizures, severe CNS depression, COPD, psychosis, and when other CNS depressants are given. Monitor patient carefully. • Use with percussion and chest vibration. • Warn patient against driving or other hazardous activities until response to drug is determined. • An antitussive; don't use when cough is a valuable diagnostic sign or is beneficial (as after thoracic surgery). • Monitor cough type and frequency. • Discourage smoking. Offer hard candy.
MAO inhibitors: hypotension, coma, hyperpyrexia, and death have occurred. Do not use together.	• Contraindicated in patients currently taking or within 2 weeks of stopping MAO inhibitors. Use cautiously in productive cough. • Produces no analgesia or addiction and little or no CNS depression. • An antitussive; don't use when cough is valuable as diagnostic sign or is beneficial (as after thoracic surgery). • Instruct patient not to take fluids immediately after taking drug. • Use with percussion and chest vibration. • Do not mix dextromethorphan syrups together with penicillins, tetracyclines, salicylates, phenobarbital, hydriodic acid, or high concentrations of sodium or potassium iodide. • Monitor cough type and frequency. • Discourage smoking. Offer hard candy. • Available in most over-the-counter cough medicines.
None significant.	• Contraindicated in acute asthma, narrow-angle glaucoma, prostatic hypertrophy, peptic ulcer, pyloroduodenal and bladder neck obstruction. Use cautiously in pregnancy, lactation, and in asthmatic, hypertensive, or cardiac patients. • Warn patient against alcoholic beverages during therapy and against driving or other hazardous activities until response to drug is determined. • Liquid preparations are recommended for antitussive affect. • Instruct patient not to take fluids immediately after taking drug. • Coffee and tea may reduce drowsiness. Gum, sour hard candy, or ice chips may relieve dry mouth. • If tolerance develops, another antihistamine may be substituted. • Warn patient to stop taking drug the evening before allergy skin tests; otherwise, accuracy of tests may be affected.

NAME	INDICATIONS & DOSAGE	SIDE EFFECTS
guaifenesin (formerly glyceryl guaiacolate) Anti-Tuss, Balminil◆◆, Bowtussin, Cosin-GG, Demo-Cineol◆◆, Dilyn, 2/G, G-100, G-200, GG-CEN, Glycotuss, Gly-O-Tussin, Glytuss, G-Tussin, Guaiatussin, Hytuss, Malotuss, Motussin◆◆, Nortussin, Proco, Recsei-Tuss, Resyl◆◆, Robitussin◆, Sedatuss◆◆, Tursen, Tussanca◆◆, Wal-Tussin DM	*Productive and nonproductive cough—* **Adults:** 100 to 200 mg P.O. q 2 to 4 hours. **Children:** 12 mg/Kg P.O. daily in 6 divided doses.	*GI:* vomiting and nausea occur with large doses.
hydriodic acid	*Chronic bronchitis, bronchial asthma—* **Adults:** 0.6 to 1.3 ml P.O. t.i.d. well diluted, or 5 to 10 ml syrup diluted in water P.O. t.i.d. or q.i.d.	*EENT:* tooth damage.
hydrocodone bitartrate Controlled substance Schedule II Coditrate, Codone, Corutol DH◆◆, Dicodethal, Dicodid, Hycodan◆, Robidone◆◆	*Nonproductive cough—* **Adults:** 5 to 10 mg P.O. q 4 to 6 hours, p.r.n. Maximum single dose 15 mg. **Children over 12 years:** 5 mg P.O. q 4 to 6 hours, p.r.n. Maximum single dose 10 mg. **Children 2 to 12 years:** 2.5 mg P.O. q 4 to 6 hours, p.r.n. Maximum single dose 5 mg. **Children under 2 years:** 1.25 mg P.O. q 4 to 6 hours, p.r.n. Maximum single dose 1.25 mg.	*CNS:* drowsiness, dizziness. *GI:* nausea, constipation. *Other:* tolerance and physical dependence after long-term use.
hydromorphone hydrochloride Controlled substance Schedule II Dilaudid cough syrup◆	*Cough—* **Adults:** 1 mg P.O. q 3 to 4 hours, p.r.n. **Children 6 to 12 years:** 0.5 mg P.O. q 3 to 4 hours, p.r.n.	*CNS:* dizziness, somnolence, respiratory depression. *CV:* hypotension. *GI:* nausea, vomiting, anorexia, constipation.

INTERACTIONS	NURSING CONSIDERATIONS
None significant.	• May interfere with certain laboratory tests for 5-hydroxyindoleacetic acid and vanillylmandelic acid. • Watch for bleeding gums, hematuria, and bruising if given to patients on heparin. Should such symptoms appear, guaifenesin should be discontinued. • Liquifies thick, tenacious sputum; maintain fluid intake. Advise patient to take with a glass of water whenever possible. • Monitor cough type and frequency. • Discourage smoking. Offer hard candy. • An expectorant. • Encourage deep-breathing exercises.
None significant.	• Dilute well. Use straw to avoid injuring teeth; syrup is very acidic. • Liquifies thick, tenacious sputum; maintain fluid intake. Advise patient to take with a glass of water whenever possible. • Don't use if syrup is deep brown color. • Monitor cough type and frequency. • Discourage smoking. Offer hard candy. • Encourage deep-breathing exercises. • An expectorant.
None significant.	• Contraindicated in glaucoma. Use cautiously in asthma, emphysema, drug dependence, after thoracotomy or laporotomy, in debilitated or dehydrated patients. • Warn patient against driving or other hazardous activities until response to drug is determined. • Evaluate patient's need for drug, which is addictive. • An antitussive; don't use when cough is valuable as diagnostic sign or is beneficial (as after thoracic surgery). • Use with percussion and chest vibration. • Monitor cough type and frequency. • Discourage smoking. Offer hard candy. • CNS depressants cause potentiation. Use together cautiously.
None significant.	• Contraindicated in increased intracranial pressure, status asthmaticus. Use cautiously in hepatic or renal disease, hypothyroidism, Addison's disease, acute alcoholism, seizures, head injury, severe CNS depression, brain tumor, bronchial asthma, chronic obstructive pulmonary disease, or psychosis. • Warn patient against driving and other hazardous activities until response to drug is determined. • Monitor respiration, pupil size, bowel function. • An antitussive; don't use when cough is a valuable diagnostic sign or is beneficial (as after thoracic surgery). • Use with percussion or chest vibration. • Monitor cough type and frequency. • Discourage smoking. Offer hard candy. • Addictive. • CNS depressants cause potentiation. Use together cautiously.

NAME	INDICATIONS & DOSAGE	SIDE EFFECTS
iodinated glycerol Organidin◆	*Bronchial asthma, bronchitis, emphysema (adjunct)*— **Adults:** 60 mg P.O. q.i.d.(tablets) or 20 drops (solution) P.O. q.i.d. with fluids or 1 teaspoonful (elixir) P.O. q.i.d. **Children:** up to ½ adult dose based on child's weight.	**After long-term use:** *CNS:* frontal headache. *EENT:* coryza; eye irritation; swollen eyelids; inflammation of pharynx, larynx, tonsils, parotid and submaxillary glands. *GI:* burning mouth and throat, metallic taste, nausea, vomiting. *Skin:* eruptions, sometimes severe. *Other:* pulmonary edema.
levopropoxyphene napsylate Novrad	*Nonproductive cough*— **Adults:** 50 to 100 mg q 4 hours. **Children 23 to 45 Kg:** 50 mg q 4 hours. **Children up to 23 Kg:** 25 mg q 4 hours.	*CNS:* drowsiness, jitteriness, dizziness, headache. *EENT:* visual disturbances. *GI:* dry mouth, nausea, vomiting, diarrhea, epigastric burning. *GU:* urinary frequency or urgency. *Skin:* rash, urticaria.
noscapine hydrochloride Noscatuss◆◆, Tusscapine	*Nonproductive cough*— **Adults:** 15 to 30 mg P.O. t.i.d. or q.i.d. as chewable tablet. **Children 6 to 12 years:** 7.5 to 15 mg P.O. t.i.d. or q.i.d. as syrup. **Children 2 to 6 years:** 5 to 10 mg P.O. t.i.d. or q.i.d. as syrup.	*CNS:* slight drowsiness. *EENT:* acute vasomotor rhinitis, conjunctivitis. *GI:* nausea.
potassium iodide KI-N, Kisol, Pima, SSKI	*Chronic bronchitis, bronchial asthma*— **Adults:** 300 to 600 mg P.O. q 2 hours until desired response obtained. **Children:** 0.25 to 1 ml of saturated solution (1 g/ml) b.i.d., t.i.d., or q.i.d.	*GI:* nonspecific small bowel lesions, nausea, vomiting, epigastric pain. *Metabolic:* goiter, hyperthyroid adenoma, hypothyroidism (with excessive use), collagen disease-like syndrome. *Prolonged use:* chronic iodine poisoning, soreness of mouth, coryza, sneezing, swelling of eyelids.
terpin hydrate Creoterp, Terp	*Excessive bronchial secretions*— **Adults:** 5 to 10 ml P.O. of elixir.	None.
tyloxapol Alevaire, Mucilose-Super	*Bronchitis, emphysema, pulmonary abscess, bronchiectasis, atelectasis*—(by inhalation only) **Adults:** up to 500 ml 0.125% solution q 12 to 24 hours by continuous aerosol inhalation, adjusting rate of flow, p.r.n.; or 10 to 20 ml 0.125% solution by intermittent inhalation for 30 to 90 minutes t.i.d. or q.i.d.	*GI:* nausea. *Local:* irritation.

INTERACTIONS	NURSING CONSIDERATIONS
None significant.	• Contraindicated in hypothyroidism, iodine sensitivity. • Skin rash or other hypersensitivity may require stopping drug. • May liquify thick, tenacious sputum; maintain fluid intake. • Monitor cough type and frequency. • Discourage smoking. Offer hard candy. • Encourage deep-breathing exercises. • Many patients complain of metallic taste. • An expectorant.
None significant.	• Contraindicated in first trimester of pregnancy. • An antitussive; don't use when cough is valuable as diagnostic sign or is beneficial (as after thoracic surgery). • Tell patient not to take fluids just after liquid preparation. • Use with percussion or chest vibration. • Monitor cough type and frequency. • Discourage smoking. Offer hard candy.
None significant.	• An antitussive; don't use when cough is valuable diagnostic sign or is beneficial (as after thoracic surgery). • Tell patient not to take fluids just after liquid preparation. • Use with percussion and chest vibration. • Monitor cough type and frequency. • Discourage smoking. Offer hard candy.
Lithium carbonate: may cause hypothyroidism. Don't use together.	• Contraindicated in iodine hypersensitivity, tuberculosis, hyperkalemia, acute bronchitis, hyperthyroidism. Use cautiously in pregnancy. • Maintain fluid intake to help liquify sputum. • Has strong, salty, metallic taste. Dilute with milk or fruit juice to reduce GI distress. • If given over long period, sudden withdrawal may precipitate thyroid storm. • Monitor cough type and frequency. • Discourage smoking. Offer hard candy. • Encourage deep-breathing exercises. • If skin rash appears, discontinue use. Contact doctor. • An expectorant.
None significant.	• Contraindicated on empty stomach, in peptic ulcer, or severe diabetes mellitus. Use cautiously in history of alcohol or drug abuse. • Don't give in large doses; high alcoholic content of elixir (42.5% or 84 proof). • Monitor cough type and frequency. • Discourage smoking. Offer hard candy. • Elixir contains 43% alcohol. Monitor for abuse.
None significant.	• A surfactant with detergent properties. • Lowers surface tension and reduces viscosity of thick, tenacious sputum to facilitate expectoration; maintain fluid intake. • Monitor cough type and frequency. • Discourage smoking. Offer hard candy. • Encourage deep-breathing exercises. • Incompatible with chlortetracycline. • If used as a vehicle, add phenylephrine or isoproterenol just before use.

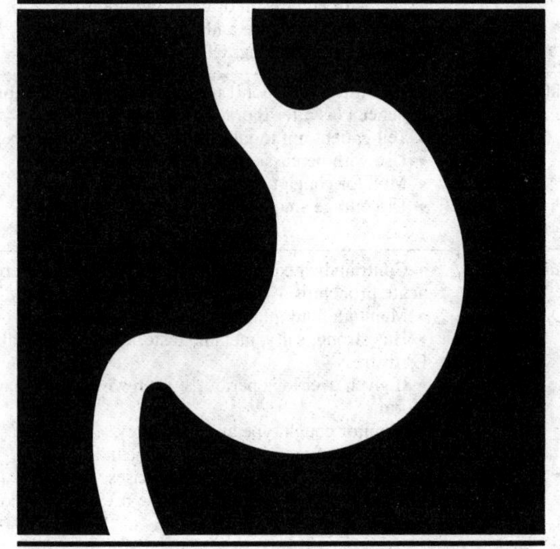

Gastrointestinal Tract

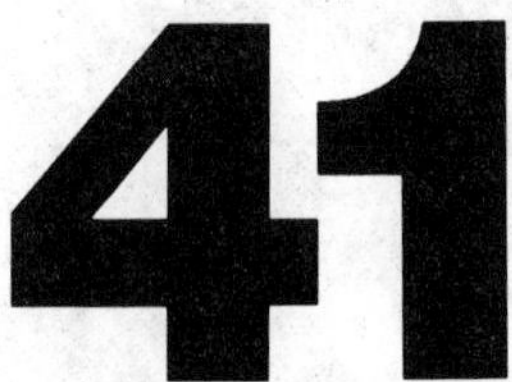

Antacids, adsorbents, and antiflatulents

activated charcoal
aluminum carbonate
aluminum hydroxide
aluminum phosphate
calcium carbonate
dihydroxyaluminum aminoacetate
dihydroxyaluminum sodium carbonate
magaldrate
magnesia magma
magnesium carbonate
magnesium oxide
magnesium trisilicate
oxethazaine
simethicone
sodium bicarbonate

Antacids are the mainstay of peptic ulcer therapy although it is not certain they actually promote ulcer healing. Adsorbents (specifically, activated charcoal) effectively inhibit gastrointestinal adsorption of a variety of drugs, chemicals, and toxins. However, activated charcoal doesn't adsorb cyanide, ethanol, methanol, iron, salt, corrosive alkalis, mineral acids, or organic solvents. Antiflatulents combine the defoaming action of simethicone with antacids to relieve hyperacidity and gas.

Major uses

- Antacids neutralize gastric acidity and help control peptic ulcer pain.
- Adsorbents serve as general purpose antidotes in certain acute oral poisonings.
- Antiflatulents relieve painful symptoms of excess gas in digestive tract.

Mechanism of action

- Antacids generally work by reducing total acid load in gastrointestinal tract and elevating intragastric pH to reduce activity of pepsin. They also strengthen the gastric mucosal barrier and increase tone of lower esophageal sphincter. They do not appear to have a coating effect on ulcers. Oxethazaine is a potent local anesthetic which may adhere to receptor sites, producing a prolonged topical anesthetic effect on the gastric mucosa.
- Adsorbents adhere to many drugs and chemicals, thereby inhibiting their absorption from the gastrointestinal tract.
- Antiflatulents use the defoaming action of simethicone to disperse or prevent the formation of mucous-surrounded gas pockets in the gastrointestinal tract. It acts in the stomach and intestine to form a film that causes gas bubbles to collapse.

Absorption, distribution, and excretion

- Antacids: Absorption varies, but antacids tend to be distributed throughout gastrointestinal tract. Prolonged use of antacids containing magnesium, calcium, or sodium may cause

systemic absorption of these ingredients in toxic quantities. Excessive aluminum antacid therapy can lead to hypophosphatemia. Antacids are mainly excreted in the feces.
• Adsorbents: Activated charcoal is neither absorbed in the gastrointestinal tract nor metabolized. It is excreted unchanged in the feces.
• Antiflatulents: Simethicone is physiologically inactive. It is not absorbed in the gastrointestinal tract and does not interfere with gastric secretion or nutrient absorption. It's excreted unchanged in the feces.

Onset and duration
• Antacids: Onset of action varies from drug to drug. Duration of action usually only 1 hour if taken on empty stomach; duration up to 3 hours if taken after meals.
• Adsorbents: Onset of action immediate. Duration varies, depending on amount of poison swallowed, dosage size of activated charcoal, and individual digestive process.
• Antiflatulents: Onset of action immediate. Duration varies.

Combination products
A-M-T: aluminum hydroxide 162 mg and magnesium trisilicate 250 mg.
CAMALOX◆: aluminum hydroxide 225 mg, magnesium hydroxide 200 mg, and calcium carbonate 250 mg.
DI-GEL and FLACID: aluminum hydroxide and magnesium carbonate 282 mg, magnesium hydroxide 85 mg, and simethicone 25 mg.
GAVISCON◆: aluminum hydroxide 80 mg, magnesium trisilicate 20 mg, sodium bicarbonate 70 mg, and alginic acid 200 mg.
GELUSIL◆: aluminum hydroxide 200 mg, magnesium hydroxide 200 mg, and simethicone 25 mg.
GELUSIL-II: aluminum hydroxide 400 mg, magnesium hydroxide 400 mg, and simethicone 30 mg.
GELUSIL-M: aluminum hydroxide 300 mg, magnesium hydroxide 200 mg, and simethicone 25 mg.
KOLANTYL TABLETS: aluminum hydroxide 300 mg and magnesium oxide 185 mg.
KOLANTYL WAFERS◆: aluminum hydroxide 180 mg and magnesium hydroxide 170 mg.
MAALOX #1: aluminum hydroxide 200 mg and magnesium hydroxide 200 mg.
MAALOX #2: aluminum hydroxide 400 mg and magnesium hydroxide 400 mg.
MAALOX PLUS◆: aluminum hydroxide 200 mg, magnesium hydroxide 200 mg, and simethicone 25 mg.

MAALOX TC: aluminum hydroxide 600 mg and magnesium hydroxide 300 mg.
MAGNATRIL: aluminum hydroxide 260 mg, magnesium hydroxide 130 mg, and magnesium trisilicate 455 mg.
MYLANTA•: aluminum hydroxide 200 mg, magnesium hydroxide 200 mg, and simethicone 20 mg.
MYLANTA-II•: aluminum hydroxide 400 mg, magnesium hydroxide 400 mg, and simethicone 30 mg.
NEUTRALOX: aluminum hydroxide 300 mg and magnesium hydroxide 150 mg.
SILAIN-GEL: aluminum hydroxide and magnesium carbonate 282 mg, magnesium hydroxide 85 mg, and simethicone 25 mg.
TRISOGEL: aluminum hydroxide 98 mg and magnesium trisilicate 293 mg.
UNIVOL••: aluminum hydroxide 300 mg, magnesium carbonate 300 mg, magnesium hydroxide, 100 mg. contains tartrazine.
WINGEL: aluminum hydroxide 180 mg and magnesium hydroxide 160 mg.

SODIUM CONTENT IN ANTACIDS

Some patients who need to take antacids also need to restrict their sodium intake. The sodium content of several common over-the-counter antacids are given below:

BiSoDol ....0.036 mg/tablet or 157 mg/5 ml

Di-Gel ....10.6 mg/tablet or 8.5 mg/5 ml

Gelusil ....9 mg/tablet or 0.8 mg/5 ml

Gelusil-II ......1.50 mg/5 ml

Maalox ....0.84 mg/tablet or 2.5 mg/5 ml

Maalox Plus ...0.84 mg/tablet or 2.5 mg/5 ml

Maalox TC ....1.25 mg/5 ml

Mylanta ....0.68 mg/5 ml

Mylanta-II .....1.36 mg/5 ml

Riopan ....0.7 mg/tablet or 5 ml

Rolaids ....53 mg/tablet

Tums ....2.7 mg/tablet

Instruct the patient to chew antacid tablets thoroughly, because the smaller the particles are when swallowed, the greater the solubility of the ingredients. Remember, though, that antacids in tablet form do not have the effectiveness, mg for mg, of those in liquid form. Liquids are easier to digest and have a greater neutralizing capability. So reserve antacid tablets for those patients who cannot tolerate liquids. With regard to effervescent tablets, tell the patient that these must be completely dissolved in water and that they should not be taken until the bubbling process stops.

NAME	INDICATIONS & DOSAGE	SIDE EFFECTS
activated charcoal Charcocaps, Charcodote, Charcotabs, Digestalin	*Flatulence or dyspepsia—* **Adults:** 600 mg to 5 g P.O. *Poisoning—* **Adults and children:** 5 to 10 times estimated weight of drug or chemical ingested. (Average dose 15 to 30 g.) Mix with water. Give orally, preferably within 30 minutes of poisoning. Larger doses are necessary if food is in the stomach. For treatment of overdosage with: acetaminophen, amphetamines, aspirin, antimony, atropine, arsenic, barbiturates, camphor, cocaine, digitalis glycosides, glutethimide, ipecac, malathion, morphine, poisonous mushrooms, opium, oxalic acid, parathion, phenol, phenothiazines, potassium permanganate, propoxyphene, quinine, stramonium, strychnine, sulfonamides, tricyclic antidepressants.	*GI:* black stools.
aluminum carbonate Basaljel◆	*As antacid—* **Adults:** suspension: 5 to 10 ml, p.r.n. Extra-strength suspension: 2.5 to 5 ml, p.r.n. Tablets: 1 to 2, p.r.n. Capsules: 1 to 2, p.r.n. *To prevent formation of urinary phosphate stones (with low phosphate diet)—* **Adults:** suspension: 15 to 30 ml suspension in water or juice 1 hour after meals and h.s.; 5 to 15 ml extra strength in water or juice 1 hour after meals and h.s.; 2 to 6 tablets or capsules 1 hour after meals or h.s.	*Blood:* hypophosphatemia. *GI:* anorexia, constipation, intestinal obstruction. *GU:* prolonged use believed to cause dialysis encephalopathy in chronic renal disease patients (with high-dose prolonged use).
aluminum hydroxide ALternaGel, Alu-Cap, Al-U-Creme, Aluminett, Amphojel◆, Basaljel◆◆, Dialume, Hydroxal, No-Co-	*Antacid—* **Adults:** 600 mg P.O. (5 to 10 ml of most products) 1 hour after meals and h.s.; 300 or 600 mg tablet, chewed before swallowing, taken with milk or water 5 to 6 times daily after meals and h.s.	*Blood:* hypophosphatemia. *GI:* anorexia, constipation, intestinal obstruction. *GU:* dialysis encephalopathy in chronic renal disease patients (with high-dose prolonged use).

◆ Also available in Canada.
◆◆ Available in Canada only.
Unmarked trade names available in United States only.

INTERACTIONS	NURSING CONSIDERATIONS
None significant.	• Because activated charcoal absorbs and inactivates syrup of ipecac, give after emesis. • Don't give in ice cream. Ice cream decreases absorptive capacity. • Powder form most effective. Mix with tap water to form consistency of thick syrup. May add small amount of fruit juice to make more palatable. • Space doses at least 1 hour apart from other drugs if activated charcoal is being used for any indication other than poisoning.
None significant.	• Use cautiously in elderly patients, especially those with decreased bowel motility (those receiving antidiarrheals, antispasmodics, or anticholinergics), dehydration, fluid restriction, chronic renal disease, and suspected intestinal obstruction. • Notify doctor if patient develops side effects. • Record amount and consistency of stools. Manage constipation with laxatives or stool softeners; alternate with magnesium-containing antacids (if not renal disease patient). • Monitor serum phosphate levels. • Shake suspension well; give with small amount of water or fruit juice to assure passage to stomach. When administering through nasogastric tube, be sure tube is placed correctly and is patent; follow antacid with water to facilitate passage. • Watch long-term, high-dose use in patient on restricted sodium intake. • Warn patient not to take aluminum carbonate indiscriminately and not to switch antacids without doctor's advice. • Because it contains aluminum, it is used in renal failure patients to help control hyperphosphatemia. Binds phosphate in GI tract. • Watch for symptoms of hypophosphatemia with prolonged use (anorexia, malaise, muscle weakness); can also lead to resorption of calcium and bone demineralization. • If patient is able, he should be responsible for taking antacid while hospitalized. • May cause enteric-coated drugs to be released prematurely in stomach. Separate doses by 1 hour.
None significant.	• Use cautiously in elderly patients, especially those with decreased bowel motility (those receiving antidiarrheals, antispasmodics, or anticholinergics), dehydration, fluid restriction, chronic renal disease, and suspected intestinal obstruction. • Notify doctor if patient develops side effects. • Record amount and consistency of stools. Manage constipation with laxatives or stool softeners; alternate with magnesium-containing antacids

(continued on following page)

NAME	INDICATIONS & DOSAGE	SIDE EFFECTS
aluminum hydroxide *(continued)* Gel, Nutrajel	*Hyperphosphatemia in renal failure—* **Adults:** 500 mg to 2 g b.i.d. to q.i.d.	
aluminum phosphate Phosphaljel	*Antacid—* **Adults:** 15 to 30 ml undiluted q 2 hours between meals and h.s.	*GI:* constipation, intestinal obstruction.
calcium carbonate Alka-2, Amitone, Calcilac, Calglycine, Dicarbosil, El-Da-Mint, Equilet, Gustalac, Mallamint, P.H. Tablets, Spentacid, Titracid, Titralac, Trialea, Tums	*Antacid—* **Adults:** 1 g tablet, 4 to 6 times daily, chewed well and taken with water; or 1 g of suspension (5 ml of most products) 1 hour after meals and h.s.	*Blood:* hypercalcemia; if taken with milk—"milk-alkali syndrome." *GI:* constipation, gastric distention, flatulence, "acid-rebound."

INTERACTIONS	NURSING CONSIDERATIONS
	(if not renal disease patient). • Monitor serum phosphate levels. • Shake suspension well; give with small amount of milk or water to assure passage to stomach. When administering through nasogastric tube, be sure tube is placed correctly and is patent. After instilling antacid, flush tube with water. • Watch long-term, high-dose use in patient on restricted sodium intake. • Warn patient not to take aluminum hydroxide indiscriminately and not to switch antacids without doctor's advice. • Because it contains aluminum, it is used in renal failure patients to help control hyperphosphatemia. Binds phosphate in the GI tract. • Watch for symptoms of hypophosphatemia with prolonged use (anorexia, malaise, muscle weakness); can also lead to resorption of calcium and bone demineralization. • If patient is able, he should be responsible for taking antacid while hospitalized. • May cause enteric-coated drugs to be released prematurely in stomach. Separate doses by 1 hour.
None significant.	• Use cautiously in elderly patients, especially those with decreased bowel motility (those receiving antidiarrheals, antispasmodics, or anticholinergics), dehydration, fluid restriction, chronic renal disease, and suspected intestinal obstruction. • Notify doctor if patient develops side effects. • Record amount and consistency of stools. Manage constipation with laxatives or stool softeners; alternate with magnesium-containing antacids (if patient does not have renal disease). • Shake well; give alone or with small amount of milk or water. When administering through nasogastric tube, be sure tube is placed correctly and is patent; follow with water to facilitate passage to stomach. • Watch long-term, high-dose use in patient on restricted sodium intake. • Warn patient not to take aluminum phosphate indiscriminately and not to switch antacids without doctor's advice. • This drug is a very weak antacid. • Can reverse hypophosphatemia induced by aluminum hydroxide. • If patient is able, he should be responsible for taking antacid while hospitalized. • May cause enteric-coated drugs to be released prematurely in stomach. Separate doses by 1 hour.
None significant.	• Contraindicated in severe renal disease. Use cautiously in elderly patients, especially those with decreased bowel motility (those receiving antidiarrheals, antispasmodics, anticholinergics), dehydration, fluid restriction, chronic renal disease, and suspected intestinal obstruction. • Do not administer with milk. Can cause milk-alkali syndrome. • Notify doctor if patient develops side effects. • Record amount and consistency of stools. Manage constipation with laxatives or stool softeners. • Watch for symptoms of hypercalcemia (nausea, vomiting, headache, mental confusion, anorexia). • Monitor serum calcium levels, especially in mild renal impairment. • Warn patient not to take calcium carbonate indiscriminately and not to switch antacids without doctor's advice. • If patient is able, he should be responsible for taking antacid while hospitalized. • Has been known to cause "rebound hyperacidity." • Emphasize that it is *not* candy. • May cause enteric-coated tablets to be released prematurely in stomach. Separate doses by 1 hour.

NAME	INDICATIONS & DOSAGE	SIDE EFFECTS
dihydroxy-aluminum aminoacetate Alkam, Hyperacid, Robalate◆	*Antacid—* **Adults:** 0.5 to 1 g (1 to 2 tablets) after meals and h.s., chewed before swallowing and taken with milk or water.	*Blood:* hypophosphatemia. *GI:* anorexia, constipation, intestinal obstruction.
dihydroxy-aluminum sodium carbonate Rolaids	*Antacid—* **Adults:** chew 1 to 2 tablets (334 to 668 mg), p.r.n.	*GI:* anorexia, constipation, intestinal obstruction.
magaldrate (aluminum-magnesium complex) Riopan◆	*Antacid—* **Adults:** suspension: 400 to 800 mg (5 to 10 ml) between meals and h.s. with water. Tablet: 400 to 800 mg (1 to 2 tablets) P.O. with water between meals and h.s. Chewable tablet: 400 to 800 mg (1 to 2 tablets) chewed before swallowing, between meals and h.s.	*GI:* mild constipation.

INTERACTIONS	NURSING CONSIDERATIONS
None significant.	• Use cautiously in elderly patients, especially those with decreased bowel motility (those receiving antidiarrheals, antispasmodics, or anticholinergics), dehydration, fluid restriction, chronic renal disease, and suspected intestinal obstruction. • Notify doctor if patient develops side effects. • Record amount and consistency of stools. Less constipating than aluminum hydroxide. Manage constipation with laxatives or stool softeners; alternate with magnesium-containing antacids (if not renal disease patient). • Watch for symptoms of hypophosphatemia with prolonged use (anorexia, malaise, muscle weakness); can also lead to resorption of calcium and bone demineralization. • Monitor serum phosphate levels. • Watch long-term, high-dose use in patient on restricted sodium intake. • Warn patient not to take dihydroxyaluminum aminoacetate indiscriminately and not to switch antacids without doctor's advice. • If patient is able, he should be responsible for taking antacid while hospitalized. • May cause enteric-coated drugs to be released prematurely in stomach. Separate doses by 1 hour.
None significant.	• Use cautiously in elderly patients, especially those with decreased bowel motility (those receiving antidiarrheals, antispasmodics, or anticholinergics), dehydration, fluid restriction, chronic renal disease, and suspected intestinal obstruction. • Has high sodium content and may increase sodium and water retention. • Notify doctor if patient develops side effects. • Record amount and consistency of stools. Manage constipation with laxatives or stool softeners; alternate with magnesium-containing antacids (if patient does not have renal disease). • Watch long-term, high-dose use in patient on restricted sodium intake. • Warn patient not to take dihydroxyaluminum sodium carbonate indiscriminately. • If patient is able, he should be responsible for taking antacid while hospitalized. • Emphasize that it is *not* candy. • May cause enteric-coated drugs to be released prematurely in stomach. Separate doses by 1 hour.
None significant.	• Contraindicated in severe renal disease. Use cautiously in elderly patients, especially those with decreased bowel motility (those receiving antidiarrheals, antispasmodics, or anticholinergics), dehydration, fluid restriction, and mild renal impairment. • Notify doctor if patient develops side effects. • Record amount and consistency of stools. Manage constipation with laxatives or stool softeners. • Shake suspension well; give with small amount of water to assure passage to stomach. When administering through nasogastric tube, be sure tube is placed properly and is patent. After instilling, flush tube with water. • Monitor serum magnesium in mild renal impairment. Symptomatic hypermagnesemia usually occurs only in severe renal failure. • Not usually used in renal failure patients (although it contains aluminum) to help control hypophosphatemia, since it contains magnesium, which may accumulate in renal failure.

(continued on following page)

NAME	INDICATIONS & DOSAGE	SIDE EFFECTS
magaldrate (aluminum-magnesium complex) *(continued)*		
magnesia magma (MOM) (magnesium hydroxide) Milk of Magnesia, Mint-O-Mag	*Antacid—* **Adults:** 5 to 10 ml or 1 to 2 tablets chewed before swallowing q.i.d., usually after meals and h.s. *Laxative—* **Adults:** 15 to 30 ml, usually h.s. **Children:** 2.5 to 5 ml h.s. *Oral replacement therapy in mild hypomagnesemia*—5 to 10 ml q.i.d., usually after meals and h.s. Monitor serum magnesium response.	*Blood:* hypermagnesemia. *GI:* diarrhea, abdominal pain, nausea.
magnesium carbonate	*Antacid—* **Adults:** 0.5 to 2 g of powder product or chewable tablets between meals with ½ glass of water. *Laxative—* **Adults:** 8 g of powder product or chewable tablets with water h.s.	*Blood:* hypermagnesemia. *GI:* diarrhea, gastric distention, flatulence, abdominal pain, nausea.
magnesium oxide Mag-Ox, Maox, Niko-Mag, Oxabid, Par-Mag, Uro-Mag	*Antacid—* **Adults:** 250 mg to 1 g with water or milk after meals and h.s. *Laxative—* **Adults:** 4 g with water or milk, usually h.s. *Oral replacement therapy in mild*	*Blood:* hypermagnesemia. *GI:* diarrhea, nausea, abdominal pain.

INTERACTIONS	NURSING CONSIDERATIONS
	• Good for patient on restricted sodium intake; very low sodium content. • Warn patient not to take magaldrate indiscriminately and not to switch antacids without doctor's advice. • If patient is able, he should be responsible for taking antacid while hospitalized. • May cause enteric-coated drugs to be released prematurely in stomach. Separate doses by 1 hour.
None significant.	• Contraindicated in severe renal disease. Use cautiously in elderly patients and in mild renal impairment. • Notify doctor if side effects develop. • Usually not used as antacid, even though it is very effective and potent, due to increased frequency of stools. Usually used as laxative. • Record amount and consistency of stools. • Shake suspension well; give with small amount of water when used as antacid, large amount of water when used as laxative. When administering through nasogastric tube, be sure tube is placed properly and is patent. After instilling, flush tube with water. • Watch for symptoms of hypermagnesemia with prolonged use and some degree of renal impairment (hypotension, nausea, vomiting, depressed reflexes, respiratory depression, coma). • Monitor serum magnesium in mild renal impairment. • When used as laxative, don't give oral drugs 1 to 2 hours before or after. • If diarrhea occurs with antacid doses, suggest alternative preparation. • Subcathartic doses also used as oral magnesium replacement therapy in hypomagnesemia. • Warn patient not to take magnesia magma indiscriminately and not to switch antacids without doctor's advice. • If patient is able, he should be responsible for taking antacid while hospitalized. • May cause enteric-coated drugs to be released prematurely in stomach. Separate doses by 1 hour.
None significant.	• Contraindicated in severe renal disease. Use cautiously in elderly patients, mild renal impairment. • Notify doctor if side effects develop. • Watch for symptoms of hypermagnesemia with prolonged use and some degree of renal impairment (hypotension, nausea, vomiting, depressed reflexes, respiratory depression, coma). • Monitor serum magnesium in mild renal impairment. • When used as laxative, do not give other oral drugs 1 to 2 hours before or after. • Record amount and consistency of stools. • Warn patient not to take magnesium carbonate indiscriminately and not to switch antacids without doctor's advice. • If patient is able, he should be responsible for taking antacid while hospitalized. • May cause enteric-coated drugs to be released prematurely in stomach. Separate doses by 1 hour.
None significant.	• Contraindicated in severe renal disease. Use cautiously in elderly patients, mild renal impairment. • Notify doctor if side effects develop. • Watch for symptoms of hypermagnesemia with prolonged use and some degree of renal impairment (hypotension, nausea, vomiting, depressed reflexes, respiratory depression, coma). • Monitor serum magnesium in mild renal impairment.

(continued on following page)

NAME	INDICATIONS & DOSAGE	SIDE EFFECTS
magnesium oxide *(continued)*	*hypomagnesemia—* **Adults:** 650 mg to 1.3 g tablet or capsule daily. Monitor serum magnesium response.	
magnesium trisilicate Trisomin	*Antacid—* **Adults:** 0.5 to 1 g tablet t.i.d. chewed well and taken with ½ glass of water.	*Blood:* hypermagnesemia. *GI:* diarrhea, gastric distention, flatulence, nausea, abdominal pain. *GU:* possible formation of silica renal calculi with prolonged use.
oxethazaine Oxaine (oxethazaine in aluminum hydroxide gel)	*Adjunct therapy for hyperacidity—* **Adults:** 10 to 20 mg suspended in 5 to 10 ml aluminum hydroxide gel (equivalent to 5 to 10 ml of commercial product) q.i.d. 15 minutes before meals and h.s.	*CNS:* with high doses (120 mg oxethazaine daily): dizziness, faintness, drowsiness. *GI:* anorexia, constipation, intestinal obstruction. *GU:* dialysis encephalopathy in renal disease patients (with high-dose prolonged use).
simethicone Mylicon, Silain	*Flatulence, functional gastric bloating—* **Adults, and children over 12:** 40 to 100 mg after each meal and h.s.	*GI:* expulsion of excessive liberated gas as belching, rectal flatus.

INTERACTIONS	NURSING CONSIDERATIONS
	• When used for laxative, do not give other oral drugs 1 to 2 hours before or after. • If diarrhea occurs on antacid doses, suggest alternate preparation. • Warn patient not to take magnesium oxide indiscriminately and not to switch antacids without doctor's advice. • If patient is able, he should be responsible for taking antacid while hospitalized. • May cause enteric-coated drugs to be released prematurely in stomach. Separate doses by 1 hour.
None significant.	• Contraindicated in severe renal disease. Use cautiously in elderly patients, mild renal impairment. • Notify doctor if side effects develop. • Watch for symptoms of hypermagnesemia with prolonged use and some degree of renal impairment (hypotension, nausea, vomiting, depressed reflexes, respiratory depression, coma). • Monitor serum magnesium in mild renal impairment. • If diarrhea occurs on antacid doses, suggest alternate preparation. • Warn patient not to take magnesium trisilicate indiscriminately and not to switch antacids without doctor's advice. • If patient is able, he should be responsible for taking antacid while hospitalized. • May cause enteric-coated drugs to be released prematurely in stomach. Separate doses by 1 hour.
None significant.	• Use cautiously in elderly patients, especially those with decreased bowel motility (those receiving antidiarrheals, antispasmodics, or anticholinergics), dehydration, fluid restriction, chronic renal disease, suspected intestinal obstructions. • Notify doctor if patient develops side effects. • Record amount and consistency of stools. Manage constipation with laxatives or stool softeners. • Shake suspension well; give with small amount of water to assure passage to stomach. When administering antacids through nasogastric tube, be sure tube is placed correctly and is patent; follow with water. • Caution: Local anesthetic can affect gastric mucosa for up to 6 hours. Prolonged use may mask extension of ulcerative disease and may lead to perforation. Also may mask symptoms of gastric neoplasm. • Warn patient not to take oxethazaine indiscriminately and not to switch antacids without doctor's advice. • If patient is able, he should be responsible for taking antacid while hospitalized. • May cause enteric-coated drugs to be released prematurely in stomach. Separate doses by 1 hour.
None significant.	• Observe patient for effectiveness. • Warn patient not to take simethicone indiscriminately. • Tablets should be chewed, not swallowed whole.

NAME	INDICATIONS & DOSAGE	SIDE EFFECTS
sodium bicarbonate Bell-ans, Soda Mint	*Antacid—* **Adults:** 300 mg to 2 g tablets chewed well and taken with full glass of water, p.r.n.	*GI:* gastric distention, belching, flatulence. *GU:* renal calculi or crystals. *Metabolic:* systemic alkalosis (prolonged use), sodium and water retention.

INTERACTIONS	NURSING CONSIDERATIONS
None significant.	• Contraindicated in congestive heart failure, hypertension, advanced renal disease, sodium restrictions, tendency toward edema, patients losing chloride from continuous GI suction, and patients receiving diuretics that cause hypochloremic alkalosis. Also contraindicated for long-term use. Use cautiously in elderly patients and in mild renal impairment. • Notify doctor if side effects develop. • Discourage use as antacid. Offer nonabsorbable alternative antacid if it is to be used repeatedly. • If patient is able, he should be responsible for taking antacid while hospitalized. • Do not administer with milk; can cause milk-alkali syndrome.

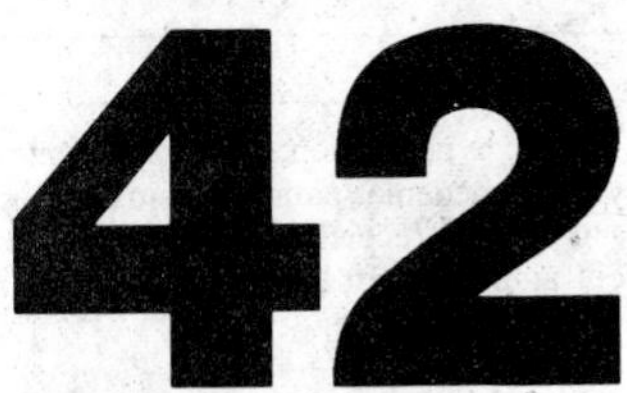

Digestants

bile salts
dehydrocholic acid
glutamic acid hydrochloride
hydrochloric acid, diluted
ketocholanic acids
pancreatin
pancrelipase

Digestants promote digestion in the gastrointestinal tract and are used when a patient lacks one or more of the specific digestive substances. They can be considered replacement therapy in specific deficiency states. The most widely used digestants are hydrochloric acid, bile salts, and stomach and pancreatic enzymes.

Major uses

Dehydrocholic and ketocholanic acids are synthetic bile salts used as an adjunct in:

- Treatment of recent or recurrent biliary tract surgery, biliary calculi or strictures (repeated episodes); recurring noncalculous cholangitis; biliary dyskinesia, chronic partial obstruction of common bile duct; prolonged drainage from biliary fistulas or from T-tube drainage of infected bile duct, and sclerosing choledochitis; and also to prevent bacterial accumulation following biliary tract surgery and partial obstruction of the common bile duct.
- Bile salts are used in uncomplicated constipation and help maintain normal solubility of cholesterol in the bile.
- Gastric acidifiers such as glutamic acid hydrochloride and diluted hydrochloric acid are used in hypochlorhydria and achlorhydria.
- Enzymes such as pancreatin and pancrelipase are used in deficiency of exocrine pancreatic secretions.

Mechanism of action

- Bile salts and synthetic bile salts stimulate the flow of bile from hepatic to aid normal digestion and absorption of fats and fat-soluble vitamins and cholesterol.
- Hydrochloric acid and glutamic acid replace gastric acid.
- Pancreatin and pancrelipase replace deficient exocrine pancreatic enzymes and aid intestinal digestion of starch, fat, and protein.

Absorption, distribution, and excretion

- Approximately 80% to 90% of bile salts are reabsorbed primarily in the ileum, returned to the liver, and reenter the bile acid pool.

Onset and duration

- Unknown.

Combination products

ACCELERASE-PB CAPSULES: lipase 4,000 units, amylase 15,000 units, protease 15,000 units cellulase 2 mg, mixed conjugated bile salts 65 mg, calcium carbonate 20 mg, 1-alkaloids of belladonna 0.2 mg, and phenobarbital 16 mg.

BILOGEN TABLETS: pancreatin 250 mg, ox bile extract 120 mg, oxidized mixed ox bile acids 75 mg, and desoxycholic acid 30 mg.
BILRON♦: bile salts and iron.
BUTIBEL-ZYME TABLETS: proteolytic enzyme 10 mg, amylolytic enzyme 20 mg, lipolytic enzyme 100 mg, cellulolytic enzyme 5 mg, iron ox bile 30 mg, belladonna extract 15 mg, and sodium butabarbital 15 mg.
CHOLAN V TABLETS: dehydrocholic acid 250 mg and homatropine methylbromide 5 mg.
CHOLAN-HMB TABLETS: dehydrocholic acid 250 mg, homatropine methylbromide 2.5 mg, and phenobarbital 8 mg.
COTAZYM-B TABLETS: lipase 4,000 units, amylase 15,000 units, protease 15,000 units, cellulase 2 mg, and mixed conjugated bile salts 65 mg.
DONNAZYME♦ tablets: pancreatin 300 mg, pepsin 150 mg, bile salts 150 mg, hyoscyamine sulfate 0.0518 mg, atropine sulfate 0.0097 mg, hyoscine hydrobromide 0.0033 mg, and phenobarbital 8.1 mg.
ENTOZYME TABLETS♦: pancreatin 300 mg, pepsin 250 mg, and bile salts 150 mg.
ENZYPAN TABLETS: pancreatin (sufficient to digest 19 g protein, 43 g starch, 10 g fat), pepsin 9 mg, and dessicated ox bile 56 mg.
FESTAL ENTERIC-COATED TABLETS♦: protease 17 units, amylase 10 units, lipase 10 units, bile constituents 25 mg, and hemicellulase 50 mg.
FESTALAN TABLETS: protease 17 units, amylase 10 units, lipase 10 units, bile constituents 25 mg, hemicellulase 50 mg, and atropine methylnitrate 1 mg.
GOURMASE CAPSULES: pancreatin 525 mg, *a*-amylase 20 mg, pepsin 150 mg, and ox bile extract 100 mg.
KANULASE TABLETS: pancreatin 500 mg, pepsin 150 mg, ox bile extract 100 mg, cellulase 9 mg, and glutamic acid hydrochloride 200 mg.
MURIPSIN TABLETS: glutamic acid hydrochloride 500 mg and pepsin 35 mg.
PHAZYME TABLETS (enteric-coated): pancreatin 240 mg and simethicone 60 mg.
PHAZYME-95 TABLETS (enteric-coated): pancreatin 240 mg and simethicone 95 mg.
PHAZYME PB TABLETS (enteric-coated): pancreatin 240 mg, phenobarbital 15 mg, and simethicone 60 mg.
PROBILAGOL LIQUID: d-sorbitol 4.5 g and homatropine methylbromide 1 mg.
RO-BILE TABLETS (enteric-coated): enzyme concentrate 75 mg, lipase equivalent to 750 mg pancreatin, amylase and protease equivalent to 300 mg pancreatin, ox bile extract 100 mg, dehydrocholic acid 30 mg, belladonna extract 8 mg, and pepsin 260 mg.
TAKA-DIASTASE TABLETS: pancreatin 130 mg, pepsin 65 mg, and amylase concentrate 130 mg.

NAME	INDICATIONS & DOSAGE	SIDE EFFECTS
bile salts Biso, Chobile, Ox-Bile Extract Enseals	*Uncomplicated constipation—* **Adults and children:** 300 to 500 mg (enteric-coated tablets) b.i.d. or t.i.d. after meals; or 150 to 450 mg capsules with or after meals.	*GI:* loose stools and mild cramping (in large doses).
dehydrocholic acid Bio-Cholin♦♦, Cholan-DH, Cholyphyl♦♦, Decholin♦, Dycholium♦♦, Hepahydrin, Idrocrine♦♦, Neocholan	*Constipation, biliary tract conditions—* **Adults:** 250 to 500 mg P.O. b.i.d. to t.i.d. after meals for 4 to 6 weeks.	None reported.
glutamic acid hydrochloride Acidulin♦	*Hypoacidity—* **Adults:** 1 to 3 capsules P.O. t.i.d. before meals.	*Metabolic:* systemic acidosis in massive overdose.
hydrochloric acid, diluted	*Hypoacidity—* **Adults:** 2 to 8 ml P.O. well diluted in 25 to 50 ml water.	*Metabolic:* systemic acidosis in massive overdose. *Other:* tooth enamel damage.
ketocholanic acids Ketochol	*Constipation, biliary tract conditions—* **Adults:** 250 mg to 500 mg P.O. t.i.d. with meals.	None reported.
pancreatin Beef Viokase Elzyme, Panteric Double Strength, Viokase	*Exocrine pancreatic secretion insufficiency, digestive aid in cystic fibrosis—* **Adults and children:** 325 mg to 1 g P.O. with meals.	*GI:* nausea, diarrhea in high doses.

♦ Also available in Canada.
♦♦ Available in Canada only.
Unmarked trade names available in United States only.

INTERACTIONS	NURSING CONSIDERATIONS
None significant.	• Contraindicated in marked hepatic dysfunction except in malnutrition with steatorrhea and vitamin K deficiency with hypoprothrombinemia. • Use Ox-Bile Extract cautiously in obstructive jaundice. • Don't use Ox-Bile Extract if other preparations are available, since it doesn't provide an adequate amount of conjugated bile salts.
None significant.	• Contraindicated in complete mechanical biliary obstruction. Use cautiously in prostatic hypertrophy, acute hepatitis, asthmatic bronchitis, elderly patients, and partial GI or GU tract obstruction. • Do not use when patient is nauseated or vomiting, or has abdominal pain. • Simultaneous administration of bile salts may be needed in biliary fistula. • Used to prevent bacterial accumulation after biliary tract surgery. • Probably much less effective than natural bile salts in lowering surface tension and promoting absorption. • Check periodically to prevent fluid and electrolytic deficiencies. • Don't use dehydrocholic acid to accelerate rate of healing in jaundice. • Frequent use may result in dependence on laxatives.
None significant.	• Contraindicated in gastric hyperacidity or peptic ulcer. • Use instead of hydrochloric acid so tooth enamel won't be damaged; however, glutamic acid HCl is not as effective in increasing gastric pH. • Gastric acidifier.
None significant.	• Contraindicated in gastric hyperacidity or peptic ulcer. • Sip, during meal, through glass straw to protect tooth enamel. • Alleviates primary functional hypoacidity or hypoacidity caused by organic disease such as pernicious anemia, certain allergies, chronic gastritis, other chronic debilitation diseases, or after gastric resection. • Gastric acidifier; usual dose not sufficient to release free acid in stomach; no evidence that even larger doses are beneficial for this.
None significant.	• Use cautiously in prostatic hypertrophy, acute hepatitis, asthmatic bronchitis, elderly patients, partial GI or GU tract obstruction. • Bile salt; derived from beef bile. • Approximately equivalent to 250 mg dehydrocholic acid. • Do not use when patient is nauseated, vomiting, or has abdominal pain. • Check periodically to prevent fluid and electrolytic deficiencies. • Frequent use may result in dependence on laxatives.
None significant.	• Use cautiously in sensitivity to pork. • Balance fat, protein, and starch intake properly to avoid indigestion. Dosage varies according to degree of maldigestion and malabsorption, amount of fat in diet, and enzyme activity of individual preparations. • Pancreatin therapy shouldn't delay or replace treatment of primary disorder. • Adequate replacement decreases number of bowel movements and improves stool consistency. • Use only after confirmed diagnosis of exocrine pancreatic insufficiency. Not effective in GI disorders unrelated to pancreatic enzyme deficiency. • Bovine preparations available for use in pork sensitivity; less effective. • For infants, mix powder with applesauce and give with meals. Older children may swallow capsules with food. • Enteric coating on some products may reduce availability or enzyme in upper portion of jejunum where it is primarily required.

NAME	INDICATIONS & DOSAGE	SIDE EFFECTS
pancrelipase Cotazym◆, Ilozyme, Ku-Zyme HP	*Dose must be titrated to patient's response. Exocrine pancreatic secretion insufficiency, cystic fibrosis, in adults and children, steatorrhea and other disorders of fat metabolism secondary to insufficient pancreatic enzymes—* **Adults and children:** dosage range 1 to 3 capsules or tablets P.O. before or with meals and 1 capsule or tablet with snack; or 1 to 2 powder packets before meals or snacks.	*GI:* nausea, diarrhea in high doses.

INTERACTIONS	NURSING CONSIDERATIONS
None significant.	• Contraindicated in severe pork sensitivity. Otherwise, use with caution. • Pancrelipase therapy shouldn't delay or replace treatment of primary disorder. • Use only after confirmed diagnosis of exocrine pancreatic insufficiency. Not effective in GI disorders unrelated to enzyme deficiency. • Lipase activity greater than with other pancreatic enzymes. • For infants, mix powder with applesauce and give at mealtime. Older children may swallow capsules with food. • Dosage varies with degree of maldigestion and malabsorption, amount of fat in diet, and enzyme activity of individual preparations. • Adequate replacement decreases number of bowel movements and improves stool consistency. • Enteric coating on some products may reduce availability of enzyme in upper portion of jejunum where it is primarily required.

43 Antidiarrheals

bismuth subcarbonate
bismuth subgallate
bismuth subsalicylate
diphenoxylate hydrochloride (with atropine sulfate)
kaolin and pectin mixtures
lactobacillus
loperamide
opium tincture
opium tincture, camphorated

Diarrhea may be caused by certain foods or drugs, allergies, endocrine dysfunction, malabsorption, neurologic or inflammatory diseases, mechanical obstruction, parasitic infestation, resectional surgery of stomach, laxative abuse, or radiation poisoning. Antidiarrheals reduce the fluidity of the stool and the frequency of defecation.

Major uses

- To treat acute, mild, or chronic nonspecific diarrhea.
- Bismuth subgallate also acts as deodorizer for fecal odors in colostomy and ileostomy patients.
- Loperamide also reduces the volume of ileostomy discharge.

Mechanism of action

- Kaolin and pectin appear to decrease the fluid content of the stool, although the total water loss seems to remain the same.
- Bismuth salts have a mild water-binding capacity; also may absorb toxins and provide protective coating for intestinal mucosa.
- Opium tinctures directly increase smooth muscle tone in the gastrointestinal tract, inhibit motility and propulsion, and diminish digestive secretions.
- Diphenoxylate hydrochloride is a synthetic opiate with action similar to the opium tinctures.
- Lactobacillus cultures may suppress the growth of pathogenic microorganisms to help reestablish normal intestinal flora.
- Loperamide also inhibits peristaltic activity, prolongs transit time of intestinal contents, and reduces daily fecal volume and fluid and electrolyte loss.

Absorption, distribution, and excretion

- Adsorbent antidiarrheals are not systemically absorbed.
- Diphenoxylate hydrochloride is well absorbed from the gastrointestinal tract and is excreted in the urine and in the feces via the bile.
- Loperamide is poorly absorbed orally and is excreted primarily in the feces.

• Opium tincture is absorbed from the gastrointestinal tract as morphine; metabolized in the liver; excreted in urine.

Onset and duration

• Diphenoxylate hydrochloride begins to act within 45 minutes to 1 hour and lasts up to 4 hours.
• Opium tinctures begin to act rapidly.
• Peak levels for loperamide occur in 4 hours; plasma half-life is about 40 hours.

Combination products

CORRECTIVE MIXTURE: zinc sulfocarbolate 10 mg, phenyl salicylate 22 mg, bismuth subsalicylate 85 mg, pepsin 45 mg, and alcohol 1.5% in 5 ml suspension.
CORRECTIVE MIXTURE WITH PAREGORIC: paregoric 0.6 ml, zinc sulfocarbolate 10 mg, phenyl salicylate 22 mg, bismuth subsalicylate 85 mg, pepsin 45 mg, and alcohol 2% in 5 ml suspension.
DONNAGEL SUSPENSION♦: kaolin 1 g, hyoscyamine sulfate 0.0173 mg, atropine sulfate 0.0032 mg, hyoscine hydrobromide 0.0011 mg, and alcohol 3.8% in 5 ml suspension.
DONNAGEL-MB♦♦: kaolin 6 g and pectin 142.8 mg.
DONNAGEL-PG♦: powdered opium 4 mg (equivalent to 1 ml paregoric), kaolin 1 g, pectin 23.8 mg, hyoscyamine sulfate 0.0173 mg, atropine sulfate 0.0032 mg, hyoscine hydrobromide 0.0011 mg, and alcohol 5% in 5 ml suspension.
KENPECTIN-P: opium 2.7 mg (equivalent to 0.6 ml paregoric), kaolin 975 mg, pectin 32.5 mg, alcohol 6%, and aluminum hydroxide 108 mg in 5 ml suspension.
MUL-SED: kaolin 860 mg, pectin 43.2 mg, bismuth magma 0.8 ml, paregoric 1.1 ml (equivalent to 4.98 mg opium), and alcohol 10.4% in 5 ml suspension.
PARELIXIR: tincture opium 0.03 ml (equivalent to 0.75 ml paregoric), pectin 24 mg, and alcohol 18% in 5 ml suspension.
PAREPECTOLIN: opium 2.0 mg (equivalent to paregoric 0.6 ml), kaolin 917 mg, pectin 27 mg, and alcohol 0.69% in 5 ml suspension.
PECTOCEL: kaolin 975 mg, pectin 48.75 mg, and zinc phenolsulfonate 12 mg in 5 ml suspension.
PEKTAMALT: kaolin 1.08 g, pectin 100 mg, and potassium gluconate and sodium citrate in 5 ml suspension.
POLYMAGMA PLAIN: activated attapulgite 500 mg, pectin 45 mg, and hydrated alumina powder 50 mg.

NAME	INDICATIONS & DOSAGE	SIDE EFFECTS
bismuth subcarbonate **bismuth subgallate** **bismuth subsalicylate** Pepto-Bismol	*Deodorize fecal odors in colostomy and ileostomy—* **Adults:** 200 mg P.O. t.i.d. after each meal. *Mild, nonspecific diarrhea—* **Adults:** 1 to 4 g suspended in water P.O. q 2 to 4 hours. *Mild, nonspecific diarrhea—* **Adults:** 600 mg to 2 g q 6 to 8 hours.	*CNS:* personality changes. Prolonged use (especially in colostomy and ileostomy patients) may lead to reversible deterioration of mental ability, confusion, tremors, and impaired coordination. *GI:* transient darkened tongue and stool (both with subgallate); fecal impaction or ulceration (in infants, elderly, or debilitated patients) after chronic use; constipation.
diphenoxylate hydrochloride (with atropine sulfate) Controlled substance Schedule V Colonil, Lofene, Loflo, Lomo-Plus, Lomotil•, Lonox, Lotrol, Ro-Diphen-Atro	*Acute, nonspecific diarrhea—* **Adults:** initially, 5 mg P.O. q.i.d., then adjust dose to individual response. **Children 2 to 12 years:** 0.3 to 0.4 mg/Kg P.O. daily in divided doses.	*CNS:* sedation, dizziness, headache, drowsiness, lethargy, restlessness, depression, malaise, numbness in extremities, euphoria, coma. *CV:* tachycardia. *EENT:* mydriasis. *GI:* dry mouth, nausea, vomiting, abdominal discomfort or distention, paralytic ileus, anorexia, fluid retention in bowel (may mask depletion of extracellular fluid and electrolytes, especially in young children treated for acute gastroenteritis). *GU:* urinary retention. *Skin:* pruritus, giant urticaria, rash. *Other:* possibly physical dependence in long-term use, angioedema, respiratory depression, dry skin, flushing, hyperthermia.
kaolin and pectin mixtures Baropectin, Kaoparin, Kaopectate•, Kapectin, Keotin, Pargel, Pecto-Kalin, Pectokay	*Mild, nonspecific diarrhea—* **Adults:** 60 to 120 ml after each bowel movement. **Children over 12 years:** 60 ml after each bowel movement. **Children 6 to 12 years:** 30 to 60 ml after each bowel movement. **Children 3 to 6 years:** 15 to 30 ml after each bowel movement.	*GI:* drug absorbs nutrients and enzymes; fecal impaction or ulceration in infants, elderly, and debilitated patients after chronic use; constipation.
lactobacillus Bacid•, DoFUS, Lactinex•	*Diarrhea, especially that caused by antibiotics—* **Adults:** 2 capsules (Bacid) P.O. b.i.d., t.i.d., or q.i.d., preferably with milk; or 4 tablets or 1 packet (Lactinex) P.O. t.i.d. or q.i.d., preferably with food, milk, or juice; or 1 tablet (DoFUS) P.O. daily before meals.	*GI:* (with Bacid and DoFUS) increased intestinal flatus at beginning of therapy; subsides with continued therapy.

• Also available in Canada.
•• Available in Canada only.
Unmarked trade names available in United States only.

INTERACTIONS	NURSING CONSIDERATIONS
None significant.	• GI adsorbent. • Don't use in place of specific therapy for underlying cause. • May reduce absorption of other P.O. drugs, requiring dosage adjustment. • Pepto-Bismol has been used successfully to treat "turista" diarrhea.
None significant.	• Contraindicated in acute diarrhea resulting from poison until toxic material is eliminated from GI tract; in acute diarrhea caused by organisms that penetrate intestinal mucosa; in diarrhea resulting from antibiotic-induced pseudomembraneous colitis; jaundiced patients. Use cautiously in children, hepatic disease, narcotic dependence, pregnancy. Use cautiously in acute ulcerative colitis. Stop therapy immediately if abdominal distention or other signs of toxic megacolon develop. • Risk of physical dependence increases with long-term use. Discourage long-term or unsupervised use. Atropine sulfate is included to discourage abuse. • Warn patient not to exceed recommended dosage. • Dehydration, especially in young children, may increase risk of delayed toxicity. Correct fluid and electrolyte disturbances before starting drug. • Dose of 2.5 mg as effective as 5 ml camphorated tincture of opium. • Not indicated in treatment of antibiotic-induced diarrhea. • For symptoms and treatment of toxicity, see p. 1119.
None significant.	• Contraindicated in suspected obstructive bowel lesions. • Don't use for more than 2 days. • Don't use in place of specific therapy for underlying cause. • May reduce absorption of other P.O. drugs, requiring dosage adjustments. • GI absorbent.
None significant.	• Bacid and DoFUS contraindicated in fever. • Don't use Bacid for more than 2 days. • Store in refrigerator. • Diet containing amounts of carbohydrate (up to 400 g), such as lactose, lactulose, and dextrin, may be more effective than lactobacillus in reestablishing normal flora after antibiotic therapy. • Controversial form of diarrhea treatment. • May be used prophylactically in history of antibiotic-induced diarrhea.

NAME	INDICATIONS & DOSAGE	SIDE EFFECTS
loperamide Controlled substance Schedule V Imodium◆	*Acute, nonspecific diarrhea—* **Adults:** initially, 4 mg P.O., then 2 mg after each unformed stool. Maximum 16 mg daily. *Chronic diarrhea—* **Adults:** initially, 4 mg P.O., then 2 mg after each unformed stool until diarrhea subsides. Adjust dose to individual response.	*CNS:* drowsiness, fatigue, dizziness. *GI:* dry mouth; abdominal pain, distention, or discomfort; constipation; nausea; vomiting. *Skin:* rash.
opium tincture **opium tincture, camphorated** Controlled substance Schedule III Paregoric◆	*Acute, nonspecific diarrhea—* **Adults:** 0.6 ml opium tincture (range 0.3 to 1 ml) P.O. q.i.d. Maximum dose 6 ml daily; or 5 to 10 ml camphorated opium tincture daily b.i.d., t.i.d., or q.i.d. until diarrhea subsides. **Children:** 0.25 to 0.5 ml/Kg camphorated opium tincture daily, b.i.d., t.i.d., or q.i.d. until diarrhea subsides.	*GI:* nausea, vomiting. *Other:* physical dependence after long-term use.

INTERACTIONS	NURSING CONSIDERATIONS
None significant.	• Contraindicated in acute diarrhea resulting from poison until toxic material is removed from GI tract, when constipation must be avoided, and in acute diarrhea caused by organisms that penetrate intestinal mucosa. Use cautiously in severe prostatic hypertrophy, hepatic disease, and history of narcotic dependence. • Stop drug immediately if abdominal distention or other symptoms develop in patients with acute ulcerative colitis. • In acute diarrhea, stop drug if no improvement within 48 hours; in chronic diarrhea, stop drug if no improvement after giving 16 mg daily for at least 10 days. • Appears to have low potential for abuse. • Warn patient not to exceed recommended dosage. • Produces antidiarrheal action similar to diphenoxylate HC1 but without as many CNS side effects; 3 times more potent than diphenoxylate HC1.
None significant.	• Contraindicated in acute diarrhea resulting from poisons until toxic material is removed from GI tract, and in acute diarrhea caused by organisms that penetrate intestinal mucosa. Use cautiously in asthma, severe prostatic hypertrophy, hepatic disease, narcotic dependence. • Risk of physical dependence increases with long-term use. Discourage long-term or unsupervised use. • An effective and prompt-acting antidiarrheal. • Opium content of opium tincture 25 times greater than camphorated tincture of opium. Camphorated opium tincture is more dilute, and teaspoonful doses easier to measure than dropper quantities of opium tincture. • Not used as widely today as in past, but unique because dose can be adjusted precisely to patient's needs. • Milky fluid forms when camphorated opium tincture is added to water. • Camphorated opium tincture 0.06 to 0.5 ml daily has been used to treat infants with mild narcotic physical dependence.

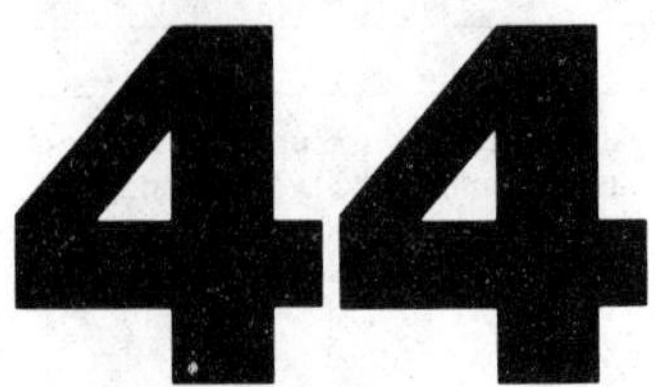

Laxatives

barley-malt extract
bisacodyl
cascara sagrada
castor oil
danthron
dioctyl calcium sulfosuccinate
dioctyl potassium sulfosuccinate
dioctyl sodium sulfosuccinate
magnesium salts
methylcellulose
mineral oil
phenolphthalein
psyllium
senna
sodium biphosphate
sodium phosphate

Laxatives are used (and often abused) to relieve constipation. Laxatives can be classified according to the way in which they act: bulk laxatives (methylcellulose, barley-malt extract, psyllium), stimulant laxatives (castor oil, cascara sagrada, senna, danthron, bisacodyl, phenolphthalein), emollient laxatives or stool softeners (dioctyl calcium sulfosuccinate, dioctyl potassium sulfosuccinate, dioctyl sodium sulfosuccinate), lubricant laxatives (mineral oil), and saline laxatives (magnesium salts, sodium biphosphate, sodium phosphate).

Major uses

- To relieve or prevent constipation.
- To evacuate bowel before rectal or bowel exam, barium enema, abdominal X-rays, or various surgical procedures.
- To soften stools and prevent straining during defecation.

Mechanism of action

- Bulk laxatives hydrate the stool, increasing its bulk and water content. They also cause mechanical distention, which promotes peristalsis and aids in stool passage.
- Castor oil undergoes hydrolysis to form ricinoleic acid, which appears to decrease the contractile activity of circular smooth muscle of the small intestine and speeds up fecal movement. Castor oil may also stimulate water and electrolyte secretion to increase fecal movement.
- Although the action of cascara sagrada, senna, and danthron is unknown, they may directly stimulate the mesenteric plexus and alter sodium transport.
- Phenolphthalein and bisacodyl are thought to act directly on the intramural nerve plexus of the colon, but they may also inhibit sodium potassium adenosinetriphosphatase (AT Pase) and glucose absorption.
- The dioctyl sulfosuccinates are anionic surface active agents with detergent activity. They lower surface tension of the stool, thereby allowing fecal material to be penetrated by

water and fat. They also may cause fluid and electrolyte accumulation in the colon.
• Mineral oil presents a barrier between the colon wall and the feces, thereby preventing colonic absorption of fecal water.
• Saline laxatives produce a hypertonic environment in the lumen of the bowel which captures fluid from the intestinal mucosa. The accumulation of fluid in the intestinal lumen produces bulk, stimulates peristalsis, and decreases fecal transit time. Saline laxatives also stimulate the release of cholecystokinin, which stimulates intestinal motility and inhibits the absorption of fluids and electrolytes from the jejunum and ileum.

Absorption, distribution, and excretion
• Bulk laxatives are not absorbed systemically.
• A small amount of ricinoleic acid formed from castor oil is absorbed systemically but is handled by the body like other fatty acids.
• Cascara sagrada, senna, and danthron are only slightly absorbed. Danthron is more readily absorbed. All are metabolized in the liver. These drugs then are either secreted into the intestines or are excreted in the urine and the milk.
• Only a small amount of bisacodyl is systemically absorbed.
• As much as 15% of phenolphthalein is systemically absorbed and undergoes enterohepatic circulation. A portion of the drug is excreted in the urine.
• Emollient laxatives are systemically absorbed and are excreted in the bile.
• As much as one half of emulsified mineral oil may be absorbed, but nonemulsified mineral oil is not significantly absorbed.
• About 20% of the magnesium in magnesium salts is systemically absorbed and excreted in the urine, with a small amount excreted in the milk.
• Up to 10% of the sodium content of sodium phosphate and of sodium biphosphate enemas may be absorbed.

Onset and duration
• Bulk laxatives usually begin to act within 12 to 24 hours, but results may be delayed up to 3 days in some patients.
• Castor oil cleanses the entire bowel in about 3 hours.
• Cascara sagrada, senna, and danthron begin to act in 6 to 24 hours.
• Bisacodyl and phenolphthalein begin to act in 6 to 8 hours when given orally or within 15 to 60 minutes when bisacodyl is given rectally.
• Dioctyl sulfosuccinates begin to act within 24 to 48 hours.
• Mineral oil begins to act in 6 to 8 hours after oral or rectal administration.
• Saline laxatives act within 3 to 6 hours.

Combination products

AGORAL: mineral oil 32% and white phenolphthalein 1.3%.
CAROID AND BILE SALTS: phenolphthalein 32.4 mg, cascara sagrada extract 48.6 mg, caroid 75 mg, capsicum 6.48 mg, and bile salts (as contained in dessicated whole bile 70 mg).
CASYLLIUM: psyllium husk powder 4.1 g, debittered fluidextract cascara sagrada 3 ml, and prune powder 1.2 g.
COMFOLOX-PLUS: dioctyl sodium sulfosuccinate 100 mg and casanthranol 30 mg.
CORRECTOL: yellow phenolphthalein 64.8 mg and dioctyl sodium sulfosuccinate 100 mg.
DIALOSE: dioctyl sodium sulfosuccinate 100 mg and sodium carboxymethylcellulose 400 mg.
DIALOSE-PLUS♦: dioctyl sodium sulfosuccinate 100 mg, sodium carboxymethylcellulose 400 mg, and casanthranol 30 mg.
DORBANTYL: dioctyl sodium sulfosuccinate 50 mg and danthron 25 mg.
DORBANTYL FORTE: dioctyl sodium sulfosuccinate 100 mg and danthron 50 mg.
DOXAN-TABLETS: dioctyl sodium sulfosuccinate 60 mg and danthron 50 mg.
DOXIDAN♦: dioctyl calcium sulfosuccinate 60 mg and danthron 50 mg.
D-S-S PLUS: dioctyl sodium sulfosuccinate 100 mg and casanthranol 30 mg.
HALEY'S M-O: mineral oil (25%) and milk of magnesia.
HYDROCIL, FORTIFIED: blond psyllium coating 40%, gum karaya 10%, and casanthranol (with dextrose) 30 mg.
KONDREMUL WITH CASCARA♦: heavy mineral oil 55%, cascara sagrada extract 660 mg, and Irish moss as emulsifier.
KONDREMUL WITH PHENOLPHTHALEIN♦: heavy mineral oil 55%, white phenolphthalein 147 mg, and Irish moss as emulsifier.
OXIPHEN: phenolphthalein 32.4 mg, cascara sagrada extract 32.4 mg, aloin 8.1 mg, sodium glycocholate 16.2 mg, and sodium taurocholate 16.2 mg.
PERI-COLACE♦ (capsules): dioctyl sodium sulfosuccinate 100 mg and casanthranol 30 mg per 15 ml.
PERI-COLACE (syrup): dioctyl sodium sulfosuccinate 60 mg and casanthranol 30 mg.
PETROGALAR WITH PHENOLPHTHALEIN: mineral oil 65% and phenolphthalein 0.3%.
PRO-LAX: refined psyllium mucilloid and dextrose (in equal amounts).
SENOKOT-S♦: dioctyl sodium sulfosuccinate 50 mg and standardized senna concentrate 187 mg.
SENOKOT WITH PSYLLIUM: psyllium 1 g and standardized senna concentrate 326 mg.
SYLLAMALT: malt-soup extract 3.5 g and powdered psyllium seed husks 3.5 g.
SYLLAMALT EFFERVESCENT: malt-soup extract 25%, powdered psyllium seeds husks 25%, sodium bicarbonate, citric acid, and sugar.

PATIENT TEACHING AID — HOW TO AVOID CONSTIPATION

Dear Patient:

You can alleviate troublesome constipation by following these suggestions:

- Get sufficient rest, at least 6 hours a night.
- Incorporate moderate exercise into your daily routine. Even walking will do; just don't be sedentary.
- Drink at least 8 to 10 glasses of liquid every day. Fluids help keep the intestinal contents in a semisolid state for easier passage. Before breakfast or in the evening, try drinking hot or cold water, plain or with lemon, for bowel stimulation. Prune juice also works well.
- Your diet should have enough fiber (see the fiber chart below) to contribute bulk to the intestines and induce peristalsis. Your richest source of fiber is whole-grain cereals and bran. But be careful; too much bran can create an irritable bowel. When buying breakfast cereals, look for ones with bran in the title or, better yet, read the label for fiber content (low fiber: 0.3 - 1 g, moderate fiber: 1.1 - 2.0 g, high fiber: 2.1 - 4.2 g). Whole wheat and whole rye are good bread choices. Some cereals to include are oatmeal, rolled oats, bran flakes, granola, grape nuts, shredded wheat, wheat flakes, and brown rice.
- Use fat-containing foods, such as bacon, butter, cream, and oil, in moderation. They produce sufficient bulk, but they sometimes cause diarrhea. If you're on a low-fat diet, you should avoid these foods anyway.
- Include an abundance of both raw and cooked vegetables and fruit in your diet, i.e., carrots, apples, oranges, lettuce, stewed fruit, potatoes cooked in skin.
- Avoid highly refined foods, such as white rice, cream of wheat, and farina; white pastries, pie, and cakes; macaroni, spaghetti, noodles; and ice cream.
- If you have any special problems or questions, don't hesitate to call your doctor.

FIBER CONTENT OF SOME COMMON FOODS

Food	Grams of fiber per ¼ cup
Bran flakes (100% bran)	2.2
Bran flakes (40% bran)	1.0
Raisin bran	0.8
Puffed wheat	0.6
Shredded wheat	0.6
Sunflower seeds (kernels)	1.1
Sesame seeds	1.8
Pumpkin seeds (kernels)	0.5
English walnuts	1.2

Food	Grams of fiber per ½ cup
Peanuts, with skins	2.7
Almonds, with skins	2.2
Pecans	1.3
Peanut butter (2 tbsp)	0.7
Whole-grain bread (1 slice)	0.4
Bran muffin (1 muffin)	0.7
Fresh fruit, with skin (1 average)	1.5
Fresh fruit, without skin	1.0
Raw vegetables	1.1

NAME	INDICATIONS & DOSAGE	SIDE EFFECTS
barley-malt extract Maltsupex	*Constipation—* **Adults:** 2 to 3 tablets P.O. with meals and at bedtime for 4 days, then 2 to 4 tablets at bedtime; or 2 tablespoonsful powder or liquid b.i.d. for 3 to 4 days, until stools become soft, then 1 to 2 tablespoonsful at bedtime. **Children over 2 months:** ½ to 2 tablespoonsful in milk or on cereal daily or b.i.d. **Infants 1 or 2 months:** ½ tablespoonful daily with milk or cereal. To prevent constipation, may add 1 to 2 teaspoonsful to each day's feeding.	*GI:* nausea, vomiting, diarrhea (all after excessive use); esophageal, gastric, small intestinal, or colonic strictures when drug is chewed or taken in dry form; abdominal cramps (especially in severe constipation). *Metabolic:* electrolyte depletion. *Other:* laxative dependence in frequent or long-term use.
bisacodyl Biscolax♦, Codylax, Dulcolax♦, Dulcolax Micro-enema♦♦, Fleet Bisacodyl, Rolax, Theralax	*Chronic constipation; preparation for delivery, surgery, or rectal or bowel examination—* **Adults:** 10 to 15 mg P.O. in evening or before breakfast. Up to 30 mg may be used for thorough evacuation needed for examinations or surgery. **Children:** 5 to 10 mg P.O. Rectal: **Adults, and children over 2 years:** 10 mg. **Under 2 years:** 5 mg. Enema: **Adults:** 1.25 oz. **Children under 6 years:** approximately ½ contents of micro enema.	*CNS:* muscle weakness in excessive use. *GI:* abdominal cramps, diarrhea in high doses, burning sensation in rectum with suppositories, nausea. *Metabolic:* alkalosis, hypokalemia, tetany, protein-losing enteropathy in excessive use. *Other:* laxative dependence in long-term or excessive use.
cascara sagrada Cas-Evac **cascara sagrada aromatic fluidextract** **cascara sagrada fluidextract**	*Acute constipation; in preparation for bowel or rectal exam—* **Adults:** 325 mg cascara sagrada tablets P.O. at bedtime; or 120 to 360 mg Bileo-Secrin P.O. at bedtime; or 1 ml fluidextract daily; or 5 ml aromatic fluidextract daily; or 1.25 to 2.5 ml Cas-Evac liquid b.i.d.; or 2.5 to 5 ml Cas-Evac liquid at bedtime. **Children 2 to 12 years:** ½ adult dose. **Children under 2 years:** ¼ adult dose.	*GI:* nausea, vomiting, diarrhea, loss of normal bowel function in excessive use; abdominal cramps, especially in severe constipation; malabsorption of nutrients, "cathartic colon" (syndrome resembling ulcerative colitis radiologically and pathologically) after chronic misuse; discoloration of rectal mucosa after long-term use. *GU:* reddish-pink discoloration in alkaline urine (harmless). *Metabolic:* hypokalemia, protein enteropathy, electrolyte imbalance in excessive use. *Other:* laxative dependence in long-term or excessive use.

♦ Also available in Canada.
♦♦ Available in Canada only.
Unmarked trade names available in United States only.

INTERACTIONS	NURSING CONSIDERATIONS
None significant.	• Contraindicated in abdominal pain, nausea, vomiting, or other symptoms of appendicitis or acute surgical abdomen, and in intestinal obstruction or ulceration, disabling adhesion, or difficulty swallowing. • In diabetics, allow for carbohydrate content of approximately 14 g/tablespoon of liquid, 13 g/tablespoon of powder, and 0.6 g/tablet. • Tell patient to take with at least 8 ounces pleasant-tasting liquids to mask grittiness. To dissolve, mix with a little hot water, then cold. Esophageal or bowel obstruction possible if not taken with sufficient liquid. • Rectal bleeding or failure to respond may indicate need for surgery. • For short-term use. Before giving, determine if patient has adequate fluid intake, lacks exercise, or follows proper diet. Tell him that dietary sources of bulk include bran and other cereals, fresh fruit, and vegetables. • Infants usually need diet change to increase bulk in addition to laxative. • Laxative effect usually takes 12 to 24 hours; may be delayed 3 days. • Bulk laxative; increases bulk and water content of stool. • Not absorbed systemically; nontoxic. • Reduces fecal pH. Especially useful in constipated postpartum mothers, debilitated patients, infants, chronic laxative abuse, irritable bowel syndrome, diverticular disease, and to empty colon before barium enema examination. • Increased intestinal motility lessens absorption of concomitantly administered P.O. drugs. Reschedule dosage.
None significant.	• Contraindicated in abdominal pain, nausea, vomiting, or other symptoms of appendicitis or acute surgical abdomen, or in rectal fissures or ulcerated hemorrhoids. • Rectal bleeding or failure to respond may indicate need for surgery. • Tell patient to swallow enteric-coated tablet whole to avoid GI irritation. Don't give with milk or antacids. Begins to act 6 to 12 hours after oral administration. • Soft, formed stool usually produced 15 to 60 minutes after rectal administration. • Tablets and suppositories may be used together to cleanse colon before and after surgery and before barium enema. • Use for short-term treatment. Stimulant laxative, class of laxative most abused. Discourage excessive use. • Before giving for constipation, determine if patient has adequate fluid intake, lacks exercise, or follows a proper diet. Tell him that dietary sources of bulk include bran and other cereals, fresh fruit, and vegetables. • Store tablets and suppositories at temperature below 86°F. (30°C).
None significant.	• Contraindicated in abdominal pain, nausea, vomiting, or other symptoms of appendicitis or acute surgical abdomen; in acute surgical delirium, fecal impaction, intestinal obstruction or perforation. Use cautiously in rectal bleeding. • Failure to respond may indicate acute condition requiring surgery. • Aromatic cascara fluid extract is less active and less bitter than nonaromatic fluidextract. • Liquid preparations more reliable than solid dosage forms. • Drug of choice among stimulant laxatives. Use for short-term treatment. • Before giving for constipation, determine if patient has adequate fluid intake, lacks exercise, or follows a proper diet. Tell him that dietary sources of bulk include bran and other cereals, fresh fruit, and vegetables.

NAME	INDICATIONS & DOSAGE	SIDE EFFECTS
castor oil Alphamul, Neoloid♦	*Preparation for rectal or bowel exam, or surgery; acute constipation (rarely)*— **Adults:** 15 to 60 ml P.O. as liquid or 1.25 to 3.7 mg P.O. as tablet. **Children over 2 years:** 5 to 15 ml P.O. **Children under 2 years:** 1.25 to 7.5 ml P.O. **Infants:** up to 4 ml P.O. Increased dose produces no greater effect.	*GI:* nausea, vomiting, diarrhea, loss of normal bowel function in excessive use; abdominal cramps, especially in severe constipation; malabsorption of nutrients, "cathartic colon" (syndrome resembling ulcerative colitis radiologically and pathologically) in chronic misuse. May cause constipation after catharsis. *GU:* pelvic congestion in menstruating women. *Metabolic:* hypokalemia, protein enteropathy, other electrolyte imbalance in excessive use. *Other:* laxative dependence in long-term or excessive use.
danthron Anavac, Danivac, Dorbane♦, Duolax, Modane♦, Modane Mild♦, Weslax	*Acute constipation, preparation for rectal or bowel exam, postsurgical and postpartum constipation*— **Adults and children:** 37.5 to 150 mg P.O. after or with evening meal.	*GI:* nausea, vomiting, diarrhea, loss of normal bowel function in excessive use; abdominal cramps, especially in severe constipation; malabsorption of nutrients, "cathartic colon" (syndrome resembling ulcerative colitis radiologically and pathologically) in chronic misuse; discoloration of rectal mucosa in long-term use. *GU:* reddish-pink discoloration in alkaline urine (harmless). *Metabolic:* hypokalemia, protein enteropathy, electrolyte imbalance in excessive use. *Other:* laxative dependence in long-term or excessive use.
dioctyl calcium sulfosuccinate Surfak♦ **dioctyl potassium sulfosuccinate** Kasof, Rectalad Enema **dioctyl sodium sulfosuccinnate** Bu-Lax, Colace, Comfolax, Disonate, Doxinate, D.S.S., Dynoctol, Laxinate, Regutol, Roctate	*Stool softener*— **Adults and older children:** 50 to 300 mg (dioctyl sodium sulfosuccinate) P.O. daily or 240 mg (dioctyl calcium sulfosuccinate and dioctyl potassium sulfosuccinate) P.O. daily until bowel movements are normal; or 5 ml (250 mg) (dioctyl potassium sulfosuccinate) enema. **Children over 12:** 2 ml (100 mg) (dioctyl potassium sulfosuccinate) as enema. **Children 6 to 12 years:** 40 to 120 mg (dioctyl sodium sulfosuccinate) P.O. daily.	*EENT:* throat irritation. *GI:* bitter taste, mild abdominal cramping. *Other:* laxative dependence in long-term or excessive use.

INTERACTIONS	NURSING CONSIDERATIONS
None significant.	• Contraindicated in ulcerative bowel lesions; during menstruation; in abdominal pain, nausea, vomiting, or other symptoms of appendicitis or acute surgical abdomen; in anal or rectal fissures, fecal impaction, intestinal obstruction or perforation. Use cautiously in rectal bleeding. • Failure to respond may indicate acute condition requiring surgery. • Give with juice or carbonated beverage to mask oily taste. Ice held in mouth before taking drug will help prevent tasting it. • Shake emulsion well. Store below 4.4° C. (40° F.). Don't freeze. • Give on empty stomach for best results. • Produces complete evacuation after 3 hours. Warn that after castor oil has emptied bowel, patient will not have bowel movement for 1 to 2 days. • Generally used for diagnostic purposes or therapy requiring thorough evacuation of GI tract. • Use for short-term treatment. Not recommended for routine use; useful for acute constipation not responsive to milder laxatives. • Before giving for constipation, determine if patient has adequate fluid intake, lacks exercise, or follows a proper diet. Tell him that dietary sources of bulk include bran and other cereals, fresh fruit, and vegetables. • Stimulant laxative. • Increased intestinal motility lessens absorption of concomitantly administered P.O. drugs. Reschedule dosage.
None significant.	• Contraindicated in abdominal pain, nausea, vomiting, or other symptoms of appendicitis or acute surgical abdomen; in intestinal obstruction or perforation; and in hepatic dysfunction. Use cautiously in rectal bleeding or fecal impaction. • Failure to respond may indicate acute condition requiring surgery. • Give with fruit juice or carbonated beverage to mask oily taste. • Give on empty stomach for best results. • Produces complete evacuation of bowel in 6 to 24 hours. Warn patient that he will not have another bowel movement for 1 to 2 days. • Generally used for diagnostic purposes or therapy requiring thorough evacuation of GI tract. • Agent of choice for cardiac patients; reduces strain of evacuation. • Use for short-term treatment. Not recommended for routine use; useful for acute constipation not responsive to milder laxatives. • Before giving for constipation, determine if patient has adequate fluid intake, lacks exercise, or follows a proper diet. Tell him that dietary sources of bulk include bran and other cereals, fresh fruit, and vegetables. • Stimulant laxative.
None significant.	• Sodium salts: contraindicated in sodium-restricted diets, edema, congestive heart failure, renal dysfunction. • Potassium salts: contraindicated in renal dysfunction. • Give liquid in milk, fruit juice, or infant formula to mask bitter taste. • Not for use in treating existing constipation but prevents constipation from developing. • Laxative of choice in patients who should not strain during defecation, such as those recovering from myocardial infarction or rectal surgery; in disease of rectum and anus, which makes passage of firm stool difficult; or postpartum constipation. • Acts within 24 to 48 hours to produce firm, semisolid stool. • Instruct patient that dietary sources of bulk include bran and other cereals, fresh fruit, and vegetables. • Emollient laxative or stool softener; doesn't stimulate intestinal peristaltic movements. • Store at 15° to 30°C. (59° to 86°F.). Protect liquid from light.

(continued on following page)

NAME	INDICATIONS & DOSAGE	SIDE EFFECTS
dioctyl sodium sulfosuccinate *(continued)*	**Children 3 to 6 years:** 20 to 60 mg (dioctyl sodium sulfosuccinate) P.O. daily. **Children under 3 years:** 10 to 40 mg (dioctyl sodium sulfosuccinate) P.O. daily. Higher doses are for initial therapy. Adjust dose to individual response. Usual dose in children and adults with minimal needs: 50 to 150 mg (calcium sulfosuccinate) P.O. daily.	
magnesium salts Concentrated Milk of Magnesia, Magnesium Citrate, Magnesium Sulfate, Milk of Magnesia	*Constipation, to evacuate bowel before surgery—* **Adults, and children over 6 years:** 15 g (magnesium sulfate) P.O. in glass of water; 10 to 20 ml concentrated milk of magnesia P.O.; or 15 to 30 ml milk of magnesia P.O., or 5 to 10 oz. magnesium citrate at bedtime.	*GI:* abdominal cramping, nausea. *Metabolic:* fluid and electrolyte disturbances if used daily. *Other:* laxative dependence in long-term or excessive use.
methylcellulose Cellothyl, Cologel, Hydrolose, Syncelose	*Chronic constipation—* **Adults:** 5 to 20 ml liquid P.O. t.i.d. with a glass of water, or 15 ml syrup P.O. morning and evening. **Children:** 5 to 10 ml P.O. daily or b.i.d.	*GI:* nausea, vomiting, diarrhea (all after excessive use); esophageal, gastric, small intestinal, or colonic strictures when drug is chewed or taken in dry form; abdominal cramps, especially in severe constipation. *Other:* laxative dependence in long-term or excessive use.
mineral oil Agoral Plain, Fleet Mineral Oil Enema, Kondremul Plain♦, Neo-Cultol, Petrogalar Plain, Saf-Tip Oil Retention Enema	*Constipation; preparation for bowel studies or surgery—* **Adults:** 15 to 30 ml P.O., usually at bedtime, or 4 oz. enema. **Children:** 5 to 15 ml P.O. at bedtime, or 1 to 2 oz. enema.	*GI:* nausea, vomiting, diarrhea in excessive use; abdominal cramps, especially in severe constipation; decreased absorption of nutrients and fat-soluble vitamins, resulting in deficiency; slowed healing after hemorrhoidectomy and increased risk of rectal infections due to seepage from rectum. *Other:* laxative dependence in long-term or excessive use.

INTERACTIONS	NURSING CONSIDERATIONS
None significant.	• Contraindicated in abdominal pain, nausea, vomiting, or other symptoms of appendicitis or acute surgical abdomen; in myocardial damage, heart block, imminent delivery, fecal impaction, rectal fissures, intestinal obstruction or perforation, renal disease. Use cautiously in rectal bleeding. • Failure to respond may indicate acute condition requiring surgery. • For short-term therapy; don't use longer than 1 week. • Saline laxative; produces watery stool in 3 to 6 hours. • Magnesium sulfate is more potent than other saline laxatives. • Before giving for constipation, determine if patient has adequate fluid intake, lacks exercise, or follows a proper diet. Tell him that dietary sources of bulk include bran and other cereals, fresh fruit, and vegetables. • Magnesium may accumulate in renal insufficiency.
None significant.	• Contraindicated in abdominal pain, nausea, vomiting, or other symptoms of appendicitis or acute surgical abdomen; and in intestinal obstruction or ulceration, disabling adhesion, or difficulty swallowing. • Laxative effect usually takes 12 to 24 hours, but may be delayed 3 days. • Tell patient to take drug with at least 8 ounces of pleasant-tasting liquid to mask grittiness. • Especially useful in postpartum constipation, debilitated patients, chronic laxative abuse, irritable bowel syndrome, diverticular disease, colostomies, and to empty colon before barium enema examinations. • Rectal bleeding or failure to respond may indicate need for surgery. • Use for short-term treatment. • Before giving for constipation, determine if patient has adequate fluid intake, lacks exercise, or follows a proper diet. Tell him that dietary sources of bulk include bran and other cereals, fresh fruit, and vegetables. • Not absorbed systemically; nontoxic. • Bulk laxative; increases bulk and water content of stool. • Instruct patient to notify doctor in 1 week about response to therapy.
None significant.	• Contraindicated in abdominal pain, nausea, vomiting, or other symptoms of appendicitis or acute surgical abdomen; in fecal impaction, intestinal obstruction or perforation. Use cautiously in young children; in elderly or debilitated patients due to susceptibility to lipid pneumonitis through aspiration, absorption, and transport from intestinal mucosa; in rectal bleeding. Enema contraindicated in children under 2 years. • Failure to respond may indicate acute condition requiring surgery. • Don't give drug with meals or immediately after, as it delays passage of food from stomach. More active on an empty stomach. • A lubricant laxative. • Give with fruit juices or carbonated drinks to disguise taste. • Use when patient needs to ease the strain of evacuation. • Before giving for constipation, determine if patient has adequate fluid intake, lacks exercise, or follows a proper diet. Tell him that dietary sources of bulk include bran and other cereals, fresh fruit, and vegetables.

NAME	INDICATIONS & DOSAGE	SIDE EFFECTS
phenolphthalein Alophen, Espotabs, Evac-U-Lac, Ex-Lax, Feen-A-Mint, Phenolax	*Constipation—* **Adults:** 60 to 200 mg P.O., preferably at bedtime.	*GI:* diarrhea, colic in large doses; factitious nausea, vomiting, loss of normal bowel function in excessive use; abdominal cramps, especially in severe constipation; malabsorption of nutrients, "cathartic colon" (syndrome resembling ulcerative colitis radiologically and pathologically) in chronic misuse. *GI:* reddish discoloration in alkaline feces. *GU:* reddish-pink discoloration in alkaline urine. *Skin:* dermatitis, pruritus. *Other:* laxative dependence in long-term or excessive use.
psyllium Effersyllium Instant Mix, Konsyl, L.A. Formula, Metamucil◆, Metamucil Instant Mix◆, Modane Bulk, Mucillium, Mucilose, Plain Hydrocil, Siblin◆, Syllact	*Constipation; bowel management—* **Adults:** 1 to 2 rounded tsp. P.O. in full glass of liquid daily, b.i.d., or t.i.d., followed by second glass of liquid; or 1 packet P.O. dissolved in water daily, b.i.d., or t.i.d. **Children over 6 years:** 1 level tsp. P.O. in ½ glass of liquid at bedtime.	*GI:* nausea, vomiting, diarrhea, all after excessive use; esophageal, gastric, small intestinal, or colonic strictures when drug taken in dry form; abdominal cramps, especially in severe constipation.
senna Black Draught, Glysennid, Senokot, X-Prep	*Acute constipation, preparation for bowel or rectal exam—* **Adults:** 2 tablets or ¼ to 1 level teaspoon granules P.O. with liquid; 12 to 24 mg calcium salts tablets h.s.; or 10 to 15 ml syrup h.s.; or 1 suppository h.s. **Children over 60 lbs.:** ½ adult dose of tablets or granules (except Black Draught tablets and granules not recommended for children).	*GI:* nausea, vomiting, diarrhea, loss of normal bowel function in excessive use; abdominal cramps, especially in severe constipation; malabsorption of nutrients, "cathartic colon" (syndrome resembling ulcerative colitis radiologically in chronic misuse; may cause constipation after catharsis), yellow, yellow-greenish cast feces, diarrhea in nursing infants of mothers on senna; darkened pigmentation of rectal mucosa in long-term use which

INTERACTIONS	NURSING CONSIDERATIONS
None significant.	• Contraindicated in abdominal pain, nausea, vomiting, or other symptoms of appendicitis or acute surgical abdomen; in fecal impaction, intestinal obstruction or perforation. Use cautiously in rectal bleeding. • Failure to respond may indicate acute condition requiring surgery. • Laxative effect may last up to 3 to 4 days. • Produces semisolid stool within 6 to 8 hours, with little or no griping. • Warn patient with rash to avoid sun and discontinue use. • Before giving for constipation, determine if patient has adequate fluid intake, lacks exercise, or follows a proper diet. Tell him that dietary sources of bulk include bran and other cereals, fresh fruit, and vegetables. • Drug is available in many dosage forms. Most popular over-the-counter laxative: a frequent constituent of chewing gum and chocolate laxatives. Stimulant laxative, class of laxative most abused.
None significant.	• Contraindicated in abdominal pain, nausea, vomiting, or other symptoms of appendicitis; and in intestinal obstruction or ulceration, disabling adhesion, or difficulty swallowing. • Metamucil Instant Mix (effervescent form) contains a significant amount of sodium and should not be used for patients on sodium-restricted diets. • Mix with at least 8 ounces of cold, pleasant-tasting liquid to mask grittiness and stir only a few seconds. Patient should drink it immediately or mixture will solidify. Follow with additional glass of liquid. • Rectal bleeding or failure to respond may indicate need for surgery. • Use for short-term treatment. Don't use for maintenance. • Frequent use of laxatives can cause drug dependence for evacuation. • Before giving for constipation, determine if patient has adequate fluid intake, lacks exercise, or follows a proper diet. Tell him that dietary sources of bulk include bran and other cereals, fresh fruit, and vegetables. • Laxative effect usually seen in 12 to 24 hours, but may be delayed 3 days. • Popular bulk laxative; increases bulk and water content of stool. • Highly refined, purified vegetable mucilloid; from seeds of platango plant. • Not absorbed systemically; nontoxic. Especially useful in postpartum constipation, debilitated patients, chronic laxative abuse, irritable bowel syndrome, diverticular disease, and in combination with other laxatives to empty colon before barium enema examinations.
None significant.	• Contraindicated in ulcerative bowel lesions; in nausea, vomiting, abdominal pain, or other symptoms of appendicitis or acute surgical abdomen; in fecal impaction, intestinal obstruction, or perforation. • Use for short-term treatment. • Failure to respond may indicate acute condition requiring surgery. • More potent than cascara sagrada; produces more griping. Acts in 6 to 10 hours. X-Prep gives thorough, strong bowel action beginning in 6 hours. • Most recommended stimulant laxative. • Before giving for constipation, determine if patient has adequate fluid intake, lacks exercise, or follows a proper diet. Tell him that dietary sources of bulk include bran and other cereals, fresh fruit, and vegetables. • After X-Prep liquid is taken, diet should be confined to clear liquids.

(continued on following page)

NAME	INDICATIONS & DOSAGE	SIDE EFFECTS
senna *(continued)*	**Children 1 month to 1 year:** 1.25 to 2.5 ml Senokot syrup P.O. h.s. X-Prep used solely as single dose for preradiographic bowel evacuation. Give ¾ oz. powder dissolved in juice or 2.5 oz. liquid between 2 to 4 p.m. on day before X-ray procedure. May be given in divided doses for elderly or debilitated patients.	is usually reversible within 4 to 12 months after stopping drug. *GU:* reddish-pink discoloration in alkaline urine; yellowish-brown color to acid urine. *Metabolic:* hypokalemia, protein enteropathy, electrolyte imbalance with excessive use. *Other:* laxative dependence in long-term or excessive use.
sodium biphosphate Enemeez, Fleet enema♦, Phospho-Soda, Saf-Tip Phosphate Enema, Travad Enema♦ **sodium phosphate** Sal-Hepatica	*Constipation:*— **Adults:** 5 to 20 ml liquid P.O. with water; or 4 g powder P.O. dissolved in warm water; or 20 to 46 ml solution mixed with 4 oz. cold water; or 2 to 4.5 oz. as enema.	*GI:* abdominal cramping. *Metabolic:* fluid and electrolyte disturbances (hypernatremia, hyperphosphatemia) if used daily. *Other:* laxative dependence in long-term or excessive use.

INTERACTIONS	NURSING CONSIDERATIONS
None significant.	• Contraindicated in abdominal pain, nausea, vomiting, or other symptoms of appendicitis or acute surgical abdomen; in intestinal obstruction or perforation; edema; congestive heart failure; megacolon; impaired renal function; and in patients on salt-restricted diets. • Failure to respond may indicate acute condition requiring surgery. • Available in oral and rectal forms. • Before giving for constipation, determine if patient has adequate fluid intake, lacks exercise, or follows a proper diet. Tell him that dietary sources of bulk include bran and other cereals, fresh fruit, and vegetables. • Saline laxative; up to 10% of sodium content may be absorbed. • Enema form elicits response within 5 to 10 minutes. • Used in preparation for barium enema and for fecal impaction.

45

Emetics and antiemetics

apomorphine hydrochloride
benzquinamide hydrochloride
buclizine hydrochloride
cyclizine hydrocholoride
cyclizine lactate
dimenhydrinate
diphenidol
ipecac syrup
meclizine hydrochloride
prochlorperazine edisylate
prochlorperazine maleate
thiethylperazine maleate
trimethobenzamide hydrochloride

Emetics are used to induce vomiting after ingestion of poisonous substances to prevent extensive absorption. The use of emetics with symptomatic and supportive care in many cases can be lifesaving. Emetics should be given immediately but may still be useful even if administration is delayed. Emetics should not be used after ingestion of corrosives and certain other substances, however, since further damage may result.

Antiemetics are used to relieve nausea and vomiting resulting from various conditions. Their use is clearly indicated whenever vomiting is severe enough to produce significant fluid, electrolyte, and nutrient losses. They are also used to prevent damage to the esophagus from violent retching, disruption of postoperative suture lines, and retching after intraocular surgery.

Major uses

- Emetics induce vomiting after poisoning from ingestion of toxic substances.
- Antiemetics are used to treat and prevent nausea, vomiting, and, occasionally, dizziness.

Mechanism of action

- Apomorphine hydrochloride induces vomiting by acting directly on the chemoreceptor trigger zone.
- Ipecac syrup induces vomiting by acting locally on the gastric mucosa and centrally on the chemoreceptor trigger zone.
- Antihistamine antiemetics, such as buclizine hydrochloride, cyclizine hydrochloride and lactate, dimenhydrinate, and meclizine hydrochloride, may affect neural pathways originating in the labyrinth to inhibit nausea and vomiting, but the exact mechanism of action is unknown.
- Phenothiazine antiemetics, such as prochlorperazine and thiethylperazine maleate, act on the chemoreceptor trigger zone to inhibit nausea and vomiting, and in larger doses

partially depress the vomiting center as well.
• Benzquinamide hydrochloride and trimethobenzamide hydrochloride may act on the chemoreceptor zone to inhibit nausea and vomiting.

Absorption, distribution, and excretion
• Apomorphine hydrochloride acts within 10 to 15 minutes after parenteral administration.
• Ipecac absorption occurs within 30 minutes.
• Benzquinamide is rapidly absorbed after intramuscular administration and is rapidly distributed throughout body tissues, with highest concentrations in the hepatic and the kidneys. It is metabolized in the hepatic and excreted in the feces and urine.
• Trimethobenzamide is less effective than other antiemetics. Its duration of action is 4 to 6 hours.
• Diphenidol is rapidly absorbed and completely excreted in the urine and feces within 3 to 4 days after administration.

Onset and duration
• Duration of action of meclizine hydrochloride is 24 to 48 hours.
• Prochlorperazine begins to act in 30 to 40 minutes after oral administration and has a duration of action of 3 to 4 hours; the extended-release form also begins to act in 30 to 40 minutes but has a duration of action of 10 to 12 hours. Prochlorperazine begins to act within 1 hour after rectal administration. After parenteral administration, it has an onset of action within 10 to 20 minutes and a duration of action of 3 to 4 hours.
• Benzquinamide hydrochloride begins to act within 15 minutes after parenteral administration and has a duration of action of 3 to 4 hours.
• Trimethobenzamide hydrochloride begins to act within 10 to 20 minutes after oral administration and has a duration of action of 3 to 4 hours. After intramuscular administration it begins to act within 15 to 30 minutes and has a duration of action of 2 to 3 hours.
• Diphenidol begins to act within 30 to 45 minutes after oral administration and within 15 minutes after parenteral administration. By either route, the duration of action is 3 to 6 hours.

Combination products
None.

NAME	INDICATIONS & DOSAGE	SIDE EFFECTS
apomorphine hydrochloride Controlled substance Schedule II	*To induce vomiting in poisoning—* **Adults:** 2 to 10 mg S.C. preceded by 200 to 300 ml water. Don't repeat. **Children over 1 year:** 0.07 mg/Kg S.C. preceded by up to 2 glasses of water. **Children under 1 year:** 0.07 mg/Kg S.C. preceded by ½ to 1 glass of water.	*CNS:* depression, euphoria, restlessness, tremors. *CV:* acute circulatory failure in elderly or debilitated patients, tachycardia. *Other:* depressed respiratory center in large or repeated doses.
benzquinamide hydrochloride Emete-Con	*Nausea and vomiting associated with anesthesia and surgery—* **Adults:** 50 mg I.M. (0.5 mg/Kg to 1 mg/Kg). May repeat in 1 hour, and thereafter q 3 to 4 hours, p.r.n.; or 25 mg (0.2 mg/Kg to 0.4 mg/Kg) I.V. as single dose, administered slowly.	*CNS:* drowsiness (common), fatigue, insomnia, restlessness, headache, excitation, tremors, twitching, dizziness. *CV:* sudden rise in blood pressure and transient arrhythmias (premature atrial and ventricular contractions, atrial fibrillation) after I.V. administration; hypertension; hypotension. *EENT:* dry mouth, salivation, blurred vision. *GI:* anorexia, nausea, hiccups. *Skin:* urticaria, rash. *Other:* muscle weakness, flushing, sweating, chills, fever. May mask signs of overdose of toxic agents or underlying conditions (intestinal obstruction, brain tumor).
buclizine hydrochloride Bucladin-S, Softran	*Motion sickness (prevention)—* **Adults:** 50 mg P.O. at least ½ hour before beginning travel. If needed, may repeat another 50 mg P.O. after 4 to 6 hours. *Nausea (treatment)—* **Adults:** 50 mg P.O., up to 150 mg P.O. daily in severe cases. Maintenance dose is 50 mg b.i.d.	*CNS:* drowsiness, headache, dizziness, jitteriness. *EENT:* blurred vision, dry mouth. *GU:* urinary retention. *Other:* may mask symptoms of ototoxicity, intestinal obstruction, or brain tumor.
cyclizine hydrochloride **cyclizine lactate** Marezine, Marzine••	*Motion sickness (prevention and treatment)—* **Adults:** 50 mg P.O. (hydrochloride) ½ hour before travel, then q 4 to 6 hours, p.r.n., to maximum of 200 mg daily; or 50 mg I.M.	*CNS:* drowsiness, dizziness, auditory and visual hallucinations. *CV:* hypotension. *EENT:* blurred vision, dry mouth. *GI:* constipation. *GU:* urinary retention.

• Also available in Canada.
•• Available in Canada only.
Unmarked trade names available in United States only.

INTERACTIONS	NURSING CONSIDERATIONS
None significant.	• Contraindicated in hypersensitivity to narcotics; impending shock; corrosive poisoning; narcosis resulting from opiates, barbiturates, alcohol, or other CNS depressants; and in patients too inebriated to stand unaided. Use cautiously in children and in patients who are debilitated, have cardiac decompensation, or are predisposed to nausea and vomiting. • Don't give after ingestion of petroleum distillates (e.g., kerosene, gasoline) or volatile oils; retching and vomiting may cause aspiration and lead to bronchospasm, pulmonary edema, or aspiration pneumonitis. Vegetable oil will delay absorption of these substances. • Don't give after ingestion of caustic substances, such as lye; additional injury to the esophagus and mediastinum can occur. • Keep narcotic antagonists, such as naloxone, available to help stop vomiting and to alleviate drowsiness. • When absorbable poison is ingested or if delay in giving emetic is expected, give activated charcoal P.O. immediately after apomorphine HCl. • Vomiting occurs in 5 to 10 minutes in adults. If vomiting doesn't occur within 15 minutes, gastric lavage should begin. Apomorphine HCl is emetic of choice when rapid removal of poisons is necessary, and when identification of enteric-coated tablets or other ingested toxic material in vomitus is important. Stomach contents are usually expelled completely; vomitus may also contain material from upper portion of intestinal tract.
None significant.	• I.V. use contraindicated in cardiovascular disease. Don't give I.V. within 15 minutes of preanesthetic or concomitant cardiovascular drugs. • Give I.M. injections in large muscle mass. Use deltoid area only if well developed. Don't inject into lower and midthird of upper arm. Aspirate syringe for I.M. injection to avoid inadvertent intravascular injection. • Reconstituted solution stable for 14 days at room temperature. Store dry powder and reconstituted solution in light-resistant container. • Monitor blood pressure frequently. • Excellent antiemetic if prochlorperazine (Compazine) is contraindicated.
None significant.	• Warn patient against driving and other hazardous activities until response to drug is established. • Tablets may be placed in mouth and allowed to dissolve without water. May also be chewed or swallowed whole. • Piperazine antihistamine.
None significant.	• Use cautiously in glaucoma, GU or GI obstruction, in elderly males with possible prostatic hypertrophy. • Warn patient against driving and other hazardous activities until response to drug is determined. • Antihistamine. • Store in cool place.

(continued on following page)

NAME	INDICATIONS & DOSAGE	SIDE EFFECTS
cyclizine *(continued)*	(lactate) q 4 to 6 hours, p.r.n. *Postop vomiting (prevention)—* 50 mg I.M. (lactate) preop or 20 to 30 minutes before expected termination of surgery; then postop 50 mg I.M. (lactate) q 4 to 6 hours, p.r.n.; or 100 mg rectally (hydrochloride) q 4 to 6 hours. *Motion sickness and postop vomiting—* **Children 6 to 12 years:** 3 mg/Kg (lactate) I.M. divided t.i.d., or 25 mg (hydrochloride) P.O. q 4 to 6 hours p.r.n.	*Other:* may mask symptoms of ototoxicity, brain tumor, or intestinal obstruction.
dimenhydrinate Dimen, Dimentabs, Dipendrate, Dramaject, Dramamine♦, Dramamine Junior, Dramocen, Dymenate, Eldodram, Gravol♦♦, Hydrate, Hypoemesis, Marmine, Nauseal♦♦, Nauseatol♦♦, Novodimenate♦♦, Ram, Reidamine, Signate, Travamine♦♦, Trav-Arex, Traveltabs, Vertiban, Wehamine	*Nausea, vomiting, dizziness of motion sickness (treatment and prevention)—* **Adults:** 50 mg P.O. q 4 hours, or 100 mg q 4 hours if drowsiness is not objectionable; or 100 mg rectally daily or b.i.d. if oral route is not practical; or 50 mg I.M., p.r.n.; or 50 mg I.V. diluted in 10 ml NaCl solution, injected over 2 minutes. **Children:** 6 mg/Kg P.O. or I.M. or rectally, divided q.i.d. Maximum 300 mg daily.	*CNS:* drowsiness, headache, incoordination, dizziness. *CV:* palpitations, hypotension. *EENT:* blurred vision, tinnitus, dry mouth and respiratory passages. *Other:* may mask symptoms of ototoxicity, brain tumor, or intestinal obstruction.
diphenidol Vontrol♦	*Peripheral (labyrinthine) dizziness; nausea and vomiting—* **Adults:** 25 to 50 mg P.O. q 4 hours, p.r.n., or 20 to 40 mg deep I.M. injection (for rapid control of acute symptoms), then another 20 mg I.M. after 1 hour if symptoms persist. Thereafter 20 to 40 mg I.M. q 4 hours, p.r.n., or 20 mg I.V. injected directly through venoclysis already in operation (for rapid control of acute symptoms). May inject another 20 mg I.V. after 1 hour if symptoms persist, then switch to P.O. or I.M. route. Total daily dosage should not exceed 300 mg. *Nausea and vomiting—* **Children:** 0.9 mg/Kg P.O. or rectally, or 0.4 mg/Kg I.M. Give children's doses no more frequently than q 4 hours unless symptoms persist after 1 dose, then repeat q 4 hours, p.r.n. Maximum children's dose 5.5 mg/Kg P.O. daily; or 3.3 mg/Kg I.M. daily.	*CNS:* drowsiness, dizziness, confusion. *CV:* transient hypotension. *EENT:* auditory and visual hallucinations, disorientation occur within 3 days of starting drug; subside within 3 days after stopping drug. *GI:* dry mouth, nausea, indigestion, heartburn, antiemetic activity. *Skin:* urticaria. *Other:* antiemetic effect may mask signs of overdose of drugs, or may obscure diagnosis of intestinal obstruction, brain tumor, or other conditions.

INTERACTIONS	NURSING CONSIDERATIONS
None significant.	• Use cautiously in seizures, narrow-angle glaucoma, enlargement of prostate gland. • Undiluted solution is irritating to veins; may sclerose. • Antihistamine. • Warn patient not to drive a car or operate dangerous machinery. • May mask ototoxicity of aminoglycoside antibiotics.
None significant.	• Contraindicated in anuria. Use cautiously in glaucoma, pyloric stenosis, pylorospasm, obstructive lesions of GI or GU tract, prostatic hypertrophy, or organic cardiospasm. • I.V. use contraindicated in children and in sinus tachycardia. • Don't give S.C. • Drug should be stopped if auditory or visual hallucinations, or disorientation or confusion occur. • Closely supervise patient. Patients are usually hospitalized when receiving this drug. • Treatment of toxicity is symptomatic and supportive. • Used in Meniere's disease, following middle and inner ear surgery, labyrinthine disturbances, and to control nausea and vomiting associated with infectious disease, malignancies, radiation sickness, general anesthetics, and antineoplastic agents.

NAME	INDICATIONS & DOSAGE	SIDE EFFECTS
ipecac syrup	*To induce vomiting in poisoning*— **Adults:** 15 to 30 ml P.O., followed by 200 to 300 ml of water. **Children 1 year or older:** 15 ml P.O., preceded by about 200 ml of water. **Children under 1 year:** 5 to 10 ml P.O., preceded by about 200 ml of water. May repeat dose once after 20 minutes, if necessary.	*CV:* cardiac disturbances, atrial fibrillation, or fatal myocarditis if drug is absorbed (e.g., if patient doesn't vomit within 30 minutes).
meclizine hydrochloride Antivert♦, Bonamine♦♦, Bonine, Lamine, Roclizine, Vertrol, Whevert	*Dizziness*— **Adults:** 25 to 100 mg P.O. daily in divided doses. Dose varies with patient response. *Motion sickness*— **Adults:** 25 to 50 mg P.O. 1 hour before travel, repeated daily for duration of journey.	*CNS:* drowsiness, fatigue. *EENT:* dry mouth, blurred vision. *Other:* may mask symptoms of ototoxicity, brain tumor, or intestinal obstruction.
prochlorperazine edisylate **prochlorperazine maleate** Compazine, Stemetil♦♦	*Preop nausea control*—5 to 10 mg I.M. 1 to 2 hours before induction of anesthetic, repeat once in 30 minutes, if necessary; or 5 to 10 mg I.V. 15 to 30 minutes before induction of anesthetic (repeat once if necessary); or 20 mg/liter isotonic solution by I.V. infusion, added to infusion 15 to 30 minutes before induction. Maximum parenteral dose 40 mg daily. *Severe nausea, vomiting*— **Adults:** 5 to 10 mg P.O. t.i.d. or q.i.d.; or 15 mg sustained-release form P.O. on arising; or 10 mg sustained-release form P.O. q 12 hours; or 25 mg rectally b.i.d. (may repeat rectal dose q 6 hours); or 5 to 10 mg I.M. injected deeply into upper outer quadrant of gluteal region. Repeat q 3 to 4 hours, p.r.n. **Children 18 to 31 Kg:** 2.5 mg P.O. or rectally t.i.d.; or 5 mg P.O. or rectally b.i.d. Maximum 15 mg daily; or 0.132 mg/Kg deep	The phenothiazines are related structurally and therefore have the potential to cause all the side effects listed; however, all may not have been reported with each drug. *Blood:* agranulocytosis and other dyscrasias. *CNS:* drowsiness, extrapyramidal reactions (akathisia, acute dystonias, parkinsonism, tardive dyskinesias), moderate incidence of sedation, EEG changes, cerebral edema, headache. *CV:* moderate incidence of orthostatic hypotension (possible shock), tachycardia, fainting, dizziness, arrhythmias, pallor. *EENT:* visual impairment, nasal congestion. *GI:* anorexia, dyspepsia, constipation, diarrhea, cholestatic jaundice, paralytic ileus, excessive salivation, increased appetite, weight changes, "oral syndrome" (dry mouth; gum changes; stomatitis; cracked lips; white or black hairy tongue; bald, red tongue; pseudomembrane in mouth).

INTERACTIONS	NURSING CONSIDERATIONS
Activated charcoal: neutralized emetic effect. Don't give together but may give activated charcoal after vomiting has occurred.	• Contraindicated in semicomatose or unconscious patients, severe inebriation, convulsions, shock, loss of gag reflex. • Don't give after ingestion of petroleum distillates (e.g., kerosene, gasoline) or volatile oils; retching and vomiting may cause aspiration and lead to bronchospasm, pulmonary edema, or aspiration pneumonitis. Vegetable oil will delay absorption of these substances. • Don't give after ingestion of caustic substances, such as lye; additional injury to the esophagus and mediastinum can occur. • Clearly indicate ipecac *syrup,* not single word "ipecac," to avoid confusion with fluidextract. Fluidextract is 14 times more concentrated and if advertently used instead of syrup may cause death. • Induces vomiting within 30 minutes in more than 90% of patients; average time usually less than 20 minutes. • Stomach is usually emptied completely; vomitus may contain some intestinal material as well. • In antiemetic toxicity, ipecac syrup is usually effective if less than 1 hour has passed since ingestion of antiemetic. • Recommend that 1 ounce of syrup be readily available in the home when child becomes 1 year old for immediate use in case of emergency. • No systemic toxicity with doses of 30 ml or less. • If 2 doses do not induce vomiting, gastric lavage is necessary.
None significant.	• Warn patient against driving and other hazardous activities until drug response is determined. • Antihistamine with a slower onset and longer duration of action than other antihistamine antiemetics.
Anticholinergics, including antidepressant and antiparkinson agents: increased anticholinergic activity, aggravated parkinson-like symptoms. Use together cautiously. *Antacids:* inhibited absorption of oral phenothiazines. Separate antacid and phenothiazine dosage by at least 2 hours. *Barbiturates:* may decrease phenothiazine effect. Monitor patient for decreased antiemetic effect.	• Contraindicated in phenothiazine hypersensitivity, coma, depression, CNS depression, bone marrow depression, subcortical damage, pediatric surgery, use of spinal or epidural anesthetic or adrenergic blocking agents, alcohol usage. Use with caution in combination with other CNS depressants, hepatic disease, elderly or debilitated patients, arteriosclerosis or cardiovascular disease (may cause sudden drop in blood pressure), exposure to extreme heat or cold (including antipyretic therapy), respiratory disorders, hypocalcemia, vomiting in children, acutely ill or dehydrated children, convulsive disorders or severe reactions to insulin or electroshock therapy, suspected brain tumor or intestinal obstruction, glaucoma or prostatic hypertrophy. • A piperazine phenothiazine. • Store in light-resistant container. Slight yellowing does not affect potency; discard markedly discolored solutions. • Since drug has a very long duration of action, timed-release capsules have no significant advantage over ordinary oral dosage forms. • Use only when vomiting can't be controlled by other measures, or when only a few doses are required. If more than 4 doses needed in 24-hour period, notify doctor. • Not effective in motion sickness. • To prevent contact dermatitis, avoid getting concentrate or injection solution on hands or clothing. • Dilute concentrate with tomato or fruit juice, milk, coffee, carbonated beverage, tea, water, soup, or pudding. • Monitor CBC and hepatic function studies. • Warn patient against driving and other hazardous activities until re-

(continued on following page)

NAME	INDICATIONS & DOSAGE	SIDE EFFECTS
prochlorperazine *(continued)*	I.M. injection. (Control usually obtained with 1 dose.) **Children 14 to 17 Kg:** 2.5 mg P.O. or rectally b.i.d. or t.i.d. Maximum 10 mg daily; or 0.132 mg/Kg deep I.M. injection. (Control usually obtained with 1 dose.) **Children 9 to 13 Kg:** 2.5 mg P.O. or rectally daily or b.i.d. Maximum 7.5 mg daily; or 0.132 mg/Kg deep I.M. injection. (Control usually obtained with 1 dose.)	*GU:* dark urine, difficult urination, incontinence, delayed ovulation, menstrual irregularities, changed libido, impotence, inhibited ejaculation, glycosuria. *Metabolic:* hyper- and hypothermia. *Skin:* photosensitivity (yellowish-brown or grayish-purple pigment deposits after sun exposure), dermatoses (erythematous and eczematous). *Other:* heat prostration, respiratory distress, fever, asthma, edema (laryngeal, angioneurotic, peripheral), gynecomastia, lactation. *After abrupt withdrawal:* gastritis, nausea, vomiting, dizziness, tremors, feeling of warmth or cold, sweating, tachycardia, headache, insomnia.
thiethylperazine maleate Torecan◆	*Nausea, vomiting*— **Adults:** 10 mg P.O., I.M., or rectally daily, b.i.d. or t.i.d.	The phenothiazines are related structurally and therefore have the potential to cause all the side effects listed; however, all may not have been reported with each drug. *Blood:* agranulocytosis and other dyscrasias. *CNS:* drowsiness, high incidence of extrapyramidal reactions (akathisia, acute dystonias, parkinsonism, tardive dyskinesias), low to moderate incidence of sedation, EEG changes, headache, cerebral edema. *CV:* orthostatic hypotension (possible shock), tachycardia, fainting, dizziness, arrhythmias, pallor. *EENT:* visual impairment, nasal congestion. *GI:* anorexia, excessive salivation, dyspepsia, constipation, diarrhea, cholestatic jaundice, paralytic ileus, increased appetite, weight gain, "oral syndrome" (dry mouth, gum changes, stomatitis, cracked lips, white or black hairy tongue, bald and beefy red tongue, pseudomembrane in mouth). *GU:* dark urine, difficult urination, incontinence, delayed ovulation, menstrual irregularities, changed libido, impotence, inhibited ejaculation, glycosuria. *Metabolic:* hyper- and hypoglycemia, hyper- and hypothermia. *Skin:* photosensitivity (yellowish-brown or grayish-purple pigment deposits after sun exposure), sweating, dermatoses (erythematous and eczematous).

INTERACTIONS	NURSING CONSIDERATIONS
	sponse to drug is determined. • Watch for orthostatic hypotension. • Do not give S.C. or mix in syringe with another drug. • For symptoms and treatment of toxicity, see p. 1120.
Anticholinergics, including antidepressants and antiparkinson agents: increased anticholinergic activity, aggravated parkinson-like symptoms. Use together cautiously. *Antacids:* inhibited absorption of oral phenothiazines. Separate antacid and phenothiazine dosage by at least 2 hours. *Barbiturates:* may decrease phenothiazine effect. Monitor for decreased antiemetic effect.	• Contraindicated in severe CNS depression, hepatic disease, coma, phenothiazine hypersensitivity. • Don't give I.V. • For nausea and vomiting associated with anesthesia and surgery, give deep I.M. injection on or shortly before terminating anesthesia. • Possibly effective in dizziness; not effective in motion sickness. • A phenothiazine. • Use only when vomiting can't be controlled by other measures, or when only a few doses are required. • If drug gets on skin, wash off at once to prevent contact dermatitis. • For symptoms and treatment of toxicity, see p. 1120.

(continued on following page)

NAME	INDICATIONS & DOSAGE	SIDE EFFECTS
thiethylperazine maleate *(continued)*		*Other:* heat prostration, respiratory distress, fever, asthma, edema (laryngeal, angioneurotic, peripheral), gynecomastia, lactation. *After abrupt withdrawal:* gastritis, nausea, vomiting, dizziness, tremors, feeling of warmth or cold, sweating, tachycardia, headache, insomnia.
trimethobenzamide hydrochloride Tigan	*Nausea and vomiting (treatment)—* **Adults:** 250 mg P.O. t.i.d. or q.i.d.; or 200 mg I.M. or rectally t.i.d. or q.i.d. *Postop nausea and vomiting (prevention)—* **Adults:** 200 mg I.M. or rectally (single dose) before or during surgery; may repeat 3 hours after termination of anesthesia, p.r.n. **Children 13 to 40 Kg:** 100 to 200 mg P.O. or rectally t.i.d. or q.i.d. **Children under 13 Kg:** 100 mg rectally t.i.d. or q.i.d. Limited to prolonged vomiting of known etiology.	*CNS:* drowsiness, dizziness (in large doses). *CV:* hypotension. *GI:* diarrhea, exaggeration of preexisting nausea (in large doses). *Local:* pain, stinging, burning, redness, swelling at I.M. injection site. *Skin:* skin hypersensitivity reactions. *Other:* antiemetic effect may mask signs of overdosage of toxic agents, or intestinal obstruction, brain tumor, or other conditions.

INTERACTIONS	NURSING CONSIDERATIONS
None significant.	• Contraindicated in children with viral illness (a possible cause of vomiting in children); may contribute to the development of Reye's syndrome, a potentially fatal acute childhood encephalopathy, characterized by fatty degeneration of the liver. • Suppositories contraindicated in hypersensitivity to benzocaine hydrochloride or similar local anesthetic. • Stop drug if allergic skin reaction occurs. • Warn patient against driving and other hazardous activities until response to drug is determined. • Give I.M. dose by deep injection into upper outer quadrant of gluteal region to reduce pain and local irritation. • Store suppositories in refrigerator. • Has little or no value in preventing motion sickness; limited value as an antiemetic.

46

Gastrointestinal anticholinergics

anisotropine methylbromide
atropine sulfate
belladonna alkaloids
belladonna leaf
clidinium bromide
dicyclomine hydrochloride
diphemanil methylsulfate
glycopyrrolate
hexocyclium methylsulfate
homatropine methylbromide
isopropamide iodide
levorotatory alkaloids of belladonna
l-hyoscyamine sulfate
mepenzolate bromide
methantheline bromide
methixene hydrochloride
methscopolamine bromide
oxyphencyclimine hydrochloride
oxyphenonium bromide
propantheline bromide
thiphenamil hydrochloride
tridihexethyl chloride

Anticholinergic agents are often used to help relieve the pain associated with peptic ulcers. They inhibit gastrointestinal smooth-muscle contraction and delay gastric emptying time, thus enhancing the action of antacids. These agents should not be used alone, or even as the basis of treatment, but should be part of a total therapeutic program. There is no concrete evidence that they help in the healing of peptic ulcers.

Drugs in this category can be divided into four distinct groups: belladonna alkaloids, quaternary derivatives, quaternary synthetics, and tertiary synthetics.

Major uses

- Adjunctive treatment of peptic ulcers (specifically, the pain associated with them).
- Irritable bowel syndrome (spastic colon, mucous colitis and acute enterocolitis), other functional gastrointestinal disorders, and neurogenic bowel disturbances (including the splenic flexure syndrome and neurogenic colon).

Mechanism of action

- Anticholinergics block the vagus nerve, thus inhibiting secretion of gastric juices, and motility of the gastrointestinal tract.

Absorption, distribution, and excretion

- The naturally occurring belladonna alkaloids are rapidly absorbed and cross the blood-brain barrier, causing central nervous system stimulation. The quaternary derivatives and synthetics are poorly and irregularly absorbed through the gastrointestinal tract, and do not cross the blood-brain barrier. The tertiary synthetics are generally readily absorbed.

- Most agents are excreted largely unchanged in the urine and bile.
- Unabsorbed drugs—mostly of the quaternary groups—are excreted in the feces.

Onset and duration

- Onset of action is usually between 30 minutes and 1 hour after oral administration.
- Duration is usually between 4 and 6 hours. Exceptions to that are isopropamide iodide and oxyphencyclimine hydrochloride, which have durations of up to 12 hours.
- When administered parenterally, onset of action is usually quicker and duration shorter.

Combination products

BARBIDONNA ELIXIR: atropine sulfate 0.034 mg/5 ml, phenobarbital 21.6 mg/5 ml, hyoscyamine hydrobromide or sulfate 0.174/5 ml, and phenobarbital 21.6 mg/5 ml alcohol 15%.
BARBIDONNA TABLETS: atropine sulfate 0.025 mg, hyoscine hydrobromide 0.0074 mg, hyoscyamine hydrobromide or sulfate 0.1286 mg, and phenobarbital 16 mg.
BARBIDONNA #2 TABLETS: atropine sulfate 0.025 mg, hyoscine hydrobromide 0.0074 mg, hyoscyamine hydrobromide or sulfate 0.1286 mg, and phenobarbital 32 mg.
BELLADENAL TABLETS♦: L-alkaloids of belladonna 0.25 mg and phenobarbital 50 mg.
BENTYL WITH PHENOBARBITAL SYRUP: dicyclomine hydrochloride 10 mg/5 ml, phenobarbital 15 mg/5 ml, and alcohol 19%.
BENTYL 10 MG WITH PHENOBARBITAL CAPSULES: dicyclomine hydrochloride 10 mg and phenobarbital 15 mg.
BENTYL 20 MG WITH PHENOBARBITAL CAPSULES: dicyclomine hydrochloride 20 mg and phenobarbital 15 mg.
BUTIBEL ELIXIR: belladonna extract 15 mg/5 ml, butabarbital sodium 15 mg/5 ml, and alcohol 7%.
BUTIBEL TABLETS: belladonna extract 15 mg and butabarbital sodium 15 mg.
CANTIL PHB LIQUID: mepenzolate bromine 25 mg/5 ml and phenobarbital 16 mg/5 ml.
CANTIL WITH PHENOBARBITAL TABLETS: mepenzolate bromide 25 mg and phenobarbital 16 mg.
CHARDONNA-2: belladonna extract 5 mg and phenobarbital 20 mg.
COMBID SPANSULES♦: isopropamine iodide 5 mg and prochlorperazine maleate 10 mg.
DARICON PB TABLETS: oxyphencyclimine hydrochloride 10 mg and phenobarbital 15 mg.
DONNATAL ELIXIR♦: atropine sulfate 0.0194 mg/5 ml, hyoscine hydrobromide 0.0065 mg/5 ml, alcohol 23%, hyoscyamine hydrobromide or sulfate 0.1037 mg/5 ml.
DONNATAL EXTENTABS♦: atropine sulfate 0.0582 mg, hyoscine hydrobromide 0.0195 mg,

hyoscyamine hydrobromide or sulfate 0.3111 mg, phenobarbital 48.6 mg.
DONNATAL TABLETS AND CAPSULES•: atropine sulfate 0.0194 mg, hyoscine hydrobromide 0.0065 mg, hyoscyamine hydrobromide or sulfate 0.1037 mg, and phenobarbital 16.2 mg.
DONNATAL #2 TABLETS: atropine sulfate 0.0194 mg, hyoscine hydrobromine 0.0065 mg, hyoscyamine hydrobromide or sulfate 0.1037 mg, phenobarbital 32.4 mg.
ENARAX 5 TABLETS: oxyphencyclimine hydrochloride 5 mg and hydroxyzine hydrochloride 25 mg.
ENARAX 10 TABLETS: oxyphencyclimine hydrochloride 10 mg and hydroxyzine hydrochloride 25 mg.
HYBEPHEN ELIXIR: atropine sulfate 0.0122 mg/5 ml, hyoscine hydrobromide 0.0094 mg/5 ml, hyoscyamine hydrobromide or sulfate 0.1277 mg/5 ml, phenobarbital 15 mg/5 ml, and alcohol 16.5%.
KINESED TABLETS: atropine sulfate 0.02 mg, hyoscine hydrobromide 0.007 mg, hyoscyamine hydrobromide or sulfate 0.1 mg, and phenobarbital 16 mg.
LIBRAX CAPSULES•: clidinium bromide 2.5 mg and chlordiazepoxide hydrochloride 5 mg.
MILPATH 200 TABLETS: tridihexethyl chloride 25 mg and meprobamate 200 mg.
MILPATH 400 TABLETS: tridihexethyl chloride 25 mg and meprobamate 400 mg.
PATHIBAMATE 200 TABLETS: tridihexethyl chloride 25 mg and meprobamate 200 mg.
PATHIBAMATE 400 TABLETS•: tridihexethyl chloride 25 mg and meprobamate 400 mg.
PATHILON WITH PHENOBARBITAL SEQUELS: tridihexethyl chloride 75 mg and phenobarbital 45 mg.
PATHILON WITH PHENOBARBITAL TABLETS: tridihexethyl chloride 25 mg and phenobarbital 15 mg.
PRO-BANTHINE WITH PHENOBARBITAL TABLETS•: propantheline bromide 15 mg and phenobarbital 15 mg.
ROBINUL PH TABLETS•: glycopyrrolate 1 mg and phenobarbital 16.2 mg.
ROBINUL PH FORTE TABLETS•: glycopyrrolate 2 mg and phenobarbital 16.2 mg.
VALPIN 50-PB TABLETS: anisotropine methylbromide 50 mg and phenobarbital 15 mg.
VISTRAX 10 TABLETS: oxyphencyclimine hydrochloride 10 mg and hydroxyzine hydrochloride 25 mg.

HOW GI ANTICHOLINERGICS WORK

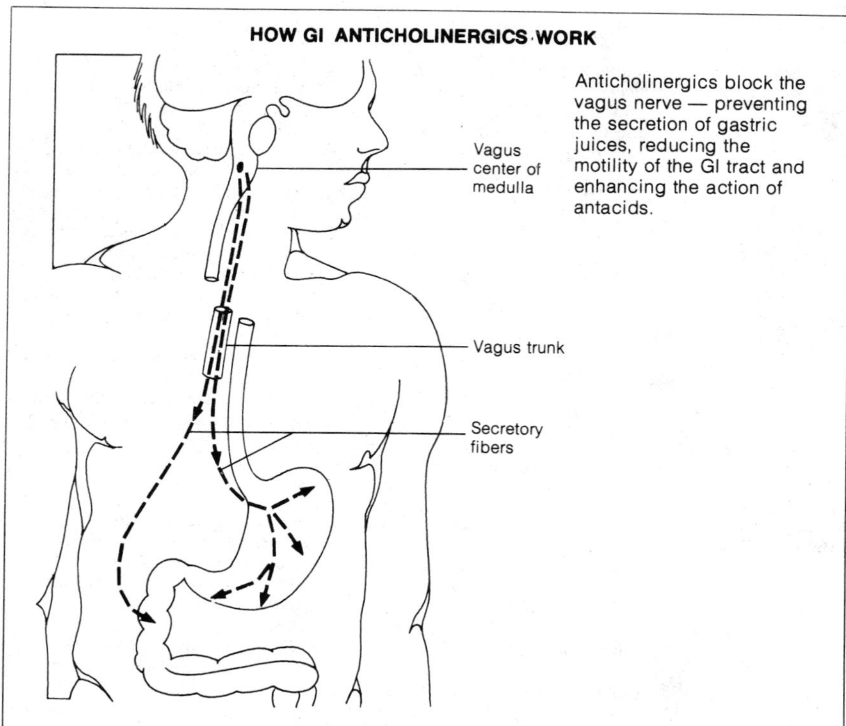

Anticholinergics block the vagus nerve — preventing the secretion of gastric juices, reducing the motility of the GI tract and enhancing the action of antacids.

NAME	INDICATIONS & DOSAGE	SIDE EFFECTS
anisotropine methylbromide Valpin 50	*Adjunctive treatment of peptic ulcer—* **Adults:** 50 mg P.O. t.i.d. To be effective should be titrated to individual patient needs.	*CNS:* headache, insomnia, drowsiness, dizziness, confusion or excitement in elderly patients, nervousness, weakness. *CV:* palpitations, tachycardia. *EENT:* blurred vision, mydriasis, increased ocular tension, cycloplegia, photophobia. *GI:* dry mouth, dysphagia, heartburn, loss of taste, nausea, vomiting, paralytic ileus, constipation. *GU:* suppression of lactation, urinary hesitancy and retention, impotence. *Skin:* urticaria, decreased sweating and possibly anhidrosis, other dermal manifestations. *Other:* fever, allergic reactions. Overdosage may cause curare-like symptoms.
atropine sulfate	*Adjunctive therapy in peptic ulcers, irritable bowel syndrome, neurogenic bowel disturbances, and functional gastrointestinal disorders—* **Adults:** 0.4 to 0.6 mg P.O. q 4 to 6 hours. **Children:** the following dosages P.O. q 4 to 6 hours: 7 to 16 lbs.—0.1 mg (1/600 gr) 17 to 24 lbs.—0.15 mg (1/400 gr) 24 to 40 lbs.—0.2 mg (1/300 gr) 40 to 65 lbs.—0.3 mg (1/200 gr) 65 to 90 lbs.—0.4 mg (1/150 gr) Over 90 lbs.—0.4 to 0.6 mg (1/150 to 1/100 gr)	*CNS:* headache, insomnia, drowsiness, dizziness, confusion or excitement in elderly patients, nervousness, weakness. *CV:* palpitations, tachycardia. *EENT:* blurred vision, mydriasis, increased ocular tension, cycloplegia, photophobia. *GI:* dry mouth, dysphagia, heartburn, loss of taste, nausea, vomiting, paralytic ileus. *GU:* suppression of lactation, urinary hesitancy and retention, impotence. *Skin:* urticaria, decreased sweating or anhidrosis, other dermal manifestations. *Other:* fever, allergic reactions. Overdosage may cause curare-like symptoms.
belladonna alkaloids Prydon Spansule (0.120 mg atropine sulfate, 0.070 mg scopolamine hydrobromide, 0.610 mg hyoscyamine sulfate in 0.8 mg Spansule, or half the above in 0.4 mg Spansule)	*Adjunctive therapy in gastric, peptic, duodenal, or intestinal ulcers to control excess motor activity, hyperirritability or spasm of the gastrointestinal tract—* **Adults:** 0.4 to 0.8 mg (timed-release capsules) P.O. q 12 hours.	*CNS:* headache, insomnia, drowsiness, dizziness, confusion or excitement in elderly patients, nervousness, weakness. *CV:* palpitations, tachycardia. *EENT:* blurred vision, mydriasis, increased ocular tension, cycloplegia, photophobia. *GI:* dry mouth, dysphagia, heartburn, loss of taste. *GU:* urinary hesitancy and retention, impotence.

♦ Also available in Canada.
♦♦ Available in Canada only.
Unmarked trade names available in United States only.

INTERACTIONS	NURSING CONSIDERATIONS
Methotrimeprazine: may produce extrapyramidal symptoms. Monitor patient carefully.	• Contraindicated in narrow-angle glaucoma, obstructive uropathy, obstructive disease of the GI tract, severe ulcerative colitis, myasthenia gravis, hypersensitivity to anticholinergics, paralytic ileus, intestinal atony, unstable cardiovascular status in acute hemorrhage, and toxic megacolon. Use cautiously in autonomic neuropathy; hyperthyroidism, coronary heart disease, cardiac arrhythmias, congestive heart failure, hypertension, hiatal hernia associated with reflux esophagitis, hepatic or renal disease, ulcerative colitis, or patients over 40 because of increased incidence of glaucoma. • Use with caution in hot or humid environments. Drug-induced heat stroke can develop. • Give 30 minutes to 1 hour before meals. • Administer smaller doses to the elderly. • Antacids may interfere with absorption; administer alternately. • Monitor patient's vital signs and urinary output carefully. • Tell patient to avoid driving and other hazardous activities if he is drowsy, dizzy, or has blurred vision; to drink plenty of fluids to help prevent constipation; to report any skin rash or local eruption. Gum or sugarless hard candy may relieve mouth dryness. • Quaternary ammonium derivative; these derivatives have fewer, less severe CNS side effects because they do not cross blood-brain barrier. • For symptoms and treatment of toxicity, see p. 1115.
Methotrimeprazine: may produce extrapyramidal symptoms. Monitor patient carefully.	• Contraindicated in narrow-angle glaucoma, obstructive uropathy, obstructive disease of GI tract, severe ulcerative colitis, myasthenia gravis, hypersensitivity to anticholinergics, paralytic ileus, intestinal atony, unstable cardiovascular status in acute hemorrhage, toxic megacolon. Use cautiously in autonomic neuropathy, hyperthyroidism, coronary heart disease, cardiac arrhythmias, congestive heart failure, hypertension, hiatal hernia associated with reflux esophagitis, hepatic or renal disease, ulcerative colitis, or patients over 40 because of increased incidence of glaucoma. • Use with caution in hot or humid environments. Drug-induced heat stroke can develop. • Give 30 minutes to 1 hour before meals and at bedtime. Bedtime dose can be larger and should be given at least 2 hours after last meal of day. • Administer smaller doses to the elderly. • Antacids may interfere with absorption; administer alternately. • Monitor patient's vital signs and urinary output carefully. • Tell patient to avoid driving and other hazardous activities if he is drowsy, dizzy, or has blurred vision; to drink plenty of fluids to help prevent constipation; to report any skin rash. Gum, sugarless hard candy, or pilocarpine syrup may relieve mouth dryness. • Other anticholinergic drugs may increase vagal blockage. • For symptoms and treatment of toxicity, see p. 1115.
Methotrimeprazine: may produce extrapyramidal symptoms. Monitor patient carefully.	• Contraindicated in narrow-angle glaucoma, obstructive uropathy, obstructive disease of GI tract, severe ulcerative colitis, myasthenia gravis, hypersensitivity to anticholinergics, paralytic ileus, intestinal atony, unstable cardiovascular status in acute hemorrhage, toxic megacolon. Use cautiously in autonomic neuropathy, hyperthyroidism, coronary heart disease, cardiac arrhythmias, congestive heart failure, hypertension, hiatal hernia with reflux esophagitis, hepatic or renal disease, ulcerative colitis, or patients over 40 because of increased incidence of glaucoma. • Use with caution in hot or humid environments. Drug-induced heat stroke can develop. • Administer smaller doses to the elderly. • Antacids may interfere with absorption; administer alternately.

(continued on following page)

NAME	INDICATIONS & DOSAGE	SIDE EFFECTS
belladonna alkaloids *(continued)*		*Skin:* urticaria, decreased sweating or anhidrosis, other dermal manifestations. *Other:* suppression of lactation, fever, allergic reactions. Overdosage may cause curare-like symptoms.
belladonna leaf (used to prepare extract, fluidextract, and tincture) Belladonna Tincture USP, Belladonna Fluidextract	*Adjunctive therapy for peptic ulcer, irritable bowel syndrome, functional gastrointestinal disorders, and neurogenic bowel disturbances—* **Adults:** 10.8 to 21.6 mg P.O. t.i.d. or q.i.d. of the extract; 0.06 ml P.O. t.i.d. or q.i.d. of the Fluidextract; 0.6 to 1 ml t.i.d. or q.i.d. of tincture.	*CNS:* headache, insomnia, drowsiness, dizziness, confusion or excitement in elderly patients, nervousness, weakness. *CV:* palpitations, tachycardia. *EENT:* blurred vision, mydriasis, increased ocular tension, cycloplegia, photophobia. *GI:* dry mouth, dysphagia, heartburn, loss of taste, constipation. *GU:* urinary hesitancy and retention, impotence. *Skin:* urticaria, decreased sweating or anhidrosis, other dermal manifestations. *Other:* suppression of lactation, fever, allergic reactions. Overdosage may cause curare-like symptoms.
clidinium bromide Quarzan	*Adjunctive therapy for peptic ulcers—* Dosage should be individualized according to severity of symptoms and occurrence of side effects. **Adults:** 2.5 to 5 mg P.O. t.i.d. or q.i.d. before meals and at bedtime. **Geriatric or debilitated patients:** 2.5 mg P.O. t.i.d. before meals.	*CNS:* headache, insomnia, drowsiness, dizziness, confusion or excitement in elderly patients; nervousness, weakness. *CV:* palpitations, tachycardia. *EENT:* blurred vision, mydriasis, increased ocular tension, cycloplegia, photophobia. *GI:* dry mouth, dysphagia, heartburn, loss of taste, nausea, vomiting, paralytic ileus. *GU:* urinary hesitancy and retention, impotence. *Skin:* urticaria, decreased sweating or anhidrosis, other dermal manifestations. *Other:* suppression of lactation, fever, allergic reactions. Overdosage may cause curare-like symptoms.

INTERACTIONS	NURSING CONSIDERATIONS
	• Monitor patient's vital signs and urinary output carefully. • Instruct patient to avoid driving and other hazardous activities if he is drowsy, dizzy, or has blurred vision; to drink plenty of fluids to help prevent constipation; and to report any skin rash. • For symptoms and treatment of toxicity, see p. 1115.
Methotrimeprazine: may produce extrapyramidal symptoms. Monitor patient carefully.	• Contraindicated in narrow-angle glaucoma, obstructive uropathy, obstructive disease of GI tract, severe ulcerative colitis, myasthenia gravis, hypersensitivity to anticholinergics, paralytic ileus, intestinal atony, unstable cardiovascular status in acute hemorrhage, and toxic megacolon. Use cautiously in autonomic neuropathy, hyperthyroidism, coronary heart disease, cardiac arrhythmias, congestive heart failure, hypertension, hiatal hernia associated with reflux esophagitis, hepatic or renal disease, ulcerative colitis, or patients over 40 because of increased incidence of glaucoma. • Give 30 minutes to 1 hour before meals and at bedtime. Bedtime dose can be larger and should be given at least 2 hours after last meal of day. • Administer smaller doses to the elderly. • Use caution in hot or humid environments. Drug-induced heat stroke can develop. • Antacids may interfere with absorption; administer alternately. • Monitor patient's vital signs and urinary output carefully. • Instruct patient to avoid driving and other hazardous activities if he is drowsy, dizzy, or has blurred vision; to drink plenty of fluids to help prevent constipation; to report any skin rash. Gum or sugarless hard candy may relieve mouth dryness. • For symptoms and treatment of toxicity, see p. 1115.
Methotrimeprazine: may produce extrapyramidal symptoms. Monitor patient carefully.	• Contraindicated in narrow-angle glaucoma, obstructive uropathy, obstructive disease of GI tract, severe ulcerative colitis, myasthenia gravis, hypersensitivity to anticholinergics, paralytic ileus, intestinal atony, unstable cardiovascular status in acute hemorrhage, and toxic megacolon. Use cautiously in autonomic neuropathy, hyperthyroidism, coronary heart disease, cardiac arrhythmias, congestive heart failure, hypertension, hiatal hernia associated with reflux esophagitis, hepatic or renal disease, ulcerative colitis, or patients over 40 because of increased incidence of glaucoma. • Give 30 minutes to 1 hour before meals and at bedtime. Bedtime dose can be larger and should be given at least 2 hours after last meal of day. • Administer smaller doses to the elderly. • Use with caution in hot or humid environments. Drug-induced heat stroke may develop. • Antacids may interfere with absorption; administer alternately. • Monitor patient's vital signs and urinary output carefully. • Tell patient to avoid driving and other hazardous activities if he is drowsy, dizzy or has blurred vision; to drink plenty of fluids to help prevent constipation; and to report any skin rash or local eruption. Gum or sugarless hard candy may relieve mouth dryness. • Quaternary ammonium derivative; these derivatives have fewer, less severe CNS side effects, since they do not cross blood-brain barrier. • For symptoms and treatment of toxicity, see p. 1115.

NAME	INDICATIONS & DOSAGE	SIDE EFFECTS
dicyclomine hydrochloride Antispas, Bentyl, Bentylol◆◆, Cyclobec◆◆, Dibent, Formulex◆◆, Meno-spasm◆◆, Nospaz, Or-Tyl, Rocyclo, Rotyl HCl, Stannitol, Viscerol◆◆	*Adjunctive therapy for peptic ulcers and other functional gastrointestinal disorders—* **Adults:** 10 to 20 mg P.O. t.i.d. or q.i.d.; 20 mg I.M. q 4 to 6 hours. **Children:** 10 mg P.O. t.i.d. or q.i.d. *Infant colic—* **Infants:** 5 mg P.O. t.i.d. or q.i.d. Always adjust dosage according to patient's needs and response.	*CNS:* headache, insomnia, drowsiness, dizziness, confusion or excitement in elderly patients, nervousness, weakness. *CV:* palpitations, tachycardia. *EENT:* blurred vision, mydriasis, increased ocular tension, cycloplegia, photophobia. *GI:* dry mouth, dysphagia, heartburn, loss of taste, nausea, constipation, vomiting, paralytic ileus. *GU:* urinary hesitancy and retention, impotence. *Skin:* urticaria, decreased sweating or anhidrosis, other dermal manifestations. *Other:* suppression of lactation, fever, allergic reactions. Overdosage may cause curare-like symptoms.
diphemanil methylsulfate Prantal	*Adjunctive therapy in gastric hypersecretion associated with duodenal ulcer—* **Adults:** 100 to 200 mg P.O. q 4 to 6 hours, between meals (initial dose). Daily dosage should be adjusted according to response and tolerance. Maintenance dose: 50 to 100 mg q 4 to 6 hours.	*CNS:* headache, insomnia, drowsiness, dizziness, confusion or excitement in elderly patients, nervousness, weakness. *CV:* palpitations, tachycardia. *EENT:* blurred vision, mydriasis, increased ocular tension, cycloplegia, photophobia. *GI:* dry mouth, dysphagia, constipation, heartburn, loss of taste, nausea, vomiting, paralytic ileus. *GU:* urinary hesitancy and retention, impotence. *Skin:* urticaria, decreased sweating, anhidrosis, other dermal manifestations. *Other:* suppression of lactation, fever, allergic reactions. Overdosage may cause curare-like symptoms.
glycopyrrolate Robinul◆, Robinul Forte◆	*Adjunctive therapy in peptic ulcers and other gastrointestinal disorders—* **Adults:** 1 to 2 mg P.O. t.i.d. or 0.1 mg I.M. t.i.d. or q.i.d. Dosage should be individualized.	*CNS:* headache, insomnia, drowsiness, dizziness, confusion or excitement, in elderly patients, nervousness, weakness. *CV:* palpitations, tachycardia. *EENT:* blurred vision, mydriasis, increased ocular tension, cycloplegia, photophobia. *GI:* dry mouth, dysphagia, constipation, heartburn, loss of taste, nausea, vomiting, paralytic ileus.

INTERACTIONS	NURSING CONSIDERATIONS
Methotrimeprazine: may produce extrapyramidal symptoms. Monitor patient carefully.	• Contraindicated in obstructive uropathy, obstructive disease of GI tract, severe ulcerative colitis, myasthenia gravis, hypersensitivity to anticholinergics, paralytic ileus, intestinal atony, unstable cardiovascular status in acute hemorrhage, and toxic megacolon. Use cautiously in autonomic neuropathy, narrow-angle glaucoma, hyperthyroidism, coronary heart disease, cardiac arrhythmias, congestive heart failure, hypertension, hiatal hernia associated with reflux esophagitis, hepatic or renal disease, ulcerative colitis. • Use with caution in hot or humid environments. Drug-induced heat stroke can develop. • Give 30 minutes to 1 hour before meals and at bedtime. Bedtime dose can be larger and should be given at least 2 hours after last meal of day. • Administer smaller doses to the elderly. • Antacids may interfere with absorption; administer alternately. • Monitor patient's vital signs and urinary output carefully. • Instruct patient to avoid driving and other hazardous activities if he is drowsy, dizzy, or has blurred vision; to drink plenty of fluids to help prevent constipation; and to report any skin rash. Gum or sugarless hard candy may relieve mouth dryness. • A synthetic tertiary derivative that is relatively free of atropine-like side effects. • For symptoms and treatment of toxicity, see p. 1115.
Methotrimeprazine: may produce extrapyramidal symptoms. Monitor patient carefully.	• Contraindicated in narrow-angle glaucoma, obstructive uropathy, obstructive disease of GI tract, severe ulcerative colitis, myasthenia gravis, hypersensitivity to the anticholinergics, paralytic ileus, intestinal atony, unstable cardiovascular status in acute hemorrhage, and toxic megacolon. Use cautiously in autonomic neuropathy, hyperthyroidism, coronary heart disease, cardiac arrhythmias, congestive heart failure, hypertension, hiatal hernia associated with reflux esophagitis, hepatic or renal disease, ulcerative colitis, or patients over 40 because of increased incidence of glaucoma. • Use with caution in hot or humid environments. Drug-induced heat stroke can develop. • Give 30 minutes to 1 hour before meals and at bedtime. Bedtime dose can be larger and should be given at least 2 hours after last meal of day. • Administer smaller doses to the elderly. • Antacids may interfere with absorption; administer alternately. • Monitor patient's vital signs and urinary output carefully. • Instruct patient to avoid driving and other hazardous activities if he is drowsy, dizzy or has blurred vision; to drink plenty of fluids to help prevent constipation; and to report any skin rash. Gum or sugarless hard candy may relieve mouth dryness. • Quaternary ammonium derivative; these derivatives have fewer, less severe CNS side effects, since they do not cross blood-brain barrier. • For symptoms and treatment of toxicity, see p. 1115.
Methotrimeprazine: may produce extrapyramidal symptoms. Monitor patient carefully.	• Contraindicated in narrow-angle glaucoma, obstructive uropathy, obstructive disease of GI tract, severe ulcerative colitis, myasthenia gravis, hypersensitivity to anticholinergics, paralytic ileus, intestinal atony, unstable cardiovascular status in acute hemorrhage, and toxic megacolon. Use cautiously in autonomic neuropathy, hyperthyroidism, coronary heart disease, cardiac arrhythmias, congestive heart failure, hypertension, hiatal hernia associated with reflux esophagitis, hepatic or renal disease, ulcerative colitis, or patients over 40 because of increased incidence of glaucoma. • Use with caution in hot or humid environments. Drug-induced heat stroke can develop.

(continued on following page)

NAME	INDICATIONS & DOSAGE	SIDE EFFECTS
glycopyrrolate *(continued)*		*GU:* urinary hesitancy and retention, impotence. *Skin:* urticaria, decreased sweating or anhidrosis, other dermal manifestations. *Other:* suppression of lactation, fever, allergic reactions. Overdosage may cause curare-like symptoms.
hexocyclium methylsulfate Tral	*Adjunctive therapy in peptic ulcer and other gastrointestinal disorders—* **Adults:** 25 mg q.i.d. before meals and at bedtime. Or with extended-release tablets, 50 mg before lunch and 50 or 75 mg at bedtime.	*CNS:* headache, insomnia, drowsiness, dizziness, confusion or excitement in elderly patients, nervousness, weakness. *CV:* palpitations, tachycardia. *EENT:* blurred vision, mydriasis, increased ocular tension, cycloplegia, photophobia. *GI:* dry mouth, dysphagia, heartburn, loss of taste, nausea, constipation, vomiting, paralytic ileus. *GU:* retention, impotence. *Skin:* urticaria, decreased sweating or anhidrosis, other dermal manifestations. *Other:* suppression of lactation, fever, allergic reactions. Overdosage may cause curare-like symptoms.
homatropine methylbromide Ru-Spas No. 2, Sed-Tens SE	*Treatment of gastrointestinal spasm, hyperchlorhydria, and other mild spastic conditions of the bile ducts and gallbladder—* **Adults:** 2.5 to 5 mg t.i.d. to q.i.d. before meals and at bedtime.	*CNS:* headache, insomnia, drowsiness, dizziness, confusion or excitement in elderly patients, nervousness, weakness. *CV:* palpitations, tachycardia. *EENT:* blurred vision, mydriasis, increased ocular tension, cycloplegia, photophobia. *GI:* dry mouth, dysphagia, constipation, heartburn, loss of taste, nausea, vomiting, paralytic ileus. *GU:* urinary hesitancy and retention, impotence. *Skin:* urticaria, decreased sweating or anhidrosis, other dermal manifestations. *Other:* suppression of lactation, fever, allergic reactions. Overdosage may cause curare-like symptoms.

INTERACTIONS	NURSING CONSIDERATIONS
	• Administer 30 minutes to 1 hour before meals. • Administer smaller doses to the elderly. • Antacids may interfere with absorption; administer alternately. • Monitor patient's vital signs and urinary output carefully. • Instruct patient to avoid driving and other hazardous activities if he is drowsy, dizzy, or has blurred vision; to drink plenty of fluids to help prevent constipation; to report any skin rash. Gum or sugarless hard candy may relieve mouth dryness. • Quaternary ammonium derivative; these derivatives have fewer, less severe CNS side effects, since they do not cross blood-brain barrier. • For symptoms and treatment of toxicity, see p. 1115.
Methotrimeprazine: may produce extrapyramidal symptoms. Monitor patient carefully.	• Contraindicated in narrow-angle glaucoma, obstructive uropathy, obstructive disease of GI tract, severe ulcerative colitis, myasthenia gravis, hypersensitivity to anticholinergics, paralytic ileus, intestinal atony, unstable cardiovascular status in acute hemorrhage, toxic megacolon. Use cautiously in autonomic neuropathy, hyperthyroidism, coronary heart disease, cardiac arrhythmias, congestive heart failure, hypertension, hiatal hernia associated with reflux esophagitis, hepatic or renal disease, ulcerative colitis, or patients over 40 because of increased incidence of glaucoma. • Use with caution in hot or humid environments. Drug-induced heat stroke can develop. • Give 30 minutes to 1 hour before meals and at bedtime. Bedtime dose can be larger and should be given at least 2 hours after last meal of day. • Administer smaller doses to the elderly. • Antacids may interfere with absorption; administer alternately. • Monitor patient's vital signs and urinary output carefully. • Instruct patient to avoid driving and other hazardous activities if he is drowsy, dizzy, or has blurred vision; to drink plenty of fluids to help prevent constipation; and to report any skin rash. Gum or sugarless hard candy may relieve mouth dryness. • Quaternary ammonium derivative; these have fewer, less severe CNS side effects, since they do not cross blood-brain barrier. • For symptoms and treatment of toxicity, see p. 1115.
Methotrimeprazine: may produce extrapyramidal symptoms. Monitor patient carefully.	• Contraindicated in narrow-angle glaucoma, obstructive uropathy, obstructive disease of GI tract, severe ulcerative colitis, myasthenia gravis, hypersensitivity to anticholinergics, paralytic ileus, intestinal atony, unstable cardiovascular status in acute hemorrhage, and toxic megacolon. Use cautiously in autonomic neuropathy, hyperthyroidism, coronary heart disease, cardiac arrhythmias, congestive heart failure, hypertension, hiatal hernia associated with reflux esophagitis, hepatic or renal disease, ulcerative colitis, or patients over 40 because of increased incidence of glaucoma. • Use with caution in hot or humid environments. Drug-induced heat stroke can develop. • Give 30 minutes to 1 hour before meals and at bedtime. Bedtime dose can be larger and should be given at least 2 hours after the last meal of the day. • Administer smaller doses to the elderly. • Antacids may interfere with absorption; administer alternately. • Monitor patient's vital signs and urinary output carefully. • Instruct patient to avoid driving and other hazardous activities if he is drowsy, dizzy, or has blurred vision; to drink plenty of fluids to help prevent constipation; and to report any skin rash. Gum or sugarless hard candy may relieve mouth dryness. • Quaternary ammonium derivative; these have fewer, less severe CNS side effects, since they do not cross blood-brain barrier. • For symptoms and treatment of toxicity, see p. 1115.

NAME	INDICATIONS & DOSAGE	SIDE EFFECTS
isopropamide iodide Darbid◆	*Adjunctive therapy for peptic ulcer, irritable bowel syndrome*— **Adults, and children over 12 years:** 5 mg P.O. q 12 hours. Some patients may require 10 mg or more b.i.d. Dose should be individualized to patient's need.	*CNS:* headache, insomnia, drowsiness, dizziness, confusion or excitement in elderly patients, nervousness, weakness. *CV:* palpitations, tachycardia. *EENT:* blurred vision, mydriasis, increased ocular tension, cycloplegia, photophobia. *GI:* dry mouth, dysphagia, heartburn, loss of taste, nausea, vomiting, paralytic ileus. *GU:* urinary hesitancy and retention, impotence. *Skin:* urticaria, decreased sweating or anhidrosis, other dermal manifestations, iodine skin rash. *Other:* suppression of lactation, fever, allergic reactions. Overdosage may cause curare-like symptoms.
levorotatory alkaloids of belladonna (as maleate salts) Bellafoline	*Adjunctive therapy for peptic ulcer, irritable bowel syndrome, and functional gastrointestinal disorders*— **Adults:** 0.25 to 0.5 P.O. t.i.d.; or 0.125 to 0.5 mg S.C. daily or b.i.d. **Children over 6 years of age:** 0.125 to 0.25 mg P.O. t.i.d.	*CNS:* headache, insomnia, drowsiness, dizziness, confusion or excitement in elderly patients, nervousness, weakness. *CV:* palpitations, tachycardia. *EENT:* blurred vision, mydriasis, increased ocular tension, cycloplegia, photophobia. *GI:* dry mouth, dysphagia, heartburn, loss of taste. *GU:* urinary hesitancy and retention, impotence. *Skin:* urticaria, decreased sweating or anhidrosis, other dermal manifestations. *Other:* suppression of lactation, fever, allergic reactions. Overdosage may cause curare-like symptoms.
l-hyoscyamine sulfate Anaspaz, Levsin◆, Levsinex, Levsinex Time Caps	*Treatment of gastrointestinal tract disorders due to spasm; adjunctive therapy for peptic ulcers*— **Adults:** 0.125 to 0.25 mg P.O. t.i.d. or q.i.d. before meals and at bedtime; sustained-release form 0.375 mg P.O. q 12 hours; or 0.25 to 0.5 mg (1 or 2 ml) I.M., I.V., or S.C. q 6 hours. (Substitute oral medication when symptoms	*CNS:* headache, insomnia, drowsiness, dizziness, confusion or excitement in elderly patients, nervousness, weakness. *CV:* palpitations, tachycardia. *EENT:* blurred vision, mydriasis, increased ocular tension, cycloplegia, photophobia. *GI:* dry mouth, dysphagia, constipation, heartburn, loss of taste, nausea,

INTERACTIONS	NURSING CONSIDERATIONS
Methotrimeprazine: may produce extrapyramidal symptoms. Monitor patient carefully.	• Contraindicated in narrow-angle glaucoma, obstructive uropathy, obstructive disease of GI tract, severe ulcerative colitis, myasthenia gravis, hypersensitivity to anticholinergics, paralytic ileus, intestinal atony, unstable cardiovascular status in acute hemorrhage, toxic megacolon. Use cautiously in autonomic neuropathy, hyperthyroidism, coronary heart disease, cardiac arrhythmias, congestive heart failure, hypertension, hiatal hernia associated with reflux esophagitis, hepatic or renal disease, ulcerative colitis, or patients over 40 because of increased incidence of glaucoma. • Use with caution in hot or humid environments. Drug-induced heat stroke can develop. • Give 30 minutes to 1 hour before meals and at bedtime. Bedtime dose can be larger and should be given at least 2 hours after the last meal of the day. • Administer smaller doses to the elderly. • Antacids may interfere with absorption; administer alternately. • Monitor patient's vital signs and urinary output carefully. • Instruct patient to avoid driving and other hazardous activities if he is drowsy, dizzy, or has blurred vision; to drink plenty of fluids to help prevent constipation; and to report any skin rash. Gum or sugarless hard candy may relieve mouth dryness. • Single dose produces 10- to 12-hour antisecretory effect and gastrointestinal antispasmodic effect. • Quaternary ammonium derivative; these have fewer, less severe CNS side effects, since they do not cross blood-brain barrier. • Discontinue 1 week before thyroid function tests. • For symptoms and treatment of toxicity, see p. 1115.
Methotrimeprazine: may produce extrapyramidal symptoms. Monitor patient carefully.	• Contraindicated in narrow-angle glaucoma, obstructive uropathy, obstructive disease of GI tract, severe ulcerative colitis, myasthenia gravis, hypersensitivity to anticholinergics, paralytic ileus, intestinal atony, unstable cardiovascular status in acute hemorrhage, and toxic megacolon. Use cautiously in autonomic neuropathy, hyperthyroidism, coronary heart disease, cardiac arrhythmias, congestive heart failure, hypertension, hiatal hernia associated with reflux esophagitis, hepatic or renal disease, ulcerative colitis, or patients over 40 because of increased incidence of glaucoma. • Use with caution in hot or humid environments. Drug-induced heat stroke can develop. • Administer 30 minutes to 1 hour before meals. • Administer smaller doses to the elderly. • Antacids may interfere with absorption; administer alternately. • Monitor patient's vital signs and urinary output carefully. • Instruct patient to avoid driving and other hazardous activities if he is drowsy, dizzy, or has blurred vision; to drink plenty of fluids to help prevent constipation; to report any skin rash. Gum or sugarless hard candy may relieve mouth dryness. • For symptoms and treatment of toxicity, see p. 1115.
Methotrimeprazine: may produce extrapyramidal symptoms. Monitor patient carefully.	• Contraindicated in narrow-angle glaucoma, obstructive uropathy, obstructive disease of GI tract, severe ulcerative colitis, myasthenia gravis, hypersensitivity to anticholinergics, paralytic ileus, intestinal atony, unstable cardiovascular status in acute hemorrhage, toxic megacolon. Use cautiously in autonomic neuropathy, hyperthyroidism, coronary heart disease, cardiac arrhythmias, congestive heart failure, hypertension, hiatal hernia associated with reflux esophagitis, hepatic or renal disease, ulcerative colitis, or patients over 40 because of the increased incidence of glaucoma. • Use with caution in hot or humid environments. Drug-induced heat stroke can develop.

(continued on following page)

NAME	INDICATIONS & DOSAGE	SIDE EFFECTS
l-hyoscyamine sulfate *(continued)*	are controlled.) **Children 2 to 10 years:** ½ adult dose P.O. **Children under 2 years:** ¼ adult dose P.O.	vomiting, paralytic ileus. *GU:* urinary hesitancy and retention, impotence. *Skin:* urticaria, decreased sweating or anhidrosis, other dermal manifestations. *Other:* suppression of lactation, fever, allergic reactions. Overdosage may cause curare-like symptoms.
mepenzolate bromide Cantil	*Adjunctive therapy in treating peptic ulcer, irritable bowel syndrome and neurological bowel disturbances—* **Adults:** 25 to 50 mg P.O. q.i.d. with meals and at bedtime. Adjust dosage to individual patient's needs.	*CNS:* headache, insomnia, drowsiness, dizziness, confusion or excitement in elderly patients, nervousness, weakness. *CV:* palpitations, tachycardia. *EENT:* blurred vision, mydriasis, increased ocular tension, cycloplegia, photophobia. *GI:* dry mouth, dysphagia, heartburn, loss of taste, nausea, constipation, vomiting, paralytic ileus. *GU:* urinary hesitancy and retention, impotence. *Skin:* urticaria, decreased sweating or anhidrosis, other dermal manifestations. *Other:* suppression of lactation, fever, allergic reactions. Overdosage may cause curare-like symptoms.
methantheline bromide Banthine	*Adjunctive therapy in peptic ulcer, pylorospasm, spastic colon, biliary dyskinesia, pancreatitis, and certain forms of gastritis—* **Adults:** 50 to 100 mg P.O. q 6 hours. If patient cannot take drug orally, may give I.M. or I.V. **Children over 1 year:** 12.5 to 50 mg q.i.d. **Children under 1 year:** 12.5 to 25 mg q.i.d.	*CNS:* headache, insomnia, drowsiness, dizziness, confusion or excitement in elderly patients, nervousness, weakness. *CV:* palpitations, tachycardia. *EENT:* blurred vision, mydriasis, increased ocular tension, cycloplegia, photophobia. *GI:* dry mouth,, dysphagia, constipation, heartburn, loss of taste, nausea, vomiting, paralytic ileus. *GU:* urinary hesitancy and retention, impotence. *Skin:* urticaria, decreased sweating or anhidrosis, other dermal manifestations. *Other:* suppression of lactation, fever, allergic reactions. Overdosage may cause curare-like symptoms.

INTERACTIONS	NURSING CONSIDERATIONS
	• Give 30 minutes to 1 hour before meals and at bedtime. Bedtime dose can be larger and should be given at least 2 hours after the last meal of the day. • Administer smaller doses to the elderly. • Antacids may interfere with absorption; administer alternately. • Monitor patient's vital signs and urinary output carefully. • Instruct patient to avoid driving and other hazardous activities if he is drowsy, dizzy, or has blurred vision; to drink plenty of fluids to help prevent constipation; and to report any skin rash. Gum or sugarless hard candy may relieve mouth dryness. • Quaternary ammonium derivative; these have fewer, less severe CNS side effects, since they do not cross blood-brain barrier. • For symptoms and treatment of toxicity, see p. 1115.
Methotrimeprazine: may produce extrapyramidal symptoms. Monitor patient carefully.	• Contraindicated in narrow-angle glaucoma, obstructive uropathy, obstructive disease of GI tract, severe ulcerative colitis, myasthenia gravis, hypersensitivity to anticholinergics, paralytic ileus, intestinal atony, unstable cardiovascular status in acute hemorrhage, toxic megacolon. Use cautiously in autonomic neuropathy, hyperthyroidism, coronary heart disease, cardiac arrhythmias, congestive heart failure, hypertension, hiatal hernia associated with reflux esophagitis, hepatic or renal disease, ulcerative colitis, or patients over 40 because of increased incidence of glaucoma. • Use with caution in hot or humid environments. Drug-induced heat stroke can develop. • Give with meals and at bedtime. • Administer smaller doses to the elderly. • Antacids may interfere with absorption; administer alternately. • Monitor patient's vital signs and urinary output carefully. • Instruct patient to avoid driving and other hazardous activities if he is drowsy, dizzy, or has blurred vision; to drink plenty of fluids to help prevent constipation; and to report any skin rash. Gum or sugarless hard candy may relieve mouth dryness. • Quaternary ammonium derivative; these have fewer, less severe CNS side effects, since they do not cross blood-brain barrier. • For symptoms and treatment of toxicity, see p. 1115.
Methotrimeprazine: may produce extrapyramidal symptoms. Monitor patient carefully.	• Contraindicated in narrow-angle glaucoma, obstructive uropathy, obstructive disease of GI tract, severe ulcerative colitis, myasthenia gravis, hypersensitivity to anticholinergics, paralytic ileus, intestinal atony, unstable cardiovascular status in acute hemorrhage, toxic megacolon. Use cautiously in autonomic neuropathy, hyperthyroidism, coronary heart disease, cardiac arrhythmias, congestive heart failure, hypertension, hiatal hernia associated with reflux esophagitis, hepatic or renal disease, ulcerative colitis, or patients over 40 because of the increased incidence of glaucoma. • Use with caution in hot or humid environments. Drug-induced heat stroke can develop. • Give 30 minutes to 1 hour before meals and at bedtime. Bedtime dose can be larger and should be given at least 2 hours after the last meal of the day. • Administer smaller doses to the elderly. • If patient is also taking antihistamines, he may experience increased dryness of mouth. • Do not mix with antacids; administer alternately. • Monitor patient's vital signs and urinary output carefully. • Instruct patient to avoid driving and other hazardous activities if he is drowsy, dizzy, or has blurred vision; to drink plenty of fluids to help prevent constipation; and to report any skin rash. Gum or sugarless hard candy may relieve mouth dryness.

(continued on following page)

NAME	INDICATIONS & DOSAGE	SIDE EFFECTS
methantheline bromide *(continued)*		
methixene hydrochloride Trest◆	*Adjunctive treatment of gastrointestinal disorders associated with hypermotility or spasm—* **Adults:** 1 or 2 mg P.O. t.i.d.	*CNS:* headache, insomnia, drowsiness, dizziness, confusion or excitement in elderly patients, nervousness, weakness. *CV:* palpitations, tachycardia. *EENT:* blurred vision, mydriasis, increased ocular tension, cycloplegia, photophobia. *GI:* dry mouth, dysphagia, constipation, heartburn, loss of taste, nausea, vomiting, paralytic ileus. *GU:* urinary hesitancy and retention, impotence. *Skin:* urticaria, decreased sweating or anhidrosis, other dermal manifestations. *Other:* suppression of lactation, fever, allergic reactions. Overdosage may cause curare-like symptoms.
methscopolamine bromide Pamine◆, Scoline	*Adjunctive therapy in peptic ulcer—* **Adults:** 2.5 to 5 mg ½ hour before meals and at bedtime.	*CNS:* headache, insomnia, dizziness, confusion or excitement in elderly patients, nervousness, weakness. *CV:* palpitations, tachycardia. *EENT:* blurred vision, mydriasis, increased ocular tension, cycloplegia, photophobia. *GI:* dry mouth, dysphagia, constipation, heartburn, loss of taste, nausea, vomiting, paralytic ileus. *GU:* urinary hesitancy and retention, impotence. *Skin:* urticaria, decreased sweating or anhidrosis, other dermal manifestations. *Other:* suppression of lactation, fever, allergic reactions. Overdosage may cause curare-like symptoms.
oxyphencyclimine hydrochloride Daricon◆	*Adjunctive treatment of peptic ulcer—* **Adults:** 10 mg b.i.d. in the morning and at bedtime, or 5 mg b.i.d. or t.i.d.	*CNS:* headache, insomnia, drowsiness, dizziness, confusion or excitement in elderly patients, nervousness, weakness. *CV:* palpitations, tachycardia. *EENT:* blurred vision, mydriasis,

INTERACTIONS	NURSING CONSIDERATIONS
	• Quaternary ammonium derivative; these have fewer, less severe CNS side effects, since they do not cross blood-brain barrier. • Therapeutic effects appear in 30 to 45 minutes; persist for 4 to 6 hours after oral administration, 2 to 4 hours after I.M. injection. • For symptoms and treatment of toxicity, see p. 1115.
Methotrimeprazine: May produce extra-pyramidal symptoms. Monitor patient carefully.	• Contraindicated in narrow-angle glaucoma, obstructive uropathy, obstructive disease of the gastrointestinal tract, severe ulcerative colitis, myasthenia gravis, hypersensitivity to the anticholinergics, paralytic ileus, intestinal atony, unstable cardiovascular status in acute hemorrhage, and toxic megacolon. Use cautiously in autonomic neuropathy, hyperthyroidism, coronary heart disease, cardiac arrhythmias, congestive heart failure, hypertension, hiatal hernia associated with reflux esophagitis, hepatic or renal disease, ulcerative colitis, or patients over 40 because of the increased incidence of glaucoma. • Use with caution in hot or humid environments. Drug-induced heat stroke can develop. • Give 30 minutes to 1 hour before meals. • Administer smaller doses to the elderly. • Antacids may interfere with absorption; administer alternately. • Monitor patient's vital signs and urinary output. • Instruct patient to avoid driving and other hazardous activities if he is drowsy, dizzy, or has blurred vision; to drink plenty of fluids to help prevent constipation; and to report any skin rash. Gum or sugarless hard candy may relieve mouth dryness. • Synthetic tertiary derivative. • For symptoms and treatment of toxicity, see p. 1115.
Methotrimeprazine: may produce extra-pyramidal symptoms. Monitor patient carefully.	• Contraindicated in narrow-angle glaucoma, obstructive uropathy, obstructive disease of GI tract, severe ulcerative colitis, myasthenia gravis, hypersensitivity to anticholinergics, paralytic ileus, intestinal atony, unstable cardiovascular status in acute hemorrhage, toxic megacolon. Use cautiously in autonomic neuropathy, hyperthyroidism, coronary heart disease, cardiac arrhythmias, congestive heart failure, hypertension, hiatal hernia associated with reflux esophagitis, hepatic or renal disease, ulcerative colitis, or patients over 40 because of increased incidence of glaucoma. • Use with caution in hot or humid environments. Drug-induced heat stroke can develop. • Give 30 minutes to 1 hour before meals and at bedtime. Bedtime dose can be larger and should be given at least 2 hours after the last meal of the day. • Administer smaller doses to the elderly. • Antacids may interfere with absorption; administer alternately. • Monitor patient's vital signs and urinary output carefully. • Instruct patient to avoid driving and other hazardous activities if he is drowsy, dizzy, or has blurred vision; to drink plenty of fluids to help prevent constipation; and to report any skin rash. Gum or sugarless hard candy may relieve mouth dryness. • Quaternary ammonium derivative; these have fewer, less severe CNS side effects, since they do not cross blood-brain barrier. • For symptoms and treatment of toxicity, see p. 1115.
Methotrimeprazine: may produce extra-pyramidal symptoms. Monitor patient carefully.	• Contraindicated in narrow-angle glaucoma, obstructive uropathy, obstructive disease of GI tract, severe ulcerative colitis, myasthenia gravis, hypersensitivity to anticholinergics, paralytic ileus, intestinal atony, unstable cardiovascular status in acute hemorrhage, toxic megacolon. Use cautiously in autonomic neuropathy, hyperthyroidism, coronary heart disease, cardiac arrhythmias, congestive heart failure, hypertension, hiatal

(continued on following page)

NAME	INDICATIONS & DOSAGE	SIDE EFFECTS
oxyphencyclimine hydrochloride *(continued)*		increased ocular tension, cycloplegia, photophobia. *GI:* dry mouth, dysphagia, constipation, heartburn, loss of taste, nausea, vomiting, paralytic ileus. *GU:* urinary hesitancy and retention, impotence. *Skin:* urticaria, decreased sweating or anhidrosis, other dermal manifestations. *Other:* suppression of lactation, fever, allergic reactions. Overdosage may cause curare-like symptoms.
oxyphenonium bromide Antrenyl	*Adjunctive treatment of peptic ulcer—* **Adults:** 10 mg P.O. q.i.d. for several days, then reduced according to patient response.	*CNS:* headache, insomnia, drowsiness, dizziness, confusion or excitement in elderly patients, nervousness, weakness. *CV:* palpitations, tachycardia. *EENT:* blurred vision, mydriasis, increased ocular tension, cycloplegia, photophobia. *GI:* dry mouth, dysphagia, constipation, heartburn, loss of taste, nausea, vomiting, paralytic ileus. *GU:* urinary hesitancy and retention, impotence. *Skin:* urticaria, decreased sweating or anhidrosis, other dermal manifestations. *Other:* suppression of lactation, fever, allergic reactions. Overdosage may cause curare-like symptoms.
propantheline bromide Banlin♦♦, Norpanth, Pro-Banthine♦, Propanthel♦♦, Robantaline, Ropanth, Spastil	*Adjunctive treatment of peptic ulcer and irritable bowel syndrome, and other gastrointestinal disorders—* **Adults:** 15 mg P.O. t.i.d. before meals, and 30 mg at bedtime up to 60 mg q.i.d. Or, with prolonged-action tablets, 30 mg P.O. q 8 to 12 hours, depending on individual response. For elderly patients, 7.5 mg P.O. t.i.d. before meals. When oral dosage not possible, 30 mg I.M. or I.V. q 6 hours, depending on individual response. Maintenance dose 15 mg I.M. q 6 hours.	*CNS:* headache, insomnia, drowsiness, dizziness, confusion or excitement in elderly patients, nervousness, weakness. *CV:* palpitations, tachycardia. *EENT:* blurred vision, mydriasis, increased ocular tension, cycloplegia, photophobia. *GI:* dry mouth, dysphagia, constipation, heartburn, loss of taste, nausea, vomiting, paralytic ileus. *GU:* urinary hesitancy and retention, impotence. *Skin:* urticaria, decreased sweating or anhidrosis, other dermal manifestations.

INTERACTIONS	NURSING CONSIDERATIONS
	hernia associated with reflux esophagitis, hepatic or renal disease, ulcerative colitis, or patients over 40 because of increased incidence of glaucoma. • Use with caution in hot or humid environments. Drug-induced heat stroke can develop. • Give 30 minutes to 1 hour before breakfast and at bedtime. • Administer smaller doses to the elderly. • Antacids may interfere with absorption; administer alternately. • Monitor patient's vital signs and urinary output carefully. • Instruct patient to avoid driving and other hazardous activities if he is drowsy, dizzy, or has blurred vision; to drink plenty of fluids to help prevent constipation; and to report any skin rash. Gum or sugarless hard candy may relieve mouth dryness. • Synthetic tertiary derivative. • For symptoms and treatment of toxicity, see p. 1115.
Methotrimeprazine: may produce extrapyramidal symptoms. Monitor patient carefully.	• Contraindicated in narrow-angle glaucoma, obstructive uropathy, obstructive disease of GI tract, severe ulcerative colitis, myasthenia gravis, hypersensitivity to anticholinergics, paralytic ileus, intestinal atony, unstable cardiovascular status in acute hemorrhage, toxic megacolon. Use cautiously in autonomic neuropathy, hyperthyroidism, coronary heart disease, cardiac arrhythmias, congestive heart failure, hypertension, hiatal hernia associated with reflux esophagitis, hepatic or renal disease, ulcerative colitis, or patients over 40 because of increased incidence of glaucoma. • Use with caution in hot or humid environments. Drug-induced heat stroke can develop. • Give 30 minutes to 1 hour before meals and at bedtime. Bedtime dose can be larger and should be given at least 2 hours after the last meal of the day. • Administer smaller doses to the elderly. • Antacids may interfere with absorption; administer alternately. • Monitor patient's vital signs and urinary output. • Instruct patient to avoid driving and other hazardous activities if he is drowsy, dizzy, or has blurred vision; to drink plenty of fluids to help prevent constipation; and to report any skin rash. Gum or sugarless hard candy may relieve mouth dryness. • Potent quaternary ammonium derivative; incidence of side effects may be greater than those produced by similiar compounds. • For symptoms and treatment of toxicity, see p. 1115.
Methotrimeprazine: may produce extrapyramidal symptoms. Monitor patient carefully.	• Contraindicated in narrow-angle glaucoma, obstructive uropathy, obstructive disease of GI tract, severe ulcerative colitis, myasthenia gravis, hypersensitivity to anticholinergics, paralytic ileus, intestinal atony, unstable cardiovascular status in acute hemorrhage, toxic megacolon. Use cautiously in autonomic neuropathy, hyperthyroidism, coronary heart disease, cardiac arrhythmias, congestive heart failure, hypertension, hiatal hernia associated with reflux esophagitis, hepatic or renal disease, ulcerative colitis, or patients over 40 because of the increased incidence of glaucoma. • Use with caution in hot or humid environments. Drug-induced heat stroke can develop. • Give 30 minutes to 1 hour before meals and at bedtime. Bedtime dose can be larger and should be given at least 2 hours after the last meal of the day. • Administer smaller doses to the elderly. • Antacids may interfere with absorption; administer alternately. • Monitor patient's vital signs and urinary output carefully. • Instruct patient to avoid driving and other hazardous activities if he is

(continued on following page)

NAME	INDICATIONS & DOSAGE	SIDE EFFECTS
propantheline bromide *(continued)*		*Other:* suppression of lactation, fever, allergic reactions. Overdosage may cause curare-like symptoms.
thiphenamil hydrochloride Trocinate	*Hypermotility and spasm of the gastrointestinal tract—* **Adults:** initially, 400 mg P.O. repeated in 4 hours, usually to maximum of 4 doses.	*CNS:* headache, insomnia, drowsiness, dizziness, confusion or excitement in elderly patients, nervousness, weakness. *CV:* palpitations, tachycardia. *EENT:* blurred vision, mydriasis, increased ocular tension, cycloplegia, photophobia. *GI:* dry mouth, dysphagia, constipation, heartburn, loss of taste, nausea, vomiting, paralytic ileus. *GU:* urinary hesitancy and retention, impotence. *Skin:* urticaria, decreased sweating or anhidrosis, other dermal manifestations. *Other:* suppression of lactation, fever, allergic reactions. Overdosage may cause curare-like symptoms.
tridihexethyl chloride Pathilon	*Adjunctive treatment of peptic ulcer, irritable bowel syndrome, and other gastrointestinal disorders—* **Adults:** initially, 25 to 50 mg P.O. t.i.d. before meals, and 50 mg at bedtime, increased to 75 mg q.i.d., if needed. With sustained-release capsules, 75 mg q 12 or q 6 hours. Maintenance dose usually half the therapeutic dose. Parenteral use: 10 to 20 mg I.V., I.M., or S.C. q 6 hours. Change to oral as soon as possible.	*CNS:* headache, insomnia, drowsiness, dizziness, confusion or excitement in elderly patients, nervousness, weakness. *CV:* palpitations, tachycardia. *EENT:* blurred vision, mydriasis, increased ocular tension, cycloplegia, photophobia. *GI:* dry mouth, dysphagia, constipation, heartburn, loss of taste, nausea, vomiting, paralytic ileus. *GU:* urinary hesitancy and retention, impotence. *Skin:* urticaria, decreased sweating or anhidrosis, other dermal manifestations. *Other:* suppression of lactation, fever, allergic reactions. Overdosage may cause curare-like symptoms.

INTERACTIONS	NURSING CONSIDERATIONS
	drowsy, dizzy, or has blurred vision; to drink plenty of fluids to help prevent constipation; and to report any skin rash. Gum or sugarless hard candy may relieve mouth dryness. • Quaternary ammonium derivative; these have fewer, less severe CNS side effects, since they do not cross blood-brain barrier. • For symptoms and treatment of toxicity, see p. 1115.
Methotrimeprazine: may produce extrapyramidal symptoms. Monitor patient carefully.	• Contraindicated in narrow-angle glaucoma, obstructive uropathy, obstructive disease of GI tract, severe ulcerative colitis, myasthenia gravis, hypersensitivity to anticholinergics, paralytic ileus, intestinal atony, unstable cardiovascular status in acute hemorrhage, toxic megacolon. Use cautiously in autonomic neuropathy, hyperthyroidism, coronary heart disease, cardiac arrhythmias, congestive heart failure, hypertension, hiatal hernia associated with reflux esophagitis, hepatic or renal disease, ulcerative colitis, or patients over 40 because of increased incidence of glaucoma. • Use with caution in hot or humid environments. Drug-induced heat stroke can develop. • Administer smaller doses to the elderly. • Antacids may interfere with absorption; administer alternately. • Monitor patient's vital signs and urinary output carefully. • Instruct patient to avoid driving and other hazardous activities if he is drowsy, dizzy, or has blurred vision; to drink plenty of fluids to help prevent constipation; and to report any skin rash. Gum or sugarless hard candy may relieve mouth dryness. • For symptoms and treatment of toxicity, see p. 1115.
Methotrimeprazine: may produce extrapyramidal symptoms. Monitor patient carefully.	• Contraindicated in narrow-angle glaucoma, obstructive uropathy, obstructive disease of GI tract, severe ulcerative colitis, myasthenia gravis, hypersensitivity to anticholinergics, paralytic ileus, intestinal atony, unstable cardiovascular status in acute hemorrhage, toxic megacolon. Use cautiously in autonomic neuropathy, hyperthyroidism, coronary heart disease, cardiac arrhythmias, congestive heart failure, hypertension, hiatal hernia associated with reflux esophagitis, hepatic or renal disease, ulcerative colitis, or patients over 40 because of increased incidence of glaucoma. • Use with caution in hot or humid environments. Drug-induced heat stroke can develop. • Give 30 minutes to 1 hour before meals and at bedtime. Bedtime dose can be larger and should be given at least 2 hours after the last meal of the day. • Administer smaller doses to the elderly. • Antacids may interfere with absorption; administer alternately. • Monitor patient's vital signs and urinary output carefully. • Instruct patient to avoid driving and other hazardous activities if he is drowsy, dizzy, or has blurred vision; to drink plenty of fluids to help prevent constipation; and to report any skin rash. Gum or sugarless hard candy may relieve mouth dryness. • Quaternary ammonium derivative; these have fewer, less severe CNS side effects, since they do not cross blood-brain barrier. • For symptoms and treatment of toxicity, see p. 1115.

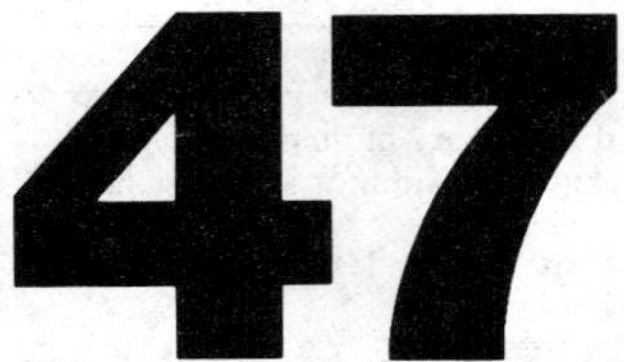

Miscellaneous gastrointestinals

choline **dexpanthenol**
cimetidine **metoclopramide hydrochloride**

Miscellaneous gastrointestinal drugs include lipotropic substances, such as choline, choline chloride, choline bitartrate, and choline dihydrogen citrate; smooth-muscle relaxants, such as dexpanthenol; and H_2 (histamine) receptor antagonists, such as cimetidine and metoclopramide.

Major uses

- Lipotropic agents decrease the fat content of the liver. They are essential for normal transport from the hepatic and are used in an attempt to treat disorders of hepatic fat-transport.
- Dexpanthenol is used prophylactically immediately after major abdominal surgery to reduce the possibility of paralytic ileus, and also to treat intestinal atony causing abdominal distention, postoperative or postpartum retention of flatus, postoperative delay in resumption of intestinal motility, and paralytic ileus.
- Cimetidine is used to treat pathologic hypersecretory conditions and duodenal ulcer.
- Metoclopramide facilitates small bowel intubation and aids in radiologic examinations.

Mechanism of action

- Lipotropic agents facilitate phospholipid turnover and enhance fat-transport from the liver to the tissues, thus decreasing the fat content of the liver.
- Dexpanthenol stimulates intestinal smooth muscles, restores tone to intestines.
- Cimetidine, an anticholinergic, competitively inhibits the action of histamine at the histamine receptors of the parietal cells and thus decreases gastric acid secretion.
- Metoclopramide stimulates motility of the upper GI tract by the antagonism of dopaminergic mechanisms.

Absorption, distribution, and excretion

- Dexpanthenol is mainly used in parenteral administration. Absorption is complete; widely distributed.
- Lipotropic substances: absorption fair after oral use, since much can be destroyed in the stomach by gastric acidity and in the intestines by bacterial action.
- Cimetidine is rapidly absorbed in the upper portion of the small intestine, widely distributed to all body tissues, and excreted in the urine.
- Metoclopramide is absorbed immediately and is distributed widely.

Onset and duration

- Lipotropic substances: unknown.
- Dexpanthenol may take up to 72 hours or longer to be effective.
- Cimetidine reaches peak blood levels within 75 minutes and has a half-life of approximately 2 hours.

• Metoclopramide acts within 1 to 3 minutes following I.V. dose and persists for 1 to 2 hours.

Combination products

GERIPLEX: choline 20 mg, vitamin A 5,000 units, vitamin E 5 units, vitamin B_1 5 mg, vitamin B_2 5 mg, vitamin B_3 15 mg, vitamin B_{12} 2 mg, vitamin C 50 mg, iron 6 mg, calcium 59 mg, and phosphorus 46 mg.
GERIZYME: inositol 100 mg, 1-lysine 100 mg, vitamin B_1 3.3 mg, vitamin B_2 3.3 mg, vitamin B_3 33.2 mg, vitamin B_5 3.3 mg, vitamin B_6 1 mg, vitamin B_{12} 3.3 mcg, iron 5 mg.
ILOPAN CHOLINE: dexpanthenol 50 mg and choline bitartrate 25 mg.
LIPOFLAVONOID: choline 111 mg, inositol 111 mg, vitamin B_1 0.3 mg, vitamin B_2 0.3 mg, vitamin B_3 3.3 mg, vitamin B_5 0.3 mg, vitamin B_6 0.3 mg, vitamin C 100 mg, and vitamin B_{12} 1.7 mcg.
LUFA: choline 111 mg, inositol 40 mg, methionine 66 mg, vitamin E 4 units, vitamin B_1 2 mg, vitamin B_2 2 mg, vitamin B_3 5 mg, vitamin B_5 1 mg, vitamin B_6 2 mg, vitamin B_{12} 1 mg, desiccated hepatic 87 mg, and unsaturated fatty acids 423 mg.
METHISCHOL: choline 115 mg, inositol 83 mg, methionine 110 mg, vitamin B_1 3 mg, vitamin B_2 3 mg, vitamin B_3 10 mg, vitamin B_5 2 mg, vitamin B_6 2 mg, vitamin B_{12} 2 mcg, and desiccated hepatic and hepatic concentrate 86 mg.

CHECKING LEVIN TUBE PLACEMENT

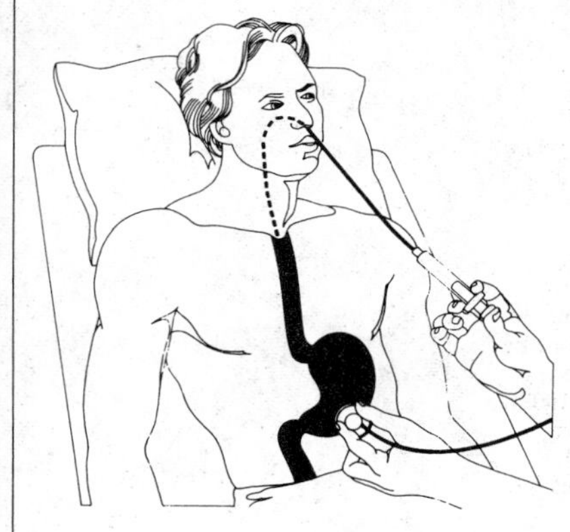

You can use the Levin (nasogastric) tube to instill medication. The first step is checking the tube for successful stomach entry (pictured at left). Connect a catheter-tip syringe to the tube, then place your stethoscope over the patient's epigastric region. Squeeze the syringe, inject about 15 ml of air and listen for the reassuring stomach "whoosh."

Now that you are sure that the Levin tube is positioned properly, attach an irrigating syringe, with plunger removed, to the Levin tube and pour in 5 ml of water.

Instill medication (diluted if necessary) and allow it to flow by gravity.

Insert 5 ml of water and clamp the Levin tube for 15 to 20 minutes.

NAME	INDICATIONS & DOSAGE	SIDE EFFECTS
choline choline bitartrate, choline chloride, choline dihydrogen citrate	*Hepatic disorders and disturbed fat metabolism*— **Adults and children:** 650 to 750 mg P.O. daily.	*GI:* irritation if taken on an empty stomach. *Metabolic:* ketosis after excessive dosages.
cimetidine Tagamet◆	*Duodenal ulcer (short-term treatment)*— **Adults, and children over 16 years:** 300 mg P.O. q.i.d. with meals and at bedtime for maximum therapy of 8 weeks. Once healing occurs, stop treatment or give bedtime dose only to control nocturnal hypersecretion. Parenteral: 300 mg diluted to 20 ml with 0.9% normal saline or other compatible I.V. solution, I.V. push over 1 to 2 minutes q 6 hours. Or 300 mg diluted in 100 ml 5% dextrose solution or other compatible I.V. solution, by I.V. infusion over 15 to 20 minutes q 6 hours. To increase dose, give 300 mg doses more frequently to maximum daily dose of 2,400 mg. *Pathological hypersecretory conditions (such as Zollinger-Ellison syndrome, systemic mastocytosis, and multiple endocrine adenomas)*— **Adults, and children over 16 years:** 300 mg P.O. with meals and at bedtime; adjust to individual needs. Maximum daily dose 2,400 mg. Parenteral: 300 mg diluted to 20 ml with 0.9% normal saline or other compatible I.V. solution, by I.V. push over 1 to 2 minutes q 6 hours. Or 300 mg diluted in 100 ml 5% dextrose solution or other compatible I.V. solution by I.V. infusion over 15 to 20 minutes q 6 hours. To increase dose, give 300 mg doses more frequently to maximum daily dose of 2,400 mg.	*Blood:* agranulocytosis, neutropenia, thrombocytopenia. *CNS:* mental confusion in higher than recommended dosages, dizziness. *GI:* mild and transient diarrhea, perforation of chronic peptic ulcers after abrupt cessation of drug. *Metabolic:* slight, transient elevation of serum transaminase levels, but no hepatic function abnormalities; slight elevation of serum creatinine levels, but no signs of renal dysfunction. *Skin:* acne-like rash, urticaria. *Other:* muscle pain, reduced sperm count; mild gynecomastia after use longer than 1 month (but no change in endocrine function); impotence.

◆ Also available in Canada.
◆◆ Available in Canada only.
Unmarked trade names available in United States only.

INTERACTIONS	NURSING CONSIDERATIONS
None significant.	• Foods supplying choline include egg yolk, beef liver, legumes, vegetables, and milk. Average diet contains from 500 to 900 mg per day. • Lipotropic agent. • Used in many multivitamin preparations, but no evidence supplemental choline intake is more beneficial for long periods than an adequate diet. • Synthesized by the body from serine, with methionine acting as a methyl-donor in the reaction. • Choline is no longer considered effective in treatment of hepatic disorders or disorders of lipid transport or metabolism. • Investigative use in treatment of tardive dyskinesia: restores cholinergic tone and decreases choreic movements. Oral choline elevates brain choline, and acetylcholine (the cholinergic neurotransmitter of the cholinergic nervous system) levels and restores cholinergic tone. • Lecithin (available in health food stores) is a source of choline.
Antacids: interfere with absorption of cimetidine. Separate cimetidine and antacids by at least 1 hour if possible.	• Contraindicated by I.M. route of administration. • I.V. solutions compatible for dilution with cimetidine: 0.9% sodium chloride, 5% and 10% dextrose (and combinations of these), lactated Ringer's solution, and 5% sodium bicarbonate injection. Do not dilute with sterile water for injection. • Hemodialysis reduces blood levels of cimetidine. Schedule cimetidine dose at end of hemodialysis treatment. • Up to 10 g overdosage has been reported without untoward effects. • Neutropenia has been reported; however, these patients were also receiving other drugs or had disease states known to produce neutropenia. • Effectiveness in treatment of gastric ulcers not as great as in duodenal ulcer. Cimetidine may prove useful but is still unapproved in pancreatic insufficiency, prevention and treatment of GI bleeding, relief of symptoms and acid sensitivity in reflux esophagitis, and to prevent gastric inactivation of oral enzyme preparations by gastric acid and pepsin. • Best to administer with meals in order to maintain blood levels. • Large parenteral doses should be avoided in asthmatics. • Elderly patients more susceptible to cimetidine-induced mental confusion. Dose should be decreased in elderly and in patients with renal insufficiency. • I.V. cimetidine often used in critically ill patients prophylactically to prevent GI bleeding.

NAME	INDICATIONS & DOSAGE	SIDE EFFECTS
dexpanthenol Ilopan◆, Intrapan, Motilyn◆◆, Tonestat	*Postop abdominal distention (resulting from flatus retention)*— **Adults and children:** 250 mg to 500 mg I.M., repeat in 2 hours and again q 6 hours until distention is relieved. May require therapy for 48 to 72 hours or longer. Or, 500 mg infused slow I.V. drip in glucose or lactated Ringer's solution. *Treatment and postop prevention of paralytic ileus*— **Adults and children:** 500 mg I.M., repeat in 2 hours; then q 4 to 6 hours until distention is relieved. May require therapy for 48 to 72 hours or longer.	*GI:* excessive passage of flatus with increased doses or prolonged use, increased frequency of bowel movements, hyperperistalsis.
metoclopramide hydrochloride Maxeran, Reglan ◆◆	*To facilitate small-bowel intubation and to aid in radiologic examinations*— **Adults:** 10 mg (2 ml) I.V. as a single dose over 1 to 2 minutes. **Children 6 to 14 years:** 2.5 to 5 mg (0.5 to 1 ml). **Children under 6 years:** 0.1 mg/Kg.	*CNS:* restlessness, drowsiness, fatigue, lassitude, insomnia, headache, dizziness. *GI:* nausea, bowel disturbances. *Other:* extrapyramidal symptoms.

INTERACTIONS	NURSING CONSIDERATIONS
None significant.	• Contraindicated in hemophilia. • Don't administer full strength solution I.V.; always dilute. • Dexpanthenol use shouldn't delay treatment of mechanical ileus if present. • A smooth-muscle stimulant; used postop against delayed resumption of intestinal motility. Also used as adjunctive treatment of peripheral neuritis and lupus erythematosus. • Hypokalemia may cause a decreased response. If this occurs, potassium supplements should be started. Increased doses of dexpanthenol may be needed. • Onset of response may take 72 hours or longer. Do not stop therapy prematurely. • May also be useful during laxative withdrawal after long-term use. • Wait 12 hours after giving parasympathomimetics before starting dexpanthenol.
Anticholinergics, narcotic analgesics: antagonized effects of metoclopramide. Use together cautiously.	• Contraindicated whenever stimulation of GI motility might be dangerous (hemorrhage, obstruction, perforation), pheochromocytoma, and epilepsy. • Speeds gastric emptying by stimulating smooth muscle in upper GI tract. • If I.V. injection is too rapid, a transient but intense feeling of anxiety and restlessness, followed by drowsiness, occurs. • Avoid activities requiring alertness for 2 hours after taking. • Oral form available in Canada only. Give with meals. • Injectable form may be useful as an antiemetic following chemotherapy. • Used investigationally to treat diabetic gastric paresis.

Hormones, Hormone Antagonists, and Synthetic Substitutes

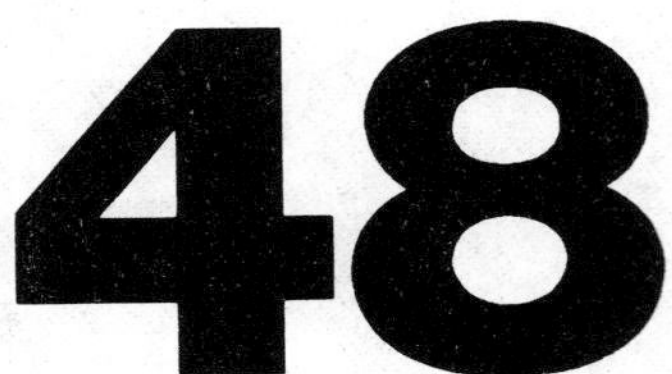

Corticosteroids

beclomethasone dipropionate
betamethasone
cortisone acetate
desoxycorticosterone
dexamethasone
fludrocortisone acetate
fluprednisolone
hydrocortisone
meprednisone
methylprednisolone
paramethasone acetate
prednisolone
prednisone
triamcinolone

Corticosteroids are hormones naturally secreted by the adrenal cortex. They can also be produced synthetically. They can be classified as glucocorticoids (which stop inflammation) and mineralocorticoids (which cause the kidneys to retain sodium and excrete potassium). They affect many metabolic functions and all organ systems.

Major uses

- Treatment of adrenal insufficiency.
- Relief of inflammation in rheumatic fever, rheumatoid arthritis, collagen diseases (lupus erythematosus, dermatomyositis, periarteritis nodosa), nephrotic syndrome. Do not affect progression of disease.
- Suppression of the inflammatory reaction in allergic dermatoses, food and drug allergies, asthma, ulcerative colitis, and vasculitis.
- Emergency treatment of shock and anaphylaxis.
- Immunosuppressive and anti-inflammatory effect in organ and tissue transplants to prevent rejection.
- Adjunctive treatment of leukemias, lymphomas, and myelomas.
- Treatment of hypercalcemia resulting from breast cancer, multiple myeloma, sarcoidosis, or vitamin D intoxication.
- Relief of cerebral edema after neurosurgery or associated with brain tumors.

Mechanism of action

- Stabilize the cell membrane, inhibiting the release of proteolytic enzymes and thereby preventing the normal inflammatory response.

- Interfere with the immune and allergic response by decreasing the number of lymphocytes, plasma cells, and eosinophils in the blood. Also decreases the conversion rate of lymphocytes into antibodies.
- Antilymphocytic actions also make them useful in treatment of some neoplasms.
- Increase the activity of the enzymes vital for glucogenesis and inhibit glycolytic enzymes. This can produce hyperglycemia and glycosuria, aggravating or precipitating diabetes mellitus.
- Retard growth in children by adverse effect on epiphyseal cartilage.
- Decrease serum calcium levels by decreasing renal excretion of calcium.
- Suppress release of adrenocorticotropic hormone (ACTH) from the pituitary which leads to suppression of adrenal cortex.
- When used to treat shock, potentiate the vasoconstrictor effect of norepinephrine.
- Mineralocorticoids act on the distal tubules of the kidneys to promote reabsorption of sodium ions and increase urinary excretion of potassium and hydrogen ions.

Absorption, distribution, and excretion

- Well absorbed after oral administration, except desoxycorticosterone, which is ineffective by this route.
- Aqueous solutions are rapidly absorbed after intramuscular injection, but aqueous suspensions and solutions in oil are slowly absorbed.
- Rapidly distributed to all body tissues when given intravenously.
- Metabolized in liver; excreted in urine.

Onset, and duration

- Oral doses usually begin to act within 6 hours.
- Aqueous suspensions and solutions in oil have slow onset and produce low, prolonged blood levels.
- Aqueous solutions by intravenous administration have rapid onset.
- Duration of action is longer than measurable physical presence or metabolic effects.

Corticosteroids	Potency in mg equivalent to 5 mg prednisone	Mineralocorticoid potency
betamethasone	0.06	0
cortisone acetate	25	1
dexamethasone	0.75	0
fludrocortisone	—	125
hydrocortisone	20	1
meprednisone	4	0
methylprednisolone	4	0.5
paramethasone	2	0
prednisolone	5	0.8
prednisone	5	0.8
triamcinolone	4	0

Dosing instructions

- To minimize adrenal insufficiency and insomnia, give ⅔ of the daily dose before 10 a.m. and ⅓ in early afternoon.
- Alternating day of therapy may reduce adverse reactions in long-term treatment.
- Short-term therapy (less than 7 days) with moderate doses (40 mg or less of prednisone or equivalent) produces few side effects and may be abruptly discontinued.
- Long-term or high-dose therapy must be discontinued gradually, or acute adrenal insufficiency may result.

Combination products

ATARAXOID: hydroxyzine hydrochloride 10 mg and prednisolone 2.5 or 5 mg.

RECOGNIZING AND TREATING CUSHINGOID SYMPTOMS

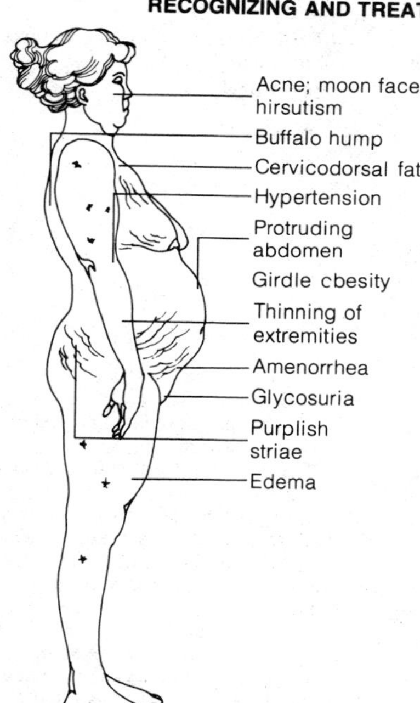

Prolonged corticosteroid therapy may cause the side effect of cushingoid syndrome, a peculiar type of obesity in which fat is distributed in pads between the shoulders — creating a buffalo hump — and around the waist — creating a girdle of fat.

RECOGNITION:

- Observe the patient for cushingoid symptoms. In addition to those listed alongside the illustration, look for: muscular weakness, wasting tissue, hyperglycemia, renal disorders, mental changes ranging from euphoria to depression, and lowered resistance to infection. Report your observations to a doctor.

TREATMENT:

- Because adrenal hormones are excreted in the urine, collect all urine.
- Record food and fluid intake.
- To keep track of the patient's emotional state, record the types of situations that disturb him.
- To relieve emotional stress, keep the patient well informed. For example, tell the woman with distressing hirsutism and a tendency toward masculinization that these changes will disappear after treatment.

NAME	INDICATIONS & DOSAGE	SIDE EFFECTS
beclomethasone dipropionate Beclovent, Vanceril◆	*Steroid-dependent asthma—* **Adults:** 2 to 4 inhalations t.i.d. or q.i.d. Maximum 20 inhalations daily. **Children 6 to 12 years:** 1 to 2 inhalations t.i.d. or q.i.d. Maximum 10 inhalations daily.	*EENT:* hoarseness, fungal infections of mouth and throat. *GI:* dry mouth.
betamethasone Betnelan◆◆, Celestone◆ **betamethasone acetate and betamethasone sodium phosphate** Celestone Soluspan◆ **betamethasone disodium phosphate** Betnesol◆◆ **betamethasone sodium phosphate** Celestone Phosphate	*Severe inflammation or immunosuppression—* **Adults:** 0.6 to 7.2 mg P.O. daily; or 0.5 to 9 mg (sodium phosphate) I.M., I.V., or into joint or soft tissue daily; or 1.5 to 12 mg (sodium phosphate-acetate suspension) into joint or soft tissue q 1 to 2 weeks, p.r.n.	*CNS:* seizures, pseudotumor cerebri, vertigo, headache. *CV:* congestive heart failure, hypertension. *EENT:* cataracts, increased intraocular pressure, glaucoma, exophthalmos. *GI:* irritation, peptic and esophageal ulcer, bleeding, pancreatitis, increased appetite. *GU:* menstrual abnormalities. *Metabolic:* growth suppression, Cushing's syndrome, suppression of hypothalamic-pituitary-adrenal axis, carbohydrate intolerance, protein catabolism, hypernatremia, hypokalemia, hypocalcemia. *Skin:* delayed wound healing, petechiae, ecchymoses, thin and shiny skin, erythema, sweating. *Other:* edema, muscle weakness, myopathy, osteoporosis, fractures, aseptic necrosis of femoral and humoral heads. May mask or exacerbate infection.
cortisone acetate Cortistan, Cortone Acetate◆	*Adrenal insufficiency, allergy, inflammation—* **Adults:** 25 to 300 mg P.O. or I.M. daily or on alternate days. Doses highly individualized, depending on severity of disease; always titrated to lowest effective dose.	*CNS:* convulsions, pseudotumor cerebri, vertigo, headache, depression or euphoria, psychotic behavior. *CV:* hypertension, congestive heart failure, thromboembolism, thrombophlebitis, thrombosis, fat embolism. *EENT:* cataracts, increased intraocular pressure, glaucoma, exophthalmos. *GI:* irritation, ulcer and perforation, pancreatitis, distention, increased appetite. *GU:* menstrual abnormalities. *Local:* atrophy at I.M. injection sites.

◆ Also available in Canada.
◆◆ Available in Canada only.
Unmarked trade names available in United States only.

INTERACTIONS	NURSING CONSIDERATIONS
None significant.	• Contraindicated in status asthmaticus. Not for asthma controlled by bronchodilators or other noncorticosteroids, or for nonasthmatic bronchial diseases. • Oral therapy should be tapered slowly. Acute adrenal insufficiency and death have occurred in asthmatics who changed abruptly from oral corticosteroids to beclomethasone. • During times of stress (trauma, surgery, infection) systemic corticosteroids may be needed to prevent adrenal insufficiency. • Instruct patient to carry a card indicating his need for supplemental systemic glucocorticoids during stress. • Patient requiring bronchodilator should use it several minutes before beclomethasone. • Don't store near heat or open flame. • Glucocorticoid with potent anti-inflammatory action. • Oral fungal infections can be prevented by following inhalations with a glass of water.
Barbiturates, phenytoin, rifampin: decreased corticosteroid effect. Corticosteroid dose may need to be increased. *Indomethacin, ASA:* increased risk of GI distress and bleeding. Give together cautiously. *Methandrostenolone:* monitor for enhanced corticosteroid response.	• Contraindicated in systemic fungal infections. • Don't use for alternate-day therapy. • Adrenal suppression may last up to 1 year after drug stopped. Gradually reduce drug dosage after long-term therapy. Tell patient not to stop drug abruptly or without doctor's consent. • To prevent muscle atrophy, give by deep I.M. injection. • Monitor serum electrolytes and blood sugar. • Warn patients who are on long-term therapy about cushingoid symptoms. • Observe for signs of infection, especially after steroid withdrawal. • Instruct patient to carry a card indicating his need for supplemental glucocorticoids during stress. • Give with milk or food to reduce gastric irritation. • Glucocorticoid with little mineralocorticoid effect. • Watch for additional potassium depletion from diuretics and amphotericin B. • Immunizations may show decreased antibody response. • Weigh patient daily; report any sudden weight gain to doctor.
Barbiturates, phenytoin, rifampin: decreased corticosteroid effect. Corticosteroid dose may need to be increased. *Indomethacin, ASA:* increased risk of GI distress and bleeding. Give together cautiously. *Methandrostenolone:* monitor for enhanced	• Contraindicated in systemic fungal infections. Use cautiously in GI ulceration or renal disease, hypertension, osteoporosis, varicella, vaccinia, exanthema, diabetes mellitus, Cushing's syndrome, thromboembolic disorders, seizures, myasthenia gravis, congestive heart failure, tuberculosis, ocular herpes simplex, hypoalbuminemia, emotional instability, or psychotic tendencies. • Gradually reduce drug dosage after long-term therapy. Tell patient not to discontinue drug abruptly or without doctor's consent. • Patient may need salt-restricted diet and potassium supplement. • I.M. route causes slow onset of action. Don't use in acute conditions where rapid effect required. • Glucocorticoid with potent mineralocorticoid effect; report sudden weight gain or edema to doctor.

(continued on following page)

NAME	INDICATIONS & DOSAGE	SIDE EFFECTS
cortisone acetate *(continued)*		*Metabolic:* growth suppression in children, hyperlipidemia, Cushing's syndrome, negative nitrogen balance, carbohydrate intolerance, hypernatremia, hypokalemia, hypercholesterolemia, hypocalcemia. *Skin:* slow wound healing, acne, thin and shiny skin, facial flushing, sweating, petechiae, ecchymoses, hyperpigmentation or hypopigmentation. *Other:* susceptibility to, or exacerbation or masking of infection; myopathy, muscle weakness, osteoporosis, compression and pathologic fractures, edema. Acute adrenal insufficiency may occur with increased stress (infection, surgery, trauma) or abrupt withdrawal after long-term therapy. *Withdrawal symptoms:* rebound inflammation, fatigue, weakness, arthralgia, fever, dizziness, lethargy, depression, fainting, orthostatic hypotension, dyspnea, anorexia, hypoglycemia. *Sudden withdrawal may be fatal.*
desoxycorticosterone acetate Cortate Acetate, Doca Acetate **desoxycorticosterone pivalate** Percorten Pivalate	*Adrenal insufficiency (partial replacement), salt-losing adrenogenital syndrome*— **Adults:** 1 to 5 mg (acetate) I.M. daily; or 25 to 75 mg (acetate) I.M. q 4 weeks; or 25 to 100 mg (pivalate) I.M. q 4 weeks.	*CNS:* headache, arthralgia, ascending paralysis, weakness. *CV:* hypertension, cardiomegaly, congestive heart failure. *Metabolic:* hypernatremia, hypokalemia, hypocalcemia. *Other:* edema, hypersensitivity.
dexamethasone Decadron◆, Dexasone◆◆, Dexone, Dezone, Hexadrol **dexamethasone acetate** Decadron-LA **dexamethasone sodium phosphate** Decadron Phosphate, Decaject, Decameth,	*Cerebral edema*— **Adults:** initially, 10 mg (phosphate) I.V. then 4 to 6 mg I.M. q 6 hours for 2 to 4 days, then taper over 5 to 7 days. **Children:** 0.2 mg/Kg P.O. daily in divided doses. *Inflammatory conditions, allergic reactions, neoplasias*— **Adults:** 0.25 to 4 mg P.O. b.i.d., t.i.d., or q.i.d.; or 4 to 16 mg (acetate) I.M. into joint or soft tissue q 1 to 3 weeks; or 0.8 to 1.6	*CNS:* convulsions, pseudotumor cerebri, vertigo, headache, depression or euphoria, psychotic behavior. *CV:* hypertension, congestive heart failure. *EENT:* cataracts, glaucoma, increased intraocular pressure, exophthalmos. *GI:* ulcer and perforation, pancreatitis, distention. *GU:* menstrual abnormalities. *Local:* atrophy at I.M. injection sites. *Metabolic:* growth suppression in children, hyperlipidemia, Cushing's

INTERACTIONS	NURSING CONSIDERATIONS
corticosteroid response.	• Observe for signs of infection, especially after steroid withdrawal. • Drug of choice for replacement therapy in adrenal insufficiency. • Used for alternate-day therapy. • Monitor serum electrolytes and blood sugar. • Warn patients on long-term therapy about cushingoid symptoms. • Give with milk or food to reduce gastric irritation. • Instruct patient to carry a card indicating his need for supplemental glucocorticoids during stress. • Not for I.V. use. • Watch for additional potassium depletion from diuretics and amphotericin B. • Immunizations may show decreased antibody response.
Barbiturates, phenytoin, rifampin: decreased corticosteroid effect. Corticosteroid dose may need to be increased. *Indomethacin, ASA:* increased risk of GI distress and bleeding. Give together cautiously. *Methandrostenolone:* monitor for enhanced corticosteroid response.	• Contraindicated in hypertension, congestive heart failure, cardiac disease. Use cautiously in Addison's disease. Patients may have exaggerated side effects. • Has no anti-inflammatory effect. • Most potent mineralocorticoid. Has little glucocorticoid effect. • Use with glucocorticoid for full treatment of adrenal insufficiency. • Report significant weight gain, edema, hypertension, or cardiac symptoms to doctor. Drug may have to be stopped. • Injection is sesame oil solution. Withdraw dose with 19-gauge needle, but give with 23-gauge needle. Inject in upper, outer quadrant of buttocks. Not for I.V. use. • Monitor sodium and potassium levels, fluid intake. Patient may need salt-restricted diet and potassium supplement. • Watch for additional potassium depletion from diuretics and amphotericin B. • Immunizations may show decreased antibody response.
Barbiturates, phenytoin, rifampin: decreased corticosteroid effect. Corticosteroid dose may need to be increased. *Indomethacin, ASA:*: increased risk of GI distress and bleeding. Give together cautiously. *Methandrostenolone:* monitor for enhanced	• Contraindicated in systemic fungal infections and for alternate-day therapy. Use cautiously in GI ulceration or renal disease, hypertension, osteoporosis, varicella, vaccinia, exanthema, diabetes mellitus, Cushing's syndrome, thromboembolic disorders, seizures, myasthenia gravis, metastatic cancer, congestive heart failure, tuberculosis, ocular herpes simplex, hypoalbuminemia, emotional instability or psychotic tendencies, and in children. • Gradually reduce drug dosage after long-term therapy. Tell patient not to discontinue drug abruptly or without doctor's consent. • Monitor patient's weight, blood pressure, serum electrolytes. • Instruct patient to carry a card indicating his need for supplemental systemic glucocorticoids during stress, especially as dose is decreased. • Teach patient signs of early adrenal insufficiency: fatigue, muscular weak-

(continued on following page)

NAME	INDICATIONS & DOSAGE	SIDE EFFECTS
dexamethasone sodium phosphate *(continued)* Dexacen-4, Dexon, Dexone, Dezone, Hexadrol Phosphate◆, Savacort-D, Solurex	mg (acetate) into lesions q 1 to 3 weeks. *Shock*— **Adults:** 1 to 6 mg/Kg (phosphate) I.V. single dose; or 40 mg I.V. q 2 to 6 hours, p.r.n.	syndrome, negative nitrogen balance, carbohydrate intolerance, hypokalemia, hypernatremia, hypocalcemia. *Skin:* slow wound healing, acne, thin and shiny skin, facial flushing, sweating, petechiae, ecchymoses, hyperpigmentation or hypopigmentation. *Other:* susceptibility to or exacerbation of infection, myopathy, muscle weakness, osteoporosis, compression and pathologic fractures, edema. Acute adrenal insufficiency may occur with increased stress (infection, surgery, trauma) or abrupt withdrawal after long-term therapy. *Withdrawal symptoms:* rebound inflammation, fatigue, weakness, arthralgia, fever, dizziness, lethargy, depression, fainting, orthostatic hypotension, dyspnea, anorexia, hypoglycemia. *Sudden withdrawal may be fatal.*
fludrocortisone acetate Florinef◆	*Adrenal insufficiency (partial replacement), salt-losing adrenogenital syndrome*— **Adults:** 0.1 to 0.2 mg P.O. daily.	*CNS:* convulsions, pseudotumor cerebri, vertigo, headache, depression or euphoria, psychotic behavior. *CV:* hypertension, congestive heart failure. *EENT:* cataracts, glaucoma, increased intraocular pressure, exophthalmos. *GI:* ulcer and perforation, pancreatitis, distention, ulcerative esophagitis. *GU:* menstrual abnormalities. *Metabolic:* growth suppression in children, hyperlipidemia, Cushing's syndrome, negative nitrogen balance, carbohydrate intolerance, hypernatremia, hypocalcemia, hypokalemia. *Skin:* slow wound healing, acne, thin and shiny skin, facial flushing, sweating, petechiae, ecchymoses, hyperpigmentation or hypopigmentation, hirsutism, acneiform eruptions. *Other:* susceptibility to or exacerbation of infection, myopathy, muscle weakness, osteoporosis, compression and pathologic fractures, edema. Acute adrenal insufficiency may occur with increased stress (infection, surgery, trauma) or abrupt withdrawal after long-term therapy. *Withdrawal symptoms:* rebound inflammation, fatigue, weakness, arthralgia, fever, dizziness, lethargy, depression, fainting, orthostatic hypotension, dyspnea, anorexia, hypoglycemia. *Sudden withdrawal may be fatal.*

INTERACTIONS	NURSING CONSIDERATIONS
corticosteroid response.	ness, joint pain, fever, anorexia, nausea, dyspnea, dizziness, fainting. • May mask or exacerbate infections. • Warn patient that mild peripheral edema is common. • Watch for depression or psychotic episodes, especially in high-dose therapy. • Inspect patient's skin for petechiae. Warn patient about easy bruising. • Diabetics may need increased insulin; monitor urine for sugar. • Monitor growth in infants and children on long-term therapy. • Give I.M. injection deep into gluteal muscle. Avoid S.C. injection, as atrophy and sterile abscesses may occur. • Give P.O. dose with food when possible. • Watch for corticosteroid effect in hypothyroidism and cirrhosis. • Warn patients on long-term therapy about cushingoid symptoms. • Watch for additional potassium depletion from diuretics and amphotericin B. • Immunizations may show decreased antibody response.
Barbiturates, phenytoin, rifampin: decreased corticosteroid effect. Corticosteroid dose may need to be increased. *Indomethacin, ASA:* increased risk of GI distress and bleeding. Give together cautiously. *Methandrostenolone:* monitor for enhanced corticosteroid response.	• Contraindicated in systemic fungal infections. Use cautiously in GI ulceration or renal disease, hypertension, osteoporosis, varicella, vaccinia, exanthema, diabetes mellitus, Cushing's syndrome, thromboembolic disorders, seizures, myasthenia gravis, metastatic cancer, congestive heart failure, tuberculosis, ocular herpes simplex, hypoalbuminemia, emotional instability or psychotic tendencies. • Gradually reduce dosage after long-term therapy. Tell patient not to discontinue drug abruptly or without doctor's consent. • Monitor patient's blood pressure, serum electrolytes. Weigh patient daily; report sudden weight gain to doctor. • May mask or exacerbate infections. • Stress (fever, trauma, surgery, emotional problems) may increase adrenal insufficiency. Dose may have to be increased. • Instruct patient to carry a card indicating his need for supplemental system glucocorticoids during stress. • Teach patient signs of early adrenal insufficiency: fatigue, muscular weakness, joint pain, fever, anorexia, nausea, dyspnea, dizziness, fainting. • Warn patient that mild peripheral edema is common. • Watch for depression or psychotic episodes, especially in high-dose therapy. • Inspect patient's skin for petechiae. Warn patient about easy bruising. • Diabetics may need increased insulin; monitor urine for sugar. • Unless contraindicated, give salt-restricted diet rich in potassium and protein. Potassium supplement may be needed. • Give P.O. dose with food when possible. • Has potent glucocorticoid and mineralocorticoid effects. • Used with cortisone or hydrocortisone in adrenal insufficiency. • Warn patients on long-term therapy about cushingoid symptoms. • Watch for additional potassium depletion from diuretics and amphotericin B. • Immunizations may show decreased antibody response.

NAME	INDICATIONS & DOSAGE	SIDE EFFECTS
fluprednisolone Alphadrol	*Severe inflammation—* **Adults:** 2.5 to 30 mg P.O. daily divided t.i.d. or q.i.d. **Children:** 0.07 to 1 mg/Kg P.O. daily divided t.i.d. or q.i.d., or 2.5 to 30 mg/m² divided t.i.d. or q.i.d.	*CNS:* convulsions, pseudotumor cerebri, vertigo, headache, depression or euphoria, psychotic behavior. *CV:* hypertension, congestive heart failure. *EENT:* cataracts, glaucoma, increased intraocular pressure, exophthalmos. *GI:* ulcer and perforation, pancreatitis, distention. *GU:* menstrual abnormalities. *Metabolic:* growth suppression in children, hyperlipidemia, Cushing's syndrome, negative nitrogen balance, carbohydrate intolerance, hypernatremia, hypocalcemia, hypokalemia. *Skin:* slow wound healing, acne, thin and shiny skin, facial flushing, sweating, petechiae, ecchymoses, hyperpigmentation or hypopigmentation. *Other:* susceptibility to or exacerbation of infection, myopathy, muscle weakness, osteoporosis, compression and pathologic fractures, edema. Acute adrenal insufficiency may occur with increased stress (infection, surgery, trauma) or abrupt withdrawal after long-term therapy. *Withdrawal symptoms:* rebound inflammation, fatigue, weakness, arthralgia, fever, dizziness, lethargy, depression, fainting, orthostatic hypotension, dyspnea, anorexia, hypoglycemia. *Sudden withdrawal may be fatal.*
hydrocortisone Bio-Cortex, Cortef◆, Hydrocortone◆ **hydrocortisone acetate** Cortril Acetate, Hydrocortone Acetate **hydrocortisone sodium phosphate** Hydrocortone phosphate **hydrocortisone sodium succinate** A-Hydrocort, S-Cortilean◆◆, Solu-Cortef◆, Solu-Ject◆◆	*Severe inflammation, adrenal insufficiency—* **Adults:** 5 to 30 mg P.O. b.i.d., t.i.d., or q.i.d. (as much as 80 mg P.O. q.i.d. may be given in acute situations); or initially, 100 to 250 mg (succinate) I.M. or I.V., then 50 to 100 mg I.M., as indicated; or 15 to 240 mg (phosphate) I.M. or I.V. q 12 hours; or 5 to 75 mg (acetate) into joints and soft tissue. Dose varies with size of joint. Often local anesthetics are injected with dose. *Shock—* **Adults:** 500 mg to 2 g (succinate) q 2 to 6 hours. **Children:** 0.16 to 1 mg/Kg (phosphate or succinate) I.M. or I.V. b.i.d. or t.i.d.	*CNS:* convulsions, pseudotumor cerebri, vertigo, headache, depression or euphoria, psychotic behavior. *CV:* hypertension, congestive heart failure. *EENT:* cataracts, glaucoma, increased intraocular pressure, exophthalmos. *GI:* ulcer and perforation, pancreatitis, distention. *GU:* menstrual abnormalities. *Local:* atrophy at I.M. injection sites. *Metabolic:* growth suppression in children, hyperlipidemia, Cushing's syndrome, negative nitrogen balance, carbohydrate intolerance, hypernatremia, hypocalcemia, hypokalemia. *Skin:* slow wound healing, acne, thin and shiny skin, facial flushing, sweating, petechiae, ecchymoses, hyperpigmentation or hypopigmentation. *Other:* susceptibility to or exacerba-

INTERACTIONS	NURSING CONSIDERATIONS
Barbiturates, phenytoin, rifampin: decreased corticosteroid effect. Corticosteroid dose may need to be increased. *Indomethacin, ASA:* increased risk of GI distress and bleeding. Give together cautiously. *Methandrostenolone:* monitor for enhanced corticosteroid response.	• Contraindicated in systemic fungal infections. Use cautiously in GI ulceration or renal disease, hypertension, osteoporosis, varicella, vaccinia, exanthema, diabetes mellitus, Cushing's syndrome, thromboembolic disorders, seizures, myasthenia gravis, metastatic cancer, congestive heart failure, tuberculosis, ocular herpes simplex, hypoalbuminemia, emotional instability or psychotic tendencies, and in children. • Gradually reduce drug dosage after long-term therapy. Tell patient not to discontinue drug abruptly or without doctor's consent. • Glucocorticoid with little mineralocorticoid effect. • Monitor patient's weight, blood pressure, serum electrolytes. • May mask or exacerbate infections. • Instruct patient to carry a card identifying his need for supplemental systemic glucocorticoids during stress. • Teach patient signs of early adrenal insufficiency: fatigue, muscular weakness, joint pain, fever, anorexia, nausea, dyspnea, dizziness, fainting. • Warn patient that mild peripheral edema is common. • Watch for depression or psychotic episodes, especially in high-dose therapy. • Inspect patient's skin for petechiae. Warn patient about easy bruising. • Diabetics may need increased insulin; monitor urine for sugar. • Monitor growth in infants and children on long-term therapy. • Unless contraindicated, give salt-restricted diet rich in potassium and protein. Potassium supplement may be needed. • Give P.O. dose with food when possible. • Warn patients on long-term therapy about cushingoid symptoms. • Watch for additional potassium depletion from diuretics and amphotericin B. • Immunizations may show decreased antibody response.

Barbiturates, phenytoin, rifampin: decreased corticosteroid effect. Corticosteroid dose may need to be increased. *Indomethacin, ASA:* increased risk of GI distress and bleeding. Give together cautiously. *Estrogens, methandrostenolone:* monitor for enhanced corticosteroid response.	• Contraindicated in systemic fungal infections. Use cautiously in GI ulceration or renal disease, hypertension, osteoporosis, varicella, vaccinia, exanthema, diabetes mellitus, Cushing's syndrome, thromboembolic disorders, seizures, myasthenia gravis, metastatic cancer, congestive heart failure, tuberculosis, ocular herpes simplex, hypoalbuminemia, emotional instability or psychotic tendencies, and in children. • Gradually reduce drug dosage after long-term therapy. Tell patient not to discontinue drug abruptly or without doctor's consent. • Glucocorticoid and mineralocorticoid effect. • Monitor patient's weight, blood pressure, serum electrolytes. • May mask or exacerbate infections. • Stress (fever, trauma, surgery, emotional problems) may increase adrenal insufficiency. Dose may have to be increased. • Instruct patient to carry a card identifying his need for supplemental systemic glucocorticoids during stress. • Teach patient signs of early adrenal insufficiency: fatigue, muscular weakness, joint pain, fever, anorexia, nausea, dyspnea, dizziness, fainting. • Warn patient that mild peripheral edema is common. • Watch for depression or psychotic episodes, especially in high-dose therapy. • Inspect patient's skin for petechiae. Warn patient about easy bruising.

(continued on following page)

NAME	INDICATIONS & DOSAGE	SIDE EFFECTS
hydrocortisone sodium succinate *(continued)*		tion of infection, myopathy, muscle weakness, osteoporosis, compression and pathologic fractures, edema. Acute adrenal insufficiency may occur with increased stress (infection, surgery, trauma) or abrupt withdrawal after long-term therapy. Withdrawal symptoms: rebound inflammation, fatigue, weakness, arthralgia, fever, dizziness, lethargy, depression, fainting, orthostatic hypotension, dyspnea, anorexia, hypoglycemia. *Sudden withdrawal may be fatal.*
meprednisone Betapar	*Severe inflammation*— **Adults:** 4 to 15 mg P.O. b.i.d., t.i.d., or q.i.d.	*CNS:* convulsions, pseudotumor cerebri, vertigo, headache, depression or euphoria, psychotic behavior. *CV:* hypertension, congestive heart failure. *EENT:* cataracts, glaucoma, increased intraocular pressure, exophthalmos. *GI:* ulcer and perforation, pancreatitis, abdominal distention, ulcerative esophagitis. *GU:* menstrual abnormalities. *Metabolic:* growth suppression in children, hyperlipidemia, Cushing's syndrome, negative nitrogen balance, carbohydrate intolerance, hypernatremia, hypokalemia, hypocalcemia. *Skin:* slow wound healing, acne, thin and shiny skin, facial flushing, sweating, petechiae, ecchymoses, hyperpigmentation or hypopigmentation. *Other:* susceptibility to or exacerbation of infection, myopathy, muscle weakness, osteoporosis, compression and pathologic fractures, edema. Acute adrenal insufficiency may occur with increased stress (infection, surgery, trauma) or abrupt withdrawal after long-term therapy. *Withdrawal symptoms:* rebound inflammation, fatigue, weakness, arthralgia, fever, dizziness, lethargy, depression, fainting, orthostatic hypotension, dyspnea, anorexia, hypoglycemia. *Sudden withdrawal may be fatal.*

INTERACTIONS	NURSING CONSIDERATIONS
	• Diabetics may need increased insulin; monitor urine for sugar. • Monitor growth in infants and children on long-term therapy. • Give I.M. injection deep into gluteal muscle. Avoid S.C. injection as atrophy and sterile abscesses may occur. • Unless contraindicated, give salt-restricted diet rich in potassium and protein. Potassium supplement may be needed. Watch for additional potassium depletion from diuretics and amphotericin B. • Give P.O. dose with food when possible. • Warn patients on long-term therapy about cushingoid symptoms. • Acetate form not for I.V. use. • Immunizations may show decreased antibody response. • Do not confuse Solu-Cortef with Solu-Medrol.
Barbiturates, phenytoin, rifampin: decreased corticosteroid effect. Corticosteroid dose may need to be increased. *Indomethacin, ASA:* increased risk of GI distress and bleeding. Give together cautiously. *Methandrostenolone:* monitor for enhanced corticosteroid response.	• Contraindicated in systemic fungal infections. Use cautiously in GI ulceration or renal disease, hypertension, osteoporosis, varicella, vaccinia, exanthema, diabetes mellitus, Cushing's syndrome, thromboembolic disorders, seizures, myasthenia gravis, metastatic cancer, congestive heart failure, tuberculosis, ocular herpes simplex, hypoalbuminemia, emotional instability or psychotic tendencies. • Gradually reduce drug dosage after long-term therapy. Tell patient not to discontinue drug abruptly or without doctor's consent. • Glucocorticoid with little mineralocorticoid effect. • Monitor patient's weight, blood pressure, serum electrolytes. • May mask or exacerbate infections. • Instruct patient to carry a card identifying his need for supplemental systemic glucocorticoids during stress. • Useful in rheumatoid and collagen diseases. • Teach patient signs of early adrenal insufficiency: fatigue, muscular weakness, joint pain, fever, anorexia, nausea, dyspnea, dizziness, fainting. • Warn patient that mild peripheral edema is common. • Watch for depression or psychotic episodes, especially in high-dose therapy. • Inspect patient's skin for petechiae. Warn patient about easy bruising. • Diabetics may need increased insulin; monitor urine for sugar. • Monitor growth in infants and children on long-term therapy. • Unless contraindicated, give salt-restricted diet rich in potassium and protein. Potassium supplement may be needed. Watch for additional potassium depletion from diuretics and amphotericin B. • Give P.O. dose with food when possible. • Warn patients on long-term therapy about cushingoid symptoms. • Immunizations may show decreased antibody response.

NAME	INDICATIONS & DOSAGE	SIDE EFFECTS
methylprednisolone Dura-Meth, Medrol◆, Mepred-40, Mepred-80 **methylprednisolone acetate** Depo-Medrol◆, D-Med, Medralone, Methydrol-40, Pre-Dep, Rep-Pred **methylprednisolone sodium succinate** Solu-Medrol◆	*Severe inflammation or immunosuppression*— **Adults:** 2 to 60 mg P.O. in 4 divided doses; or 40 to 80 mg (acetate) daily, I.M. or 10 to 250 mg (succinate) I.M. or I.V. q 4 hours; or 4 to 30 mg (acetate) into joints and soft tissue, p.r.n. *Shock*—100 to 250 mg (succinate) I.V. at 2- to 6-hour intervals.	*CNS:* convulsions, pseudotumor cerebri, vertigo, headache, depression or euphoria, psychotic behavior. *CV:* hypertension, congestive heart failure. *EENT:* cataracts, glaucoma, increased intraocular pressure, exophthalmos. *GI:* ulcer and perforation, pancreatitis, distention. *GU:* menstrual abnormalities. *Local:* atrophy at I.M. injection sites. *Metabolic:* growth suppression in children, hyperlipidemia, Cushing's syndrome, negative nitrogen balance, carbohydrate intolerance, hypernatremia, hypokalemia, hypocalcemia. *Skin:* slow wound healing, acne, thin and shiny skin, facial flushing, sweating, petechiae, ecchymoses, hyperpigmentation or hypopigmentation. *Other:* susceptibility to or exacerbation of infection, myopathy, muscle weakness, osteoporosis, compression and pathologic fractures, edema. Acute adrenal insufficiency may occur with increased stress (infection, surgery, trauma) or abrupt withdrawal after long-term therapy. *Withdrawal symptoms:* rebound inflammation, fatigue, weakness, arthralgia, fever, dizziness, lethargy, depression, fainting, orthostatic hypotension, dyspnea, anorexia, hypoglycemia. *Sudden withdrawal may be fatal.*
paramethasone acetate Haldrone	*Inflammatory conditions*— **Adults:** 0.5 to 6 mg P.O. t.i.d. or q.i.d. **Children:** 58 to 800 mcg/Kg daily divided t.i.d. or q.i.d.	*CNS:* convulsions, pseudotumor cerebri, vertigo, headache, depression or euphoria, psychotic behavior. *CV:* hypertension, congestive heart failure. *EENT:* cataracts, glaucoma, increased intraocular pressure, exophthalmos. *GI:* ulcer and perforation, pancreatitis, distention. *GU:* menstrual abnormalities. *Metabolic:* growth suppression in children, hyperlipidemia, Cushing's syndrome, negative nitrogen balance, carbohydrate intolerance, hypernatremia, hypokalemia, hypocalcemia. *Skin:* slow wound healing, acne, thin

INTERACTIONS	NURSING CONSIDERATIONS
Barbiturates, phenytoin, rifampin: decreased corticosteroid effect. Corticosteroid dose may need to be increased. *Indomethacin, ASA:* increased risk of GI distress and bleeding. Give together cautiously. *Methandrostenolone:* monitor for enhanced corticosteroid response.	• Contraindicated in systemic fungal infections. Use cautiously in GI ulceration or renal disease, hypertension, osteoporosis, varicella, vaccinia, exanthema, diabetes mellitus, Cushing's syndrome, thromboembolic disorders, seizures, myasthenia gravis, metastatic cancer, congestive heart failure, tuberculosis, ocular herpes simplex, hypoalbuminemia, emotional instability or psychotic tendencies. • Gradually reduce drug dosage after long-term therapy. Tell patient not to discontinue drug abruptly or without doctor's consent. • Glucocorticoid with little mineralocorticoid effect. • Discard reconstituted solutions after 48 hours. • Don't use acetate salt when immediate onset of action needed. • Dermal atrophy may occur with large doses of acetate salt. Use multiple small injections into lesions. • Monitor weight, blood pressure, sleep patterns, serum electrolytes. • May mask or exacerbate infections. • Instruct patient to carry a card identifying his need for supplemental systemic glucocorticoids during stress. • Teach patient signs of early adrenal insufficiency: fatigue, muscular weakness, joint pain, fever, anorexia, nausea, dyspnea, dizziness, fainting. • Warn patient that mild peripheral edema is common. • Watch for depression or psychotic episodes, especially in high-dose therapy. • Inspect patient's skin for petechiae. Warn patient about easy bruising. • Diabetics may need increased insulin; monitor urine for sugar. • Give I.M. injection deep into gluteal muscle. Avoid S.C. injection as atrophy and sterile abscesses may occur. • Unless contraindicated, give salt-restricted diet rich in potassium and protein. Potassium supplement may be needed. Watch for additional potassium depletion from diuretics and amphotericin B. • Give P.O. dose with food when possible. • Give I.V. dose slowly over 1 minute; in shock, give massive I.V. doses over 3 to 15 minutes to prevent cardiac arrhythmias and circulatory collapse. • Warn patients on long-term therapy about cushingoid symptoms. • Acetate form not for I.V. use. • Do not confuse Solu-Medrol with Solu-Cortef. • Immunizations may show decreased antibody response.
Barbiturates, phenytoin, rifampin: decreased corticosteroid effect. Corticosteroid dose may need to be increased. *Indomethacin, ASA:* increased risk of GI distress and bleeding. Give together cautiously *Methandrostenolone:* monitor for enhanced corticosteroid response.	• Contraindicated in systemic fungal infections and alternate-day therapy. Use cautiously in GI ulceration or renal disease, hypertension, osteoporosis, varicella, vaccinia, exanthema, diabetes mellitus, Cushing's syndrome, thromboembolic disorders, seizures, myasthenia gravis, metastatic cancer, congestive heart failure, tuberculosis, ocular herpes simplex, hypoalbuminemia, emotional instability or psychotic tendencies. • Gradually reduce drug dosage after long-term therapy. Tell patient not to discontinue drug abruptly or without doctor's consent. • Glucocorticoid with little mineralocorticoid effect. • Monitor patient's weight, blood pressure, serum electrolytes. • May mask or exacerbate infections. • Instruct patient to carry a card identifying his need for supplemental systemic glucocorticoids during stress. • Teach patient signs of early adrenal insufficiency: fatigue, muscular weakness, joint pain, fever, anorexia, nausea, dyspnea, dizziness, fainting. • Warn patient that mild peripheral edema is common.

(continued on following page)

NAME	INDICATIONS & DOSAGE	SIDE EFFECTS
paramethasone acetate *(continued)*		and shiny skin, facial flushing, sweating, petechiae, ecchymoses, hyperpigmentation or hypopigmentation. *Other:* susceptibility to or exacerbation of infection, myopathy, muscle weakness, osteoporosis, compression and pathologic fractures, edema. Acute adrenal insufficiency may occur with increased stress (infection, surgery, trauma) or abrupt withdrawal after long-term therapy. *Withdrawal symptoms:* rebound inflammation, fatigue, weakness, arthralgia, fever, dizziness, lethargy, depression, fainting, orthostatic hypotension, dyspnea, anorexia, hypoglycemia. *Sudden withdrawal may be fatal.*
prednisolone Cordrol, Delta-Cortef◆, Prednis, Predoxine, Ropred-lone, Ster 5, Sterane **prednisolone acetate** **prednisolone sodium phosphate** **prednisolone sodium succinate** **prednisolone tebutate**	*Severe inflammation (for immunosuppression)*— **Adults:** 2.5 to 15 mg P.O. b.i.d., t.i.d., or q.i.d.; 2 to 30 mg I.M. (acetate, phosphate, or succinate) or I.V. (succinate) q 12 hours; or 2 to 30 mg (phosphate) into joints, lesions, and soft tissue; or 4 to 40 mg (tebutate) into joints and lesions; or 0.25 to 1 ml (acetate-phosphate suspension) into joints weekly, p.r.n.	*CNS:* convulsions, pseudotumor cerebri, vertigo, headache, depression or euphoria, psychotic behavior. *CV:* hypertension, congestive heart failure. *EENT:* cataracts, glaucoma, increased intraocular pressure, exophthalmos. *GI:* ulcer and perforation, pancreatitis, distention. *GU:* menstrual abnormalities. *Local:* atrophy at I.M. injection sites. *Metabolic:* growth suppression in children, hyperlipidemia, Cushing's syndrome, negative nitrogen balance, carbohydrate intolerance, hypernatremia, hypokalemia, hypocalcemia. *Skin:* slow wound healing, acne, thin and shiny skin, facial flushing, sweating, petechiae, ecchymoses, hyperpigmentation or hypopigmentation. *Other:* susceptibility to or exacerbation of infection, myopathy, muscle weakness, osteoporosis, compression and pathologic fractures, edema. Acute adrenal insufficiency may occur with increased stress (infection, surgery, trauma) or abrupt withdrawal after long-term therapy. Withdrawal symptoms: rebound inflammation, fatigue, weakness, arthralgia, fever, dizziness, lethargy, depression, fainting, orthostatic hypotension, dyspnea, anorexia, hypoglycemia. *Sudden withdrawal may be fatal.*

INTERACTIONS	NURSING CONSIDERATIONS
	• Watch for depression or psychotic episodes, especially in high-dose therapy. • Inspect patient's skin for petechiae. Warn patient about easy bruising. • Diabetics may need increased insulin; monitor urine for sugar. • Monitor growth in infants and children on long-term therapy. • Unless contraindicated, give salt-restricted diet rich in potassium and protein. Potassium supplement may be needed. Watch for additional potassium depletion for diuretics and amphotericin B. • Give P.O. dose with food when possible. • Warn patients on long-term therapy about cushingoid symptoms. • Immunizations may show decreased antibody response.
Barbiturates, phenytoin, rifampin: decreased corticosteroid effect. Corticosteroid dose may need to be increased. *Indomethacin, ASA:* increased risk of GI distress and bleeding. Give together cautiously. *Methandrostenolone:* monitor for enhanced corticosteroid response.	• Contraindicated in systemic fungal infections. Use cautiously in GI ulceration or renal disease, hypertension, osteoporosis, varicella, vaccinia, exanthema, diabetes mellitus, Cushing's syndrome, thromboembolic disorders, seizures, myasthenia gravis, metastatic cancer, congestive heart failure, tuberculosis, ocular herpes simplex, hypoalbuminemia, emotional instability or psychotic tendencies. • Gradually reduce drug dosage after long-term therapy. Tell patient not to discontinue drug abruptly or without doctor's consent. • Glucocorticoid with slight mineralocorticoid action. • Prednisolone salts (acetate, sodium phosphate, sodium succinate, and tebutate) are used parenterally less often than other corticosteroids that have more potent anti-inflammatory action. • May use for alternate-day therapy. • Monitor patient's weight, blood pressure, serum electrolytes. • May mask or exacerbate infections. • Instruct patient to carry a card identifying his need for supplemental systemic glucocorticoids during stress. • Teach patient signs of early adrenal insufficiency: fatigue, muscular weakness, joint pain, fever, anorexia, nausea, dyspnea, dizziness, fainting. • Warn patient that mild peripheral edema is common. • Watch for depression or psychotic episodes, especially in high-dose therapy. • Inspect patient's skin for petechiae. Warn patient about easy bruising. • Diabetics may need increased insulin; monitor urine for sugar. • Give I.M. injection deep into gluteal muscle. Avoid S.C. injection, as atrophy and sterile abscesses may occur. • Unless contraindicated, give salt-restricted diet rich in potassium and protein. Potassium supplement may be needed. Watch for additional potassium depletion from diuretics and amphotericin B. • Give P.O. dose with food when possible. • Warn patients on long-term therapy about cushingoid symptoms. • Acetate form not for I.V. use. • Immunizations may show decreased antibody response.

NAME	INDICATIONS & DOSAGE	SIDE EFFECTS
prednisone Colisone◆◆, Deltasone◆, Fernisone, Meticorten, Orasone, Paracort◆	*Severe inflammation (for immunosuppression)*— **Adults:** 2.5 to 15 mg P.O. b.i.d., t.i.d., or q.i.d. **Children:** 0.14 to 2 mg/Kg daily P.O. divided q.i.d.	*CNS:* convulsions, pseudotumor cerebri, vertigo, headache, depression or euphoria, psychotic behavior. *CV:* hypertension, congestive heart failure. *EENT:* cataracts, glaucoma, increased intraocular pressure, exophthalmos. *GI:* ulcer and perforation, pancreatitis, distention. *GU:* menstrual abnormalities. *Metabolic:* growth suppression in children, hyperlipidemia, Cushing's syndrome, negative nitrogen balance, carbohydrate intolerance, hypernatremia, hypokalemia, hypocalcemia. *Skin:* slow wound healing, acne, thin and shiny skin, facial flushing, sweating, petechiae, ecchymoses, hyperpigmentation or hypopigmentation. *Other:* susceptibility to or exacerbation of infection, myopathy, muscle weakness, osteoporosis, compression and pathologic fractures, edema. Acute adrenal insufficiency may occur with increased stress (infection, surgery, trauma) or abrupt withdrawal after long-term therapy. *Withdrawal symptoms:* rebound inflammation, fatigue, weakness, arthralgia, fever, dizziness, lethargy, depression, fainting, orthostatic hypotension, dyspnea, anorexia, hypoglycemia. *Sudden withdrawal may be fatal.*
triamcinolone Artistocort◆, Kenacort◆, Spencort, Tricilone **triamcinolone acetonide** Kenalog◆ **triamcinolone diacetate** Amcort, Aristocort◆, Cenocort Forte, Cino-40, Tracilon, Triam-Forte, Tristoject	*Severe inflammation (for immunosuppression)*— **Adults:** 4 to 48 mg P.O. daily divided b.i.d., t.i.d., or q.i.d., or 40 mg I.M. (diacetate) weekly; or 5 to 48 mg (diacetate) into lesions; or 2 to 40 mg (diacetate) into joints and soft tissue; or up to 0.5 mg (hexacetonide) per square inch of affected skin intralesional; or 2 to 20 mg (hexacetonide) intra-articular or intrasynovial, into soft tissue, or into joint or lesion. Often, a local anesthetic is injected into the joint with triamcinolone.	*CNS:* convulsions, pseudotumor cerebri, vertigo, headache, depression or euphoria, psychotic behavior. *CV:* hypertension, congestive heart failure. *EENT:* cataracts, glaucoma, increased intraocular pressure, exophthalmos. *GI:* ulcer and perforation, pancreatitis, distention. *GU:* menstrual abnormalities. *Local:* atrophy at I.M. injection sites. *Metabolic:* growth suppression in children, hyperlipidemia, Cushing's syndrome, negative nitrogen balance, carbohydrate intolerance, hypernatremia, hypokalemia, hypocalcemia.

INTERACTIONS	NURSING CONSIDERATIONS
Barbiturates, phenytoin, rifampin: decreased corticosteroid effect. Corticosteroid dose may need to be increased. *Indomethacin, ASA:* increased risk of GI distress and bleeding. Give together cautiously. *Methandrostenolone:* monitor for enhanced corticosteroid response.	• Contraindicated in systemic fungal infections. Use cautiously in GI ulceration or renal disease, hypertension, osteoporosis, varicella, vaccinia, exanthema, diabetes mellitus, Cushing's syndrome, thromboembolic disorders, seizures, myasthenia gravis, metastatic cancer, congestive heart failure, tuberculosis, ocular herpes simplex, hypoalbuminemia, emotional instability or psychotic tendencies • Gradually reduce drug dosage after long-term therapy. Tell patient not to discontinue drug abruptly or without doctor's consent. • Monitor patient's blood pressure, sleep patterns, serum potassium levels. • Weigh patient daily; report sudden weight gain to doctor. • May mask or exacerbate infections. • Instruct patient to carry a card identifying his need for supplemental systemic glucocorticoids during stress. • Teach patient signs of early adrenal insufficiency: fatigue, muscular weakness, joint pain, fever, anorexia, nausea, dyspnea, dizziness, fainting. • Warn patient that mild peripheral edema is common. • Watch for depression or psychotic episodes, especially in high-dose therapy. • Inspect patient's skin for petechiae. Warn patient about easy bruising. • Diabetics may need increased insulin; monitor urine for sugar. • Monitor growth in infants and children on long-term therapy. • Give salt-restricted diet rich in potassium and protein. Potassium supplement may be needed. Watch for additional potassium depletion from diuretics and amphotericin B. • Unless contraindicated, give P.O. dose with food when possible. • May use for alternate-day therapy. • Warn patients on long-term therapy about cushingoid symptoms. • Immunizations may show decreased antibody response.
Barbiturates, phenytoin, rifampin: decreased corticosteroid effect. Corticosteroid dose may need to be increased. *Indomethacin, ASA:* increased risk of GI distress and bleeding. Give together cautiously. *Methandrostenolone:* monitor for enhanced corticosteroid response.	• Contraindicated in systemic fungal infections. Use cautiously in GI ulceration or renal disease, hypertension, osteoporosis, varicella, vaccinia, exanthema, diabetes mellitus, Cushing's syndrome, thromboembolic disorders, seizures, myasthenia gravis, metastatic cancer, congestive heart failure, tuberculosis, ocular herpes simplex, hypoalbuminemia, emotional instability or psychotic tendencies. • Gradually reduce drug dosage after long-term therapy. Tell patient not to discontinue drug abruptly or without doctor's consent. • Monitor patient's weight, blood pressure, serum electrolytes. • May mask or exacerbate infections. • Instruct patient to carry a card identifying his need for supplemental systemic glucocorticoids during stress. • Teach patient signs of early adrenal insufficiency: fatigue, muscular weakness, joint pain, fever, anorexia, nausea, dyspnea, dizziness, fainting. • Warn patient that mild peripheral edema is common. • Watch for depression or psychotic episodes, especially in high-dose therapy.

(continued on following page)

NAME	INDICATIONS & DOSAGE	SIDE EFFECTS
triamcinolone *(continued)* **triamcinolone hexacetonide** Aristospan◆		*Skin:* slow wound healing, acne, thin and shiny skin, facial flushing, sweating, petechiae, ecchymoses, hyperpigmentation or hypopigmentation. *Other:* susceptibility to exacerbation or masking of infection, myopathy, muscle weakness, osteoporosis, compression and pathologic fractures, edema. Acute adrenal insufficiency may occur with increased stress (infection, surgery, trauma) or abrupt withdrawal after long-term therapy. Withdrawal symptoms: rebound inflammation, fatigue, weakness, arthralgia, fever, dizziness, lethargy, depression, fainting, orthostatic hypotension, dyspnea, anorexia, hypoglycemia. *Sudden withdrawal may be fatal.*

INTERACTIONS	NURSING CONSIDERATIONS
	• Inspect patient's skin for petechiae. Warn patient about easy bruising. • Diabetics may need increased insulin; monitor urine for sugar. • Give I.M. injection deep into gluteal muscle. Avoid S.C. injection, as atrophy and sterile abscesses may occur. • Unless contraindicated, give salt-restricted diet rich in potassium and protein. Potassium supplement may be needed. Watch for additional potassium depletion from diuretics and amphotericin B. • Give P.O. dose with food when possible. • Glucocorticoid with very little mineralocorticoid effect. • Discard unused diluted suspension within 7 days. • Don't use diluents that contain preservatives. Flocculation may occur. • Warn patients on long-term therapy about cushingoid symptoms. • Not for I.V. use. • Immunizations may show decreased antibody response.

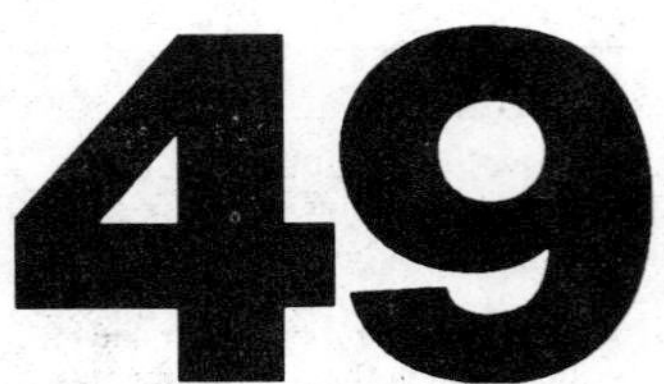

Androgens

danazol
ethylestrenol
fluoxymesterone
methandrostenolone
methyltestosterone
nandrolone decanoate
nandrolone phenpropionate
oxandrolone
oxymetholone
stanozolol
testosterone
testosterone cypionate
testosterone enanthate
testosterone propionate

The male hormone testosterone and its derivatives are called androgens because they aid the development of male secondary sex characteristics, such as facial and body hair, deep voice, and muscle development. They also have anabolic properties which stimulate the building and repair of body tissues through retention of nitrogen, potassium, and phosphorus, and a decrease in amino-acid catabolism. Some synthetic androgens exert greater androgenic effect than testosterone. Others have increased anabolic properties and are used to reverse debilitating conditions; these, too, exert some virilizing activity. Other modifications have produced steroids which are orally effective.

Major uses

- Treatment of the androgen-deficient male (primary hypogonadism, hypopituitarism, eunuchism, Klinefelter's syndrome, impotence, oligospermia or climacteric symptoms).
- Refractory anemias (aplastic, associated with chronic disease and in patients undergoing renal dialysis).
- Menstrual disorders (menorrhagia, metrorrhagia, premenstrual tension, functional dysmenorrhea, menopausal symptoms) and endometriosis.
- Suppression of lactation and postpartum breast engorgement.
- Osteoporosis, burns, decubitus ulcers, delayed healing of fractures.
- Protein depletion from long-term corticosteroid therapy, debilitating disease and convalescence, postoperative states, and chronic malnutrition.
- To promote weight gain and feeling of well-being.
- In children with retarded growth and development.
- To relieve pain in advanced metastatic mammary carcinoma in women.
- To oppose estrogen effects in estrogen-dependent tumors and hyperestrogenic conditions.

Mechanism of action

- Restores hormone in androgen-deficiency states.
- Stimulates synthesis of cellular protein and establishes positive nitrogen balance.
- Promotes production of erythrocytes by stimulating renal or extrarenal sources of erythropoietin.

Absorption, distribution, and excretion

- Well absorbed from GI tract, metabolized in liver, excreted in urine (rapid breakdown by

---

---

liver limits oral use of some androgens).
- Crosses placenta; appears in breast milk.
- Injections in oil slow absorption and prolong duration of action.
- Buccal or sublingual absorption bypasses rapid metabolic breakdown usually seen with oral administration and may allow lowered dosages.

Onset and duration
- Onset difficult to determine because subjective response is so variable.
- Hematologic and other objective responses are not apparent for at least 3 months.
- I.M. injection prolongs action.
- Subcutaneous implantation of pellets prolongs action up to 6 months.
- Testosterone propionate is of shorter duration than testosterone itself and is not suited for long-term therapy.
- Cypionate and enanthate derivatives of testosterone provide therapeutic effects for up to 4 weeks.
- Nandrolone phenpropionate—1 to 2 weeks duration; nandrolone decanoate—3 to 4 weeks duration.

Combination products
DELADUMONE INJECTION (oil)◆: testosterone enanthate 90 mg, estradiol valerate 4 mg, and chlorobutanol 0.5%.
DEPO-TESTADIOL (oil): testosterone cyclopenlylpropionate 50 mg, estradiol cypionate 2 mg, and chlorobutanol 5 mg.
DITATE: estradiol valerate 4 mg, and testosterone enanthate 90 mg.
DITATE-DS: estradiol valerate 8 mg, and testosterone enanthate 180 mg.
ESTRATEST H.S.: esterified estrogens 0.625 mg, and methyltestosterone 1.25 mg.
FORMATRIX: conjugated estrogens 1.25 mg, methyltestosterone 10 mg, and absorbic acid 400 mg.
GYNETONE "0.02": ethinyl estradiol 0.02 mg, and methyltestosterone 5 mg.
GYNETONE "0.04": ethinyl estradiol 0.04 mg, and methyltestosterone 10 mg.
LACTOSTAT (oil)◆◆: testosterone enanthate benzilic acid hydrazone 300 mg, estradiol dienanthate 15 mg, and estradiol benzoate 6 mg.
MAL-O-FEM CYP: estradiol cypionate 2 mg, and testosterone cypionate 50 mg.
MEDIATRIC: conjugated estrogens 0.25 mg, methyltestosterone 2.5 mg, methamphetamine MCL 1 mg, vitamin C 100 mg, thiamine mononitrate 10 mg, vitamin B_{12} 2.5 mcg, ferrous sulfate 30 mg, vitamin B_2 5 mg, vitamin B_6 3 mg, nicotinamide 50 mg.
OS-CALMONE: calcium 400 mg, methyltestosterone 2.67 mg, and ethinyl estradiol 5.33 mcg.
PREMARIN WITH METHYLTESTOSTERONE◆: conjugated estrogens 0.625 mg, and thyltestosterone 5 mg.

NAME	INDICATIONS & DOSAGE	SIDE EFFECTS
danazol Cyclomen••, Danocrine	*Endometriosis—* **Women:** 400 mg P.O. b.i.d. uninterrupted for 3 to 6 months; may continue for 9 months.	*Androgenic:* acne, edema, weight gain, hirsutism, hoarseness, clitoral enlargement, decrease in breast size, changes in libido, male pattern baldness, oiliness of skin or hair. *CNS:* dizziness, headache, sleep disorders, fatigue, tremor, irritability, excitation, lethargy, mental depression, chills, paresthesias. *CV:* elevated blood pressure. *EENT:* visual disturbances. *GI:* gastric irritation, nausea, vomiting, diarrhea, constipation, change in appetite. *GU:* hematuria. *Hypoestrogenic:* flushing; sweating; vaginitis, including itching, dryness, burning, and vaginal bleeding; nervousness, emotional lability. *Other:* muscle cramps or spasms in back, neck, or legs; cholestatic jaundice, skin rashes.
ethylestrenol Maxibolin•	*Promote weight gain and combat tissue depletion, refractory anemias, catabolic effects of corticosteroid therapy, osteoporosis, prolonged immobilization, and debilitative states—* **Adults:** 4 to 8 mg P.O. daily, reduced to minimum levels at first evidence of clinical response. **Children:** 1 to 3 mg P.O. daily, highly individualized. A single course of therapy in both adults and children should not exceed 6 weeks; may be reinstituted after 4-week interval.	*Androgenic:* in females—acne, edema, oily skin, weight gain, hirsutism, hoarseness, clitoral enlargement, changes in libido. In males—prepubertal: premature epiphyseal closure, acne, priapism, growth of body and facial hair, phallic enlargement; postpubertal: testicular atrophy, oligospermia, decreased ejaculatory volume, impotence, gynecomastia, epididymitis. *GI:* gastroenteritis, nausea, vomiting, diarrhea, constipation, change in appetite. *GU:* bladder irritability. *Hypoestrogenic:* in females—flushing; sweating; vaginitis with itching, drying, burning, or bleeding menstrual irregularities. *Other:* hypercalcemia, cholestatic jaundice, edema.
fluoxymesterone Android-F, Halotestin•, Oratestin••, Oratestryl	*Tissue repair and other anabolic effects—* **Adults:** 4 to 10 mg P.O. daily. *Menstrual symptoms—* **Adults:** 5 to 10 mg P.O. daily for 1 week before menses or until symptoms are controlled. *Hypogonadism—*	*Androgenic:* in females—acne, edema, oily skin, weight gain, hirsutism, deepening of voice, clitoral enlargement, change in libido. In males—prepubertal: premature epiphyseal closure, acne, priapism, growth of body and facial hair, phallic enlargement; postpubertal: testicular atrophy,

• Also available in Canada.
•• Available in Canada only.
Unmarked trade names available in United States only.

INTERACTIONS	NURSING CONSIDERATIONS
None significant.	• Contraindicated in undiagnosed abnormal genital bleeding; impaired renal, cardiac, or hepatic function. Use cautiously in epilepsy or migraines. • Amenorrhea is common; reassure patient that menses will resume 2 to 3 months after drug is discontinued. • Use with diet high in calories and protein unless contraindicated. • Monitor closely for signs of virilization. Some androgenic effects may not be reversible upon discontinuation of drug.
None significant.	• Contraindicated in prostatic hypertrophy with obstruction; carcinoma of male breast; hypercalcemia; prostatic cancer; cardiac, hepatic, or renal decompensation; nephrosis; premature infants. Use cautiously in prepubertal males; patients with diabetes or coronary disease; patients taking ACTH, corticosteroids, or anticoagulants. • Hypercalcemic symptoms may be difficult to distinguish from symptoms of condition being treated, unless anticipated and thought of as a symptom cluster. Hypercalcemia is particularly likely to occur in patients with metastatic breast cancer and may indicate bone metastases. • Instruct females to report menstrual irregularities; therapy should be discontinued pending etiologic determination. • Watch for virilizing effects; may be irreversible despite prompt stopping of therapy. Doctor must decide if benefits outweigh effects. • Closely monitor boys under 7 for precocious development of male sexual characteristics. • In children: therapy should be preceded by X-ray of wrist bones to establish level of bone maturation. During treatment, bone maturation may proceed more rapidly than linear growth; dosage should be intermittent. • Edema is generally controllable with salt restriction and/or diuretics. • Watch for symptoms of jaundice. Dose adjustment may reverse condition. If hepatic function tests are abnormal, therapy should be discontinued. • Observe patient on concomitant anticoagulant therapy for ecchymotic areas, petechiae, or abnormal bleeding. Monitor prothrombin time. • Watch for symptoms of hypoglycemia in diabetics. Dosage of antidiabetic drug may need adjustment. • Use with diet high in calories and protein unless contraindicated.
None significant.	• Contraindicated in prostatic hypertrophy with obstruction; carcinoma of male breast; prostatic cancer; cardiac, hepatic, or renal decompensation; nephrosis; hypercalcemia. Use cautiously in prepubertal males; patients with diabetes or coronary disease; and patients taking ACTH, corticosteroids, or anticoagulants. • Hypercalcemic symptoms may be difficult to distinguish from symptoms associated with condition being treated, unless anticipated and thought of as a symptom cluster. Hypercalcemia is particularly likely to occur in

(continued on following page)

NAME	INDICATIONS & DOSAGE	SIDE EFFECTS
fluoxymesterone *(continued)*	**Adults:** 2 to 10 mg P.O. daily. *Palliation of breast cancer in women*—15 to 30 mg P.O. daily in divided dosages. All dosage should be individualized and reduced to minimum when effect is noted.	oligospermia, decreased ejaculatory volume, impotence, gynecomastia, epididymitis. *GI:* gastroenteritis, nausea, vomiting, constipation, change in appetite, diarrhea. *GU:* bladder irritability. *Hypoestrogenic:* in females—flushing; sweating; vaginitis with itching, drying, burning, or bleeding; menstrual irregularities; emotional lability. *Other:* hypercalcemia, edema, cholestatic jaundice, edema.
methandrostenolone Danabol♦♦, Dianabol	*Senile and postmenopausal osteoporosis*— **Adults:** initially 5 mg P.O. daily. Maintenance 2.5 to 5 mg P.O. daily. *Anabolic effect*— **Adults:** 5 to 10 mg P.O. daily. *Severe debilitation*— **Adults:** 10 to 20 mg P.O. daily for 3 weeks, reduced to 5 to 10 mg P.O. daily for maintenance. *Severe maturational delay when growth hormone is unavailable*— **Children:** (postpubertal) up to 0.05 mg/Kg P.O. daily. Intermittent therapy is recommended in prolonged use.	*Androgenic:* in females—acne, edema, oily skin, weight gain, hirsutism, deepening of voice, clitoral enlargement, changes in libido. In males—prepubertal: premature epiphyseal closure, acne, priapism, growth of body and facial hair, phallic enlargement; postpubertal: testicular atrophy, oligospermia, decreased ejaculatory volume, impotence, gynecomastia, epididymitis. *EENT:* burning of tongue. *GI:* gastroenteritis, nausea, vomiting, change in appetite, diarrhea, anorexia, constipation. *GU:* bladder irritability. *Hypoestrogenic:* in females—flushing; sweating; vaginitis with itching, drying, burning, or bleeding; menstrual irregularities. *Other:* hypercalcemia, cholestatic jaundice, edema.
methyltestosterone Android-5, Android-10, Metandren♦, Oreton-Methyl, Testred	**Adults:** *Breast engorgement of nonnursing mothers*—80 mg P.O. daily; or 40 mg buccal daily. *Breast cancer in women 1 to 5 years postmenopausal*—200 mg P.O. daily; or 100 mg buccal daily. *Eunuchoidism and eunuchism, male climacteric symptoms*—10 to 40 mg P.O. daily; or 5 to 20 mg buccal daily. *Postpubertal cryptorchidism*—30 mg P.O. daily; or 15 mg buccal daily.	*Androgenic:* in females—acne, edema, oily skin, weight gain, hirsutism, deepening of voice, clitoral enlargement, changes in libido. In males—prepubertal: premature epiphyseal closure, acne, priapism, growth of body and facial hair, phallic enlargement; postpubertal: testicular atrophy, oligospermia, decreased ejaculatory volume, impotence, gynecomastia, epididymitis. *CNS:* dizziness, fatigue, headache, sleep disorders, tremor, irritability,

INTERACTIONS	NURSING CONSIDERATIONS
	patients with metastatic breast cancer and may indicate bone metastases. • Explain to patient on drug for palliation of breast cancer that virilization usually occurs at dosage used. Give emotional support. Tell patient to report androgenic effects immediately. Stopping drug will prevent further androgenic changes but will probably not reverse those already existing. • When used in breast cancer, subjective effects may not be seen for about 1 month; objective symptoms not for 3 months. • Instruct females to report menstrual irregularities; therapy should be discontinued pending etiologic determination. • Edema is generally controllable with salt restriction and/or diuretics. • Watch for symptoms of jaundice. Dose adjustment may reverse condition. If hepatic function tests are abnormal, therapy should be discontinued. • Observe patient on concomitant anticoagulant therapy for ecchymotic areas, petechiae, or abnormal bleeding. Monitor prothrombin time. • Watch for symptoms of hypoglycemia in diabetics. Dosage of antidiabetic drug may need adjustment. • Use with diet high in calories and protein unless contraindicated.
None significant.	• Contraindicated in prostatic hypertrophy with obstruction, carcinoma of male breast, prostatic cancer; cardiac, hepatic, or renal decompensation; nephrosis. Use cautiously in prepubertal males; patients with diabetes or coronary disease; patients taking ACTH, corticosteroids, or anticoagulants. • Hypercalcemic symptoms may be difficult to distinguish from symptoms of condition being treated, unless anticipated and thought of as a cluster. Hypercalcemia is particularly likely to occur with metastatic breast cancer and may indicate bone metastases. Therapy should be discontinued. • Instruct females to report menstrual irregularities; therapy should be discontinued pending etiologic determination. • Watch closely for virilizing effects; they may be irreversible despite prompt discontinuation of therapy. • In children, therapy should be preceded by X-ray of wrist bones to establish level of bone maturation. During treatment, bone maturation may proceed more rapidly than linear growth; dosage should be intermittent. • Edema is generally controllable with salt restriction and/or diuretics. • Watch for symptoms of jaundice. Dose adjustment may reverse condition. If hepatic function tests are abnormal, therapy should be discontinued. • Watch for ecchymotic areas, petechiae, or abnormal bleeding in patients on concomitant anticoagulant therapy. Monitor prothrombin time. • Watch for symptoms of hypoglycemia in diabetics. Dosage of antidiabetic drug may need adjustment. • May lower fasting blood sugar in both diabetic and nondiabetic patients. • Does not enhance athletic ability.
None significant.	• Contraindicated in women of childbearing potential (possible masculinization of female infant); hypercalcemia; cardiac, hepatic, or renal decompensation; prostatic or breast cancer in male; benign prostatic hypertrophy with obstruction; elderly, asthenic males who may react adversely to androgen overstimulation; conditions aggravated by fluid retention; hypertension. Use cautiously in myocardial infarction or coronary artery disease. • Treatment of breast cancer usually restricted to patients 1 to 5 years postmenopausal. • Sodium and water retention respond to diuretics. • Periodic serum cholesterol and calcium determinations, and cardiac and hepatic function tests recommended. Watch closely for jaundice. • In metastatic breast cancer, hypercalcemia may indicate progression of bone metastases. Report signs of hypercalcemia.

(continued on following page)

NAME	INDICATIONS & DOSAGE	SIDE EFFECTS
methyltestosterone *(continued)*		lethargy, mental depression, chills, excitation. *GI:* gastroenteritis, constipation, nausea, vomiting, diarrhea, change in appetite. *GU:* bladder irritability. *Hypoestrogenic:* in females—flushing; sweating; vaginitis with itching, drying, burning, or bleeding; menstrual irregularities. *Local:* irritation of oral mucosa with buccal administration. *Other:* hypercalcemia, edema, cholestatic jaundice, anaphylactoid reactions.
nandrolone decanoate Deca-Durabolin◆	*Severe debility or disease states*— **Adults:** 100 to 200 mg I.M. weekly. Therapy should be intermittent. *Tissue-building*— **Adults:** 50 to 100 mg I.M. q 3 to 4 weeks. **Children 2 to 13 years:** 25 to 50 mg I.M. q 3 to 4 weeks.	*Androgenic:* in females—acne, edema, oily skin, weight gain, hirsutism, deepening of voice, clitoral enlargement, decreased or increased libido. In males—prepubertal: premature epiphyseal closure, acne, priapism, growth of body and facial hair, phallic enlargement; postpubertal: testicular atrophy, oligospermia, decreased ejaculatory volume, impotence, gynecomastia, epididymitis. *CNS:* dizziness, headache, sleep disorders, fatigue, tremor, irritability, lethargy, mental depression, chills, excitation, paresthesia. *GI:* gastroenteritis, nausea, vomiting, diarrhea, change in appetite. *GU:* bladder irritability. *Hypoestrogenic:* in females—flushing; sweating; vaginitis with itching, drying, burning, or bleeding; menstrual irregularities with large doses. *Local:* pain at injection site, induration. *Other:* hypercalcemia, hypercalciuria, edema, cholestatic jaundice.
nandrolone phenpropionate Durabolin◆	*Severe debility or disease states*— **Adults:** 50 to 100 mg I.M. weekly. **Children 2 to 13 years:** 12.5 to 25 mg I.M. q 2 to 4 weeks. **Children under 2 years:** 12.5 mg I.M. q 2 to 4 weeks. Therapy should be intermittent, based on therapeutic response. *Tissue building and/or erythropoietic effects*— **Adults:** 25 to 50 mg I.M. weekly.	
oxandrolone Anavar	*To combat catabolic effects of corticosteroid therapy, osteoporosis, prolonged immobilization and debilitative states*— **Adults:** 2.5 mg P.O. b.i.d., t.i.d., or q.i.d. up to 20 mg daily for 2 to 4 weeks. **Children:** 0.25 mg/Kg/daily P.O. for 2 to 4 weeks. Continuous therapy should not exceed 3 months.	*Androgenic:* in females—acne, edema, oily skin, weight gain, hirsutism, deepening of voice, clitoral enlargement, decreased or increased libido. In males—prepubertal: premature epiphyseal closure, acne, priapism, growth of body and facial hair, phallic enlargement; postpubertal: testicular atrophy, oligospermia, decreased ejaculatory volume, impotence, gynecomastia, epididymitis.

INTERACTIONS	NURSING CONSIDERATIONS
	• Therapeutic response in breast cancer is usually apparent within 3 months. Therapy should be stopped if signs of disease progression appear. • Enhances hypoglycemia; tell patient to report signs of hyperinsulinism. • Watch for ecchymoses, petechiae, and abnormal bleeding in patients receiving concomitant anticoagulants. • Promptly report signs of virilization in females. • Use with diet high in calories and protein unless contraindicated. • Buccal tablets twice as potent as oral tablets. Tell patient to avoid eating, drinking, chewing, or smoking while buccal tablet is in place, and that tablet is not to be swallowed. • Does not enhance athletic ability.
None significant.	• Contraindicated in prostatic hypertrophy with obstruction; male breast and prostatic cancer; cardiac, hepatic, or renal decompensation; nephrosis. Use cautiously in prepubertal males; patients with diabetes or coronary disease; patients taking ACTH, corticosteroids, or anticoagulants. • Inject drug deep I.M., preferably into upper outer quadrant of gluteal muscle in adults. • Monitor serum cholesterol in cardiac patients. • Hypercalcemia is most likely to occur in patients with mammary carcinoma; these patients should have quantitative urinary and serum calcium level determinations. • Instruct females to report menstrual irregularities; therapy should be discontinued pending etiologic determination. • Watch for virilizing effects; they may be irreversible despite prompt discontinuation of therapy. • Closely observe boys under 7 for precocious development of male sexual characteristics. • In children, therapy should be preceded by X-ray of wrist bones to establish level of bone maturation. During treatment, bone maturation may proceed more rapidly than linear growth; dosage should be intermittent. • Edema is generally controllable with salt restrictions and/or diuretics. • Watch for symptoms of jaundice. Dose adjustment may reverse condition. If hepatic function tests are abnormal, therapy should be discontinued. • Observe patients receiving concomitant anticoagulant therapy for ecchymotic areas, petechiae, or abnormal bleeding. Monitor prothrombin time. • Watch for symptoms of hypoglycemia in diabetics. Dosage of antidiabetic drug may need adjustment. • Use with diet high in calories and protein unless contraindicated. • Does not enhance athletic ability. • Considered an adjunctive therapy.
None significant.	• Contraindicated in prostatic hypertrophy with obstruction; prostatic and male breast cancer; cardiac, hepatic, or renal decompensation; nephrosis; premature infants. Use cautiously in prepubertal males; patients with diabetes or coronary disease; patients taking ACTH, corticosteroids or anticoagulants. • Hypercalcemia symptoms may be difficult to distinguish from symptoms of condition being treated unless anticipated and thought of as a cluster. Hypercalcemia most likely to occur with metastatic breast cancer and may indicate bone metastases. • Instruct females to report menstrual irregularities; therapy should be discontinued pending etiologic determination.

(continued on following page)

NAME	INDICATIONS & DOSAGE	SIDE EFFECTS
oxandrolone *(continued)*		*CNS:* dizziness, headache, sleep disorders, fatigue, tremor, irritability, lethargy, mental depression, chills, excitation. *GI:* gastroenteritis, nausea, vomiting, constipation or diarrhea, change in appetite. *GU:* bladder irritability. *Hypoestrogenic:* in females—flushing; sweating; vaginitis with itching, drying, burning, or bleeding; menstrual irregularities. *Other:* hypercalcemia, edema.
oxymetholone Adroyd◆, Anadrol-50, Anapolon 50◆◆	*Aplastic anemia—* **Adults and children:** 1 to 5 mg/Kg P.O. daily. Dose highly individualized; response not immediate. Trial of 3 to 6 months required. *Osteoporosis, catabolic conditions—* **Adults:** 5 to 15 mg P.O. daily or up to 30 mg P.O. daily. **Children over 6 years:** up to 10 mg P.O. daily. **Children under 6 years:** 1.25 mg P.O. daily or up to q.i.d. Continuous therapy should not exceed 30 days in children; 90 days in any patient.	*Androgenic:* in females—acne, edema, oily skin, weight gain, hirsutism, deepening of voice, clitoral enlargement, decreased or increased libido, male pattern hair loss. In males—prepubertal: premature epiphyseal closure, acne, priapism, growth of body and facial hair, phallic enlargement; postpubertal: testicular atrophy, oligospermia, decreased ejaculatory volume, impotence, gynecomastia, epididymitis. *CNS:* dizziness, headache, sleep disorders, fatigue, tremor, irritability, lethargy, mental depression, chills, excitation, paresthesia. *GI:* gastroenteritis, nausea, vomiting, constipation, diarrhea, change in appetite. *GU:* bladder irritability. *Hypoestrogenic:* in females—flushing; sweating; vaginitis with itching, drying, burning or bleeding; menstrual irregularities. *Other:* hypercalcemia, liver toxicity, muscle cramps, edema.

INTERACTIONS	NURSING CONSIDERATIONS
	• Watch for virilizing effects; may be irreversible despite prompt stopping of therapy. Doctor must decide if benefits outweigh effects. • Boys under 7 should be closely observed for precocious development of male sexual characterisitics.. • In children, therapy should be preceded by X-ray of wrist bones to establish level of bone maturation. During treatment, bone maturation may proceed more rapidly than linear growth; dosage should be intermittent. • Edema is generally controllable with salt restriction and/or diuretics. • Watch for symptoms of jaundice. Dose adjustment may reverse condition. Periodic hepatic functions tests are recommended. • Observe patient on concomitant anticoagulant therapy for ecchymotic areas, petechiae or abnormal bleeding. Monitor prothrombin time. • Watch for symptoms of hypoglycemia in diabetics. Change of dosage in antidiabetic drug may be required. • Use with diet high in calories and protein unless contraindicated. • Monitor serum cholesterol levels. • Does not enhance athletic ability.
None significant.	• Contraindicated in prostatic hypertrophy with obstruction; prostatic and male breast cancer; cardiac, hepatic, or renal decompensation; nephrosis; premature infants. Use cautiously in prepubertal males; patients with diabetes or coronary diseases; patients taking ACTH, corticosteroids, or anticoagulants. • Hypercalcemia symptoms may be difficult to distinguish from symptoms of condition being treated unless anticipated and thought of as a cluster. Hypercalcemia most likely to occur in metastatic breast cancer and may indicate bone metastases. • Supportive treatment of anemias (transfusions, correction of iron, folic acid, vitamin B_{12} or pyroxidine deficiency). Give 3 to 6 months for response. • Effects in osteoporosis usually seen in 4 to 6 weeks. • Instruct females to report menstrual irregularities; therapy should be discontinued pending etiologic determination. • Watch for virilizing effects; may be irreversible despite prompt stopping of therapy. Doctor must decide if benefits outweigh effects. • Boys under 7 should be closely observed for precocious development of male sexual characteristics. • In children, therapy should be preceded by X-ray of wrist bones to establish level of bone maturation. During treatment, bone maturation may proceed more rapidly than linear growth; dosage should be intermittent. Epiphyseal development may continue 6 months after stopping therapy. • Edema is generally controllable with salt restriction and/or diuretics. • Watch for symptoms of jaundice. Dose adjustment may reverse condition; if hepatic function tests are abnormal, therapy should be discontinued. • Observe patient on concomitant anticoagulant therapy for ecchymotic areas, petechiae, or abnormal bleeding. Monitor prothrombin time. • Watch for symptoms of hypoglycemia in diabetics. Change of dosage in antidiabetic drug may be required. • Use with diet high in calories and protein unless contraindicated. • Monitor serum chloesterol and blood cell counts. • Does not enhance athletic ability.

NAME	INDICATIONS & DOSAGE	SIDE EFFECTS
stanozolol Winstrol◆	*To increase hemoglobin in some cases of aplastic anemia—* **Adults:** 2 mg P.O. t.i.d. **Children 6 to 12 years:** up to 2 mg P.O. t.i.d. **Children under 6 years:** 1 mg P.O. b.i.d. Therapy should be intermittent.	*Androgenic:* in females—acne, edema, oily skin, weight gain, hirsutism, deepening of voice, clitoral enlargement, decreased or increased libido. In males— prepubertal: premature epiphyseal closure, acne, priapism, growth of body and facial hair, phallic enlargement; postpubertal: testicular atrophy, oligospermia, decreased ejaculatory volume, impotence, gynecomastia, epididymitis. *CNS:* dizziness, headache, sleep disorders, fatigue, tremor, irritability, lethargy, mental depression, chills, excitation, paresthesia. *GI:* gastroenteritis, nausea, vomiting, constipation, diarrhea, change in appetite. *GU:* bladder irritability. *Hypoestrogenic:* in females—flushing; sweating; vaginitis with itching, drying, burning or bleeding; menstrual irregularities. *Other:* hypercalcemia, edema.
testosterone Android-T, Androlan, Andronaq, Dura-Testrone, Histerone, Homogen-S, Malogen◆, Nendron, Oreton, Tesone, Testaqua, Testoject, Testolin, Testo-Med, Testrone	*Eunuchoidism, eunuchism, and male climacteric symptoms—* **Adults:** 25 mg I.M. 2 to 5 times weekly; or 2 to 6 pellets (75 mg each) implanted subcutaneously q 3 to 6 months. *Breast engorgement of nonnursing mothers*—25 to 50 mg I.M. daily 3 to 4 days, starting at delivery. *Breast cancer in women 1 to 5 years postmenopausal*—100 to 300 mg I.M. 3 times weekly as long as improvement maintained.	*Androgenic:* in females—acne, edema, oily skin, weight gain, hirsutism, deepening of voice, clitoral enlargement, decreased or increased libido. In males— prepubertal: premature epiphyseal closure, acne, priapism, growth of body and facial hair, phallic enlargement; postpubertal: testicular atrophy, oligospermia, decreased ejaculatory volume, impotence, gynecomastia, epididymitis. *CNS:* dizziness, headache, sleep disorders, fatigue, tremor, irritability, lethargy, mental depression, chills, excitation, paresthesia. *GI:* gastroenteritis, nausea, vomiting, constipation, diarrhea, change in appetite. *GU:* bladder irritability. *Hypoestrogenic:* in females—flushing; sweating; vaginitis with itching, drying, burning or bleeding; men-

INTERACTIONS	NURSING CONSIDERATIONS
None significant.	• Contraindicated in prostatic hypertrophy with obstruction; prostatic and male breast cancer; cardiac, hepatic, or renal decompensation; nephrosis; premature infants. Use cautiously in prepubertal males; patients with diabetes or coronary disease; patients taking ACTH; corticosteroids or anticoagulants. • Hypercalcemia symptoms may be difficult to distinguish from symptoms of condition being treated unless anticipated and thought of as a cluster. Hypercalcemia most likely to occur in metastatic breast cancer and may indicate bone metastases. • Instruct females to report menstrual irregularities; therapy should be discontinued pending etiologic determination. • Smaller dose (2 mg b.i.d.) is used in females to avoid virilizing effects. Watch for virilizing effects; may be irreversible despite prompt stopping of therapy. Doctor must decide if benefits outweigh effects. • Boys under 7 should be closely observed for precocious development of male sexual characteristics. • In children, therapy should be preceded by X-ray of wrist bones to establish level of bone maturation. During treatment, bone maturation may proceed more rapidly than linear growth; dosage should be intermittent. • Edema is generally controllable with salt restriction and/or diuretics. • Watch for symptoms of jaundice. Dose adjustment may reverse condition; check hepatic function tests regularly. If abnormal, therapy should be discontinued. • Observe patient on concomitant anticoagulant therapy for ecchymotic areas, petechiae, or abnormal bleeding. Monitor prothrombin time. • Watch for symptoms of hypoglycemia in diabetics. Change of dosage in antidiabetic drug may be required. • Use with diet high in calories and protein unless contraindicated. • Administer before or with meals to minimize GI distress. • Monitor serum cholesterol in cardiac patients. • Does not enhance athletic ability.
None significant.	• Contraindicated in women of childbearing potential (possible masculinization of female infant); hypercalcemia; cardiac, hepatic, or renal decompensation; prostatic or breast cancer in male; benign prostatic hypertrophy with obstruction; elderly, asthenic males who may react adversely to androgen overstimulation; conditions aggravated by fluid retention; hypertension. Use cautiously in myocardial infarction or coronary artery disease, prepubertal males. • When dosage is stabilized, check edema. Sodium and water retention respond to diuretics and/or salt restriction. • Periodic serum cholesterol and calcium determinations, and cardiac and hepatic function tests should be performed. • In metastatic breast cancer, hypercalcemia usually indicates progression of bone metastases. Report signs of hypercalcemia. • Therapeutic response in breast cancer is usually apparent within 3 months. Stop therapy if signs of disease progression appear. • Enhances hypoglycemia; tell patient to report signs of hyperinsulinism. • Instruct males to report priapism, reduced ejaculatory volume, and gynecomastia. Withdraw drug. • Watch for signs of ecchymoses, petechiae with concomitant anticoagulants. Monitor prothrombin time. • Report signs of virilization in females; reevaluate treatment. • Monitor prepubertal males by X-ray for rate of bone maturation.

(continued on following page)

NAME	INDICATIONS & DOSAGE	SIDE EFFECTS
testosterone *(continued)*		strual irregularities. *Local:* pain at injection site, induration; irritation and sloughing with pellet implantation, edema.
testosterone cypionate Andro-Cyp, Androgen-860, D-Test, Depotest, Depo-Test, Depo-Testosterone♦, Durandro, Duratest, Jactatest, Malogen Cyp	*Eunuchism, eunuchoidism, deficiency after castration and male climacteric—* **Adults:** 200 to 400 mg I.M. q 4 weeks. *Oligospermia—* **Adults:** 100 to 200 mg I.M. q 4 to 6 weeks for development and maintenance of testicular function.	*Androgenic:* in males —prepubertal: premature epiphyseal closure, acne, priapism, growth of body and facial hair, phallic enlargement; postpubertal: testicular atrophy, oligospermia, decreased ejaculatory volume, impotence, gynecomastia, epididymitis. *CNS:* dizziness, headache, sleep disorders, fatigue, tremor, irritability, lethargy, mental depression, chills, excitation, paresthesia. *GI:* gastroenteritis, nausea, vomiting, constipation, diarrhea, change in appetite. *GU:* bladder irritability. *Local:* pain at injection site, induration; postinjection furunculosis. *Other:* hypercalcemia, edema.
testosterone enanthate Android-T, Andryl, Anthatest, Arderone, Delatest, Delatestry♦, Dura-Testate, Everone, Malogen LA, Malogex♦♦, Repo-Testro Med, Retandros, Span-Test, Tesone, Testate, Testone LA, Testostroval-P.A., Testrin-P.A.	*Eunuchism, eunuchoidism, deficiency after castration and male climacteric—* **Adults:** 200 to 400 mg I.M. q 4 weeks. *Oligospermia—* **Adults:** 100 to 200 mg I.M. q 4 to 6 weeks for development and maintenance of testicular function.	
testosterone propionate Androlan, Androlin, Malogen in Oil♦♦, Oreton Propionate, Testex, Vulvan	*Eunuchism and eunuchoidism, male climacteric, impotency—* **Adults:** 10 to 25 mg I.M. daily 2 to 4 times weekly; or 5 to 20 mg buccal daily (strictly individualized). *Breast engorgement of nonnursing mothers*—40 mg buccal daily, 3 to 5 days starting at delivery. *Metastatic breast cancer in women*—50 to 100 mg I.M. 3 times weekly; or 200 mg buccal daily as long as improvement maintained. *Postpubertal cryptorchidism—* 15 mg buccal daily.	

INTERACTIONS	NURSING CONSIDERATIONS
	• Use with diet high in calories and protein unless contraindicated. • Inject deep into upper outer quadrant of gluteal muscle. • Watch for irritation and sloughing with pellet implantation. • Watch for ecchymotic areas, petechiae, or abnormal bleeding in patients on concomitant anticoagulant therapy. Monitor prothrombin time. • Implantation of pellets may take place in physician's office in a minor surgical procedure with aseptic precautions observed.
None significant.	• Contraindicated in women of childbearing potential (possible masculinization of female infant); hypercalcemia; cardiac, hepatic, or renal decompensation; prostatic or breast cancer in male; benign prostatic hypertrophy with obstruction; elderly, asthenic males who may react adversely to androgen overstimulation; conditions aggravated by fluid retention; hypertension. Use cautiously in myocardial infarction or coronary artery disease, prepubertal males. • Periodic serum cholesterol and calcium determinations, and cardiac and hepatic function tests should be performed. • In metastatic breast cancer, hypercalcemia usually indicates progression of bone metastases. Report signs of hypercalcemia. • Response in breast cancer is usually apparent within 3 months. Stop therapy if signs of disease progression appear. • Enhances hypoglycemia; tell patient to report signs of hyperinsulinism. • Instruct males to report priapism, reduced ejaculatory volume, and gynecomastia. Withdraw drug. • Watch ecchymoses, petechiae with concomitant anticoagulants. Monitor prothrombin time. • Inject deep into upper outer quadrant of gluteal muscle. Report soreness at site; possibility of postinjection furunculosis. • Report signs of virilization in females; reevaluate treatment. • Monitor prepubertal males by X-ray for rate of bone maturation. • Use with diet high in calories and protein unless contraindicated. • Good oral hygiene decreases possibility of irritation from buccal tablet. Patient shouldn't eat, drink, chew, or smoke while tablet is in place. • Daily requirements best administered in divided doses.

50

Oral contraceptives

estrogen with progestogen

Estrogen-progestogen combinations were introduced as oral contraceptives in the United States in 1960. Although they are the most effective contraceptives available, they have potentially hazardous side effects. (For oral contraceptives that contain progestogen alone, see Chapter 52.) Side effects with high-dose combinations may be more serious, frequent, and rapid in onset than with low-dose combinations. The estrogenic component of combination oral contraceptives is mestranol or ethinyl estradiol, which are synthetic estrogens. The progestogen component is norethynodrel, norethindrone, or norgestrel, which are also synthetics.

Major uses

- Contraception.
- Correction of menstrual disorders, such as endometriosis and hypermenorrhea.

Mechanism of action

- Cause thickening of cervical mucus, which inhibits sperm movement.
- Produce atrophic changes in endometrium, reducing chance of implantation of fertilized ovum. In endometriosis, high-dose combinations cause thinning of endometrial tissue after several dosing cycles.
- Inhibit release of hypothalamic gonadotropin. This inhibition prevents ovulation.

Absorption, distribution, and excretion

- Rapidly and completely absorbed after oral administration.
- Distributed to all body tissues.
- Metabolized in liver.
- Excreted in urine.
- Cross placenta.

Onset and duration

- Act shortly after administration; effect lasts 1 day.
- Provide maximum contraceptive protection after 7 consecutive daily doses.
- Several monthly dosing cycles may be needed to regulate complex endocrine and metabolic disorders.

Combination products
None.

TEACHING PATIENTS ABOUT CONTRACEPTIVES

- Assess patient's understanding of human sexuality.
- Offer information on:
  —biology of sexuality
  —consequences of sexual activity
  —advantages and disadvantages of the various methods of contraception.
- Determine need for contraception. It is needed if patient has:
  —an active sex life or plans to have one
  —a disorder incompatible with pregnancy (renal failure)
  —recently delivered a child.
- Give the patient nonjudgmental support so he can decide:
  —whether or not to use contraception
  —which method to use.
- Make sure that the contraceptive chosen:
  —is safe for that particular patient (patient with thromboembolic disorder should not take the pill)
  —is compatible with patient's life-style (if the patient doesn't want to become pregnant in the future, tubal ligation would be a possible choice)
  —is consistent with the patient's religion or moral philosophy.
- Give the patient supportive, nonjudgmental care by:
  —carefully explaining all procedures
  —reducing discomfort
  —using gentle touch
  —speaking in a gentle voice tone
  —moving close to the patient to show interest
  —showing respect for the patient's privacy
  —allowing a family member or friend to be present, if patient desires.
- Arrange for follow-up care with the patient (periodic examinations for patient on the pill).
- Keep records as a basis for continuing care.

NAME	INDICATIONS & DOSAGE	SIDE EFFECTS
estrogen with progestogen Brevicon, Demulen◆, Enovid, Enovid-E, Loestrin 1/20, Loestrin 1.5/30◆, Lo/Ovral, Min-Ovral◆◆, Modicon, Norinyl 1 + 50◆, Norinyl 1 + 80◆, Norinyl 2 mg◆, Norlestrin◆, Ortho-Novum 1/50◆, Ortho-Novum 1/80◆, Ortho-Novum 2 mg◆, Ortho-Novum 10 mg, Ovcon 35, Ovcon 50, Ovral, Ovulen◆	*Contraception—* **Women:** 1 tablet P.O. daily, beginning on day 5 of menstrual cycle (first day of menstrual flow is day 1). With 20- and 21-tablet packages, new dosing cycle begins 7 days after last tablet taken. With 28-tablet packages, dosage is 1 tablet daily without interruption; extra tablets are placebos or contain iron. If only 1 or 2 doses are missed, dosage may continue on schedule. If 3 or more doses are missed, remaining tablets in monthly package must be discarded and another contraceptive method substituted. If next menstrual period doesn't begin on schedule, rule out pregnancy before starting new dosing cycle. If menstrual period begins, start new dosing cycle 7 days after last tablet was taken. If all doses have been taken on schedule and 1 menstrual period is missed, continue dosing cycle. If 2 consecutive menstrual periods are missed, pregnancy test is required before new dosing cycle. *Hypermenorrhea—* **Women:** use high-dose combinations only. Dose same as for contraception. *Endometriosis—* **Women:** Cyclic therapy: 1 tablet Ortho-Novum 10 mg P.O. daily for 20 days from day 5 to day 24 of menstrual cycle. Suppressive therapy: 1 tablet Ortho-Novum 10 mg P.O. daily for 3 to 9 months. May increase to 20 to 30 mg daily if breakthrough bleeding occurs. Enovid 5 mg or 10 mg—1 tablet P.O. daily for 2 weeks starting on day 5 of menstrual cycle. Continue without interruption for 6 to 9 months, increasing dose by 5 to 10 mg q 2 weeks, up to 20 mg daily. Up to 40 mg daily may be needed if breakthrough bleeding occurs.	*CNS:* headache, dizziness, chorea, depression, libido changes, lethargy. *CV:* thrombophlebitis, thromboembolism, hypertension. *EENT:* worsening of myopia or astigmatism, intolerance to contact lenses. *GI:* nausea, vomiting, abdominal cramps, bloating, diarrhea, constipation, anorexia, increased appetite, weight changes, bowel ischemia. *GU:* breakthrough bleeding, dysmenorrhea, amenorrhea, cervical erosion or abnormal secretions, enlargement of uterine fibromas, vaginal candidiasis, bacteriuria. *Metabolic:* hyperglycemia, hypercalcemia, folic acid deficiency. *Skin:* melasma, rash, acne, seborrhea, oily skin. *Other:* edema, migraine, cholestatic jaundice, leg cramps, breast changes, tenderness, enlargement, secretion. Adverse effects may be more serious, frequent, and rapid in onset with high-dose than with low-dose combinations.

◆ Also available in Canada.
◆◆ Available in Canada only.
Unmarked trade names available in United States only.

INTERACTIONS	NURSING CONSIDERATIONS
Ampicillin, barbiturates, anticonvulsants, rifampin: may diminish contraceptive effectiveness. Use supplemental form of contraception.	• Contraindicated in thromboembolic disorders, cerebrovascular or coronary artery disease, myocardial infarction, known or suspected cancer of breasts or reproductive organs, benign or malignant hepatic tumors, undiagnosed abnormal vaginal bleeding, known or suspected pregnancy, lactation. Also contraindicated in women 35 years or older who smoke over 15 cigarettes a day, and in all women over 40. Use cautiously in hypertension, mental depression, migraine, epilepsy, diabetes mellitus, amenorrhea. Report development or worsening of these conditions to doctor. • If 1 menstrual period is missed and tablets have been taken on schedule, tell patient to continue taking them. If 2 consecutive menstrual periods are missed, tell patient to stop drug and to have pregnancy test. Progestogens may cause birth defects if taken early in pregnancy. • Missed doses in midcycle greatly increase likelihood of pregnancy. • Warn patient that headache, nausea, dizziness, breast tenderness, spotting, and breakthrough bleeding are common at first. These should diminish after 3 to 6 dosing cycles. However, breakthrough bleeding in patients taking high-dose estrogen-progestogen combinations for menstrual disorders may require dosage adjustment. • Warn patient to immediately report abdominal pain; numbness, stiffness or pain in legs or buttocks; pressure or pain in chest; shortness of breath; severe headache; visual disturbances, such as blind spots, blurriness, or flashing lights; undiagnosed vaginal bleeding or discharge; 2 consecutive missed menstrual periods; lumps in the breast; swelling of hands or feet. • Tell patient to take tablets at same time each day; nighttime dosing may reduce nausea and headaches. • Stress importance of semiannual Pap smears and annual gynecologic exams while taking estrogen-progestogen combinations.

51

Estrogens

chlorotrianisene
dienestrol
diethylstilbestrol
diethylstilbestrol diphosphate
esterified estrogens
estradiol
estradiol benzoate
estradiol cypionate
estradiol valerate
estrogenic substances, conjugated
estrone
ethinyl estradiol

Estrogens include the natural hormone secreted by the ovaries and the synthetic derivative. In females, this hormone is essential for normal sexual maturation at puberty, for maintaining the normal menstrual cycle, and for balancing the secretions of the anterior pituitary and the ovaries.

Major uses

- Correction of hormonal imbalances.
- Replacement therapy in menopause and after complete hysterectomy.
- Palliative effect in prostatic and postmenopausal breast cancer.
- Relief from postpartum breast engorgement.

Mechanism of action

- Stimulate or inhibit secretion of hypothalamic, pituitary, and gonadal hormones which control sexual, endocrine, and metabolic processes.

Absorption, distribution, and excretion

- Rapidly absorbed after oral or parenteral administration, and topically from skin and mucous membranes.
- Distributed to all body tissues; concentrations may occur in fat deposits.
- Metabolized primarily in liver; excreted in urine.
- Crosses placental barrier.

Onset and duration

- Begin to act immediately.
- Oral estrogens (except chlorotrianisene) have short duration of action; daily doses are usually needed.
- Parenteral estrogens have longer duration of action; effect may last several days.

Combination products
DELUTEVAL 2X: solution in oil—estradiol valerate 5 mg/ml and hydroxyprogesterone caproate 25 mg/ml.
MENRIUM 5-2♦: chlordiazepoxide 5 mg and esterified estrogens 0.2 mg.
MENRIUM 5-4♦: chlordiazepoxide 5 mg and esterified estrogens 0.4 mg.
MENRIUM 10-4♦: chlordiazepoxide 10 mg, and esterified estrogens 0.4 mg.
MILPREM-200: conjugated estrogens 0.45 mg and meprobamate 200 mg.
MILPREM-400: conjugated estrogens 0.45 mg and meprobamate 400 mg.
PMB-200: conjugated estrogens 0.45 mg and meprobamate 200 mg.
PMB-400: conjugated estrogens 0.45 mg and meprobamate 400 mg.
See also chapter 50, for oral contraceptives and other estrogen-progestogen combinations.

PROVIDING SUPPORT FOR ESTROGEN-THERAPY PATIENTS

- Encourage the patient to report any discomforting side effects:
  - — mood changes, especially depression
  - — thrombophlebitis (warmth or pain in the calf)
  - — excessive fluid retention
  - — jaundice
  - — excessive nausea and vomiting
  - — dizziness and frequent headaches (which point to an elevated blood pressure)
  - — loss of scalp hair
  - — hirsutism
  - — indigestion after eating fatty foods, or stomach pain.
- Stress the need for the patient to regularly visit — at least yearly — the gynecologist. (Visits should include a Pap smear.)
- Instruct the patient to perform self-breast examinations monthly.
- If a patient raises questions concerning the possibility of estrogens causing cancer, assure her of the safety of these hormones for women who have first had a full physical examination.
- Explain that bleeding after estrogen withdrawal is expected. Inform the postmenopausal woman that her bleeding is pseudomenstruation and does not mean that fertility has been regained.
- Instruct the diabetic woman to make frequent urine checks.

NAME	INDICATIONS & DOSAGE	SIDE EFFECTS
chlorotrianisene Tace◆	**Men:** *Prostatic cancer*—12 to 25 mg P.O. daily. **Nonnursing mothers:** *Postpartum breast engorgement*—72 mg P.O. b.i.d. for 2 days; or 50 mg q 6 hours for 6 doses; or 12 mg q.i.d. for 7 days. Start dosing within 8 hours after delivery. **Women:** *Menopausal symptoms*—12 to 25 mg P.O. daily for 30 days or cyclic (3 weeks on, 1 week off). *Female hypogonadism*—12 to 25 mg P.O. for 21 days, followed by 1 dose of progesterone 100 mg I.M. or 5 days of oral progestogen given concurrently with last 5 days of chlorotrianisene (i.e., medroxyprogesterone 5 to 10 mg).	*CNS:* headache, dizziness, chorea, migraine, depression, libido changes. *CV:* thrombophlebitis; thromboembolism; hypertension; increased risk of stroke, pulmonary embolism, and myocardial infarction. *EENT:* worsening of myopia or astigmatism, intolerance to contact lenses. *GI:* nausea, vomiting, abdominal cramps, bloating, diarrhea, constipation, anorexia, increased appetite, excessive thirst, weight changes. *GU:* breakthrough bleeding, altered menstrual flow, dysmenorrhea, amenorrhea, cervical erosion or abnormal secretions, enlargement of uterine fibromas, vaginal candidiasis; *in males:* gynecomastia, testicular atrophy, impotence. *Metabolic:* hyperglycemia, hypercalcemia, folic acid deficiency. *Skin:* melasma, urticaria, acne, seborrhea, oily skin, hirsutism or loss of hair. *Other:* edema, cholestatic jaundice, leg cramps, purpura, breast changes (tenderness, enlargement, secretion).
dienestrol Dienestrol cream◆ Available in combination with sulfanilamide and aminacrine as AVC/Dienestrol, cream or suppositories	**Postmenopausal women:** *Atrophic vaginitis and kraurosis vulvae*—1 to 2 applicatorsful of cream daily for 2 weeks, then half that dose for 2 more weeks; or 1 to 2 vaginal suppositories daily through 1 complete menstrual cycle. *Atrophic and senile vaginitis and kraurosis vulvae when complicated by infection*—1 applicatorful AVC/Dienestrol cream intravaginally daily or b.i.d. for 1 to 2 weeks, then every other day for 1 to 2 weeks.	*GU:* vaginal discharge; with excessive use, uterine bleeding. *Local:* increased discomfort, burning sensation. Systemic effects possible. *Other:* breast tenderness.
diethylstilbestrol DES, Stibilium◆◆, Synestrin	**Women:** *Atrophic vaginitis or kraurosis vulvae*—0.1 to 1 mg as suppository daily for 10 to 14 days concurrently with oral therapy; or up to 5 mg weekly as suppository. *Hypogonadism, castration, primary ovarian failure*—0.2 to 0.5 mg P.O. daily. *Menopausal symptoms*—0.1 to 2 mg P.O. daily in cycles of 3 weeks on and 1 week off.	*CNS:* headache, dizziness, chorea, depression, lethargy. *CV:* thrombophlebitis; thromboembolism; hypertension; increased risk of stroke, pulmonary embolism, and mycardial infarction. *EENT:* worsening of myopia or astigmatism, intolerance to contact lenses. *GI:* nausea, vomiting, abdominal cramps, bloating, diarrhea, constipation, anorexia, increased appetite, excessive thirst, weight changes.

◆ Also available in Canada.
◆◆ Available in Canada only.
Unmarked trade names available in United States only.

INTERACTIONS	NURSING CONSIDERATIONS
None significant.	• Contraindicated in thrombophlebitis or thromboembolic disorders; cancer of breast, reproductive organs, or genital tract; undiagnosed abnormal genital bleeding. Use cautiously in hypertension, asthma, mental depression, bone diseases, blood dyscrasias, gallbladder disease, migraine, seizures, diabetes mellitus, amenorrhea, cardiac failure, hepatic or renal dysfunction. Development or worsening of these conditions may require stopping drug. • Long-term therapy contraindicated in menopause. • FDA regulations require that female patients receive package insert explaining possible estrogen side effects before first dose. • Warn patient to report immediately abdominal pain; pain, numbness, or stiffness in legs or buttocks; pressure or pain in chest; shortness of breath; severe headaches; visual disturbances, such as blind spots, flashing lights, blurriness; undiagnosed vaginal bleeding or discharge; breast lumps; swelling of hands or feet. • Tell male patients on long-term therapy about possible gynecomastia and impotence. • Not used for menstrual disorders because duration of action is very long. • Pathologist should be advised of estrogen therapy when specimen sent. • Diabetics should report positive urine tests so diabetic medication dose can be adjusted. • Hepatic or endocrine function tests may be abnormal during estrogen therapy. Repeat tests 2 months after discontinuing estrogen.
None significant.	• Contraindicated in thrombophlebitis or thromboembolic disorders; cancer of breast, reproductive organs, or genital tract; undiagnosed abnormal genital bleeding. Use cautiously in menstrual irregularities or endometriosis. • Prolonged therapy with estrogen-containing products is contraindicated. • FDA regulations require that female patients receive package insert, explaining possible estrogen side effects before first dose. • Systemic reactions possible with normal intravaginal use. Monitor closely. • Warn patient not to exceed dose. • Withdrawal bleeding may be precipitated if estrogen is suddenly stopped.
None significant.	• Contraindicated in thrombophlebitis or thromboembolic disorders; undiagnosed abnormal genital bleeding. Use cautiously in hypertension, asthma, mental depression, bone disease, migraine, seizures, blood dyscrasias, diabetes mellitus, gallbladder disease, amenorrhea, cardiac failure, hepatic or renal dysfunction. Development or worsening of these conditions may require stopping drug. • Long-term therapy contraindicated in menopause; linked with increased risk of endometrial cancer in premenopausal women. • FDA regulations require that all female patients receive package insert explaining possible estrogen side effects before first dose. • Only 25 mg tablet approved by FDA as the "morning-after pill." To be effective it must be taken within 72 hours after coitus.

(continued on following page)

NAME	INDICATIONS & DOSAGE	SIDE EFFECTS
diethylstilbestrol *(continued)*	*Postcoital contraception ("morning-after pill")*—25 mg P.O. b.i.d. for 5 days, starting within 72 hours after coitus. *Postpartum breast engorgement*—5 mg P.O. daily or t.i.d. up to total dose of 30 mg. **Men:** *Prostatic cancer*—1 to 3 mg P.O. daily, initially; may be reduced to 1 mg P.O. daily, or 5 mg I.M. twice weekly initially, followed by up to 4 mg I.M. twice weekly. **Men and postmenopausal women:** *Breast cancer*—15 mg P.O. daily.	*GU:* breakthrough bleeding, altered menstrual flow, dysmenorrhea, amenorrhea, cervical erosion, altered cervical secretions, enlargement of uterine fibromas, vaginal candidiasis, loss of libido; *in males:* gynecomastia, testicular atrophy, impotence. *Metabolic:* hyperglycemia, hypercalcemia, folic acid deficiency. *Skin:* melasma, urticaria, acne, seborrhea, oily skin, hirsutism or loss of hair. *Other:* edema, migraine, cholestatic jaundice, leg cramps, breast tenderness or enlargement.
diethylstilbestrol diphosphate Honvol••, Stilphostrol	**Men:** *Prostatic cancer*— 50 to 200 mg P.O. t.i.d.; or 0.25 to 1 g I.V. once or twice weekly.	
esterified estrogens Amnestrogen, Climestrone••, Estratab, Estrofol, Evex, Glyestrin, Menest, Menotrol••, Ms-Med, Neo-Estrone••, Zeste	**Men:** *Prostatic cancer*—1.25 to 2.5 mg P.O. daily. **Men and postmenopausal women:** *Breast cancer*—10 mg P.O. t.i.d. for 3 or more months. **Women:** *Hypogonadism, castration, primary ovarian failure*—2.5 to 7.5 mg P.O. b.i.d. or t.i.d. in cycles of 3 weeks on, 1 week off. *Menopausal symptoms*—average 0.3 to 3.75 mg P.O. daily in cycles of 3 weeks on, 1 week off.	*CNS:* headache, dizziness, chorea , depression, libido changes, lethargy. *CV:* thrombophlebitis; thromboembolism; hypertension; increased risk of stroke, pulmonary embolism, and myoc ardial infarction. *EENT:* worsening of myopia or astigmatism, intolerance to contact lenses. *GI:* nausea, vomiting, abdominal cramps, bloating, diarrhea, constipation, anorexia, increased appetite, weight changes. *GU:* breakthrough bleeding, altered menstrual flow, dysmenorrhea, amenorrhea, cervical erosion, altered cervical secretions, enlargement of uterine fibromas, vaginal candidiasis; *in males:* gynecomastia, testicular atrophy, impotence. *Metabolic:* hyperglycemia, hypercalcemia, folic acid deficiency. *Skin:* melasma, rash, acne, hirsutism or hair loss, seborrhea, oily skin. *Other:* breast changes (tenderness, enlargement, secretion), edema, migraine, cholestatic jaundice.
estradiol Aquagen, Estrace•, Progynon **estradiol benzoate**	**Women:** *Menopausal symptoms, hypogonadism, castration, primary ovarian failure*—1 to 2 mg P.O. daily, in cycles of 21 days on and 7 days off, or cycles of 5 days on and 2 days off; or 1 mg (estradiol benzoate) I.M.	*CNS:* headache, dizziness, chorea, depression, libido changes, lethargy. *CV:* thrombophlebitis, thromboembolism, hypertension. *EENT:* worsening of myopia or astigmatism, intolerance to contact lenses. *GI:* nausea, vomiting, abdominal cramps, bloating, diarrhea, constipa-

INTERACTIONS	NURSING CONSIDERATIONS
	• Warn patient to stop taking drug immediately if she becomes pregnant since it can affect the fetus adversely. • Warn patient to report immediately abdominal pain; pain, numbness, or stiffness in legs or buttocks; pressure or pain in chest; shortness of breath; severe headache; visual disturbances, such as blind spots, flashing lights, or blurriness; undiagnosed vaginal bleeding or discharge; breast lumps; swelling of hands or feet. • Pathologist should be advised of estrogen therapy when specimen sent. • Diabetics should report positive urine tests so diabetic medication dose can be adjusted. • Hepatic or endocrine function studies may be abnormal during estrogen therapy. Repeat test 2 months after discontinuing estrogen. • High incidence of gross nonmalignant genital changes in offspring of women taking drug during pregnancy. Female offspring also have higher than normal risk of developing cervical and vaginal adenocarcinoma. • Increased number of cardiovascular deaths reported in men taking diethylstilbestrol tablet (5 mg daily) for prostatic cancer over long period of time. This effect not associated with 1 mg daily dose.
None significant.	• Contraindicated in thrombophlebitis or thromboembolic disorders; undiagnosed abnormal genital bleeding. Use cautiously in history of hypertension, mental depression, gallbladder disease, migraine, seizure, diabetes mellitus, or amenorrhea. Development or worsening of these conditions may necessitate discontinuing drug. • Long-term therapy contraindicated in menopause. • FDA regulations require that female patients receive package insert explaining possible estrogen side effects before first dose. • Warn patient to report immediately abdominal pain; pain, numbness, or stiffness in legs or buttocks; pressure or pain in chest; shortness of breath; severe headaches; visual disturbances, such as blind spots, flashing lights, or blurriness; undiagnosed vaginal bleeding or discharge; breast lumps; swelling of hands or feet. • Pathologist should be advised of estrogen therapy when specimen sent. • Diabetics should report positive urine tests so diabetic medication dose can be adjusted. • Liver or endocrine function studies may be abnormal during estrogen therapy. Repeat tests 2 months after discontinuing estrogen.
None significant.	• Contraindicated in thrombophlebitis or thromboembolic disorders; cancer of breast, reproductive organs; undiagnosed abnormal genital bleeding. Use cautiously in hypertension, mental depression, bone diseases, blood dyscrasias, migraine, seizures, diabetes mellitus, amenorrhea, cardiac failure, hepatic or renal dysfunction. Development or worsening of these conditions may require stopping drug. • FDA regulations require that female patients receive package insert explaining possible estrogen side effects before first dose.

(continued on following page)

NAME	INDICATIONS & DOSAGE	SIDE EFFECTS
estradiol *(continued)*	weekly in divided doses for 2 to 3 weeks, then reduce dose to minimum requirement; or 1.5 mg (estradiol benzoate) I.M. 3 times weekly. *Kraurosis vulvae*—1 to 1.5 mg (estradiol benzoate) I.M. once or more per week. **Men:** *Prostatic cancer*—25 mg S.C. pellet implants (Progynon) q 3 to 4 months, or 50 mg q 4 to 6 months.	tion, anorexia, increased appetite, weight changes. *GU:* breakthrough bleeding, altered menstrual flow, dysmenorrhea, amenorrhea, cervical erosion, altered cervical secretions, enlargement of uterine fibromas, vaginal candidiasis; *in males:* gynecomastia, testicular atrophy, impotence. *Metabolic:* hyperglycemia, hypercalcemia, folic acid deficiency. *Skin:* melasma, urticaria, acne, seborrhea, oily skin, hirsutism or hair loss.
estradiol cypionate D-Est 5, Dep-Estradiol, Depo-Estradiol Cypionate, Depogen, Duraestrin, E-lonate P.A., Estro-Cyp, Estro-Depot, Estrogen-810, Estroject-L.A., Estro-Med, Femogen-Cyp◆◆, Hormogen Depot, Span-F	**Women:** *Kraurosis vulvae*—5 to 10 mg I.M. q 2 to 3 weeks. *Menopausal symptoms*—1 to 5 mg I.M. q 2 to 3 weeks.	*Other:* breast changes (tenderness, enlargement, secretion), edema, migraine, cholestatic jaundice, leg cramps.
estradiol valerate Ardefem, Atladiol, Del-estrogen◆◆, Depogen, Dioval◆, Dura-Estate, Dura-Estradiol, Duragen, Duratrad, Estate, Estratab, Estraval, Rep Estra, Repo-EstroMed, Reposo-E, Retestrin, Valergen	**Women:** *Menopausal symptoms*—5 to 20 mg I.M. repeated once after 2 to 3 weeks. *Postpartum breast engorgement*—10 to 25 mg I.M. at end of first stage of labor. **Men:** *Prostatic cancer*—30 mg I.M. q 1 to 2 weeks.	
estrogenic substances, conjugated Amnestrogen, Co-Estro, Conest, Co-Estro, Conestron, Estrofol, Estroate, Estrocon, Fem-H, Glyestrin, Kestrin, Menogen, Menotab, Ovest, Palopause, Premarin◆, Sodestrin-H, Theogen	**Women:** *Abnormal uterine bleeding (hormonal imbalance)*—25 mg I.V. or I.M. Repeat in 6 to 12 hours. *Breast cancer (at least 5 years after menopause)*—10 mg P.O. t.i.d. for 3 months or more. *Castration, primary ovarian failure, and osteoporosis*—1.25 mg P.O. daily in cycles of 3 weeks on, 1 week off. *Hypogonadism*—2.5 to 7.5 mg P.O. b.i.d. or t.i.d. for 20	*CNS:* headache, dizziness, chorea, depression, libido changes, lethargy. *CV:* thrombophlebitis; thromboembolism; hypertension; increased risk of stroke, pulmonary embolism, and myocardial infarction. *EENT:* worsening of myopia or astigmatism, intolerance to contact lenses. *GI:* nausea, vomiting, abdominal cramps, bloating, diarrhea, constipation, anorexia, increased appetite, weight changes.

INTERACTIONS	NURSING CONSIDERATIONS
	• Warn patient to report immediately abdominal pain; pain, numbness, or stiffness in legs or buttocks; pressure or pain in chest; shortness of breath; severe headaches; visual disturbances, such as blind spots, flashing lights, or blurriness; undiagnosed vaginal bleeding or discharge; breast lumps; swelling of hands or feet. • Risk of endometrial cancer is increased in postmenopausal women who take estrogens for more than 1 year. • Diabetics should report positive urine tests so diabetic medication dose can be adjusted. • Pathologist should be advised of estrogen therapy when specimen sent. • Estradiol available as aqueous suspension or solution in peanut oil. • Estradiol cypionate available as solution in cottonseed oil or vegetable oil. • Estradiol valerate available as solution in castor oil, sesame oil, and vegetable oil. Check for allergy. • Make sure drug is well suspended by rolling vial between palms. • Hepatic and endocrine function studies may be abnormal during estrogen therapy. Repeat tests 2 months after discontinuing estrogen.
None significant.	• Contraindicated in thrombophlebitis or thromboembolic disorders; undiagnosed abnormal genital bleeding. Use cautiously in hypertension, gallbladder disease, bone diseases, blood dyscrasias, migraine, seizures, diabetes mellitus, amenorrhea, cardiac failure, hepatic or renal dysfunction. Development or worsening of these conditions may require stopping drug. • Long-term therapy contraindicated in menopause. • FDA regulations require that female patients receive package insert explaining possible estrogen side effects before first dose. • Warn patient to report any unusual symptoms immediately, especially abdominal pain; pain, numbness, or stiffness in legs or buttocks; pressure or pain in chest; shortness of breath; severe headaches; visual disturbances, such as blind spots, flashing lights, or blurriness; undiagnosed vaginal bleeding or discharge; breast lumps; swelling of hands or feet.

(continued on following page)

NAME	INDICATIONS & DOSAGE	SIDE EFFECTS
estrogenic substances, conjugated *(continued)*	consecutive days each month. *Menopausal symptoms*—0.3 to 1.25 mg P.O. daily in cycles of 3 weeks on. 1 week off. *Postpartum breast engorgement*—3.75 mg P.O. q 4 hours for 5 doses or 1.25 mg q 4 hours for 5 days. **Men:** *Prostatic cancer*—1.25 to 2.5 mg P.O. t.i.d.	*GU:* breakthrough bleeding, altered menstrual flow, dysmenorrhea, amenorrhea, cervical erosion, altered cervical secretions, enlargement of uterine fibromas, vaginal candidiasis; *in males:* gynecomastia, testicular atrophy, impotence. *Metabolic:* hyperglycemia, hypercalcemia, folic acid deficiency. *Skin:* melasma, urticaria, acne, seborrhea, oily skin, flushing (when given rapidly I.V.), hirsutism or loss of hair. *Other:* breast changes (tenderness, enlargement, secretion), edema, migraine, cholestatic jaundice, leg cramps.
estrone Estrovarin, Estrugenone, Estrusol, Femogen♦♦, Follestrol, Foygen, Gravigen, Hormonin, Menagen, Ogen♦, Theelin, Wynestron	**Women:** *Atrophic vaginitis*—0.2 mg intravaginal suppository daily or apply cream to vagina once nightly. *Hypogonadism, castration, ovarian failure*—1.25 to 7.5 mg P.O. daily for 20 consecutive days each month; or 0.1 to 2 mg I.M. weekly. *Menopausal symptoms*—0.625 to 5 mg P.O. daily in cycle of 3 weeks on, 1 week off; or 0.1 to 0.5 mg I.M. 2 to 3 times weekly. **Men:** *Prostatic cancer*—2 to 4 mg I.M. 2 to 3 times weekly.	*CNS:* headache, dizziness, chorea, depression, libido changes, lethargy. *CV:* thrombophlebitis, thromboembolism, hypertension. *EENT:* worsening of myopia or astigmatism, intolerance to contact lenses. *GI:* nausea, vomiting, abdominal cramps, bloating, diarrhea, constipation, anorexia, increased appetite, weight changes. *GU:* breakthrough bleeding, altered menstrual flow, dysmenorrhea, amenorrhea, cervical erosion, altered cervical secretions, enlargement of uterine fibromas, vaginal candidiasis; *in males:* gynecomastia, testicular atrophy, impotence. *Metabolic:* hyperglycemia, hypercalcemia, folic acid deficiency. *Skin:* melasma, urticaria, acne, seborrhea, oily skin, hirsutism or hair loss. *Other:* breast changes (tenderness, enlargement, secretion), edema, migraine, cholestatic jaundice, leg cramps.
ethinyl estradiol Estinyl♦, Feminone, Lynoral, Menolyn, Roldiol, Ylestrol	**Women:** *Breast cancer (at least 5 years after menopause)*—1 mg P.O. t.i.d. *Hypogonadism*—0.02 to 0.15 mg daily to t.i.d. for 2 weeks a month; followed by 2 weeks progesterone therapy; continue for 3 to 6 monthly dosing cycles, followed by 2 months off.	*CNS:* headache, dizziness, chorea, depression, libido changes, lethargy. *CV:* thrombophlebitis, thromboembolism, hypertension. *EENT:* worsening of myopia or astigmatism, intolerance to contact lenses. *GI:* nausea, vomiting, abdominal cramps, bloating, diarrhea, constipation, anorexia, increased appetite, weight changes.

INTERACTIONS	NURSING CONSIDERATIONS
	• I.M. or I.V. use preferred for rapid treatment of dysfunctional uterine bleeding or reduction of surgical bleeding. • Refrigerate before reconstituting. Agitate gently after adding diluent. • Pathologist should be advised of estrogen therapy when specimen sent. • Diabetics should report positive urine tests so diabetic medication dose can be adjusted. • Hepatic or endocrine function studies may be abnormal during estrogen therapy. Repeat test 2 months after discontinuing estrogen. • Use associated with increased risk of endometrial cancer.
None significant.	• Contraindicated in thrombophlebitis or thromboembolic disorders; cancer of breast or reproductive organs; undiagnosed abnormal genital bleeding. Use cautiously in hypertension, mental depression, migraine, seizures, diabetes mellitus, amenorrhea, hepatic or renal dysfunction. Development or worsening of these may require stopping drug. • I.V. use contraindicated. • Long-term therapy contraindicated in menopause. • FDA regulations require that female patients receive package insert explaining possible estrogen side effects before first dose. • Warn patient to report any unusual symptoms immediately, especially abdominal pain; pain, numbness, or stiffness in legs or buttocks; pressure or pain in chest; shortness of breath; severe headaches; visual disturbances, such as blind spots, flashing lights, or blurriness; undiagnosed vaginal bleeding or discharge; breast lumps; swelling of hands or feet. • Oil preparation may become cloudy if chilled. Warm solution until clear before use. Also available in aqueous suspension. • Pathologist should be advised of estrogen therapy when specimen sent. • Diabetics should report positive urine test so diabetic medication dose can be adjusted. • Hepatic or endocrine function studies may be abnormal during estrogen therapy. Repeat test 2 months after discontinuing estrogen.
None significant.	• Contraindicated in thrombophlebitis or thromboembolic disorders; undiagnosed abnormal genital bleeding. Use cautiously in hypertension, mental depression, bone diseases, migraine, seizures, blood dyscrasias, diabetes mellitus, amenorrhea, cardiac failure, hepatic or renal dysfunction. Development or worsening of these conditions may require stopping drug. • FDA regulations require that female patients receive package insert explaining possible estrogen side effects before first dose. • Warn patient to report any unusual symptoms immediately, especially abdominal pain; pain, numbness, or stiffness in legs or buttocks; pressure or pain in chest; shortness of breath; severe headaches; visual disturbances,

(continued on following page)

NAME	INDICATIONS & DOSAGE	SIDE EFFECTS
ethinyl estradiol *(continued)*	*Menopausal symptoms*—0.02 to 0.05 mg P.O. daily for cycles of 3 weeks on, 1 week off. *Postpartum breast engorgement*—0.5 to 1 mg P.O. daily for 3 days, then taper over 7 days to 0.1 mg and discontinue. **Men:** *Prostatic cancer*—0.15 to 2 mg P.O. daily.	*GU:* breakthrough bleeding, altered menstrual flow, dysmenorrhea, amenorrhea, cervical erosion, altered cervical secretions, enlargement of uterine fibromas, vaginal candidiasis; *in males:* gynecomastia, testicular atrophy, impotence. *Metabolic:* hyperglycemia, hypercalcemia, folic acid deficiency. *Skin:* melasma, urticaria, acne, seborrhea, oily skin, hirsutism or hair loss. *Other:* breast changes (tenderness, enlargement, secretion), edema, migraine, cholestatic jaundice, leg cramps.

INTERACTIONS	NURSING CONSIDERATIONS
	such as blind spots, flashing lights, or blurriness; undiagnosed vaginal bleeding or discharge; breast lumps; swelling of hands or feet. • Pathologist should be advised of estrogen therapy when specimen sent. • Diabetics should report positive urine test so diabetic medication dose can be adjusted. • Hepatic or endocrine function studies may be abnormal during estrogen therapy. Repeat test 2 months after discontinuing estrogen.

52
Progestogens

dydrogesterone
ethisterone
hydroxyprogesterone caproate
medroxyprogesterone acetate
norethindrone
norethindrone acetate
norgestrel
progesterone

Progesterone and its synthetic derivatives are called progestogens or progestins. Progesterone is an ovarian hormone secreted primarily by the corpus luteum during the last half of the menstrual cycle. It causes swelling and development of the endometrium, necessary to prepare the uterus for implantation of a fertilized ovum. If implantation does not occur, the sharp drop in the progesterone level at the end of the menstrual cycle helps bring about menstruation. During pregnancy, the placenta secretes about 10 times the normal monthly amount of progesterone to help maintain the pregnancy. Progestogens are used mainly for menstrual disorders needing exogenous progesterone and for contraception.

Major uses
- Treatment of dysfunctional uterine bleeding, amenorrhea, dysmenorrhea.
- Treatment of endometriosis.
- Palliative effect in endometrial cancer.
- Contraception.

Mechanism of action
- Produce secretory changes in endometrium.
- Cause withdrawal bleeding when estrogen present.
- Inhibit pituitary gonadotropin secretion and possibly conception.
- Relax uterine smooth muscle which helps prevent expulsion of implanted ovum.

Absorption, distribution, and excretion
- Rapidly absorbed.
- Widely distributed to all body tissues.
- Metabolized in liver and excreted in urine.

Onset and duration
- Onset is immediate.
- Duration varies with drug and condition being treated.

Combination products
See Oral Contraceptives (Chapter 50) for estrogen-progestogen combinations.

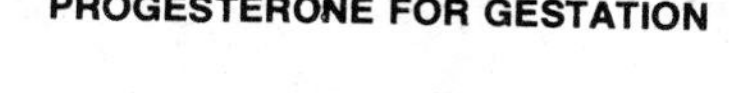

PROGESTERONE FOR GESTATION

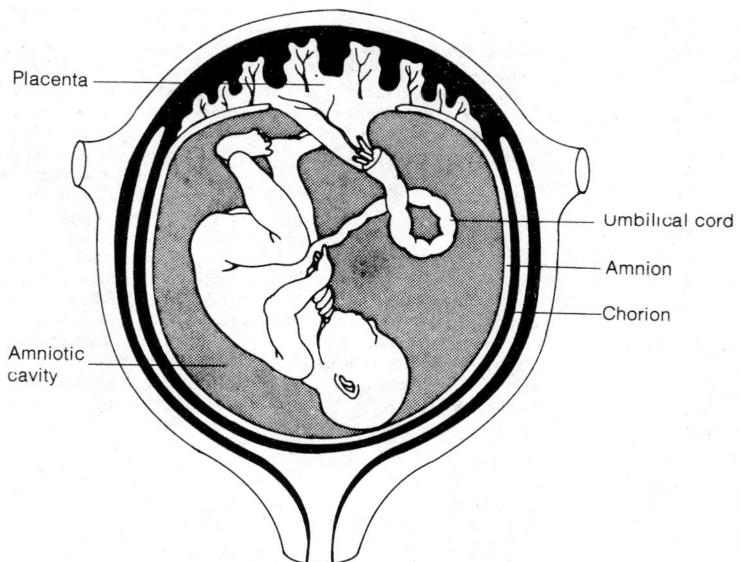

Progesterone, meaning *for gestation*, is secreted in large amounts by the placenta during pregnancy and promotes certain necessary adaptations in the pregnant woman.
Progesterone....

- contributes (along with estrogen) to increasing the thickness of the endometrium, with deposits of glycogen and mucin.
- causes cells to develop in the endometrium which nourish the young embryo
- decreases uterine contractions which prevent spontaneous abortion
- prepares the breasts for lactation.

NAME	INDICATIONS & DOSAGE	SIDE EFFECTS
dydrogesterone Duphaston , Gynorest	**Women:** *primary and secondary amenorrhea—* 5 mg P.O. b.i.d. or q.i.d. from day 15 to day 25 of menstrual cycle. *Oligomenorrhea—* 5 mg P.O. b.i.d. for 5 days. *Abnormal uterine bleeding—* 5 mg P.O. b.i.d. or q.i.d. for 5 to 10 days before usual menses. Thereafter, 5 mg P.O. b.i.d. to q.i.d. for 5 days on the 21st to 25th day of cycle.	*CNS:* dizziness, headache, lethargy, depression, decreased libido, cerebral thrombosis. *CV:* hypertension, thrombophlebitis, pulmonary embolism. *GI:* nausea, vomiting, abdominal cramps, bloating, weight changes. *GU:* breakthrough bleeding, dysmenorrhea, amenorrhea; cervical erosion and abnormal secretions; uterine fibromas; vaginal candidiasis. *Metabolic:* hyperglycemia. *Skin:* melasma, rash, pruritus. *Other:* breast tenderness, enlargement, or secretion; edema, migraine, jaundice.
ethisterone Lutocylol, Pranone, Progestolets, Progestoral	**Women:** *abnormal uterine bleeding—* 10 to 20 mg P.O. b.i.d. or q.i.d. *Functional dysmenorrhea—* 25 mg P.O. daily 3 to 8 days prior to menses.	*CNS:* dizziness, headache, lethargy, depression, decreased libido. *GI:* nausea, vomiting, abdominal cramps, bloating, weight changes. *GU:* breakthrough bleeding, dysmenorrhea, amenorrhea; cervical erosion and abnormal secretions; uterine fibromas; vaginal candidiasis. *Metabolic:* hyperglycemia. *Skin:* melasma, rash. *Other:* breast tenderness, enlargement, or secretion; edema, migraine, cholestatic jaundice.
hydroxyprogesterone caproate Corlutin L.A., Delalutin◆, Dura-Lutin	**Women:** *menstrual disorders—* 125 to 375 mg I.M. q 4 weeks. Stop after 4 cycles. *Endometrial cancer—* 1 to 5 g I.M. weekly.	*CNS:* dizziness, headache, lethargy, depression, decreased libido. *GI:* nausea, vomiting, abdominal cramps, bloating, weight changes. *GU:* breakthrough bleeding, dysmenorrhea, amenorrhea; cervical erosion or abnormal secretions; uterine fibromas; vaginal candidiasis. *Local:* irritation, pain. *Metabolic:* hyperglycemia. *Skin:* melasma, rash. *Other:* breast tenderness, enlargement, or secretion; edema, migraine, cholestatic jaundice.
medroxyprogesterone acetate Amen, depCorlutin, Depo-Provera◆, P-Medrate-P.A., Provera◆	**Women:** *abnormal uterine bleeding due to hormonal imbalance—* 5 to 10 mg P.O. daily for 5 to 10 days beginning on the 16th day of cycle. If patient has received estrogen—10 mg P.O. daily for 10 days beginning on 16th day of cycle. *Secondary amenorrhea—* 5 to 10 mg P.O. daily for 5 to 10 days.	*CNS:* dizziness, headache, lethargy, depression, decreased libido. *GI:* nausea, vomiting, abdominal cramps, bloating, weight changes. *GU:* breakthrough bleeding, dysmenorrhea, amenorrhea; cervical erosion or abnormal secretions; uterine fibromas, vaginal candidiasis. *Metabolic:* hyperglycemia. *Skin:* melasma, rash. *Other:* breast tenderness, enlargement, or secretion; edema, migraine, cholestatic jaundice, pulmonary embolism, thrombophlebitis.

◆ Also available in Canada.
◆◆ Available in Canada only.
Unmarked trade names available in United States only.

INTERACTIONS	NURSING CONSIDERATIONS
None significant.	• Contraindicated in thromboembolic disorders, breast cancer, undiagnosed abnormal vaginal bleeding, pregnancy, missed abortion, liver dysfunction. Use cautiously in diabetes mellitus, seizure disorder, migraine, cardiac or renal disease, asthma, or of mental illness. • FDA regulations require that patients receive patient package insert explaining possible progestogen side effects before first dose. Patient should report any unusual symptoms immediately and should stop drug and call doctor if visual disturbances or migraine occur. • Don't use as test for pregnancy; drug may cause birth defects. • Preliminary estrogen treatment usually needed in menstrual disorders. • Not approved by FDA for use as contraceptive in U.S.A. • Use to prevent abortion not advised in first 4 months of pregnancy.
None significant.	• Contraindicated in thromboembolic disorders, breast cancer, undiagnosed abnormal vaginal bleeding, severe liver disease, missed abortion, or pregnancy. Use cautiously in diabetes mellitus, seizure disorder, migraine, cardiac or renal disease, asthma, or mental illness. • FDA regulations require that patients receive package insert explaining possible progestogen side effects before first dose. Patient should report any unusual symptoms immediately and should stop drug and call doctor if visual disturbances or migraine occur. • Don't use as test for pregnancy; drug may cause birth defects. • Preliminary estrogen treatment usually needed in menstrual disorders. • Use to prevent abortion not advised in first 4 months of pregnancy.
None significant.	• Contraindicated in thromboembolic disorders, breast cancer, undiagnosed abnormal vaginal bleeding, severe liver disease, missed abortion, or pregnancy. Use cautiously in diabetes mellitus, seizure disorder, migraine, cardiac or renal disease, asthma, or mental illness. • FDA regulations require that patients receive package insert explaining possible progestogen side effects before first dose. Patient should report any unusual symptoms immediately and should stop drug and call doctor if visual disturbances or migraine occur. • Don't use as test for pregnancy; drug may cause birth defects. • Warn patient that edema and weight gain are likely. • Give oil solutions (sesame oil and castor oil) deep I.M.; in gluteal muscle. • Preliminary estrogen treatment usually needed in menstrual disorders. • Effect lasts 7 to 14 days. • For I.M. use only.
None significant.	• Contraindicated in thromboembolic disorders, breast cancer, undiagnosed abnormal vaginal bleeding, pregnancy, missed abortion, hepatic dysfunction. Use cautiously in diabetes mellitus, seizure disorder, migraine, cardiac or renal disease, asthma, or mental illness. • FDA regulations require that patients receive package insert explaining possible progestogen side effects before first dose. Patient should report any unusal symptoms immediately and should stop drug and call doctor if visual disturbances or migraine occur. • Don't use as test for pregnancy, drug may cause birth defects. • Use to prevent abortion not advised in first 4 months of pregnancy.

NAME	INDICATIONS & DOSAGE	SIDE EFFECTS
norethindrone Norlutin◆	**Women:** *amenorrhea; abnormal uterine bleeding*— 5 to 20 mg P.O. daily on days 5 to 25 of menstrual cycle; *Endometriosis*—10 mg P.O. daily for 14 days, then increase by 5 mg P.O. daily q 2 weeks up to 30 mg daily.	*CNS:* dizziness, headache, lethargy, depression, decreased libido. *GI:* nausea, vomiting, abdominal cramps, bloating, weight changes. *GU:* breakthrough bleeding, dysmenorrhea, amenorrhea; cervical erosion or abnormal secretions; uterine fibromas; vaginal candidiasis. *Metabolic:* hyperglycemia. *Skin:* melasma, rash. *Other:* breast tenderness, enlargement, or secretion; edema, migraine, cholestatic jaundice.
norethindrone acetate Norlutate◆	**Women:** *amenorrhea, abnormal uterine bleeding*— 2.5 to 10 mg P.O. daily on days 5 to 25 of menstrual cycle. *Endometriosis*—5 mg P.O. daily for 14 days, then increase by 2.5 mg daily q 2 weeks up to 15 mg daily.	*CNS:* dizziness, headache, lethargy, depression, decreased libido. *GI:* nausea, vomiting, abdominal cramps, bloating, weight changes. *GU:* breakthrough bleeding, dysmenorrhea, amenorrhea; cervical erosion or abnormal secretions; uterine fibromas; vaginal candidiasis. *Metabolic:* hyperglycemia. *Skin:* melasma, rash. *Other:* breast tenderness, enlargement, or secretion; edema, migraine, cholestatic jaundice.
norgestrel Ovrette	**Women:** *contraception*— 1 tablet P.O. daily.	*CNS:* cerebral thrombosis or hemorrhage, headache, lethargy, depression. *CV:* hypertension, thrombophlebitis, coronary thrombosis. *GI:* nausea, vomiting, abdominal cramps, bloating, weight change, gallbladder disease. *GU:* breakthrough bleeding, change in menstrual flow, dysmenorrhea, spotting, amenorrhea; cervical erosion, vaginal candidiasis. *Skin:* melasma, rash. *Other:* breast tenderness, enlargement, or secretions; edema, migraine, pulmonary embolism, cholestatic jaundice.
progesterone Lipo-Lutin, Profac-O, Progelan, Progestasert◆, Progestilin◆◆, Progestin	**Women:** *amenorrhea*—5 mg I.M. daily for 6 to 8 days. *Dysmenorrhea*— 10 to 25 mg I.M. daily during last week of cycle. *Abnormal uterine bleeding*— 5 to 10 mg I.M. daily for 6 doses. *Threatened spontaneous abortion*— 5 to 20 mg I.M. daily for 1 week.	*CNS:* dizziness, headache, lethargy, depression, decreased libido. *GI:* nausea, vomiting, abdominal cramps, bloating, weight changes. *GU:* breakthrough bleeding, dysmenorrhea, amenorrhea; cervical erosion or abnormal secretions; uterine fibromas; vaginal candidiasis. *Local:* pain at injection site. *Metabolic:* hyperglycemia. *Skin:* melasma, rash. *Other:* breast tenderness, enlargement or secretion; edema, migraine, cholestatic jaundice.

INTERACTIONS	NURSING CONSIDERATIONS
None significant.	• Contraindicated in thromboembolic disorders, breast cancer, undiagnosed abnormal vaginal bleeding, severe liver disease, missed abortion, or pregnancy. Use cautiously in diabetes mellitus, seizure disorder, migraine, cardiac or renal disease, asthma, or mental illness. • Don't use as test for pregnancy; drug may cause birth defects. • FDA regulations require that patients receive package insert explaining possible progestogen side effects before first dose. Patient should report any unusual symptoms immediately and should stop drug and call doctor if visual disturbances or migraine occur. • Give with milk to prevent GI distress. • Watch patient carefully for signs of edema. • Preliminary estrogen treatment usually needed in menstrual disorders.
None significant.	• Contraindicated in thromboembolic disorders, breast cancer, undiagnosed abnormal vaginal bleeding, severe liver disease, missed abortion, or pregnancy. Use cautiously in diabetes mellitus, seizure disorder, migraine, cardiac or renal disease, asthma, or mental illness. • FDA regulations require that patients receive package insert explaining possible progestogen effects before first dose. Patient should report any unusual symptoms immediately and should stop drug and call doctor if visual disturbances or migraine occur. • Don't use as test for pregnancy; drug may cause birth defects. • Preliminary estrogen treatment usually needed in menstrual disorders. • Twice as potent as norethindrone.
None significant.	• Contraindicated in thromboembolic disorders, breast cancer, undiagnosed abnormal vaginal bleeding, severe liver disease, missed abortion, or pregnancy. Use cautiously in diabetes mellitus, seizure disorder, migraine, cardiac or renal disease, asthma, or mental illness. • FDA regulations require that patients receive package insert explaining possible progestogen effects before first dose. Patient should report any unusual symptoms immediately and should stop drug and call doctor if visual disturbances or migraine occur. • Tell patient to take pill every day even if menstruating. • Progestogen—only oral contraceptive known as "mini-pill."
None significant.	• Contraindicated in thromboembolic disorders, breast cancer, undiagnosed abnormal vaginal bleeding, severe liver disease, or missed abortion. Use cautiously in diabetes mellitus, seizure disorder, migraine, cardiac or renal disease, asthma, or mental illness. • FDA regulations require that patients receive package insert explaining possible progestogen side effects before first dose. Patient should report any unusual symptoms immediately. • Give oil solutions (peanut oil or sesame oil) deep I.M. • A progesterone-containing IUD (Progestasert) available which releases 65 mcg progesterone daily for 1 year. • The only progestogen safely given in pregnancy. • Preliminary estrogen treatment usually needed in menstrual disorders.

53

Gonadotropins

chorionic gonadotropin, human
menotropins

Gonadotropins are purified preparations of hormones extracted from urine of pregnant or postmenopausal women. The gonadotropin menotropins contains both luteinizing hormone and follicle-stimulating hormone.

Major uses

- Treatment of gonadal deficiencies (e.g., cryptorchism and hypogonadism).
- Induction of ovulation in anovulatory conditions.

Mechanism of action

- Stimulate secretions of gonadal hormones.
- Stimulate ovarian follicle growth and maturation (follicle-stimulating hormone effect).
- Stimulate ovulation and development of corpus luteum (luteinizing hormone effect).

Absorption, distribution, and excretion

- Parenteral doses well absorbed; oral doses destroyed by digestive enzymes.
- Concentrated in ovaries and testes.
- Excreted in urine.

Onset and duration

Serum levels peak 6 hours after injection.

Combination products

None.

CHOOSING AND SUPPORTING GONADOTROPIN THERAPY PATIENTS

Gonadotropins are used to induce ovulation in anovulatory women. When ovulation dysfunction has been demonstrated, gonadotropins are initially given in sufficient doses to induce follicular growth and maturation.

• Preliminary steps before treatment include a thorough gynecological and endocrinological evaluation:

— Urinary gonadotropin determination to rule out primary ovarian failure. (Urinary gonadotropin varies according to a woman's age. Gonadotropin hormone secretion begins in puberty, signaling the onset of adult sexual maturation. Normally, a woman's total urinary gonadotropin secretion increases at a steady upward rate till menopause when her gonadotropin decline begins.)

— Meticulous physical examination to rule out pathologic conditions of the uterus and fallopian tubes, pregnancy, endometrial cancer, and other organic causes of abnormal bleeding.

— Similar evaluation of the patient's sexual partner.

(Approximately 15% of all couples are faced with infertility. The causes of infertility are multiple, but relatively more female abnormalities are responsible for the infertility of the population at large.)

Before treatment:

• Provide the patient with the support she needs. Many women appear anxious and tense, sensitive to real or imagined criticism of their desire for a child in this overpopulated world. The natural desire for motherhood combined with societal pressures places a great deal of stress on the infertile woman.

• Advise the patient that gonadotropin-induced ovulation may be difficult to achieve; is expensive; and is likely to produce multiple birth.

• Meanwhile counsel her on her alternatives: adoption or artificial insemination.

NAME	INDICATIONS & DOSAGE	SIDE EFFECTS
chorionic gonadotropin, human Android HCG, Antuitrin-S◆, A.P.L. ◆, CG10, Chorex, Chorigon, Follutein, Glucotropin-Forte, Gonadex, Khorion, Libigen, Luton, Pregnyl, Pre-Ine, Rochoric, Stemultrolin	*Anovulation and infertility*— **Women:** 10,000 units I.M. 1 day after last dose of menotropins. *Hypogonadism*— **Men:** 500 to 1,000 units I.M. 3 times weekly for 3 weeks, then twice weekly for 3 weeks; or 4,000 units I.M. 3 times weekly for 6 to 9 months, then 2,000 units 3 times weekly for 3 more months. *Nonobstructive cryptorchism*— **Boys 4 to 9 years:** 500 to 4,000 units I.M. q 2 to 3 days for up to 6 weeks, or 5,000 units I.M. every other day for 4 doses.	*CNS:* headache, fatigue, irritability, restlessness, depression. *GU:* early puberty (growth of testes, penis, pubic and axillary hair, voice change, down on upper lip, growth of body hair). *Other:* gynecomastia, edema, pain at injection site.
menotropins Pergonal	**Women:** *Anovulation*— 75 IU (international units) each FSH and LH I.M. daily for 9 to 12 days, followed by 10,000 units chorionic gonadotropin I.M. 1 day after last dose of menotropins. Repeat for 1 to 3 menstrual cycles until ovulation occurs. *Infertility with ovulation*— 75 IU each of FSH and LSH I.M. daily for 9 to 12 days, followed by 10,000 units chorionic gonadotropin I.M. 1 day after last dose of menotropins. Repeat for 2 menstrual cycles and then increase to 150 IU each FSH and LH I.M. daily for 9 to 12 days, followed by 10,000 units chorionic gonadotropin I.M. 1 day after last dose of menotropins. Repeat for 2 menstrual cycles. Menotropins available in amps containing 75 IU each FSH (follicle-stimulating hormone) and LH (luteinizing hormone).	*Blood:* hemoconcentration with fluid loss into abdomen. *GI:* nausea, vomiting, diarrhea. *GU:* ovarian enlargement with pain and abdominal distention, multiple pregnancies, ovarian hyperstimulation syndrome (sudden ovarian enlargement, ascites with or without pain, or pleural effusion). *Other:* fever.

◆ Also available in Canada.
◆◆ Available in Canada only.
Unmarked trade names available in United States only.

INTERACTIONS	NURSING CONSIDERATIONS
None significant.	• Contraindicated in pituitary hypertrophy or tumor, prostatic cancer, and early puberty (usual onset between 10 and 13 years of age). Use cautiously in epilepsy, migraine, asthma, cardiac or renal disease. • Not for obesity control. • When used with menotropins to induce ovulation, multiple births possible. • In infertility, encourage daily intercourse from day before chorionic gonadotropin is given until ovulation occurs. • Inspect genitalia of boys for signs of early puberty. Notify doctor, who may discontinue drug if early puberty occurs.
None significant.	• Contraindicated in high urinary gonadotropin levels, thyroid or adrenal dysfunction, pituitary tumor, abnormal uterine bleeding, ovarian cysts or enlargement, and pregnancy. • Tell patient that there is a possibility of multiple births. • Encourage daily intercourse from day before chorionic gonadotropin is given until ovulation occurs. • Reconstitute with 1 to 2 ml sterile saline injection. Use immediately.

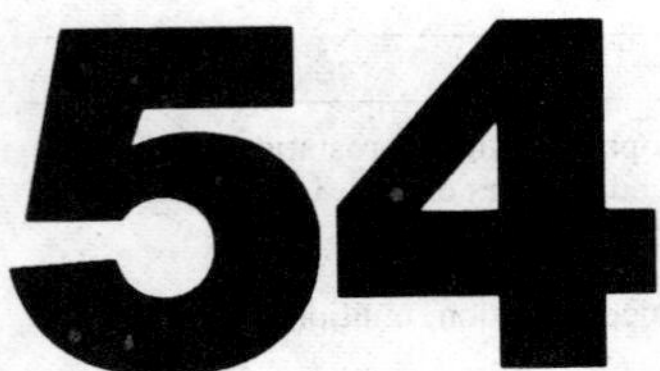

Antidiabetic agents

acetohexamide
chlorpropamide
glucagon
insulins
phenformin
tolazamide
tolbutamide

Antidiabetic drugs are used in the management of diabetes mellitus to supply insulin or to stimulate insulin production when the natural supply is insufficient. Phenformin neither supplies insulin nor stimulates production of insulin, but it does lower blood sugar in diabetes mellitus. Unlike other drugs in this group, glucagon raises blood sugar and is used to counteract hypoglycemic reactions in diabetic patients receiving insulin or in psychiatric patients during insulin shock therapy.

Major uses

• Complete or partial supplementation of endogenous insulin in the treatment of diabetes mellitus.

• Treatment of juvenile-onset diabetes mellitus (insulin only).

• Treatment of maturity-onset diabetes mellitus inadequately controlled by diet alone. Insulin is necessary if oral hypoglycemics are ineffective.

• Emergency treatment of insulin-induced hypoglycemia (glucagon only).

Mechanism of action

• Insulin

—Increases glucose transport across muscle and fat cell membranes to reduce blood sugar.

—Promotes conversion of glucose to its storage form, glycogen.

—Stimulates amino acid uptake and conversion to protein in muscle cells and inhibits protein degradation.

—Increases conversion of free fatty acids to triglycerides and inhibits triglyceride breakdown to free fatty acids.

—Stimulates lipoprotein lipase activity, which converts circulating lipoproteins to fatty acids.

• Sulfonylureas (acetohexamide, chlorpropamide, tolazamide, and tolbutamide) stimulate

insulin secretion from the beta cells of the pancreas.
• Phenformin may reduce sugar levels by promoting the breakdown of glucose into simpler compounds, primarily pyruvate and lactate, and by decreasing the absorption of glucose from the gastrointestinal tract.
• Glucagon raises blood sugar levels by activating enzymes that convert glycogen into glucose in the liver.

Absorption, distribution, and excretion
• Insulin is destroyed in the gastrointestinal tract. It is absorbed directly into the blood stream from the injection site and is distributed throughout the extracellular fluid.
• Insulin absorption rate depends on insulin type, concentration, dose and volume, administration route and rate, vascularity at injection site, and patient's physical exercise pattern. Vigorous exercise accelerates absorption and metabolism of insulin from a thigh injection but apparently not from an arm injection.
• Insulin is metabolized primarily in the liver but partially in the kidneys and muscle tissue. Only small quantities are normally excreted in urine.
• Acetohexamide, chlorpropamide, tolazamide, and tolbutamide are well absorbed from the gastrointestinal tract (tolazamide more slowly than the others), are distributed throughout the extracellular fluid in both free and bound forms, and are metabolized and excreted through the kidneys.
• Phenformin (IND exemption) is adequately absorbed from the gastrointestinal tract, is metabolized in the liver, and is excreted in the urine.
• Glucagon is rapidly absorbed after parenteral administration and is metabolized primarily in the liver.

Onset and duration
See chart below.

Combination products
Drugs may be administered in combinations or insulin mixtures but are commercially available only as individual components.

Drug	Onset (hours)	Peak (hours)	Duration (hours)
RAPID-ACTING			
regular insulin	½ to 1	2 to 3	5 to 7
prompt insulin zinc suspension (semilente)	½ to 1	4 to 7	12 to 16
INTERMEDIATE-ACTING			
globin zinc insulin	2	8 to 16	18 to 24
isophane insulin suspension (NPH)	1 to 2	8 to 12	24 to 28
insulin zinc suspension (lente)	1 to 2	8 to 12	24 to 28
LONG-ACTING			
protamine zinc insulin suspension (PZI)	4 to 8	14 to 20	over 36
extended insulin zinc suspension (ultralente)	4 to 8	16 to 18	over 36
tolbutamide	1	4 to 6	6 to 12
acetohexamide	1	4 to 5	12 to 24
tolazamide	4 to 6	4 to 6	10 to 14
chlorpropamide	1	3 to 6	36
phenformin	rapid after initial loading (3 to 4 days)	—	12 (timed-disintegration form)
glucagon	½	—	1 to 2

HOW TO CHOOSE AN INSULIN INJECTION SITE

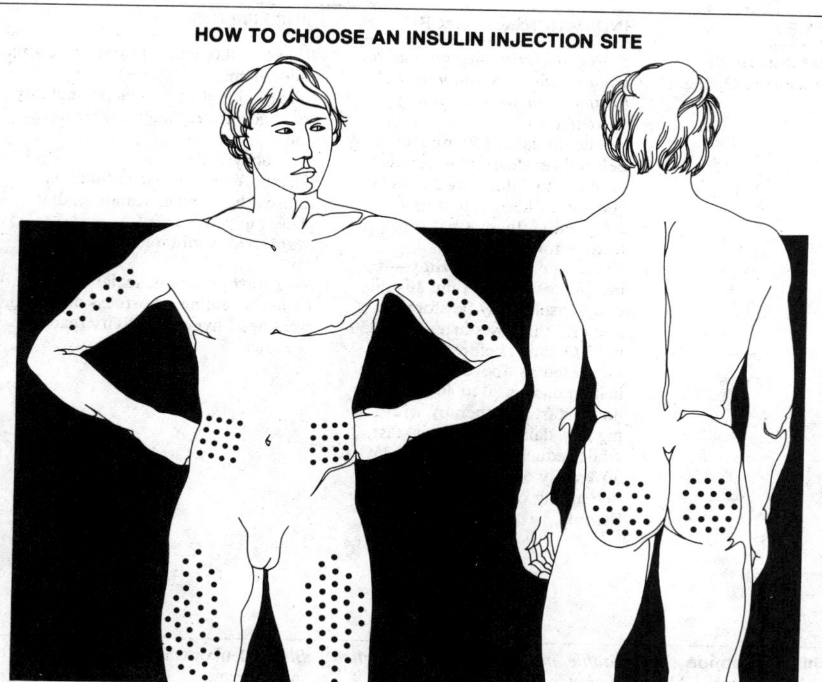

To effectively inject insulin without creating unwanted lipodystrophy (dimpling), hypertrophy (thickening), or abscess formation, instruct your patient to: keep a daily record so that he can systematically rotate all viable injection sites — subcutaneous tissue of both deltoids, anterior and lateral thighs, abdomen, and buttocks (pictured above) — maintaining a 6- to 8-week cycle before repeating; and to use all designated points in one body area, with a 1-inch space between injections, before proceeding to the next body area.

NAME	INDICATIONS & DOSAGE	SIDE EFFECTS
acetohexamide Dimelor••, Dymelor	*Stable, maturity-onset nonketotic diabetes mellitus uncontrolled by diet alone and previously untreated*— **Adults:** initially, 250 mg P.O. daily before breakfast; may increase dose q 5 to 7 days (by 250 to 500 mg) as needed to maximum 1.5 g daily, divided b.i.d. to t.i.d. before meals. *To replace insulin therapy*—if insulin dose is less than 20 units daily, insulin may be stopped and oral therapy started with 250 mg P.O. daily, before breakfast, increased as above if needed. If insulin dose is 20 to 40 units daily, start oral therapy with 250 mg P.O. daily, before breakfast, while reducing insulin dose 25% to 30% daily or every other day, depending on response to oral therapy.	*Blood:* leukopenia, thrombocytopenia, mild anemia. *CNS:* irritability, headache, inability to concentrate, fatigue, dizziness, coma. *CV:* tachycardia. *GI:* anorexia, epigastric fullness, nausea, heartburn, vomiting, diarrhea, hunger. *Metabolic:* sodium loss, hypoglycemia. *Skin:* rash, pruritus, facial flushing. *Other:* sweating, shortness of breath, weakness, hypersensitivity reactions, jaundice.
chlorpropamide Chloromide••, Chloronase••, Diabinese•, Novopropamide••, Stabinol••	*Stable, maturity-onset nonketotic diabetes mellitus uncontrolled by diet alone and previously untreated*— **Adults:** 250 mg P.O. daily with breakfast or in divided doses if GI disturbances occur. First dosage increase may be made after 5 to 7 days, then dose may be increased q 3 to 5 days by 50 to 125 mg, if needed, to maximum 750 mg daily. Start with dose of 100 to 125 mg in older patients. *To change from insulin to oral therapy*—If insulin dose less than 40 units daily, insulin may be stopped and oral therapy started as above. If insulin dose is 40 units or more daily, start oral therapy as above with insulin dose reduced 50%. Further insulin reductions should be made according to patient response.	*Blood:* leukopenia, thrombocytopenia, mild anemia. *CNS:* irritability, headache, inability to concentrate, dizziness, coma. *CV:* tachycardia. *GI:* anorexia, epigastric fullness, nausea, heartburn, vomiting, diarrhea, clay-colored stool, abdominal cramps, constipation, hunger. *GU:* tea-colored urine. *Metabolic:* sodium loss, prolonged hypoglycemia. *Skin:* rash, pruritus, facial flushing. *Other:* sweating, shortness of breath, weakness, hypersensitivity reactions, jaundice, alterations in hepatic function.

• Also available in Canada.
•• Available in Canada only.
Unmarked trade names available in United States only.

INTERACTIONS	NURSING CONSIDERATIONS
Acetazolamide, adrenergic agents, alcohol, corticosteroids, glucagon, rifampin, thiazide diuretics, thyroxine: decreased hypoglycemic response. Monitor blood glucose. *Allopurinol, anabolic steroids, clofibrate, guanethidine, halofenate, MAO inhibitors, phenylbutazone, salicylates, sulfonamides, oral anticoagulants:* increased hypoglycemic activity. Monitor blood glucose. *Metoprolol, propranolol, clonidine:* prolonged hypoglycemic effect and masked symptoms of hypoglycemia. Use together cautiously.	• Contraindicated in treatment of juvenile, growth-onset, brittle, and severe diabetes; in diabetes mellitus adequately controlled by diet and in maturity-onset diabetes complicated by ketosis, acidosis, diabetic coma, Raynaud's gangrene, renal or hepatic impairment, thyroid or other endocrine dysfunction. Use cautiously in sulfonamide hypersensitivity. • Instruct patient about nature of disease; importance of following therapeutic regimen and adhering to specific diet, weight reduction, exercise, personal hygiene, and avoiding infection; how and when to test for glycosuria and ketonuria; recognition of hypoglycemia. • Be sure patient knows that therapy relieves symptoms but doesn't cure disease. • Patient transferring from another oral sulfonylurea antidiabetic drug usually needs no transition period. • Monitor patient transferring from insulin therapy to an oral antidiabetic for urinary glucose and ketones at least t.i.d.; patient may require hospitalization during transition. • During periods of increased stress, such as infection, fever, surgery, or trauma, patient may require insulin therapy. Monitor patient closely for hyperglycemia in these situations. • Oral contraceptives may alter diabetic control. Use another form of birth control. • Advise patient to avoid moderate to large intake of alcohol; antabuse reaction possible. • For symptoms and treatment of toxicity, see p. 1118.
Acetazolamide, adrenergic agents, alcohol, corticosteroids, glucagon, rifampin, thiazide diuretics: decreased hypoglycemic response. Monitor blood glucose. *Allopurinol, anabolic steroids, chloramphenicol, clofibrate, guanethidine, halofenate, MAO inhibitors, phenylbutazone, salicylates, sulfonamides, oral anticoagulents:* increased hypoglycemic activity. Monitor blood glucose. *Metoprolol, propranolol, clonidine:* prolonged hypoglycemic effect and masked symptoms of hypoglycemia. Use together cautiously.	• Contraindicated in the treatment of juvenile, growth-onset, brittle, and severe diabetes. • Contraindicated in diabetes mellitus adequately controlled by diet and in maturity-onset diabetes complicated by fever, ketosis, acidosis, diabetic coma, major surgery, severe trauma, Raynaud's gangrene, renal or hepatic impairment, thyroid or other endocrine dysfunction. • Use cautiously in sulfonamide hypersensitivity. • Instruct patient about nature of the disease; importance of following therapeutic regimen and adhering to specific diet, weight reduction, exercise, personal hygiene, avoiding infection; how and when to test for glycosuria and ketonuria; and recognition of hypoglycemia. • Make sure patient understands that therapy relieves symptoms but does not cure the disease. • Side effects, especially hypoglycemia, may be more frequent or severe than with some other sulfonylurea drugs (acetohexamide, tolazamide, and tolbutamide) because of its long duration of effect (36 hours). • If hypoglycemia occurs, patient should be monitored closely for a minimum of 3 to 5 days. • Patient transferring from another oral sulfonylurea antidiabetic drug usually needs no transition period. • Monitor patient transferring from insulin therapy to an oral antidiabetic for urinary glucose and ketones at least t.i.d.; patient may require hospitalization during transition. • May accumulate in renal insufficiency. • Oral contraceptives may alter diabetic control. Use another form of birth control. • Advise patient to avoid moderate to large intake of alcohol; antabuse reaction possible. • For symptoms and treatment of toxicity, see p. 1118.

NAME	INDICATIONS & DOSAGE	SIDE EFFECTS
glucagon	*Coma of insulin-shock therapy—* **Adults:** 0.5 to 1 mg S.C., I.M., or I.V. 1 hour after coma develops; may repeat within 25 minutes, if necessary. In very deep coma, also give glucose 10% to 50% I.V. for faster response. When patient responds, give additional carbohydrate immediately. *Severe insulin-induced hypoglycemia during diabetic therapy—* **Adults and children:** 0.5 to 1 mg S.C., I.M., or I.V.; may repeat q 20 minutes for 2 doses, if necessary. If coma persists, give glucose 10% to 50% I.V.	*GI:* nausea, vomiting. *Other:* hypersensitivity.
insulins **regular insulin** Beef Regular Iletin (acid neutral CZI), Insulin-Toronto (beef or pork)◆◆, Pork Regular Iletin **regular insulin concentrated** Regular (concentrated) Iletin **prompt insulin zinc suspension** Semilente Iletin, Semilente Insulin◆ **isophane insulin suspension (NPH)** Beef NPH Iletin, NPH Iletin, NPH Insulin◆◆, Pork NPH Iletin **insulin zinc suspension** Beef Lente Iletin, Lente Iletin, Lente Insulin◆, Pork Lente Iletin **globin zinc insulin** **protamine zinc insulin suspension (PZI)**	*Diabetic ketoacidosis (use regular insulin only)—* **Adults:** 25 to 150 units I.V. stat, then additional doses may be given q 1 hour based on blood sugar levels until patient is out of acidosis; then give S.C. q 6 hours thereafter. Alternative dosage schedule: 50 to 100 units I.V. and 50 to 100 units S.C. stat; additional doses may be given q 2 to 6 hours based on blood sugar levels; or 0.33 units/Kg I.V. bolus, followed by 7 to 10 units/hour I.V. by continuous infusion. Continue infusion until blood sugar drops to 250 mg%, then start S.C. insulin q 6 hours. **Children:** 0.5 to 1 unit/Kg divided into 2 doses, 1 given I.V. and the other S.C., followed by 0.5 to 1 unit/Kg I.V. q 1 to 2 hours; or 0.1 unit/Kg I.V. bolus, then 0.1 unit/Kg/hour continuous I.V. infusion until blood sugar drops to 250 mg%, then start S.C. insulin. Preparation of infusion: add 100 units regular insulin and 1 g albumin to 100 ml 0.9% saline solution. Insulin concentration will be 1 unit/ml. *Ketosis-prone and juvenile-onset diabetes mellitus, diabetes mellitus inadequately controlled by diet, and oral hypoglycemics—* **Adults and children:** therapeutic regimen prescribed by doctor and adjusted according to patient's	*CNS:* uncontrollable yawning, tingling in fingers, confusion, agitation, lethargy, fatigue, personality changes, tremor, headache, nightmares, ataxia, irritability, muscle weakness, inability to concentrate, hypothermia, shallow breathing, aphasia, stupor, coma. *CV:* tachycardia. *EENT:* blurred vision. *GI:* increased appetite, nausea, vomiting, numbness of mouth. *Local:* lipoatrophy, lipohypertrophy, itching, swelling, redness, stinging, warmth at site of injection. *Metabolic:* hypoglycemia, hyperglycemia (rebound or Somogyi effect). *Skin:* sweating, urticaria, pallor. *Other:* anaphylaxis. *Note:* most of the side effects listed above are associated with insulin overdose and are signs of hypoglycemia. Obtain blood sugar level stat and notify doctor.

INTERACTIONS	NURSING CONSIDERATIONS
Phenytoin: inhibited glucagon-induced insulin release. Use cautiously.	• Use glucagon only under medical supervision. • Hypoglycemic juvenile or unstable diabetics usually do not respond to glucagon. Give dextrose I.V. instead. • It is vital to arouse the patient from coma as quickly as possible and to give additional carbohydrates to prevent secondary hypoglycemic reactions. • For I.V. drip infusion, glucagon is compatible with dextrose solution but forms a precipitate in chloride solutions. • Instruct patient and family in proper glucagon use, recognition of hypoglycemia, and urgency of calling doctor immediately in emergencies. • May be stored for 3 months at 2° to 15° C. (35.6° to 59° F.) after reconstitution.
Metoprolol, propranolol: hyperglycemia or hypoglycemia may occur. Symptoms of hypoglycemia may be masked. Use together cautiously. *Acetazolamide, adrenergic agents, alcohol, corticosteroids, glucagon, rifampin, thiazide diuretics, thyroxine:* decreased insulin response. Monitor blood glucose. *Allopurinol, anabolic steroids, clofibrate, guanethidine, halofenate, MAO inhibitors, phenylbutazone, salicylates, sulfonamides, oral anticoagulants:* increased insulin response. Monitor for blood glucose.	• Use only regular insulin in patients with circulatory collapse, diabetic ketoacidosis. or hyperkalemia. Do not use regular insulin concentrated, I.V. Do not use intermediate or long-acting insulins for coma or other emergency requiring rapid drug action. • Observe closely until dosage is established. • Accuracy of measurement is very important, especially with regular insulin concentrated. • With regular insulin concentrated, a deep secondary hypoglycemic reaction may occur 18 to 24 hours after injection. • Dosage is always expressed in USP units. • Regular, intermediate, and long-acting insulin may be mixed to meet patient's needs. All components should have same concentration. • Store insulin in a cool area. Refrigeration is desirable but not essential, except with regular insulin concentrated. • Don't use insulin that has changed color. • Check expiration date on vial before using contents. • Administration route is S.C. because absorption rate and pain are less than with I.M. injections. Ketosis-prone juvenile-onset, severely ill, and newly diagnosed diabetics with very high blood sugar levels may require hospitalization and I.V. treatment with regular fast-acting insulin. Ketosis-resistant diabetics may be treated as outpatients with intermediate-acting insulin and instructions on how to alter dosage according to self-performed urine glucose determinations. • Press but do not rub site after injection. Rotate injection sites. Chart sites to avoid overuse of one area. • To mix insulin suspension, swirl vial gently or rotate between palms. Don't shake vigorously. • Insulin requirements increase, sometimes drastically, in pregnant diabetics and then decline immediately postpartum. • Be sure patient knows that therapy relieves symptoms but doesn't cure disease. • Tell patient about nature of disease, importance of following therapeutic regimen and specific diet, weight reduction, exercise, personal hygiene, avoiding infection, and timing of injection and eating. Teach that urine tests are essential guides to dosage and success of therapy; important to recognize hypoglycemic symptoms because insulin-induced hypoglycemia is hazardous and may cause brain damage if prolonged; most side effects are self-limiting and temporary.

(continued on following page)

NAME	INDICATIONS & DOSAGE	SIDE EFFECTS
protamine zinc insulin suspension (PZI) *(continued)* Beef Protamine Zinc Iletin, Pork Protamine Zinc Iletin, Protamine Zinc Iletin **extended insulin zinc suspension** Ultralente Iletin, Ultralente Insulin◆	blood and urine glucose concentrations. *Marked insulin resistance (when daily requirements more than 200 units; 1 to 3 injections daily)—regular insulin concentrated.* *Mild or stable diabetes*—isophane insulin suspension, insulin zinc suspension, and globin zinc insulin: 1 S.C. injection daily in a.m. before breakfast or ⅔ dose before breakfast and ⅓ dose before dinner. *Mild to moderately severe but stable diabetes (not recommended for use in children)*—protamine zinc insulin and extended insulin zinc suspension: dosage and frequency of administration must be carefully individualized; usual dose 1 S.C. injection in a.m. before breakfast. *Severe, unstable complicated diabetes*—regular insulin and prompt insulin zinc suspension: 1 S.C. injection before meals and at bedtime with snack.	
phenformin (available only through U.S. Food and Drug Administration by Investigational New Drug Application. Formerly known as DBI).	*Maturity-onset diabetes mellitus in nonketosis-prone patient with high blood sugar and polydipsia for whom other therapy is ineffective or impractical and for whom benefits outweigh risks*— **Adults:** 25 mg P.O. daily up to q.i.d. given with meals, or 50 mg timed-release capsule daily with breakfast or b.i.d. with breakfast and supper.	*GI:* nausea, diarrhea, anorexia, metallic taste, abdominal pain. *Other:* lactic acidosis, hyperventilation, hypovolemia, hypotension, confusion, coma, death.
tolazamide Tolinase	*Stable, maturity-onset nonketotic diabetes mellitus uncontrolled by diet alone and previously untreated*— **Adults:** initially, 100 mg P.O. daily with breakfast if fasting blood sugar (FBS) under 200 mg%, or 250 mg if FBS is over 200 mg%. May adjust dose at weekly intervals by 100 to 250 mg.	*Blood:* leukopenia, thrombocytopenia, agranulocytosis. *CNS:* headache, weakness, fatigue, dizziness, malaise. *GI:* anorexia, nausea, vomiting, flatus. *Metabolic:* hypoglycemia. *Skin:* rash, urticaria. *Other:* hypersensitivity reactions, cholestatic jaundice.

INTERACTIONS	NURSING CONSIDERATIONS
	• Advise patient to wear medical I.D. always; to carry ample insulin supply and syringes on trips; to have carbohydrates (lump of sugar or candy) on hand for emergency; to take note of time zone changes for dose schedule when traveling. • Marijuana may increase insulin requirements. • For symptoms and treatment of toxicity, see p. 1118.
Metoprolol, propranolol, clonidine: prolonged hypoglycemic effect and masked symptoms of hypoglycemia. Use together cautiously.	• Not commercially available because of high incidence of lactic acidosis associated with its use. Doctor must file Investigational New Drug Application with U.S. Food and Drug Administration to obtain drug. • Contraindicated in juvenile or growth-onset diabetes, insulin-dependent diabetics, hemorrhage, myocardial infarction, congestive heart failure, alcoholism, septicemia, shock, surgery, starvation, renal failure, hypoxia-related disease, ischemia, hepatic disease, lactic acidosis, or diabetes mellitus with complications (acidosis, infection, gangrene, coma). • Patient must be informed of risks and must sign investigational new drug consent form before start of therapy. • Nurse and patient should be familiar with symptoms of lactic acidosis (nausea, vomiting, diarrhea, hyperventilation, hypotension, confusion). Notify doctor immediately if they occur. Alcohol ingestion may contribute to lactic acidosis. • Development of GI upset requires stopping drug. • For symptoms and treatment of toxicity, see p. 1118.
Acetazolamide, adrenergic agents, alcohol, corticosteroids, glucagon, rifampin, thiazide diuretics, thyroxine: decreased hypoglycemic response. Monitor blood glucose.	• Contraindicated in juvenile, growth-onset, and severe diabetes mellitus; diabetes mellitus adequately controlled by diet or in maturity-onset diabetes mellitus complicated by fever, ketosis, acidosis, or coma; major surgery; severe trauma; Raynaud's gangrene; renal or hepatic impairment; thyroid or other endocrine dysfunction. Use cautiously in sulfonamide hypersensitivity and in elderly, debilitated, or malnourished patients. • Tell patient about nature of disease; importance of following therapeutic regimen and specific diet, weight reduction, exercise, personal hygiene, avoiding infection; how and when to test for glycosuria and ketonuria; and recognition of hypoglycemia.

(continued on following page)

NAME	INDICATIONS & DOSAGE	SIDE EFFECTS
tolazamide *(continued)*	Maximum dose 500 mg b.i.d. **Elderly or debilitated patients:** increase dose by 50 to 125 mg at weekly intervals. *To change from insulin to oral therapy*—if insulin dose under 20 units daily, insulin may be stopped and oral therapy started at 100 mg P.O. daily with breakfast. If insulin dose is 20 to 40 units daily, insulin may be stopped and oral therapy started at 250 mg P.O. daily with breakfast. If insulin dose is over 40 units daily, decrease insulin dose 50% and start oral therapy at 250 mg P.O. daily with breakfast. Increase doses as above.	
tolbutamide Mellitol♦♦, Mobenol♦♦, Neo-Dibetic♦♦, Novobutamide♦♦, Oramide♦♦, Orinase♦, Tolbutone♦♦	*Stable, maturity-onset nonketotic diabetes mellitus uncontrolled by diet alone and previously untreated*— **Adults:** initially, 1 to 2 g P.O. daily as single dose or divided b.i.d. to t.i.d. May adjust dose to maximum 3 g daily. *To change from insulin to oral therapy*—if insulin dose is under 20 units daily, insulin may be stopped and oral therapy started at 1 to 2 g daily. If insulin dose is 20 to 40 units daily, insulin dose is reduced 30% to 50% and oral therapy started as above. If insulin dose is over 40 units daily, insulin dose is decreased 20% and oral therapy started as above. Further reductions in insulin dose are based on patient's response to oral therapy.	*Blood:* agranulocytosis, pancytopenia, aplastic anemia, leukopenia, thrombocytopenia, hemolytic anemia. *CNS:* headache. *GI:* epigastric fullness, nausea, heartburn. *Metabolic:* hypoglycemia. *Skin:* rash, pruritus, erythema. *Other:* hypersensitivity, reactions, cholestatic jaundice.

INTERACTIONS	NURSING CONSIDERATIONS
Allopurinol, anabolic steroids, clofibrate, guanethidine, halofenate, MAO inhibitors, phenylbutazone, salicylates, sulfonamides, oral anticoagulants: increased hypoglycemic activity. Monitor blood glucose. *Metoprolol, propranolol, clonidine:* prolonged hypoglycemic effect and masked symptoms of hypoglycemia. Use together cautiously.	• Be sure patient knows that therapy relieves symptoms but doesn't cure disease. • Patient transferring from another oral sulfonylurea antidiabetic drug usually needs no transition period. • Patient transferring from insulin therapy to an oral hypoglycemic should test urine for glucose and ketones at least t.i.d.; hospitalization may be required during the transition. • Oral contraceptives may alter diabetic control. Use another form of birth control. • Advise patient to avoid moderate to large intake of alcohol; antabuse reaction possible. • For symptoms and treatment of toxicity, see p. 1118.
Acetazolamide, adrenergic agents, alcohol, corticosteroids, glucagon, rifampin, thiazide diuretics, thyroxine: decreased hypoglycemic response. Monitor blood glucose. *Allopurinol, anabolic steroids, chloramphenicol, clofibrate, guanethidine, halofenate, MAO inhibitors, phenylbutazane, salicylates, sulfonamides, oral anticoagulants:* increased hypoglycemic activity. Monitor blood glucose. *Metoprolol, propranolol, clonidine:* prolonged hypoglycemic effect and masked symptoms of hypoglycemia. Use together cautiously.	• Contraindicated in juvenile, growth-onset, brittle, and severe diabetes; diabetes mellitus adequately controlled by diet or in maturity-onset diabetes mellitus complicated by fever, ketosis, acidosis, or coma; major surgery; severe trauma; Raynaud's gangrene; renal or hepatic impairment; thyroid or other endocrine dysfunction; or pregnancy. Use cautiously in sulfonamide hypersensitivity. • Tell patient about nature of disease; importance of following therapeutic regimen and specific diet, weight reduction, exercise, personal hygiene, and avoiding infection; how and when to test for glycosuria and ketonuria; and recognition of hypoglycemia. • Be sure patient knows that therapy relieves symptoms but doesn't cure disease. • Patient transferring from another oral sulfonylurea antidiabetic drug usually needs no transition period. • Patient transferring from insulin therapy to an oral hypoglycemic should test urine for glucose and ketones at least t.i.d.; hospitalization may be required during the transition. • Oral contraceptives may alter diabetic control. Use another form of birth control. • Advise patient to avoid moderate to large intake of alcohol: antabuse reaction possible. • For symptoms and treatment of toxicity, see p. 1118.

55

Thyroid hormones

levothyroxine sodium (T_4)
liothyronine sodium (T_3)
liotrix
thyroglobulin
thyroid USP (desiccated)
thyrotropin

Thyroid extract is the prototype of the substances used to treat hypothyroidism. This substance, the desiccated thyroid gland of animals, contains T_3 (liothyronine) and T_4 (tetraiodothyronine or thyroxine), as well as other organic materials. The cells of the thyroid gland produce these hormones from iodine in the serum by iodination of the amino acid tyrosine; the resulting hormones are stored in thyroglobulin. Synthetic salts of the pure thyroid hormones include sodium levothyroxine, sodium liothyronine, and a mixture of the two synthetic salts, liotrix. Because of their uniform potency, most doctors prefer to prescribe one of the synthetic salts.

Major uses

- Replacement therapy in treatment of primary and secondary myxedema, myxedemic coma, cretinism, and simple nontoxic goiter.
- Treatment of confirmed hypothyroidism.
- Prevention of goitrogenesis and hypothyroidism in patients receiving antithyroid drugs for thyrotoxicosis.
- Treatment of autonomous thyroid tumors and chronic thyroiditis.
- Differential diagnosis of subclinical hypothyroidism or low thyroid reserve.

Mechanism of action

Thyroid hormones affect the rate of metabolism, growth, and development via calorigenic and protein anabolic effects. They increase the rate of oxidation in the cells, thereby increasing energy expenditure and heat production. This, in turn, affects the metabolism of vitamins, proteins, carbohydrates, lipids, electrolytes, and water.

Absorption, distribution, and excretion

- Gastrointestinal absorption is satisfactory with sodium liothyronine, sodium levothyroxine, thyroglobulin, and thyroid extract.
- Levothyroxine is distributed to most body tissues, with higher concentration in the hepatic and kidneys.
- Thyroid hormones cross the placenta slowly.
- Levothyroxine conjugates with glucuronic acid and sulfuric acid in the hepatic and may be excreted in bile into the intestine, along with a small amount of free levothyroxine, which is then returned to the liver.

• Levothyroxine is excreted in the feces primarily unchanged; in the urine as inorganic iodide.

Onset and duration

• Onset of full effect of thyroid, thyroglobulin, and sodium levothyroxine takes 1 to 3 weeks. Their effect lasts for the same length of time.
• Onset of full effect of sodium liothyronine takes 1 to 3 days and lasts for up to 3 days.
• Mean half-life of levothyroxine is 6.5 days; mean half-life of liothyronine is less than 3 days.

Combination products

EUTHROID-½: sodium levothyroxine 30 mg and sodium liothyronine 7.5 mg.
EUTHROID-1: sodium levothyroxine 60 mg and sodium liothyronine 15 mg.
EUTHROID-2: sodium levothyroxine 120 mg and sodium liothyronine 30 mg.
EUTHROID-3: sodium levothyroxine 180 mg and sodium liothyronone 45 mg.
THYROLAR-¼: sodium levothyroxine 12.5 mg and sodium liothyronine 3.1 mg.
THYROLAR-½◆: sodium levothyroxine 25 mg and sodium liothyronine 6.25 mg.
THYROLAR-1◆: sodium levothyroxine 50 mg and sodium liothyronine 12.5 mg.
THYROLAR-2◆: sodium levothyroxine 100 mg and sodium liothyronine 25 mg.
THYROLAR-3◆: sodium levothyroxine 150 mg and sodium liothyronine 37.5 mg.

THYROTOXICOSIS ALERT

Hyperthyroid crisis or thyrotoxicosis is a life-threatening disorder that requires early recognition and immediate medical intervention.

SIGNS AND SYMPTOMS:

Hyperpyrexia — 100° F. (38° C.) to 106° F. (41° C.).
Cardiac arrhythmia — sinus tachycardia, atrial fibrillation
Gastrointestinal — nausea, vomiting, profuse diarrhea
CNS — nervousness, tremors, agitation
Palpable goiter
Unusually rapid speech
Elevated blood pressure — with wide pulse pressure; may suddenly fall to shock levels.

NAME	INDICATIONS & DOSAGE	SIDE EFFECTS
levothyroxine sodium (T_4) Cytolen, Eltroxin◆◆, Levoid, Levothroid, Noroxine, Ro-Thyroxine, Roxstan, Synthroid◆	*Cretinism in children younger than 1 year*— initially, 0.025 to 0.05 mg P.O. daily, increased by 0.025 to 0.05 mg P.O. q 2 to 3 weeks to total daily dose 0.1 to 0.3 mg P.O. *Myxedematous coma*— **Adults:** 0.2 to 0.5 mg I.V. If no response in 24 hours, additional 0.1 to 0.3 mg I.V. After condition stabilized, oral maintenance. *Thyroid hormone replacement*— **Adults:** initially, 0.025 mg to 0.1 mg P.O. daily, increased by 0.05 to 0.1 mg P.O. q 1 to 4 weeks until desired response. Maintenance dose 0.1 to 0.4 mg daily. **Children:** initially, maximum 0.05 mg P.O. daily, gradually increased by 0.025 to 0.05 mg P.O. q 1 to 4 weeks until desired response. Maintenance dose 0.3 to 0.4 mg daily.	*Side effects of thyroid hormones are extensions of their pharmacologic properties and reflect patient sensitivity to them.* *Signs of overdosage:* *CNS:* nervousness, insomnia, tremor. *CV:* tachycardia, palpitations, angina pectoris. *GI:* change in appetite, nausea, diarrhea. *Other:* headache, leg cramps, weight loss, sweating, heat intolerance, fever, menstrual irregularities.
liothyronine sodium (T_3) Cytomel◆, Ro-Thyronine	*Cretinism*— **Children 3 years and older:** 50 to 100 mcg P.O. daily. **Children under 3 years:** 5 mcg P.O. daily, increased by 5 mcg q 3 to 4 days until desired response. **Infants:** up to approximately 20 mcg P.O. daily. *Male infertility due to hypothyroidism*—initially, 5 mcg daily. Based on sperm count and motility, dose may be increased by 5 or 10 mcg q 2 to 4 weeks. Maintenance dose 25 mcg daily, not to exceed 50 mcg. *Myxedema*— **Adults:** initially 5 mcg daily, increased by 5 to 10 mcg q 1 or 2 weeks. Maintenance dose 50 to 100 mcg daily. *Nontoxic goiter*— **Adults:** initially, 5 mcg P.O. daily; may be increased by 5 to 10	*Side effects of thyroid hormones are extensions of their pharmacologic properties and reflect patient sensitivity to them.* *CNS:* hyperirritability, nervousness, insomnia, twitching, tremors, headache. *CV:* increased cardiac output, tachycardia, cardiac arrhythmias, angina pectoris, increased pulse rate and blood pressure, cardiac decompensation and collapse. *GI:* diarrhea, abdominal cramps, vomiting. *Other:* weight loss, heat intolerance, hyperhidrosis, menstrual irregularities; in infants and children—accelerated rate of bone maturation.

◆ Also available in Canada.
◆◆ Available in Canada only.
Unmarked trade names available in United States only.

INTERACTIONS	NURSING CONSIDERATIONS
Cholestyramine: levothyroxine absorption impaired. Separate doses by 4 to 5 hours. *I.V. phenytoin:* free thyroid released. Monitor for tachycardia.	• Contraindicated in myocardial infarctions, thyrotoxicosis (except with antithyroid drugs), or uncorrected adrenal insufficiency (thyroid hormones increase tissue demand for adrenocortical hormone and may cause acute adrenal crisis). Use with extreme caution in angina pectoris, hypertension, or other cardiovascular disorders; renal insufficiency; or ischemic states. • Use carefully in myxedema; patients unusually sensitive to thyroid hormone. • Rapid replacement in patients with arteriosclerosis may precipitate angina, coronary occlusion, or stroke. Use cautiously in such patients. • In patients with coronary artery disease who must receive thyroid, observe carefully for possible coronary insufficiency if catecholamines must be given. • Potentially dangerous; not indicated to relieve vague symptoms, such as physical and mental sluggishness, irritability, depression, nervousness, and ill-defined pains; to treat obesity in euthyroid persons; to treat metabolic insufficiency not associated with thyroid insufficiency; or to treat menstrual disorders or male infertility, unless associated with hypothyroidism. • When changing from levothyroxine to liothyronine, stop levothyroxine and begin liothyronine. Increase in small increments after residual effects of levothyroxine have disappeared. When changing from liothyronine to levothyroxine, start levothyroxine several days before withdrawing liothyronine to avoid relapse. • Warn patient to tell doctor at once if chest pain (especially in elderly), palpitations, sweating, nervousness, or other overdosage signs occur. Also notify doctor immediately if any signs of aggravated cardiovascular disease develop (chest pain, dyspnea, tachycardia). • Tell patient to take thyroid hormones regularly, at the same time each day, to maintain constant hormone levels. • Suggest morning dosage to prevent insomnia. • Monitor pulse rate and blood pressure. • Protect from moisture and light. Prepare I.V. dose immediately before injection.
Cholestyramine: liothyronine absorption impaired. Separate doses by 4 to 5 hours. *I.V. phenytoin:* free thyroid released. Monitor for tachycardia.	• Contraindicated in myocardial infarction, thyrotoxicosis (except with antithyroid drugs), or uncorrected adrenal insufficiency (thyroid hormones increase tissue demand for adrenocortical hormone and may cause acute adrenal crisis). Use with extreme caution in angina pectoris, hypertension, or other cardiovascular disorders; renal insufficiency; or ischemic states. • Rapid replacement in patients with arteriosclerosis may precipitate angina, coronary occlusion, or stroke. Use cautiously in such patients. • In patients with coronary artery disease who must receive thyroid, observe carefully for possible coronary insufficiency if catecholamines must be given. • Use carefully in myxedema; patients unusually sensitive to thyroid hormone. • Potentially dangerous; not indicated to relieve vague symptoms, such as physical and mental sluggishness, irritability, depression, nervousness, and ill-defined aches and pains; to treat obesity in euthyroid persons; to treat metabolic insufficiency; or to treat menstrual disorders or male infertility, unless associated with hypothyroidism. • When changing from levothyroxine to liothyronine, stop levothyroxine and begin liothyronine. Increase in small increments after residual effects of levothyroxine have disappeared. When changing from liothyronine to levothyroxine, start levothyroxine several days before withdrawing liothyronine to avoid relapse. • Warn patient to tell doctor at once if chest pain (especially in elderly), palpitations, sweating, nervousness, or other overdosage signs occur. Also

(continued on following page)

NAME	INDICATIONS & DOSAGE	SIDE EFFECTS
liothyronine sodium (T_3) *(continued)*	mcg daily q 1 to 2 weeks. Usual maintenance dose 75 mcg daily. **Elderly:** initially, 5 mcg P.O. daily, increased by 5 mcg increments at weekly intervals until desired response. **Children:** initially, 5 mcg P.O. daily, increased by 5 mcg increments at weekly intervals until desired response. *Thyroid hormone replacement—* **Adults:** initially, 25 mcg P.O. daily, increased by 12.5 to 25 mcg q 1 to 2 weeks until satisfactory response. Usual maintenance dose 25 to 75 mcg daily.	
liotrix Euthroid, Thyrolar◆	*Hypothyroidism*— dosages must be individualized to approximate the deficit in the patient's thyroid secretion. **Adults and children:** initially, 15 mg to 30 mg P.O. daily, increasing by 15 mg to 30 mg q 1 to 2 weeks to desired response; increments in children's dose q 2 weeks. **Elderly:** initially, 15 mg to 30 mg. Usual adult dose doubled q 6 to 8 weeks to desired response.	*Side effects of thyroid hormones are extensions of their pharmacologic properties and reflect patient sensitivity to them.* *CNS:* hyperirritability, nervousness, insomnia, twitching, tremors. *CV:* increased cardiac output, tachycardia, cardiac arrhythmia, angina pectoris, increased pulse rate and blood pressure, cardiac decompensation and collapse. *GI:* diarrhea, abdominal cramps, vomiting. *Other:* weight loss, menstrual irregularities, heat intolerance, hyperhidrosis; infants and children— accelerated rate of bone maturation.
thyroglobulin Proloid◆	*Cretinism and juvenile hypothyroidism—* **Children 1 year and older:** dosage may approach adult dose (60 to 180 mg P.O. daily), depending on response. **Children 4 to 12 months:** 60 to 80 mg P.O. daily.	*Side effects of thyroid hormones are extensions of their pharmacologic properties and reflect patient sensitivity to them.* *CNS:* hyperirritability, nervousness, insomnia, twitching, tremors, headache. *CV:* increased cardiac output, tachy-

INTERACTIONS	NURSING CONSIDERATIONS
	notify doctor immediately if any signs of aggravated cardiovascular disease develop (chest pain, dyspnea, tachycardia). • Tell patient to take thyroid hormones regularly, at the same time each day, to maintain constant hormone levels. • Suggest morning dosage to prevent insomnia. • Monitor pulse rate and blood pressure.
Cholestyramine: liotrix absorption impaired. Separate doses by 4 to 5 hours. *I.V. phenytoin:* free thyroid released. Monitor for tachycardia.	• Contraindicated in myocardial infarction, thyrotoxicosis (except with antithyroid drugs), or uncorrected adrenal insufficiency (thyroid hormones increase tissue demand for adrenocortical hormone and may cause acute adrenal crisis). Use with extreme caution in angina pectoris, hypertension, or other cardiovascular disorders; renal insufficiency; or ischemic states. • Rapid replacement in patients with arteriosclerosis may precipitate angina, coronary occlusion, or stroke. Use cautiously in such patients. • Use carefully in myxedema; patients are unusually sensitive to thyroid hormone. • In patients with coronary artery disease who must receive thyroid, observe carefully for possible coronary insufficiency if catecholamines must be given. Also observe carefully during surgery, since cardiac arrhythmias can be precipitated. • Potentially dangerous; not indicated to relieve vague symptoms, such as physical and mental sluggishness, irritability, depression, nervousness, and ill-defined pains; to treat obesity in euthyroid persons; to treat metabolic insufficiency not associated with thyroid insufficiency; or to treat menstrual disorders or male infertility, unless associated with hypothyroidism. • Tell patient to take thyroid hormones regularly, at the same time each day, preferably before breakfast, to maintain constant hormone levels. • Warn patient to tell doctor at once if chest pain (especially in elderly), palpitations, sweating, nervousness, or other overdosage signs occur. Also notify doctor immediately if any signs of aggravated cardiovascular disease develop (chest pain, dyspnea, tachycardia). • The two commercially prepared liotrix drugs contain different amounts of each ingredient; do not change from one brand to the other without considering the differences in potency: Thyrolar-½ contains 25 mcg T_4 and 6.25 mcg T_3; Euthroid-½ contains 30 mcg T_4 and 7.5 mcg T_3. • Monitor pulse rate and blood pressure. • Protect from heat, light, and moisture.
Cholestyramine: thyroglobulin absorption impaired. Separate doses by 4 to 5 hours. *I.V. phenytoin:* free thyroid released. Monitor for tachycardia.	• Contraindicated in myocardial infarction, thyrotoxicosis (except with antithyroid drugs), or uncorrected adrenal insufficiency (thyroid hormones increase tissue demand for adrenocortical hormone and may cause acute adrenal crisis). Use with extreme caution in angina pectoris, hypertension, or other cardiovascular disorders; renal insufficiency; or ischemic states. • In patients with coronary artery disease who must receive thyroid, observe carefully for possible coronary insufficiency if catecholamines must be given.

(continued on following page)

NAME	INDICATIONS & DOSAGE	SIDE EFFECTS
(continued)	**Children 1 to 4 months:** initially, 15 to 30 mg P.O. daily, increased at 2-week intervals. Usual maintenance dose 30 to 45 mg P.O. daily. *Hypothyroidism or myxedema*— **Adults:** initially, 15 to 30 mg P.O. daily, increased by 15 to 30 mg at 2-week intervals until desired response. Usual maintenance dose 60 to 180 mg P.O. daily, as a single dose. **Elderly:** initially 7.5 to 15 mg P.O. daily; the dose is doubled at 6- to 8-week intervals until desired response is obtained.	cardia, cardiac arrhythmias, angina pectoris, increased pulse rate and blood pressure, cardiac decompensation and collapse. *GI:* diarrhea, abdominal cramps, vomiting. *Other:* weight loss, heat intolerance, hyperhidrosis, menstrual irregularities; in infants and children—accelerated rate of bone maturation.
thyroid USP (desiccated) Dathroid, Delcoid, S-P-T, Thyrar, Thyrocrine, Thyro-Teric	*Adult hypothyroidism or myxedema*— **Adults:** initially, 60 mg P.O. daily, increased by 60 mg q 30 days until desired response. Usual maintenance dose 60 to 180 mg P.O. daily, as a single dose. **Elderly:** 7.5 to 15 mg P.O. daily; the dose is doubled at 6- to 8-week intervals. *Cretinism and juvenile hypothyroidism*— **Children 1 year and older:** dosage may approach adult dose (60 to 180 mg) daily, depending on response. **Children 4 to 12 months:** 30 to 60 mg P.O. daily. **Children 1 to 4 months:** initially, 15 to 30 mg P.O. daily, increased at 2-week intervals. Usual maintenance dose 30 to 45 mg P.O. daily. *Suppressive therapy*— **Adults:** 120 to 180 mg P.O. daily; initial dose should not exceed 60 mg, increased as indicated by response.	*Side effects of thyroid hormones are extensions of their pharmacologic properties and reflect patient sensitivity to them.* *CNS:* hyperirritability, nervousness, insomnia, twitching, tremors, headache. *CV:* increased cardiac output, tachycardia, cardiac arrhythmias, angina pectoris, increased pulse rate and blood pressure, cardiac decompensation and collapse. *GI:* diarrhea, abdominal cramps, vomiting. *Other:* weight loss, heat intolerance, hyperhidrosis, menstrual irregularities; in infants and children—accelerated rate of bone maturation.

INTERACTIONS	NURSING CONSIDERATIONS
	• Use carefully in myxedema; patients unusually sensitive to thyroid hormone. • Potentially dangerous; not indicated to relieve vague symptoms, such as physical and mental sluggishness, irritability, depression, nervousness, and ill-defined pains; to treat obesity in euthyroid persons; to treat metabolic insufficiency not associated with thyroid insufficiency; or to treat menstrual disorders or male infertility, unless associated with hypothyroidism. • Tell patient to take thyroid hormones regularly, at the same time each day, to maintain constant hormone levels. • Warn patient to tell doctor at once if chest pain (especially in elderly), palpitations, sweating, nervousness, or other signs of overdosage occur. Also notify doctor immediately if any signs of aggravated cardiovascular disease develop (chest pain, dyspnea, tachycardia). • Suggest morning dosage to prevent insomnia. • Monitor pulse rate and blood pressure. • Will alter thyroid function studies.
Cholestyramine: thyroid absorption impaired. Separate doses by 4 to 5 hours. *I.V. phenytoin:* free thyroid released. Monitor for tachycardia.	• Contraindicated in myocardial infarction, thyrotoxicosis (except with antithyroid drugs), or uncorrected adrenal insufficiency (thyroid hormones increase tissue demand for adrenocortical hormone and may cause acute adrenal crisis). Use with extreme caution in angina pectoris, hypertension, or other cardiovascular disorders; renal insufficiency; or ischemic states. • In patients with coronary artery disease who must receive thyroid, observe carefully for possible coronary insufficiency if catecholamines must be given. • Potentially dangerous; not indicated to relieve vague symptoms, such as physical and mental sluggishness, irritability, depression, nervousness, and ill-defined pains; to treat obesity in euthyroid persons; to treat metabolic insufficiency not associated with thyroid insufficiency; or to treat menstrual disorders or male infertility, unless associated with hypothyroidism. • Tell patient to take thyroid hormones regularly, at the same time each day, to maintain constant hormone levels. • Warn patient to tell doctor at once if chest pain (especially in elderly), palpitations, sweating, nervousness, or other signs of overdosage occur. Also notify doctor immediately if any signs of aggravated cardiovascular disease develop (chest pain, dyspnea, tachycardia). • Suggest morning dosage to prevent insomnia. • Monitor pulse rate and blood pressure. • In children, the sleeping pulse and basal morning temperature are guides to treatment. • Will alter thyroid function tests.

NAME	INDICATIONS & DOSAGE	SIDE EFFECTS
thyrotropin Thyrotron♦♦, Thytropar♦	*Diagnosis of thyroid cancer remnant with ^{131}I after surgery*—10 international units I.M. or S.C. for 3 to 7 days. *Differential diagnosis of primary and secondary hypothyroidism*—10 units I.M. or S.C. for 1 to 3 days. *In PBI or ^{131}I uptake determinations for differential diagnosis of subclinical hypothyroidism or low thyroid reserve*—10 units I.M. or S.C. *Therapy of thyroid carcinoma (local or metastatic) with ^{131}I*—10 units I.M. or S.C. for 3 to 8 days. *To determine thyroid status of patient receiving thyroid*—10 units I.M. or S.C. for 1 to 3 days.	*CNS:* headache. *CV:* tachycardia, auricular fibrillation, angina pectoris, congestive failure, hypotension. *GI:* nausea, vomiting. *Other:* thyroid hyperplasia (large doses), fever, menstrual irregularities, allergic reactions (postinjection flare, urticaria, anaphylaxis, transitory hypotension).

INTERACTIONS	NURSING CONSIDERATIONS
None significant.	• Contraindicated in coronary thrombosis, untreated Addison's disease. Use cautiously in angina pectoris, cardiac failure, hypopituitarism, adrenocortical suppression. • Purified thyrotropic hormone (TSH) is isolated from bovine anterior pituitary. It stimulates the formation and secretion of thyroid hormone and increases thyroidal uptake of iodine: May cause thyroid hyperplasia. • Diagnostic use: to identify subclinical hypothyroidism or low thyroid reserve, to evaluate need for thyroid therapy, to distinguish between primary and secondary hypothyroidism, and to detect thyroid remnants and metastases of thyroid carcinoma. • Therapeutic use: management of certain types of thyroid carcinoma and resulting metastases, and in conjunction with radioactive ^{131}I to enhance the uptake of ^{131}I by the thyroid. • 3-day dosage schedule may be used in long-standing pituitary myxedema or with prolonged use of thyroid medication. • Will alter thyroid function studies. • For treatment of anaphylaxis, see p. 1114.

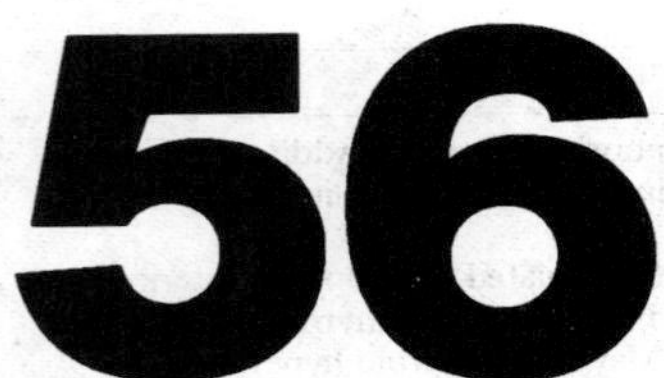

Thyroid hormone antagonists

iodine
radioactive iodine ^{131}I
methimazole
methylthiouracil
propylthiouracil

Antithyroid drugs, mainly iodine and thionamide derivatives (methimazole, methylthiouracil, and propylthiouracil), suppress excessive thyroid hormone production. Radioiodine ^{131}I is used in selective cases.

Major uses

- To treat hyperthyroidism in Graves' disease, multinodular goiter, and thyroiditis.
- To prepare patients for surgery or to treat thyrotoxic crisis.
- The thionamides precede or follow treatment with radioactive iodine.
- Iodine is used to treat potentially fatal thyrotoxic crisis in adults and neonates and preoperatively to decrease vascularity of the thyroid gland.
- Radioactive iodine is used when surgery is contraindicated.

Mechanism of action

- Thionamides block the organic binding of iodide into thyroglobulin to form thyroid hormone; they do not affect thyroid hormone that has been previously formed and stored.
- Iodine inhibits the formation of thyroid hormone by blocking iodothyrosine and iodothyronine synthesis; and also limits iodide transport into the thyroid gland.
- Iodine blocks the release of thyroid hormone.
- Radioactive iodine limits thyroid hormone secretion by damaging and destroying thyroid tissue.

Absorption, distribution, and excretion

- All the thionamides are readily absorbed from the gastrointestinal tract.
- Propylthiouracil and methylthiouracil are rapidly metabolized.
- Approximately 35% of propylthiouracil is excreted unchanged in the urine within 24 hours; approximately 40% of methylthiouracil is excreted in the urine within 24 hours.

Onset and duration

- Onset of response to thionamides may take days or weeks because effect doesn't become apparent until stored supply of thyroid hormone is consumed.
- Severe cases respond most rapidly, usually in 1 to 2 days.
- Thionamides do not permanently affect the thyroid gland but control hormone production until spontaneous remission occurs during the course of the disease.

- The half-life of propylthiouracil is 1 to 1.6 hours; of methimazole, 6 to 9 hours.
- Onset of radioiodine therapy may take months.

Combination products
None.

PATIENT TEACHING AID — POSTOPERATIVE THYROIDECTOMY MANAGEMENT

Dear Patient:

After your thyroidectomy, to prevent strain on your neck muscles when raising yourself to a sitting position, support your head with a pillow and put your hands together behind your head (as illustrated).

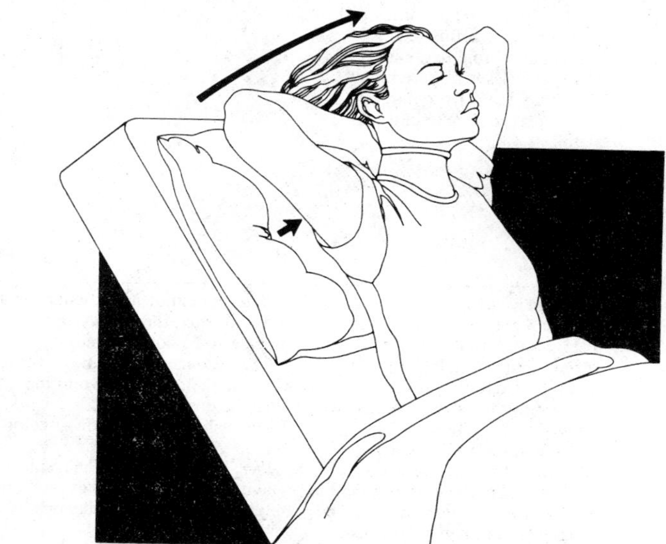

NAME	INDICATIONS & DOSAGE	SIDE EFFECTS
iodine Potassium Iodide Solution, U.S.P.; Sodium Iodide, U.S.P.; Strong Iodine Solution, U.S.P. (Lugol's Solution), containing 5% iodine and 10% potassium iodide	*Preparation for thyroidectomy*— **Adults and children:** Strong Iodine Solution, U.S.P., 0.1 to 0.3 ml t.i.d., or Potassium Iodide Solution, U.S.P., 5 drops in water t.i.d. after meals for 2 to 3 weeks before surgery. *Thyroid crises*— **Adults and children:** Strong Iodine Solution, U.S.P., 1 ml in water P.O. t.i.d. after meals in refractory cases; Sodium Iodide, U.S.P., 250 to 500 mg (or up to 2 g) daily, by slow I.V. infusion with antithyroid drugs and propranolol.	*EENT:* acute rhinitis, inflammation of salivary glands, periorbital edema, conjunctivitis, hyperemia. *GI:* burning, irritation, nausea, vomiting, metallic taste. *Skin:* acneiform rash, mucous membrane ulceration. *Other:* fever, frontal headache; with I.V. use (sodium iodide): acute iodism, colloidoclastic shock, pulmonary edema.
radioactive iodine **^{131}I**	*Hyperthyroidism*— **Adults:** usual dose is 5 to 15 millicuries P.O. Dose based on estimated weight of thyroid gland and thyroid uptake. Treatment may be repeated after 6 weeks, according to serum thyroxine levels. *Thyroid cancer*— **Adults:** 50 to 150 millicuries P.O. Dose based on estimated malignant thyroid tissue and metastatic tissue as determined by total body scan. Dose may be repeated according to clinical status.	*EENT:* radiation thyroiditis. *Endocrine:* hypothyroidism, exacerbation of symptoms of hyperthyroidism.
methimazole Tapazole	*Hyperthyroidism*— **Adults:** 5 mg P.O. t.i.d. if mild; 10 to 15 mg P.O. t.i.d. if moderately severe; and 20 mg P.O. t.i.d. if severe. Continue until patient euthyroid, then start maintenance dose of 5 mg daily to t.i.d. Maximum dose 150 mg daily. **Children:** 0.4 mg/Kg/day divided q 8 hours. Continue until patient euthyroid, then start maintenance dose of 0.2 mg/Kg/day divided q 8 hours. *Preparation for thyroidectomy*— **Adults and children:** same doses as for hyperthyroidism until patient is euthyroid; then iodine is added for 10 days before surgery.	*Blood:* agranulocytosis, leukopenia, granulopenia, thrombocytopenia (appear to be dose-related). *CNS:* headache, drowsiness, vertigo. *GI:* diarrhea, nausea, vomiting (may be dose-related). *Skin:* rash, urticaria, skin discoloration. *Other:* arthralgias, myalgia, salivary gland enlargement, loss of taste, drug fever, jaundice, lymphadenopathy.

♦ Also available in Canada.
♦♦ Available in Canada only.
Unmarked trade names available in United States only.

INTERACTIONS	NURSING CONSIDERATIONS
Lithium carbonate: hypothyroidism may occur. Use with caution.	• Contraindicated in tuberculosis, iodide hypersensitivity, hyperkalemia, after meals that contain excessive starch; in laryngeal edema, swelling of salivary glands. • Generally use I.V. route only if patient is vomiting or cannot receive anything by mouth. Some prefer I.V. route to prevent GI side effects, especially during critical time at beginning of treatment. • Dilute oral doses in milk to prevent gastric irritation, to hydrate the patient, and to mask the very salty taste. • Tell patient to ask doctor about using iodized salt or eating shellfish during treatment. • Warn patient that sudden withdrawal may precipitate thyroid storm. • Store in light-resistant container. • Give iodides through straw to avoid tooth discoloration. • Usually given with other antithyroid drugs.
Lithium carbonate: hypothyroidism may occur. Use with caution.	• Contraindicated in pregnancy and lactation unless used to treat thyroid cancer. • Stop all antithyroid medications, thyroid preparations, and iodine-containing preparations 1 week before ^{131}I dose. If medications are not stopped, patient may receive thyroid-stimulating hormone for 3 days prior to ^{131}I. When treating women of childbearing age, give dose during menstruation or within 7 days after menstruation. • Treatment for hyperthyroidism may be done as outpatient. • Patient must be hospitalized for thyroid cancer treatment. • After therapy for hyperthyroidism, do not resume antithyroid drugs. However, patient should continue propranolol or other drugs used to treat symptoms of hyperthyroidism until full effect of ^{131}I seen (usually 6 weeks). • Monitor thyroid function with serum thyroxine levels. • After dose for hyperthyroidism, tell patient to use good toilet habits and to avoid coughing or expectorating because urine and saliva are slightly radioactive for 24 hours. • After dose for thyroid cancer, patient's urine and saliva remain radioactive for 3 days. Isolate patient and observe following precautions: pregnant personnel should not take care of patient; use disposable eating utensils and linens; stress good bathroom habits (urine may be flushed down toilet). Limit contact with patient to 30 minutes per shift per person the first day. May increase time to 1 hour second day and longer on third day.
None significant.	• Contraindicated in nursing mothers; passes placental barrier and appears in human milk. Use cautiously in pregnancy. Pregnant women may require less drug as pregnancy progresses. Monitor thyroid function studies closely. Thyroid may be added to regimen. Drugs may be stopped during last few weeks of pregnancy. • Watch for signs of hypothyroidism (mental depression, cold intolerance, hard nonpitting edema). Dose may need to be adjusted. • Monitor CBC periodically to detect impending leukopenia, thrombocytopenia, and agranulocytosis. • Warn patient to report immediately fever, sore throat, or mouth sores (possible signs of developing agranulocytosis). Agranulocytosis can develop too rapidly to be detected by periodic blood cell counts. Tell him also to report immediately any skin eruptions (sign of hypersensitivity). • Drug should be stopped if severe rash or enlarged cervical lymph nodes occur. • Tell patient to ask doctor about using iodized salt or eating shellfish during treatment. • Warn against over-the-counter cough medicines; many contain iodine.

(continued on following page)

NAME	INDICATIONS & DOSAGE	SIDE EFFECTS
methimazole *(continued)*	*Thyrotoxic crisis—* **Adults and children:** same doses as for hyperthyroidism with concomitant iodine therapy and propranolol.	
methylthiouracil Methiocil	*Hyperthyroidism (in patients refractory to or intolerant of other antithyroid drugs)—* **Adults:** 50 mg P.O. q.i.d. Dosage should generally not exceed 300 mg daily. Maintenance dose is based on basal metabolic rate, usually after 2 months of therapy if symptoms controlled.	*Blood:* agranulocytosis, leukopenia, thrombocytopenia (appear to be dose-related). *CNS:* headache, drowsiness, vertigo. *EENT:* visual disturbances. *GI:* nausea, diarrhea, vomiting (may be dose-related). *Skin:* rash, urticaria, pruritus. *Other:* drug fever, arthralgias, myalgias, salivary gland enlargements, jaundice, lymphadenopathy.
propylthiouracil (PTU) Propacil, Propyl-Thyracil♦♦	*Hyperthyroidism—* **Adults:** 100 mg P.O. t.i.d. up to 300 mg q 8 hours has been used in severe cases. Continue until patient euthyroid, then start maintenance dose of 50 mg daily to t.i.d. **Children over 10 years:** 100 mg P.O. t.i.d. Continue until patient euthyroid, then start maintenance dose of 25 mg t.i.d. to 100 mg b.i.d. **Children 6 to 10 years:** 50 to 150 mg P.O. divided doses q 8 hours. *Preparation for thyroidectomy—* **Adults and children:** same doses as for hyperthyroidism, with iodine added 10 days before surgery. *Thyrotoxic crisis—* **Adults and children:** same doses as for hyperthyroidism, with concomitant iodine therapy and propranolol.	*Blood:* agranulocytosis, leukopenia, thrombocytopenia (appear to be dose-related). *CNS:* headache, drowsiness, vertigo. *EENT:* visual disturbances. *GI:* diarrhea, nausea, vomiting (may be dose-related). *Skin:* rash, urticaria, skin discoloration, pruritus. *Other:* arthralgias, myalgias, salivary gland enlargements, loss of taste, drug fever, lymphadenopathy, jaundice.

INTERACTIONS	NURSING CONSIDERATIONS
	• Check prothrombin time before surgery. Rare cases of hypoprothrombinemia have been reported. • Give with meals to reduce GI side effects. • Teach patient and family to take pulse and to report tachycardia. Tell patient to weigh himself twice a week and to report sudden weight gain. • Store in light-resistant container.
None significant.	• Contraindicated in nursing mothers; passes placental barrier and appears in human milk. Use cautiously in pregnancy. Pregnant women may require less drug as pregnancy progresses. Monitor thyroid function studies closely. Thyroid may be added to regimen. Drugs may be stopped during last few weeks of pregnancy. • Watch for signs of hypothyroidism (mental depression, cold intolerance, hard nonpitting edema). Dose may need to be adjusted. • Monitor CBC periodically to detect impending leukopenia, thrombocytopenia, and agranulocytosis. • Warn patient to report immediately fever, sore throat, or mouth sores (possible signs of developing agranulocytosis). Agranulocytosis can develop too rapidly to be detected by periodic blood cell counts. Tell him also to report immediately any skin eruptions (sign of hypersensitivity). • Drug should be stopped if severe rash or enlarged cervical lymph nodes occur. • Tell patient to ask doctor about using iodized salt or eating shellfish during treatment. • Warn against over-the-counter cough medicines; many contain iodine. • Check prothrombin time before surgery. Rare cases of hypoprothrombinemia have been reported. • Give with meals to reduce GI side effects. • Teach patient and family to take pulse and to report tachycardia. Tell patient to weigh himself twice a week and to report sudden weight gain. • Store in light-resistant container.
None significant.	• Contraindicated in nursing mothers; passes placental barrier and appears in human milk. Use cautiously in pregnancy. Pregnant women may require less drug as pregnancy progresses. Monitor thyroid function studies closely. Thyroid may be added to regimen. Drugs may be stopped during last few weeks of pregnancy. • Watch for signs of hypothyroidism (mental depression, cold intolerance, hard nonpitting edema). Dose may need to be adjusted. • Monitor CBC periodically to detect impending leukopenia, thrombocytopenia, and agranulocytosis. • Warn patient to report immediately fever, sore throat, or mouth sores (possible signs of developing agranulocytosis). Agranulocytosis can develop too rapidly to be detected by periodic blood cell counts. Tell him also to report immediately any skin eruptions (sign of hypersensitivity). • Drug should be stopped if severe rash or enlarged cervical lymph nodes occur. • Tell patient to ask doctor about using iodized salt or eating shellfish during treatment. • Warn against over-the-counter cough medicines; many contain iodine. • Check prothrombin time before surgery. Rare cases of hypoprothrombinemia have been reported. • Give with meals to reduce GI side effects. • Teach patient and family to take pulse and to report tachycardia. Tell patient to weigh himself twice a week and to report sudden weight gain. • Store in light-resistant container.

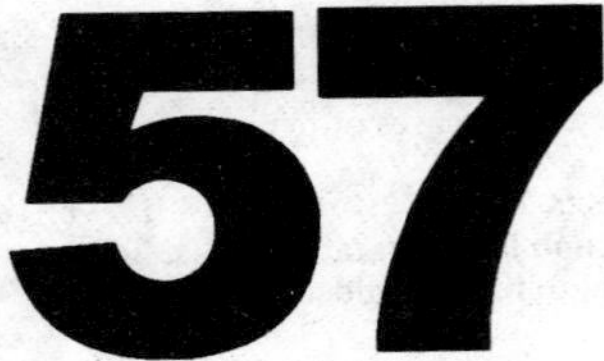

Pituitary hormones

corticotropin
cosyntropin
desmopressin
lypressin
somatropin
vasopressin
vasopressin tannate

The anterior and posterior pituitary glands secrete many different hormones. Those used in therapy are either natural extracts or synthetic derivatives. All have a variety of clinical uses and are specifically formulated for inpatient and outpatient use.

Major uses

- As a diagnostic agent in determining the source of adrenocortical insufficiency (corticotropin, cosyntropin).
- Treatment of growth impairment due to growth hormone deficiency (somatropin).
- Treatment of symptoms of neurohypophyseal or central diabetes insipidus (vasopressin, lypressin, desmopressin).

Mechanism of action

- Stimulate an increase in cyclic AMP and water permeability by acting on the renal tubular epithelium, where it promotes the reabsorption of water and produces a concentrated urine. This is an antidiuretic hormone (ADH) effect (vasopressin, lypressin, desmopressin).
- Contract smooth muscle in the vascular bed, a vasopressor effect (vasopressin, lypressin).
- Stimulate linear growth in patients with pituitary growth deficiency by a number of mechanisms, including intracellular transport of amino acids; increasing intestinal absorption and urinary excretion of calcium; increasing renal tubular absorption of phosphorus and decreasing calcium; increasing synthesis of collagen and chondroitin, which form cartilage; and by other metabolic effects such as inhibition of intracellular glucose metabolism (somatropin).
- Cause contraction of smooth muscles of the gastrointestinal tract, and on all parts of the vascular bed.

Absorption, distribution, and excretion

• Vasopressin is inactivated by the enzyme trypsin in the GI tract and must be administered intramuscularly, subcutaneously, or intranasally. I.V. administration is minimal unless by constant infusion due to rapid inactivation. Vasopressin is distributed throughout the extracellular fluid; metabolized in the liver and kidneys; and excreted in the urine.

• Lypressin and desmopressin are inactivated in the GI tract by the enzyme trypsin and are usually given intranasally. Absorption is adequate through the nasal mucosa but is decreased in the presence of nasal congestion, rhinitis, or upper respiratory infections. Both drugs are distributed unchanged to the extracellular fluid and are metabolized in the liver and the kidneys. They are excreted in the urine.

• Somatropin is destroyed in the GI tract after oral administration. After intramuscular administration, it is distributed well into plasma. It is metabolized by the liver and excreted in the urine.

• Corticotropin is destroyed in the GI tract after oral administration. It is readily absorbed parenterally, rapidly distributed, and inactivated in the tissues before being excreted in the urine.

Onset and duration

• Following S.C. or I.M. administration of aqueous vasopressin, the duration of antidiuretic activity is maintained for 2 to 8 hours.

• Vasopressin tannate in oil is absorbed more slowly and has a longer duration of action, about 48 to 96 hours after injection.

• Following intranasal administration, ADH effects of vasopressin last for 6 to 12 hours.

• Lypressin intranasally has an onset of 1 hour and a duration of 3 to 8 hours.

• Desmopressin has an onset similar to lypressin, with a duration that is longer to allow for once-daily doses in some patients.

• Somatropin has an almost immediate onset and peak, and a duration of several days.

Combination products

None.

NAME	INDICATIONS & DOSAGE	SIDE EFFECTS
corticotropin (ACTH) ACTH-Actest, Acthar◆, Acton "X"◆◆, Cortigel-80, Cortrophin Gel, Cortrophin Zinc, Duracton◆◆, H.P. Acthar Gel	*Diagnostic test of adrenocortical function—* **Adults:** up to 80 units I.M. or S.C. in divided doses; or a single dose of repository form; or 10 to 25 units (aqueous form) in 500 ml dextrose 5% in water I.V. over 8 hours, between blood samplings. Individual dosages generally vary with adrenal glands' sensitivity to stimulation as well as with specific disease. Infants and younger children require larger doses per kilogram than do older children and adults. *Therapeutic dose—* 10 units I.M. q 6 hours (aqueous); 40 units q 12 to 24 hours (repository), or 10 units S.C. of aqueous q 6 hours; 40 units of gel q 24 to 72 hours. *Average dose—*20 units I.M. or S.C. q.i.d. Start with low dose, gradually increasing until clinical effect is noted, to maximum of 25 units q.i.d.	*CNS:* convulsions, dizziness, increased intracranial pressure, papilledema, headache, euphoria, insomnia, mood swings, personality changes, depression, psychosis. *CV:* hypertension, inflammation of arteries, congestive heart failure. *EENT:* bulging eyes, cataracts, glaucoma. *GI:* peptic ulcer with perforation and hemorrhage, pancreatitis, abdominal distention, ulcerative esophagitis, nausea, vomiting. *GU:* menstrual irregularities. *Metabolic:* sodium and fluid retention, calcium and potassium loss, hypokalemic alkalosis, negative nitrogen balance. *Skin:* impaired wound healing, thin fragile skin, petechiae, ecchymoses, facial erythema, increased sweating, acne, hyperpigmentation, allergic skin reactions, hirsutism. *Other:* muscle weakness, steroid myopathy, loss of muscle mass, osteoporosis, vertebral compression fractures, aseptic necrosis of femoral and humeral heads, fracture of long bones, cushingoid state, suppression of growth in children, activation of latent diabetes mellitus, abscess, progressive increase in antibodies and loss of ACTH stimulatory effect.
cosyntropin Cortrosyn◆, Synacthen Depot◆◆	*Diagnostic test of adrenocortical function—* **Adults and children:** 0.25 to 1 mg I.M. or I.V. (unless label prohibits I.V. administration) between blood samplings. **Children younger than 2 years:** 0.125 mg I.M. or I.V.	*Skin:* pruritus (rare). *Other:* flushing (rare).
desmopressin DDAVP	*Nonnephrogenic diabetes insipidus, temporary polyuria and polydipsia associated with pituitary trauma—* **Adults:** 0.1 to 0.4 ml intranasally daily in 1 to 3 doses. Adjust morning and evening doses separately for adequate diurnal rhythm of water turnover. **Children 3 months to 12 years:** 0.05 to 0.3 ml intranasally daily in 1 or 2 doses.	*CNS:* headache. *CV:* slight rise in blood pressure at high dosage. *EENT:* nasal congestion, rhinitis. *GI:* abdominal cramps, nausea. *GU:* vulval pain. *Other:* flushing.

◆ Also available in Canada.
◆◆ Available in Canada only.
Unmarked trade names available in United States only.

INTERACTIONS	NURSING CONSIDERATIONS
None significant.	• Contraindicated in scleroderma, osteoporosis, systemic fungal infections, ocular herpes simplex, recent surgery, peptic ulcer, congestive heart failure, hypertension, sensitivity to pork and pork products, concomitant smallpox vaccination, adrenocortical hyperfunction or primary insufficiency, or Cushing's syndrome. Use with caution in pregnant women or nursing mothers and in women of childbearing age; patients being immunized; latent tuberculosis or tuberculin reactivity; hypothyroidism, cirrhosis, infection (use anti-infective therapy during and after ACTH treatment); acute gouty arthritis (limit ACTH treatment to a few days and use conventional therapy during and for several days after ACTH treatment); emotional instability or psychotic tendencies; diabetes, abscess, pyogenic infections, renal insufficiency, myasthenia gravis. • ACTH treatment should be preceded by verification of adrenal responsiveness and test for hypersensitivity and allergic reactions. • ACTH should be adjunctive; not sole therapy. • Unusual stress may require additional use of rapidly acting corticosteroids. Reduce ACTH dosage gradually when reduction is possible to minimize induced adrenocortical insufficiency. Reinstitute therapy if stressful situation occurs shortly after stopping drug. • Watch neonates of ACTH-treated mothers for signs of hypoadrenalism. Carefully check growth and development of children on long-term ACTH therapy. • Counteract edema by low-sodium, high-potassium intake; nitrogen loss by high-protein diet; and psychotic changes by reducing ACTH dosage or administering sedatives. • ACTH may mask signs of chronic disease and decrease host resistance and ability to localize infection. • Note and record weight changes, fluid exchange, and resting blood pressures until minimal effective dose is achieved. • Refrigerate reconstituted solution and use within 24 hours.
None significant.	• Use cautiously in hypersensitivity to natural corticotropin. • Drug is synthetic duplication of the biologically active part of the ACTH molecule. It is less likely to produce sensitivity than natural ACTH from animal sources.
None significant.	• Use with caution in patients with coronary artery insufficiency or hypertensive cardiovascular disease. • Adjust fluid intake to reduce risk of water intoxication and sodium depletion, especially in very young or old patients. • Titrate dosage to allow patient sufficient sleep. • Give intranasally only. • Overdose may cause oxytocic or vasopressor activity. Withhold drug until effects subside. Furosemide may be used if fluid retention is excessive. • Not effective in nephrogenic diabetes insipidus. • Drug of choice for central (neurogenic) diabetes insipidus.

NAME	INDICATIONS & DOSAGE	SIDE EFFECTS
lypressin Diapid	*Nonnephrogenic diabetes insipidus; control or prevention of polydipsia, polyuria, and dehydration—* **Adults and children:** 1 or 2 sprays (approximately 2 USP posterior pituitary pressor units per spray) in either or both nostrils q.i.d. and an additional dose at bedtime, if needed, to prevent nocturia. If usual dosage is inadequate, increase frequency rather than number of sprays.	*CNS:* headache, dizziness. *CV:* coronary artery constriction due to large doses. *EENT:* nasal congestion or ulceration, irritation, pruritus of nasal passages, rhinorrhea, conjunctivitis. *GI:* heartburn due to drip of excess spray into pharynx, abdominal cramps, more frequent bowel movements. *GU:* possible transient fluid retention due to overdose. *Skin:* hypersensitivity reaction.
somatropin Asellacrin	*Growth failure due to pituitary growth hormone deficiency—* **Children:** 2 I.U. (1 ml) I.M. 3 times weekly, with a minimum of 48 hours between injections. Double dose if growth doesn't exceed 1 inch in 6 months, or recheck diagnosis. Discontinue when epiphyses close, patient achieves satisfactory adult height, or patient fails to respond.	*GU:* excess calcium in urine. *Metabolic:* hyperglycemia.
vasopressin Pitressin◆ **vasopressin tannate** Pitressin Tannate	*Nonnephrogenic, nonpsychogenic diabetes insipidus—* **Adults:** 5 to 10 units I.M. or S.C. b.i.d. to q.i.d., p.r.n.; or intranasally (spray or cotton balls) in individualized doses, based on response. For chronic therapy, inject 2.5 to 5 units Pitressin Tannate in oil suspension I.M. every 2 to 3 days. **Children:** 2.5 to 10 units I.M. or S.C. b.i.d. to q.i.d., p.r.n.; or intranasally (spray or cotton balls) in individualized doses. For chronic therapy, inject 1.25 to 2.5 units Pitressin Tannate in oil suspension I.M. every 2 to 3 days. *Postop abdominal distention—* **Adults:** 5 units I.M. initially, then q 3 to 4 hours, increasing dose to 10 units, if needed. Reduce dose for children proportionately. *To expel gas before abdominal X-ray—* **Adults:** inject 10 units S.C. at 2 hours, then again at 30 minutes before X-ray. Enema before first dose may also help to eliminate gas.	*CNS:* tremor, dizziness, headache. *CV:* angina in patients with vascular disease, vasoconstriction. Large doses may cause hypertension, electrocardiographic changes, coronary insufficiency, myocardial infarction. *GI:* abdominal cramps, nausea, vomiting, diarrhea, intestinal hyperactivity. *GU:* uterine cramps, anuria. *Skin:* circumoral pallor. *Other:* water intoxication (drowsiness, listlessness, headache, confusion, weight gain), hypersensitivity reactions (urticaria, angioneurotic edema, bronchoconstriction, fever, rash, wheezing, dyspnea, circulatory collapse, cardiac arrest, anaphylaxis), sweating.

INTERACTIONS	NURSING CONSIDERATIONS
None significant.	• Use with caution in patients with coronary artery disease. • Particularly useful if diabetes insipidus is unresponsive to other therapy, or if antidiuretic hormones of animal origin cause adverse reactions. • Nasal congestion, allergic rhinitis, or upper respiratory infections may diminish drug absorption and require larger dose or adjunctive therapy. • Inadvertent spray inhalation may cause tightness in chest, coughing, and transient dyspnea. • Test patients sensitive to antidiuretic hormone for sensitivity to lypressin • To administer a uniform, well-diffused spray, hold bottle upright while patient in vertical position holds head upright.
None significant.	• Contraindicated in closed epiphyses or intracranial lesions. Use with caution in diabetics or in patients with family history of diabetes. Regular urine testing for glycosuria should be done. • S.C. administration not recommended. • Should be used only by doctors experienced in treating patients with pituitary growth hormonal deficiency. • Concurrent thyroid hormone or androgen therapy may accelerate epiphyseal closure and limit duration of somatropin treatment. • Monitor bone age progression annually. • Store powder at or below room temperature. • Reconstitute with 5 ml of bacteriostatic water per 10-I.U. vial. Refrigerate unused portion; discard after 1 month. Rotate injection sites.
Lithium, demeclocycline: reduced antidiuretic activity. Use together cautiously. *Chloropropamide:* increased antidiuretic response. Use together cautiously.	• Contraindicated in chronic nephritis with nitrogen retention. Use cautiously in children, the elderly, pregnant women, and patients with epilepsy, migraine, asthma, cardiovascular disease, or fluid overload. • Never inject during first stage of labor; may cause ruptured uterus. • Monitor specific gravity of urine. • Shake tannate in oil thoroughly or warm in hands to make suspension uniform before withdrawing I.M. injection dose. Use absolutely dry syringe to avoid dilution. • Give with 1 to 2 glasses of water to reduce side effects and to improve therapeutic response. • To prevent convulsions, coma, and death, observe patient closely for early signs of water intoxication. • Overhydration more likely with long-acting tannate oil suspension than with aqueous vasopressin solution. • Use minimum effective dose to reduce side effects. • May be used for transient polyuria due to antidiuretic hormone deficiency related to neurosurgery or head injury. • Synthetic desmopressin is sometimes preferred because of longer duration and less frequent side effects. • For treatment of anaphylaxis, see p. 1114.

58

Parathyroid and parathyroid-like agents

calcitonin (Salmon)
calcitriol
dihydrotachysterol
etidronate disodium
parathyroid hormone

Calcitonin is a hormone secreted by the parafollicular cells of the thyroid gland. Calcitonin and parathyroid hormone work on a feedback system. As serum calcium levels increase, calcitonin secretion increases and causes an immediate lowering of serum calcium levels. Dihydrotachysterol and calcitriol, which are activated forms of vitamin D, have actions similar to parathyroid hormone in mobilizing calcium from bone. This results in a reduction of parathyroid hormone levels. Etidronate, a synthetic substance, lowers serum calcium by acting primarily on bone, with little effect on parathyroid hormone levels. Parathyroid hormone regulates serum calcium and phosphorous levels in the body. It does this by altering the renal excretion, intestinal, and bone absorption of calcium and phosphate. Bone is the major site of parathyroid activity.

Major uses

- Management of hypocalcemia in renal failure.
- Treatment of Paget's disease of the bone (osteitis deformans).
- Reduction of plasma phosphate and increase of plasma calcium in hypoparathyroidism.
- Reduction of serum calcium in acute hypercalcemia.

Mechanism of action

- Calcitonin and etidronate decrease osteoclastic activity, inhibit osteocytic osteolysis, and decrease mineral release and matrix or collagen breakdown in bone.
- Dihydrotachysterol and calcitriol stimulate calcium absorption from GI tract and bone calcium mobilization to raise calcium levels and may also increase urinary excretion of inorganic phosphate.
- Parathyroid hormone enhances phosphate excretion by inhibiting tubular reabsorption of phosphate, mobilizing bone calcium, and increasing gastrointestinal absorption of calcium.

Absorption, distribution, and excretion

- Calcitonin and parathyroid hormone are destroyed in gastrointestinal tract so they must be given parenterally. They are well absorbed after I.M. or S.C. injection. Calcitonin is metabolized by kidneys and excreted in urine.
- Dihydrotachysterol, calcitriol, and etidronate are absorbed from GI tract. Dihydrotachsterol and calcitriol are metabolized in liver. Dihydrotachysterol is secreted in bile and excreted via feces; also reported to be excreted in breast milk. Etidronate is excreted unmetabolized in the urine with a small amount of unabsorbed drug excreted in feces.

Onset and duration

- Calcitriol's effect lasts for 3 to 5 days.

- Therapeutic onset of etidronate appears after 1 to 3 months.
- Dihydrotachysterol's maximum hypercalcemic effects occur within 2 weeks after chronic administration; within 1 week if loading dose is used. Calcium levels markedly decrease within 4 to 5 days after discontinuation and completely disappear after 2 weeks.
- After I.V. administration, parathyroid hormone effect begins within 15 minutes; serum calcium rises in 1 hour. After I.M. or S.C. injection, calcium level rises within 4 hours, peaks in 12 to 18 hours, and lasts from 20 to 24 hours (much shorter after I.V. administration).

Combination products
None.

PREVENTING FRACTURES IN PAGET'S DISEASE

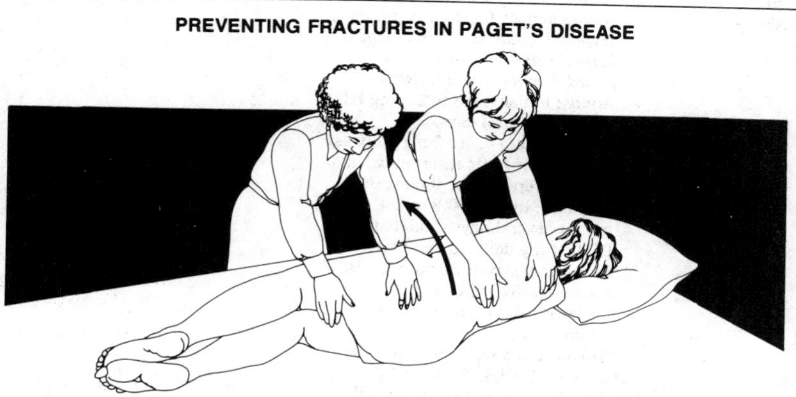

Paget's disease occurs when there is overactivity in building up and breaking down bone accompanied by an altered bone chemical pattern. The patient with Paget's disease has brittle bones that are easily broken.

To prevent pathologic fractures, be particularly gentle when caring for one of these patients. Orient the patient to the unit so that he will not fall by bumping into unfamiliar objects. To turn the patient, enlist the assistance of another nurse. Do not attempt turning the patient by yourself.

NAME	INDICATIONS & DOSAGE	SIDE EFFECTS
calcitonin (Salmon) Calcimar◆	*Paget's disease of bone (osteitis deformans)*— **Adults:** initially, 100 MRC units daily, S.C. or I.M. Maintenance: 50 to 100 units daily or every other day. *Hypercalcemia*— **Adults:** 100 to 400 MRC units I.M. once or twice daily.	*CNS:* headaches. *GI:* transient nausea with or without vomiting, diarrhea. *GU:* transient diuresis. *Local:* inflammation at injection site, skin rashes. *Other:* facial flushing; hypocalcemia; swelling, tingling, and tenderness of hands; unusual taste sensation.
calcitriol (1,25-dihydroxychole-calciferol) Rocaltrol	*Management of hypocalcemia in patients undergoing chronic dialysis*— **Adults:** initially, 0.25 mcg daily. Dosage may be increased by 0.25 mcg/day at 2- to 4-week intervals. Maintenance: 0.25 mcg every other day up to 0.5 to 1.25 mcg daily.	Vitamin D intoxication associated with hypercalcemia: *CNS:* headache, somnolence. *EENT:* conjunctivitis, photophobia, rhinorrhea. *GI:* nausea, vomiting, constipation, metallic taste, dry mouth. *GU:* polyuria. *Other:* weakness, bone and muscle pain.
dihydrotachysterol (AT-10) Hytakerol◆	*Familial hypophosphatemia*— **Adults:** 0.5 to 2 mg P.O. daily. Maintenance: 0.3 to 1.5 mg daily. *Hypocalcemia associated with hypoparathyroidism and pseudohypoparathyroidism*— **Adults:** initially, 0.8 to 2.4 mg P.O. daily for several days. Maintenance: 0.2 to 2 mg daily as required for normal serum calcium levels. Average dose 0.6 mg daily. **Children:** initially, 0.8 to 2.4 mg for several days. Maintenance: 0.2 to 1 mg daily, as required for normal serum calcium levels. *Postoperative hypocalcemic tetany refractory to calcium administration*— **Adults:** Loading dose 4 mg P.O. daily for 2 days, followed by 2 mg daily for 2 days, then 1 mg daily until normal serum calcium levels attained. *Renal osteodystrophy in chronic uremia*— **Adults:** 0.25 to 0.5 mg P.O. daily. *Suppression of hyperparathyroidism in chronic renal failure*— **Adults:** 0.25 to 0.375 mg P.O. daily.	None.

◆ Also available in Canada.
◆◆ Available in Canada only.
Unmarked trade names available in United States only.

INTERACTIONS	NURSING CONSIDERATIONS
None significant.	• Not recommended for nursing mothers, or women who are or may become pregnant. • Periodic serum alkaline phosphatase and 24-hour urinary hydroxyproline levels should be determined to evaluate drug effect. • Skin test is usually done before beginning therapy. • Systemic allergic reactions possible since hormone is protein. Keep epinephrine available when administering. • Monitor calcium levels closely. Watch for signs of hypercalcemic relapse: bone pain, renal calculi, polyuria, anorexia, nausea, vomiting, thirst, constipation, lethargy, bradycardia, muscle hypotonicity, pathologic fracture, psychosis, and coma. • Periodic examinations of urine sediment advisable. • Solution should be refrigerated.
None significant.	• Contraindicated in hypercalcemia or vitamin D toxicity. Withhold all preparations containing vitamin D in patients taking calcitriol. Not recommended in nursing mothers. Use cautiously in patients on digitalis; hypercalcemia may precipitate cardiac arrhythmias. • Monitor serum calcium; serum calcium times serum phosphate should not exceed 70. During titration, determine serum levels twice weekly. If hypercalcemia occurs, discontinue, but resume after serum calcium returns to normal. Patient should receive adequate daily intake of calcium, 1,000 mg RDA. • Protect from heat and light. • Instruct patient to adhere to diet and calcium supplementation and to avoid unapproved nonprescription drugs.
None significant.	• Contraindicated in hypercalcemia, hypocalcemia associated with renal insufficiency and hyperphosphatemia, renal stones, hypersensitivity to vitamin D, and in nursing mothers. • Monitor serum and urinary calcium. Watch for signs of hypercalcemia. • Adequate dietary calcium intake is necessary; usually supplemented with 10 to 15 g oral calcium lactate or gluconate daily. • Report hypercalcemia reactions to doctor. • Store in tightly closed, light-resistant containers. Don't refrigerate.

NAME	INDICATIONS & DOSAGE	SIDE EFFECTS
etidronate disodium Didronel	*Symptomatic Paget's disease—* **Adults:** 5 mg/Kg/day P.O. as a single dose 2 hours before a meal with water or juice. Patient should not eat for 2 hours after dose. May give up to 10 mg/Kg/day in severe cases. Maximum dose 20 mg/Kg/day.	*GI:* (seen most frequently at 20 mg/Kg/day) diarrhea, increased frequency of bowel movements, nausea. *Other:* increased or recurrent bone pain at Pagetic sites, pain at previously asymptomatic sites, increased risk of fracture, elevated serum phosphate.
parathyroid hormone Para-thor-mone, Paroidin	*Acute hypoparathyroidism with tetany—* **Adults:** 20 to 40 units S.C., I.M., or I.V. q 12 hours. **Infants:** (with transient congenital idiopathic true hypopara, thyroidism) 25 to 50 units I.M. q 12 hours for 1 to 3 days.	*Allergic:* anaphylactic reactions (parathyroid hormone is a foreign protein). *Other:* hypercalcemia (muscle weakness, bone and flank pain), lethargy, headache, anorexia, nausea, vomiting, diarrhea, abdominal cramps, vertigo, tinnitus, ataxia.

INTERACTIONS	NURSING CONSIDERATIONS
None significant.	• Use cautiously in enterocolitis, impaired renal function. • Therapy should not last more than 6 months. After 3 months, resume if needed. Don't give longer than 3 months at doses above 10 mg/Kg/day. • Don't give drug with food, milk, or antacids; may reduce absorption. • Monitor renal function before and during therapy. • Monitor drug effect by serum alkaline phosphatase and urinary hydroxyproline excretion (both lowered if therapy effective). • Tell patient that improvement may not occur for up to 3 months but may continue for months after drug stopped. Stress importance of good nutrition, especially high in calcium and vitamin D.
None significant.	• Contraindicated in hypercalcemia, hypercalciuria, tetany unrelated to parathyroid failure, and I.V. administration when serum calcium levels are above normal. Use cautiously in sarcoidosis, renal or cardiac disease, and in digitalized patients. • Rarely used because calcium salts often effective alone. • S.C. injections may produce moderate inflammatory reaction. • Therapy lasts only a few days; patients may soon become refractory to it. • If given I.V., skin-test for sensitivity. If positive, desensitize patient. • Keep epinephrine injection available when giving parathyroid hormone. • Monitor serum calcium and serum phosphate levels, intake and output. • Know and watch for signs of hypoparathyroidism and calcium deficiency. Test for Chvostek's and Trousseau's signs. Watch for drug-induced hypercalcemia. • Use seizure precautions in patients with calcium deficiency: padded rails, soft light, no irritating noises until normal calcium level restored. • Do not dilute with saline solution as a precipitate will form. • Store ampules at 2° C. to 8° C. (36° F. to 46° F.); do not freeze.

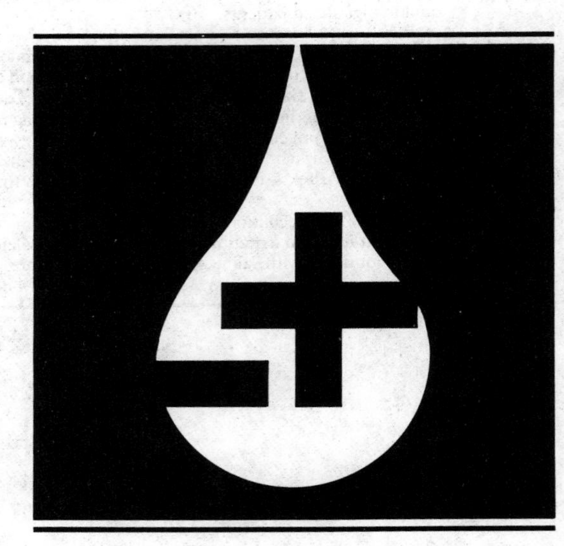

Fluid and Electrolyte Balance

59

Diuretics

acetazolamide
bendroflumethiazide
benzthiazide
chlorothiazide
chlorthalidone
cyclothiazide
dichlorphenamide
ethacrynate sodium
ethacrynic acid
ethoxzolamide
furosemide
hydrochlorothiazide
hydroflumethiazide
mannitol
mercaptomerin sodium
methazolamide
methyclothiazide
metolazone
polythiazide
quinethazone
spironolactone
triamterene
trichlormethiazide
urea

Diuretics increase urinary excretion of water and sodium. They enhance the activity of the kidneys but do not stimulate diseased kidneys. Diuretics are used primarily in excess fluid retention or in hypertension. They are usually classified according to their action and structure.

Major uses

- Treatment of edema.
- Treatment of hypertension.
- Carbonic anhydrase inhibitors and osmotic diuretics also reduce intracranial and intraocular pressure.

Mechanism of action

- Carbonic anhydrase inhibitors inhibit action of the enzyme carbonic anhydrase, resulting in increased excretion of sodium, potassium, bicarbonate, and water in the kidneys. Independent of diuretic action, they decrease formation of aqueous humor in the eye, thereby lowering intraocular pressure.
- Loop diuretics inhibit reabsorption of sodium and chloride at the ascending loop of Henle in the kidneys, enhancing water excretion.
- Osmotic diuretics increase the osmotic pressure of glomerular filtrate, resulting in inhibited tubular reabsorption of water and electrolytes.
- Spironolactone antagonizes the hormone aldosterone in the distal tubule, increasing excretion of sodium and water but conserving potassium.
- Triamterene also spares potassium. It depresses reabsorption of sodium and secretion of potassium by direct action on the distal tubule in the kidneys.

• Thiazide and mercurial diuretics inhibit renal tubular reabsorption of sodium, chloride, and water in the cortical diluting segment.

Absorption, distribution, and excretion

• Carbonic anhydrase inhibitors are absorbed from the gastrointestinal tract after oral administration and are distributed throughout body tissues. Acetazolamide is excreted unchanged in the urine, but other carbonic anhydrase inhibitors are partially metabolized and excreted in the urine and by other routes.
• Ethacrynic acid is rapidly absorbed after oral administration, metabolized and excreted by the kidneys and the liver.
• Approximately 60% of furosemide is absorbed from the gastrointestinal tract; a small amount is metabolized and excreted with the unchanged remainder in the urine.
• Mannitol is administered intravenously, remains in the extracellular compartment, is filtered by the glomeruli, and is excreted unchanged in urine.
• Mercurial diuretics are rapidly and completely absorbed after intramuscular or subcutaneous administration, distributed mainly to the kidneys, and excreted almost entirely in the urine.
• Spironolactone is absorbed from the gastrointestinal tract, metabolized in the liver, and excreted in the urine and feces.
• Triamterene is rapidly absorbed from the gastrointestinal tract, partially bound to plasma proteins, distributed to body tissues, and rapidly excreted in the urine.
• Thiazides and related diuretics are absorbed from the gastrointestinal tract in varying degree and are excreted in the urine. They cross the placenta and are present in breast milk.
• Urea is rapidly absorbed after oral administration, although it is seldom used orally because of its unpleasant taste. Following I.V. administration it is distributed to intracellular and extracellular fluids, including cerebrospinal fluid, partially hydrolyzed in the gastrointestinal tract by bacterial ureas (even intravenous forms), and excreted by the kidneys. It crosses the placenta and can be found in breast milk.

Onset and duration

• Carbonic anhydrase inhibitors begin to act within 1 to 3 hours after oral administration and have a duration of 8 to 12 hours, except for acetazolamide (timed-release form), which acts up to 24 hours, and methazolamide, which acts up to 18 hours. After intravenous administration, acetazolamide begins to act within 2 minutes and has a duration of 4 to 5 hours.
• Ethacrynic acid begins to act 30 minutes after oral administration and has a duration of

up to 12 hours when given by this route. It begins to act within 5 minutes after intravenous administration and has a duration of 2 hours by this route.

• Furosemide begins to act 30 to 60 minutes after oral administration and has a duration of 6 to 8 hours by this route. It begins to act 5 minutes after intravenous administration and has a duration of 2 hours when given by this route. It begins to act within 30 minutes, with a duration of 6 to 8 hours, after intramuscular administration.

• Mannitol begins to act 15 to 30 minutes after intravenous administration; diuresis occurs in 1 to 3 hours. Duration is 4 to 6 hours and may extend to 8 hours in reduction of cerebrospinal fluid pressure.

• Urea begins to act 1 to 2 hours after intravenous administration and has a duration of 3 to 10 hours.

• Mercurial diuretics begin to work 1 to 3 hours after intramuscular or subcutaneous administration and have a duration of 12 to 24 hours.

• Spironolactone begins to act gradually over 2 to 3 days, but a loading dose may be used for a faster onset of action. It continues to act for 2 to 3 days.

• Triamterene begins to act in 2 to 4 hours and has a duration of up to 24 hours. Maximum therapeutic effect may not occur during initial few days of therapy.

• Thiazides and related diuretics begin to act within 1 to 2 hours after oral administration. Most have a duration of action of 12 to 24 hours, except polythiazide, which acts up to 48 hours, and chlorthalidone, which acts for 48 to 72 hours. Intravenous chlorothiazide sodium begins to act within 15 minutes of administration and has a duration of 2 hours.

Combination products

ALDACTAZIDE◆: spironolactone 25 mg and hydrochlorothiazide 25 mg.
DYAZIDE◆: triamterene 50 mg and hydrochlorothiazide 25 mg.

EVALUATING EDEMA

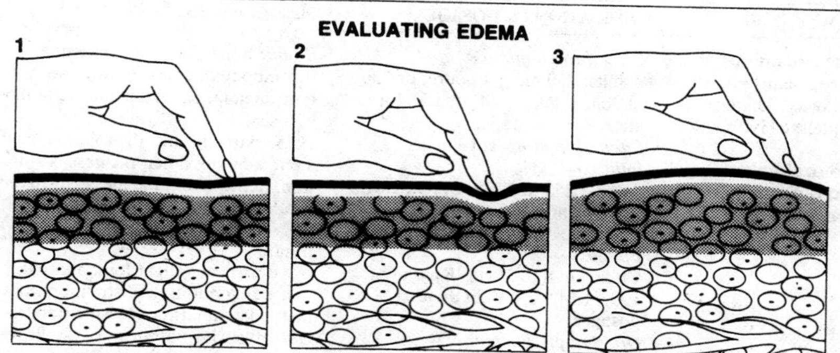

Pitting edema is evaluated on a 4-point scale: from +1 (a barely detectable pit, as in Figure 1) to +4 (a deep and persistent pit, approximately 1 inch or 25.4 mm deep, as in Figure 2). An adult patient can accumulate up to 10 lb (4.5 Kg) of fluid before you will be able to detect a pit. The skin pits against a bony surface, such as the subcutaneous aspect of the tibia, fibula, sacrum, or sternum.

Edema can become so severe that pitting is not possible; the tissue becomes so full that fluid can't be displaced. Subcutaneous tissue becomes fibrotic and as a result, the surface tissue feels rock hard. In time, this condition can develop into brawny edema (Figure 3). For example, a mastectomy patient whose axillary nodes have been removed may develop brawny edema in her affected arm. The patient's skin looks like a pig's skin, and her arm becomes hard or gelatinous to the touch. Brawny edema can also indicate lymphatic obstruction. Protect all edematous extremities from injury. Edema makes the skin prone to sloughing and ulceration.

NAME	INDICATIONS & DOSAGE	SIDE EFFECTS
acetazolamide Acetazolam◆◆, Diamox◆, Diamox sequels◆, Hydrazol **acetazolamide sodium** Diamox parenteral◆	*Closed-angle glaucoma—* **Adults:** 250 mg q 4 hours; or 250 mg b.i.d. P.O., I.M. or I.V. for short-term therapy. *Edema, in congestive heart failure—* **Adults:** 250 to 375 mg P.O., I.M., or I.V. daily in a.m. **Children:** 5 mg/Kg daily in a.m. *Epilepsy—* **Children:** 8 to 30 mg/Kg/daily P.O., I.M. or I.V. in divided dosages. *Open-angle glaucoma—* **Adults:** 250 mg daily to 1 g P.O., I.M., or I.V. divided q.i.d.	*Blood:* bone marrow depression, thrombocytopenia, leukopenia, hemolytic anemia, pancytopenia, agranulocytosis. *CNS:* paresthesias, drowsiness, confusion, weakness, nervousness, sedation, depression, dizziness, vertigo, headache. *EENT:* transient myopia, anosmia, tinnitus. *GI:* diarrhea, weight loss, anorexia, nausea, vomiting, constipation, loss of taste, dry mouth, excessive thirst. *GU:* dysuria, polyuria, crystalluria, renal calculi, urinary frequency, ureteral colic. *Metabolic:* acidosis, hyperuricemia, hypokalemia. *Skin:* urticaria and pruritus in hypersensitivity; rash. *Other:* fever in hypersensitivity, hepatitis.
bendroflumethiazide Naturetin◆	*Edema, hypertension—* **Adults:** 5 to 20 mg P.O. daily or b.i.d. in divided doses. **Children:** initially, 0.1 to 0.4 mg/Kg daily in 1 or 2 doses. Maintenance: 0.05 to 0.1 mg/Kg daily in 1 or 2 doses.	*Blood:* leukopenia, agranulocytosis, thrombocytopenia, aplastic anemia. *CNS:* dizziness, vertigo, paresthesias, headache, restlessness, weakness. *CV:* orthostatic hypotension. *EENT:* transient blurred vision, xanthopsia. *GI:* anorexia, GI irritation, nausea, vomiting, cramping, diarrhea, constipation, pancreatitis. *GU:* glycosuria, allergic glomerulonephritis. *Metabolic:* hyperuricemia, decreased calcium excretion, hypokalemia, fluid or electrolyte imbalances, mild chloride deficit, hyperglycemia, acidosis in diabetic patients, dilutional hyponatremia. *Skin:* purpura, photosensitivity, rash, urticaria, necrotizing angiitis. *Other:* jaundice, fever, respiratory distress, anaphylaxis, muscle spasm.
benzthiazide Aquapres, Aqua-Scrip, Aquasec, Aquastat, Aquatag, Diretic, Diucen, Exna◆, Hydrex, Lemazide, Marazide, Proaqua, Rid-ema, S-Aqua, Urazide	*Edema—* **Adults:** 50 to 200 mg P.O. daily or in divided doses. **Children:** 1 to 4 mg/Kg daily in 3 divided doses. *Hypertension—* **Adults:** 50 mg P.O. daily b.i.d., t.i.d., or q.i.d., adjusted to patient's response.	*Blood:* leukopenia, agranulocytosis, thrombocytopenia, aplastic anemia. *CNS:* dizziness, vertigo, paresthesias, headache, restlessness, weakness. *CV:* orthostatic hypotension. *EENT:* transient blurred vision, xanthopsia. *GI:* anorexia, GI irritation, nausea,

◆ Also available in Canada.
◆◆ Available in Canada only.
Unmarked trade names available in United States only.

INTERACTIONS	NURSING CONSIDERATIONS
None significant.	• Contraindicated in long-term therapy for chronic noncongestive angle-closure glaucoma; also in depressed sodium or potassium blood serum levels, kidney or liver disease or dysfunction, adrenal gland failure, and hyperchloremic acidosis. Use cautiously in respiratory acidosis, emphysema, chronic lung disease, or patients receiving other diuretics. • Monitor intake/output and electrolytes, especially serum potassium. When used in diuretic therapy, consult with doctor and dietitian to provide high-potassium diet. • Weigh patient daily. Rapid weight loss may cause hypotension. • Diuretic effect decreased when acidosis occurs but can be reestablished by withdrawing drug for several days and then restarting, or by utilizing intermittent administration schedules. • Reconstitute 500 mg vial with at least 5 ml sterile water for injection. Use within 24 hours of reconstitution. • I.M. injection painful because of alkalinity of solution. Direct I.V. administration preferred (100 to 500 mg/minute). • Elderly patients are especially susceptible to excessive diuresis. • May cause false positive urine protein tests by alkalinizing the urine. • A carbonic anhydrase inhibitor. Its acidotic effects limit usefulness for daily treatment of edema.
Cholestyramine, colestipol: intestinal absorption of thiazides decreased. Keep doses as separate as possible. *Diazoxide:* increased antihypertensive, hyperglycemic, and hyperuricemic effects. Use together cautiously.	• Contraindicated in anuria; hypersensitivity to other thiazides or other sulfonamide-derived drugs. Use cautiously in severe renal disease, impaired hepatic function. • Monitor intake/output, weight, and serum electrolytes regularly. Monitor serum creatinine and BUN levels regularly. Not effective if these levels are more than twice normal. • Monitor serum potassium levels; consult with doctor and dietitian to provide high-potassium diet. Watch for signs of hypokalemia (e.g., muscle weakness, cramps). May use with potassium-sparing diuretic to prevent potassium loss. • Monitor blood sugar. Check insulin requirements in diabetics. May treat severe hyperglycemia with oral antidiabetic agents. • Monitor blood uric acid levels, especially in patients with a history of gout. • Give in a.m. to prevent nocturia. • Elderly patients are especially susceptible to excessive diuresis. • In hypertension, therapeutic response may be delayed several days. • A thiazide diuretic. • For treatment of anaphylaxis, see p. 1114.
Cholestyramine, colestipol: intestinal absorption of thiazides decreased. Keep doses as separate as possible. *Diazoxide:* increased antihypertensive, hyperglycemic, and	• Contraindicated in anuria; hypersensitivity to other thiazides or other sulfonamide-derived drugs. Use cautiously in severe renal disease, impaired hepatic function. • Monitor intake/output, weight, and serum electrolytes regularly. Monitor serum potassium levels; consult with doctor and dietitian to provide high-potassium diet. Watch for signs of hypokalemia (e.g., muscle weakness, cramps). May use with potassium-sparing diuretic to prevent potassium loss. • Monitor serum creatinine and BUN levels regularly. Not effective if these

(continued on following page)

NAME	INDICATIONS & DOSAGE	SIDE EFFECTS
benzthiazide *(continued)*		vomiting, cramping, diarrhea, constipation, pancreatitis. *GU:* glycosuria, allergic glomerulonephritis. *Metabolic:* fluid or electrolyte imbalances, hypokalemia, dilutional hyponatremia, hypochloremic alkalosis, hyperuricemia, decreased calcium excretion, hyperglycemia. *Skin:* purpura, photosensitivity, rash, urticaria, necrotizing angiitis. *Other:* jaundice, fever, respiratory distress, anaphylaxis.
chlorothiazide Diuril◆, Ro-Chlorozide	*Diuresis—* **Children over 6 months:** 20 mg/Kg P.O. or I.V. daily in divided doses. **Children under 6 months:** may require 30 mg/Kg P.O. or I.V. daily in 2 divided doses. *Edema, hypertension—* **Adults:** 500 mg to 2 g P.O. or I.V. daily or in 2 divided doses.	*Blood:* leukopenia, agranulocytosis, thrombocytopenia, aplastic anemia. *CNS:* paresthesias, headache, dizziness, vertigo, restlessness, weakness. *CV:* orthostatic hypotension. *EENT:* transient blurred vision, xanthopsia. *GI:* anorexia, gastric distress, nausea, vomiting, cramping, diarrhea, constipation, pancreatitis. *GU:* glycosuria, allergic glomerulonephritis. *Metabolic:* fluid or electrolyte imbalances, hypokalemia (in 30% to 50% of patients), dilutional hyponatremia, hypochloremic alkalosis, hyperuricemia (40% in male patients, less common in females), frank gout, hyperglycemia, decreased calcium excretion. *Skin:* purpura, photosensitivity, rash, urticaria, necrotizing angiitis. *Other:* jaundice, fever, respiratory distress, anaphylaxis, muscle spasm.
chlorthalidone Hygroton◆, Novothalidone◆◆, Uridon◆◆	*Edema, hypertension—* **Adults:** 50 to 100 mg P.O. daily, or 100 mg 3 times weekly or on alternate days. Occasionally, up to 200 mg daily may be needed. **Children:** 2 mg/Kg P.O. 3 times weekly.	*Blood:* leukopenia, agranulocytosis, thrombocytopenia, aplastic anemia. *CNS:* dizziness, paresthesias, headache, restlessness, weakness. *CV:* orthostatic hypotension. *EENT:* transient blurred vision, xanthopsia. *GI:* anorexia, GI irritation, nausea, vomiting, cramping, diarrhea, constipation, pancreatitis. *GU:* glycosuria, allergic glomerulonephritis, impotence. *Metabolic:* hyperuricemia, decreased calcium excretion, hypokalemia, fluid imbalance, mild chloride deficit, hyperglycemia, dilutional hyponatremia. *Skin:* purpura, photosensitivity, rash, urticaria, necrotizing angiitis. *Other:* jaundice, fever, respiratory distress, anaphylaxis, muscle spasm.

INTERACTIONS	NURSING CONSIDERATIONS
hyperuricemic effects. Use together cautiously.	levels are more than twice normal. • Monitor blood sugar. Check insulin requirements in diabetics. May treat severe hyperglycemia with oral antidiabetic agents. • Monitor blood uric acid levels, especially in patients with a history of gout. • Give in a.m. to prevent nocturia. • Elderly patients are especially susceptible to excessive diuresis. • In hypertension, therapeutic response may be delayed several days. • A thiazide diuretic. • For treatment of anaphylaxis, see p. 1114.
Cholestyramine, colestipol: intestinal absorption of thiazides decreased. Keep doses as separate as possible. *Diazoxide:* increased antihypertensive, hyperglycemic, and hyperuricemic effects. Use together cautiously.	• Contraindicated in anuria; hypersensitivity to other thiazides or other sulfonamide-derived drugs; impaired hepatic function; progressive liver disease. Use cautiously in severe renal disease. • Monitor intake/output, weight, and serum electrolytes regularly. • Monitor potassium levels; consult with doctor and dietitian to provide high-potassium diet. Watch for signs of hypokalemia (e.g., muscle weakness, cramps). May use with potassium-sparing diuretic to prevent potassium loss. • Monitor blood sugar. Check insulin requirements in diabetes. May treat severe hyperglycemia with oral antidiabetic agents. • Monitor serum creatinine and BUN levels regularly. Not effective if these levels are more than twice normal. • Monitor blood uric acid levels, especially in patients with a history of gout. • Watch for decreased calcium excretion and progressive renal impairment. • Only injectable thiazide. For I.V. use only—not I.M. or S.C. Reconstitute with 18 ml of sterile water for injection/500 mg vial. May store reconstituted solutions at room temperature up to 24 hours. Compatible with dextrose or sodium chloride solutions intravenously. • Avoid I.V. infiltration; can be very painful. • Give in a.m. to prevent nocturia. • In hypertension, therapeutic response may be delayed several days. • Elderly patients especially susceptible to excessive diuresis. • A thiazide diuretic. • For treatment of anaphylaxis, see p. 1114.
Cholestyramine, colestipol: intestinal absorption of thiazides decreased. Keep doses as separate as possible. *Diazoxide:* increased antihypertensive, hyperglycemic, and hyperuricemic effects. Use together cautiously.	• Contraindicated in anuria; hypersensitivity to thiazides or other sulfonamide-derived drugs. Use cautiously in severe renal disease, progressive liver disease, impaired hepatic function. • Monitor intake/output, weight, and serum electrolytes regularly. • Monitor serum potassium levels; consult with doctor and dietitian to provide high-potassium diet. Watch for signs of hypokalemia (e.g., muscle weakness, cramps). May use with potassium-sparing diuretic to prevent potassium loss. • Monitor serum creatinine and BUN levels regularly. Not effective if these levels are more than twice normal. • Monitor blood uric acid levels, especially in patients with a history of gout. • Monitor blood sugar. Check insulin requirements in diabetics. May treat severe hyperglycemia with oral antidiabetic agents. • In hypertension, therapeutic response may be delayed several days. • Give in a.m. to prevent nocturia. • Elderly patients are especially susceptible to excessive diuresis. • A thiazide-like diuretic. • For treatment of anaphylaxis, see p. 1114.

NAME	INDICATIONS & DOSAGE	SIDE EFFECTS
cyclothiazide Anhydron	*Edema—* **Adults:** 1 to 2 mg P.O. daily. May be used on alternate days as maintenance dose. **Children:** 0.02 to 0.04 mg/Kg P.O. daily. *Hypertension—* **Adults:** 2 mg P.O. daily; up to 2 mg b.i.d. or t.i.d.	*Blood:* leukopenia, agranulocytosis, thrombocytopenia, aplastic anemia. *CNS:* dizziness, paresthesias, headache, restlessness, weakness. *CV:* orthostatic hypotension. *EENT:* transient blurred vision, xanthopsia. *GI:* anorexia, GI irritation, nausea, vomiting, cramping, diarrhea, constipation, pancreatitis. *GU:* glycosuria, allergic glomerulonephritis. *Metabolic:* hyperuricemia, decreased calcium excretion, hypokalemia, fluid or electrolyte imbalances, mild chloride deficit, hyperglycemia, frank gout, dilutional hyponatremia. *Skin:* purpura, photosensitivity, rash, urticaria, necrotizing angiitis. *Other:* jaundice, fever, respiratory distress, anaphylaxis, muscle spasm.
dichlorphenamide Daranide◆, Oratrol	*Adjunct in glaucoma—* **Adults:** initially, 100 to 200 mg P.O., followed by 100 mg q 12 hours until desired response obtained. Maintenance: 25 to 50 mg P.O. daily b.i.d. or t.i.d. Give miotics concomitantly.	*Blood:* bone marrow depression, thrombocytopenia, leukopenia, hemolytic anemia, pancytopenia, agranulocytosis. *CNS:* nervousness, sedation, depression, dizziness, vertigo, fatigue, confusion, headache, paresthesias, ataxia. *EENT:* transient myopia, tinnitus, loss of smell. *GI:* anorexia, nausea, vomiting, constipation, loss of taste, dry mouth, excessive thirst. *GU:* dysuria, ureteral colic, renal calculi, crystalluria. *Metabolic:* acidosis, hypokalemia, hyperuricemia. *Skin:* urticaria, pruritus in hypersensitivity. *Other:* fever in hypersensitivity.
ethacrynate sodium Sodium Edecrin **ethacrynic acid** Edecrin◆	*Acute pulmonary edema—* **Adults:** 50 to 100 mg of ethacrynate sodium I.V. slowly over several minutes. *Edema—* **Adults:** 50 to 200 mg P.O. daily. Refractory cases may require up to 200 mg b.i.d. **Children:** initial dose 25 mg P.O., cautiously, increased in 25 mg increments daily until desired effect is obtained.	*Blood:* thrombocytopenia, neutropenia, agranulocytosis. *CNS:* weakness, paresthesias in excessive use; dizziness, headache, fatigue, apprehension, confusion. *EENT:* deafness (usually reversible), tinnitus, fullness in ears, vertigo, blurred vision. *GI:* anorexia, abdominal discomfort or pain, dysphagia, nausea, vomiting, diarrhea, sudden onset of profuse watery diarrhea, GI bleeding. *GU:* hematuria.

INTERACTIONS	NURSING CONSIDERATIONS
Cholestyramine, colestipol: intestinal absorption of thiazides decreased. Keep doses as separate as possible. *Diazoxide:* increased antihypertensive, hyperglycemic, and hyperuricemic effects. Use together cautiously.	• Contraindicated in anuria; hypersensitivity to other thiazides or other sulfonamide-derived drugs. Use cautiously in severe renal disease, impaired hepatic function, progressive liver disease. • Monitor intake/output, weight, and serum electrolytes regularly. • Monitor serum potassium levels; consult with doctor and dietitian to provide high-potassium diet. Watch for signs of hypokalemia (e.g., muscle weakness, cramps). May use with potassium-sparing diuretic to prevent potassium loss. • Monitor blood sugar. Check insulin requirements in diabetics. May treat severe hyperglycemia with oral antidiabetic agents. • Monitor serum creatinine and BUN levels regularly. Not effective if these levels are more than twice normal. • Monitor blood uric acid levels, especially in patients with a history of gout. • In hypertension, therapeutic response may be delayed several days. • Give in a.m. to prevent nocturia. • Elderly patients are especially susceptible to excessive diuresis. • A thiazide diuretic. • For treatment of anaphylaxis, see p. 1114.
None significant.	• Contraindicated in hepatic insufficiency, renal failure, adrenocortical insufficiency, hyperchloremic acidosis, depressed sodium or potassium levels, severe pulmonary obstruction with inability to increase alveolar ventilation, Addison's disease. Long-term use contraindicated in severe, absolute, or chronic noncongestive angle-closure glaucoma. Use cautiously in respiratory acidosis, monitoring blood pH and blood gases. • Monitor electrolytes, especially serum potassium in initial treatment. Usually no problem in long-term glaucoma therapy unless risk for hypokalemia from other causes; potassium supplements may be necessary. • May cause false positive results in urine protein tests. • A carbonic anhydrase inhibitor.
Aminoglycoside antibiotics: potentiated ototoxic side effects of both ethacrynic acid and aminoglycosides. Use together cautiously.	• Contraindicated in anuria, and infants. Use cautiously in electrolyte abnormalities. If electrolyte imbalance, azotemia, or oliguria develop, may require discontinuing drug. • Monitor intake/output, weight, and serum electrolytes regularly. • Monitor serum potassium levels; consult with doctor and dietitian to provide high-potassium diet. Watch for signs of hypokalemia (e.g., muscle weakness, cramps). • I.V. injection painful; may cause thrombophlebitis. Don't give S.C. or I.M. Give slowly through tubing of running infusion over several minutes. • Salt and potassium chloride supplement may be necessary during therapy. • Reconstitute vacuum vial with 50 ml of 5% dextrose injection or NaCl injection. Discard unused solution after 24 hours. Don't use cloudy or

(continued on following page)

NAME	INDICATIONS & DOSAGE	SIDE EFFECTS
ethacrynic acid *(continued)*		*Local:* local irritation and pain after I.V. *Metabolic:* reversible hyperuricemia, acute gout, hyperglycemia, dilutional hyponatremia, hypokalemia, hypochloremic alkalosis, hypovolemia. *Other:* muscle cramps after excessive use, fever, chills, malaise, jaundice.
ethoxzolamide Cardrase, Ethamide	*Edema (from congestive heart failure)*— **Adults:** 62.5 to 125 mg P.O. daily in a.m. for 3 consecutive days each week or every other day. Refractory cases may require 250 mg/day. *Glaucoma*— **Adults:** 62.5 to 250 mg P.O. b.i.d., t.i.d., or q.i.d. Give miotics concomitantly.	*Blood:* bone marrow depression, thrombocytopenia, leukopenia, hemolytic anemia, pancytopenia, agranulocytosis. *CNS:* nervousness, sedation, depression, dizziness, vertigo, fatigue, confusion, headache, paresthesias. *EENT:* transient myopia, anosmia, tinnitus. *GI:* anorexia, nausea, vomiting, constipation, dry mouth, loss of taste, excessive thirst, diarrhea, weight loss. *GU:* urinary frequency, urethral colic, dysuria, renal calculi, crystalluria. *Metabolic:* hypokalemia, acidosis. *Skin:* urticaria, pruritus in hypersensitivity. *Other:* fever in hypersensitivity.
furosemide Lasix◆, Novosemide◆◆, Uritol◆◆	*Acute pulmonary edema*— **Adults:** 40 mg I.V. injected slowly; then 40 mg I.V. in 1 to 1½ hours if needed. *Edema*— **Adults:** 20 to 80 mg P.O. daily in a.m., second dose can be given in 6 to 8 hours; carefully titrated up to 600 mg daily if needed; or 20 to 40 mg I.M. or I.V. Increase by 20 mg q 2 hours until desired response is achieved. I.V. dose should be given slowly over 1 to 2 minutes. **Infants and children:** 2 mg/Kg P.O. daily; dose increased by 1 to 2 mg/Kg in 6 to 8 hours if needed; carefully titrated up to 6 mg/Kg daily if needed. *Hypertensive crisis, acute renal failure*— **Adults:** 100 to 200 mg I.V. over 1 to 2 minutes. *Chronic renal failure*— **Adults:** initially, 80 mg P.O. daily. Increase by 80 to 120 mg daily until desired response is achieved.	*Blood:* hypovolemia with excessive diuresis, anemia, leukopenia, aplastic anemia, thrombocytopenia, agranulocytosis. *CNS:* weakness, fatigue, lethargy, light-headedness, dizziness, paresthesias, postural hypotension. *EENT:* tinnitus, reversible hearing impairment in I.V. administration; blurred vision. *GI:* nausea, vomiting, diarrhea, thirst, abdominal pain and cramping (children). *GU:* urinary bladder spasm, urinary frequency. *Metabolic:* dehydration in excessive diuresis; electrolyte depletion and imbalances, alkalosis, asymptomatic hyperuricemia. *Skin:* dermatitis, urticaria, pruritus. *Other:* muscle cramps, sweating.

INTERACTIONS	NURSING CONSIDERATIONS
	opalescent solutions. • Elderly patients are especially susceptible to excessive diuresis. • Give P.O. doses in a.m. to prevent nocturia. • Monitor blood uric acid levels, especially in patients with history of gout. • A loop diuretic; especially strong.
None significant.	• Contraindicated in hyperchloremic acidosis, renal failure, hepatic insufficiency, adrenal failure, depressed sodium or potassium blood levels, and long-term therapy for chronic noncongestive angle-closure glaucoma. Use with caution in advanced pulmonary disease, respiratory acidosis, and concomitantly with other diuretics. • Monitor electrolytes, especially serum potassium; consult with doctor and dietitian to provide high-potassium diet. Monitor intake/output and weight. • May cause false positive results in urine protein tests. • Watch for dehydration, especially in elderly patients. • A carbonic anhydrase inhibitor. When used on a daily basis for edema, its acidotic effects limit its usefulness.
Aminoglycoside antibiotics: potentiated ototoxicity. Use together cautiously. *Chloral hydrate:* sweating, flushing with I.V. furosemide. Observe patient. *Clofibrate:* enhanced furosemide effects. Use cautiously. *Indomethacin:* inhibited diuretic response. Use cautiously.	• Contraindicated in anuria, hepatic coma, or electrolyte imbalances. Use cautiously in cardiogenic shock complicated by pulmonary edema. • Potent loop diuretic; can lead to profound water and electrolyte depletion. Monitor blood pressure and pulse during rapid diuresis. • Sulfonamide-sensitive patients may have allergic reaction to furosemide. • If oliguria or azotemia increase or develop, may require stopping drug. • Monitor serum electrolytes, BUN, and CO_2 frequently. • Monitor serum potassium levels. Watch for signs of hypokalemia (e.g., muscle weakness, cramps). Consult with doctor and dietitian to provide high-potassium diet. • Monitor blood sugar levels in diabetics. May treat severe hyperglycemia with oral antidiabetic agents. • Monitor blood uric acid levels, especially in patients with a history of gout. • Give I.V. doses over 1 to 2 minutes. For doses over 100 mg, give at 10 mg/minute to prevent tinnitus associated with rapid infusion of large doses. In decreased renal function, give I.V. doses at rate of 10 mg/minute or less. • Don't use parenteral route in infants and children unless oral dosage form is not practical. • I.M. injection causes transient pain; moderate by using "Z" track to limit leakage into S.C. tissues. • Give P.O. and I.M. preparations in a.m. to prevent nocturia. • Elderly patients are especially susceptible to excessive diuresis, with potential for circulatory collapse and thromboembolic complications. • Store tablets in light-resistant container to prevent discoloration (doesn't affect potency). Don't use discolored (yellow) injectable preparation. • Promotes calcium excretion. I.V. furosemide often used to treat hypercalcemia.

NAME	INDICATIONS & DOSAGE	SIDE EFFECTS
hydrochlorothiazide Chlorzide, Delco-Retic, Diuchlor-H◆◆, Diu-Scrip, Esidrix◆, Hydrid◆◆, Hydro-Aquil◆◆, Hydro-Diuril◆, Hydromal, Hydro-Z-25, Hydro-Z-50, Hydrozide◆◆, Hyperetic, Kena-zide, Lexor, Neo-Codema◆◆, Novohydrazide◆◆, Oretic, Ro-Hydrazide, Thiu-retic, Urozide◆◆, Zide	*Edema—* **Adults:** initially, 25 to 100 mg P.O. daily or intermittently for maintenance to minimize electrolyte imbalance. **Children over 6 months:** 2.2 mg/Kg P.O. daily divided b.i.d. **Children under 6 months:** up to 3.3 mg/Kg P.O. daily divided b.i.d. *Hypertension—* **Adults:** 25 to 100 mg P.O. daily or divided dosage. Daily dosage increased or decreased according to blood pressure.	*Blood:* leukopenia, agranulocytosis, thrombocytopenia, aplastic anemia. *CNS:* dizziness, vertigo, paresthesias, headache, restlessness, weakness. *CV:* orthostatic hypotension. *EENT:* transient blurred vision, xanthopia. *GI:* anorexia, irritation, nausea, vomiting, cramping, diarrhea, constipation, pancreatitis. *GU:* glycosuria, allergic glomerulonephritis. *Metabolic:* fluid or electrolyte imbalances, dilutional hyponatremia, hypochloremia, hypokalemia, hyperuricemia, decreased calcium excretion, hyperglycemia. *Skin:* purpura, photosensitivity, rash, urticaria, necrotizing angiitis. *Other:* jaundice, fever, pulmonary edema and allergic pneumonitis, anaphylaxis, muscle spasm.
hydroflumethiazide Diucardin◆, Saluron	*Edema—* **Adults:** 25 mg to 200 mg P.O. daily in divided doses. Maintenance doses may be on intermittent or alternate day schedule. **Children:** 1 mg/Kg P.O. daily. *Hypertension—* **Adults:** 50 to 100 mg P.O. daily or b.i.d.	*Blood:* leukopenia, agranulocytosis, thrombocytopenia, aplastic anemia. CNS: dizziness, vertigo, paresthesias, headache, restlessness, weakness. *CV:* orthostatic hypotension. *EENT:* transient blurred vision, xanthopsia. *GI:* anorexia, irritation, nausea, vomiting, cramping, diarrhea, constipation, pancreatitis. *GU:* glycosuria, allergic glomerulonephritis. *Metabolic:* fluid imbalance, hypokalemia (in 30% to 50% of patients), dilutional hyponatremia, hypochloremic alkalosis, hyperuricemia (in 40% of males, less common in females), decreased calcium excretion, hyperglycemia. *Skin:* purpura, photosensitivity, rash, urticaria, necrotizing angiitis. *Other:* jaundice, fever, respiratory distress, anaphylaxis, muscle spasm.
mannitol Osmitrol◆	**Adults, and children over 12:** *Test dose for marked oliguria or suspected inadequate renal function*—200 mg/Kg or 12.5 g as a 15% or 20% solution I.V. over 3 to 5 minutes. Response adequate if 30 to 50 ml urine/hr is	*CNS:* rebound increase in intracranial pressure 8 to 12 hours after osmotic diuresis, headache, dizziness, confusion. *CV:* thrombophlebitis; hypotension; hypertension; tachycardia; angina-like chest pain; transient expansion of

INTERACTIONS	NURSING CONSIDERATIONS
Cholestyramine, colestipol: intestinal absorption of thiazides decreased. Keep doses as separate as possible. *Diazoxide:* increased antihypertensive, hyperglycemic, and hyperuricemic effects. Use together cautiously.	• Contraindicated in anuria; hypersensitivity to other thiazides or other sulfonamide derivatives. Use cautiously in severe renal disease, impaired hepatic function, progressive liver disease. • Monitor intake/output, weight, and serum electrolytes regularly. • Monitor serum potassium levels; consult with doctor and dietitian to provide high-potassium diet. Watch for hypokalemia (e.g., muscle weakness, cramps). May use with potassium-sparing diuretic to prevent potassium loss. • Monitor serum creatinine and BUN levels regularly. Not effective if these levels are more than twice normal. • Monitor blood uric acid levels, especially in patients with a history of gout. • Check insulin requirements in diabetics. May treat severe hyperglycemia with oral antidiabetic agents. • In hypertension, therapeutic response may be delayed several days. • Give in a.m. to prevent nocturia. • Elderly patients are especially susceptible to excessive diuresis. • A thiazide diuretic. • For treatment of anaphylaxis, see p. 1114.
Cholestyramine, colestipol: intestinal absorption of thiazides decreased. Keep doses as separate as possible. *Diazoxide:* increased antihypertensive, hyperglycemic, and hyperuricemic effects. Use together cautiously.	• Contraindicated in anuria; hypersensitivity to other thiazides or other sulfonamide-derived drugs. Use cautiously in severe renal disease, impaired hepatic function, progressive liver disease. • Monitor intake/output, weight, and serum electrolytes regularly. • Monitor serum potassium levels; consult with doctor and dietitian to provide high-potassium diet. Watch for hypokalemia (e.g., muscle weakness, cramps). May use with potassium-sparing diuretic to prevent potassium loss. • Monitor serum creatinine and BUN levels regularly. Not effective if these levels are more than twice normal. • Monitor blood uric acid levels, especially in patients with history of gout. • Check insulin requirements in diabetics. May treat severe hyperglycemia with oral antidiabetic agents. • Give in a.m. to prevent nocturia. • In hypertension, therapeutic response may be delayed several days. • Elderly patients are especially susceptible to excessive diuresis. • A long-acting thiazide diuretic. • For treatment of anaphylaxis, see p. 1114.
None significant.	• Contraindicated in anuria, severe pulmonary congestion, frank pulmonary edema, severe congestive heart disease, severe dehydration, metabolic edema, progressive renal disease or dysfunction, progressive heart failure during administration, active intracranial bleeding except during craniotomy. • Monitor vital signs (including CVP) at least hourly; intake/output hourly (report increasing oliguria); weight daily; renal function, fluid balance,

(continued on following page)

NAME	INDICATIONS & DOSAGE	SIDE EFFECTS
mannitol *(continued)*	excreted over 2 to 3 hours. *Treatment of oliguria*— 50 to 100 g I.V. as a 15% to 20% solution over 90 minutes to several hours. *Prevention of oliguria or acute renal failure*— 50 to 100 g I.V. of a concentrated (5% to 25%) solution. Exact concentration is determined by fluid requirements. *Edema*— 100 g as a 10% to 20% solution over 2- to 6-hour period. *To reduce intraocular pressure or intracranial pressure*—1.5 to 2 g/Kg as a 15% to 25% solution I.V. over 30 to 60 minutes. *To promote diuresis in drug intoxication*—5% to 10% solution continuously up to 200 g I.V., while maintaining 100 to 500 ml urinary output/hour and a positive fluid balance.	plasma volume during infusion, causing circulatory overload and pulmonary edema. *EENT:* blurred vision, rhinitis. *GI:* dry mouth, thirst, nausea, vomiting. *GU:* uricosuria, urinary retention. *Metabolic:* hyponatremia, hypokalemia, hyperkalemia, acidosis, cellular dehydration, water intoxication if unable to excrete. *Skin:* urticaria. *Other:* arm pain, lethargy, backache, chills, fever, transient muscle rigidity, cramps, weakness.
mercaptomerin sodium Thiomerin Sodium◆	*Edema*— **Adults:** 125 to 250 mg I.M. or S.C. daily. Maintenance with 1 to 2 times weekly dose. **Children:** 125 mg/m² I.M.	*Blood:* bone marrow depression, neutropenia, agranulocytosis. *CNS:* weakness, somnolence, dizziness, faintness, mental confusion, headache, paresthesia in excessive use. *CV:* orthostatic hypotension. *GI:* stomatitis, nausea, vomiting, thirst, anorexia, diarrhea (sometimes with bloody stools). *GU:* hematuria, albuminuria, casts in urine, related to nephrotoxicity. *Metabolic:* hypokalemia, hypochloremic alkalosis. *Skin:* pruritus, urticaria, rash, local ecchymoses and induration, cutaneous eruptions. *Other:* mercurialism (stomatitis, metallic taste, proteinuria, diarrhea) in excessive use; muscle cramps, hypersensitivity reactions, anaphylaxis, fever, chills, flushing, liver toxicity.
methazolamide Neptazane	*Glaucoma (open-angle, or preop in obstructive or closed-angle)*— **Adults:** 50 to 100 mg b.i.d. or t.i.d.	*Blood:* bone marrow depression, thrombocytopenia, leukopenia, hemolytic anemia, pancytopenia, agranulocytosis. *CNS:* paresthesias, drowsiness, confusion, weakness, nervousness, sedation, depression, dizziness, vertigo, headache.

INTERACTIONS	NURSING CONSIDERATIONS
	serum and urine Na+ and K+ levels. • Solution often crystallizes, especially at low temperatures. To redissolve, warm bottle in hot water bath, shake vigorously. Cool to body temperature before giving. Concentrations greater than 15% have greater tendency to crystallize. Do not use solution with undissolved crystals. • Infusions should always be given I.V. via an in-line filter. • Avoid infiltration; observe for inflammation, edema, potential necrosis. • For maximum pressure reduction before surgery, give 1 to 1½ hours preop. • Can be used to measure glomerular filtration rate. • Give frequent mouth care or fluids as permitted to relieve thirst. • An osmotic diuretic.
None significant.	• Contraindicated in renal insufficiency, acute or subacute nephritis. Use cautiously in impaired hepatic function. • Rarely used; agents available with less severe side effects. • Mercurial diuretic. Test for mercury hypersensitivity with 0.5 ml 24 hours before initiating therapy. Watch for signs of mercurialism. • Monitor urine for albumin, blood cells, and casts. Regularly monitor weight and serum electrolyte levels, especially potassium. Consult with doctor and dietitian to provide high-potassium diet. • Give in the morning for diuresis within 1 to 2 hours. • Rotate site of injections, massage gently; avoid edematous or adipose tissue; areas of poor circulation. Do not use I.V. • Good oral hygiene important to limit or prevent stomatitis. • Elderly patients are more susceptible to excessive dehydration with potential for circulatory collapse or thromboembolic phenomena. • For symptoms and treatment of anaphylaxis, see p. 1114.
None significant.	• Contraindicated in severe or absolute glaucoma; for long-term use in chronic noncongestive angle-closure glaucoma; in patients with depressed sodium or potassium serum levels, renal or hepatic disease or dysfunction, adrenal gland dysfunction, and hyperchloremic acidosis. Use cautiously in respiratory acidosis, emphysema, chronic lung disease. • Monitor intake/output, weight, and serum electrolytes frequently. • May cause false positive urine protein tests by alkalinizing urine. • A carbonic anhydrase inhibitor.

(continued on following page)

NAME	INDICATIONS & DOSAGE	SIDE EFFECTS
methazolamide *(continued)*		*EENT:* transient myopia, anosmia, tinnitus. *GI:* anorexia, nausea, vomiting, constipation, dry mouth, excessive thirst, loss of taste, diarrhea, weight loss. *GU:* dysuria, polyuria, crystalluria, renal calculi, urinary frequency, urethral colic. *Metabolic:* acidosis, hyperuricemia. *Skin:* urticaria and pruritus in hypersensitivity; rash. *Other:* malaise, pancreatitis, fever in hypersensitivity.
methyclothiazide Aquatensen, Duretic◆◆, Enduron	*Edema, hypertension*— **Adults:** 2.5 to 10 mg P.O daily.	*Blood:* leukopenia, agranulocytosis, thrombocytopenia, aplastic anemia. *CNS:* dizziness, vertigo, paresthesias, headache, restlessness, weakness. *CV:* orthostatic hypotension. *EENT:* transient blurred vision, xanthopsia. *GI:* anorexia, irritation, nausea, vomiting, cramping, diarrhea, constipation, pancreatitis. *GU:* glycosuria, allergic glomerulonephritis. *Metabolic:* fluid or electrolyte imbalances, hypokalemia, mild chloride deficit, hyperuricemia, frank gout, hyperglycemia, decreased calcium excretion, dilutional hyponatremia. *Skin:* purpura, photosensitivity, rash, urticaria, necrotizing angiitis. *Other:* jaundice, fever, respiratory distress, anaphylaxis, muscle spasm.
metolazone Diulo, Zaroxolyn◆	*Edema (cardiac failure)*— **Adults:** 5 to 10 mg P.O. daily. *Edema (renal disease)*— **Adults:** 5 to 20 mg P.O. daily. *Hypertension*— **Adults:** 2.5 to 5 mg P.O. daily. Maintenance dose determined by patient's blood pressure.	*Blood:* leukopenia. *CNS:* dizziness, drowsiness, fainting, vertigo, headache, weakness, restlessness. *CV:* orthostatic hypotension, excessive fluid loss, hemoconcentration, venous thrombosis, palpitations, chest pain. *EENT:* transient blurred vision. *GI:* constipation, nausea, vomiting, anorexia, diarrhea, abdominal bloating, epigastric distress, dry mouth. *GU:* glycosuria. *Metabolic:* hypokalemia, dilutional hyponatremia, hypochloremia, hypochloremic alkalosis, hyperuricemia, hyperglycemia, increase in creatinine or BUN, acute gouty attacks. *Skin:* urticaria, rash. *Other:* fatigue, muscle cramps or spasm, hepatitis, jaundice, chills.

INTERACTIONS	NURSING CONSIDERATIONS
	• Elderly patients are especially susceptible to excessive diuresis. • Diuretic effect decreases in acidosis.
Cholestyramine, colestipol: intestinal absorption of thiazides decreased. Keep doses as separate as possible. *Diazoxide:* increased antihypertensive, hyperglycemic, and hyperuricemic effects. Use together cautiously.	• Contraindicated in renal decompensation; anuria; hypersensitivity to other thiazides or other sulfonamide-derived drugs. Use cautiously in potassium depletion, renal disease or dysfunction, impaired hepatic function, progressive liver disease. • Monitor intake/output, weight, and serum electrolytes regularly. • Monitor serum potassium levels; consult with doctor and dietitian to provide high-potassium diet. Watch for hypokalemia (e.g., muscle weakness, cramps). May use with potassium-sparing diuretic to prevent potassium loss. • Check insulin requirements in diabetics. May treat severe hyperglycemia with oral antidiabetic agents. • Monitor serum creatinine and BUN levels regularly. Not effective if these levels are more than twice normal. • Monitor blood uric acid levels, especially in patients with a history of gout. • In hypertension, therapeutic response may be delayed several days. • Give in a.m. to prevent nocturia. • Elderly patients are especially susceptible to excessive diuresis. • A thiazide diuretic. • For treatment of anaphylaxis, see p. 1114.
Cholestyramine, colestipol: intestinal absorption of thiazides decreased. Keep doses as separate as possible. *Diazoxide:* increased antihypertensive, hyperglycemic, and hyperuricemic effects. Use together cautiously.	• Contraindicated in anuria; hepatic coma or pre-coma; hypersensitivity to thiazides or other sulfonamide-derived drugs. Use cautiously in hyperuricemia or gout and severely impaired renal function. • Monitor intake/output, weight, and serum electrolytes regularly. • Monitor serum potassium levels; consult with doctor and dietitian to provide high-potassium diet. Watch for hypokalemia (e.g., muscle weakness, cramps). May use with potassium-sparing diuretic to prevent potassium loss. • Check insulin requirements in diabetics. May treat severe hyperglycemia with oral antidiabetic agents. • Monitor blood uric acid levels, especially in patients with a history of gout. • In hypertension, therapeutic response may be delayed several days. • Give in a.m. to prevent nocturia. • Elderly patients are especially susceptible to excessive diuresis. • A thiazide-related diuretic. However, unlike thiazide diuretics, metolazone is effective in patients with decreased renal function. • Used as an adjunct in furosemide-resistant edema.

NAME	INDICATIONS & DOSAGE	SIDE EFFECTS
polythiazide Renese◆	*Hypertension—* **Adults:** 2 to 4 mg P.O. daily. *Edema (heart failure, renal failure)—* **Adults:** 1 to 4 mg P.O. daily.	*Blood:* leukopenia, agranulocytosis, thrombocytopenia, aplastic anemia. *CNS:* dizziness, vertigo, paresthesias, headache, restlessness, weakness. *CV:* orthostatic hypotension. *EENT:* transient blurred vision, xanthopsia. *GI:* anorexia, gastric irritation, nausea, vomiting, cramping, diarrhea, constipation, pancreatitis. *GU:* glycosuria, allergic glomerulonephritis. *Metabolic:* fluid or electrolyte imbalances, hypokalemia, mild chloride deficit, hyperuricemia, hyperglycemia, decreased calcium excretion, dilutional hyponatremia. *Skin:* purpura, photosensitivity, rash, urticaria, necrotizing angiitis. *Other:* jaundice, fever, respiratory distress, anaphylaxis, muscle spasm.
quinethazone Aquamox◆◆, Hydromox	*Edema—* **Adults:** 50 to 100 mg P.O. daily or 50 mg P.O. b.i.d. Occasionally, up to 150 to 200 mg P.O. daily may be needed.	*Blood:* leukopenia, agranulocytosis, thrombocytopenia, aplastic anemia. *CNS:* dizziness, vertigo, paresthesias, headache, restlessness, weakness. *CV:* orthostatic hypotension. *EENT:* transient blurred vision, xanthopsia. *GI:* anorexia, gastric irritation, nausea, vomiting, cramping, diarrhea, constipation, pancreatitis. *GU:* glycosuria, allergic glomerulonephritis. *Metabolic:* fluid imbalance, hypokalemia, mild chloride deficit, hyperuricemia, decreased calcium excretion, hyperglycemia, dilutional hyponatremia. *Skin:* purpura, photosensitivity, rash, urticaria, necrotizing angiitis. *Other:* jaundice, fever, respiratory distress, anaphylaxis, muscle spasm.
spironolactone Aldactone◆	*Edema—* **Adults:** 25 to 200 mg P.O. daily in divided doses. **Children:** initially, 3.3 mg/Kg P.O. daily in divided doses. *Hypertension—* **Adults:** 50 to 100 mg P.O. daily in divided doses. *Treatment of diuretic-induced hypokalemia—*	*CNS:* drowsiness, lethargy, confusion, headache, ataxia. *GI:* dry mouth, thirst, cramping, diarrhea. *Metabolic:* hyperkalemia, dehydration, hyponatremia, transient rise in BUN, acidosis. *Skin:* maculopapular and erythematous rashes, urticaria. *Other:* drug fever, gynecomastia,

INTERACTIONS	NURSING CONSIDERATIONS
Cholestyramine, colestipol: intestinal absorption of thiazides decreased. Keep doses as separate as possible. *Diazoxide:* increased antihypertensive, hyperglycemic, and hyperuricemic effects. Use together cautiously.	• Contraindicated in anuria; hypersensitivity to other thiazides or other sulfonamide-derived drugs. Use cautiously in severe renal disease, impaired hepatic function, allergies. • Monitor intake/output, weight, and serum electrolytes regularly. • Monitor serum potassium levels; consult with doctor and dietitian to provide high-potassium diet. Watch for hypokalemia (e.g., muscle weakness, cramps). May use with potassium-sparing diuretic to prevent potassium loss. • Monitor serum creatinine and BUN levels regularly. Not effective if these levels are more than twice normal. • Monitor blood uric acid levels, especially in patients with a history of gout. • Check insulin requirements in diabetics. May treat severe hyperglycemia with oral antidiabetic agents. • In hypertension, therapeutic response may be delayed several days. • Give in a.m. to prevent nocturia. • Elderly patients are especially susceptible to excessive diuresis. • A long-acting thiazide diuretic. • For treatment of anaphylaxis, see p. 1114.
Cholestyramine, colestipol: intestinal absorption of thiazides decreased. Keep doses as separate as possible. *Diazoxide:* increased antihypertensive, hyperglycemic, and hyperuricemic effects. Use together cautiously.	• Contraindicated in anuria; hypersensitivity to quinethazones, thiazides, or other sulfonamide-derived drugs. Use cautiously in severe renal disease, impaired hepatic function, allergies. • Monitor intake/output, weight, and serum electrolytes regularly. • Monitor serum potassium levels; consult with doctor and dietitian to provide high-potasium diet. Watch for hypokalemia (e.g., muscle weakness, cramps). May use with potassium-sparing diuretic to prevent potassium loss. • Monitor serum creatinine and BUN levels regularly. Not effective if these levels are more than twice normal. • Check insulin requirements in diabetics. May treat severe hyperglycemia with oral antidiabetic agents. • Monitor blood uric acid levels, especially in patients with a history of gout. • In hypertension, therapeutic response may be delayed several days. • Give in a.m. to prevent nocturia. • Elderly patients are especially susceptible to excessive diuresis. • A long-acting sulfonamide similar to thiazide diuretics. • For treatment of anaphylaxis, see p. 1114.
Aspirin: possible blocked spironolactone effect. Watch for diminished spironolactone response.	• Contraindicated in anuria, acute or progressive renal insufficiency, hyperkalemia. Use cautiously in fluid or electrolyte imbalances, impaired renal function, hepatic disease, pregnancy, lactation. If essential, nursing mother should stop breastfeeding infant. • Monitor serum potassium levels, electrolytes, intake/output, weight, and blood pressure regularly. • Potassium-sparing diuretic; useful as an adjunct to other diuretic therapy. Less potent diuretic than thiazide and loop types. Diuretic effect delayed 2 to 3 days when used alone. • Maximum antihypertensive response may be delayed up to 2 weeks.

(continued on following page)

NAME	INDICATIONS & DOSAGE	SIDE EFFECTS
spironolactone *(continued)*	**Adults:** 25 to 100 mg P.O. daily when oral potassium supplements are considered inappropriate. *Detection of primary hyperaldosteronism—* **Adults:** 400 mg P.O. daily for 4 days (short test) or for 3 to 4 weeks (long test). If hypokalemia and hypertension are corrected, a presumptive diagnosis of primary hyperaldosteronism is made.	decreased libido in males, impotence, irregular menses, amenorrhea, postmenopausal bleeding, hirsutism, deepened voice.
triamterene Dyrenium◆	*Diuresis—* **Adults:** initially, 100 mg P.O. b.i.d. after meals. Total daily dosage should not exceed 300 mg.	*Blood:* eosinophilia, leukopenia, megaloblastic anemia related to low folic acid levels. *CNS:* dizziness, drowsiness, weakness, headache. *CV:* hypotension. *EENT:* sore throat. *GI:* dry mouth, foul breath, diarrhea, nausea, vomiting. *Metabolic:* electrolyte imbalances (hyperkalemia, hyponatremia, hyperchloremic acidosis, mild nitrogen retention, hyperuricemia, magnesium depletion). *Skin:* photosensitivity, rash. *Other:* anaphylaxis, fever, muscle cramps.
trichlormethiazide Aquazide, Aquex, Diurese, Metahydrin, Naqua, Rochlomethiazide	*Edema—* **Adults:** 1 to 4 mg P.O. daily or in 2 divided dosages. *Hypertension—* **Adults:** 2 to 4 mg P.O. daily.	*Blood:* leukopenia, agranulocytosis, thrombocytopenia, aplastic anemia. *CNS:* dizziness, vertigo, paresthesias, headache, restlessness, weakness. *CV:* orthostatic hypotension. *EENT:* transient blurred vision, xanthopsia. *GI:* anorexia, gastric irritation, nausea, vomiting, cramping, diarrhea, constipation, pancreatitis. *GU:* glycosuria, allergic glomerulonephritis. *Metabolic:* fluid or electrolyte imbalances, hypokalemia, mild chloride deficit, hyperuricemia, decreased calcium excretion, dilutional hyponatremia, hyperglycemia. *Skin:* purpura, photosensitivity, rash, urticaria, necrotizing angiitis. *Other:* jaundice, fever, respiratory distress, anaphylaxis, muscle spasm.

INTERACTIONS	NURSING CONSIDERATIONS
	• Warn patient to avoid excessive ingestion of potassium-rich foods. • Elderly patients are more susceptible to excess diuresis. • Protect drug from light. • Breast cancer reported in some patients taking spironolactone, but cause-and-effect relationship not confirmed. Warn against taking drug indiscriminately. • Give with meals to enhance absorption. • Concomitant potassium supplement can lead to serious hyperkalemia.
None significant.	• Contraindicated in anuria, severe or progressive renal disease or dysfunction, severe hepatic disease, hyperkalemia. Use cautiously in impaired hepatic function, diabetes mellitus, pregnancy or lactation. • Watch for blood dyscrasias. • Monitor BUN and serum potassium, electrolytes. • A potassium-sparing diuretic, useful as an adjunct to other diuretic therapy. Less potent than thiazides and loop diuretics. Full diuretic effect delayed 2 to 3 days. • Warn patients to avoid excessive ingestion of potassium-rich foods. • Give medication after meals to prevent nausea. • Should be withdrawn gradually to prevent excessive rebound potassium excretion. • Concomitant potassium supplement can lead to serious hyperkalemia. • For treatment of anaphylaxis, see p. 1114.
Cholestyramine, colestipol: intestinal absorption of thiazides decreased. Keep doses as separate as possible. *Diazoxide:* increased antihypertensive, hyperglycemic, and hyperuricemic effects. Use together cautiously.	• Contraindicated in anuria; hypersensitivity to other thiazides, or other sulfonamide-derived drugs. Use cautiously in severe renal disease, impaired hepatic function. • Monitor intake/output, weight, and electrolytes regularly. • Monitor serum potassium levels; consult with doctor and dietitian to provide high-potassium diet. Watch for hypokalemia (e.g., muscle weakness, cramps). May use with potassium-sparing diuretic to prevent potassium loss. • Monitor serum creatinine and BUN levels regularly. Not effective if these levels are more than twice normal. • Check insulin requirements in diabetics. May treat severe hyperglycemia with oral antidiabetic agents. Monitor blood sugar. • Monitor blood uric acid levels, especially in patients with a history of gout. • In hypertension, therapeutic response may be delayed several days. • Give in a.m. to prevent nocturia. • Elderly patients are especially susceptible to excessive diuresis. • A long-acting thiazide diuretic. • For treatment of anaphylaxis, see p. 1114.

NAME	INDICATIONS & DOSAGE	SIDE EFFECTS
urea (carbamide) Ureaphil	*Intracranial or intraocular pressure—* **Adults:** 1 to 1.5 g/Kg as a 30% solution by slow I.V. infusion over 1 to 2.5 hours. **Children over 2 years:** 0.5 to 1.5 g/Kg slow I.V. infusion. **Children under 2 years:** as little as 0.1 g/Kg slow I.V. infusion. Maximum 4 ml/min. Maximum adult daily dose 120 g. To prepare 135 ml 30% solution, mix contents of 40 g vial of urea with 105 ml dextrose 5% or 10% in water or 10% invert sugar in water. Each ml of 30% solution provides 300 mg urea.	*Blood:* electrolyte depletion, especially sodium and potassium. *CNS:* fainting, disorientation, headache, agitation, nervousness. *CV:* hypotension, tachycardia. *GI:* nausea, vomiting. *Local:* irritation or necrotic sloughing may occur with extravasation.

INTERACTIONS	NURSING CONSIDERATIONS
None significant.	• Contraindicated in severely impaired renal function, marked dehydration, frank liver failure, active intracranial bleeding. Use cautiously in pregnancy, lactation, cardiac disease, liver impairment, or sickle cell damage with CNS involvement. • Avoid rapid I.V. infusion; may cause hemolysis or increased capillary bleeding. Avoid extravasation; may cause reactions ranging from mild irritation to necrosis. • Don't administer through the same infusion as blood. • Don't infuse into leg veins; may cause phlebitis or thrombosis, especially in the elderly. • Watch for hyponatremia or hypokalemia (muscle weakness, lethargy); may indicate electrolyte depletion before serum levels are reduced. • Maintain adequate hydration; monitor fluid and electrolyte balance. • In kidney disease, monitor BUN frequently. • Indwelling urethral catheter should be used in comatose patients to assure bladder emptying. • If satisfactory diuresis does not occur in 6 to 12 hours, urea should be discontinued and renal function reevaluated.

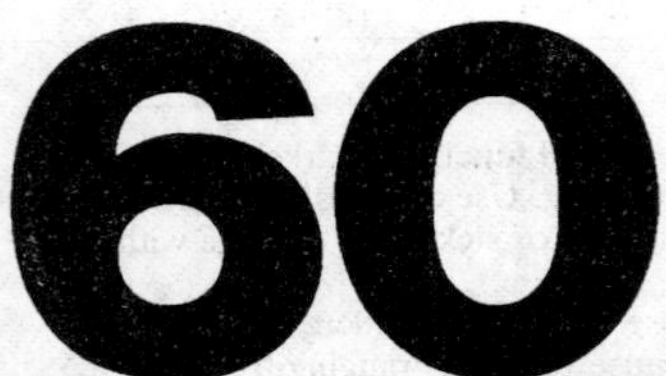

Electrolytes and replacement solutions

calcium salts
dextrans
magnesium sulfate
potassium acetate
potassium bicarbonate
potassium chloride
potassium gluconate
potassium phosphate
Ringer's injection
Ringer's injection lactated
sodium salts

These electrolyte solutions are used to replace lost anions or cations, or to prevent their depletion. Dextrans, however, are used mainly to expand plasma volume and early fluid replacements.

Major uses

- Replacement of specific anion or cation.
- Dextran is used as plasma volume expander and early fluid replacement.

Mechanism of action

- Replacement therapy.

Absorption, distribution, and excretion

- All are readily absorbed after I.V. administration.
- Soluble, ionized calcium is readily absorbed from the duodenum and proximal jejunum when the pH is 5 to 7, if parathyroid hormone and vitamin D levels are adequate.
- Potassium is slowly but well absorbed from the gastrointestinal tract.
- Dextran, magnesium, potassium and Ringer's solution are excreted by the kidneys.
- Calcium salts are excreted mainly in the feces; to a lesser degree, in urine.

Onset and duration

- Dextran effect on plasma volume occurs in several minutes after the end of infusion and lasts no longer than 24 hours.
- Onset of magnesium sulfate is 30 minutes after I.V. administration; 1 hour after I.M. Duration is 3 to 4 hours.
- With I.V. calcium, serum calcium levels rise immediately and return to normal in 30 minutes to 2 hours.
- Onset and duration of potassium varies according to form used.

Combination products

CALCIUM-SANDOZ FORTE♦♦: calcium lactate-gluconate 2.94 g, calcium carbonate 0.3 g, elemental sodium 275.8 mg, and 500 mg elemental calcium.
DUO-K: 20 mEq potassium, 3.3 mEq chloride (from potassium gluconate, and potassium chloride).
GRAMCAL♦♦: calcium lactate gluconate 3,080 mg, calcium carbonate 1,500 mg, and potassium 390 mg provides 1,000 mg of elemental calcium.

KAOCHLOR-EFF: 20 mEq potassium, 20 mEq chloride (from potassium chloride, potassium citrate, potassium bicarbonate, and betaine hydrochloride).
KEFF: 20 mEq each potassium and chloride (potassium chloride, potassium carbonate, potassium bicarbonate, and betaine hydrochloride).
KLORVESS: 20 mEq each potassium and chloride (from potassium chloride, potassium bicarbonate, and l-lysine mono-hydrochloride).
KOLYUM: 20 mEq potassium, 3.3 mEq chloride (from potassium gluconate and potassium chloride).
NEUTRA-PHOS: phosphorus 250 mg, sodium 164 mg, potassium 278 mg, through dibasic and monobasic sodium and potassium phosphate.
POTASSIUM-SANDOZ♦♦: potassium chloride 23.1% and potassium bicarbonate 15.4% (12 mEq potassium and 8 mEq chloride).
POTASSIUM TRIPLEX: 15 mEq potassium (from potassium acetate, potassium bicarbonate, and potassium citrate).
THERMOTABS: 450 mg sodium chloride and 30 mg potassium chloride, and 18 mg calcium carbonate and 200 mg dextrose.
TWIN-K: 20 mEq potassium (as potassium gluconate and potassium citrate).

POINTERS FOR POTASSIUM REPLACEMENT

LIQUIDS

- Never switch potassium products without a doctor's order.
- Give potassium in 2 to 4 doses per day over several days to avoid severe hyperkalemia. Give it with or after meals with a full glass of water or fruit juice to minimize GI irritation. Follow the manufacturer's recommendations for dilution. Tell patients to sip liquid potassium products slowly to minimize GI irritation. Give to patients on fluid restriction at mealtime.

EFFERVESCENT TABLETS

- Tell the patient to drink the solution after effervescence has subsided to minimize ingestion of HCO_3. Make sure the patient drinks all of the solution.

POWDERS

- Make sure powder is completely dissolved.
- A helpful tip: If patient's diet allows, mix total daily dose of potassium powder in boiling water and then add one packet of gelatin dessert, adding usual amount of cold water to the gelatin. Once the mixture sets, it can be divided into four servings or "doses."

PARENTERAL

- Always administer slowly as dilute solutions (not to exceed 80 mEq/L); do not exceed 20 mEq/hour. Do not exceed 150 mEq/day in adults; 3 mEq/Kg in children.
- EKG monitoring best indicates tissue potassium levels. Also monitor plasma potassium levels. Never use until urine flow is established.
- Don't administer to any patient with acute dehydration or severe renal impairment.
- Observe for pain and redness at injection site.

NAME	INDICATIONS & DOSAGE	SIDE EFFECTS
calcium salts **calcium chloride** **calcium gluceptate** **calcium gluconate** **calcium lactate**	*Hypocalcemia, hypocalcemic tetany, hypocalcemia during exchange transfusions, cardiac resuscitation for inotropic effect when epinephrine has failed; magnesium intoxication*— **Adults and children:** initially 500 mg to 1 g elemental calcium I.V. with further dosage based on serum calcium determinations. Dosage with calcium chloride (1 g [10 ml] yields 13.5 mEq Ca++): *Magnesium intoxication*— **Adults and children:** initially 500 mg I.V. with further doses based on calcium and magnesium determination. *Cardiac arrest*—0.5 to 1 g I.V. not to exceed 1 ml/min or 200 to 800 mg into the ventricular cavity. *Hypocalcemia*—500 mg to 1 g I.V. at intervals of 1 to 3 days, determined by serum calcium levels. Dosage with calcium gluconate (1 g [10 ml] yields 4.5 mEq Ca++): *Hypocalcemia*— **Adults:** 500 mg to 1 g I.V., repeated q 1 to 3 days p.r.n. as determined by serum calcium levels. Further doses depend on serum calcium determination. **Children:** 500 mg/Kg I.V. daily. Rate of infusion should not exceed 0.5 ml/min. Dosage with calcium gluceptate (1.1 g [5 ml] yields 4.5 mEq Ca++) and calcium salts (18 mg [1 ml] yields 0.898 mEq Ca++): *Hypocalcemia*— **Adults:** initially, 5 to 20 ml I.V. with further doses based on serum calcium determinations. If I.V. injection is impossible, 2 to 5 ml I.M. Average adult oral dose 1 to 2 g/day P.O. in divided doses, t.i.d. or q.i.d. Average oral dose for children 45 to 65 mg/Kg P.O. daily, in divided doses, t.i.d. or q.i.d. *During exchange transfusions*— **Adults and children:** 0.5 ml I.V. after each 100 ml blood exchanged.	*CNS:* from I.V. use, tingling sensations, sense of oppression or heat waves; with rapid I.V. injection, syncope. *CV:* mild fall in blood pressure; with rapid I.V. injection, vasodilation, bradycardia, cardiac arrhythmias, and cardiac arrest. *GI:* with oral ingestion, irritation, hemorrhage, constipation; with I.V. administration chalky taste; with oral calcium chloride, gastrointestinal hemorrhage, nausea, vomiting, thirst, abdominal pain. *GU:* hypercalcemia, polyuria, renal calculi. *Local:* with S.C. injection, pain and irritation; with I.V., venous irritation. *Skin:* local reaction if calcium salts given I.M.: burning, necrosis, sloughing of tissue, cellulitis, soft tissue calcification.

• Also available in Canada.
•• Available in Canada only.
Unmarked trade names available in United States only.

INTERACTIONS	NURSING CONSIDERATIONS
Digitalis glycosides: increased digitalis toxicity; administer calcium very cautiously (if at all) to digitalized patients.	• Contraindicated in ventricular fibrillation, hypercalcemia, renal calculi. Use cautiously in sarcoidosis, renal or cardiac disease, and digitalized patients. Use calcium chloride cautiously in cor pulmonale, respiratory acidosis, or respiratory failure. • Monitor EKG when giving calcium I.V. Such injections should not exceed 0.7 to 1.5 mEq/minute. Stop if patient complains of discomfort. Following I.V. injection, patient should remain recumbent for a short while. • I.M. injection should be given in the gluteal region, adults; lateral thigh, infants. I.M. route used only in emergencies when no I.V. route available. • Monitor blood calcium levels frequently. Report abnormalities. • Hypercalcemia may result after large doses in chronic renal failure. • I.V. route generally recommended in children, but not by scalp vein. • Solutions should be warmed to body temperature. • Calcium chloride and calcium gluconate should be given I.V. only. • Severe necrosis and sloughing of tissues follow extravasation. • Give oral calcium products 1 to 1½ hours after meals or with milk. • Oxalic acid (found in rhubarb and spinach), phytic acid (in bran and whole cereals), and phosphorus (in milk and dairy products) may interfere with absorption of calcium. Monitor calcium levels.

NAME	INDICATIONS & DOSAGE	SIDE EFFECTS
dextrans (low molecular weight dextran) Dextran 40, Gentran 40, LMVD, Rheomacrodex◆	*Plasma volume expansion*— Dosage of 10% solution by I.V. infusion depends on amount of fluid loss. First 500 ml of Dextran 40 may be infused rapidly with central venous pressure monitoring. Infuse remaining dose slowly. Total daily dose not to exceed 2 g/Kg body weight. If therapy continued past 24 hours, do not exceed 1 g/Kg daily. Continue for no longer than 5 days. *Reduction of blood sludging*— 500 ml of 10% solution by I.V. infusion.	*Blood:* decreased level of hemoglobin and hematocrit; with higher doses, increased bleeding time. *CV:* fluid shift from extravascular space, headache. *GI:* hypersensitivity reaction, increased specific gravity, and viscosity of urine. *GU:* tubular stasis and blocking, possible renal failure. *Skin:* hypersensitivity reaction, urticaria. *Other:* increased SGPT and SGOT levels, anaphylaxis.
dextrans (high molecular weight dextran) Dextran 70, Dextran 75◆, Gentran 75, Macrodex◆	*Plasma expander*— **Adults:** usual dose 30 g (500 ml of 6% solution) I.V. In emergency situations, may be administered at rate of 1.2 to 2.4 g (20 to 40 ml) per minute. In normovolemic or nearly normovolemic patients, rate of infusion should not exceed 240 mg (4 ml per minute). Total dose during first 24 hours not to exceed 1.2 g/Kg; actual dose depends on amount of fluid loss and resultant hemoconcentration and must be determined for each patient.	*Blood:* decreased level of hemoglobin and hematocrit; with doses of 15 ml/Kg body weight, prolonged bleeding time and significant suppression of platelet function. *CV:* fluid shift from extravascular space. *GI:* nausea, vomiting. *GU:* increases specific gravity and viscosity of urine, tubular stasis and blocking, possible renal failure. *Skin:* hypersensitivity reaction, urticaria. *Other:* fever, arthralgia, increased SGPT and SGOT levels, nasal congestion, anaphylaxis.
magnesium sulfate	*Hypomagnesemia*— **Adults:** 1 g or 8.12 mEq of 50% solution (2 ml) I.M. q 6 hours for 4 doses, depending on serum magnesium level. *Severe hypomagnesemia (serum magnesium 0.8 mEq/liter or less, with symptoms)*—6 g or 50 mEq of 50% solution I.V. in 1 liter of solution over 4 hours. Subsequent doses depend on serum magnesium levels. *Magnesium supplementation in hyperalimentation*— **Adults:** 8 to 24 mEq/day added to hyperalimentation solution.	*CNS:* toxicity: weak or absent deep-tendon reflexes, flaccid paralysis, hypothermia, drowsiness, respiratory depression or paralysis; hypocalcemia (perioral paresthesias, twitching carpopedal spasm, tetancy seizures). *CV:* slow, weak pulse; hypocalcemia (cardiac arrhythmias), hypotension. *Skin:* flushing, sweating.

INTERACTIONS	NURSING CONSIDERATIONS
None significant.	• Contraindicated in marked hemostatic defects; marked cardiac decompensation or pulmonary edema; renal disease with severe oliguria or anuria; or extreme dehydration. Use cautiously in active hemorrhage; may cause additional blood loss. • Hazardous when given to patients with heart failure, especially if in saline solution. Use dextrose solution instead. • Works as plasma expander via colloidal osmotic effect, thereby drawing fluid from interstitial to intravascular space. Provides plasma expansion slightly greater than volume infused. Watch for circulatory overload. • Monitor urine flow rate during administration. If oliguria or anuria occur or are not relieved by infusion, stop dextran and give osmotic diuretic. • Hydration should be assessed before starting therapy; otherwise, use urine or serum osmolarity, because urine specific gravity is affected by urine dextran concentration. • Check hemoglobin and hematocrit; don't allow to fall below 30% by volume. • Draw blood samples *before* starting infusion. • Store at constant 25° C. (77° F.). May precipitate in storage but can be heated to dissolve if necessary.
None significant.	• Contraindicated in marked hemostatic defects; marked cardiac decompensation or pulmonary edema; renal disease with severe oliguria or anuria; and extreme dehydration. Use cautiously in active hemorrhage; may cause additional blood loss. • Hazardous when given to patients with heart failure, especially if in saline solution. Use dextrose solution instead. • Works as plasma expander via colloidal osmotic effect, thereby drawing fluid from interstitial to intravascular space. Provides plasma expansion slightly greater than volume infused. Watch for circulatory overload. • Monitor urine flow rate during administration. If oliguria or anuria occur or are not relieved by infusion, stop dextran and give osmotic diuretic. • Hydration should be assessed before starting therapy; otherwise, use urine or serum osmolarity, because urine specific gravity is affected by the urine dextran concentration. • Check hemoglobin and hematocrit; don't allow to fall below 30% by volume. • Draw blood samples *before* starting infusion. • May precipitate in storage but can be heated to dissolve if necessary. • Dextran 70 and Dextran 75 can be used interchangeably. Differ significantly from Dextran 40—do not interchange.
None significant.	• Contraindicated in impaired renal function, myocardial damage, heart block, and in actively progressing labor. Use parenteral magnesium with extreme caution in patients receiving digitalis preparations. Treating magnesium toxicity with calcium in such patients could cause serious alterations in cardiac conduction and heart block may result. • Maximum infusion rate 150 mg/min. Rapid drip causes feeling of heat. • Keep I.V. calcium available to reverse magnesium intoxication. • Monitor vital signs every 15 minutes when giving I.V. for severe hypomagnesemia. Watch for respiratory depression and signs of heart block. Respirations should be about 16 per minute before dose is given. • Monitor intake/output. Output should be 100 ml or more during 4-hour period before dose. • Test knee jerk and patellar reflexes before each additional dose. If absent, give no more magnesium until reflexes return; otherwise, patient may develop temporary respiratory failure and need artificial respiration or I.V. administration of calcium.

(continued on following page)

NAME	INDICATIONS & DOSAGE	SIDE EFFECTS
magnesium sulfate *(continued)*	**Children over 6 years:** 2 to 10 mEq/day added to hyperalimentation solution. Each 2 ml of 50% solution contains 1 g or 8.12 mEq magnesium sulfate.	
potassium acetate	*Potassium replacement*—I.V. should be used for life-threatening hypokalemia or when oral replacement not feasible. Give no more than 20 mEq/hour in concentration of 40 mEq/liter or less. Total 24-hour dose should not exceed 150 mEq (3 mEq/Kg in children). Potassium replacement should be done with EKG monitoring and frequent serum K+ determinations. *Prevention of hypokalemia*— **Adults and children:** 20 mEq P.O. daily, in divided doses b.i.d., t.i.d., or q.i.d. *Potassium depletion*— **Adults and children:** usual dose 40 to 100 mEq P.O. daily, in divided doses b.i.d., t.i.d., or q.i.d.	*Signs of hyperkalemia*— *CNS:* paresthesias of the extremities, listlessness, mental confusion, weakness or heaviness of legs, flaccid paralysis. *CV:* peripheral vascular collapse with fall in blood pressure, cardiac arrhythmias, heart block, possible cardiac arrest, EKG changes (prolonged P-R intervals, wide QRS, S-T segment depression; tall tented T wave). *GI:* nausea, vomiting, abdominal pain, diarrhea, bowel ulceration after enteric-coated tablets. *GU:* oliguria. *Skin:* cold skin, gray pallor.
potassium bicarbonate K-Lyte, K-Lyte DS	*Hypokalemia*— 25 mEq or 50 mEq tablet dissolved in water 1 to 4 times a day.	*CNS:* paresthesias of the extremities, listlessness, mental confusion, weakness or heaviness of legs, flaccid paralysis. *CV:* peripheral vascular collapse with fall in blood pressure, cardiac arrhythmias, heart block, possible cardiac arrest, EKG changes (prolonged P-R interval, wide QRS, S-T segment depression, tall tented T waves). *GI:* nausea, vomiting, abdominal pain, diarrhea, ulcerations, hemorrhage, obstruction, perforation. *GU:* oliguria. *Skin:* cold skin, gray pallor.
potassium chloride K-Lor, K-Lyte/ Cl, K-10◆, Kaochlor S-F 10%, Kaochlor 10%, Kaon, Kaon-Cl, Kaon-Cl 20%, Kato Powder, KayCiel◆, Klor-10%, Kloride, Klorvess, Pfiklor, Slow K◆	*Hypokalemia*— 40 to 100 mEq P.O. divided into 3 to 4 doses daily for treatment; 20 mEq for prevention. Further dose based on serum potassium determinations. I.V. route when oral replacement not feasible or when hypokalemia life-threatening. Usual dose 20 mEq/hour in concentration of 40	*Signs of hyperkalemia:* *CNS:* paresthesias of the extremities, listlessness, mental confusion, weakness or heaviness of legs, flaccid paralysis. *CV:* peripheral vascular collapse with fall in blood pressure, cardiac arrhythmias, heart block, possible cardiac arrest, EKG changes (prolonged P-R interval, wide QRS; S-T segment

INTERACTIONS	NURSING CONSIDERATIONS
	• Check magnesium levels after repeated doses. • After giving to toxemic mothers within 24 hours before delivery, watch newborn for signs of magnesium toxicity, including neuromuscular and respiratory depression.
None significant.	• Contraindicated in severe renal impairment with oliguria, anuria, azotemia, and untreated Addison's disease; acute dehydration, hyperkalemia, hyperkalemic form of familial periodic paralysis, and conditions associated with extensive tissue breakdown. Use cautiously in cardiac disease, patients receiving potassium-sparing diuretics, and those with renal impairment. • Monitor: EKG for signs of hypokalemia or hyperkalemia; serum potassium level, renal function, BUN, and serum creatinine; intake/output. Never give potassium postop until urine flow is established. • Give slowly as diluted solution; potentially fatal hyperkalemia may result from too rapid infusion. • Observe for pain and redness at injection site. Large-bore needle reduces local irritation. • Parenteral potassium given by infusion only; never I.V. push, or I.M. • Watch for signs of GI ulceration: obstruction, hemorrhage, pain, distention, severe vomiting, bleeding. • Reconstitute potassium acetate powder with liquids; give after meals.
None significant.	• Contraindicated in severe renal impairment with oliguria, anuria, azotemia, and untreated Addison's disease; also in acute dehydration, hyperkalemia, hyperkalemic familial periodic paralysis, and conditions associated with extensive tissue breakdown. Use with caution in cardiac disease, and patients receiving potassium-sparing diuretics. • Monitor serum potassium level, BUN, serum creatinine, and intake/output. • Never switch potassium products without a doctor's order. • Dissolve potassium bicarbonate tablets in 6 to 8 ounces of cold water. • Take with meals and sip slowly over a 5- to 10- minute period. • Potassium bicarbonate cannot be given instead of potassium chloride. • Potassium bicarbonate does not correct hypokalemic alkalosis. • Available in lime or orange flavor. Check for patient flavor preference.
None significant.	• Contraindicated in severe renal impairment with oliguria, anuria, azotemia and untreated Addison's disease; also in acute dehydration, hyperkalemia, hyperkalemic form of familial periodic paralysis, conditions associated with extensive tissue breakdown. Use with caution in cardiac disease, patients receiving potassium-sparing diuretics. • Potassium should not be given during immediate postoperative period until urine flow is established. • Parenteral potassium given by infusion only; never I.V. push or I.M. • Give slowly as dilute solution; potentially fatal hyperkalemia may result from too rapid infusion.

(continued on following page)

NAME	INDICATIONS & DOSAGE	SIDE EFFECTS
potassium chloride *(continued)*	mEq/liter or less. Total daily dose not to exceed 150 mEq (3 mEq/Kg in children). Potassium replacement should be done only with EKG monitoring and frequent serum K+ determinations.	depression, tall, tented T waves). *GI:* nausea, vomiting, abdominal pain, diarrhea, *GI* ulcerations (possible stenosis, hemorrhage, obstruction, perforation). *GU:* oliguria. *Skin:* cold skin, gray pallor.
potassium gluconate Kalinate Elixir, Kaon Liquid, Kaon Tablets♦, Potassium Rougier♦♦	*Hypokalemia*—40 to 200 mEq P.O. divided into 3 to 4 doses daily for treatment; 20 mEq/day for prevention. Further dose based on serum potassium determinations.	*Signs of hyperkalemia*— *CNS:* paresthesias of the extremities, listlessness, mental confusion, weakness or heaviness of legs, flaccid paralysis. *CV:* peripheral vascular collapse with fall in blood pressure, cardiac arrhythmias, heart block, possible cardiac arrest, EKG changes (prolonged P-R interval, wide QRS, S-T segment depression, tall tented T waves). *GI:* nausea, vomiting, abdominal pain, diarrhea, GI ulcerations with oral products (especially enteric coated tablets); ulcerations may be accompanied by stenosis, hemorrhage obstruction, perforation. *GU:* oliguria. *Skin:* cold skin, gray pallor.
potassium phosphate	*Hypokalemia*—I.V. should be used when oral replacement not feasible or when hypokalemia life-threatening. Dosage up to 20 mEq/hour in concentration of 60 mEq/liter or less. Total daily dose not to exceed 150 mEq. Should be done only with EKG monitoring and frequent serum K determinations. Average P.O. dose: 40 to 200 mEq.	*Signs of hyperkalemia*— *CNS:* paresthesias of the extremities, listlessness, mental confusion, weakness or heaviness of legs, flaccid paralysis; hypocalcemia—perioral paresthesias, twitching, carpopedal spasm, tetany and seizures. *CV:* peripheral vascular collapse with fall in blood pressure, cardiac arrhythmias, heart block, possible cardiac arrest, EKG changes (prolonged P-R interval wide QRS, S-T segment depression, tall tented T waves). *GI:* nausea, vomiting, abdominal pain, diarrhea. *GU:* oliguria. *Skin:* cold skin, gray pallor. *Other:* soft tissue calcification.

INTERACTIONS	NURSING CONSIDERATIONS
	• Give oral potassium supplements with extreme caution because its many forms deliver varying amounts of potassium. Never switch products without a doctor's order. Tell the doctor if the patient tolerates one product better than another. • Sugar-free liquid available (Kaochlor S-F 10%). • Have patient sip liquid potassium slowly to minimize GI irritation. • Give with or after meals with full glass of water or fruit juice to lessen GI distress. • Make sure powders are completely dissolved before giving. • Enteric-coated tablets not recommended due to potential GI bleeding and small bowel ulcerations. • Tablets in wax matrix sometimes lodge in esophagus and cause ulceration in cardiac patients who have esophageal compression due to enlarged left atrium. In such patients and in those with esophageal stasis or obstruction, use liquid form. • Often used orally with diuretics that cause potassium excretion. Potassium chloride most useful since diuretics waste chloride ion. Hypokalemic alkalosis treated best with potassium chloride.
None significant.	• Contraindicated in severe renal impairment with oliguria, anuria, azotemia, and untreated Addison's disease; also in acute dehydration, hyperkalemia, hyperkalemic form of familial periodic paralysis, and conditions associated with extensive tissue breakdown. Use with caution in cardiac disease; patients receiving potassium-sparing diuretics. • Monitor serum potassium level, BUN, serum creatinine, and intake/output. • Give oral potassium supplements with extreme caution because its many forms deliver varying amounts of potassium. Never switch products without doctor's order. If one product is tolerated better than another, tell doctor so brand and dosage can be changed. • Have patient sip liquid potassium slowly to minimize GI irritation. • Give with or after meals with full glass of water or fruit juice to lessen GI distress. • Enteric-coated tablets not recommended due to potential for GI bleeding and small-bowel ulcerations.
None significant.	• Contraindicated in severe renal impairment with oliguria, anuria, azotemia, and untreated Addison's disease; also acute dehydration, hyperkalemia, hyperkalemic form of familial periodic paralysis, extensive tissue damage, hypocalcemia. Use with caution in cardiac disease, patients receiving potassium-sparing diuretics. • Never give potassium postop until urine flow is established. • Monitor: EKG for indications of tissue potassium levels; plasma potassium and calcium levels as well as BUN and creatinine for renal function; inorganic phosphorus levels; intake/output. • Give slowly as dilute solution; potentially fatal hyperkalemia may result from too rapid an infusion. • Observe for pain and redness at injection site. • Parenteral potassium given by infusion only; never I.V. push or I.M. • Rarely used due to major side effects of hypocalcemia, renal damage, shock, and soft tissue calcification. • Reconstitute powder in juice. Give after meals.

NAME	INDICATIONS & DOSAGE	SIDE EFFECTS
Ringer's injection	*Fluid and electrolyte replacement—* **Adults and children:** dose highly individualized but generally, 1.5 to 3 liters (2 to 6% body weight) infused I.V. over 18 to 24 hours.	*CV:* fluid overload.
Ringer's injection, lactated (Hartmann's solution)	*Fluid and electrolyte replacement—* **Adults and children:** dose highly individualized, but generally 1.5 to 3 liters (2 to 6 % body weight) infused I.V. over 18 to 24 hours.	*CV:* fluid overload.
sodium salts **sodium chloride**	*Highly individualized fluid and electrolyte replacement in hyponatremia due to electrolyte loss or in severe salt depletion—* 400 ml of 3% or 5% solutions only with frequent electrolyte determination and only if given slowly intravenously; *with .45% solution:* 3 to 8% of body weight, according to deficiencies, over 18 to 24 hours; *with 0.9% solution:* 2 to 6% of body weight, according to deficiencies, over 18 to 24 hours. *Management of "heat cramp" due to excessive perspiration—* **Adults:** 1 g P.O. with every glass of water.	*CV:* aggravation of congestive heart failure; edema and pulmonary edema if too much given, or given too rapidly. *Metabolic:* aggravation of existing acidosis with excessive infusion. *Other:* hypernatremia with excessive infusion; serious electrolyte disturbance, loss of potassium.

INTERACTIONS	NURSING CONSIDERATIONS
None significant.	• Contraindicated in renal failure, except as emergency volume expander. Use cautiously in CHF, circulatory insufficiency, kidney dysfunction, hypoproteinemia, or pulmonary edema. • Ringer's injection contains sodium, 147 mEq/liter, potassium, 4 mEq/liter; calcium 4.5 mEq liter; and chloride, 155.5 mEq/liter. This electrolyte content is insufficient for treating severe electrolyte deficiencies. • May be given with dextrose injection.
None significant.	• Contraindicated in renal failure, except as emergency volume expander. Use cautiously in CHF, circulatory insufficiency, kidney dysfunction, hypoproteinemia, and pulmonary edema. • Ringer's injection, lactated contains sodium 130 mEq/liter; potassium 4 mEq/liter; calcium 2.7 mEq/liter; chloride 109.7 mEq/liter; and lactate 27 mEq/liter. • Approximates more closely the electrolyte concentration in blood plasma than Ringer's injection. • May be given with dextrose injection.
None significant.	• Use with caution in congestive heart failure, circulatory insufficiency, kidney dysfunction, hypoproteinemia. • Infuse 3% and 5% solutions very slowly and with caution to avoid pulmonary edema. Use only for critical situations. Observe patient constantly. • Concentrates available for addition to parenteral nutrient solutions. Don't confuse these small volumes of parenterals with sodium chloride injection isotonic 0.9%. READ LABEL carefully.

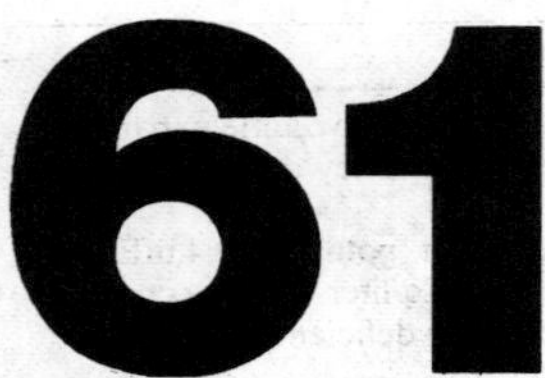

Potassium-removing resin

sodium polystyrene sulfonate

This potassium-removing resin is useful for reducing excessive potassium levels.

Major uses

• Treatment of hyperkalemia; useful in chronic renal failure. Because it is slow-acting and gives a variable response, sodium polystyrene sulfonate should not be used as primary treatment of acute renal failure or burns where there is rapid tissue breakdown.

Mechanism of action

• Ion exchange: sodium ions of resin partially released in intestines, replaced by up to 1 milliequivalent of potassium (plus some calcium, magnesium, and ammonium) per gram of resin.
• Potassium excretion: potassium-bearing resin excreted in feces.

Absorption, distribution, and excretion

• Distribution through intestines (especially large intestine) where exchange occurs.
• Excretion via feces.

Onset and duration

• Ion exchange requires approximately 6 hours in intestines.
• Action slow, unpredictable, variable.

Combination products

None.

FOODS FOR A LOW-POTASSIUM DIET

A low-potassium diet provides no more than 2 g (50 mEq) of potassium daily. Foods low in potassium include the following:

DAIRY PRODUCTS	MG PER 100 GRAMS
Cheese, cheddar	82
Cheese, cream	85
Eggs	98
Butter	23

FRUITS AND VEGETABLES	
Applesauce	65
Blueberries	81
Cranberry juice	10
Pears, canned	84
Pineapple, canned	96
Beans, snap	95
Corn, canned	97
Peas, canned	96

MEAT, FISH, POULTRY	MG PER 100 GRAMS
	350 (approximately)

BREAD AND CEREAL	
Rice	28
Noodles	44
Macaroni	61
Bread, cracked wheat	134
Bread, white	105
Bread, rye	115
Oatmeal	61
Cornflakes	120
Corn grits	11
Farina	188

MANAGING HYPERKALEMIA

It's time to count potassium grams when serum potassium is above 5.5 mEq/liter causing severe muscle weakness, paralysis, abdominal distention, diarrhea, oliguria, and anuria.

You can expect potassium excess to develop in patients with inadequate renal function; adrenocortical insufficiency; potassium-sparing diuretics; and increased potassium load, as in severe tissue damage, metabolic acidosis, or overtreatment with potassium salts.

One way to control hyperkalemia is to withhold dietary potassium. Use the chart above as a guide for measuring and minimizing potassium intake.

NAME	INDICATIONS & DOSAGE	SIDE EFFECTS
sodium polystyrene sulfonate Kayexalate◆	*Hyperkalemia—* **Adults:** 15 g daily to q.i.d. in water or sorbitol (3 to 4 ml/g of resin). **Children:** 1 g of resin for each mEq of potassium to be removed. Oral administration preferred since drug should remain in intestine for at least 6 hours; otherwise consider nasogastric administration. Nasogastric administration: mix dose with appropriate medium: aqueous suspension, or diet appropriate for renal failure; instill in plastic tube. Rectal administration: **Adults:** 30 to 50 g/100 ml of sorbitol q 6 hours as warm emulsion deep into sigmoid colon (20 cm). In persistent vomiting or paralytic ileus, high-retention enema of sodium polystyrene sulfonate (30 g) suspended in 200 ml of 10% methylcellulose, 10% dextrose, or 25% sorbitol.	*GI:* constipation, fecal impaction (in elderly), anorexia, gastric irritation, nausea, vomiting, diarrhea (with sorbitol emulsions). *Other:* hypokalemia, hypocalcemia, hypomagnesemia, sodium retention.

◆ Also available in Canada.
◆◆ Available in Canada only.
Unmarked trade names available in United States only.

INTERACTIONS	NURSING CONSIDERATIONS
Antacids and laxatives (nonabsorbable cation-donating type, including magnesium hydroxide): systemic alkalosis, reduced potassium exchange capability. Don't use together.	• Use with caution in elderly patients and those on digitalis therapy, with severe congestive heart failure, severe hypertension, and marked edema. • Treatment may result in potassium deficiency. Monitor serum potassium at least once daily. Usually stopped when potassium level is reduced to 4 or 5 mEq/liter. Watch for other signs of hypokalemia: irritability, confusion, cardiac arrhythmias, EKG changes, severe muscle weakness and sometimes paralysis, and digitalis toxicity in digitalized patients. • Monitor for symptoms of other electrolyte deficiencies (magnesium, calcium) since drug is nonselective. Monitor serum calcium determination in patients receiving sodium polystyrene therapy for more than 3 days. Supplementary calcium may be needed. • Watch for sodium overload. About ⅓ of resin's sodium stays in body. • Use only fresh suspensions. Stir just before use. Discard unused portions after 24 hours. • Do not heat resin. This will impair effectiveness of drug. • Chill oral suspension for greater palatability. • If sorbitol is given, it may be mixed with resin suspension. • Consider solid form. Resin cookie recipe is available; perhaps pharmacist or dietitian can supply. • Watch for constipation in oral or nasogastric administration. Use sorbitol (10 to 20 ml of 70% syrup every 2 hours as needed) to produce 1 or 2 watery stools daily. • Mix polystyrene-resin only with water and sorbitol for oral or rectal use. Do not use other vehicles (i.e., mineral oil) for rectal administration to prevent impactions. Ion exchange requires aqueous medium. Sorbitol content prevents impaction. • Prevent fecal impaction in elderly by administering resin rectally. Give cleansing enema before rectal administration. Explain necessity of retaining enema to patient. Retention for 6 to 10 hours is ideal, but 30 to 60 minutes is acceptable. • Prepare rectal dose at room temperature. Stir emulsion gently during administration. • Use French 28 rubber tube for rectal dose; insert 20 cm into sigmoid colon. Tape tube in place. Alternately consider a 30 ml Foley catheter with balloon inflated distal to anal sphincter to aid in retention. Use gravity flow. Drain returns constantly through Y-tube connection. When giving rectally, place patient in knee-chest position or with hips on pillow for a while if back-leakage occurs. • After rectal administration, flush with 50 to 100 ml of nonsodium fluid. • If hyperkalemia is severe, more drastic modalities can be added; for example, dextrose 50% with regular insulin I.V. push. Do not depend solely on polystyrene-resin to lower serum potassium levels in severe hyperkalemia.

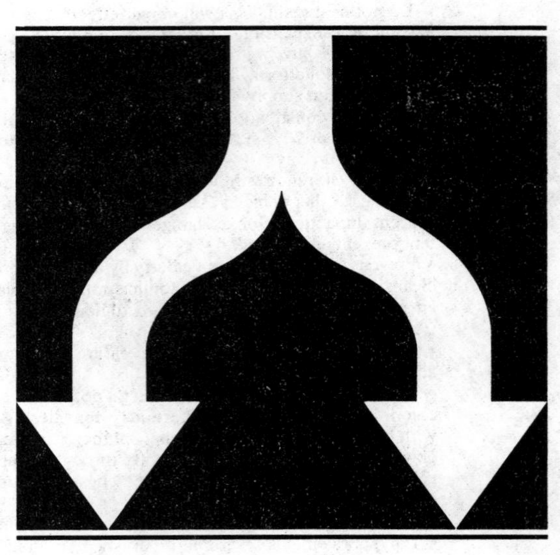

Blood

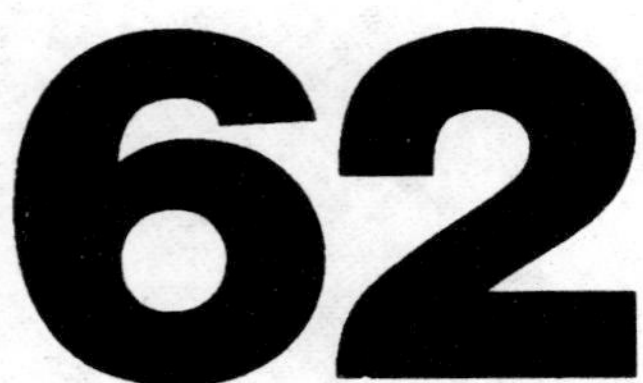

Hematinics

ferrocholinate
ferrous fumarate
ferrous gluconate
ferrous sulfate
iron dextran

Iron is needed to maintain enough hemoglobin within red blood cells to transport and deliver adequate oxygen. Iron deficiency results in decreased hemoglobin synthesis, decreased red blood cell production, and consequent anemia.

Major uses

• Iron preparations supplement depleted iron stores, thereby arresting the anemic process. As a dietary supplement, 10 to 18 mg elemental iron daily for adults and 4 to 8 mg of elemental iron for children is sufficient.
• In iron deficiency, 90 to 200 mg elemental iron may be required daily.

Mechanism of action

• Absorbed iron is taken up into the bone marrow tissues that form blood cells, where it's used to synthesize hemoglobin.

Absorption, distribution, and excretion

• Iron is best absorbed in the ferrous form. Absorption occurs mainly in the duodenum, although in normal patients a small amount is absorbed in the proximal jejunum. Only 5% of the iron ingested is actually absorbed. Anemic patients may absorb as much as 20%.
• On the basis of diet (6 mg iron/100 calories—approximately 18 mg total iron per day) 1 mg iron is absorbed while 1 mg is excreted in the urine, feces, sweat, and desquamated tissue.
• Iron is distributed in the bone marrow (2,400 mg) and in the liver (males 800 mg, females 300 mg). The remainder of body iron is bound to serum proteins and is contained in muscles and certain enzymes.

Onset and duration

• When administered to iron deficient patients, hematinics increase the hemoglobin concentration by approximately 0.1 g/100 ml/day, or 1 g/100 ml per week. To correct iron deficiency anemias, storage iron in the liver must be replaced. This takes approximately 3 months of therapy, with dosages of elemental iron ranging from 100 to 180 mg/day.

Combination products

FEROCYL: iron (as fumarate) 50 mg and dioctyl sodium sulfosuccinate 100 mg.

FER-REGULES: iron (as fumarate) 50 mg and dioctyl sodium sulfosuccinate 100 mg.
FERRO-SEQUELS: iron (as fumarate) 50 mg and dioctyl sodium sulfosuccinate 100 mg.
Many vitamin preparations contain iron.
SIMRON: iron (as gluconate) 10 mg and polysorbate 20, 400 mg.

HOW TO INJECT IRON SOLUTIONS

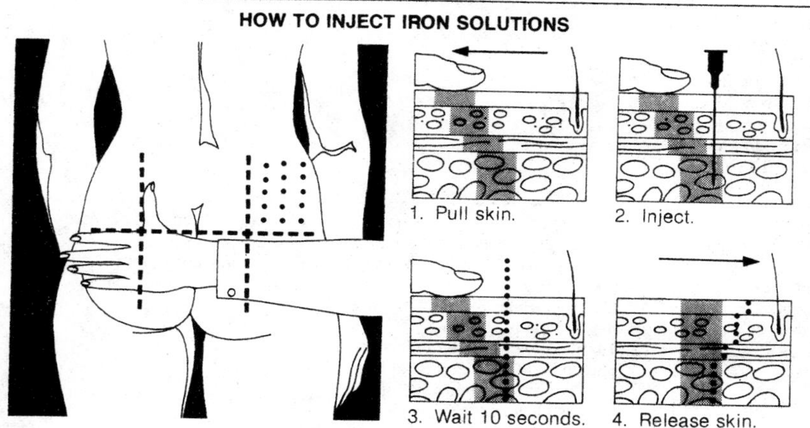
1. Pull skin.
2. Inject.
3. Wait 10 seconds.
4. Release skin.

Use 19 or 20 gauge, 1½" to 3" needle (depending on patient's size). Change to a fresh needle after medication is drawn to avoid tracking the iron solution through to subcutaneous tissue. Allow 0.5 ml air in syringe. Position patient prone or lateral. Locate and expose injection site. Displace the skin firmly to one side. Cleanse area; insert needle. Withdraw plunger to check against entry into blood vessel. Inject medication slowly, into upper outer quadrant of buttocks, followed by the air in syringe. Wait 10 seconds. Withdraw needle; release skin.

NAME	INDICATIONS & DOSAGE	SIDE EFFECTS
ferrocholinate Chel-Iron, Ferrolip, Firon, Kelex	*Iron deficiency—* **Adults:** 333 mg tablet P.O. t.i.d. **Children:** 6 mg/Kg P.O. daily in divided doses t.i.d. *Prevention of iron deficiency—* **Children:** 1 mg/Kg P.O. daily as single dose or divided.	*GI:* nausea, vomiting, constipation, black stools. *Other:* stained tooth enamel.
ferrous fumarate Eldofe, F&B Caps, Farbegen, Feco-T, Feostat, Feroton◆◆, Ferranol, Ferrofume◆◆, Fersamal◆◆, Fumarin, Fumasorb, Hematon◆◆, Hemocyte, Ircon, Laud-Iron, Maniron, Novofumar◆◆, Palafer◆◆, Palmiron, Span-FF, Toleron	*Iron deficiency states—* **Adults:** 200 mg P.O. daily t.i.d. or q.i.d.	*GI:* nausea, vomiting, constipation, black stools. *Other:* stained tooth enamel.
ferrous gluconate Entron, Fergon◆, Ferralet, FerrousG, Fertinic◆◆, Novoferrogluc◆◆	*Iron deficiency—* **Adults:** 200 to 600 mg P.O., t.i.d. **Children 6 to 12 years:** 300 to 900 mg P.O. daily. **Children under 6 years:** 100 to 300 mg P.O. daily. 1 tablet contains 320 mg ferrous gluconate (37 mg elemental iron). 5 ml of elixir contains 300 mg ferrous gluconate (35 mg elemental iron).	*GI:* nausea, vomiting, constipation, black stools. *Other:* elixir may stain teeth.

◆ Also available in Canada.
◆◆ Available in Canada only.
Unmarked trade names available in United States only.

INTERACTIONS	NURSING CONSIDERATIONS
Antacids, cholestyramine resin, pancreatic extracts, vitamin E: decreased iron absorption. Separate doses if possible. *Chloramphenicol:* watch for delayed response to iron therapy. *Vitamin C:* may increase iron absorption. Beneficial drug interaction.	• Contraindicated in hemosiderosis, hemochromatosis, and hemolytic anemia. Usually contraindicated in peptic ulcer or ulcerative colitis. Use cautiously on long-term basis. • GI upset related to dose. Between-meal dosing preferable but can be given with some foods although absorption may be decreased. Enteric-coated products reduce GI upset but also reduce amount of iron absorbed. • Iron is toxic; parents should be aware of iron poisoning in children. • Dilute liquid preparations in juice or water, but not in milk or antacids. • Check for constipation; record color and amount of stool. Teach dietary measures for preventing constipation. • Instruct patient to get frequent blood tests. • To avoid staining teeth, give liquid iron preparations with glass straw.
Antacids, cholestyramine resin, pancreatic extracts, vitamin E: decreased iron absorption. Separate doses if possible. *Chloramphenicol:* watch for delayed response to iron therapy. *Vitamin C:* may increase iron absorption. Beneficial drug interaction.	• Contraindicated in peptic ulcer, regional enteritis, ulcerative colitis, hemosiderosis, and hemochromatosis. Use cautiously on long-term basis and in anemic patients. • GI upset related to dose. Between-meal dosing preferable but can be given with some foods although absorption may be decreased. Enteric-coated products reduce GI upset but also reduce amount of iron absorbed. • Iron is toxic; parents should be aware of iron poisoning in children. • Dilute liquid preparations in juice or water, but not in milk or antacids. • Check for constipation; record color and amount of stool. Teach dietary measures for preventing constipation. • Instruct patient to get frequent blood tests. • Combination products Simron, Ferro-Sequels, Ferocyl, Fer-Regules contain stool softeners to help prevent constipation. Fermalox contains antacids to help relieve GI upset, if present; don't use this product unless absolutely necessary because of decreased iron absorption.
Antacids, cholestyramine resin, pancreatic extracts, vitamin E: decreased iron absorption. Separate doses if possible. *Chloramphenicol:* watch for delayed response to iron therapy. *Vitamin C:* may increase iron absorption. Beneficial drug interaction.	• Contraindicated in peptic ulcer, regional enteritis, ulcerative colitis, hemosiderosis, and hemochromatosis. Use cautiously on long-term basis, and in patients with anemia. • GI upset related to dose. Between-meal dosing preferable but can be given with some foods although absorption may be decreased. Enteric-coated products reduce GI upset but also reduce amount of iron absorbed. • Iron is toxic; parents should be aware of iron poisoning in children. • Dilute liquid preparations in juice or water, but not in milk or antacids. • Check for constipation; record color and amount of stool. Teach dietary measures for preventing constipation. • Instruct patient to get frequent blood tests.

NAME	INDICATIONS & DOSAGE	SIDE EFFECTS
ferrous sulfate Arne Modified Caps, Feosol, Fer-In-Sol♦, Fero-Grad♦♦, Fero-Gradumet, Ferolix, Ferospace, Ferralyn, Fesofor♦♦, Fesotyme, Irospan, Mol-Iron, Novo-ferrosulfa♦♦, Slow-Fe♦♦, Telefon	*Iron deficiency—* **Adults:** 750 mg to 1.5 g P.O. daily divided t.i.d.; or 225 to 525 mg P.O. sustained-release preparations once daily or q 12 hours. **Children 6 to 12 years:** 600 mg P.O. daily in divided doses. *Prophylaxis for iron-deficiency anemia—* **Pregnant women:** 300 to 600 mg P.O. daily in divided doses. **Premature or undernourished infants:** 3 to 6 mg/Kg P.O. daily in divided doses.	*GI:* nausea, vomiting, constipation, black stools. *Other:* elixir may stain teeth.
iron dextran Ferrodex, Hematran, Hydextran, Imferon♦, K-FeRON	*Iron deficiency anemia—* **Adults:** I.M. or I.V. injections of iron are advisable only for patients for whom oral administration is impossible or ineffective. Test dose (0.5 ml) required before administration. I.M. (by Z track): inject 0.5 ml test dose. If no reactions, next daily dose should ordinarily not exceed 0.5 ml (25 mg) for infants under 10 lbs.; 1 ml (50 mg) for children under 20 lbs.; 2 ml (100 mg) for patients under 110 lbs.; 5 ml (250 mg) for patients over 110 lbs. I.V. push: inject 0.5 ml test dose. If no reactions, within 2 to 3 days the dosage may be raised to 2 ml per day I.V., 1 ml/min undiluted and infused slowly until total dose is achieved. No single dose should exceed 100 mg of iron. I.V. infusion: dosages expressed in terms of elemental iron. A dosage guide based on body weight and the severity of the anemia. Dilute in 250 to 1,000 ml of normal saline solution; dextrose increases local vein irritation. Infuse test dose of 25 mg slowly over 5 minutes. If no reaction occurs in 5 minutes, infusion may be started. Infuse total dose slowly over approximately 6 to 12 hours. 1 ml iron dextran = 50 mg elemental iron.	*CNS:* headache, transitory paresthesias, arthralgia, myalgia, dizziness, malaise, syncope. *CV:* local phlebitis at injection site (I.V. injection), hypotensive reaction, peripheral vascular flushing with overly rapid I.V. administration, tachycardia. *GI:* nausea, vomiting, metallic taste, transient loss of taste perception. *Local:* soreness and inflammation at injection site (I.M.); brown skin discoloration at injection site (I.M.). *Other:* anaphylaxis.

INTERACTIONS	NURSING CONSIDERATIONS
Antacids, cholestyramine resin, pancreatic extracts, vitamin E: decreased iron absorption. Separate doses if possible. *Chloramphenicol:* watch for delayed response to iron therapy. *Vitamin C:* may increase iron absorption. Beneficial drug interaction.	• Contraindicated in peptic ulcer, ulcerative colitis, regional enteritis, hemosiderosis and hemochromatosis. Use cautiously on long-term basis and in patients with anemia. • GI upset related to dose. Between-meal dosing preferable but can be given with some foods although absorption may be decreased. Enteric-coated products reduce GI upset but also reduce amount of iron absorbed. • Iron is toxic; parents should be aware of iron poisoning in children. • Dilute liquid preparations in juice or water, but not in milk or antacids. • Check for constipation; record color and amount of stool. Teach dietary measures for preventing constipation. • Instruct patient to get frequent blood tests.
None significant.	• Contraindicated in all anemias other than iron deficiency anemia. Use with extreme caution in impaired hepatic function and rheumatoid arthritis. • Watch vital signs for drug reaction. Reactions are varied and severe, ranging from pain, inflammations, myalgias to hypotension, shock, and death. • Inject deeply into upper outer quadrant of buttock—never into arm or other exposed area—with a 2- to 3-inch, 19- or 20-gauge needle. Use Z-track technique to avoid leakage into subcutaneous tissue and tattooing of skin. • Hemoglobin concentration, hematocrit, and reticulocyte count should be determined periodically. • Use I.V. in these situations: insufficient muscle mass for deep intramuscular injection; impaired absorption from muscle due to stasis or edema; possibility of uncontrolled intramuscular bleeding from trauma (as may occur in hemophilia); where massive and prolonged parenteral therapy is indicated (as may be necessary in cases of chronic substantial blood loss). • Patient should rest 15 to 30 minutes after I.V. administration. • Check hospital policy before administering I.V. In some hospitals, only doctor may administer iron I.V. • Not removed by hemodialysis. • For treatment of anaphylaxis, see p. 1114.

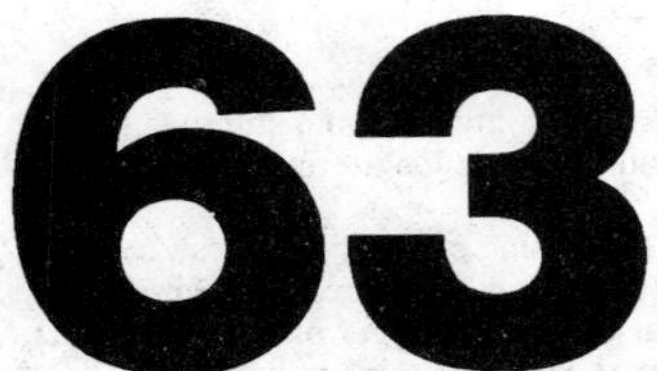

Anticoagulants and heparin antagonist

anisindione
dicumarol
heparin sodium
phenindione
phenprocoumon
protamine sulfate
warfarin potassium
warfarin sodium

Oral anticoagulants include the coumarin derivatives, such as warfarin sodium, warfarin potassium, dicumarol, and phenprocoumon, and the indandione derivatives, such as anisindione, diphenadione, and phenindione. Heparin sodium, a parenteral anticoagulant, is antagonized by protamine sulfate, a weak anticoagulant. Heparin, the coumarin derivatives, and the indandione derivatives alter the clotting system to prevent the formation of fibrin. Anticoagulants are used in patients who are at risk of developing clots and for the treatment of an active clot to prevent extension of the thrombus.

Major uses

- All anticoagulants are used in the treatment of pulmonary emboli, to prevent and treat deep-vein thrombosis, and to reduce the formation of thrombi after myocardial infarction.
- Oral anticoagulants are also used in rheumatic heart disease with heart valve damage, and in atrial arrhythmias that alter hemodynamics.
- Protamine sulfate neutralizes the effects of heparin.

Mechanism of action

- Oral anticoagulants inhibit vitamin K-dependent synthesis activation of clotting factors II, VII, IX, and X, which are formed in the liver.
- Heparin sodium acts directly with Antithrombin III to prevent formation of thrombin and fibrin. Low dosages of heparin diminish production of clotting factor X and in this way limit the clotting factor substrates available to form thrombin and fibrin.
- Protamine sulfate is highly basic and forms a complex with heparin sodium, which is highly acidic. This complex is physiologically inert.

Absorption, distribution, and excretion

- Oral anticoagulants are absorbed from the upper gastrointestinal tract, metabolized by microsomal enzymes in the liver, and are excreted in the urine.
- Heparin sodium is absorbed parenterally but not orally. It is distributed into the plasma volume, metabolized by the reticuloendothelial cells and heparinase enzymes in the serum, and excreted primarily in the urine. But it does not cross the placenta.
- The metabolic fate of protamine sulfate is not clear.

Onset and duration

• Oral anticoagulants require 1 to 3 days to produce therapeutic anticoagulation, even though they alter the prothrombin time the first day of therapy. The average course of anticoagulant therapy lasts 3 to 6 months, but these drugs should be used for the shortest duration necessary. Their duration of action varies from 1 to 20 days.

• Heparin sodium begins to act immediately, with peak effects occuring within minutes. The clotting time returns to normal within 2 to 6 hours.

• Protamine sulfate neutralizes heparin within 5 minutes after intravenous administration.

Combination products

None.

INJECTION TIPS

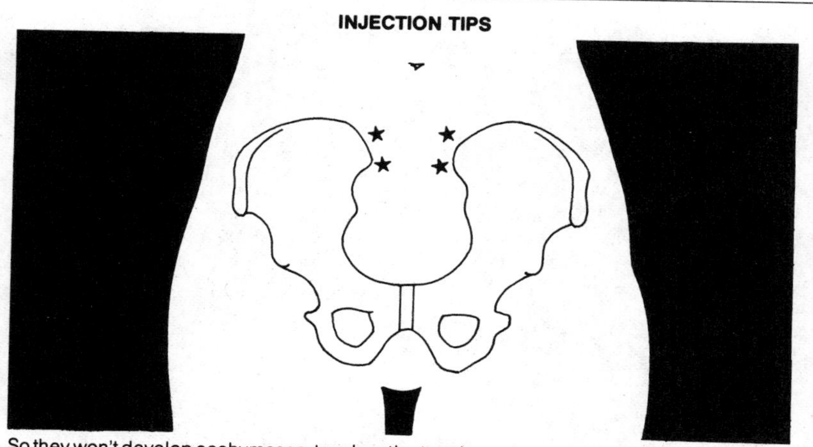

So they won't develop ecchymoses, teach patients using subcutaneous heparin to rotate the injection sites along the abdominal fat pad above the iliac crest. Make sure patients don't rub the site with an alcohol sponge, as this increases the absorption time. Instead, after an injection have the patient merely hold the sponge on the site for a few seconds.

NAME	INDICATIONS & DOSAGE	SIDE EFFECTS
anisindione Miradon	*Treatment of pulmonary emboli; prevention and treatment of deep-vein thrombosis, myocardial infarction, rheumatic heart disease with heart valve damage, and atrial arrhythmias*— **Adults:** 300 mg P.O. first day, 200 mg P.O. second day, 100 mg P.O. third day. Maintenance dose: 25 to 250 mg daily based on prothrombin times.	*Blood:* agranulocytosis, leukopenia, leukocytosis, eosinophilia, anemia. *CNS:* headache. *CV:* myocarditis, tachycardia. *EENT:* conjunctivitis, blurred vision, paralysis of ocular accommodation. *GI:* diarrhea, sore mouth and throat. *GU:* nephropathy with renal tubular necrosis, albuminuria, red-orange urine. *Skin:* rash, severe exfoliative dermatitis. *Other:* jaundice, massive generalized edema, hepatitis, alopecia, fever, malaise.

INTERACTIONS	NURSING CONSIDERATIONS
Allopurinol, clofibrate dextrothyroxine, thyroid drugs, heparin, anabolic steroids, disulfiram, aminosalicylic acid, glucagon, inhalation anesthetics, sulfonamides: increased prothrombin time. Monitor patient carefully. Consider anticoagulant dose reduction. *Ethacrynic acid, indomethacin, mefenamic acid, oxyphenbutazone, phenylbutazone, salicylates:* increased prothrombin time; ulcerogenic effects. Don't use together. *Antipyrine, carbamezepine, antacids, griseofulvin, haloperidol, paraldehyde, rifampin:* decreased prothrombin time. Monitor patient carefully. *Phenytoin, glutethimide, chloral hydrate, triclofos sodium, alcohol, diuretics:* increased or decreased prothrombin time. Avoid use if possible; or monitor patient carefully. *Barbiturates:* inhibition of hypoprothrombinemic effect of anticoagulants. If barbiturates are withdrawn, reduce anticoagulant dose; inhibition may last for weeks after anticoagulant is withdrawn, but fatal hemorrhage can occur when inhibiting effect disappears. *Cholestyramine:* decreased response when administered too close together. Give 6 hours after oral anticoagulants.	• Contraindicated in hemophilia, thrombocytopenic purpura, leukemia with pronounced bleeding tendency, open wounds or ulcers, impaired hepatic or renal function, severe hypertension, acute nephritis, subacute bacterial endocarditis. Use cautiously in pregnancy, lactation, during menses, during use of any drainage tube in any orifice, and in any patient in whom slight bleeding is dangerous. Use with extreme caution (if at all) in psychiatric patients, debilitated patients, or cachectic patients. • Use caution when adding or stopping any drug for patient receiving anticoagulants. May change the clotting status and result in hemorrhage. • Fever and skin rash signal severe complications. • Give drug at same time daily. Stress importance of complying with recommended dosage and keeping follow-up appointments. Patient should carry a card that identifies him as a potential bleeder. • Regularly inspect patient for bleeding gums, bruises on arms or legs, petechiae, nosebleeds, melena, tarry stools, hematuria, hematemesis. Tell patient and family to watch for these signs and notify doctor immediately. • Warn patient to avoid over-the-counter products containing aspirin, other salicylates, or drugs which may interact with anisindione. • Because onset of action is delayed, heparin sodium is often given during first few days of treatment. When heparin is being given simultaneously, don't draw blood for prothrombin times within 5 hours of I.V. heparin administration. • Schedule doses according to prothrombin time (P.T.). Doctors usually try to maintain P.T. at 1.5 to 2 times normal. Numerical P.T. values depend on procedure and reagents used in individual laboratory. • Tell patient to notify doctor if menses is heavier than usual. May require adjusting dose. • Tell patient to use electric razor when shaving to avoid scratching skin, and to brush teeth with a soft toothbrush. • Warn patient that urine may turn red-orange. • An indandione derivative. • Duration of action 1.5 to 5 days. • Light to moderate alcohol intake does not significantly affect prothrombin times. • For symptoms and treatment of toxicity, see p. 1120.

NAME	INDICATIONS & DOSAGE	SIDE EFFECTS
dicumarol Dufalone◆◆	*Treatment of pulmonary emboli; prevention and treatment of deep-vein thrombosis, myocardial infarction, rheumatic heart disease with heart valve damage, and atrial arrhythmias*— **Adults:** 200 to 300 mg P.O. on first day, 25 to 200 mg P.O. daily thereafter, based on prothrombin times.	*Blood:* hemorrhage with excessive dosage; leukopenia, agranulocytosis. *GI:* anorexia, nausea, vomiting, cramps, diarrhea, mouth ulcers. *GU:* red-orange urine, hematuria. *Skin:* dermatitis, urticaria, rash. *Other:* alopecia, fever.

INTERACTIONS

Allopurinol, clofibrate dextrothyroxine, thyroid drugs, heparin, anabolic steroids, disulfiram, aminosalicylic acid, glucagon, inhalation anesthetics, sulfonamides: increased prothrombin time. Monitor patient carefully. Consider anticoagulant dose reduction.

Ethacrynic acid, indomethacin, mefenamic acid, oxyphenbutazone, phenylbutazone, salicylates: increased prothrombin time; ulcerogenic effects. Don't use together.

Antipyrine, carbamezepine, antacids, griseofulvin, haloperidol, paraldehyde, rifampin: decreased prothrombin time. Monitor patient carefully.

Phenytoin, glutethimide, chloral hydrate, triclofos sodium: increased or decreased prothrombin time. Avoid use if possible; or monitor patient carefully.

Barbiturates: inhibition of hypoprothrombinemic effect of anticoagulants. If barbiturates are withdrawn, reduce anticoagulant dose; inhibition may last for weeks after anticoagulant is withdrawn, but fatal hemorrhage can occur when inhibiting effect disappears.

Cholestyramine: decreased response when administered too close together. Give 6 hours after oral anticoagulants.

NURSING CONSIDERATIONS

- Contraindicated in hemophilia, thrombocytopenic purpura, leukemia with pronounced bleeding tendency, open wounds or ulcers, impaired hepatic or renal function, severe hypertension, acute nephritis, subacute bacterial endocarditis. Use cautiously in pregnancy, lactation, during menses, during use of any drainage tube; and in any patient in whom slight bleeding is dangerous. Use with extreme caution (if at all) in psychiatric patients, debilitated patients, or cachectic patients.
- Use caution when adding or stopping any drug for patient receiving anticoagulants. May change the clotting status and result in hemorrhage.
- Fever and skin rash signal severe complications.
- Give drug at same time daily. Stress importance of complying with recommended dosage and keeping follow-up appointments. Patient should carry a card that identifies him as a potential bleeder.
- Regularly inspect patient for bleeding gums, bruises on arms or legs, petechiae, nosebleeds, melena, tarry stools, hematuria, hematemesis. Tell patient and family to watch for these signs and notify doctor immediately.
- Warn patient to avoid over-the-counter products containing aspirin, other salicylates, or drugs which may interact with dicumarol.
- Because onset of action is delayed, heparin sodium is often given during first few days of treatment. When heparin is being given simultaneously, don't draw blood for prothrombin times within 5 hours of I.V. heparin administration.
- Dose given depends on prothrombin times (P.T.). Doctors usually try to maintain P.T. at 1.5 to 2 times normal. P.T. values depend on procedure and reagents used in individual laboratory.
- Tell patient to notify doctor if menses is heavier than usual. May require adjusting dose.
- Tell patient to use electric razor when shaving to avoid scratching skin, and to brush teeth with a soft toothbrush.
- Duration of action 2 to 6 days.
- Light to moderate alcohol intake does not significantly affect prothrombin times.
- For symptoms and treatment of toxicity, see p. 1120.

NAME	INDICATIONS & DOSAGE	SIDE EFFECTS
heparin sodium Hepalean◆◆, Heprinar, Lipo-Hepin, Liquaemin Sodium, Panheprin	*Treatment of deep vein thrombosis, myocardial infarction—* **Adults:** initially, 5,000 to 7,500 units I.V. push, then adjust dose according to P.T.T. results and give dose I.V. q 4 hours (usually 4,000 to 5,000 units); or 5,000 to 7,500 units I.V. bolus, then 1,000 units/hour by I.V. infusion pump. Wait 8 hours following bolus dose, and adjust hourly rate according to P.T.T. *Treatment of pulmonary embolism—* **Adults:** initially, 7,500 to 10,000 units I.V. push, then adjust dose according to P.T.T. results and give dose I.V. q 4 hours (usually 4,000 to 5,000 units); or 7,500 to 10,000 units I.V. bolus, then 1,000 units/ hour by I.V. infusion pump. Wait 8 hours following bolus dose, and adjust hourly rate according to P.T.T. *Prophylaxis of embolism—* **Adults:** 5,000 units S.C. q 12 hours. *Open heart surgery—* **Adults:** (total body perfusion) 150 to 300 units/Kg continuous I.V infusion. *Treatment of pulmonary emboli; prevention and treatment of deep-vein thrombosis—* **Children:** initially, 50 units/Kg I.V. drip. Maintenance dose 100 units/Kg I.V. drip q 4 hours. Constant infusion: 20,000 units/M^2 daily. Dosages adjusted according to P.T.T. Heparin dosing is highly individualized, depending upon disease state, age, renal and hepatic status.	*Blood:* hemorrhage, overly prolonged clotting time, minor bleeding, acute reversible thrombocytopenia. *Local:* irritation, mild pain. *Other:* hypersensitivity reactions include chills, fever, pruritus, rhinitis, burning of feet, conjunctivitis, lacrimation, arthralgia, urticaria.

INTERACTIONS	NURSING CONSIDERATIONS
Salicylates: increased anticoagulant effect. Don't use together. *Anticoagulants, oral:* additive anticoagulation. Monitor prothrombin time and partial thromboplastin time.	• Conditionally contraindicated in active bleeding, blood dyscrasias or bleeding tendencies such as hemophilia, thrombocytopenia, or hepatic disease with hypoprothrombinemia; suspected intracranial hemorrhage; suppurative thrombophlebitis; inaccessible ulcerative lesions (especially of GI tract); open ulcerative wounds; extensive denudation of skin; ascorbic acid deficiency and other conditions causing increased capillary permeability; during or after brain, eye, or spinal cord surgery; during continuous tube drainage of stomach or small intestine; in subacute bacterial endocarditis; shock; advanced kidney disease; threatened abortion; severe hypertension. While the use of heparin is clearly hazardous in these conditions, a decision to use it depends on the comparative risk in failure to treat the coexisting thromboembolic disorder. • Use cautiously during menses; in mild hepatic or renal disease; alcoholism; in patients in occupations with the risk of physical injury; immediately postpartum; in past history of allergies, asthma, or GI ulcers. • Measure partial thromboplastin time (PTT) carefully and regularly. Anticoagulation present when PTT values are 1½ to 2 times control values. • Drug requirements are higher in early phases of thrombogenic diseases and febrile states; lower when patient becomes stabilized. • Regularly inspect patient for bleeding gums, bruises on arms or legs, petechiae, nosebleeds, melena, tarry stools, hematuria, hematemesis. Tell patient and family to watch for these signs and notify doctor immediately. • Tell patient to avoid over-the-counter medications containing aspirin, other salicylates, or drugs that may interact with heparin. • Heparin comes in various concentrations. Check order and vial carefully. • Low-dose injections given sequentially between iliac crest in lower abdomen deep into S.C. fat. Inject S.C. in fat pad; withdraw plunger. If no blood present, inject drug slowly. Leave needle in place for 10 seconds; withdraw needle. Alternate site every 12 hours—right for a.m., left for p.m. • Don't massage after S.C. injection. Watch for signs of bleeding at injection site. Rotate sites and keep accurate record. • Check constant I.V. infusions regularly, even when pumps are in good working order, to prevent over- or underdosage. • I.M. administration not recommended. • I.V. administration preferred because of long-term effect and irregular absorption when given S.C. Whenever possible, administer I.V. heparin in infusion pump to provide maximum safety. • Concentrated heparin solutions (greater than 100 units/ml) can irritate blood vessels. • Place sign above patient's bed to inform I.V. team or lab personnel to apply pressure dressings after taking blood. • Avoid excessive I.M. injections to avoid or minimize hematomas. If possible, don't give I.M. injections at all. • Elderly patients should usually start at lower doses. • When I.V. intermittent therapy is utilized, always draw blood ½ hour before next scheduled dose to avoid falsely elevated PTTs. • PTTs can be drawn any time after 8 hours of initiation of continuous I.V. heparin therapy. Never draw blood for P.T.T.'s from the IV tubing of the heparin infusion, or from vein of infusion. Falsely elevated PTT will result. Always draw blood from opposite arm. • Give on time; try not to skip a dose. If I.V. is out, get it restarted as soon as possible, and reschedule dose immediately. • Never piggyback other drugs into an infusion line while heparin infusion is running. Many antibiotics and other drugs inactivate heparin. Never mix any drug with heparin in syringe when bolus therapy is used. • For symptoms and treatment of toxicity, see p. 1118.

NAME	INDICATIONS & DOSAGE	SIDE EFFECTS
phenindione Danilone◆◆, Eridione, Hedulin	*Treatment of pulmonary emboli; prevention and treatment of deep-vein thrombosis, myocardial infarction, rheumatic heart disease with heart valve damage, atrial arrhythmias—* **Adults:** 300 mg P.O. first day; 200 mg P.O. second day. Maintenance dose: 50 to 150 mg daily, based on prothrombin times.	*Blood:* agranulocytosis, leukopenia, leukocytosis, eosinophilia, anemia. *CNS:* headache. *CV:* myocarditis, tachycardia. *EENT:* conjunctivitis, blurred vision, paralysis of ocular accommodation. *GI:* diarrhea, sore mouth and throat. *GU:* nephropathy with renal tubular necrosis, albuminuria, red-orange urine. *Skin:* rash, severe exfoliative dermatitis. *Other:* jaundice, massive generalized edema, hepatitis, alopecia, fever, malaise.

INTERACTIONS

Allopurinol, clofibrate dextrothyroxine, thyroid drugs, heparin, anabolic steroids, disulfiram, aminosalicylic acid, glucagon, inhalation anesthetics, sulfonamides: increased prothrombin time. Monitor patient carefully. Consider anticoagulant dose reduction.

Ethacrynic acid, indomethacin, mefenamic acid, oxyphenbutazone, phenylbutazone, salicylates: increased prothrombin time; ulcerogenic effects. Don't use together.

Antipyrine, carbamezepine, antacids, griseofulvin, haloperidol, paraldehyde, rifampin: decreased prothrombin time. Monitor patient carefully.

Phenytoin, glutethimide, chloral hydrate, triclofos sodium, alcohol, diuretics: increased or decreased prothrombin time. Avoid use if possible; or monitor patient carefully.

Barbiturates: inhibition of hypoprothrombinemic effect of anticoagulants. If barbiturates are withdrawn, reduce anticoagulant dose; inhibition may last for weeks after anticoagulant is withdrawn, but fatal hemorrhage can occur when inhibiting effect disappears.

Cholestyramine: decreased response when administered too close together. Give 6 hours after oral anticoagulants.

NURSING CONSIDERATIONS

- Contraindicated in hemophilia, thrombocytopenic purpura, leukemia with pronounced bleeding tendency, open wounds or ulcers, impaired hepatic or renal function, severe hypertension, acute nephritis and subacute bacterial endocarditis. Use cautiously in pregnancy, lactation, during menses, during use of any drainage tube in any orifice, and in any patient in whom slight bleeding is dangerous. Use with extreme caution (if at all) in psychiatric patients, debilitated patients, or cachectic patients.
- Use caution when adding or stopping any drug. May cause alteration in clotting status and result in hemorrhage.
- Fever and skin rash signal severe complications.
- Give drug at same time daily. Stress importance of complying with recommended dosage and keeping follow-up appointments. Patient should carry a card that identifies him as a potential bleeder.
- Regularly inspect patient for bleeding gums, bruises on arms or legs, petechiae, nosebleeds, melena, tarry stools, hematuria, hematemesis. Tell patient and family to watch for these signs and notify doctor immediately.
- Warn patient to avoid over-the-counter products containing aspirin, or salicylates, or other drugs which may interact with phenindione.
- Because onset of action is delayed, heparin sodium is often given during first few days of treatment. When heparin is being given simultaneously, don't draw blood for prothrombin times within 5 hours of I.V. heparin administration.
- Dose given depends on prothrombin times (P.T.) Doctors usually try to maintain P.T. at 1.5 to 2 times normal. Numerical P.T. values depend on procedure and reagents used in individual laboratory.
- Tell patient to notify doctor if menses is heavier than usual. May require adjusting dose.
- Tell patient to use electric razor when shaving to avoid scratching skin, and to brush teeth with a soft toothbrush.
- Warn patient that urine may turn red-orange.
- Indandione derivative.
- Duration of action is 2 to 4 days.
- Light to moderate alcohol intake does not significantly affect prothrombin times.
- For symptoms and treatment of toxicity, see p. 1120.

NAME	INDICATIONS & DOSAGE	SIDE EFFECTS
phenprocoumon Liquamar, Marcumar◆◆	*Treatment of pulmonary emboli; prevention and treatment of deep-vein thrombosis, myocardial infarction, rheumatic heart disease with heart valve damage, and atrial arrhythmias*— **Adults:** initially, 24 mg, P.O. maintenance dose: 0.75 to 6 mg daily, based on prothrombin time.	*Blood:* agranulocytosis, leukopenia. *GI:* paralytic ileus and intestinal obstruction (both resulting from hemorrhage), nausea, vomiting, cramps, diarrhea, mouth ulcers. *GU:* nephropathy, red-orange urine, hematuria. *Skin:* rash. *Other:* alopecia, fever.

INTERACTIONS	NURSING CONSIDERATIONS
Allopurinol, clofibrate dextrothyroxine, thyroid drugs, heparin, anabolic steroids, disulfiram, aminosalicylic acid, glucagon, inhalation anesthetics, sulfonamides: increased prothrombin time. Monitor patient carefully. Consider anticoagulant dose reduction. *Ethacrynic acid, indomethacin mefenamic acid, oxyphenbutazone, phenylbutazone, salicylates:* increased prothrombin time; ulcerogenic effects. Don't use together. *Antipyrine, carbamezepine, antacids, griseofulvin, haloperidol, paraldehyde, rifampin:* decreased prothrombin time. Monitor patient carefully. *Phenytoin, glutethimide, chloral hydrate, triclofos sodium:* increased or decreased prothrombin time. Avoid use if possible; or monitor patient carefully. *Barbiturates:* inhibition of hypoprothrombinemic effect of anticoagulants. If barbiturates are withdrawn, reduce anticoagulant dose; inhibition may last for weeks after anticoagulant is withdrawn, but fatal hemorrhage can occur when inhibiting effect disappears. *Cholestyramine:* decreased response when administered too close together. Give 6 hours after oral anticoagulants.	• Contraindicated in hemophilia, thrombocytopenic purpura, leukemia with pronounced bleeding tendency, open wounds or ulcers, impaired hepatic or renal function, severe hypertension, acute nephritis and subacute bacterial endocarditis. Use cautiously in pregnancy, lactation, during menses, during use of any drainage tube in any orifice, and in any patient in whom slight bleeding is dangerous. Use with extreme caution (if at all) in psychiatric, debilitated, or cachectic patients. • Use caution when adding or stopping any drug for patient receiving anticoagulants. May change the clotting status and result in hemorrhage. • Fever and skin rash signal severe complications. • Give drug at same time daily. Stress importance of complying with recommended dosage and keeping follow-up appointments. Patient should carry a card that identifies him as a potential bleeder. • Do periodic blood and hepatic function test. • Regularly inspect patient for bleeding gums, bruises on arms or legs, petechiae, nosebleeds, melena, tarry stools, hematuria, hematemesis. Tell patient and family to watch for these signs and notify doctor immediately. • Warn patient to avoid over-the-counter products containing aspirin, other salicylates, or drugs which may interact with phenprocoumon. • Because onset of action is delayed, heparin sodium is often given during first few days of treatment. When heparin is being given simultaneously, don't draw blood for protrombin times within 5 hours of I.V. heparin administration. • Dose given depends on prothombin times (P.T.). Doctors usually try to maintain P.T. at 1.5 to 2 times normal. Numerical P.T. values depend on procedure and reagents used in individual laboratory. • Tell patient to notify doctor if menses is heavier than usual. May require adjusting dose. • Tell patient to use electric razor when shaving to avoid scratching skin, and to brush teeth with a soft toothbrush. • A coumarin derivative. • Duration of action is 4 to 7 days. • Light to moderate alcohol intake does not significantly affect prothrombin times. • For symptoms and treatment of toxicity, see p. 1120.

NAME	INDICATIONS & DOSAGE	SIDE EFFECTS
protamine sulfate	*Heparin overdose—* **Adults:** dosage based on venous blood coagulation studies, generally 1 mg for each 78 to 95 units of heparin. Give diluted to 1% (10 mg/ml) slow I.V. injection over 1 to 3 minutes. Maximum 50 mg/10 minutes.	*CV:* fall in blood pressure, bradycardia. *Other:* transitory flushing, feeling of warmth, dyspnea.
warfarin potassium Athrombin-K◆ **warfarin sodium** Coumadin◆, Panwarfin, Warfilone Sodium◆◆, Warnerin Sodium◆◆	*Treatment of pulmonary emboli; prevention and treatment of deep-vein thrombosis, myocardial infarction, rheumatic heart disease with heart valve damage, and atrial arrhythmias—* **Adults:** 10 to 15 mg P.O. for 3 days, then dosage based on daily prothrombin times. Usual maintenance dose 2 to 10 mg P.O. daily. Alternate regimen: initially, 40 to 60 mg P.O. daily; then 2 to 10 mg daily based on P.T. determinations.	*Blood:* leukopenia. *GI:* paralytic ileus, intestinal obstruction (both resulting from hemorrhage); diarrhea, vomiting, cramps, nausea. *GU:* excessive uterine bleeding, hemorrhagic necrosis of female breast. *Skin:* dermatitis, urticaria, rash. *Other:* fever, alopecia.

INTERACTIONS	NURSING CONSIDERATIONS
None significant.	• Use cautiously in allergy to fish or after cardiac surgery. • Doctor gives this drug. Should be given slowly to reduce side effects. Have equipment available to treat shock. • Monitor patient continually. Check vital signs frequently. • Watch for spontaneous bleeding, especially dialysis patients and patients after cardiac surgery (heparin "rebound"). • Protamine sulfate may act as anticoagulant in very high doses. • One mg of protamine neutralizes 78 to 95 units of heparin. • Heparin antagonist.
Allopurinol, clofibrate dextrothyroxine, thyroid drugs, heparin, anabolic steroids, cimetidine, disulfiram, aminosalicylic acid, glucagon, inhalation anesthetics, sulfonamides: increased prothrombin time. Monitor patient carefully. Consider anticoagulant dose reduction. *Ethacrynic acid, indomethacin, mefenamic acid, oxyphenbutazone, phenylbutazone, salicylates:* increased prothrombin time; ulcerogenic effects. Don't use together. *Griseofulvin, haloperidol, paraldehyde, rifampin:* decreased prothrombin time. Monitor patient carefully. *Glutetimide, chloral hydrate, triclofos sodium:* increased or decreased prothrombin time. Avoid use if possible; or monitor patient carefully.	• Contraindicated in bleeding or hemorrhagic tendencies resulting from open wounds, visceral cancer, GI ulcers, severe hepatic or renal disease, severe uncontrolled hypertension, subacute bacterial endocarditis, vitamin K deficiency; after recent operations in eye, brain, or spinal cord. Use cautiously in diverticulitis, colitis, mild or moderate hypertension, mild or moderate hepatic or renal disease, lactation, in presence of drainage tubes in any orifice, with regional or lumbar block anesthesia, or any condition increasing risk of hemorrhage. • Observe nursing infants of mothers on drug for unexpected bleeding. • P.T. determinations essential for proper control. High incidence of bleeding when P.T. exceeds 2½ times control values. Doctors usually try to maintain P.T. at 1.5 to 2 times normal. • May divide large doses to reduce GI distress. • Give at same time daily. Stress importance of complying with recommended dosage and keeping follow-up appointments. Patient should carry a card that identifies him as a potential bleeder. • Elderly patients and patients in renal or hepatic failure are especially sensitive to warfarin effect. • Half-life of warfarin is 36 to 44 hours. • Warfarin effect can be neutralized by vitamin K injections. • Regularly inspect patient for bleeding gums, bruises on arms of legs, petechiae, nosebleeds, melena, tarry stools, hematuria, hematemesis.. Tell patient and family to watch for these signs and notify doctor immediately. • Warn patient to avoid over-the-counter products containing aspirin, other salicylates, or drugs which may interact with warfarin potassium or warfarin sodium. • Because onset of action is delayed, heparin sodium is often given during first few days of treatment. When heparin is being given simultaneously, don't draw blood for prothrombin times within 5 hours of I.V. heparin administration. • Fever and skin rash signal severe complications. • Tell patient to notify doctor if menses is heavier than usual. May require adjusting dose. • Tell patient to use electric razor when shaving to avoid scratching skin, and to brush teeth with a soft toothbrush. • Best oral anticoagulant. When patient must receive antacids or phenytoin.

(continued on following page)

NAME	INDICATIONS & DOSAGE	SIDE EFFECTS
warfarin sodium *(continued)*		

INTERACTIONS	NURSING CONSIDERATIONS
Barbiturates: inhibition of hypoprothrombinemic effect of anticoagulants. If barbiturates are withdrawn, reduce anticoagulant dose; inhibition may last for weeks after anticoagulant is withdrawn, but fatal hemorrhage can occur when inhibiting effect disappears. *Cholestyramine:* decreased response when administered too close together. Give 6 hours after oral anticoagulants.	• Light to moderate alcohol intake does not significantly affect prothrombin times. • For symptoms and treatment of toxicity, see p. 1120.

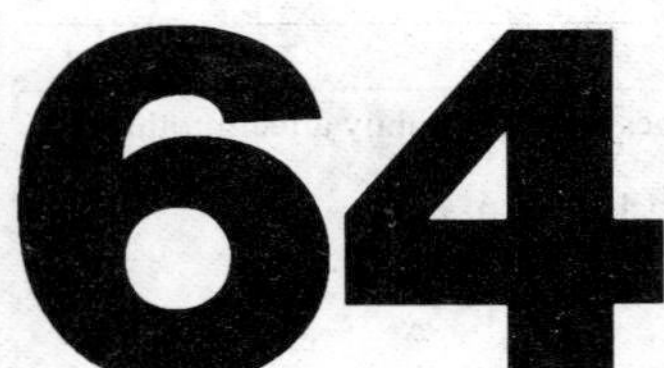

Hemostatics

absorbable gelatin sponge
aminocaproic acid
antihemophilic factor
carbazochrome salicylate
Factor IX complex
microfibrillar collagen hemostat
negatol
oxidized cellulose
thrombin

Hemostatics arrest the flow of blood or reduce capillary bleeding. Some of these drugs are of human or animal origin, while others are synthetically derived.

Major uses

- Antihemophilic factor is used in the correction of hemophilia A (Factor VIII deficiency).
- Factor IX complex contains factors II, VII, IX, and X. It is used in the treatment of Factor IX deficiency (hemophilia B or Christmas disease) and in anticoagulant overdose.
- Thrombin is used to treat bleeding from parenchymatous tissue, cancellous bone, dental sockets, nasal and laryngeal surgery, and in plastic surgery and skin-grafting procedures, and acute GI hemorrhages.
- Microfibrillar collagen hemostat, absorbable gelatin sponge, and oxidized cellulose are used as adjuncts to provide hemostasis during various kinds of surgery. Absorbable gelatin sponge is also used to aid healing of decubitus ulcers.
- Negatol acts as a styptic and hemostatic and is used for oral ulcers and cervical bleeding.
- Aminocaproic acid is used in the treatment of excessive bleeding resulting from hyperfibrinolysis and as an antidote for streptokinase and urokinase toxicity.
- Carbazochrome salicylate corrects excessive capillary permeability during surgery in conditions with excessive oozing.

Mechanism of action

- Antihemophilic factor directly replaces deficient clotting factors.
- Thrombin clots to form fibrin in the presence of fibrinogen.
- Microfibrillar collagen hemostat attracts and aggregates platelets.
- Oxidized cellulose and absorbable gelatin sponge absorb and hold many times their weight in blood. Absorbable gelatin sponge also provides a framework for the growth of granulation tissue.
- Negatol is an astringent and protein denaturant.
- Aminocaproic acid inhibits plasminogen activator substances and, to a lesser degree, antiplasmin activity, to inhibit fibrinolysis.
- Carbazochrome salicylate corrects excessive capillary permeability.

Absorption, distribution, and excretion

- Antihemophilic factor is distributed to the plasma volume after injection. It is metabolized and excreted as a normal physiological substance.

• Aminocaproic acid is rapidly absorbed after oral administration and excreted mostly unmetabolized in the urine.

Onset and duration

• Antihemophilic factor begins to act immediately. Its duration of action is related to the level of factor deficiency that exists and the presence of antibodies against it.
• The onset and duration of thrombin are dependent on concentration.
• Aminocaproic acid has an extremely rapid onset and very short duration of action.

Combination products

None.

HEMOPHILIA AND HEREDITY

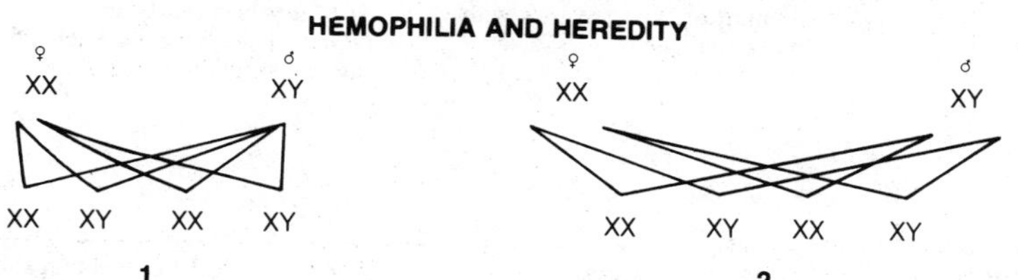

Figure 1 (above, left): A female carrier XX marries a normal male XY. There is a 50-percent chance that their daughters will be carriers or normal XX, and a 50-percent chance that their sons will have hemophilia XY or be normal.

Figure 2 (above, right): A noncarrier female XX marries a hemophiliac male XY. All the daughters are carriers XX, and all the sons are normal.

WHEN HEMOPHILIA STRIKES

Because hemophilia is a chronic disease, the young patient is likely to remember past bleeding episodes and be very nervous. To counteract his anxiety, remain gentle, calm, and patient.

Do not confine the child to bed unnecessarily. If such confinement is really necessary, be creative in providing safe sensory stimuli. You can insure safety and comfort by checking toys and padding the sides of the crib.

NAME	INDICATIONS & DOSAGE	SIDE EFFECTS
absorbable gelatin sponge Gelfoam	**Adults:** *Decubitus ulcers*—place aseptically deep into ulcer. Don't disturb or remove; may add extra p.r.n. *To provide hemostasis in surgery (adjunct)*— apply saturated with isotonic NaCl injection or thrombin solution. Hold in place for 10 to 15 seconds. When bleeding is controlled, allow material to remain in place.	None reported.
aminocaproic acid Amicar◆	*Excessive bleeding resulting from hyperfibrinolysis*— **Adults:** initially, 5 g P.O. or slow I.V. infusion, followed by 1 to 1.25 g hourly until bleeding is controlled. Maximum dose 30 g daily.	*CNS:* dizziness, headache. *EENT:* tinnitus, nasal stuffiness, conjunctival suffusion. *GI:* nausea, cramps, diarrhea. *Skin:* rash. *Other:* malaise.
antihemophilic factor (AHF) Antihemophilic Globulin (AHG), Factorate, Hemofil, Humafac Koate, Profilate	*Hemophilia A (Factor VIII deficiency)*— **Adults and children:** 10 to 20 units/Kg I.V. push or infusion q 8 to 24 hours. Maintenance doses may be less. Infusion rate usually 10 to 20 ml reconstituted solution per 3 minutes. Dosage varies with individual needs.	*CNS:* headache, paresthesias, clouding or loss of consciousness. *CV:* tachycardia, hypotension, possible intravascular hemolysis in patients with blood type A, B, or AB. *EENT:* disturbed vision. *GI:* nausea, vomiting. *Skin:* erythema, urticaria. *Other:* chills, fever, backache, flushing, constriction in chest, hepatitis.
carbazochrome salicylate Adrenosem Salicylate	*Surgery with excessive capillary bleeding or oozing*— **Adults, and children over 12 years:** 10 mg I.M. preoperatively on night before surgery and with on-call medication, and 5 mg P.O. or I.M. postop q 2 to 4 hours. **Children under 12 years:** 5 mg I.M. preoperatively on night before surgery and with on-call medication, and 2.5 mg P.O. or I.M. postop q 2 to 4 hours.	*Local:* pain at I.M. injection site.

◆ Also available in Canada.
◆◆ Available in Canada only.
Unmarked trade names available in United States only.

INTERACTIONS	NURSING CONSIDERATIONS
None significant.	• Contraindicated in frank infection, as sole hemostatic agent in abnormal bleeding, or in postpartum bleeding or hemorrhage. • Avoid overpacking when placed into body cavities or closed tissue spaces. • Systemically absorbed; no need to remove.
Oral contraceptives: increased probability of hypercoagulability. Use together cautiously.	• Contraindicated in active intravascular clotting. Use cautiously in thrombophlebitis, or cardiac, hepatic, or renal disease. • Don't give without definite diagnosis or lab results indicating hyperfibrinolysis. • Monitor coagulation studies, pulse rate, heart rhythm, and blood pressure. Notify doctor of any change immediately. • Also used as antidote for streptokinase or urokinase toxicity. • Dilute solution with sterile water for injection, normal saline injection, 5% dextrose water, or Ringer's injection.
None significant.	• Use cautiously in neonates, infants, and patients with liver disease because of susceptibility to hepatitis, which may be transmitted in antihemophilic factor. • Have blood typed and crossmatched to treat possible hemorrhage. • Monitor vital signs regularly. Take pulse rate before I.V. administration. If pulse rate increases significantly, flow rate should be reduced or administration stopped. • Monitor patient for allergic reactions. • For I.V. use only. Use plastic syringe; drug may interact with glass syringe, causing binding of ground-glass surface. • Refrigerate concentrate until ready to use, but not after reconstituted. Before reconstituting, concentrate and diluent bottles should be warmed to room temperature. Reconstituted solution unstable; use within 3 hours. Store away from heat. Don't shake or mix with other I.V. solutions. • Monitor coagulation studies before and during therapy.
None significant.	• Contraindicated in hypersensitivity to salicylates. • Obtain patient history concerning allergies, especially to salicylates. • Has no effect on blood-clotting time, prothrombin, or vitamin K levels.

NAME	INDICATIONS & DOSAGE	SIDE EFFECTS
Factor IX complex Konyne, Proplex	*Factor IX deficiency (hemophilia B or Christmas disease), anticoagulant overdosage—* **Adults and children:** units required equal 0.6 x body weight in Kg x percentage of desired increase of Factor IX level, by slow I.V. infusion. Dosage is highly individualized, depending on degree of deficiency, level of Factor IX desired, weight of patient, and severity of bleeding.	*CNS:* headache. *CV:* possible intravascular hemolysis in patients with blood type A, B, or AB. *Other:* transient fever, chills, flushing, tingling, hepatitis.
microfibrillar collagen hemostat Avitene	*To provide hemostasis in surgery (adjunct)—* **Adults and children:** amount depends on severity of bleeding. Compress area with dry sponges. Apply drug directly to bleeding site for 1 to 5 minutes. Gently remove excess. Reapply if needed.	*Blood:* hematoma. *Local:* wound dehiscence, abscess formation, foreign body reaction, adhesion formation. *Other:* advanced infection in contaminated wounds, mediastinitis, hypersensitivity.
negatol Negatan	*Cervical bleeding—* **Women:** apply 1-inch gauze dipped in 1:10 dilution of drug; insert in cervical canal. If tolerated, may increase to full strength solution. Remove pack after 24 hours; give 2-quart douche of dilute negatol or vinegar. *Oral ulcers—* **Adults and children:** apply to dried lesion with applicator, leave for 1 minute, then neutralize with large amounts of water.	*Local:* burning sensation. *Skin:* erythema, superficial desquamation when applied to skin.
oxidized cellulose Oxycel◆, Surgicel	*To provide hemostasis in surgery (adjunct)—* **Adults and children:** apply with sterile technique, p.r.n. Remove after hemostasis, if possible, with dry sterile forceps. May be left in place if necessary.	*CNS:* headache when used as packing for epistaxis, or after rhinological procedures or application to surface wounds. *EENT:* sneezing, epistaxis or stinging, burning when used as packing for rhinological procedures; nasal membrane necrosis or septal perforation. *Local:* encapsulation of fluid; foreign body reaction; burning or stinging after application to surface wounds. *Other:* possible prolongation of drainage in cholecystectomies.

INTERACTIONS	NURSING CONSIDERATIONS
None significant.	• Contraindicated in hepatic disease, intravascular coagulation, or fibrinolysis. Use cautiously in neonates and infants because of susceptibility to hepatitis, which may be transmitted with Factor IX complex. • Have blood typed and crossmatched to treat possible hemorrhage. If given to patients with blood types A, B, AB, intravascular hemolysis may occur. • Monitor patient for allergic reactions and vital signs regularly. • Avoid rapid infusion. If tingling sensation develops during I.V. infusion, decrease flow rate. • Reconstitute with 20 ml sterile water for injection for each vial of lyophilized drug. Keep refrigerated until ready to use; warm to room temperature before reconstituting. Use within 3 hours of reconstitution. Unstable in solution. Don't shake, refrigerate, or mix reconstituted solution with other I.V. solutions. Store away from heat.
None significant.	• Contraindicated in closure of skin incisions. • Not for injection. • Don't spill on nonbleeding surfaces. • Don't dilute. Always apply dry. • Adheres to wet gloves, instruments, or tissue surfaces. Handle and apply with smooth, dry forceps. Apply directly to source of bleeding.
None significant.	• Grayish vaginal membrane after vaginal use. • When used in vagina, patient should wear a perineal pad to prevent soiling of clothing. • When used for oral ulcers, may apply topical anesthetic first to prevent burning sensation. • Always clean and dry area to be treated. • Astringent, styptic, and protein denaturant; highly acidic.
None significant.	• Contraindicated in controlling hemorrhage from large arteries; in nonhemorrhagic, serous, oozing surfaces; in implantation in bone defects. • Don't pack or wad unless it will be removed after hemostasis. Don't apply too tightly when used as wrap sheet in vascular surgery. Apply loosely against bleeding surface. • Always remove after hemostasis when used in laminectomies or near optic nerve chain. • Don't autoclave this product. • Use only amount needed to produce hemostasis. Remove excess before surgical closure. • Use minimal amounts in urologic procedures. • In large wounds, don't overlap skin edges. • Remove with sterile technique from open wounds after hemostasis. • Don't moisten. Hemostatic effect is greater when applied dry. • Should not be used for permanent packing in fractures because it may result in cyst formation.

NAME	INDICATIONS & DOSAGE	SIDE EFFECTS
thrombin Fibrindex	*Bleeding from parenchymatous tissue, cancellous bone, dental sockets, nasal and laryngeal surgery, and in plastic surgery and skin-grafting procedures—* **Adults:** apply 100 units per ml of sterile isotonic NaCl solution or sterile distilled water to area where clotting is needed (or may apply dry powder in bone surgery); in major bleeding, apply 1,000 to 2,000 units/ml of sterile isotonic NaCl solution. Sponge blood from area before application, but avoid sponging area after application. *GI hemorrhage—* **Adults:** give 2 oz of milk, followed by 2 oz of milk containing 10,000 to 20,000 units thrombin. Repeat t.i.d. for 4 to 5 days or until bleeding is controlled.	*Systemic:* hypersensitivity and fever.

INTERACTIONS	NURSING CONSIDERATIONS
None significant.	• Contraindicated in hypersensitivity to thrombin or bovine products. • Obtain patient history of past reactions to thrombin or bovine products. • Monitor vital signs regularly. • Have blood typed and crossmatched to treat possible hemorrhage. • Don't inject topical thrombin or allow it to enter large blood vessels. I.V. injection may cause death because of severe intravascular clotting. • May be used with absorbable gelatin sponge but not with oxidized cellulose. Consult sponge labeling before use. • Neutralize stomach acids before oral use in GI hemorrhage. • Keep refrigerated, preferably frozen, until ready to use. Unstable in solution. Use within 24 hours of reconstitution; discard after 48 hours. Store away from heat. • Broken down by diluted acid, alkali, and salts of heavy metals.

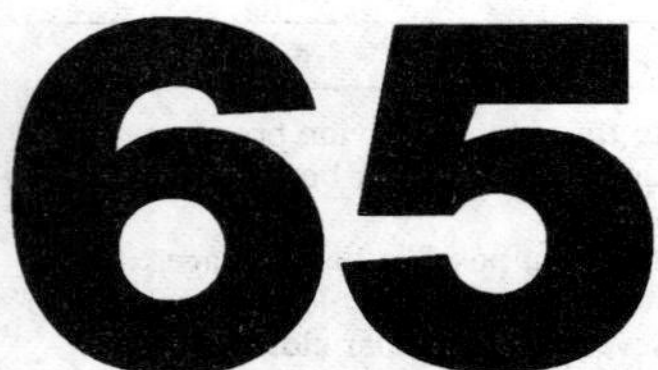

Blood derivatives

normal serum albumin
plasma protein fraction

Normal serum albumin and plasma protein fraction provide a mechanism to maintain hemodynamics in hypovolemic shock or hypoproteinemia. These preparations are made from pooled normal human blood, plasma, or serum. Albumin is also obtained from human placentas.

Major uses

• Treatment of shock associated with burns, trauma, sepsis, or surgery.
• Treatment of hypoproteinemia associated with malnutrition, hepatic cirrhosis, nephrotic syndrome, toxemia of pregnancy, or prematurity.
• Hyperbilirubinemia and erythroblastosis fetalis.

Mechanism of action

• Normal serum albumin 25% provides intravascular oncotic pressure in a 5:1 ratio; causes shift of fluid from interstitial spaces into the circulation; also slightly increases concentration of plasma proteins.
• Plasma protein fraction and normal serum albumin 5% provide colloid to the blood and expand plasma volume.

Absorption, distribution, and excretion

• Given only by I.V. route so absorption is 100% complete.
• Distributed rapidly throughout circulating blood volume.

Onset and duration

• Adequate patient response to normal serum albumin is usually obtained within 15 to 30 minutes. Duration of therapy with albumin and plasma protein fraction varies with patient response and condition being treated.

Combination products

None.

HOW TO CORRECT SLUGGISH I.V. FLOW

1.

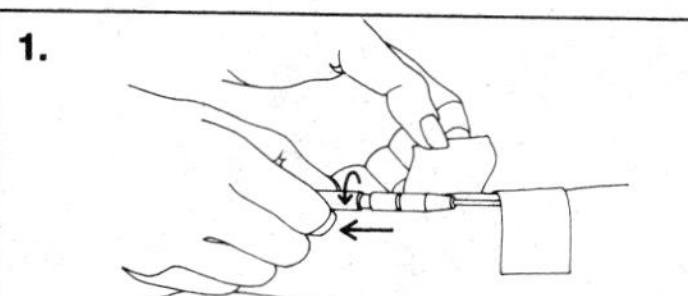

Pull back on the catheter and rotate needle slightly.

2.

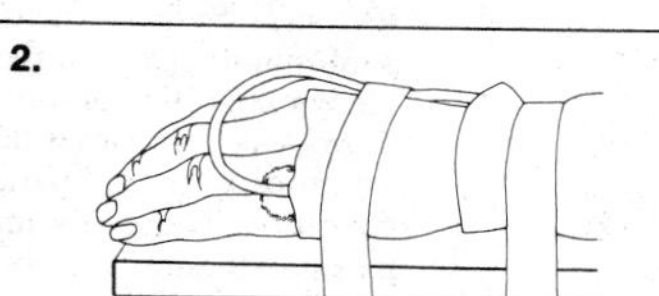

Place a piece of cotton underneath the needle and catheter.

3.

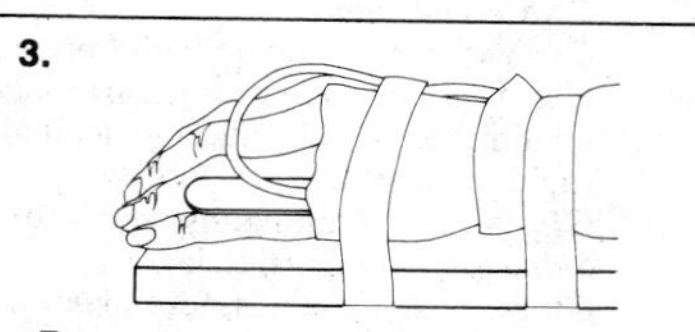

For an alternative, place and tape a tongue blade underneath the needle.

4.

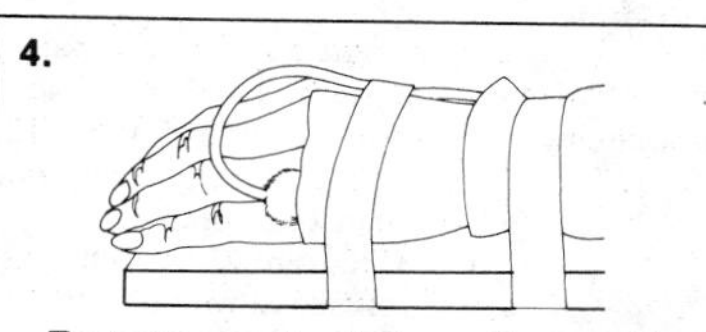

To permanently depress the needle, place a cotton ball on the I.V. site.

5.

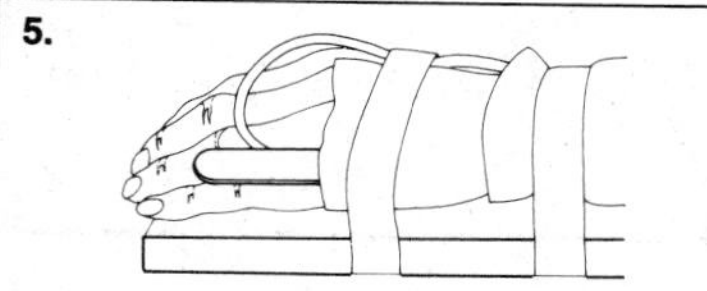

Taping a tongue blade on top of the I.V. site also works.

6.

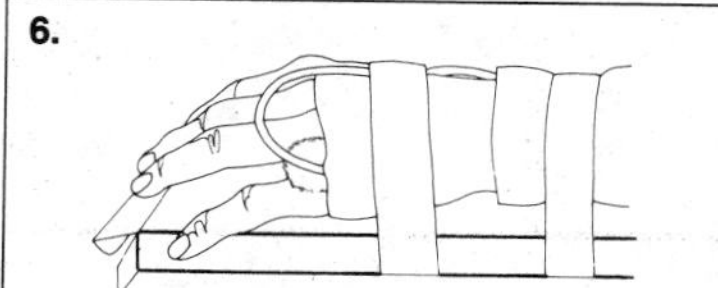

Take care not to tape too tightly, lest you restrict fluid flow.

NAME	INDICATIONS & DOSAGE	SIDE EFFECTS
normal serum albumin 5% Albuminar5, Albumisol 5%, Albuspan 5%, Albutein 5%, Buminate 5% **normal serum albumin 25%** Albuminar25, Albumisol 25%, Buminate 25%	*Shock*— **Adults:** initially, 500 ml (5% solution) by I.V. infusion, repeat q 30 minutes, p.r.n. Dose varies with patient's condition and response. **Children:** 25% to 50% adult dose in nonemergency. *Hypoproteinemia*— **Adults:** 1,000 to 1,500 ml 5% solution by I.V. infusion daily, maximum rate 5 to 10 ml/minute, or 25 to 100 g 25% solution by I.V. infusion daily, maximum rate 3 ml/minute. Dose varies with patient condition and response. *Burns*—dosage varies according to extent of burn and patient's condition. Generally maintain plasma albumin at 2 to 3 g/100 ml. *Hyperbilirubinemia*— **Infants:** 1 g albumin (4 ml. 25%) per Kg before transfusion.	*CV:* vascular overload after rapid infusion, hypotension, altered pulse rate. *GI:* increased salivation, nausea, vomiting. *Skin:* urticaria. *Other:* chills, fever, altered respiration.
plasma protein fraction Plasmanate, Plasma-Plex, Plasmatein, Protenate	*Shock*— **Adults:** varies with patient's condition and response, but usual dose is 250 to 500 ml (12.5 to 25 g protein), usually not faster than 10 ml/min. **Children:** 22 to 33 ml/Kg I.V. infused at rate of 5 to 10 ml/min. *Hypoproteinemia*— **Adults:** 1,000 to 1,500 ml I.V. daily. Maximum infusion rate 8 ml/hour.	*CNS:* headache. *CV:* variable effects on blood pressure after rapid infusion or intra-arterial administration; vascular overload after rapid infusion. *GI:* nausea, vomiting, hypersalivation. *Skin:* erythema, urticaria. *Other:* flushing, chills, fever, back pain, dyspnea.

♦ Also available in Canada.
♦♦ Available in Canada only.
Unmarked trade names available in United States only.

INTERACTIONS	NURSING CONSIDERATIONS
None significant.	• Contraindicated in severe anemia, cardiac failure. Use cautiously in low cardiac reserve, absence of albumin deficiency, restricted salt intake. • Do not give more than 250 g in 48 hours. • Watch for hemorrhage or shock if used after surgery or injury. • Monitor vital signs carefully. • Watch for signs of hypervolemia, (cardiac failure or pulmonary edema). • Patient should be properly hydrated before infusion of 25% solution. • Avoid rapid I.V. infusion. • Dilute with sterile water for injection, 0.9% NaCl, or 5% dextrose injection. Use solution promptly; contains no preservatives. Discard unused solution. • Don't use cloudy solutions or those containing sediment. Solution should be clear amber color. • Freezing may cause the bottle to break. Follow storage instructions on bottle. • One volume of 25% albumin is equivalent to 5 volumes of 5% albumin in producing hemodilution and relative anemia. • This product is very expensive and random supply shortages occur often.
None significant.	• Contraindicated in severe anemia, cardiac failure, patients undergoing cardiac bypass. Use cautiously in hepatic or renal failure, low cardiac reserve, restricted salt intake. • Monitor blood pressure. Infusion should be slowed or stopped if sudden hypotension occurs. • Vital signs should return to normal gradually; monitor hourly. • Watch for signs of vascular overload (cardiac failure or pulmonary edema). • Monitor intake and output. Watch for decreased urinary output. • Check expiration date on container before using. Discard solutions in containers which have been opened for more than 4 hours. Solution contains no preservatives. • Don't use solutions that are cloudy, contain sediment, or have been frozen. • If patient is dehydrated, give additional fluids either P.O. or I.V. • Do not give more than 250 g (5,000 ml 5%) in 48 hours. • Contains 130 to 160 mEq sodium per liter.

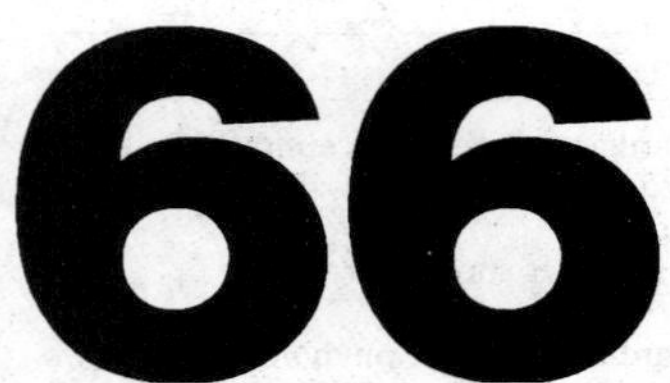

Thrombolytic enzymes

streptokinase
urokinase

Thrombolytic enzymes have been proven effective for the treatment of acute extensive, life-threatening thrombotic disorders. However, before considering therapy with these agents, one must consider the increased risk of hemorrhage accompanying their use.

Major uses

• Treatment of acute massive pulmonary emboli, extensive deep-vein thrombosis, arterial embolic syndrome, and for clearing arteriovenous cannulas.

Mechanism of action

• Thrombolytic enzymes stimulate physiological substances in the body, converting plasminogen to plasmin. Once formed, plasmin degrades fibrin clots, fibrinogen, and other plasma proteins.

Absorption, distribution, and excretion

• Urokinase and streptokinase are administered only by I.V. infusion and are distributed throughout the body.
• They are excreted in the urine.

Onset and duration

• Both streptokinase and urokinase begin to act immediately.
• They must be infused at a constant dosage level to maintain therapeutic effectiveness. Their action ceases when the I.V. infusion is discontinued, but residual effects on coagulation may last up to 12 hours.

Combination products

None.

SITES OF OCCLUSION

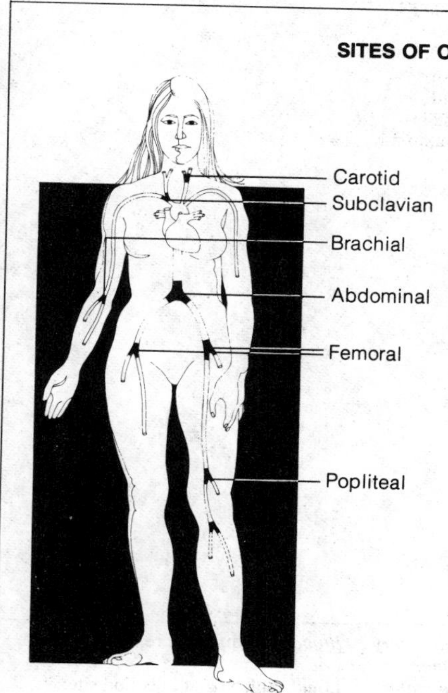

Thrombolytic enzymes are used to treat emboli that develop in these common sites. By watching for respiratory distress, pulse changes, temperature drops, and skin color changes from mottled to blue that appear distal to the site, you can help detect occlusive problems early and report them to the doctor.

NAME	INDICATIONS & DOSAGE	SIDE EFFECTS
streptokinase Kabikinase, Streptase	*Arteriovenous cannula occlusion—* **Adults:** 250,000 I.U. in 2 ml I.V. solution by I.V. pump infusion into each occluded limb of the cannula over 25 to 35 minutes. Clamp off cannula for 2 hours. Then aspirate contents of cannula; flush with saline and reconnect. *Venous thrombosis and pulmonary embolism—* **Adults:** loading dose: 250,000 I.U. I.V. infusion over 30 minutes. Sustaining dose: 100,000 I.U./hour I.V. infusion for 72 hours for deep venous thrombosis and 100,000 I.U. per hour over 24 to 72 hours by I.V. infusion pump for pulmonary embolism.	*Blood:* bleeding, decreased hematocrit. *EENT:* periorbital swelling. *Local:* phlebitis at injection site. *Skin:* urticaria. *Other:* hypersensitivity to drug, anaphylaxis, musculoskeletal pain, minor breathing difficulty, bronchospasms, angioneurotic edema.
urokinase Abbokinase, Win-Kinase	*Lysis of acute massive pulmonary emboli and lysis of pulmonary emboli accompanied by unstable hemodynamics—* **Adults:** for I.V. infusion only by constant infusion pump which will deliver a total volume of 195 ml. Priming dose: 4,400 I.U./Kg/hour of urokinase-normal saline admixture given over 10 minutes. Follow with 4,400 I.U./Kg/hour for 12 to 24 hours. Total volume should not exceed 200 ml. Follow therapy with continuous	*Blood:* bleeding, decreased hematocrit. *Local:* phlebitis at injection site. *Other:* hypersensitivity (not as frequent as streptokinase), musculoskeletal pain, bronchospasm, anaphylaxis.

◆ Also available in Canada.
◆◆ Available in Canada only.
Unmarked trade names available in United States only.

INTERACTIONS	NURSING CONSIDERATIONS
Anticoagulants: concurrent use of anticoagulants with streptokinase is not recommended. Reversing the effects of oral anticoagulants must be considered before beginning therapy, and heparin must be stopped and its effect allowed to diminish. *Aspirin, indocin, phenylbutazone, drugs, affecting platelet activity:* increased risk of bleeding. Do not use together.	• Contraindicated in ulcerative wounds; recent trauma with possible internal injuries; visceral or intracranial malignancy; ulcerative colitis; diverticulitis or any bleeding lesions of GI or GU tract; severe hypertension; acute or chronic hepatic or renal insufficiency; uncontrolled hypocoagulable state; chronic lung disease with cavitation; subacute bacterial endocarditis or rheumatic valvular disease; recent cerebral embolism, thrombosis, or hemorrhage. Also contraindicated within 10 days after intra-arterial diagnostic procedure or any surgery, including liver or kidney biopsy, lumbar puncture, thoracentesis, paracentesis, or extensive or multiple cutdowns. • I.M. injections contraindicated during streptokinase therapy. • Before initiating therapy, draw blood to determine PTT and prothrombin time. Rate of I.V. infusion depends on thrombin time and streptokinase resistance. • If the patient has had a recent streptococcal infection or recent treatment with streptokinase, a higher loading dose may be necessary. • Preparation of I.V. solution: reconstitute each vial with 5 ml sodium chloride for injection. Further dilute to 45 ml. Don't shake; roll gently to mix. Use within 24 hours. Store at room temperature. • Monitor patient for excessive bleeding; if evident, stop therapy. Pretreatment with heparin or drugs affecting platelets causes high risk of bleeding. • Have crossmatched and typed packed red cells and whole blood available to treat possible hemorrhage. • Keep aminocaproic acid (Amicar) and corticosteroids available to treat adverse reactions not responding to blood replacement. • Before using streptokinase to clear an occluded arteriovenous cannula, try flushing with heparinized saline solution. • Bruising more likely during therapy; avoid unnecessary handling. • Keep puncture sites to a minimum; use pressure dressing on puncture sites for at least 15 minutes. • Monitor vital signs frequently. • Watch for signs of hypersensitivity. Notify doctor immediately. • Heparin by continuous infusion is usually started within an hour after stopping streptokinase. Use infusion pump to administer heparin. • Should be used only by doctors with wide experience in thrombotic diseases management, where clinical and laboratory monitoring can be performed. • Store at room temperature. • For symptoms and treatment of anaphylaxis, see p. 1114.
Anticoagulants: concurrent use of anticoagulants with urokinase is not recommended. Reversing the effects of oral anticoagulants must be considered before beginning therapy, and heparin must be stopped and its effect allowed to diminish.	• Contraindicated in ulcerative wounds; recent trauma with possible internal injuries; visceral or intracranial malignancy; pregnancy and first 10 days postpartum; ulcerative colitis; diverticulitis or any bleeding lesions of GI or GU tract; severe hypertension; acute or chronic hepatic or renal insufficiency; uncontrolled hypocoagulation; chronic lung disease with cavitation; subacute bacterial endocarditis or rheumatic valvular disease; and recent cerebral embolism, thrombosis, or hemorrhage. Also contraindicated within 10 days after intra-arterial diagnostic procedure or any surgery, including liver or kidney biopsy, lumbar puncture, thoracentesis, paracentesis, or extensive or multiple cutdowns. • I.M. injections are contraindicated during urokinase therapy. • Preparation of I.V. solution: add 5.2 ml sterile water for injection to vial. Dilute further with 0.9% saline solution before infusion. Don't use bacteriostatic water for injection to reconstitute; it contains preservatives.

(continued on following page)

NAME	INDICATIONS & DOSAGE	SIDE EFFECTS
urokinase *(continued)*	I.V. infusion of heparin, then oral anticoagulants.	

INTERACTIONS	NURSING CONSIDERATIONS
Aspirin, indocin, phenylbutazone, other drugs affecting platelet activity: increased risk of bleeding. Do not use together.	• Monitor patient for bleeding. Pretreatment with drugs affecting platelets puts patient at high risk of bleeding. • Have crossmatched and typed red cells and whole blood available to treat possible hemorrhage. • Keep aminocaproic acid (Amicar) and corticosteroids available to treat adverse reactions not responding to blood replacement. • Watch for signs of hypersensitivity. Notify doctor immediately. • Monitor vital signs. • Keep puncture sites to a minimum; use pressure dressing on puncture sites for at least 15 minutes. • Heparin by continuous infusion usually started within an hour after urokinase has been stopped. Use an infusion pump to administer heparin. • Bruising during therapy more likely; avoid unnecessary handling of patient. • Should only be used by doctors with wide experience in thrombotic diseases management, where clinical and laboratory monitoring can be performed. • For symptoms and treatment of anaphylaxis, see p. 1114.

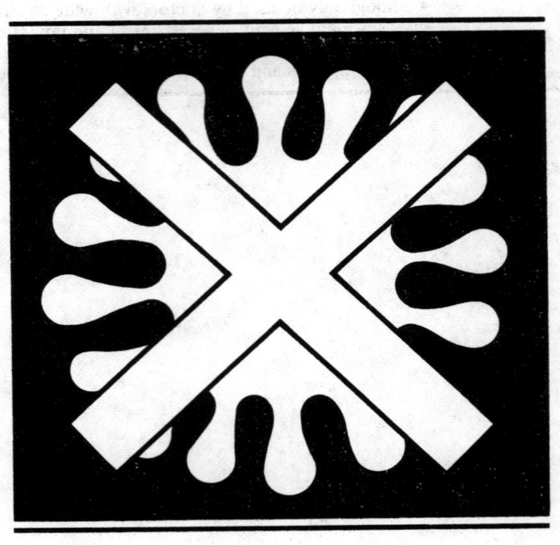

Antineoplastics

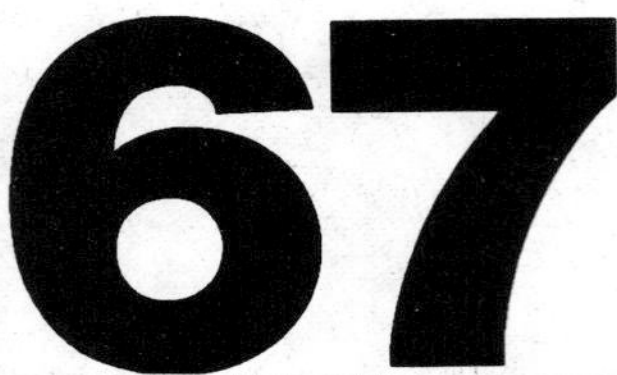

Nursing implications of chemotherapy

In the past, chemotherapy was reserved as a last resort for cancer patients after radiation or surgery had failed. Today, however, chemotherapy is widely used to prolong the lives of more patients, usually in combination with surgery and/or radiation.

The goal of chemotherapy is to destroy every cancer cell in the patient's body by interfering with neoplastic cell division. However, each dose of an antineoplastic drug destroys only a fraction of neoplastic cells, since only a fraction of the cells are dividing when the drug is given. Therefore, to eradicate all neoplastic cells, either a very large dose of an antineoplastic must be given, or treatment must begin very early, when there are still few cancer cells, and it must be prolonged. The doses needed to obtain maximum therapeutic response are quite toxic. Cells that are actively dividing, such as bone marrow, skin, gastrointestinal mucosa, hair follicles, and fetal tissues, are most susceptible to this toxicity.

The benefits of using chemotherapy in pregnant or lactating women should be weighed against risks of probable teratogenicity, mutagenicity, and carcinogenicity in infant or fetus.

Common terminology

Myelosuppression: suppression of bone marrow function.

Nadir: point at which blood count (mainly WBC, platelets, granulocytes) reach their lowest level as a result of chemotherapy (usually 7 to 10 days after dose). It's important to know when to expect the nadir because the patient is then at greatest risk of developing complications, such as infections.

Pancytopenia: decreased level of all blood components—WBC, platelets, granulocytes.

Stomatitis: inflamed, painful mouth ulcers—may often appear as white patches on oral mucosa.

Response Rate:

1. Complete (CR)—complete disappearance of all measurable and evaluable disease.
2. Partial (PR)—50% decrease of all measurable and evaluable disease except for hepatomegaly, where there need only be a 30% decrease.
3. No change—less than 50% decrease in all measurable and evaluable disease.
4. Progression—appearance of any new lesions, or increase by 25% of any previously measurable disease.

Supportive Therapy: treatment given with systemic chemotherapy (steroids, radiation).

Adjuvant Therapy: chemotherapy and radiation therapy used in addition to surgery even though there is no evidence of metastasis and patient is asymptomatic.

Dosing antineoplastics

- Dosage is often based on m^2 (body surface area in meters squared) because edema may make the patient's weight an unreliable measure of body mass.
- Weigh the patient carefully, since dosage is based on lean (ideal) body weight or actual weight, whichever is less.
- Fat tissue absorbs drugs at a different rate than other tissues. For all these reasons, m^2 (body surface area) is used to calculate drug dosages. This requires the use of a mathematical table and some careful mathematical calculations.
- Protein-binding occurs to some extent with most antineoplastic drugs. This means that a certain percentage of the drug binds temporarily with serum proteins. The doctor takes this into consideration in calculating the drug dose.
- Some non-antineoplastic drugs may compete for protein-binding sites with the antineoplastic drug. If this occurs and has not been accounted for, more of the antineoplastic drug will be free in the blood serum, causing toxic effects. Phenothiazines are one such group of drugs which can compete for protein-binding sites with some antineoplastic drugs. Keep this in mind if administering a phenothiazine antiemetic (prochlorperazine) before antineoplastic therapy.

Combination therapy

In many cases, the best way to destroy cancer cells with chemotherapy is to combine several different antineoplastic drugs. This is done to delay the development of neoplastic cells resistant to specific antineoplastic agents and to obtain an additive or complementary therapeutic effect with minimum toxicity. In some cancers, such as leukemia, different antineoplastic agents are given in a specific order for optimum results. For instance, one drug may induce a remission, but not maintain it; so this drug is followed by another more effective at maintaining the remission.

When combining antineoplastic agents, the doctor must consider the scheduling of the drugs and the serious side effects, such as bone marrow depression, which they may cause. Drugs with different side effects, or with the same side effects occurring at different times, are usually combined.

Some common protocols for combination chemotherapy follow. Remember, all dosages for chemotherapy are subject to change because of constant research. Always check the latest protocols or current literature for dosing information.

OAP (regulated according to the degree of bone marrow depression)
vincristine (Oncovin): 1.4 mg/m^2 I.V. push on day 1 (2 mg maximum).
cytarabine (Cytosar): 200 mg/m^2 daily for 5 days as continuous I.V. infusion.
prednisone: 100 mg total dose daily (25 mg q.i.d.) for 5 days.

POMP (regulated according to the degree of bone marrow depression)
mercaptopurine (Purinethol): 500 mg/m^2 daily for 5 days.
vincristine (Oncovin): 1.4 mg/m^2 I.V. push on days 1 and 7.
methotrexate: 7.5 mg/m^2 I.V. daily for 5 days.
prednisone: 100 mg daily (25 mg q.i.d.) for 5 days.

MOPP (repeated every 28 days)
mechlorethamine (Mustargen): 6 mg/m^2 I.V. push on days 1 and 8.
vincristine (Oncovin): 1.4 mg/m^2 I.V. push on days 1 and 8.
procarbazine (Matulane): 100 mg/m^2 daily P.O. for 14 days.
prednisone: 40 mg/m^2 daily P.O. for 14 days.

COP (repeated every 15 days)
cyclophosphamide (Cytoxan): 800 mg/m^2 I.V. push on day 1.
vincristine (Oncovin): 1.4 mg/m^2 on day 1.
prednisone: 100 mg total daily dose (25 mg q.i.d.) for 5 days.

MAC (repeated every 21 days)
methotrexate: 4 mg/m^2 I.V. daily for 5 days.
dactinomycin (Cosmegen): 0.5 mg I.V. daily for 5 days.
cyclophosphamide (Cytoxan): 120 mg/m^2 I.V. daily for 5 days.

COMFU-P (repeated monthly)
cyclophosphamide (Cytoxan): 120 mg/m^2 I.V. daily for 5 days.
vincristine (Oncovin): 0.625 mg/m^2 I.V. push on days 1 and 5.
methotrexate: 4 mg/m^2 I.V. daily for 5 days.
fluorouracil (5-FU): 180 mg/m^2 I.V. daily for 5 days.
prednisone: 40 mg/m^2 daily in divided doses for 5 days.

CODFU (repeated monthly)
cyclophosphamide (Cytoxan): 120 mg/m^2 I.V. daily for 5 days.
vincristine (Oncovin): 0.625 mg/m^2 I.V. push on days 1 and 5.
dactinomycin (Cosmegen): 0.25 mg I.V. daily for 5 days.
fluorouracil (5-FU): 180 mg/m^2 I.V. daily for 5 days.

COAP (regulated according to the degree of bone marrow depression)
cyclophosphamide (Cytoxan): 100 mg/m^2 I.V. daily for 5 days.
vincristine (Oncovin): 1.4 mg/m^2 as I.V. push on day 1 (2 mg maximum).
cytarabine (Cytosar): 100 mg/m^2 daily for 5 days as continuous infusion.
prednisone: 100 mg total daily dose (25 mg q.i.d.) for 5 days.

A wide range of side effects is common with antineoplastic agents, but good patient care and close monitoring can prevent many of these or make the patient more comfortable.

Bone marrow depression critical

This remains the most important factor limiting the dosage of an antineoplastic. Dosages should be reduced in the presence of bone marrow depression.

White blood cells (WBC) and platelets are indicators of bone marrow depression. When the WBC count falls below 4,000 cells/mm^3, or the platelet count falls below 120,000 cells/mm^3, the dose of most drugs is reduced by 50%. Further dosage reductions are made as the counts drop. When the WBC count falls below 2,500 cells/mm^3, or the platelets fall below 80,000 cells/mm^3, all drugs except bleomycin are usually withheld. Once the bone marrow recovers (WBC over 4,000 cells/mm^3 and platelets over 120,000 cells/mm^3), therapy is resumed.

Monitor carefully for bone marrow depression, keeping the following in mind:

- Question the patient carefully about signs of infection, such as sore throat or increased temperature. Report these immediately to doctor.
- Be especially careful in watching for bone marrow depression in patients undergoing concurrent radiation therapy, as this may potentiate the problem.
- A fever that develops when the granulocyte count drops below 500/mm^3 is especially ominous. Take temperature frequently. Call doctor immediately if fever develops.
- The destruction of WBCs by antineoplastic agents interferes with the patient's normal immune response, making him highly susceptible to infection. Patients with bone marrow depression should be placed in reverse isolation and should always be in a private room.
- If possible, the same nurse, or a few nurses, should be assigned to the patient daily to limit the number of people going in and out of his room.
- Antineoplastic destruction of platelets also can cause spontaneous bleeding that is difficult to stop. Watch for signs of bleeding and easy bruising.
- To avoid infection, prepare injection sites carefully with iodophor or similar solutions.
- Avoid routine blood cultures whenever possible, because they can ruin good veins that may be needed for I.V. sites, and because they increase the chance of infection. Do cultures only when the patient develops a fever over 101° F. (38.3° C.).
- Myelosuppression is generally cumulative with antineoplastic agents, so patients don't tolerate subsequent courses of treatment as well as they did the first.

GI side effects troublesome

Nausea, vomiting, and anorexia are very common with most antineoplastic agents, yet they must, if possible, be reduced or avoided so the patient can better tolerate chemotherapy.

- Check hospital policy as to whether or not informed consent is needed before giving first dose.
- Call the doctor immediately if a patient vomits after receiving an antineoplastic drug orally, since the drug may be lost and the dosage may need to be adjusted.
- Giving an antiemetic and small amounts of bland food half an hour before giving antineoplastics will help reduce nausea and vomiting. An antiemetic is more effective when given before, rather than after, chemotherapy.
- To speed recovery and lessen toxicity, patient must be encouraged to eat well despite

anorexia. The dietitian may be able to work out a diet the patient likes. (He's most likely to accept food without an overpowering aroma.) Suggest that the patient's family bring his favorite soups or stews, or other foods that can be warmed easily. Be flexible concerning meal times. Postpone tiring patient-care until after the patient has eaten.

• Erythema of buccal mucosa is an early sign of bone marrow toxicity. The antineoplastic dosage should be lowered or stopped in order to prevent oral ulceration. If stopped, drug may be restarted at a lower dose about 7 to 10 days after ulcer heals.

• Excellent mouth care can help prevent oral side effects. Mucosal deterioration sets in when more than 6 hours pass without giving patient mouth care. Use soft rayon-tipped swabs for mouth care. To avoid gum irritation, use a soft-bristled tooth brush.

• Rinse sore and ulcerated mouth with hydrogen peroxide and water (1:1). To further reduce discomfort, have the patient, before he eats, use lidocaine viscous as an oral rinse. Apply petrolatum jelly to cracked, dry lips.

• Patient with stomatitis should avoid spicy, hot, and rough-textured foods.

• Diarrhea and constipation should be prevented to avoid further irritation of lower gastrointestinal tract. Question patient frequently about stools. If patient has diarrhea, give small feedings, decrease roughage; if constipated, increase roughage in diet. See that a laxative or antidiarrheal is ordered as needed.

• Use of a rectal thermometer may be irritating to rectal mucosa.

• Pharmacy can prepare a popsicle of nystatin for fungal overgrowth in mouth. The cold popsicle is also anesthetizing.

• If a patient develops a dietary deficiency from chemotherapy, request some dietary supplements and ask the dietitian to add more calories and protein to his menu. Freezing the supplements and serving them like ice cream in sundaes and shakes may make them more palatable.

Fluids prevent dehydration

• Maintain good hydration, especially before giving an antineoplastic. Patient may not be able to hold down food for several days after treatment, and dehydration must be avoided. Force fluids to 2 to 3 liters daily. Sometimes carbonated beverages are well tolerated.

• Record fluid intake/output, since drug excretion depends on good urine outflow.

• Watch for an elevated BUN. Destroyed neoplastic cells are excreted through the kidneys and may affect patient's kidney function.

Hair and skin damage

Alopecia is common with certain antineoplastic drugs, and many patients find it quite distressing. Antineoplastics damage hair follicles perhaps even more than they do malignant cells. A patient may lose some or all of his hair, including scalp hair, eyelashes, eyebrows, and underarm and pubic hair. Warn patient that alopecia is likely, but reassure him that the hair should grow back about 8 weeks after therapy is stopped. With some drugs, new hair may even grow during maintenance therapy. However, the new hair may be of a different texture and color. Suggest that a hairpiece be obtained before treatment, or have the patient's family provide scarves.

• Check the patient's skin carefully for petechiae, ecchymoses (especially over chest and antecubital surfaces). Report these to the doctor. If the same nurse or a few nurses are assigned to the same patient, they can keep a continuous daily record of skin changes.

• During administration of sclerosing drugs, such as carmustine, dacarbazine, dactinomycin, doxorubicin, mechlorethamine, mithramycin, mitomycin, thio-tepa, vinblastine sulfate, and vincristine sulfate, extravasation may cause chemical cellulitis, necrosis, or secondary infection. In case of extravasation, apply ice pack and notify doctor immediately and at regular intervals throughout the next 24 hours. After 24 hours, apply warm, moist soak.

HOW TO ANSWER PATIENTS' QUESTIONS ABOUT CHEMOTHERAPY

Before speaking to the patient about chemotherapy, assess his knowledge about his illness. He may not accept or recognize his illness as cancer. For instance, he may speak of "my tumor." Only after he himself tells you he has cancer, should you use this word. If needed, modify the following answers to use the patient's own terms for his illness.

What is chemotherapy?
Chemotherapy literally means treatment with chemicals. However, it's commonly accepted to mean drug treatment of cancer.

Is there more than one type of chemotherapy?
Yes. Many drugs can be given many ways (orally, by injection into a muscle or subcutaneous tissue, or by intravenous infusion). Your doctor will select one that is correct for you and your condition.

Will it hurt?
Not usually. However, with some intravenous drugs, you may experience a temporary burning or cold sensation. You will be told this beforehand, so you won't be alarmed if it happens.

How long will each treatment take?
That will depend on the kind and number of drugs. Some drugs are given directly into the vein; others are given with a running I.V. solution; still others are added to an I.V. solution and dripped in over a specified time. Check with your doctor or nurse for some idea of how long the treatment will take.

Will I have to be hospitalized?
Most drugs can be given in your doctor's office or at a hospital's out-patient department. But, if you are taking a drug which requires close medical supervision, you may have to be hospitalized.

How long will I have to take these drugs and how often?
Length of treatment varies according to the kind and number of drugs you receive. Check with your doctor or nurse for a time estimate. Usually, the duration of treatment varies from several months to 2 years depending on the type of cancer, the type of drug, and your response to the drug (including adverse reactions). Most drugs are given weekly or monthly. Between times, you may take an oral form at home.

Will I be sick when I get chemotherapy?
Remember, *everyone responds differently.* With many of the drugs, you may experience nausea or vomiting. If you do, you will be given another drug to relieve it.

Will I be able to continue working or taking care of my family?
Again, this depends on the kind of cancer and response to treatment. You will probably be able to resume normal activities without problems. But if you feel a little tired after treatment, relax for the rest of the day.

Will I be able to take alcoholic drinks while I'm undergoing chemotherapy?
Usually, a cocktail or glass of wine will not be harmful. But with some conditions, you must avoid alcohol; so ask your doctor.

Will my diet be restricted?
No. As long as you're not having any problems eating normally, continue to do so. If you have any problems, your doctor may suggest a diet change. You may tolerate chemotherapy better if you eat a light meal before and after the procedure. Also, increase your fluid intake before, during, and after chemotherapy by 2 to 4 glasses daily.

Should I discontinue other drugs I'm taking?
Tell your doctor about all other drugs you're taking, how much and how often. He needs to know this because some drugs can interfere with your reaction to chemotherapy. Some examples of such drugs: anticoagulants, antibiotics, aspirin, barbiturates, diuretics, hormones, cough medicines, and medications for diabetes and high blood pressure. The doctor will adjust your prescriptions as needed.

Is chemotherapy really worthwhile?
Patients *really do benefit* from chemotherapy, with increased chances of survival and enhanced quality of life. Ultimately based on your condition and the kind of chemotherapy, only you and your family can decide how worthwhile it is for you.

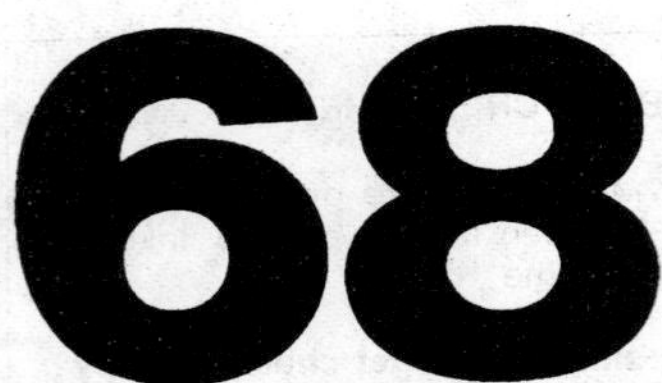

Alkylating agents

busulfan
carmustine (BCNU)
chlorambucil
cis-platinum or cisplatin
cyclophosphamide
dacarbazine (DTIC)
lomustine (CCNU)
mechlorethamine hydrochloride (nitrogen mustard)
melphalan
pipobroman
thiotepa
uracil mustard

The alkylating agents were developed as a result of military research into mustard gases. Because these compounds cause bone marrow depression and atrophy of lymphoid tissue, they were first used for treating malignant lymphomas and leukemias. But since the introduction of mechlorethamine, the first nitrogen mustard used clinically, an intense search for more effective and less toxic antineoplastic alkylating agents has been under way. Alkylating agents can act during any phase of a cell's life cycle; this gives them an advantage over more specific antineoplastics which are only effective during a single phase of the cycle, and also makes their toxicity nonspecific to the cells, as well.

Major uses

- For treatment of sarcomas, lymphomas, and some leukemias and carcinomas.

Mechanism of action

- Cause chromosome breakage by cross-linking strands of DNA and inhibit replication.
- Interfere with many cell functions, such as synthesis and respiration.

Absorption, distribution, and excretion

- Oral absorption is good with busulfan, chlorambucil, cyclophosphamide, lomustine, melphalan, pipobroman, and uracil mustard.
- Distributed to all body tissues.
- Carmustine and lomustine rapidly diffuse into cerebrospinal fluid and cross the blood-brain barrier.

• Metabolized by liver.
• Excreted in urine within 1 to 2 days.
• Cis-platinum, or cisplatin, concentrates in liver, kidneys, large and small intestines after intravenous administration. Full urinary excretion of dose takes 5 days.

Onset and duration
• Varies with drug, disease, and patient response.

Combination products
• None.

HOW ALKYLATING AGENTS AFFECT DNA

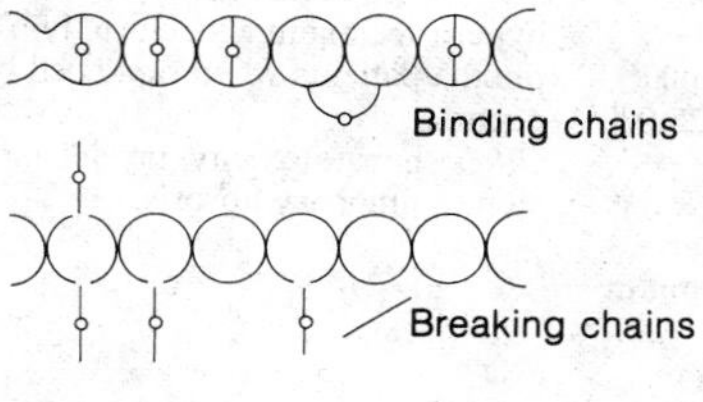

Alkylating agents settle in the cell nucleus, where they attack DNA by binding its chains together, or by breaking them apart. They act at all phases of the cell cycle and so are called cell-cycle nonspecific agents. Because of their inability to selectively attack cancer cells, they also affect other rapidly dividing cells, such as those in the gastrointestinal mucosa, the hair follicles, and the bone marrow. Consequently, their common side effects include gastrointestinal irritation, alopecia, and pancytopenia.

NAME	INDICATIONS & DOSAGE	SIDE EFFECTS
busulfan Myleran◆	*Chronic myelocytic (granulocytic) leukemia—* **Adults:** 4 to 6 mg P.O. daily up to 8 mg P.O. daily or 4 to 6 mg/m^2 until WBC falls to 10,000/mm^3; stop drug until WBC rises to 50,000/mm^3, then resume treatment as before; or 4 to 8 mg P.O. daily until WBC falls to 10,000 to 20,000/mm^3, then reduce daily dose as needed to maintain WBC at this level (usually 2 mg daily). **Children:** 0.06 to 0.12 mg/Kg or 2.3 to 4.6 mg/m^2/day P.O.; adjust dose to maintain WBC at 20,000/mm^3, but never less than 10,000/mm^3.	*Blood:* WBC begins to fall after about 10 days and continues for 2 weeks after stopping drugs; thrombocytopenia, pancytopenia, anemia. *GI:* nausea, vomiting, diarrhea, cheilosis, glossitis. *GU:* amenorrhea, testicular atrophy, uric acid nephropathy, impotence. *Metabolic:* Addison-like wasting syndrome. Profound hyperkalemia may occur in patients with very high WBCs, and cell lysis. Profound hyperuricemia due to increased cell lysis. *Skin:* transient hyperpigmentation, anhidrosis. *Other:* gynecomastia; alopecia; myelosuppression; irreversible pulmonary fibrosis, commonly termed "busulfan lung."
carmustine (BCNU) BiCNU◆	*Brain, colon, and stomach cancer; Hodgkin's disease; non-Hodgkin's; lymphomas; melanomas; multiple myeloma; and hepatoma—* **Adults:** 100 mg/m^2 I.V. by slow infusion daily for 2 days; repeat q 6 weeks if platelets are above 100,000/mm^3 and WBC is above 4,000/mm^3. Dose is reduced 50% when WBC less than 2,000/mm^3 and platelets less than 25,000/mm^3. Alternate therapy: 200 mg/m^2 I.V. slow infusion as a single dose, repeat q 6 to 8 weeks; or 40 mg/m^2 I.V. slow infusion for 5 consecutive days, repeated q 6 weeks.	*Blood:* cumulative bone marrow depression, delayed 4 to 6 weeks, lasts 1 to 2 weeks; leukopenia; thrombocytopenia. *GI:* nausea 2 to 6 hours after giving (can be severe). *GU:* uric acid nephropathy. *Local:* intense pain at injection site. *Metabolic:* profound hyperkalemia, hyperuricemia may occur in lymphoma patients when rapid cell lysis occurs. *Other:* hepatotoxicity, myelosuppression, pulmonary fibrosis.

◆ Also available in Canada.
◆◆ Available in Canada only.
Unmarked trade names available in United States only.

INTERACTIONS	NURSING CONSIDERATIONS
None significant.	• Use cautiously in patients recently given other myelosuppressive drugs or radiation treatment, and in those with depressed neutrophil or platelet counts. • Isolate patient. Watch for signs of infection (fever, sore throat). • Warn patient that side effects may be delayed for 4 to 6 months. • Persistent cough, progressive dyspnea with alveolar exudate may result from drug toxicity, not pneumonia. • Monitor serum potassium, uric acid, and CBC. • To prevent hyperuricemia with resulting uric acid nephropathy, allopurinol may be used with adequate hydration and alkalinization of urine. • Screen urine for stones. • Patient response usually begins within 1 to 2 weeks (increased appetite, sense of well-being, decreased total leukocyte, reduction in size of spleen). • Can cause false positive cytology in all body secretions. • Anticoagulants should be used cautiously. Watch closely for signs of bleeding. • Avoid all I.M. injections when platelets are low.
None significant.	• To reduce pain on injection, 50 to 75 mg meperidine I.M. or P.O. should be given before injection. • Warn patient to watch for signs of infection and bone marrow toxicity (fever, sore throat, anemia, fatigue, easy bruising, nose or gum bleeds, melena). Take temperature daily. • Monitor serum potassium, uric acid, CBC. • Isolate patient when bone marrow depression occurs. • To reduce nausea, give antiemetic before administering. • Don't mix with other drugs during administration. • To reconstitute, dissolve 100 mg carmustine in 3 ml absolute alcohol. Dilute solution with 27 ml sterile water for injection. Resultant solution contains 3.3 mg carmustine/ml in 10% alcohol. Dilute in normal saline solution or dextrose 5% in water for I.V. infusion. • Protect from light; wrap bottle in aluminum foil. Keep dry powder. May store reconstituted solution in refrigerator for 24 hours. • If powder liquifies or appears oily, it is sign of decomposition. Discard. • Can cause false positive cytology in all body secretions. • To prevent hyperuricemia with resulting uric acid nephropathy, allopurinol may be used with adequate hydration and alkalinization of urine. Screen urine for stones. • Avoid contact with skin, as carmustine will cause a brown stain. If drug comes into contact with skin, wash off thoroughly. • Anticoagulants should be used cautiously. Watch closely for signs of bleeding. • Avoid all I.M. injections when platelets are low.

NAME	INDICATIONS & DOSAGE	SIDE EFFECTS
chlorambucil Leukeran◆	*Chronic lymphocytic leukemia, lymphosarcoma, giant follicular lymphoma, Hodgkin's disease, ovarian carcinoma, mycosis fungoides—* **Adults:** 0.1 to 0.2 mg/Kg P.O. daily for 3 to 6 weeks, then adjust for maintenance (usually 2 mg daily). **Children:** 0.1 to 0.2 mg/Kg/day or 4.5 mg/m^2/day P.O. as single dose or in divided doses.	*Blood:* leukopenia, delayed up to 3 weeks, lasts up to 10 days after last dose; thrombocytopenia; anemia; myelosuppression (usually moderate, gradual, and rapidly reversible). *GU:* may cause sterility at cumulative doses of 400 mg or more; uric acid nephropathy. *Metabolic:* profound hyperkalemia may occur in leukemia patients with very high WBCs, and in lymphoma patients when rapid cell lysis occurs; hyperuricemia. *Skin:* exfoliative dermatitis. *Other:* allergic febrile reactions.
cis-platinum or cisplatin Platinol	*Adjunctive therapy in metastatic testicular cancer—* **Adults:** 20 mg/m^2 I.V. daily for 5 days. Repeat every 3 weeks for 3 cycles or longer. *Adjunctive therapy in metastatic ovarian cancer—*100 mg/m^2 I.V. Repeat every 4 weeks; or 50 mg/m^2 I.V. every 3 weeks with concurrent doxorubicin HCl therapy. Give as I.V. infusion in 2 liters 5% dextrose in 0.45% normal saline or 5% dextrose in 0.3% normal saline with 37.5 g mannitol over 6 to 8 hours.	*Blood:* reversible myelosuppression in 25% to 30% of patients, leukopenia, thrombocytopenia, anemia; nadirs in circulating platelets and leukocytes on days 18 to 23 with recovery by day 39. *CNS:* peripheral neuritis, loss of taste, seizures. *EENT:* tinnitus, hearing loss, both in up to 31% of patients. *GI:* nausea, vomiting, beginning 1 to 4 hours after dose and lasting 24 hours. *GU:* renal toxicity (in 28% to 36% of patients), becomes more prolonged and severe with repeated courses of therapy. *Other:* anaphylactoid reaction, hyperuricemia.
cyclophosphamide Cytoxan◆, Procytox◆◆	*Breast, colon, head, neck, lung, ovarian and prostatic cancer; Hodgkin's disease; chronic lymphocytic leukemia; chronic myelocytic leukemia; acute lymphoblastic leukemia; neuroblastoma; retinoblastoma; non-Hodgkin's lymphomas; multiple myeloma; mycosis fungoides; sarcomas—* **Adults:** 40 to 50 mg/Kg P.O., I.V. in single dose or in 2 to 8 daily doses, then adjust for maintenance; or 2 to 4 mg/Kg P.O. daily for 10 days, then adjust for maintenance. Maintenance dose	*Blood:* leukopenia, nadir between days 8 to 15, lasts 17 to 28 days; thrombocytopenia, anemia. *CV:* cardiotoxicity (with very high doses). *GI:* anorexia, nausea, and vomiting begin within 6 hours, lasts 4 hours; stomatitis; mucositis. *GU:* gonadal suppression (may be irreversible), hemorrhagic cystitis, bladder fibrosis, sterility, nephrotoxicity. *Metabolic:* profound hyperkalemia may occur in leukemia patients with very high WBCs and in lymphoma patients when rapid cell lysis occurs; hyperuricemia; syndrome of inappro-

INTERACTIONS	NURSING CONSIDERATIONS
None significant.	• Don't give for at least 4 weeks after radiation or other chemotherapy. • Myelosuppression reversible up to cumulative dose of 6.5 mg/kg. • Monitor serum potassium, uric acid, CBC. • Give before breakfast or at bedtime to reduce nausea. • To prevent hyperuricemia with resulting uric acid nephropathy, allopurinol may be used with adequate hydration and alkalinization of urine. Screen urine for stones. • Can cause false positive cytology in all body secretions. • Avoid I.M. injections when platelets are low. • Used with dactinomycin and methotrexate in treatment of testicular cancer. • Anticoagulants should be used cautiously. Watch closely for signs of bleeding.
None significant.	• Contraindicated in preexisting renal impairment, myelosuppression, and hearing impairment. • Hydrate patient with 5% dextrose in 0.45% normal saline before giving drug. Maintain urine output of 100 ml/hour for 4 consecutive hours before therapy and for 24 hours after therapy. • Mannitol may be given as 12.5 g I.V. bolus before starting cis-platinum infusion. Follow by infusion of mannitol 20% at rate up to 5 g/hour p.r.n. to maintain urine output during and 6 hours after cis-platinum infusion. • Do not repeat dose unless platelets are over 100,000/mm^3, WBC are over 4,000/mm^3, creatinine is under 1.5 mg%, or BUN is under 25 mg%. • Monitor CBC, platelets, and renal function studies before initial and subsequent doses. • Tell patient to report tinnitus immediately to prevent permanent hearing loss. Do audiometry before and during treatment. • Nausea and vomiting may be severe and protracted (up to 24 hours). Continue I.V. hydration until patient can tolerate adequate oral intake. • May give allopurinol for hyperuricemia. • Reconstitute with sterile water for injection. Stable for 8 hours at room temperature. Don't refrigerate. • Given with bleomycin and vinblastine for testicular cancer and with doxorubicin hydrochloride for ovarian cancer. • Renal toxicity becomes more severe with repeated doses. Renal function must return to normal before next dose can be given. • Avoid I.M. injections when platelets are low.
Corticosteroids, chloramphenicol: reduced activity of cyclophosphamide. Use cautiously. *Allopurinol:* may produce excessive cyclophosphamide effect. Monitor for enhanced toxicity.	• Use cautiously in severe leukopenia, thrombocytopenia, malignant cell infiltration of bone marrow, recent radiation therapy or chemotherapy, hepatic or renal disease. • Advise male and female patients to practice contraception while taking this drug and for 4 months after; drug is potentially teratogenic. • Monitor serum potassium, uric acid, CBC, renal and hepatic functions. • To reduce nausea, give antiemetic before administering. • Give excellent mouth care to help prevent stomatitis. • Push fluid (3 liters daily) to prevent hemorrhagic cystitis. Don't give drug at bedtime, since voiding is too infrequent to avoid cystitis. If hemorrhagic cystitis occurs, drug is usually decreased by half; if it persists, drug is stopped. Cystitis can occur months after therapy has been stopped. • Reconstituted solution is stable 6 days refrigerated or 24 hours at room temperature. • Can cause false positive cytology in all body secretions. • Avoid I.M. injections when platelets are low.

(continued on following page)

NAME	INDICATIONS & DOSAGE	SIDE EFFECTS
cyclophosphamide *(continued)*	1.5 to 3 mg/Kg/day P.O.; or 10 to 15 mg/Kg q 7 to 10 days I.V.; or 3 to 5 mg/Kg twice weekly I.V. **Children:** 2 to 8 mg/Kg/day or 60 to 250 mg/m²/day P.O. or I.V. for 6 days (dose depends on susceptibility of neoplasm); divide oral dosages; give I.V. dosages once weekly. Maintenance dose 2 to 5 mg/Kg or 50 to 150 mg/m² twice weekly P.O.	priate secretion of ADH (with high doses). *Other:* alopecia in 50% of patients, especially with high doses; secondary malignancies, pulmonary fibrosis (high doses); hepatitis.
dacarbazine DTIC-Dome◆	*Hodgkin's disease, metastatic malignant melanoma, neuroblastoma, sarcomas—* **Adults:** 2 to 4.5 mg/Kg or 70 to 160 mg/m² I.V. daily for 10 days; then repeat q 4 weeks as tolerated; or 250 mg/m² I.V. daily for 5 days, repeated at 3-week intervals.	*Blood:* WBC falls for up to 5 weeks, recovers in 2 weeks; thrombocytopenia, anemia. *GI:* severe nausea and vomiting begin within 1 to 3 hours in 90% of patients, last 1 to 12 hours; anorexia, metallic taste in mouth. *Local:* severe pain if I.V. infiltrates; tissue damage. *Metabolic:* profound hyperkalemia may occur in lymphoma patients when rapid cell lysis occurs. *Other:* flu-like syndrome (fever, malaise, myalgia begin 7 days after treatment stopped and may last 7 to 21 days), edema (in children), alopecia, facial flushing, paresthesias, hepatic enzyme elevation.
lomustine (CCNU) CeeNU◆	*Brain, colon, lung and renal cell cancer; Hodgkin's disease; lymphomas; melanomas; multiple myeloma—* **Adults and children:** 130 mg/m² P.O. as single dose q 6 weeks. Reduce dose according to bone marrow depression. Repeat doses should not be given until WBC is more than 4,000/mm³, and platelet count is more than 100,000/mm³.	*Blood:* leukopenia, delayed up to 6 weeks, lasts 1 to 2 weeks; thrombocytopenia, delayed up to 4 weeks, lasts 1 to 2 weeks; anemia. *CNS:* lethargy, ataxia, dysarthria. *GI:* nausea and vomiting begin within 4 to 5 hours, last 24 hours, stomatitis. *Metabolic:* profound hyperkalemia may occur in lymphoma patients when rapid cell lysis occurs. *Other:* alopecia, hepatotoxicity.
mechlorethamine hydrochloride Mustargen◆	*Breast, lung, and ovarian cancer; Hodgkin's disease; chronic myelocytic and acute leukemia; non-Hodgkin's lymphomas; lymphosarcoma—* **Adults:** 0.4 mg/Kg or 10 mg/m² I.V. as single or divided dose q 3 to 6 weeks. Give through running I.V. infusion. Dose reduced in prior radiation or chemotherapy to 0.2 to 0.4 mg/Kg. Dose based on ideal or actual	*Blood:* nadir of leukopenia, thrombocytopenia; myelosuppression occurs by days 4 to 10, lasts 10 to 21 days; mild anemia begins in 2 to 3 weeks, may last 7 weeks. *CNS:* temporary aphasia, paresis, convulsions, progressive muscular paralysis. *EENT:* tinnitus, metallic taste, immediately after dose; deafness in high doses. *GI:* nausea, vomiting, and anorexia

INTERACTIONS	NURSING CONSIDERATIONS
	• Can be given by direct I.V. push into a running I.V. line or by infusion in normal saline solution or dextrose 5% in water. • To prevent hyperuricemia with resulting uric acid nephropathy, keep patient well hydrated; alkalinize the urine. • Warn patient that alopecia is likely to occur. • Anticoagulants should be used cautiously. Watch closely for signs of bleeding. • Has been used successfully to treat systemic necrotizing vasculitis.
None significant.	• Use lower dose if renal function or bone marrow is impaired. Stop drug if WBC falls to 3,000/mm^3 or platelets drop to 100,000/mm^3. • Don't give food for 2 to 6 hours before giving drug. • Take temperature daily. • Isolate patient when WBC drops. • Watch for increased BUN; readily reversible when dose is decreased. • Monitor serum potassium, uric acid, CBC, hepatic and renal function. • Discard refrigerated solution after 72 hours, room temperature solution after 8 hours. • Can cause false positive cytology in all body secretions. • Avoid I.M. injections when platelets are low. • Give I.V. infusion in 50 to 100 ml dextrose 5% in water over 30 minutes. Make sure drug does not infiltrate. • For Hodgkin's disease, usually given with bleomycin, vinblastine, doxorubicin. • Anticoagulants should be used cautiously. Watch closely for signs of bleeding.
None significant.	• Give 2 to 4 hours after meals. To avoid nausea, give antiemetic before administering. • May be useful in cancer involving CNS, since CSF level equals 30% to 50% of plasma level 1 hour after administration. • Monitor blood counts weekly. Don't give more often than every 6 weeks; bone marrow toxicity is cumulative and delayed. • Monitor serum potassium, uric acid, CBC, hepatic function. • Can cause false positive cytology in all body secretions. • Avoid I.M. injection when platelets are low. • For Hodgkin's disease, usually given with mechlorethamine. • Anticoagulants should be used cautiously. Watch closely for signs of bleeding.
None significant.	• Use cautiously in severe anemia, depressed neutrophil or platelet counts, patients recently treated with radiation or chemotherapy. • Avoid contact with skin or mucous membranes. If contact occurs, wash with copious amounts of water and an alkali solution. • Giving antiemetic before drug not always effective in reducing nausea. • Be sure I.V. doesn't infiltrate. If drug extravasates, apply cold compresses; area should be infiltrated with sodium thiosulfate. • When given intracavitarily, turn patient from side to side every 15 minutes to 1 hour to distribute drug. • Monitor serum potassium, uric acid, CBC. • Pretreatment hearing evaluation recommended. • Severe herpes zoster may require stopping drug.

(continued on following page)

NAME	INDICATIONS & DOSAGE	SIDE EFFECTS
mechlorethamine hydrochloride *(continued)*	body weight, whichever is less. *Neoplastic effusions—* **Adults:** 10 to 20 mg intracavitarily.	begin within minutes, last 8 to 24 hours. *GU:* uric acid nephropathy. *Local:* thrombophlebitis, slough, severe irritation if drug extravasates or touches skin. *Metabolic:* profound hyperkalemia may occur in leukemia patients with very high WBCs, and in lymphoma patients when rapid cell lysis occurs, hyperuricemia. *Other:* may precipitate herpes zoster, maculopapular rash, alopecia.
melphalan Alkeran◆	*Multiple myeloma, malignant melanoma, testicular seminoma, reticulum cell sarcoma, osteogenic sarcoma, breast and ovarian cancer—* **Adults:** 6 mg P.O. daily for 2 to 3 weeks, then stop drug for up to 4 weeks or until WBC and platelets stop dropping and begin to rise again; resume with maintenance dose of 2 to 4 mg daily. Stop drug if WBC below 3,000/mm³ or platelets below 100,000/mm³. Alternate therapy 0.15 mg/Kg/day P.O. for 7 days, wait for WBC and platelets to recover, then resume with 0.05 mg/Kg/day P.O.	*Blood:* thrombocytopenia, leukopenia, anemia, agranulocytosis. *GI:* anorexia, nausea, vomiting, stomatitis, oral ulcers. *Metabolic:* profound hyperkalemia may occur in lymphoma patients when rapid cell lysis occurs.
pipobroman Vercyte◆	*Polycythemia vera—* **Adults, and children over 15 years:** 1 mg/Kg P.O. daily for 30 days; may increase to 1.5 to 3 mg/Kg P.O. daily until hematocrit reduced 50% to 55%, then 0.1 to 0.2 mg/Kg daily maintenance. *Chronic myelocytic leukemia—* **Adults, and children over 15 years:** 1.5 to 2.5 mg/Kg P.O. daily until WBC drops to 10,000/mm³, then start maintenance 7 to 175 mg daily. Stop drug if WBC below 3,000/mm³, or platelets below 150,000/mm³.	*Blood:* leukopenia and thrombocytopenia, delayed up to 4 weeks or longer; anemia, hemolysis with reticulocytosis, elevated bilirubin and sudden drop in hemoglobin. *GI:* nausea, vomiting, cramping, diarrhea, anorexia. *Metabolic:* profound hyperkalemia may occur in leukemia patients with very high WBCs. *Skin:* rash.

INTERACTIONS	NURSING CONSIDERATIONS
	• Very unstable solution. Prepare immediately before injection. Use within 15 minutes. Discard unused solution. • To prevent hyperuricemia with resulting uric acid nephropathy, allopurinol may be given; keep patient well hydrated; alkalinize the urine. • Can cause false positive cytology in all body secretions. • Avoid I.M. injections when platelets are low. • One of the most effective drugs in treatment of Hodgkin's disease. • Has been used topically in treatment of mycosis fungoides. • Anticoagulants should be used cautiously. Watch closely for signs of bleeding.
None significant.	• Contraindicated in severe leukopenia, thrombocytopenia, or anemia, chronic lymphocytic leukemia, patients with suppurative inflammation. • To reduce nausea, give antiemetic before administering. • Monitor serum potassium, uric acid, CBC. • Give excellent mouth care to help prevent stomatitis. • Can cause false positive cytology in all body secretions. • Avoid I.M. injections when platelets are low. • May need dose reduction in renal impairment. • Drug of choice in multiple myeloma. • Anticoagulants should be used cautiously. Watch closely for signs of bleeding.
None significant.	• Contraindicated in bone marrow depression. • Do WBC and platelet count until desired response or toxicity occurs (platelets less than 150,000/mm³ or WBC less than 3,000/mm³). • Stop drug if hemolysis occurs. May require blood replacement. • Monitor serum potassium, uric acid, CBC, hepatic and renal function. • Anticoagulants should be used cautiously. Watch closely for signs of bleeding.

NAME	INDICATIONS & DOSAGE	SIDE EFFECTS
thiotepa Thiotepa◆	**Adults, and children over 12 years:** *Breast, lung, and ovarian cancer; Hodgkin's disease, lymphomas*—0.2 mg/Kg I.V. daily for 5 days; then maintenance dose of 0.2 mg/Kg I.V. q 1 to 3 weeks. *Bladder tumor*—60 mg in 60 ml water instilled in bladder once weekly for 4 weeks. *Neoplastic effusions*—10 to 15 mg intracavitarily, p.r.n. Stop drug or decrease dosage if WBC below 4,000/mm³, or if platelets below 150,000/mm³.	*Blood:* leukopenia begins within 5 to 30 days; thrombocytopenia, anemia, neutropenia, mild erythrocyte depression, lymphopenia. *GI:* nausea, vomiting, anorexia. *GU:* amenorrhea, decreased spermatogenesis. *Local:* intense pain at injection site. *Metabolic:* profound hyperkalemia may occur in lymphoma patients when rapid cell lysis occurs; hyperuricemia. *Skin:* hives, rash. *Other:* headache, fever, tightness of throat, dizziness.
uracil mustard	*Chronic lymphocytic and myelocytic leukemia; Hodgkin's disease; reticulum cell sarcoma; lymphomas; mycosis fungoides; polycythemia vera; cancer of ovaries, cervix, and lungs*— **Adults:** 1 to 2 mg P.O. daily for 3 months or until desired response obtained, or toxicity; maintenance 1 mg daily for 3 out of 4 weeks until optimum response or relapse; or 3 to 5 mg P.O. for 7 days (total dose 0.5 mg/Kg), then 1 mg daily for 3 out of 4 weeks.	*Blood:* bone marrow depression, delayed 2 to 4 weeks; thrombocytopenia, leukopenia, anemia. *CNS:* irritability, nervousness, mental cloudiness and depression. *GI:* nausea, vomiting, diarrhea, epigastric distress, abdominal pain, anorexia. *GU:* uric acid nephropathy, amenorrhea, decreased spermatogenesis. *Metabolic:* profound hyperkalemia may occur in leukemia patients with very high WBCs, and in lymphoma patients when rapid cell lysis occurs; hyperuricemia. *Skin:* pruritus, dermatitis, hyperpigmentation, alopecia.

INTERACTIONS	NURSING CONSIDERATIONS
None significant.	• Use cautiously in bone marrow depression, chronic lymphocytic leukemia, renal or hepatic dysfunction. • Do WBC, RBC counts weekly for at least 3 weeks after last dose. Warn patient to report even mild infections. • GU side effects reversible in 6 to 8 months. • May require use of local anesthetic at injection site if intense pain occurs. • For bladder instillation: dehydrate patient 8 to 10 hours before therapy. Instill drug into bladder by catheter; ask patient to retain solution for 2 hours. Volume may be reduced to 30 ml if discomfort is too great with 60 ml. Reposition patient every 15 minutes for maximum area contact. • Toxicity delayed and prolonged because drug binds to tissue and stays in body several hours. • Monitor serum potassium, uric acid, CBC. • Refrigerate dry powder, protect from light. • Use only sterile water for injection to reconstitute. Refrigerated solution stable 5 days. • To prevent hyperuricemia with resulting uric acid nephropathy, allopurinol may be given; keep patient well hydrated; alkalinize the urine. • Can cause false positive cytology in all body secretions. • Avoid I.M. injections when platelets are low. • Can be given by all parenteral routes, including direct injection into the tumor. • Anticoagulants should be used cautiously. Watch closely for signs of bleeding.
None significant.	• Contraindicated in severe thrombocytopenia, aplastic anemia or leukopenia, acute leukemias. • Keep accurate daily record of total cumulative dose. Toxicity may be irreversible at total doses of 1 mg/Kg. • Give at bedtime to reduce nausea. • Watch for signs of ecchymoses, easy bruising, petechiae. • Monitor serum potassium and uric acid. Do regular platelet count. Do CBC 1 to 2 times weekly for 4 weeks; then 4 weeks after stopping drug. • Don't give drug within 2 to 3 weeks after maximum bone marrow depression from past radiation or chemotherapy. • Screen urine for stones. • To prevent hyperuricemia and resulting uric acid nephropathy, allopurinol can be given; keep patient hydrated; alkalinize the urine. • Can cause false positive cytology in all body secretions. • Avoid I.M. injections when platelets are low. • Anticoagulants should be used cautiously. Watch closely for signs of bleeding.

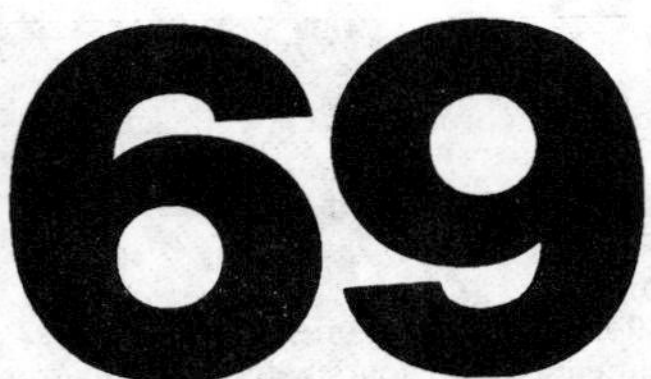

Antimetabolites

azathioprine
cytarabine
floxuridine
fluorouracil
hydroxyurea
mercaptopurine
methotrexate
methotrexate sodium
thioguanine

Antimetabolites represent the first group of antineoplastics designed specifically as antitumor agents. They function in one of two ways. They may substitute for a component in a necessary cellular chemical compound. The resultive cell product, however, fails to function and thereby blocks cell division. Antimetabolites may also inhibit a key enzyme function, thereby interfering with the normal cellular metabolism. Antimetabolites can be divided into three groups: folic acid antagonists (methotrexate and methotrexate sodium); purine antagonists (azathioprine, thioguanine, and mercaptopurine); and pyrimidine antagonists (floxuridine, fluorouracil, and cytarabine). Hydroxyurea is also thought to function as an antimetabolite.

Major uses

- Treatment of choriocarcinomas, leukemias, medulloblastomas, osteogenic sarcomas, and other carcinomas.
- Immunosuppression in renal transplants (azathiprine).

Mechanism of action

- Folic acid antagonists prevent reduction of folic acid to tetrahydrofolic acid by inhibiting production of a needed enzyme.
- Purine and pyrimidine antagonists interfere with nucleic acid biosynthesis.
- Cytarabine and hydroxyurea interfere with conversion of RNA into DNA.

Absorption, distribution, and excretion

- Azathioprine, hydroxyurea, mercaptopurine, methotrexate, methotrexate sodium, and thioguanine are well absorbed orally.
- Cytarabine, floxuridine, and fluorouracil must be given parenterally.
- Distributed widely into body fluids.
- Metabolized in liver.

• Excreted in urine.

Onset and duration
• Varies with drug, disease, and patient response.

Combination products
None.

HOW ANTIMETABOLITES WORK

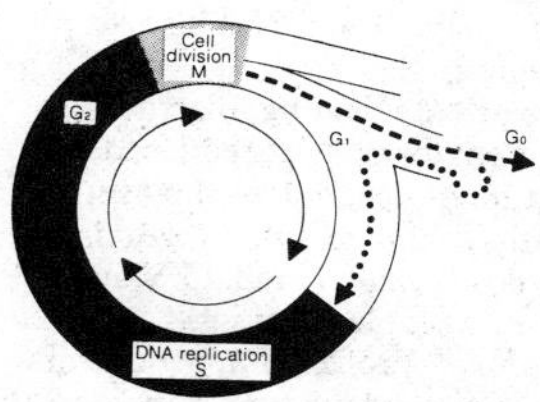

Antimetabolites are cell-cycle specific antineoplastics. Like all antineoplastics, by interrupting protein synthesis they prevent cells, including cancer cells, from reproducing and surviving.

A cell's various proteins are manufactured at specific points during the cell-cycle, which is divided into several distinct phases: Phase G_1 is the period immediately before DNA synthesis (at that time, the cell may also become dormant, a state designated G_0); DNA synthesis takes place at Phase S and RNA synthesis at Phase G_2; Phase M includes the four stages of mitosis — prophase, metaphase, anaphase, and telophase. The duration of a cell's life cycle differs according to its tissue of origin, but the average length of the process, excluding mitosis, is 10 hours.

Antimetabolites act only at Phases S and G_2. They are divided into folic acid antagonists, and purine and pyrimidine antagonists. The former interfere with biosynthetic enzymes, and the latter take the place of normal components during DNA and RNA synthesis. Antimetabolites destroy healthy as well as diseased cells; their limited toxicity can be attributed to the different rates at which different cells grow. The degree of their toxicity is such, however, that they have the narrowest range of application of all antineoplastics.

NAME	INDICATIONS & DOSAGE	SIDE EFFECTS
azathioprine Imuran◆	*Immunosuppression in renal transplants—* **Adults and children:** initially, 3 to 5 mg/Kg P.O. daily. Maintain at 1 to 2 mg/Kg/day (dose varies considerably according to patient response).	*Blood:* leukopenia, bone marrow depression, anemia, pancytopenia, thrombocytopenia. *EENT:* retinopathy. *GI:* nausea, vomiting, anorexia, pancreatitis, ascites, steatorrhea, mouth ulceration, esophagitis. *Skin:* rash. *Other:* Raynaud's disease, immunosuppression (possibly profound), arthralgia, muscle wasting, pulmonary edema, alopecia, hepatitis, jaundice.
cytarabine (ARA-C, cytosine arabinoside) Cytosar◆	*Acute myelocytic and other acute leukemias—* **Adults:** 2 to 3 mg/Kg (100 mg/m²) I.V. or SC b.i.d. for 7 days; 2 to 3 mg/Kg (100 mg/m²) daily for 7 days by 24-hour continuous infusion; or 10 to 30 mg/m² intrathecally, up to 3 times weekly. Maintenance 2 to 3 mg/Kg I.V. or S.C. b.i.d. for 5 days. **Children:** initially, 2 mg/Kg/day I.V. for 10 days; 0.5 to 1 mg/Kg in 1-to-24 hour infusions for 10 days. Maintenance 1 mg/Kg S.C. twice weekly.	*Blood:* WBC nadir occurs days 5 to 7 and may continue after drug stopped; leukopenia, anemia, thrombocytopenia, reticulocytopenia; platelet nadir occurs day 10; megaloblastosis (common). *GI:* nausea, vomiting, diarrhea are common; dysphagia; reddened area at juncture of lips, followed by sore mouth, oral ulcers in 5 to 10 days; high dose given via rapid I.V. may cause projectile vomiting. *Metabolic:* profound hyperkalemia may occur in leukemia patients with very high WBCs when rapid cell lysis occurs; hyperuricemia. *Other:* phlebitis, hepatotoxicity (usually mild and reversible).
floxuridine FUDR	*Brain, breast, head, neck, liver, gallbladder, and bile duct cancer—* **Adults:** 0.1 to 0.6 mg/Kg daily by intra-arterial infusion (use pump for continuous, uniform rate); or 0.4 to 0.6 mg/Kg daily into hepatic artery.	*Blood:* leukopenia, anemia, thrombocytopenia. *CNS:* cerebellar ataxia, vertigo, nystagmus, convulsions, depression, hemiplegia, hiccups, lethargy. *EENT:* blurred vision. *GI:* stomatitis, cramps, nausea, vomiting, diarrhea, bleeding, enteritis, gastritis, duodenal ulcer. *Metabolic:* hypoadrenalism. *Skin:* erythema most common; also dermatitis, excoriation, maceration, pruritus, rash. *Other:* hepatotoxicity.

◆ Also available in Canada.
◆◆ Available in Canada only.
Unmarked trade names available in United States only.

INTERACTIONS	NURSING CONSIDERATIONS
Allopurinol: impaired inactivation of azathioprine. Decrease azathioprine dose to ¼ or ⅓ normal dose.	• Use cautiously or avoid in hepatic or renal dysfunction. • Watch for clay-colored stools, dark urine, pruritus, yellow skin, sclera, and for increased alkaline phosphatase, bilirubin, SGOT, SGPT. • In renal homotransplants, start drug 1 to 5 days before surgery; continue 24 to 96 hours after surgery. • Hemoglobin, WBC, and platelet count should be done at least once a week; more often at beginning of treatment. Drug should be stopped immediately when WBC is less than 3,000/mm³ to prevent extension to irreversible bone marrow depression. • This is a potent immunosuppressant. Warn patient to report even mild infections (coryza, fever, sore throat, malaise). • To reduce nausea, give an antiemetic before administering. • Excretion of urine metabolites delayed up to 17 days. • Patient should avoid conception during and up to 4 months after stopping therapy. • Warn patient that alopecia may occur. • Avoid I.M. injections in patients with severely depressed platelet counts (thrombocytopenia) to prevent bleeding.
None significant.	• Contraindicated in inadequate bone marrow reserve. Use cautiously in renal or hepatic disease and after other chemotherapy or radiation. • Watch for signs of infection (leukoplakia, fever, sore throat). • Excellent mouth care can help prevent oral side effects. • Monitor intake/output carefully. Maintain high fluid intake and give allopurinol to avoid urate nephropathy. • Check serum potassium, uric acid, CBC with platelets, and liver function. • Use preservative-free water for intrathecal use. • Optimum schedule is continuous infusion. • To reduce nausea, give antiemetic before administering. • Store dry powder in refrigerator; refrigerated, reconstituted solution stable 12 hours. Discard cloudy reconstituted solution. • Avoid I.M. injections in patients with severely depressed platelet count (thrombocytopenia) to prevent bleeding. • Modify or discontinue therapy if polymorphonuclear granulocyte count is 1,000/mm³ or if platelet count is 50,000/mm³.
None significant.	• Contraindicated in poor nutritional state, bone marrow depression, serious infection. Use cautiously following high-dose pelvic irradiation or use of alkylating agent, and in impaired hepatic or renal function. • Severe skin and GI side effects require stopping drug. Use of antacid eases but probably won't prevent GI distress. • Excellent mouth care can help prevent oral side effects. • May be difficult to distinguish between drug side effects and CNS metastasis, if present. • Supplemental corticosteroids may be needed in infection, surgery, stress. • Monitor intake/output, CBC, and renal and hepatic function. • Discontinue if WBC falls below 3,500/mm³ or if platelet count below 100,000/mm³. • Therapeutic effect may be delayed 1 to 6 weeks. • 10% to 30% of drug excreted in urine; the remainder is exhaled. • Reconstitute with sterile water for injection. Dilute further in 5% dextrose in water or normal saline for actual infusion. • Always use infusion pump. • Avoid I.M. injections in patients with thrombocytopenia to prevent bleeding. • Refrigerated solution stable no more than 2 weeks. • Observe precautions for catheter line care in arterial perfused area. Check line for bleeding, blockage, displacement, or leakage.

NAME	INDICATIONS & DOSAGE	SIDE EFFECTS
fluorouracil (5-fluorouracil) Adrucil, 5-FU	*Colon, rectal, breast, ovarian, cervical, bladder, liver, and pancreatic cancer—* **Adults:** 12.5 mg/Kg I.V. daily for 3 to 5 days q 4 weeks; or 15 mg/Kg weekly for 6 weeks. (Doses recommended based on lean body weight.) Maximum single recommended dose is 800 mg, although higher single doses (up to 1.5 g) have been used. The injectable form has been given orally but is not recommended.	*Blood:* leukopenia, granulocytopenia, thrombocytopenia, anemia. WBC nadir occurs days 9 to 14 after first dose; nadir lasts 30 days; platelets nadir occurs days 7 to 14. *CNS:* cerebellar ataxia in 5% of patients. *CV:* angina. *EENT:* eye irritation and watering, blurred vision, photophobia. *GI:* stomatitis and GI ulcer may precede leukopenia, nausea, vomiting in 30% to 50% of patients; diarrhea (signs of toxicity). *Skin:* dermatitis, hyperpigmentation (especially in blacks), nail changes, pigmented palmar creases. *Other:* alopecia in 5% to 20% of patients, weakness, malaise.
hydroxyurea Hydrea	*Melanoma; resistant chronic myelocytic leukemia; recurrent, metastatic, or inoperable ovarian cancer—* **Adults:** 80 mg/Kg P.O. as single dose q 3 days; or 20 to 30 mg/Kg P.O. daily.	*Blood:* leukopenia, thrombocytopenia, anemia. WBC, RBC, and platelets nadir occurs in 1 to 2 days; megaloblastosis; bone marrow depression is dose-limiting and dose-related; recovery rapid. *CNS:* drowsiness. *GI:* anorexia, nausea, vomiting, diarrhea, stomatitis. *Metabolic:* profound hyperkalemia may occur in leukemia patients with very high WBCs; hyperuricemia. *Skin:* rash, pruritus. *Other:* increased BUN and serum creatinine; potential mutagenic effect on offspring.
mercaptopurine Purinethol◆	*Acute lymphoblastic leukemia (in children), acute myeloblastic leukemia, chronic myelocytic leukemia—* **Adults and children:** 2.5 mg/Kg P.O. daily, or 70 mg/m² P.O. daily as single dose up to 5 mg/Kg	*Blood:* WBC and platelets nadir occurs day 7; decreased RBC; eosinophilia; leukopenia, thrombocytopenia, bone marrow hypoplasia; all may persist several days after drug is stopped. *GI:* nausea, vomiting, and anorexia in

INTERACTIONS	NURSING CONSIDERATIONS
None significant.	• Contraindicated following major surgery, in poor nutritional state, serious infections, bone marrow depression. Use cautiously following high-dose pelvic irradiation or use of alkylating agents, in impaired hepatic or renal function, or widespread neoplastic infiltration of bone marrow. • Watch for stomatitis or diarrhea (signs of toxicity). May use topical oral anesthetic to soothe lesions. • Give antiemetic before administering to reduce GI side effects. • Do WBC and platelet counts daily. Drug should be stopped when WBC is less than 3,500/mm³. Watch for ecchymoses, petechiae, easy bruising, and anemia. Drug should be stopped if platelets are less than 100,000/mm³. Patient may require reverse isolation. • Skin and ocular side effects reversible when drug is stopped. Patient should use highly protective sun blockers to avoid inflammatory erythematous dermatitis. • Therapeutic concentrations don't reach cerebrospinal fluid. • Side effects more prominent after adrenalectomy. • Slowing infusion rate so it takes from 2 to 8 hours lessens toxicity but also lessens efficacy compared with rapid injection; avoid extravasation. • Monitor intake/output, CBC, and renal and hepatic functions. • Do not refrigerate 5-FU. Protect from light. • Don't use cloudy solution. If crystals form, redissolve by warming. • Sometimes ordered as 5-FU. The number 5 is part of the drug name and should not be confused with dosage units. • Sometimes administered via hepatic arterial infusion in treatment of hepatic metastases. • Question patient about chest pains. • Warn patient that alopecia may occur but is reversible. • Avoid excessive I.M. injections in patients with thrombocytopenia to prevent bleeding. • 5-FU toxicity is delayed for 1 to 3 weeks.
None significant.	• Use cautiously following other chemotherapy or radiation therapy, and in renal disease. • Use with caution in renal dysfunction. Discontinue if WBC is less than 2,500/mm³ or if platelet count is less than 100,000 mm³. • If patient can't swallow capsule, he may empty contents into water and take immediately. • Monitor intake/output; keep patient hydrated. • Routinely measure BUN, uric acid, serum creatinine, and potassium. • Drug passes blood-brain barrier. • Auditory and visual hallucinations, and blood toxicity when decreased renal function exists. • May exacerbate postirradiation erythema. • Avoid I.M. injections when platelets are low.
Allopurinol: slowed inactivation of mercaptopurine. Decrease mercaptopurine to ¼ or ⅓ normal dose.	• Use cautiously following chemotherapy or radiation therapy, in depressed neutrophil or platelet count, impaired hepatic or renal function. • Observe for signs of bleeding and infection. • Nausea and vomiting signal toxicity. Discontinue drug. • Hepatic dysfunction reversible when drug is stopped. Watch for jaundice, clay-colored stools, frothy dark urine. Drug should be stopped if liver tenderness occurs.

(continued on following page)

NAME	INDICATIONS & DOSAGE	SIDE EFFECTS
mercaptopurine *(continued)*	until response or toxicity occurs; adjust for maintenance.	25% of patients; painful oral ulcers. *GU:* renal dysfunction, oliguria, uric acid nephrotoxicity. *Metabolic:* profound hyperkalemia may occur in leukemia patients with very high WBCs; hyperuricemia. *Skin:* rash. *Other:* jaundice.
methotrexate **methotrexate sodium** Mexate	*Trophoblastic tumors (choriocarcinoma, hydatidiform mole)*— **Adults:** 15 to 30 mg P.O. or I.M. daily for 5 days. Repeat after 1 or more weeks, according to response or toxicity. *Acute lymphoblastic and lymphatic leukemia*— **Adults and children:** 3.3 mg/m^2 P.O., I.M., or I.V. daily for 4 to 6 weeks or until remission occurs; then 20 to 30 mg/m^2 P.O. or I.M. twice weekly. *Meningeal leukemia*— **Adults and children:** 0.2 to 0.5 mg/Kg intrathecally every 2 to 5 days until cerebrospinal fluid is normal. Use only 25 mg/ml concentration, and dilute to concentration of 1 mg/ml using 0.9% NaCl injection *without* preservatives. Use only new vials of drug and diluent. Use immediately. *Burkitt's lymphoma* (Stage I or II)— **Adults:** 10 to 25 mg P.O. daily for 4 to 8 days with 1-week rest intervals. *Burkitt's lymphoma* (Stage III)— **Adults:** up to 1 g/m^2/day with cyclophosphamide and prednisolone. *Lymphosarcoma* (Stage III)— **Adults:** 0.625 to 2.5 mg/Kg daily P.O., I.M., or I.V. *Mycosis fungoides*— **Adults:** 2.5 to 10 mg P.O. daily or 50 mg I.M. weekly; or I.M. 25 mg twice weekly. *Psoriasis*— **Adults:** 10 to 25 mg P.O., I.M., or I.V. as single weekly dose. To detect idiosyncratic reactions, 5 to 10 mg test dose recommended 1 week before methotrexate regimen.	*Blood:* WBC and platelets nadir occurs day 7; anemia, leukopenia, thrombocytopenia (all dose-related). *CNS:* arachnoiditis within hours of intrathecal use; subacute neurotoxicity may begin a few weeks later; necrotizing demyelinating leukoencephalopathy a few years later. *GI:* stomatitis (common); diarrhea leading to hemorrhagic enteritis and intestinal perforation. *GU:* tubular necrosis. *Metabolic:* profound hyperkalemia may occur in leukemia patients with very high WBCs and lymphoma patients when rapid cell lysis occurs; hyperuricemia. *Skin:* dermatitis; exposure to sun may aggravate psoriatic lesions or hyperpigmented skin. *Other:* alopecia; pulmonary interstitial bleeding (reversible when drug is stopped); long-term use in children may cause osteoporosis; hepatic dysfunction leading to cirrhosis or hepatic fibrosis; chromosome damage.

INTERACTIONS	NURSING CONSIDERATIONS
	• Do weekly blood counts; watch for precipitous fall. • Monitor serum potassium and intake/output. Push fluids (3 liters daily). • Drug is less effective with each successive treatment. • Sometimes ordered as 6-mercaptopurine or 6-MP. The number 6 is part of drug name and does not signify number of dosage units. • Improvement may take 2 to 4 weeks or longer. • Avoid I.M. injections when platelets are low.
Alcohol: increased hepatotoxicity; warn patient not to drink alcoholic beverages. Don't give patient cough preparations that contain alcohol. *Probenecid, phenylbutazone, salicylates, sulfonamides:* increased methotrexate toxicity; don't use together if possible.	• Contraindicated in impaired hepatic or renal function, bone marrow depression, aplasia, leukopenia, thrombocytopenia, anemia. Use cautiously in infection, peptic ulcer, ulcerative colitis, and in very young, old, or debilitated patients. • Warn patient to avoid conception during and immediately following therapy because of potential chromosome damage. • GI side effects may require stopping drug. • Weigh patient weekly. • Rash, redness, or ulcerations in mouth or pulmonary side effects may signal serious complications. • Monitor blood sugar, serum potassium, and uric acid. • Monitor intake/output daily. Force fluids (2 to 3 liters daily). Check thirst and urinary frequency. • Alkalinize urine by giving $NaHCO_3$ tablets to prevent precipitation of drug, especially with high doses. Maintain urine pH at more than 6.5. Reduce dose if BUN 20 to 30 mg% or creatinine 1.2 to 2 mg%. Stop drug if BUN more than 30 mg% or creatinine more than 2 mg%. • Watch SGOT, SGPT, alkaline phosphatase; may signal hepatic dysfunction. • Watch for bleeding (especially GI) and infection. • Warn patient to use highly protective sun blocker when exposed to sun. • Take temperature daily, and watch for cough, dyspnea, cyanosis; corticosteroids may help reduce pulmonary side effects. • Leucovorin rescue: Leucovorin calcium (folinic acid) is given within 4 hours of administration of methotrexate. Don't confuse with folic acid. This rescue technique is effective against systemic toxicity but does not interfere with the tumor cells' absorption of the methotrexate. • Avoid I.M. injections in patients with thrombocytopenia.

NAME	INDICATIONS & DOSAGE	SIDE EFFECTS
thioguanine Lanvis◆◆	*Acute leukemia, chronic granulocytic leukemia*— **Adults and children:** initially, 2 mg/Kg daily P.O. (usually calculated to nearest 20 mg); then increased gradually to 3 mg/Kg/day if no toxic effects occur.	*Blood:* leukopenia, anemia, thrombocytopenia (occurs slowly over 2 to 4 weeks). *GI:* nausea, vomiting, stomatitis, diarrhea, anorexia. *Metabolic:* profound hyperkalemia may occur in leukemia patients with very high WBCs; hyperuricemia. *Other:* jaundice.

INTERACTIONS	NURSING CONSIDERATIONS
None significant.	• Use cautiously in renal or hepatic dysfunction. • Stop drug if hepatotoxicity or liver tenderness occurs. Watch for jaundice; may reverse if drug stopped promptly. • Do CBC daily during induction, then weekly during maintenance therapy. • Monitor serum potassium and serum uric acid. • Usually used after patient has developed resistance or severe side effects to mercaptopurine or busulfan. • Sometimes ordered as 6-thioguanine. The number 6 is part of drug name and does not signify dosage units. • Avoid I.M. injections when platelets are low.

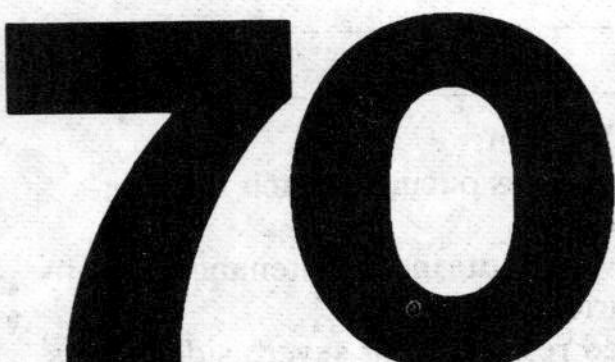

Antibiotic antineoplastic agents

bleomycin sulfate
dactinomycin (actinomycin D)
doxorubicin hydrochloride
mithramycin
mitomycin
procarbazine hydrochloride

Antineoplastic antibiotics are isolated from naturally occurring microorganisms that can inhibit bacterial growth. But unlike the anti-infective drugs they're related to, antineoplastic antibiotics can disrupt the functioning of host as well as bacterial cells. Procarbazine hydrochloride is not an antibiotic, but it's included here because it acts in a similar manner. Dosage and indications may vary, so consult the doctor about the patient's protocol.

Major uses
- Treatment of lymphomas, leukemias, sarcomas, and some carcinomas.
- Mithramycin is also used to treat hypercalcemia.

Mechanism of action
- Inhibit DNA or RNA synthesis, thereby inhibiting proper cell division.

Absorption, distribution, and excretion
- Procarbazine is well absorbed orally. All others must be given parenterally.
- Widely distributed to most body tissues and organs, especially liver, spleen, kidneys, lungs, and heart.
- Do not cross blood-brain barrier.
- Metabolized in liver.
- Excreted in feces and urine.

Onset and duration
- Varies with drug, disease, and patient response.

Combination products
None.

ANTIBIOTICS INHIBIT NUCLEAR SYNTHESIS

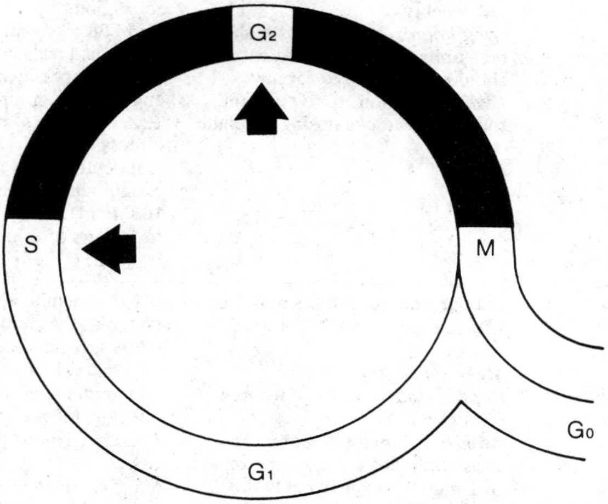

Antineoplastic drugs stop cancer cell production by interrupting protein synthesis. Each of the many cell proteins is manufactured at a specific point within the cell cycle, which is divided into several stages: Phase$_1$ is the period before DNA synthesis (at which time the cell may also become dormant, a state designated G_0); Phase S represents DNA synthesis; Phase G_2 includes RNA synthesis; and Phase M represents mitosis. The exact mechanism of action is not known; however, antibiotics are mostly cell-cycle nonspecific, but inhibit DNA synthesis (S) and RNA synthesis (G_2).

NAME	INDICATIONS & DOSAGE	SIDE EFFECTS
bleomycin sulfate Blenoxane◆	Dosage and indications may vary. Check patient's protocol with doctor. *Cervical, esophageal, head, neck, and testicular cancer—* **Adults:** 10 to 20 units/m² I.V., I.M. or S.C. 1 or 2 times weekly to total of 300 to 400 mg. *Hodgkin's disease—* 10 to 20 units/m² I.V., I.M. or S.C. weekly or twice weekly. After 50% response, maintenance 1 unit I.M. or I.V. daily or 5 units I.M. or I.V. weekly. *Lymphomas—* first 2 doses should be 2 units or less, and patient should be monitored for any adverse reaction. If no reaction, then follow above dosing schedule.	Blood: thrombocytopenia, leukopenia. *CNS:* hyperesthesia of scalp and fingers, headache. *GI:* stomatitis in 22% to 50% of patients, prolonged anorexia in 13% of patients, nausea, vomiting, diarrhea. *Metabolic:* profound hyperkalemia may occur in lymphoma patients when rapid cell lysis occurs. *Skin:* brawny edema, erythema, vesiculation, and hardening and discoloration of palmar and plantar skin in 8% of patients; desquamation of hands, feet, and pressure areas. *Other:* alopecia; swelling of interphalangeal joints; pulmonary fibrosis in 10% of patients; pulmonary side effects (fine rales, fever, dyspnea); leukocytosis and non-productive cough; allergic reaction (fever up to 106° F. [41.1° C.], with chills up to 5 hours after injection; anaphylaxis in 1% to 6% of patients; hypotension).
dactinomycin (actinomycin D) Cosmegen◆	Dosage and indications may vary. Check patient's protocol with doctor. *Melanomas, sarcomas, trophoblastic tumors in women, testicular cancer—* **Adults:** 500 mcg I.V. daily for 5 days; wait 2 to 4 weeks and repeat; or 2 mg I.V. single weekly dose for 3 weeks; wait for bone marrow recovery, then repeat in 3 to 4 weeks. *Wilms' tumor, rhabdomyosarcoma—* **Children:** 15 mcg/Kg I.V. daily for 5 days. Maximum dose 500 mcg daily. Wait for marrow recovery, then repeat q 6 to 12 weeks.	*Blood:* anemia, aplastic anemia, leukopenia, thrombocytopenia, agranulocytosis, pancytopenia. *GI:* anorexia, nausea, vomiting, abdominal pain, diarrhea, stomatitis, cheilitis, glossitis, proctitis. *Local:* phlebitis, severe damage to soft tissue. *Skin:* erythema, desquamation, hyperpigmentation of skin, especially in previously irradiated areas; acne-like eruptions (reversible); viral infections such as chicken pox can become widely disseminated systemic diseases. *Other:* reversible alopecia, malaise, fatigue, fever, myalgia.
doxorubicin hydrochloride Adriamycin◆	Dosage and indications may vary. Check patient's protocol with doctor. *Bladder, breast, cervical, head, neck, liver, lung, ovarian, prostatic, stomach, testicular, and thyroid cancer; Hodgkin's disease; acute lymphoblastic and myeloblastic leukemia; Wilms' tumor; neuroblastomas;*	*Blood:* leukopenia, especially agranulocytosis, during days 10 to 15, with recovery by day 21; thrombocytopenia. *CV:* cardiac depression, seen in such EKG changes as sinus tachycardia, T wave flattening, S-T segment depression, voltage reduction; arrhythmias in 11% of patients; congestive heart failure (sometimes with pulmonary

◆ Also available in Canada.
◆◆ Available in Canada only.
Unmarked trade names available in United States only.

INTERACTIONS	NURSING CONSIDERATIONS
None significant.	• Contraindicated in renal or pulmonary impairment. • Glutathione and vitamin C may help relieve skin side effects. • Drug concentrates in keratin of squamous epithelium. To prevent linear streaking, don't use adhesive dressings on skin. • Allergic reactions may be delayed 6 to 15 hours, especially in lymphoma. • Monitor serum potassium. • Pulmonary function tests should be performed to establish baseline. Drug should be stopped if pulmonary function test shows a marked decline. • Pulmonary side effects common in patients over 70 years and in patients who receive a total dose of more than 400 mg/m^2. • Warn patient that alopecia may occur. • Refrigerated, reconstituted solution stable 4 weeks; at room temperature stable 2 weeks. Solutions prepared in ampules should be discarded if not used immediately. • Fatal pulmonary fibrosis occurs in 1% of patients, especially when cumulative dose exceeds 500 mg. • Bleomycin-induced fever is common and may be treated with antipyretics.
None significant.	• Contraindicated in renal, hepatic, or bone marrow impairment; viral infection. Use cautiously in metastatic testicular tumors, in combination therapy with chlorambucil and methotrexate therapy. Extreme bone marrow and GI toxicity can occur with this combined therapy. • Stomatitis, diarrhea, leukopenia, thrombocytopenia may require stopping therapy. • Give antiemetic before administering to reduce nausea. • Monitor renal and hepatic functions. • Monitor CBCs daily and platelet counts every third day. • Observe for signs of bleeding. Avoid contact with skin or mucous membranes. Wash hands and contaminated surfaces thoroughly. • Warn patient that alopecia may occur but is usually reversible. • Use only sterile water (without preservatives) as diluent for injection. • Administer through a running I.V. infusion. Avoid infiltration.
None significant.	• Contraindicated in myelosuppression, impaired cardiac function. • Stop drug or slow rate of infusion if tachycardia develops. • Stop drug immediately in signs of congestive heart failure. Prevent by limiting cumulative dose to 550 mg/m^2. • Monitor EKG before treatment, monthly during therapy. • Note if resting pulse is high: a signal of cardiac side effects. • *Avoid extravasation;* inject into tubing of freely flowing I.V. • Monitor CBC, serum potassium, and liver function. • Warn patient urine will be red for 1 to 2 days. • Dose should be reduced in hepatic dysfunction.

(continued on following page)

NAME	INDICATIONS & DOSAGE	SIDE EFFECTS
doxorubicin hydrochloride *(continued)*	*lymphomas; sarcomas—* **Adults:** 60 to 75 mg/m² I.V. as single dose q 3 weeks; or 30 mg/m² I.V. in single daily dose, days 1 to 3 of 4-week cycle. Maximum cumulative dose 550 mg/m².	edema) with mortality rate of 30% to 75%. *GI:* nausea, vomiting, diarrhea, stomatitis, esophagitis. *GU:* red-colored urine. *Local:* severe cellulitis or tissue slough if drug extravasates. *Metabolic:* profound hyperkalemia may occur in leukemia patients with very high WBCs and in lymphoma patients when rapid cell lysis occurs. *Other:* hyperpigmentation of nails and dermal creases, complete alopecia within 3 to 4 weeks; hair may regrow 2 to 5 months after drug is stopped.
mithramycin Mithracin	Dosage and indications may vary. Check patient's protocol with doctor. *Hypercalcemia—* **Adults:** 25 mcg/Kg I.V. daily for 3 to 4 days. *Testicular cancer—* **Adults:** 25 to 30 mcg/Kg I.V. daily for up to 8-10 days (based on ideal body weight or actual weight, whichever is less). I.V. infusions should be in 5% dextrose in water or 0.9% normal saline solution (1,000 ml over 4 to 6 hours).	*Blood:* thrombocytopenia; bleeding syndrome, from epistaxis to generalized hemorrhage. *CNS:* drowsiness, irritability, weakness, dizziness, headache, depression, facial flushing. *EENT:* conjunctivitis. *GI:* nausea, vomiting, anorexia, diarrhea, stomatitis. *GU:* proteinuria. *Local:* extravasation causes irritation, cellulitis. *Metabolic:* decreased serum calcium, potassium, and phosphorus; increased BUN, serum creatinine. *Skin:* erythema of face, neck, upper thorax; periorbital pallor, usually the day before toxic symptoms occur. *Other:* malaise, fever.
mitomycin Mutamycin◆	Dosage and indications may vary. Check patient's protocol with doctor. *Breast, colon, head, neck, lung, pancreatic, and stomach cancer; malignant melanoma—* **Adults:** 2 mg/m² I.V. daily for 5 days. Stop drug for 2 days, then repeat dose for 5 more days; or 20 mg/m² as a single dose. Repeat cycle 6 to 8 weeks. Stop drug if WBC less than 4,000/mm³ or platelets less than 75,000/mm³.	*Blood:* thrombocytopenia, leukopenia, hemorrhage in 14% of patients. *CNS:* paresthesias. *GI:* nausea, vomiting, anorexia, stomatitis. *GU:* renal failure (may be delayed several months on high dose). *Local:* desquamation, induration, pruritus, pain at site of injection. Extravasation causes cellulitis, ulceration, sloughing. *Other:* alopecia, fever, hemoptysis, dyspnea, cough, interstitial pneumonia.

INTERACTIONS	NURSING CONSIDERATIONS
	• Warn patient that alopecia will occur. • Refrigerated, reconstituted solution stable 48 hours; at room temperature, stable 24 hours. • If cumulative dose exceeds 550 mg/m² body surface area, 30% of patients develop cardiac side effects, which begin 2 weeks to 6 months after stopping drug. • Decrease dose if serum bilirubin is increased: 50% dose when bilirubin is 1.2 to 3 mg/100 ml; 25% dose when bilirubin is > 3 mg/100 ml. • Esophagitis very common in patients who have also received radiation therapy.
None significant.	• Contraindicated in thrombocytopenia; coagulation and bleeding disorders; renal, hepatic, or bone marrow impairment. • Slow infusion reduces nausea that develops with I.V. push. • Monitor LDH, BUN, SGOT, SGPT, alkaline phosphatase, BUN, creatinine, potassium. • Monitor platelet count and prothrombin time before and during therapy. • Observe for signs of bleeding. • Give antiemetic before administering to reduce nausea. • Avoid extravasation. If I.V. infiltrates, stop immediately; apply warm, moist soaks. Restart I.V. • Avoid contact with skin or mucous membranes. • Therapeutic effect in hypercalcemia may not be seen for 24 to 48 hours; may last 3 to 15 days. • Precipitous drop in calcium possible. Monitor patient for tetany, carpopedal spasm, Chvostek's sign, muscle cramps; check serum calcium levels. • Store lyophilized powder in refrigerator. Reconstitute immediately before giving; discard unused portions.
None significant.	• Contraindicated when platelet count is less than 75,000/mm³, WBC is less than 4,000/mm³, in coagulation or bleeding disorders, serious infections, impaired renal function. • Continue CBC and blood studies at least 7 weeks after therapy is stopped. Observe for signs of bleeding. • Monitor intake/output. Drug is nephrotoxic. Push fluids to 2 to 2.5 liters daily. • Stop drug if BUN rises or if creatinine rises above 1.7 mg%. • Warn patient that alopecia may occur. • Reconstituted solution stable 1 week at room temperature, 2 weeks refrigerated. • Recently discovered to cause serious pulmonary toxicity. Monitor carefully for pneumonitis.

NAME	INDICATIONS & DOSAGE	SIDE EFFECTS
procarbazine hydrochloride Matulane, Natulan♦♦	Dosage and indications may vary. Check patient's protocol with doctor. *Hodgkin's disease, lymphomas, brain and lung cancer—* **Adults:** 2 to 4 mg/Kg daily for 1 week, then 4 to 6 mg/Kg daily until WBC falls below 4,000/mm^3 or platelets fall below 100,000/mm^3. After bone marrow recovers, resume maintenance dose 1 to 2 mg/Kg P.O. daily. **Children:** 50 mg P.O. daily for first week, then 100 mg/m^2 until response or toxicity occurs. Maintenance dose 50 mg P.O. daily after bone marrow recovery.	*Blood:* bleeding tendency, leukopenia, anemia. *CNS:* headache, dizziness, nervousness, flushing, paresthesias, neuropathies, depression, insomnia, nightmares, hallucinations, confusion, ataxia, coma, convulsions, tremors, decreased reflexes, weakness, lethargy. *EENT:* retinal hemorrhage, nystagmus, photophobia, hoarseness. *GI:* nausea, vomiting, anorexia, stomatitis, dry mouth, dysphagia, diarrhea, constipation. *Metabolic:* profound hyperkalemia may occur in lymphoma patients when rapid cell lysis occurs. *Skin:* dermatitis, pruritus, herpes, hyperpigmentation. *Other:* alopecia, jaundice, myalgia, arthralgia, excessive sweating, pleural effusion, edema, cough, intercurrent infections.

INTERACTIONS	NURSING CONSIDERATIONS
Alcohol: disulfiram (Antabuse)-like reaction. Warn patient not to drink alcohol or use cough syrups, mouthwashes, etc. that contain alcohol.	• Contraindicated in inadequate bone marrow reserve. Use cautiously in leukopenia, thrombocytopenia, anemia, impaired hepatic or renal function. • Monitor serum potassium. • Observe for signs of bleeding. • Wait at least 1 month after radiation or chemotherapy before starting. • Give antiemetic before administering to reduce nausea. • Warn patient that alopecia may occur. • May increase effects of CNS depressants.

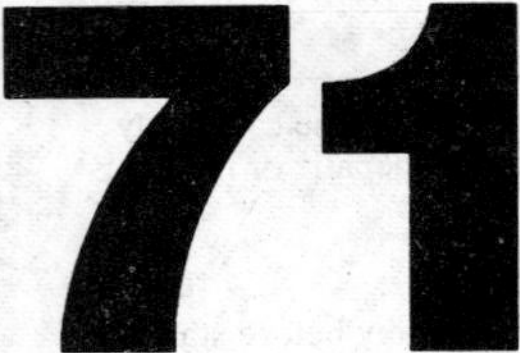

Antineoplastics altering hormone balance

calusterone
dromostanolone propionate
megestrol acetate
mitotane
tamoxifen citrate
testolactone

Sex hormones such as megestrol acetate, calusterone, dromostanolone propionate and testolactone counterbalance the hormonal effect of endometrial, breast, and other sex hormone-related cancers. Mitotane, which is not a hormone, selectively attacks adrenal cortical cells and alters extra-adrenal metabolism of cortisal. Tamoxifen citrate is an estrogen antagonist. These drugs are especially useful in treating cancer because they inhibit neoplastic cell growth in specific tissues without a direct cytotoxic effect.

Major use

- Palliative effect in breast, endometrial, and adrenal cortical cancer.

Mechanism of action

- Inhibit or stimulate changes in hormonal balance of the body.
- Inhibit neoplastic and normal cell growth in specific tissues.

Absorption, distribution, and excretion

- Most are absorbed orally and distributed widely in body tissues.
- Mitotane is about 40% absorbed orally; dromostanolone propionate must be given I.M.
- Metabolized in liver.
- Excreted in urine.

Onset and duration

Varies with drug, disease, and patient response.

Combination products

None.

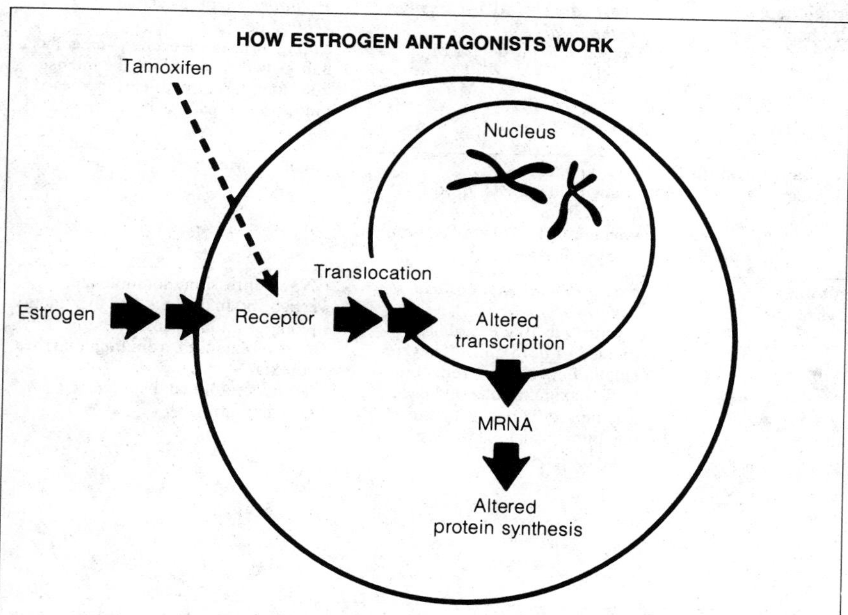

Upon entry into target cells, estrogens combine within 10 to 15 seconds with a "receptor" protein in the cytoplasm, and then, in combination enter the nucleus. Tamoxifen is thought to interact with the cytoplasmic and nuclear estrogen receptor, thereby preventing proliferation of cancer cells.

NAME	INDICATIONS & DOSAGE	SIDE EFFECTS
calusterone Methosarb•	*Postmenopausal breast cancer—* **Women:** 50 mg P.O. q.i.d. up to 300 mg/day.	*GI:* nausea, vomiting. *GU:* clitoral enlargement. *Metabolic:* hypercalcemia. *Skin:* acne, oily skin. *Other:* virilism (hirsutism, deepened voice, facial hair) in 25% of patients, increased libido, alopecia, hepatic dysfunction, cholestatic jaundice, edema, fever. Brief exacerbation of pain from osseous metastases.
dromostanolone propionate Drolban	*Advanced, inoperable metastatic breast cancer, 1 to 5 years post-menopausal—* **Women:** 100 mg deep I.M. 3 times weekly.	*GU:* clitoral enlargement. *Metabolic:* hypercalcemia. *Skin:* acne. *Other:* virilism (deepened voice, facial hair growth), which may be intense after long-term treatment; increased libido, edema, pain at injection site.
megestrol acetate Megace•	*Breast cancer—* **Women:** 40 mg P.O. q.i.d. *Endometrial cancer—* **Women:** 40 to 320 mg P.O. daily in divided dosages.	None reported.
mitotane Lysodren•	*Inoperable adrenal cortical cancer—* **Adults:** 9 to 10 g P.O. daily, divided t.i.d. to q.i.d. If severe side effects appear, reduce dose until maximum tolerated dose is achieved (varies from 2 to 16 g/day but is usually 8 to 10 g/day).	*CNS:* depression, somnolence, vertigo; brain damage and dysfunction in long-term, high-dose therapy. *GI:* severe nausea, vomiting, diarrhea, anorexia. *Metabolic:* adrenal insufficiency. *Skin:* dermatitis.
tamoxifen citrate Nolvadex•	*Advanced pre-and postmenopausal breast cancer—* **Women:** 10 to 20 mg P.O. b.i.d.	*Blood:* transient fall in WBC or platelets. *GI:* nausea in 10% of patients, vomiting, anorexia. *GU:* vaginal discharge and bleeding. *Skin:* rash. *Other:* temporary bone or tumor pain, hot flashes in 7% of patients, lactation in premenopausal women.

• Also available in Canada.
•• Available in Canada only.
Unmarked trade names available in United States only.

INTERACTIONS	NURSING CONSIDERATIONS
None significant.	• Contraindicated in premenopausal women (unless ovarian function has been terminated) and male breast cancer. • Monitor hepatic function and serum calcium regularly. • Take temperature daily. • Monitor for signs of tumor progression. • Therapy usually lasts for at least 3 months.
None significant.	• Contraindicated by any route other than I.M.; in male breast cancer and premenopausal women. Use cautiously in hepatic disease, cardiac decompensation, nephritis, nephrosis, and prostatic cancer. • If severe hypercalcemia develops or disease accelerates, drug should be stopped. • Therapeutic effect may be delayed 8 to 12 weeks. Reassure patient that results are not immediate. • Do not store in refrigerator; drug precipitates at cold temperatures.
None significant.	• Use cautiously in history of thrombophlebitis. • Adequate trial is 2 months. Reassure patient that therapeutic response isn't immediate.
None significant.	• Contraindicated immediately following shock or severe trauma. Use cautiously in hepatic disease. • Drug should be stopped if shock or trauma occur. Use of corticosteroids may avoid acute adrenocorticoid insufficiency. • Assess and record behavioral and neurological signs for baseline data and daily throughout therapy. • Give antiemetic before administering to reduce nausea. • Dosage may be reduced if GI or skin side effects are severe. • Obese patients may need higher dosage and may have longer-lasting side effects, since drug distributes mostly to body fat. • Warn patient of CNS side effects if he performs hazardous tasks requiring mental alertness or physical coordination. • Monitor effectiveness by reduction in pain, weakness, anorexia. • Adequate trial is at least 3 months, but therapy can continue if clinical benefits are observed.
None significant.	• Use cautiously in preexisting leukopenia, thrombocytopenia. • Use analgesic to relieve pain. • Monitor WBC and platelet counts. • Acts as an "anti-estrogen." Best results in patients with positive estrogen receptors. • Side effects are usually minor and are well tolerated.

NAME	INDICATIONS & DOSAGE	SIDE EFFECTS
testolactone Teslac◆	*Advanced postmenopausal breast cancer—* **Women:** 100 mg deep I.M. 3 times weekly; or 250 mg P.O. q.i.d.	*Local:* pain, inflammation at injection site.

INTERACTIONS	NURSING CONSIDERATIONS
None significant.	• Contraindicated in male breast cancer and in premenopausal females. • Adequate trial is 3 months. Reassure patient that therapeutic response isn't immediate. • Monitor fluids and electrolytes, especially calcium levels. • Immobilized patients more prone to hypercalcemia. Exercise may prevent it. Push fluids to aid calcium excretion. • Shake vial vigorously before drawing up injections. Do not refrigerate. • Use 1.5 inch-needle and inject into upper outer quadrant of gluteal region. Rotate injection sites. • No advantage over testosterone, except less virilization. • Higher than recommended doses do not increase incidence of remission.

72
Vinca alkaloids and asparaginase

asparaginase (L-asparaginase)
vinblastine sulfate
vincristine sulfate

Vincristine sulfate and vinblastine sulfate are closely related drugs derived from the periwinkle plant. Their potential for serious neurotoxicity limits their usefulness. Asparaginase, derived from Escherichia coli, is used in combination with other antineoplastic agents.

Major uses
- Treatment of lymphomas, leukemias, sarcomas, and some carcinomas (vinca alkaloids).
- Adjunctive treatment of acute lymphocytic leukemia (asparaginase and vinca alkaloids).

Mechanism of action
- Thought to arrest cell division by binding nuclear protein in the cell (vinca alkaloids).
- High concentrations of vinca alkaloids alter nucleic acids and protein synthesis.
- Asparaginase breaks down the amino acid asparagine in tumor cells, resulting in cell death.

Absorption, distribution, and excretion
- Asparaginase given intravenously or intramuscularly.
- Vinca alkaloids given intravenously only.
- Rapidly cleared from blood and localized in body tissue.
- Doesn't penetrate blood-brain barrier.
- Metabolized in liver.
- Excreted in feces and urine.

Onset and duration
- Varies with indication, disease, and patient response (vinca alkaloids).
- Accumulates in body tissue and is detectable up to 3 weeks after injection (asparaginase).

Combination products
None.

PERIWINKLE PLANT DERIVATIVE

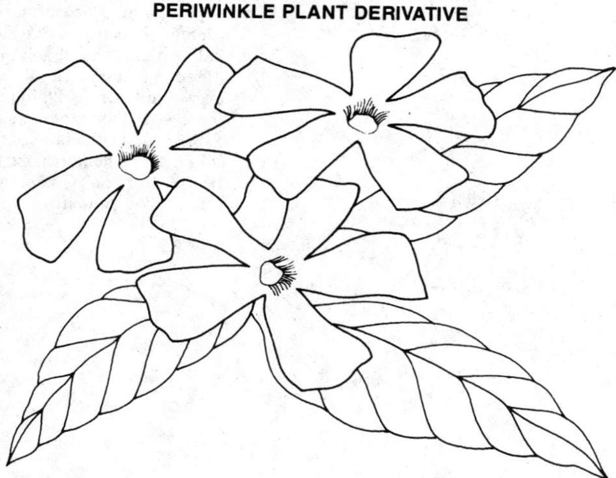

The vinca alkaloids, commonly used in cancer treatment, are derived from the periwinkle plant, vinca rosea, a species of myrtle. For many years, the beneficial properties of the periwinkle have been described in worldwide medicinal folklore.

In 1949, an alleged activity as an oral hypoglycemic agent prompted research on crude fractions obtained from the plant. Working with periwinkle extracts, in 1958, Noble and co-workers were unable to back up the claims for hypoglycemic activity in experimental animals. They did, however, see granulocytopenia and bone marrow suppression in rats—effects that led to the extraction and purification of an active alkaloid; originally termed vincaleukoblastine. Other investigations by Johnson and associates supplemented this work.

A frequent side effect with vinca alkaloid usage is peripheral neuropathy, especially prevalent in fingers and hands. This side effect generally subsides several weeks after discontinuation of the drug treatment.

NAME	INDICATIONS & DOSAGE	SIDE EFFECTS
asparaginase (or L-asparaginase) Elspar	*Acute lymphocytic leukemia (when used along with other drugs)*— **Adults and children:** 1,000 international units (I.U.)/Kg/I.V. daily for 10 days, injected over 30 minutes or by slow I.V. push; or 6,000 I.U./m^2 I.M. at intervals specified in protocol. Sole induction agent—200 I.U./Kg/I.V. daily for 28 days.	*Blood:* hypofibrinogenemia and depression of other clotting factors, thrombocytopenia, leukopenia, depression of serum albumin. *CNS:* depression, somnolence, fatigue, coma, confusion, agitation, hallucinations, headache, irritability. *GI:* vomiting (may last up to 24 hours), anorexia, nausea, cramps, weight loss, malabsorption. *GU:* azotemia, renal failure, uric acid nephropathy, glucosuria, polyuria. *Metabolic:* elevated SGOT, SGPT, alkaline phosphatase, and bilirubin (direct and indirect); increase or decrease in total lipids, hyperglycemia, increased blood ammonia. *Skin:* rash, urticaria. *Other:* fever, hemorrhagic pancreatitis, hepatotoxicity, anaphylaxis (relatively common).
vinblastine sulfate (VLB) Velban, Velbe••	*Breast or testicular cancer, generalized Hodgkin's disease, choriocarcinoma, lymphosarcoma, neuroblastoma, mycosis fungoides, histiocytosis*— **Adults and children:** 0.1 mg/Kg or 3.7 mg/m^2 I.V. weekly or q 2 weeks. May be increased to maximum dose (adults) of 0.5 mg/Kg or 18.5 mg/m^2 I.V. weekly according to response. Dose should not be repeated if WBC less than 4,000/mm^3.	*Blood:* leukopenia (nadir days 5 to 7, lasts 7 to 14 days), thrombocytopenia, agranulocytosis. *CNS:* depression, paresthesias, peripheral neuropathy and neuritis, numbness, loss of deep tendon reflexes, muscle pain and weakness, dizziness, convulsions, headache. *CV:* tachycardia, orthostatic hypotension. *EENT:* pharyngitis. *GI:* nausea, vomiting, stomatitis, ulcer and bleeding, constipation, diarrhea, ileus, anorexia, weight loss, abdominal pain. *GU:* oligospermia, aspermia, urinary retention. *Local:* irritation, phlebitis, cellulitis,

• Also available in Canada.
•• Available in Canada only.
Unmarked trade names available in United States only.

INTERACTIONS	NURSING CONSIDERATIONS
None significant.	• Contraindicated in pancreatitis, previous hypersensitivity unless desensitized. Use cautiously in preexisting hepatic dysfunction. • Should be administered in hospital setting with close supervision. • Don't use as sole agent to induce remission unless combination therapy is inappropriate. Not recommended for maintenance therapy. • Risk of hypersensitivity increases with repeated doses. Patient should be desensitized, but this doesn't rule out risk of allergic reactions. Routine administration of 50 unit I.V. test dose may identify high-risk patients. A test dose of 500 units may identify additional allergy-prone patients. • Intravenous administration of asparaginase with or immediately before vincristine or prednisone may increase toxicity reactions. • Give I.V. injection over 30-minute period through arm of a running infusion of sodium chloride injection or 5% dextrose injection. • For I.M. injection, limit dose at single injection site to 2 ml. • Due to vomiting, patient may need parenteral fluids for 24 hours or until oral fluids are tolerated. • Take temperature before administering and routinely thereafter. Fever may signal allergic reaction. • Monitor blood count and bone marrow levels. Bone marrow regeneration may take 5 to 6 weeks. • Obtain frequent serum amylase determinations to check pancreatic status. If elevated, asparaginase should be stopped. • Watch for uric acid nephropathy. Prevent occurrence by increasing fluid intake, alkalinization of urine. Allopurinol may be ordered. • Watch for signs of bleeding, such as petechiae and melena. • Monitor blood sugar and test urine for sugar before and during therapy. Watch for signs of hyperglycemia such as glucosuria, polyuria. • Reconstitute with 2 to 5 ml sterile water for injection or sodium chloride injection. • Don't shake vial. May cause loss of potency. Don't use cloudy solutions. • Refrigerate unopened dry powder. Reconstituted solution stable 6 hours at room temperature, 24 hours refrigerated. • Keep epinephrine, diphenhydramine, and I.V. corticosteroids available for treatment of anaphylaxis. • For treatment of anaphylaxis, see. p. 1114.
None significant.	• Contraindicated in severe leukopenia bacterial infection. Use cautiously in jaundice or hepatic dysfunction. • Give antiemetic before administering to reduce nausea. • Drug should be stopped if stomatitis occurs. • Give laxatives as needed. • Don't repeat dose more frequently than every 7 days or severe leukopenia will develop. • Patients, especially elderly, with cachexia or skin ulcers are more susceptible to leukopenia. • Less neurotoxic than vincristine. • Should be injected directly into vein or tubing of running I.V. over 1 minute. If extravasation occurs, stop infusion; moderate heat and local injection of hyaluronidase 150 units S.C. may decrease reaction. • Monitor serum potassium. • Allopurinol prevents nephropathy caused by cell death. Often used prophylactically. Check serum uric acid and urine for stones. Push fluids and alkalinize urine to help prevent uric acid nephropathy. • Warn patient that alopecia may occur but is usually reversible.

(continued on following page)

NAME	INDICATIONS & DOSAGE	SIDE EFFECTS
vinblastine sulfate (VLB) *(continued)*		necrosis if I.V. extravasates. *Skin:* dermatitis, vesiculation, phototoxicity. *Other:* reversible alopecia in 5% to 10% of patients; pain in tumor site, low fever, hyperuricemia.
vincristine sulfate Oncovin◆	*Acute lymphoblastic and other leukemias, Hodgkin's disease, lymphosarcoma, reticulum-cell sarcoma, neuroblastoma, rhabdomyosarcoma, Wilms' tumor, osteogenic and other sarcomas, lung and breast cancer—* **Adults:** 1 to 2 mg/m² I.V. weekly. **Children:** 1.5 to 2 mg/m² I.V. weekly. Maximum single dose (adults and children) is 2 mg.	*Blood:* rapidly reversible mild anemia, leukopenia (nadir day 4), thrombocytopenia. *CNS:* peripheral neuropathy, sensory loss, deep tendon reflex loss, paresthesias, wrist and foot drop, ataxia, cranial nerve palsies (headache, jaw pain, hoarseness, vocal cord paralysis, visual disturbances), muscle weakness and cramps, depression, agitation, insomnia, hallucinations, convulsions, coma. *CV:* orthostatic hypotension, hypertension. *EENT:* diplopia, optic and extraocular neuropathy, ptosis. *GI:* constipation, cramps, ileus which mimics surgical abdomen, nausea, vomiting, anorexia, stomatitis, weight loss, dysphagia. *GU:* polyuria, dysuria. *Local:* phlebitis, cellulitis. *Metabolic:* severe hyperkalemia in leukemia patients with very high WBCs and in lymphoma patients when rapid cell lysis occurs. *Other:* reversible alopecia (up to 71% of patients), hyperuricemia, muscle wasting, respiratory depression.

INTERACTIONS	NURSING CONSIDERATIONS
	• Adequate trial 12 weeks; reassure patient that therapeutic response isn't immediate. • Reconstitute 10 mg vial with 10 ml of sodium chloride injection or sterile water. This yields 1 mg/ml. • Refrigerate reconstituted solution. Discard after 30 days. Protect from light. • Don't confuse vinblastine with vincristine.
None significant.	• Use cautiously in jaundice or hepatic dysfunction, neuromuscular disease, infection, or with other neurotoxic drugs. • Because of neurotoxicity, don't give drug more than once a week. Children more resistant to neurotoxicity than adults. • Should be given directly into vein or tubing of running I.V. slowly over 1 minute. If drug infiltrates, local injection of hyaluronidase 150 units S.C. and heat application may decrease reaction. Use care in applying heat because of sensory loss. • Allopurinol prevents nephropathy caused by cell death. Often used prophylactically. Check serum uric acid and urine for stones. • Check for depression of Achilles tendon reflex, numbness, tingling, foot or wrist drop, difficulty in walking, ataxia, slapping gait. Also check ability to walk on heels. Support patient when walking. • Monitor serum potassium and bowel function. Give stool softener, laxative, or water before dosing. • Reconstitute with sodium chloride injection, physiologic saline, or sterile water. • Refrigerate reconstituted solution. Discard after 14 days. • Warn patient that alopecia may occur but is usually reversible. • Be extremely careful about doses. Don't confuse vincristine with vinblastine.

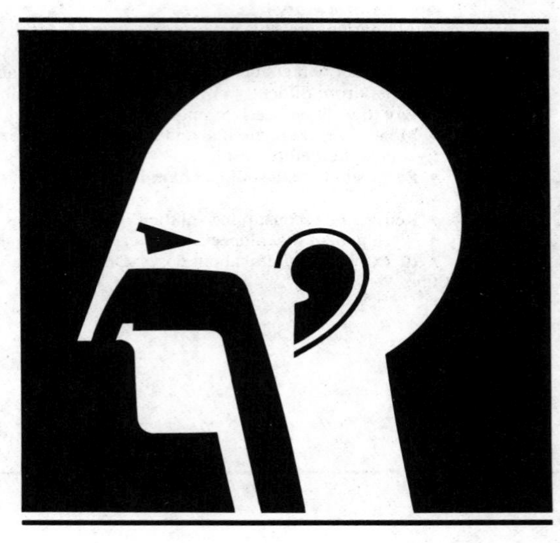

Eye, Ear, Nose, and Throat

73

Ophthalmic anti-infectives

bacitracin
benzalkonium chloride
boric acid
chloramphenicol
chlortetracycline hydrochloride
erythromycin
gentamicin sulfate
idoxuridine (IDU)
natamycin
neomycin sulfate
polymyxin B sulfate
silver nitrate 1%
sulfacetamide sodium
tetracycline hydrochloride
vidarabine

Ophthalmic anti-infectives have antibacterial, antiviral, or antifungal activity. Most are antibiotics, but others, such as boric acid or benzalkonium chloride, have weak bacteriostatic or germicidal effects. Sulfacetamide sodium is also an anti-infective, but antibiotics have replaced it except for minor infections. Vidarabine and idoxuridine (IDU) are specific antiviral agents. Ophthalmic anti-infectives are available in solutions, suspensions, or ointments; and in combinations with other ophthalmic drugs, especially corticosteroids.

Major uses

- Treatment of surface bacterial infections involving the conjunctiva or cornea, with organisms such as *Chlamydia trachomatis, Pseudomonas, Staphylococcus,* and other ocular pathogens.
- Treatment of acute keratoconjunctivitis or recurrent epithelial keratitis caused by herpes simplex types I and II (vidarabine and idoxuridine [IDU]).
- Silver nitrate is used to prevent gonorrheal ophthalmia neonatorum; boric acid is a bacteriostatic and fungistatic irrigating solution; and benzalkonium chloride is a weak germicide used as a wetting solution, a preservative, and to facilitate transcorneal penetration of other ophthalmic drugs.
- Natamycin is used to treat ophthalmic fungal infections.

Mechanism of action

- Antibiotics inhibit bacterial protein synthesis in susceptible microorganisms.
- Idoxuridine (IDU) and vidarabine interfere with viral DNA synthesis.
- Sulfacetamide sodium prevents uptake of para-aminobenzoic acid (PABA), a metabolite used in bacterial folic acid synthesis.
- Benzalkonium chloride is a bacteriostatic, surface-active agent which increases corneal permeability, enabling greater drug penetration.
- Silver nitrate causes protein denaturation which prevents gonorrheal ophthalmia neonatorum.
- Natamycin increases fungal cell membrane permeability.

Absorption, distribution, and excretion

- Bacitracin, chloramphenicol, and neomycin sulfate penetrate the cornea and conjunctiva, and are excreted by the nasolacrimal system.
- Polymyxin B sulfate, gentamicin sulfate, erythromycin, chlortetracycline hydrochloride,

and tetracycline hydrochloride are poorly absorbed through an intact cornea but are well absorbed in corneal abrasions. Chloramphenicol also penetrates the aqueous humor. Chloramphenicol and gentamicin sulfate are excreted through the nasolacrimal system.
• Idoxuridine (IDU) and boric acid are poorly absorbed topically; benzalkonium chloride is not absorbed at all.
• Trace amounts of vidarabine are found in the aqueous humor when topically applied to a cornea with an epithelial defect, but vidarabine is not absorbed systemically.
• Natamycin is not absorbed from the mucosa; does not reach measurable levels in the deeper layers of the cornea unless there is a defect in the epithelium.
• Intraocular penetration of sulfacetamide sodium varies.
• Long-term use of silver nitrate may cause silver deposits in the conjunctiva.

Onset and duration
• Bacitracin, neomycin sulfate, and polymyxin B sulfate begin to act quickly.
• Benzalkonium chloride begins to act within 5 minutes and has a long duration of action.
• Chloramphenicol and gentamicin sulfate begin to act within 1 hour.
• Chlortetracycline hydrochloride, tetracycline hydrochloride, sulfacetamide sodium, and silver nitrate have a slow onset of action. Silver nitrate also has a short duration of action.
• Vidarabine, idoxuridine (IDU), and natamycin have a short duration of action, requiring repeated instillations.
• Neomycin sulfate and polymyxin B sulfate have a duration of action of 4 to 6 hours.
• Bacitracin has a variable duration of action and is usually instilled 2 to 4 times daily.
• Erythromycin has a duration of action of approximately 4 hours.

Combination products
BLEPHAMIDE LIQUIFILM SOLUTION: sulfacetamide 10%, prednisolone acetate 0.2%, and phenylephrine hydrochloride 0.12%.
BLEPHAMIDE S.O.P. OPHTHALMIC OINTMENT: sulfacetamide 10% and prednisolone acetate 0.2%.
B.N.P. OPHTHALMIC OINTMENT: bacitracin 400 units, polymyxin B sulfate 5,000 units, and neomycin sulfate 5 mg.
CETAPRED OINTMENT♦: sulfacetamide 10% and prednisolone acetate 0.25%.
CHLOROMYCETIN-HYDROCORTISONE OPHTHALMIC♦: chloramphenicol 0.25% and hydrocortisone acetate 0.5%.
CHLOROMYXIN OPHTHALMIC♦: chloramphenicol 10 mg and polymyxin B sulfate 5,000 units.
CHLOROPTIC-P S.O.P.: chloramphenicol 1% and prednisolone alcohol 0.5%.
CORTISPORIN OPHTHALMIC OINTMENT♦: polymyxin B sulfate 5,000 units, bacitracin zinc 400 units, neomycin sulfate 5 mg, and hydrocortisone 1%.
CORTISPORIN OPHTHALMIC SUSPENSION♦: polymyxin B sulfate 10,000 units, neomycin sulfate 5 mg, and hydrocortisone 1%.
EPIMYCIN 2 OINTMENT: polymyxin B sulfate 10,000 units and bacitracin 500 units.
ISOPTO CETAPRED SUSPENSION♦: sulfacetamide 10% and prednisolone acetate 0.25%.
MAXITROL OPHTHALMIC OINTMENT/SUSPENSION♦: dexamethasone alcohol 0.1%, neomycin

sulfate 3.5 mg, and polymyxin B sulfate 6,000 units.
METIMYD OPHTHALMIC OINTMENT/SUSPENSION: sulfacetamide 10% and prednisolone acetate 0.5%.
MYCITRACIN OPHTHALMIC: polymyxin B sulfate 5,000 units, neomycin sulfate 5 mg, and bacitracin 500 units.
NEO-CORTEF OPHTHALMIC♦: hydrocortisone 0.5% or 1.5% and neomycin sulfate 0.5%.
NEODECADRON OPHTHALMIC OINTMENT: dexamethasone phosphate 0.5 mg and neomycin sulfate 3.5 mg.
NEODECADRON OPHTHALMIC SOLUTION♦: dexamethasone phosphate 1 mg and neomycin sulfate 3.5 mg.
NEO-DELTA-CORTEF OINTMENT: prednisolone acetate 0.25% or 0.5% and neomycin sulfate 3.5 mg.
NEO-DELTA CORTEF SUSPENSION: prednisolone acetate 2.5 mg and neomycin sulfate 3.5 mg.
NEO-DELTEF SOLUTION: prednisolone 2 mg and neomycin sulfate 5 mg.
NEO-MEDROL OINTMENT: methylprednisolone 1 mg and neomycin sulfate 5 mg.
NEO-POLYCIN OPHTHALMIC OINTMENT: neomycin sulfate 5 mg, polymyxin B sulfate 10,000 units, and bacitracin zinc 500 units.
NEO-POLYCIN OPHTHALMIC SOLUTION: polymyxin B sulfate 5,000 units, neomycin sulfate 1.75 mg, and gramicidin 0.025 mg.
NEOSPORIN OPHTHALMIC OINTMENT♦: polymyxin B sulfate 5,000 units, neomycin sulfate 5 mg, and bacitracin zinc 400 units.
NEOSPORIN OPHTHALMIC SOLUTION♦: polymyxin B sulfate 5,000 units, neomycin sulfate 2.5 mg, and gramicidin 0.025 mg.
NEOTAL OPHTHALMIC OINTMENT: polymyxin B sulfate 5,000 units, neomycin sulfate 5 mg, and bacitracin zinc 400 units.
OPHTHA P/S OPHTHALMIC DROPS: prednisolone acetate 0.5% and sulfacetamide 10%.
OPHTHOCORT OINTMENT: chloramphenicol 1.0%, polymyxin B sulfate 5,000 units, and hydrocortisone acetate 0.5%.
OPTIMYD SOLUTION: prednisolone phosphate 0.5% and sodium sulfacetamide 10%.
POLYSPECTRIN LIQUIFILM OPHTHALMIC SOLUTION: polymyxin B sulfate 5,000 units and neomycin sulfate 5 mg.
POLYSPECTRIN S.O.P. OPHTHALMIC OINTMENT: polymyxin B sulfate 5,000 units, neomycin sulfate 5 mg, and bacitracin zinc 400 units.
POLYSPORIN OPHTHALMIC OINTMENT♦: polymyxin B sulfate 10,000 units and bacitracin zinc 500 units.
PYOCIDIN OPHTHALMIC OINTMENT: polymyxin B sulfate 5,000 units, neomycin sulfate 5 mg, and bacitracin zinc 400 units.
STATROL OPHTHALMIC OINTMENT: neomycin sulfate 5 mg and polymyxin B sulfate 6,000 units.
STATROL OPHTHALMIC SOLUTION: neomycin sulfate 5 mg and polymyxin B sulfate 16,250 units.
SULFAPRED OPHTHALMIC SUSPENSION: sodium sulfacetamide 10%, prednisolone acetate 0.25%, and phenylephrine HCl 0.125%.
VASOCIDIN OINTMENT: sulfacetamide 10%, prednisolone phosphate 0.2%, and phenylephrine HCl 0.125%.
VASOCIDIN SOLUTION♦: sodium sulfacetamide 10%, prednisolone phosphate 0.2%, and phenylephrine 0.125%.
VASOSULF SOLUTION♦: sodium sulfacetamide 15% and phenylephrine HCl 0.125%.

INSTILLING EYE DROPS

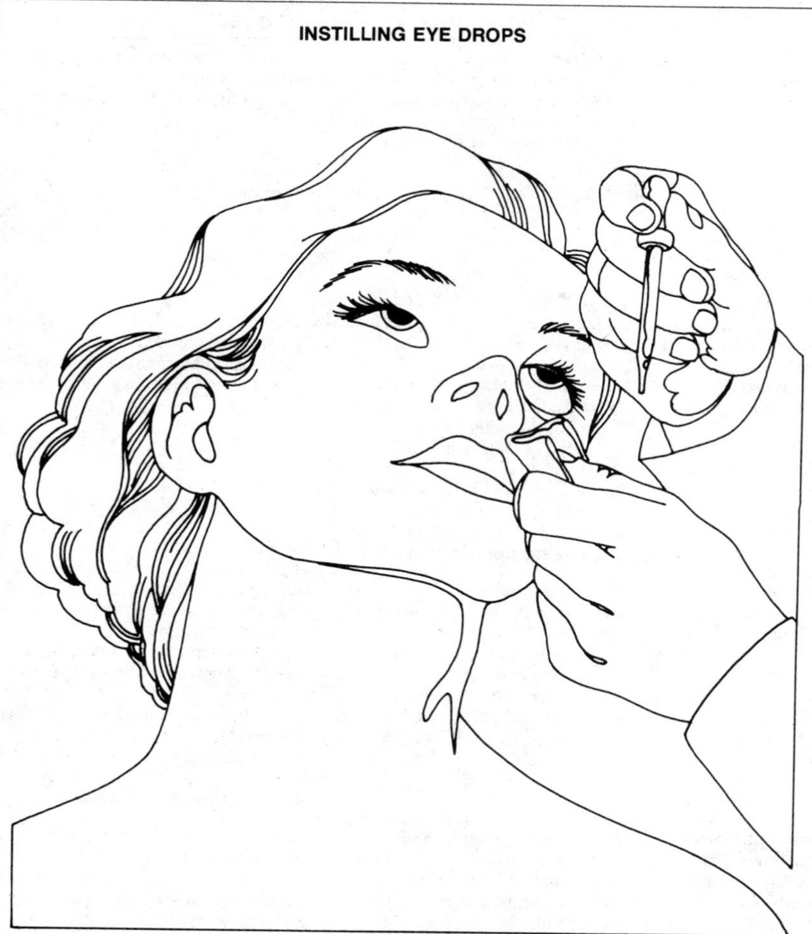

Always wash your hands just before instilling any eye medication. Position the patient with head tilted back and to the side with the unaffected eye uppermost. Instruct patient to open eyes and look up. Pull down lower eyelid of eye to be treated and instill drops in conjunctival sac — never on the eyeball itself. Always work carefully and gently, especially when the eyes are swollen, inflamed, and tender.

NAME	INDICATIONS & DOSAGE	SIDE EFFECTS
bacitracin Baciguent Ophthalmic Ointment◆	*Ocular infections—* **Adults and children:** apply small amount into conjunctival sac several times a day or p.r.n. until favorable response is observed.	*Eye:* slowed corneal wound healing, temporary visual haze. *Other:* overgrowth of nonsusceptible organisms.
benzalkonium chloride Spensomide, Zephiran◆	*To increase transcorneal penetration of drugs—* **Adults and children:** 1:5,000 to 1:2,000 concentration used in some irrigating solutions for its antiseptic as well as its surface-active qualities. *To sterilize ophthalmic solutions:* use 1:5,000 concentration. An ingredient in germicidal cleaning solutions for contact lens.	*Eye:* toxic to abraded cornea and to endothelial cells of cornea if introduced into anterior chamber.
boric acid Blinx, Collyrium, Dacriose, Neo-Flo	*For irrigation following tonometry, gonioscopy, foreign body removal, or use of fluorescein; used to soothe and cleanse the eye; used in conjunction with contact lens—* **Adults:** irrigate eye with 2% solution, or apply 5% or 10% ointment, p.r.n.	Note: toxic if absorbed from abraded skin areas, granulating wounds, or ingestion. *CNS:* headache, restlessness, weakness, delirium, convulsions, hypothermia, coma. *CV:* tachycardia, cyanosis, circulatory collapse. *GI:* nausea, vomiting, diarrhea, anorexia. *Skin:* erythematous skin lesions.
chloramphenicol Antibiopto, Chloromycetin Ophthalmic◆, Chloroptic Ophthalmic◆, Chloroptic S.O.P., Econochlor Ophthalmic, Fenicol◆◆, Isopto Fenicol◆◆, Nova-Phenicol◆◆, Ophthoclor Ophthalmic, Pentamycetin◆◆	*Surface bacterial infection involving conjunctiva or cornea—* **Adults and children:** instill 2 drops of solution in eye q 1 hour until condition improves, or instill q.i.d., depending on severity of infection. Apply small amount of ointment to lower conjunctival sac at bedtime as supplement to drops. May use ointment alone by applying a small amount of ointment to lower conjunctival sac q 3 to 6 hours or more frequently, if necessary. Continue until condition improves.	Note: systemic adverse reactions have not been reported with short-term topical use. *Blood:* bone marrow hypoplasia with prolonged use. *Eye:* slowed corneal wound healing, optic atrophy in children, stinging or burning of eye after instillation. *Other:* overgrowth of nonsusceptible organisms; hypersensitivity, including itching and burning eye, dermatitis, angioedema.

◆ Also available in Canada.
◆◆ Available in Canada only.
Unmarked trade names available in United States only.

INTERACTIONS	NURSING CONSIDERATIONS
Heavy metals (silver nitrate): inactivate bacitracin. Don't use together.	• Use cautiously in patients with hereditary predisposition to antibiotic hypersensitivity. • Warn patient to avoid sharing washcloths, etc. with family members. • Always wash hands before and after applying ointment. • Tell patient to watch for signs of sensitivity, such as itching lids or constant burning. Patient should stop drug and notify doctor immediately. • Show patient how to apply. For instillation instructions, see p. 811. Stress importance of compliance with recommended therapy. • Don't touch tip of tube to any part of eye or surrounding tissue. • Solution not commercially available but may be prepared by pharmacy. May be stored up to 3 weeks in refrigerator. • Bactericidal or bacteriostatic, depending on concentration and infection. • Store in tightly closed, light-resistant container.
Fluorescein: destroyed benzalkonium chloride antibacterial activity. May cause corneal staining. Don't use together. *Sulfonamides (ophthalmic):* incompatible. Don't apply at same time.	• Never prepare a straight benzalkonium chloride solution for use in eye. • Warn patient to avoid sharing washcloths, etc. with family members. • Don't use concentrations greater than 1:2,000 in the eye; may be irritating. • Tell patient to watch for signs of sensitivity, such as itching lids or constant burning. Patient should stop drug and notify doctor immediately. • Don't touch applicator to eye or surrounding tissue. • Always wash hands before and after applying drug. • Present in majority of combination topical eye preparations commercially available. • For instillation instructions, see p. 841.
Polyvinyl alcohol (Liquifilm): may form insoluble complex. Check with pharmacy on contents in eye drugs and contact lens wetting solutions.	• Contraindicated in eye abrasions. • Don't apply to abraded cornea or skin. • Lethal dose is 5 to 6 g in infants and 15 to 20 g in adults. • Always wash hands before and after instilling solution or ointment. • Not for use with soft contact lenses. • Weak bacteriostatic, fungistatic agent. • For instillation instructions, see pp. 811 and 841.
None significant.	• Not for long-term use. Notify doctor if no improvement in 3 days. • If patient has more than a superficial infection, systemic therapy should be used also. • Bacteriostatic. • One of the safest topical ocular antibiotics, especially for endophthalmitis. • Warn patient to avoid sharing washcloths, etc. with family members. • Always wash hands before and after applying ointment or solution. • Tell patient to watch for signs of sensitivity, such as itching lids or constant burning. Patient should stop drug and notify doctor immediately. • Show patient how to instill. For instillation instructions, see pp. 801 and 811. Stress importance of compliance with recommended therapy. • Warn patient not to touch tip of applicator to eye or surrounding tissue. • If chloramphenicol drops are to be given q 1 hour, then tapering, follow order closely to ensure adequate anterior chamber levels. • Store in tightly closed, light-resistant container.

NAME	INDICATIONS & DOSAGE	SIDE EFFECTS
chlortetracycline hydrochloride Aureomycin Ophthalmic	*Superficial ocular infection—* **Adults and children:** apply 1% ointment to eye q 2 hours or more, p.r.n.	*Local:* itching, dermatitis. *Other:* overgrowth of nonsusceptible organisms with long-term use.
erythromycin Ilotycin Ophthalmic◆	*Acute and chronic conjunctivitis, other eye infections—* **Adults and children:** apply 0.5% ointment 1 or more times daily, depending upon severity of infection.	*Eye:* slowed corneal wound healing. *Other:* overgrowth of nonsusceptible organisms with long-term use; hypersensitivity, including itchy and burning eye, urticaria, dermatitis, angioedema.
gentamicin sulfate Garamycin Ophthalmic◆	*External ocular infections (conjunctivitis, keratoconjunctivitis, corneal ulcers, blepharitis, blepharoconjunctivitis, meibomianitis, and dacryocystitis) due to susceptible organisms, especially Pseudomonas aeruginosa, Proteus sp., Klebsiella pneumoniae, Escherichia coli.—* **Adults and children:** instill 1 to 2 drops in eye q 4 hours. In severe infections, may use up to 2 drops q 1 hour. Apply ointment to lower conjunctival sac b.i.d. to t.i.d.	Note: systemic absorption from excessive use which may cause systemic toxicities. *Eye:* photosensitivity, burning or stinging with ointment, transient irritation from solution. *Other:* hypersensitivity, overgrowth of nonsusceptible organisms with long-term use.

INTERACTIONS	NURSING CONSIDERATIONS
None significant.	• Contraindicated in tetracycline hypersensitivity. • *Pseudomonas, Proteus,* and *Staphylococcus* resistant to drug. Used mainly for trachoma in conjunction with oral therapy. Trachoma treatment may continue 2 months or more. Trachoma may cause blindness if left untreated or if treated improperly. • Warn patient to avoid sharing washcloths, etc. with family members. • Always wash hands before and after applying ointment. • Tell patient to watch for signs of sensitivity, such as itching lids or constant burning. Patient should stop drug and notify doctor immediately. • Show patient how to instill. For instillation instructions, see p. 811. Stress importance of compliance with recommended therapy. • Warn patient not to touch tip of tube to eye or surrounding tissue. • Bacteriostatic. • Store in tightly closed, light-resistant container.
None significant.	• Bacteriostatic but may be bactericidal in high concentrations or against highly susceptible organisms. • Has a limited antibacterial spectrum. Use only when sensitivity studies show it is effective against infecting organisms. Don't use in infections of unknown etiology. • Warn patient to avoid sharing washcloths, etc. with family members. • Always wash hands before and after applying ointment. • Tell patient to watch for signs of sensitivity, such as itching lids or constant burning. Patient should stop drug and notify doctor immediately. • Show patient how to apply. For instillation instructions, see p. 811. Stress importance of compliance with recommended therapy. • Warn patient not to touch tube to eye or surrounding tissue. • Store at room temperature in tightly closed, light-resistant container.
None significant.	• Contraindicated in aminoglycoside hypersensitivity. Use cautiously in impaired renal function. • Have culture taken before giving drug. • Stress importance of following recommended therapy. *Pseudomonas* infections can cause complete vision loss within 24 hours if infection is not controlled. • Warn against excessive exposure to sunlight. Recommend sunglasses. • Warn patient to avoid sharing washcloths, etc. with family members. • Always wash hands before and after applying ointment or solution. • Tell patient to watch for signs of sensitivity, such as itching lids or constant burning. Patient should stop drug and notify doctor immediately. • Show patient how to instill. For instillation instructions, see pp. 801 and 811. • Warn patient not to touch tip of tube or dropper to eye or surrounding tissue. • Store away from heat.

NAME	INDICATIONS & DOSAGE	SIDE EFFECTS
idoxuridine (IDU) Dendrid, Stoxil◆	*Herpes simplex keratitis*— **Adults and children:** instill 1 drop of solution into conjunctival sac q 1 hour during day and q 2 hours at night, or apply ointment to conjunctival sac q 4 hours or 5 times daily, with last dose at bedtime. A response should be seen in 7 days; if not, discontinue and begin alternate therapy. Therapy should not be continued longer than 21 days.	*Eye:* temporary visual haze; irritation, pain, burning, or inflammation of eye; mild edema of eyelid or cornea; photosensitivity; small punctate defects in corneal epithelium; slowed corneal wound healing with ointment. *Other:* hypersensitivity.
natamycin Natacyn	*Treatment of fungal keratitis*— **Adults:** initial dosage 1 drop instilled in conjunctival sac q 1 to 2 hours. After 3 to 4 days, reduce dosage to 1 drop 6 to 8 times daily.	*Eye:* ocular edema, hyperemia.
neomycin sulfate Myciguent Ophthalmic	*Used alone or in combination with other antibiotics in treating superficial ocular infections involving conjunctiva or cornea*— **Adults and children:** apply ointment to lower conjunctival sac daily to t.i.d.	*Skin:* sensitization in 5% to 10% of patients. *Other:* hypersensitivity reactions (itching and burning eye, erythema, dermatitis, urticaria, anaphylaxis); after long-term use, overgrowth of nonsusceptible organisms.
polymyxin B sulfate Aerosporin◆	*Used alone or in combination with other agents for treating corneal ulcers resulting from Pseudomonas infection or other gram-negative organism infections*— **Adults and children:** instill 1 to 3 drops of 0.1% to 0.25% (10,000 to 25,000 units per ml) q 1 hour. Increase interval according to patient response; or up to 10,000 units subconjunctivally daily by doctor.	*Eye:* eye irritation, conjunctivitis. *Other:* overgrowth of nonsusceptible organisms, hypersensitivity (local burning, itching).

INTERACTIONS	NURSING CONSIDERATIONS
None significant.	• Contraindicated in deep ulceration. • Not for long-term use. • Idoxuridine should not be mixed with other medications. • Don't use old solution; causes ocular burning and has no antiviral activity. • Warn patient to avoid sharing washcloths, etc. with family members. • Always wash hands before and after applying ointment or solution. • Tell patient to watch for signs of sensitivity, such as itching lids or constant burning. Patient should stop drug and notify doctor immediately. • Show patient how to apply. For instillation instructions, see pp. 801 and 811. Stress importance of compliance with recommended therapy. • Warn patient not to touch tip of tube or dropper to eye or surrounding tissue. • Refrigerate idoxuridine 0.1% solution. Store in tightly closed, light-resistant container. • Boric acid increases irritation. Don't use together.
None significant.	• Only antifungal available as ophthalmic preparation. • Treatment of choice for fungal keratitis. May also be used to treat fungal blepharitis and conjunctivitis. • Therapy should be continued for 14 to 21 days, or until active disease subsides. • Reduce dosage gradually at 4- to 7-day intervals to assure that organism has been eliminated. • If infection does not improve with 7 to 10 days of therapy, clinical reevaluation and more laboratory studies are recommended.
None significant.	• Contraindicated in aminoglycide hypersensitivity. • Effective against gram-positive and gram-negative organisms. • Warn patient to avoid sharing washcloths, etc. with family members. • Always wash hands before and after applying ointment. • Tell patient to watch for signs of sensitivity, such as itching lids or constant burning. Patient should stop drug and notify doctor immediately. • Show patient how to apply. For instillation instructions, see p. 811. Stress importance of compliance with recommended therapy. • Warn patient not to touch tip of tube to eye or surrounding tissue. • Bactericidal. • For symptoms and treatment of anaphylaxis, see p. 1114.
None significant.	• One of the most effective antibiotics against gram-negative organisms, especially *Pseudomonas.* • Often used in combination with neomycin sulfate. • Warn patient to avoid sharing washcloths, etc. with family members. • Always wash hands before and after instilling solution. • Tell patient to watch for signs of sensitivity, such as itching lids and lashes or constant burning. Patient should stop drug and notify doctor immediately. • Show patient how to instill. For instillation instructions, see p. 801. Stress importance of compliance with recommended therapy. • Warn patient not to touch tip of dropper to eye or surrounding tissue. • Bactericidal. • Not commercially available. Polymyxin B sulfate powder must be reconstituted with sterile water for injection or normal saline solution. Refrigerated solutions stable for 6 months.

NAME	INDICATIONS & DOSAGE	SIDE EFFECTS
silver nitrate 1%	*Prevention of gonorrheal ophthalmia neonatorum*— **Neonates:** cleanse lids thoroughly; instill 1 drop of 1% solution into each eye.	*Eye:* periorbital edema, temporary staining of lids and surrounding tissue, conjunctivitis (with concentrations greater than 1%).
sulfacetamide sodium 10% Bleph-10 Liquifilm Ophthalmic◆, Cetamide Ophthalmic◆, 10% sodium Sulamyd ophthalmic, Sulf-10 Ophthalmic◆ **sulfacetamide sodium 15%** Isopto Cetamide Ophthalmic◆, Sulfacel-15 Ophthalmic **sulfacetamide sodium 30%** Bleph-30 Liquifilm Ophthalmic, sodium Sulamyd 30% ophthalmic◆	*Inclusion conjunctivitis, corneal ulcers, trachoma, prophylaxis to ocular infection*— **Adults and children:** instill 1 to 2 drops of 10% solution into lower conjunctival sac q 2 to 3 hours during day, less often at night; or instill 1 to 2 drops of 15% solution into lower conjunctival sac q 1 to 2 hours initially, increasing interval as condition responds; or instill 1 drop of 30% solution into lower conjunctival sac q 2 hours. Instill ½ to 1 inch of 10% ointment into conjunctival sac q.i.d. and at bedtime. May use ointment at night along with drops during the day.	*Eye:* slowed corneal wound healing, pain on instilling eye drop. *Other:* hypersensitivity (including itching or burning), overgrowth of nonsusceptible organisms.
tetracycline hydrochloride Achromycin Ophthalmic◆	**Adults and children:** *Superficial ocular infections, trachoma, and inclusion conjunctivitis*—instill 1 to 2 drops in eye b.i.d., q.i.d., or more often, depending on severity of infection. *Trachoma*—instill 2 drops in each eye b.i.d., t.i.d., or q.i.d. Continue for 1 to 2 months or longer, or use 1% ointment t.i.d. to q.i.d. for 30 days.	*Eye:* itching. *Other:* hypersensitivity (eye itching and dermatitis), overgrowth of nonsusceptible organisms with long-term use.
vidarabine Vira-A Ophthalmic◆	*Acute keratoconjunctivitis, superficial keratitis, and recurrent epithelial keratitis resulting from herpes simplex types I and II*— **Adults and children:** instill ½ inch ointment into lower conjunctival sac 5 times daily at 3-hour intervals.	*Eye:* temporary visual burning, itching, mild irritation of eye, lacrimation, foreign body sensation, conjunctival injection, superficial punctate keratitis, eye pain, photosensitivity. *Other:* hypersensitivity.

INTERACTIONS	NURSING CONSIDERATIONS
Bacitracin: inactivated silver nitrate. Don't use together.	• Legally required for neonates in most states. • Don't use repeatedly. • If 2% solution is accidentally used in eye, prompt irrigation with isotonic sodium chloride is advised to prevent eye irritation. • May delay instillation slightly to allow neonate to bond with mother. • Always wash hands before instilling solution. • Store wax ampules away from light and heat. • Bacteriostatic, germicidal, and astringent. • For instillation instructions, see p. 801. • Don't irrigate eyes following instillation.
Local anesthetics (procaine, tetracaine), p-aminobenzoic acid derivatives: decreased sulfacetamide sodium action. Wait for ½ to 1 hour after instilling anesthetic or *p*-aminobenzoic acid derivative before instilling sulfacetamide.	• Contraindicated in sulfonamide hypersensitivity. • Often used with systemic tetracycline in treating trachoma and inclusion conjunctivitis. • Replaced by antibiotics in treating major ocular infections; still used in minor ocular infections. • Purulent exudate interferes with sulfacetamide action. Remove as much exudate as possible from lids before instilling sulfacetamide. • Incompatible with silver preparations. • Warn patient that eye drop is painful. • Warn patient to avoid sharing washcloths, etc. with family members. • Always wash hands before and after applying ointment or solution. • Tell patient to watch for signs of sensitivity, such as itching lids or constant burning. Patient should stop drug and notify doctor immediately. • Show patient how to instill. For instillation instructions, see pp. 801 and 811. Stress importance of compliance with recommended therapy. • Warn patient not to touch tip of tube or dropper to eye or surrounding tissue. • Store in tightly closed, light-resistant container away from heat. • Don't use discolored (dark brown) solution.
None significant.	• Tell patient or family that trachoma therapy should continue for 1 to 2 months or longer. Trachoma may cause blindness if left untreated or if not treated properly. • Warn patient to avoid sharing washcloths, etc. with family members. • Always wash hands before and after applying solution. • Tell patient to watch for signs of sensitivity, such as itching lids or constant burning. Patient should stop drug and notify doctor immediately. • Show patient how to instill. For instillation instructions, see pp. 801 and 811. Stress importance of compliance with recommended therapy. • Warn patient not to touch tip of dropper to eye or surrounding tissue. • Store in tightly closed, light-resistant container.
None significant.	• Not for long-term use. • A relatively new alternative in treating herpes simplex ocular infections. • Warn patient not to exceed recommended frequency or duration of dosage. • Not effective against RNA virus or adenoviral ocular infections, or against bacterial, fungal, or chlamydial infections. • Warn patient to avoid sharing washcloths, etc. with family members. • Always wash hands before and after applying ointment. • Tell patient to watch for signs of sensitivity, such as itching lids or constant burning. Patient should stop drug and notify doctor immediately. • Show patient how to instill. For instillation instructions, see p. 811. • Warn patient not to touch tip of tube to eye or surrounding tissue. • Available in 3% ointment. • Store in tightly closed, light-resistant container.

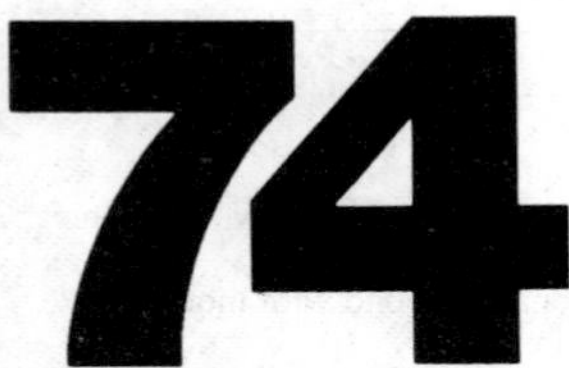

Ophthalmic anti-inflammatory agents

dexamethasone
dexamethasone sodium phosphate
fluorometholone
hydrocortisone
hydrocortisone acetate
medrysone
prednisolone acetate
prednisolone sodium phosphate

Corticosteroids are used topically in the eye to treat inflammatory ophthalmic conditions. They are potent drugs, however, and should only be used with medical supervision.

Major uses

- Treatment of inflammatory disorders of the eyelids, conjunctiva, cornea, and anterior segment of globe.
- Dexamethasone is also used to prevent corneal scarring.

Mechanism of action

- Exact mechanism of action is unknown.

Absorption, distribution, and excretion

- Absorption through intact cornea is not great; absorption is usually greater in corneal abrasion.

Onset and duration

- Onset of action is moderate and variable.
- Therapeutic effects of dexamethasone are maintained approximately 3 to 4 hours.

Combination products

- Corticosteroids for the eye are commonly combined with antibiotics and sulfonamides. See pp. 799-800.

HOW TO INSTILL EYE OINTMENT

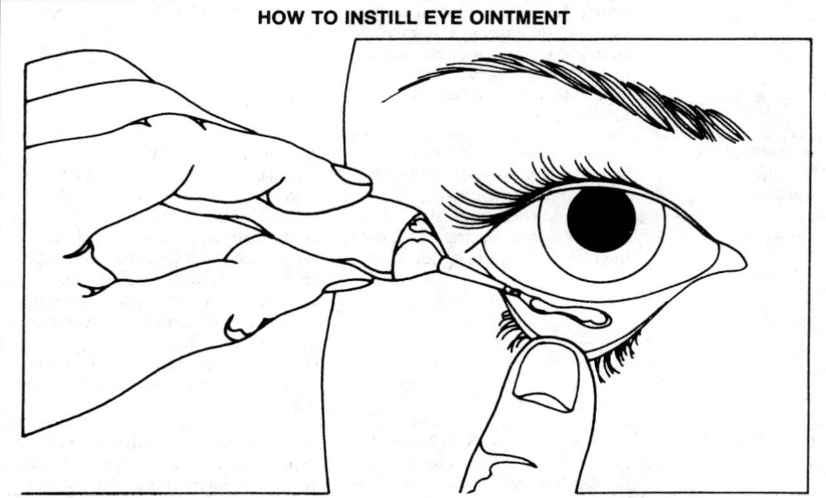

When instilling eye ointment, first cleanse the patient's eyelid and lashes with saline or irrigating solution. Take care not to contaminate the applicator end by touching it against anything as you remove the cap from the tube and apply the ointment. Squeeze a small ribbon of medication along the inside of the lower eyelid. The patient should then keep the eyelids closed for 1 to 2 minutes to allow the medicine to spread and be absorbed.

NAME	INDICATIONS & DOSAGE	SIDE EFFECTS
dexamethasone Maxidex Ophthalmic Suspension◆ **dexamethasone sodium phosphate** Decadron Phosphate Ophthalmic◆, Maxidex Ophthalmic◆, Novadex◆◆, Opto-Methasone◆◆	*Uveitis; iridocyclitis; inflammatory condition of eyelids, conjunctiva, cornea, anterior segment of globe; to prevent corneal scarring in visual axis; corneal injury from chemical or thermal burns, or penetration of foreign bodies; allergic conjunctivitis—* **Adults and children:** instill 1 to 2 drops into conjunctival sac. In severe disease, drops may be used hourly, tapering to discontinuation as condition improves. In mild conditions, drops may be used up to 4 to 6 times daily. Treatment may extend from a few days to several weeks.	*Eye:* increased intraocular pressure, especially in elderly patients; thinning of cornea, interference with corneal wound healing, increased susceptibility to viral or fungal corneal infection, corneal ulceration; with excessive or long-term use, glaucoma exacerbations, cataracts, visual acuity and visual field defects, optic nerve damage. *Other:* systemic effects and adrenal suppression with excessive or long-term use.
fluorometholone FML Liquifilm Ophthalmic◆	*Inflammatory and allergic conditions of cornea, conjunctiva, sclera, anterior uvea—* **Adults and children:** instill 1 to 2 drops q 1 hour for first 1 to 2 days, then b.i.d., t.i.d., or q.i.d.	*Eye:* increased intraocular pressure, especially in elderly patients; thinning of cornea, interference with corneal wound healing, corneal ulceration, increased susceptibility to viral or fungal corneal infections; with excessive or long-term use, glaucoma exacerbations, cataracts, decreased visual acuity, diminished visual field; optic nerve damage. *Other:* systemic effects and adrenal suppression in excessive or long-term use.
hydrocortisone Optef **hydrocortisone acetate** Cortamed◆◆, Hydrocortone◆	*Uveitis, iridocyclitis, inflammatory condition of eyelids, conjunctiva, cornea, anterior segment of globe; to prevent corneal scarring in visual axis; corneal injury from chemical or thermal burns, or penetration of foreign bodies; allergic conjunctivitis—* **Adults and children:** instill 1 to 3 drops into conjunctival sac q hour during the day and q 2 hours during the night in acute situations. May be decreased to 1 drop t.i.d. or q.i.d.; or instill ointment t.i.d. to q.i.d. initially. May decrease to daily or b.i.d.	*Eye:* increased intraocular pressure, especially in elderly patients; thinning of cornea, interference with corneal wound healing, increased susceptibility to viral or fungal corneal infection, corneal ulceration; with excessive or long-term use, glaucoma exacerbations, cataracts, visual acuity and visual field defects, optic nerve damage. *Other:* systemic effects and adrenal suppression with excessive or long-term use.

◆ Also available in Canada.
◆◆ Available in Canada only.
Unmarked trade names available in United States only.

INTERACTIONS	NURSING CONSIDERATIONS
None significant.	• Contraindicated in acute superficial herpes simplex (dendritic keratitis), vaccinia, varicella, or other fungal or viral diseases of cornea and conjunctiva; presence of active diabetes; ocular tuberculosis, or any acute, purulent, untreated infection of the eye. Use cautiously in corneal abrasions, since these may be infected (especially herpes); glaucoma patients (any form), due to possibility of increasing intraocular pressure (miotic medication drug regimen may need to be increased to compensate). • Viral and fungal infections of the cornea may be exacerbated by the application of steroids. • Warn patient to call doctor immediately and to stop drug if visual acuity changes or visual field diminishes. • Not for long-term use. • May use eye pad with ointment for increased effect. • Watch for corneal ulceration; may require stopping drug. • Dexamethasone has greater anti-inflammatory effect than dexamethasone sodium phosphate. • For instillation instructions, see p. 801.
None significant.	• Contraindicated in vaccinia, varicella, acute superficial herpes simplex (dendritic keratitis), or other fungal or viral eye diseases; ocular tuberculosis; or any acute, purulent, untreated eye infection. Use cautiously in corneal abrasions, since they are commonly contaminated (i.e., herpes). • Not for long-term use. • Less likely to cause increased intraocular pressure with long-term use than other ophthalmic anti-inflammatory drugs (except medrysone). • Store in tightly covered, light-resistant container. • Warn patient to call doctor immediately and to stop drug if visual acuity decreases or visual field diminishes. • For instillation instructions, see p. 801.
None significant.	• Contraindicated in acute superficial herpes simplex (dendritic keratitis), vaccinia, varicella, or other fungal or viral diseases of cornea and conjunctiva; presence of active diabetes; ocular tuberculosis; or any acute, purulent, untreated eye infection. Use cautiously in corneal abrasions, since they are commonly contaminated (i.e., herpes). • Viral and fungal infections of the cornea may be exacerbated by the application of steroids. • Keep in mind possibility of increasing intraocular pressure. • Warn patient to call doctor immediately and to stop drug if visual acuity changes or visual field diminishes. • Not for long-term use. • May use eye pad with ointment for increased effect. • Watch for corneal ulceration; may require stopping drug. • For instillation instructions, see p. 801.

NAME	INDICATIONS & DOSAGE	SIDE EFFECTS
medrysone HMS Liquifilm Ophthalmic◆	*Allergic conjunctivitis, vernal conjunctivitis, episcleritis, ophthalmic epinephrine sensitivity reaction—* **Adults and children:** instill 1 drop in conjunctival sac b.i.d. to q.i.d. May use q hour during first 1 to 2 days if needed.	*Eye:* thinning of cornea, interference with corneal wound healing, increased susceptibility to viral or fungal corneal infection, corneal ulceration; with excessive or long-term use, glaucoma exacerbations, cataracts, visual acuity and visual field defects, optic nerve damage. *Other:* systemic effects and adrenal suppression with excessive or long-term use.
prednisolone acetate (suspensions) Econopred Ophthalmic, Econopred Plus Ophthalmic, Pred-Forte◆, Pred Mild Ophthalmic◆, Prednicon◆◆, Predulose Ophthalmic **prednisolone sodium phosphate (solutions)** Hydeltrasol Ophthalmic, Inflamase Forte◆, Inflamase Ophthalmic◆, Metreton Ophthalmic, Nova-Pred Forte◆◆	*Inflammation of palpebral and bulbar conjunctiva, cornea, and anterior segment of globe—* **Adults and children:** instill 2 drops in eye. In severe conditions, may be used hourly, tapering to discontinuation as inflammation subsides. In mild conditions, may be used up to 4 to 6 times daily.	*Eye:* increased intraocular pressure, especially in elderly patients; thinning of cornea, interference with corneal wound healing, increased susceptibility to viral or fungal corneal infection, corneal ulceration; with excessive or long-term use, glaucoma exacerbations, cataracts, visual acuity and visual field defects, optic nerve damage. *Other:* systemic effects and adrenal suppression with excessive or long-term use.

INTERACTIONS	NURSING CONSIDERATIONS
None significant.	• Contraindicated in vaccinia, varicella, acute superficial herpes simplex (dendritic keratitis), viral diseases of conjunctiva and cornea, ocular tuberculosis, fungal or viral eye diseases, iritis, uveitis, or any acute, purulent, untreated eye infection. Use cautiously in corneal abrasions, since they are commonly contaminated (i.e., herpes). • Shake well before using. Don't freeze. • For instillation instructions, see p. 801.
None significant.	• Contraindicated in acute untreated purulent ocular infections, acute superficial herpes simplex (dendritic keratitis), vaccinia, varicella, or other viral or fungal eye diseases, ocular tuberculosis. Use cautiously in corneal abrasions, since they are commonly contaminated (i.e., herpes). • Instruct patient on long-term therapy to have frequent tonometric exams. • Shake before using and store in tightly covered container. • Don't stop therapy prematurely. • For instillation instructions, see p. 801.

Miotics

acetylcholine chloride
carbachol
demecarium bromide
echothiophate iodide
isoflurophate
physostigmine salicylate
pilocarpine hydrochloride
pilocarpine nitrate

Miotics cause pupillary constriction (miosis) and are used in chronic conditions such as glaucoma and during or after ocular surgery.

Major uses

- Treatment of open-angle, narrow-angle, acute-angle closure, and chronic simple glaucoma.
- Treatment of accommodative esotropia.
- In iridectomy, anterior segment surgery, and other ocular surgery.
- Prevents adhesions after ocular surgery when used with mydriatics.

Mechanism of action

- Cholinergics, such as acetylcholine chloride, carbachol, and pilocarpine hydrochloride, cause contraction of the sphincter muscles of the iris, resulting in pupillary constriction (miosis). They also cause ciliary spasm, deepening of the anterior chamber, and vasodilation of conjunctival vessels of outflow tract.
- Anticholinesterase drugs, such as isoflurophate, demecarium bromide, echothiophate iodide, and physostigmine salicylate, inhibit the enzymatic destruction of acetylcholine by inactivating cholinesterase. This leaves acetylcholine free to act on the effector cells of the iris sphincter and ciliary muscles, causing pupillary constriction and spasm of accommodation.

Absorption, distribution, and excretion

- Acetylcholine cannot penetrate cornea if applied topically. It is used intraocularly at the end of surgical procedures. It is rapidly destroyed and does not accumulate.
- Carbachol is poorly absorbed unless wetting agents such as benzalkonium chloride are added to enhance corneal penetration.
- All others are well absorbed after topical instillation.
- Accumulation of echothiophate iodide is possible.

Onset and duration

- Acetylcholine chloride produces, in 10 to 15 seconds, miosis that lasts about 10 minutes.
- Carbachol produces maximal miosis in 2 to 5 minutes. Duration varies from 4 to 8 hours, to more than 2 days.
- Demecarium bromide produces miosis within 45 minutes, reaches a maximum within 2 to 4 hours, and lasts from 3 to 10 days.
- Echothiophate iodide has a slow onset and long duration of action.
- Isoflurophate produces, in 5 to 10 minutes, miosis that lasts from 2 to 4 weeks.

• Physostigmine salicylate produces, within 30 minutes, miosis that lasts 12 to 36 hours.
• Pilocarpine produces miosis in 15 to 30 minutes, reaches a maximum within 90 minutes, and lasts from 4 to 8 hours. Onset of spasm of accommodation occurs within 15 minutes and lasts 2 to 3 hours.

Combination products

E-CARPINE♦: epinephrine bitartrate 0.5% and pilocarpine hydrochloride 1%, 2%, 3%, 4%, or 6%.
EPICAR: epinephrine hydrochloride 0.65% and pilocarpine hydrochloride 1%, 2%, 3%, 4%, or 6%.
E-PILO♦: epinephrine bitartrate 1% and pilocarpine hydrochloride 1%, 2%, 3%, 4%, or 6%.
ISOPTO P-ES: pilocarpine hydrochloride 2% and eserine salicylate 0.25%.
MIOCEL: pilocarpine hydrochloride 2% and physostigmine salicylate 0.125%.
PE: epinephrine bitartrate 1% and pilocarpine hydrochloride 1%, 2%, 3%, 4%, or 6%.
PILOFRIN: phenylephrine hydrochloride 0.12% and pilocarpine nitrate 0.5%, 1%, 2%, 3%, 4%, or 6%.

RECOGNIZING HIGH-RISK GLAUCOMA PATIENTS

Do you know when your patient has glaucoma? You won't know for certain until he's been tested. But you can help detect vulnerable patients. Elevated intraocular pressure may be the first sign of glaucoma, so early tonometry screening is essential. Vulnerable patients who should be screened at least every 2 years are:

• *Everyone between ages 55 and 65.*
• *Diabetics:* Primary open-angle glaucoma occurs approximately three times more frequently in diabetics; and visual field loss appears to develop at lower pressures in diabetics. Therefore, urge your diabetic patients to see an ophthalmologist regularly.
• *Blacks:* Reportedly, the black population has eight times more glaucoma-related blindness than the white population. No physiological cause is known, but some attribute the increased incidence to poor preventive care.
• *Hypertensive patients with primary open-angle glaucoma:* In these patients, lowering of blood pressure may reduce the blood flow to the optic nerve, making it more vulnerable to damage.
• *Patients with a family history of glaucoma:* The genetic factor is so strongly indicated (about one third of patients with chronic open-angle glaucoma have relatives with the disease) that any patient with glaucoma in the family within two generations should be regularly screened from age 25 on.
• *"Large-eyed" children:* If a child has frequent tearing, photophobia (light sensitivity), or blepharospasm (continual blinking), and seems to have exceptionally large corneas (normal corneal diameter is approximately 11.5 mm), these could be indications of congenital glaucoma. (However, this is a rare variation of the disease.)
• *Patients who've suffered eye injuries:* Be especially alert for glaucoma in patients who've had eye injuries caused by the blow of a tennis ball, a fist, or blunt instruments.

NAME	INDICATIONS & DOSAGE	SIDE EFFECTS
acetylcholine chloride Miochol◆	*Anterior segment surgery—* **Adults and children:** doctor instills 0.5 to 2 ml of 0.5% to 1% solution gently in anterior chamber of eye.	None reported with 1% concentration. Iris atrophy possible with higher concentrations.
carbachol (intraocular) Miostat **carbachol (topical)** Carbacel, Isopto Carbachol◆	*Ocular surgery (to produce pupillary miosis)—* **Adults:** doctor should gently instill 0.5 ml into the anterior chamber for production of satisfactory miosis. It may be instilled before or after securing sutures. *Open-angle or narrow-angle glaucoma—* **Adults:** instill 1 drop into eye daily, b.i.d., t.i.d., or q.i.d. An ointment form is also available with b.i.d. dosage.	*CNS:* headache. *Eye:* accommodative spasm, conjunctival vasodilation, eye and brow pain. *GI:* abdominal cramps, diarrhea. *Other:* sweating, flushing, asthma.
demecarium bromide Humorsol	*Glaucoma, postiridectomy—* **Adults:** instill 1 drop 0.125% or 0.25% solution in eyes twice weekly up to b.i.d., depending on intraocular pressure. *Accommodative esotropia—* **Children:** instill 1 drop 0.125% solution in each eye daily for 2 to 3 weeks, taper to 1 drop q 2 days for 3 to 4 weeks, then 1 drop twice weekly. Therapy should be discontinued after 4 months if control of condition still requires q other day therapy or if patient shows no response.	*CNS:* headache. *CV:* hypotension, bradycardia. *Eye:* iris cysts (reversible with discontinuation), lens opacity, ciliary or accommodative spasm, blurred vision, eye or brow pain, photosensitivity, eyelid twitching, congestive iritis, iridocyclitis, conjunctival and intraocular hyperemia, ocular pain, photophobia, acute attack of congestive glaucoma. *GI:* nausea, vomiting, abdominal pain, diarrhea, excessive salivation. *GU:* frequent urination. *Skin:* contact dermatitis. *Other:* flushing, bronchial constriction.

◆ Also available in Canada.
◆◆ Available in Canada only.
Unmarked trade names available in United States only.

INTERACTIONS	NURSING CONSIDERATIONS
None significant.	• Shake vial gently until clear solution is obtained. • Reconstitute immediately before using. • Discard any unused solution. • Complete miosis within seconds. • Don't gas sterilize vial. Ethylene oxide may produce formic acid.
None significant.	• Contraindicated in acute iritis, corneal abrasion. Use cautiously in acute cardiac failure, bronchial asthma, peptic ulcer, hyperthyroidism, GI spasm, urinary tract obstruction, Parkinson's disease. • A cholinergic agent. • Used in glaucoma, especially when patient is resistant or allergic to pilocarpine HC1 or nitrate. • Warn patient not to exceed recommended dosage. • For single-dose intraocular use only. Premixed; discard unused portions. • Warn patient not to touch tip of dropper to eye or surrounding tissue. • Tell glaucoma patient that long-term use may be necessary. Stress compliance. Tell him to remain under medical supervision for periodic tonometric readings. • In case of toxicity, atropine should be given parenterally. • Show patient how to instill. For instillation instructions, see p. 801.
Systemic anticholinesterase for myasthenia gravis: additive effects. Monitor for signs of toxicity. *Echothiophate iodide:* decreased duration of miosis if demecarium bromide is given first. Give echothiophate iodide first. *Organophosphate insecticides:* additive effects. Warn patient exposed to these insecticides of this danger. *Pilocarpine:* interfered with miosis. Do not use together. *Succinylcholine:* respiratory or cardiovascular collapse. Don't use together.	• Contraindicated in active uveal inflammation, narrow-angle glaucoma, secondary glaucoma resulting from iridocyclitis, ocular hypertension, vasomotor instability, bronchial asthma, spastic GI conditions, peptic ulcer, severe bradycardia, hypotension, recent myocardial infarction, epilepsy, parkinsonism, history of retinal detachment. Use cautiously in myasthenia gravis patients on systemic anticholinesterase therapy; in patients exposed to organophosphate insecticides. • Systemic absorption may be minimized by compressing inner canthus of eye for 1 to 2 minutes after instilling drops. • Dangerous drug capable of producing cumulative systemic side effects. It is essential that nurse follow closely the prescribed concentration and dosage schedule, and that patient be closely monitored. • Atropine sulfate S.C. or I.V. or pralidoxine chloride is antidote of choice. • Tell patient to stop drug and report immediately if excessive salivation, diaphoresis, urinary incontinence, diarrhea, or muscle weakness occurs. • Instruct patient to take at bedtime since drug blurs vision. • Warn patient not to exceed recommended dosage. • Warn patient not to touch tip of dropper to eye or surrounding tissue. • Stop drug at least 2 weeks preop. • If solution comes into contact with skin, wash promptly with large amount of water. • Wash hands immediately before and after administering. • Monitor patient for lenticular opacities every 6 months. • Instruct patient that close and constant medical supervision is vital. • Treat any extraocular pressure changes with rapid instillation of 1% to 2% epinephrine at 5-minute intervals. • Antidote for atropine for glaucoma or preglaucoma patients, and to control pre- and postop intraocular pressure tension of glaucoma. • Store in tightly closed container. • An extremely potent, long-acting anticholinesterase drug. • Show patient how to instill. For instillation instructions, see p. 801.

NAME	INDICATIONS & DOSAGE	SIDE EFFECTS
echothiophate iodide Echodide, Phospholine Iodide◆	*Open-angle glaucoma, conditions obstructing aqueous outflow, accommodative esotropia*— **Adults and children:** instill 1 drop 0.03% to 0.125% solution into conjunctival sac daily. Maximum 1 drop b.i.d. Use lowest possible dosage to continuously control intraocular pressure.	*CNS:* fatigue, muscle weakness, paresthesias, headache. *CV:* bradycardia, hypotension. *Eye:* ciliary or accommodative spasm, ciliary or conjunctival injection, nonreversible cataract formation (time- and dose-related), reversible iris cysts, pupillary block, blurred or dimmed vision, eye or brow pain, lid-twitching, hyperemia, photosensitivity, lens opacities, lacrimation, retinal detachment. *GI:* diarrhea, nausea, vomiting, abdominal pain, intestinal cramps, salivation. *GU:* frequent urination. *Metabolic:* reduced serum pseudocholinesterases. *Other:* reversible tolerance with long-term use, flushing, sweating, bronchial constriction, chest tightness.
isoflurophate Floropryl	*Glaucoma*— **Adults and children:** instill ¼-inch strip 0.025% ointment in conjunctival sac q 8 to 72 hours. *Esotopia uncomplicated by amblyopia or anisometropia*— 1 drop of 0.025% solution or ¼-inch of ointment every night for 2 weeks.	*CNS:* headache. *Eye:* moderate conjunctival hyperemia, eye pain, ciliary spasm causing discomfort, iris cysts, cataract formation, retinal detachment, paradoxical increase in intraocular pressure; precipitate attacks of acute congestive glaucoma.

INTERACTIONS	NURSING CONSIDERATIONS
Organophosphate insecticides (parathion, malathion): may have an additive effect that could cause systemic effects. Warn patient exposed to these insecticides of this danger. *Succinylcholine:* respiratory and cardiovascular collapse. Don't use together. *Systemic anticholinesterase for myasthenia gravis:* effects may be additive. Monitor patient for signs of toxicity.	• Contraindicated in narrow-angle glaucoma, angle-closure glaucoma, epilepsy, vasomotor instability, parkinsonism, iodide hypersensitivity, active uveal inflammation, ocular hypertension with intraocular inflammatory processes, bronchial asthma, spastic GI conditions, urinary tract obstruction, peptic ulcer, severe bradycardia or hypotension, vascular hypertension, myocardial infarction, history of retinal detachment. Use cautiously in patients routinely exposed to organophosphate insecticides. May cause nausea, vomiting, and diarrhea, progressing to muscle weakness and respiratory difficulty. Use cautiously in myasthenia gravis patients on anticholinesterase therapy. • Toxicity is cumulative. Toxic systemic symptoms don't appear for weeks or months after initiating therapy. • Reconstitute powder carefully to avoid contamination. Use only diluent provided. Discard refrigerated, reconstituted solution after 6 months; solution at room temperature after 1 month. • Warn patient that transient browache or dimmed or blurred vision are common at first but usually disappear within 5 to 10 days. • Systemic absorption may be minimized by compressing inner canthus of eye for 1 to 2 minutes after instilling drops. • Instill at bedtime, since drug causes transient blurred vision. • Tell patient to remain under constant medical supervision. Warn him not to exceed recommended dosage. • Report salivation, diarrhea, profuse sweating, urinary incontinence, or muscle weakness. • Stop drug at least 2 weeks preop. • Atropine sulfate (S.C., I.M., or I.V.) is antidote of choice. • A potent long-acting irreversible anticholinesterase. • Warn patient not to touch tip of dropper to eye or surrounding tissue. • Show patient how to instill. For instillation instructions, see p. 801.
Demecarium, physostigmine: competitive action decreased duration of miosis if isoflurophate given second. Give isoflurophate first instead. *Pilocarpine:* interfered with miosis. Use cautiously or therapeutically for ciliary spasm. *Succinylcholine:* respiratory or cardiovascular collapse. Don't use together. *Systemic anticholinesterase for myasthenia gravis:* additive effects. Monitor patient for signs of toxicity.	• Contraindicated in hypersensitivity to organophosphorous compounds and to peanut oil and polyethylene mineral oil, uveal inflammation, narrow-angle glaucoma, ocular hypertension, bronchial asthma, peptic ulcer, severe bradycardia, hypotension, recent MI, epilepsy, parkinsonism, or history of retinal detachment. Use cautiously in patients exposed to organophosphate insecticides; myasthenia gravis patients on concurrent anticholinesterase drugs. • Tell glaucoma patient to use at bedtime if possible because of blurred vision and ciliary spasm. • Don't touch tip of tube to eye, surrounding tissues, or any moist surface. • Warn patient that close, constant medical supervision is vital and not to exceed prescribed dosage. • Treat paradoxical pressure changes with rapid instillation of 1% to 2% epinephrine at 5-minute intervals. • Instruct patient to stop therapy at once if he experiences excessive salivation, diarrhea, sweating, muscle weakness and notify doctor. • Systemic absorption may be minimized by compressing inner canthus of eye for 1 to 2 minutes after instilling drops. • Unstable and inactivated in the presence of water. • Store in tightly closed container. • Rapidly absorbed through skin. • A potent parasympathomimetic or anticholinesterase drug. • Show patient how to instill. For instillation instructions, see pp. 801 and 811.

NAME	INDICATIONS & DOSAGE	SIDE EFFECTS
physostigmine salicylate Eserine Salicylate, Isopto Eserine	*Atropine mydriasis, acute angle-closure glaucoma—* **Adults and children:** instill ¼ inch 0.25% ophthalmic ointment in conjunctival sac, or instill 1 to 2 drops 0.25% to 0.5% solution in conjunctival sac t.i.d. Repeat p.r.n. to obtain miosis.	*CNS:* headache. *Eye:* twitching of eyelids, conjunctival irritation, reversible depigmentation of lid skin in blacks allergic to ointment, eye and brow pain, marked miosis, lacrimation, dimmed or blurred vision, follicular cysts. *Skin:* allergic dermatitis.
pilocarpine hydrochloride Adsorbocarpine♦, Almocarpine, Isopto Carpine♦, Miocarpine♦♦, Nova-Carpine♦♦, Ocusert Pilo♦, Opto-Pilo♦♦, Pilocar, Pilocel, Pilomiotin **pilocarpine nitrate** P.V. Carpine Liquifilm♦	*Chronic simple glaucoma, prior to emergency surgery in acute narrow-angle glaucoma—* **Adults and children:** instill 2 drops in eye daily b.i.d., t.i.d., q.i.d., or as directed by doctor.	*CV:* hypertension, tachycardia. *Eye:* suborbital headache, myopia, ciliary spasm, blurred vision, conjunctival irritation, lacrimation, changes in visual field, brow pain. *GI:* nausea, vomiting, abdominal cramps, diarrhea, GI distress, salivation. *Other:* bronchiolar spasm, pulmonary edema, hypersensitivity.

INTERACTIONS	NURSING CONSIDERATIONS
Isoflurophate: decreased miosis if isoflurophate given second. Give isoflurophate first. *Organophosphate insecticides:* additive effect. Warn patient exposed to these insecticides of this danger. *Pilocarpine:* prolonged miosis. May be used together therapeutically. *Succinylcholine:* caused additive effects. Don't use together.	• Contraindicated in inflammatory diseases of iris or ciliary body, asthma, diabetes mellitus, gangrene, cardiovascular disease, mechanical obstruction of intestinal or urogenital tract, vagotonia, secondary glaucoma. Use cautiously in bradycardia, epilepsy, parkinsonism, and in patients exposed to organophosphate insecticides. • Glaucoma therapy is long-term. Stress patient compliance. Warn him not to exceed dosage. • Lid-twitching, temporarily blurred vision, and difficulty in seeing in the dark are common side effects. • Irritating to eye. Watch for signs of conjunctivitis or allergic reactions. • Don't touch dropper or tip of tube to eye or surrounding tissue. • Systemic absorption may be minimized by compressing inner canthus of eye for 1 to 2 minutes after instilling drops. • Discard discolored (rusty or pink-colored) solution or ointment. Aqueous solutions oxidize on exposure to light or air. • Anticholinesterase. • Used in ocular myasthenia gravis. • May be used alternately with atropine as a miotic to break adhesions between the iris and lens. • Show patient how to instill. For instillation instructions, see pp. 801 and 811.
Carbachol: additive effect. Do not use together. *Phenylephrine HCl:* decreased amount of dilation by phenylephrine HCl. Don't use together.	• Contraindicated in acute iritis, acute inflammatory disease of anterior segment of eye, secondary glaucoma. Use cautiously in bronchial asthma, hypertension. • Warn patient that vision will be temporarily blurred. • Transient browache and myopia are common at first; usually disappear in 10 to 14 days. • Warn patient not to exceed recommended dosage. • Warn patient not to touch dropper to eye or surrounding tissue. • Glaucoma therapy is long-term. Stress compliance. Warn that glaucoma can cause blindness. • Most widely used drug in initial treatment of chronic, simple glaucoma. • Systemic absorption may be minimized by compressing inner canthus of eye for 1 to 2 minutes after instilling drops. • Also used to counteract effects of mydriatics and cycloplegics after surgery or ophthalmoscopic examination. • May be used alternately with atropine to break adhesions between iris and lens. • In acute narrow-angle glaucoma prior to surgery, may be used alone or with physostigmine or mannitol, urea, or glycerol. • Show patient how to instill. For instillation instructions, see p. 801.

76

Mydriatics

atropine sulfate
cyclopentolate hydrochloride
epinephrine bitartrate
epinephrine hydrochloride
epinephryl borate
homatropine hydrobromide
hydroxyamphetamine hydrobromide
phenylephrine hydrochloride
scopolamine hydrobromide
tropicamide

Mydriasis (dilation of the pupil) and cycloplegia (paralysis of accommodation) are produced when anticholinergic drugs are applied topically to the eye. Adrenergics produce mydriasis without cycloplegia.

Major uses

- Diagnostic procedures requiring mydriasis or cycloplegia.
- To dilate pupil in acute iris inflammation (iritis) or uveal tract inflammation (uveitis).
- Epinephrine is used with miotics to lower intraocular pressure of open-angle glaucoma, to diagnose episcleritis, and to control local bleeding in eye surgery.

Mechanism of action

- Anticholinergics block acetylcholine, leaving the pupil under the unopposed influence of its sympathetic or adrenergic nerve supply. This causes pupil dilation.
- Contraction of the ciliary muscle allows the lens to become more convex.
- Adrenergics dilate the pupil by contraction of the dilator muscle of the iris.

Absorption, distribution, and excretion

- All mydriatics, except the adrenergics, are well absorbed transconjunctivally.
- Adrenergics are slowly absorbed, but absorption is increased in the traumatized eye or during surgery; metabolized in the liver and excreted in urine.
- Anticholinergics are all hydrolyzed in the liver and excreted in the urine.

Onset and duration

- Atropine sulfate produces mydriasis in 30 to 40 minutes; the condition lasts up to 12 to 14 days before complete recovery. Cycloplegia is produced by atropine sulfate within a few hours, and lasts for 2 weeks or longer before complete recovery.
- Cyclopentolate hydrochloride produces mydriasis in 15 to 30 minutes that lasts up to 24 hours. Cyclopentolate HCl produces cycloplegia in 15 to 45 minutes that lasts up to 24 hours.
- Epinephrine produces, in 5 minutes, a vasoconstriction that lasts for 1 hour. Mydriasis occurs within a few minutes and lasts several hours. Epinephrine's duration of action on intraocular pressure varies (maximum effect 4 to 8 hours; recovery in 12 to 24 hours or more).
- Homatropine hydrobromide has a shorter action than atropine as a mydriatic. Cycloplegia begins in 30 to 90 minutes, and recovery takes from 10 to 48 hours. Maximum cycloplegia occurs within 1 hour; recovery, 1 to 3 days.

• Hydroxyamphetamine hydrobromide produces maximum mydriasis within 40 minutes. The mydriasis continues for several hours. Cycloplegia begins in 30 to 60 minutes, and recovery takes 20 hours for adults, several days in children.
• Phenylephrine hydrochloride 2.5% produces mydriasis within minutes. Maximum dilation occurs in 15 to 60 minutes and lasts up to 3 hours.
• Scopolamine hydrobromide produces maximum mydriasis within 40 minutes; recovery 3 to 7 days, and cycloplegia in 10 to 30 minutes, reaching a maximum within 30 to 45 minutes. Complete recovery may take several days.
• Tropicamide produces, in 20 to 25 minutes, maximum mydriasis and cycloplegia that last approximately 20 minutes, with complete recovery in about 6 hours.

Combination products

CYCLOMYDRIL: cyclopentolate hydrochloride 0.2% and phenylephrine hydrochloride 1%.

MYDRIATICS FACILITATE EYE EXAM

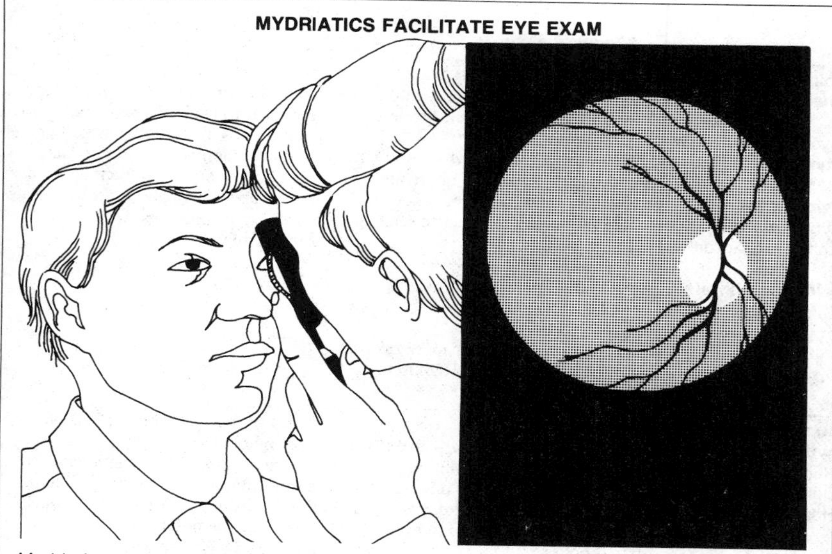

Mydriatics and cycloplegics are used to dilate the pupil and paralyze the muscles of accommodation so that the eyegrounds can be visualized during ophthalmic examination.

NAME	INDICATIONS & DOSAGE	SIDE EFFECTS
atropine sulfate Atropisol, BufOpto Atropine, Isopto Atropine◆, Opto-Tropinal◆◆	*Acute iris inflammation (iritis)*— **Adults:** 1 to 2 drops of 1% solution or small amount of ointment 2 to 3 times daily, b.i.d., or t.i.d. **Children:** instill 1 to 2 drops of 0.5% solution daily, b.i.d., or t.i.d. *Cycloplegic refraction*— **Adults:** instill 1 to 2 drops of 1% solution 1 hour before refracting. **Children:** instill 1 to 2 drops of 0.5% solution to each eye b.i.d. for 1 to 3 days before eye exam and 1 hour before refraction, or instill small amount ointment daily or b.i.d. 2 to 3 days before exam.	*Eye:* increased intraocular pressure, ocular congestion in long-term use, conjunctivitis, contact dermatitis edema, blurred vision, eye dryness, photophobia. *Systemic:* flushing, dry skin and mouth, fever, tachycardia, abdominal distention in infants, hallucinations, ataxia, irritability, confusion, delirium, somnolence.
cyclopentolate hydrochloride Cyclogyl◆, Mydplegic◆◆, Nova-Cyclo◆◆, Opto-Pentolate◆◆	*Diagnostic procedures requiring mydriasis and cycloplegia*— **Adults:** instill 1 drop 1% solution in eye, followed by 1 more drop in 5 minutes. Use 2% solution in heavily pigmented irises. **Children:** instill 1 drop of 0.5%, 1%, or 2% solution in each eye, followed in 5 minutes with 1 drop 0.5% or 1% solution, if necessary. Not recommended for children under 6.	*Eye:* burning sensation on instillation, increased intraocular pressure, blurred vision, eye dryness, photophobia, ocular congestion, contact dermatitis, conjunctivitis. *Systemic:* flushing, tachycardia, urinary retention, dry skin, fever, hallucinations, ataxia, irritability, confusion, delirium, somnolence, convulsions.
epinephrine bitartrate E1, E2, Epitrate◆, Lyophrin, Murocoll, Mytrate **epinephrine hydrochloride** Epifrin◆, Glaucon◆ **epinephryl borate** Epinal◆, Eppy◆	**Adults and children:** *Intraocular injection:* 0.1 to 0.2 ml of 0.01% or 0.1% epinephrine HCl by doctor. *Open-angle glaucoma*—instill 1 to 2 drops of 1% or 2% bitartrate solution in eye with frequency determined by tonometric readings (once q 2 to 4 days up to q.i.d.) or instill 1 drop 0.5%, 1%, or 2% HCl solution (or 0.25%, 0.5%, or 1% epinephryl borate solution) in eye b.i.d. *During surgery*—1 or more drops of 0.1% epinephrine HCl up to 3 times.	*Eye:* corneal or conjunctival pigmentation or corneal edema in long-term use; follicular hypertrophy; chemosis; conjunctivitis; iritis; hyperemic conjunctiva; maculopapular rash; severe stinging, burning, and tearing upon instillation; browache. *Systemic:* palpitations, tachycardia, extrasystoles.
homatropine hydrobromide Homatrocel Ophthalmic, Isopto Homatropine◆	**Adults and children:** *Cycloplegic refraction*—instill 1 to 2 drops 2% or 5% solution in eye; repeat in 5 to 10 minutes. *Uveitis*—instill 1 to 2 drops 2% or 5% solution in eye up to every 3 to 4 hours.	*Eye:* eye irritation, blurred vision, photophobia. *Systemic:* flushing, dry skin and mouth, fever, tachycardia, hallucinations, ataxia, irritability, confusion, delirium, somnolence.

◆ Also available in Canada.
◆◆ Available in Canada only.
Unmarked trade names available in United States only.

INTERACTIONS	NURSING CONSIDERATIONS
None significant.	• Contraindicated in primary glaucoma (shallow anterior chamber or narrow-angle), increased intraocular pressure. Use cautiously in infants, children, elderly or debilitated patients. • Warn patient that vision will be temporarily blurred. Dark glasses should be worn to decrease photophobia. • Not for internal use. Treat drops and ointment as poison. Keep physostigmine available as antidote for poisoning. • Don't touch dropper or tip of tube to eye or surrounding tissue. • Watch for signs of glaucoma: increased intraocular pressure, ocular pain, headache, blurred vision. • Most potent mydriatic and cycloplegic available; long duration of action. • Warn patient not to exceed recommended dosage. • Systemic absorption may be minimized by compressing inner canthus of eye for 1 to 2 minutes after instilling drops. • Show patient how to instill. For instillation instructions, see pp. 801 and 811. • For symptoms and treatment or toxicity (if ingested), see p. 1115.
None significant.	• Contraindicated in narrow-angle glaucoma. Use cautiously in elderly patients. • Systemic absorption may be minimized by compressing inner canthus of eye for 1 to 2 minutes after instilling drops. • Close container after each use to avoid contamination. • Potent drug with mydriatic and cycloplegic effect; superior to homatropine hydrobromide and has shorter duration of action. • Instruct patient to wear dark glasses to decrease photophobia. • Warn patient drug will burn when instilled. • For instillation instructions, see p. 801.
Cyclopropane or halogenated hydrocarbons: arrhythmias, tachycardia. Use cautiously, if at all. *Tricyclic antidepressants, antihistamines (diphenhydramine, dexchlorpheniramine):* potentiated cardiac effects of epinephrine. Use together cautiously.	• Contraindicated in shallow anterior chamber or narrow-angle glaucoma. Use cautiously in diabetes mellitus, hypertension, Parkinson's disease, hyperthyroidism, aphakia (eye without lens), cardiac disease, cerebral arteriosclerosis, elderly patients, or pregnancy. • May stain soft contact lenses. • Use with pilocarpine: additive effect in lowering intraocular pressure. • Monitor blood pressure and other systemic effects. • Protect from light and heat. • Don't use darkened solution. • Also used during surgery to control local bleeding, or injected into the anterior chamber to produce rapid mydriasis during cataract removal. • Warn patient not to touch dropper to eye or surrounding tissue. • For instillation instructions, see p. 801.
None significant.	• Contraindicated in primary glaucoma (shallow anterior chamber or narrow-angle). Use cautiously in infants, elderly or debilitated patients, or in hypertension, cardiac disease, or increased intraocular pressure. • Warn patient vision will be temporarily blurred after instillation. Dark glasses should be worn to decrease photophobia. • Long-term frequent use may produce symptoms of atropine SO_4 poisoning, such as dryness of mouth, increase in heart rate. • Not for internal use. Treat as poison. Keep physostigmine available as antidote for poisoning.

(continued on following page)

NAME	INDICATIONS & DOSAGE	SIDE EFFECTS
hydroxyamphetamine hydrobromide Paredrine	*Diagnostic in Horner's syndrome*— **Adults, and children over 12:** instill 1 to 2 drops 1% solution into conjunctival sac.	*Eye:* increased intraocular pressure, blurred vision, photophobia.
phenylephrine hydrochloride Neo-Synephrine♦	**Adults and children:** *Mydriasis (without cycloplegia)*—instill 1 drop 2.5% or 10% solution in eye before exam. *Posterior synechiae (adhesion of iris)*—instill 1 drop 10% solution in eye. Do not use 10% concentration in infants; use cautiously in elderly.	*Eye:* transient burning or stinging on instillation, blurred vision, reactive hyperemia, allergic conjunctivitis, iris floaters, angle-closure glaucoma, rebound miosis, allergic conjunctivitis, dermatitis, browache. *CNS:* headache, browache. *CV:* arrythmias, hypertension. tachycardia, palpitations, premature ventricular contractions. *Eye:* transient burning or stinging on instillation, blurred vision, reactive hyperemia, allergic conjunctivitis, iris floaters, angle-closure glaucoma, rebound miosis, allergic conjunctivitis, dermatitis. *Other:* pallor, trembling, sweating.
scopolamine hydrobromide Isopto Hyoscine	*Cycloplegic refraction*— **Adults:** instill 1 to 2 drops 0.5% to 1% solution in eye 1 hour before refraction. **Children:** instill 1 drop 0.2% or 0.25% solution or ointment b.i.d. for 2 days before refraction. *Iritis*— **Adults:** 1 to 2 drops of 0.1% solution daily, b.i.d., or t.i.d.	*Eye:* ocular congestion with prolonged use; conjunctivitis, blurred vision, eye dryness, increased intraocular pressure, photophobia, contact dermatitis. *Systemic:* flushing, fever, dry skin and mouth, tachycardia, hallucinations, ataxia, irritability, confusion, delirium, somnolence.

INTERACTIONS	NURSING CONSIDERATIONS
	• Systemic absorption may be minimized by compressing inner canthus of eye for 1 to 2 minutes after instilling drops. • Show patient how to instill. For instillation instructions, see p. 801. • Warn patient not to touch dropper tip to eye or surrounding tissue. • Similar to atropine SO_4 but weaker, with a shorter duration of action. • For symptoms and treatment of toxicity (if ingested), see p. 1115.
None significant.	• Contraindicated in narrow-angle glaucoma. Use cautiously in hypertension, hyperthyroidism, diabetes mellitus, increased intraocular pressure. • Instruct patient to wear dark glasses to decrease photophobia. • Store in tightly closed container. Do not use discolored solution. • If ingested, toxic symptoms include arrhythmias, headache, nausea, vomiting. Contact doctor immediately. • For instillation instructions, see p. 801.
Guanethidine: increased mydriatic and pressor effects of phenylephrine HC1. Use together cautiously. *Levodopa (systemic):* reduced mydriatic effect of phenylephrine HCl. Use together cautiously. *MAO inhibitors:* may cause arrhythmias due to increased pressor effect. Use together cautiously. *Tricyclic antidepressants:* potentiated cardiac effects of epinephrine. Use together cautiously.	• Contraindicated in narrow-angle glaucoma, soft contact lens use. Use cautiously in marked hypertension, cardiac disorders, and in children of low body weight. • Should be avoided in patients with idiopathic orthostatic hypotension. May produce high blood pressure response. • Protect from light and heat. • Warn patient not to exceed recommended dosage. Systemic effects can result. Monitor blood pressure and pulse. • Warn patient not to touch dropper tip to eye or surrounding tissue. • Systemic absorption can be minimized by compressing inner canthus of eye for 1 to 2 minutes after instilling drops. • Potential for systemic side effects less severe with 2.5% solution. • Show patient how to instill. For instillation instructions, see p. 801.
None significant.	• Contraindicated in primary glaucoma (shallow anterior chamber or narrow-angle). Use cautiously in cardiac disease, increased intraocular pressure, and in patients over 40 years. • Observe patient closely for systemic effects (disorientation, delirium). • Warn patient vision will be temporarily blurred. • Instruct patient to wear dark glasses to decrease photophobia. • Not for internal use. • May be used when patient is sensitive to atropine. Faster acting and has shorter duration of action. • Warn patient not to touch dropper tip to eye or surrounding tissue. • Systemic absorption may be minimized by compressing inner canthus of eye for 1 to 2 minutes after instilling drops. • For instillation instructions, see pp. 801 and 811. • For symptoms and treatment of toxicity (if ingested), see p. 1115.

NAME	INDICATIONS & DOSAGE	SIDE EFFECTS
tropicamide Mydriacyl♦	**Adults and children:** *Cycloplegic refractions*—instill 1 to 2 drops of 1% solution in each eye, repeat in 5 minutes. Additional drop may be instilled in 20 to 30 minutes. *Fundus exams*—instill 1 to 2 drops 0.5% solution in each eye 15 to 20 minutes before exam.	*EENT:* transient stinging on instillation, increased intraocular pressure (less than with other mydriatic agents because of shorter duration of action), blurred vision, photophobia, dry mouth and throat.

INTERACTIONS	NURSING CONSIDERATIONS
None significant.	• Contraindicated in narrow-angle and shallow anterior chamber glaucoma. Use cautiously in elderly patients. • Shortest acting cycloplegic, but mydriatic effect greater than cycloplegic effect. • Causes transient stinging; vision temporarily blurred. • Instruct patient to wear dark glasses if photosensitivity occurs (lasts about 2 hours). • Store at room temperature in tightly closed container. • For installation instructions, see p. 801.

Ophthalmic vasoconstrictors

epinephrine hydrochloride
naphazoline hydrochloride
phenylephrine hydrochloride
tetrahydrozoline hydrochloride
zinc sulfate

Ophthalmic vasoconstrictors relieve the itching and reduce the redness associated with irritations and inflammations of the eye. They are available as eye drops, and many are available without a prescription.

Major uses

- Treatment of ocular congestion, irritation, itching.

Mechanism of action

- Naphazoline hydrochloride, tetrahydrozoline hydrochloride, and phenylephrine hydrochloride produce vasoconstriction by local adrenergic action on the blood vessels of the conjunctiva.
- Zinc sulfate produces astringent action on mucous membranes.
- Epinephrine produces localized vasoconstriction.

Absorption, distribution, and excretion

- Naphazoline hydrochloride and tetrahydrozoline hydrochloride have variable absorption. They may, however, be absorbed in high enough concentrations to cause systemic side effects, especially in young children.
- Zinc sulfate is not absorbed and has a local effect only.
- Epinephrine hydrochloride and phenylephrine hydrochloride well absorbed via the eye.

Onset and duration

- Epinephrine acts in 5 minutes, and its effect lasts for 1 hour.
- Naphazoline hydrochloride and tetrahydrozoline hydrochloride begin to act rapidly.
- Naphazoline hydrochloride acts for as long as 3 to 4 hours; the effect of tetrahydrozoline hydrochloride is noticeably shorter.
- Phenylephrine begins to act within minutes and continues to act for up to 3 hours.
- Zinc sulfate has a moderate onset and duration of action.

Combination products

ALBALON-A◆: naphazoline hydrochloride 0.05% and antazoline phosphate 0.5%.
BLEPHAMIDE◆: phenylephrine hydrochloride 0.12%, sulfacetamide 10%, and prednisolone acetate 0.2%.
DEGEST 2: naphazoline hydrochloride 0.012% and antipyrine 0.1%.

EYEPHRINE: phenylephrine hydrochloride 0.12% and zinc sulfate 0.1%.
M-Z: phenylephrine hydrochloride 0.12%, zinc sulfate 0.25%, and piperocaine hydrochloride 0.75%.
NEOZIN OPHTH: phenylephrine hydrochloride 0.125% and zinc sulfate 0.25%.
PHENYLZIN DROPS: zinc sulfate 0.25% and phenylephrine hydrochloride 0.12%.
PREFRIN-A◆: phenylephrine hydrochloride 0.12% and pyrilamine maleate 0.1%.
PREFRIN-Z: phenylephrine hydrochloride 0.12% and zinc sulfate 0.25%.
VASOCIDIN◆: phenylephrine hydrochloride 0.12%, sulfacetamide 10%, and prednisolone sodium phosphate 0.25%.
VASOCON-A◆: naphazoline hydrochloride 0.05% and antazoline phosphate 0.5%.
ZINCFRIN◆: phenylephrine hydrochloride 0.12% and zinc sulfate 0.25%.

RECOGNIZE CAUSES OF CONJUNCTIVITIS

	VIRAL	BACTERIAL PURULENT	BACTERIAL NON-PURULENT	FUNGAL AND PARASITIC	ALLERGIC
DISCHARGE	Minimum	Copious	Minimum	Minimum	Minimum
TEARING	Copious	Moderate	Moderate	Minimum	Moderate
ITCHING	Minimum	Minimum	None	None	Marked
LOCALIZED CONJUNCTIVAL LESIONS	None	None	Frequent	Frequent	None
PREAURICULAR NODES	Common	Uncommon	Common	Common	None
ASSOCIATED SORE THROAT AND FEVER	Occasionally	Seldom	None	None	None

Reproduced, with permission, from Vaughan D, Asbury T: General Ophthalmology, 8th ed. Copyright 1977 by Lange Medical Publications, Los Altos, California.

NAME	INDICATIONS & DOSAGE	SIDE EFFECTS
epinephrine hydrochloride Adrenalin chloride 0.1%, Epinephrine 1:1,000 0.1%	*Preop to control bleeding and conjunctivitis—* **Adults and children:** 1 or 2 drops of 0.1% solution or injected by doctor intracamerally 0.01% to 0.1%. Frequency individualized. See mydriatic dosage, p. 826	*Eye:* corneal or conjunctival pigmentation or corneal edema in long-term use; follicular hypertrophy; chemosis; conjunctivitis; iritis; hyperemic conjunctiva; maculopapular rash; severe stinging, burning, and tearing upon instillation; browache. *Systemic:* palpitations, tachycardia, extrasystoles.
naphazoline hydrochloride 0.012%, 0.1% Albalon Liquifilm Ophthalmic◆, Clear Eyes, Naphcon, Naphcon Forte Ophthalmic◆, Opto-Zoline◆◆, Vasocon Regular Ophthalmic◆	*Ocular congestion, irritation, itching—* **Adults:** instill 1 to 2 drops in eye every 3 to 4 hours.	*Eye:* transient stinging, pupillary dilation, increased intraocular pressure, irritation.
phenylephrine hydrochloride Isopto Frin, Prefrin, Tear-Efrin	*Decongestant minor eye irritations—* **Adults and children:** 2 drops of 0.12% or 0.25% in affected eye. May repeat in 3 to 4 hours, p.r.n. See mydriatic dosage, p. 828	*CNS:* headache. *Eye:* transient stinging, iris floaters, angle-closure glaucoma, blurred vision, reactive hyperemia, browache. *Systemic:* none with 0.12% concentration.
tetrahydrozoline hydrochloride Clear & Bright, Murine 2, Tetrasine, Visine	*Ocular congestion, irritation, and allergic conditions—* **Adults, and children over 2 years:** instill 1 to 2 drops in eye b.i.d. or t.i.d., or as directed by doctor.	*Eye:* transient stinging, pupillary dilation, increased intraocular pressure, irritation, iris floaters in elderly. *Systemic:* drowsiness, CNS depression, cardiac irregularities, headache, dizziness, tremors, insomnia.
zinc sulfate Bufopto Zinc Sulfate, Eye-Sed Ophthalmic, Op-Thal-Zin	*Ocular congestion, irritation—* **Adults and children:** solution 0.2%—instill 1 to 2 drops in eye b.i.d. or t.i.d. Ointment 0.5%.	*Eye:* irritation.

◆ Also available in Canada.
◆◆ Available in Canada only.
Unmarked trade names available in United States only.

INTERACTIONS	NURSING CONSIDERATIONS
Pilocarpine: additive effect on decreasing intraocular pressure. Monitor blood pressure and side effects.	• Contraindicated in shallow anterior eye chamber, narrow-angle glaucoma. Use with caution in cardiac disease, hyperthyroidism, hypertension, diabetes mellitus, and the elderly. • May cause staining of soft contact lenses. • Keep container tightly sealed, away from light, and in a cool place. • Discard solution if it is brown or contains precipitate. • If signs of hypersensitivity (edema of lids, itching, discharge, crusting eyelids) occur, stop drops and contact doctor. • If administering in conjunction with miotic, miotic should be instilled 2 to 10 minutes before epinephrine.
MAO inhibitors: hypertensive crisis if naphazoline HCl is systemically absorbed. Use together cautiously.	• Contraindicated in narrow-angle glaucoma, hypersensitivity to any ingredients. Use cautiously in hyperthyroidism, heart disease, hypertension, diabetes mellitus, elderly patients. • Can produce marked sedation and coma if ingested by child. • Advise patient that photophobia from pupil dilation may occur if he is sensitive to drug. Tell patient to report this to the doctor if it occurs. • Warn patient not to exceed recommended dosage. Rebound congestion and rhinitis may occur with frequent or prolonged use. • Notify doctor if blurred vision, pain, or lid edema develop. • Store in tightly closed container. • Most effective and widely used ocular decongestant. • Show patient how to instill. For instillation instructions, see p. 801.
MAO inhibitors: may cause hypertensive crisis. Give cautiously.	• Contraindicated in narrow-angle glaucoma, in patients taking tricyclic antidepressants or MAO inhibitors, and in hypersensitivity to any ingredient. • Should be avoided in patients with idiopathic orthostatic hypotension. May produce hypertension. • Do not use butacaine drops as local anesthetic, since phenylephrine and butacaine are incompatible. • Do not exceed prescribed dose. • Monitor blood pressure and pulse; watch for overdosage. • Do not use if solution is dark brown or contains precipitate. • Keep container tightly sealed and away from light.
MAO inhibitors: hypertensive crisis if tetrahydrozoline HCl is systemically absorbed. Use together cautiously.	• Contraindicated in patients receiving MAO inhibitors, hypersensitivity to any ingredients, narrow-angle glaucoma. Use cautiously in hyperthyroidism, heart disease, hypertension, diabetes mellitus, elderly patients. • Do not exceed recommended dosage. Rebound congestion and rhinitis may occur with frequent or prolonged use. • Warn patient to stop drug and notify doctor if relief is not obtained within 48 hours, or if redness or irritation persists or increases. • Available without prescription. • Available in 0.05% concentration; less effective than naphazoline hydrochloride 0.1%. • Warn patient not to touch dropper tip to eye or surrounding tissue. • Show patient how to instill. See instructions on p. 801.
None significant.	• Use cautiously in patients with a shallow anterior chamber, predisposition to narrow-angle glaucoma. • A decongestant astringent. • Store in tightly closed container. • Warn patient not to touch dropper tip to eye or surrounding tissue. • Show patient how to instill drops or ointment. See instructions on pp. 801 and 811.

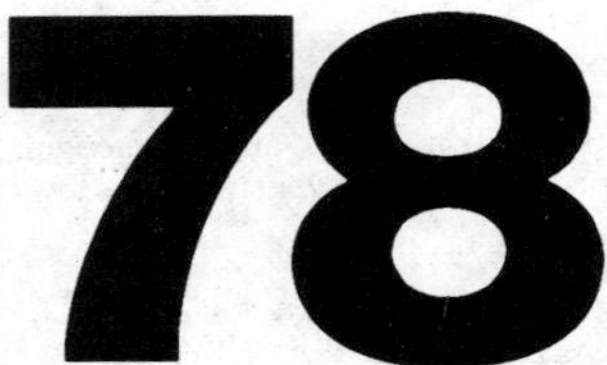

Topical ophthalmic anesthetics

benoxinate hydrochloride
cocaine hydrochloride
proparacaine hydrochloride
tetracaine hydrochloride

Topical ophthalmic anesthetics are used for a variety of diagnostic and minor surgical procedures. They are not for self-medication and should only be used under a doctor's supervision.

Major uses

• Anesthesia in tonometry, gonioscopy, suture removal from cornea, removal of corneal foreign bodies, and other diagnostic or minor surgical procedures.
• Cocaine hydrochloride is also used to diagnose Horner's syndrome.

Mechanism of action

• Topical ophthalmic anesthetics produce anesthesia by preventing initiation and transmission of nerve impulses at the cell membrane.
• Cocaine hydrochloride also exerts an adrenergic effect which produces mydriasis and constriction of conjunctival vessels.

Absorption, distribution, and excretion

• All are absorbed rapidly from the cornea and conjunctiva.
• Recommended doses of benoxinate hydrochloride, proparacaine hydrochloride, and tetracaine hydrochloride are not absorbed systemically.
• Cocaine hydrochloride is absorbed systemically, metabolized in the liver, and excreted in the urine.

Onset and duration

• Benoxinate hydrochloride and proparacaine hydrochloride begin to act within 20 seconds, cocaine hydrochloride within 30 seconds, and tetracaine hydrochloride within 1 minute.
• Benoxinate hydrochloride and proparacaine hydrochloride provide anesthesia up to 15 minutes, tetracaine hydrochloride up to 20 minutes.
• Cocaine hydrochloride provides complete anesthesia for 10 minutes, and incomplete anesthesia for another 5 to 10 minutes, and some degree of anesthesia up to 2 hours.

Combination products

None.

HOW TO PROTECT THE ANESTHETIZED EYE

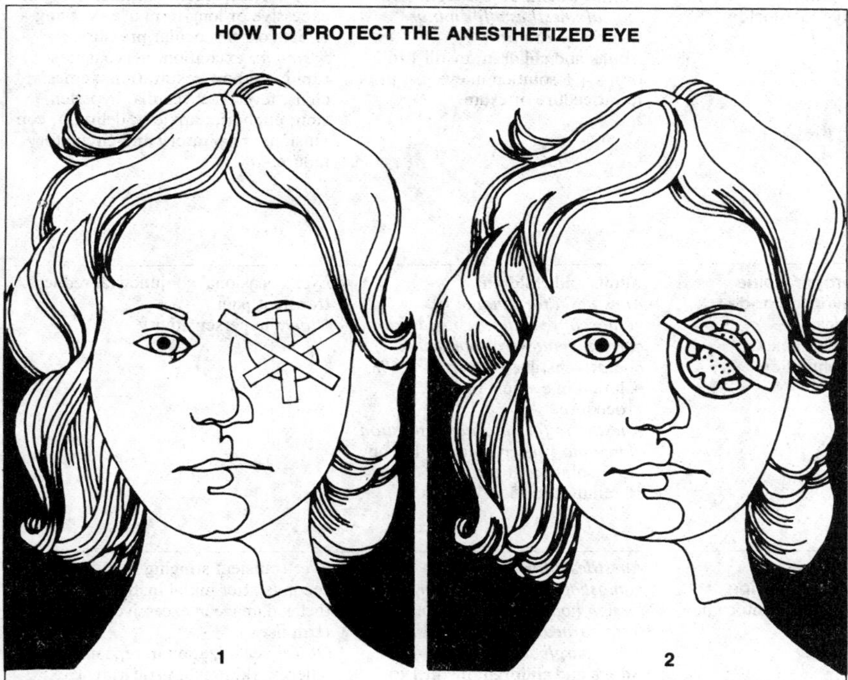

After applying topical ophthalmic anesthetics, be sure to protect the patient's eye from further injury from dust, smoke, or other irritants by applying an eyepad — an oval layer of absorbent cotton between two layers of gauze. Hold the pad in place with three narrow strips of ordinary transparent tape or nonallergenic plastic adhesive tape (Figure 1). For added protection, you may want to add an eye shield, bent so it rests upon bony prominences of the brow, cheek, and nose without touching the underlying dressing. Then, tape the shield in place as shown (Figure 2).

NAME	INDICATIONS & DOSAGE	SIDE EFFECTS
benoxinate hydrochloride Dorsacaine	*Procedures requiring rapid short-acting anesthesia—* **Adults and children:** instill 1 to 2 drops 0.4% solution just before procedure. For greater anesthesia, instill 2 drops at 90-second intervals, up to 3 doses.	*Eye:* slight conjunctival irritation.
cocaine hydrochloride	*Horner's syndrome (diagnosis), topical anesthesia for minor surgery or exams—* **Adults and children:** instill 1 to 2 drops 4% solution in eye just prior to procedure or exam.	*Eye:* corneal ulceration or scarring in excessive or long-term use. Varying effects on intraocular pressure. *Systemic:* excitation; nervousness; rapid, shallow respirations; emesis; chills; fever; tachycardia; hypertension; euphoria; anxiety; delirium; convulsions; respiratory and circulatory failure.
proparacaine hydrochloride Alcaine◆, Ophthaine◆, Ophthetic◆	**Adults and children:** *Anesthesia for tonometry, gonioscopy; suture removal from cornea, removal of corneal foreign bodies*—instill 1 to 2 drops 0.5% solution in eye just before procedure. *Anesthesia for cataract extraction; glaucoma surgery*—instill 1 drop 0.5% solution in eye every 5 to 10 minutes for 5 to 7 doses.	*Eye:* occasional conjunctival redness, transient pain. *Other:* hypersensitivity.
tetracaine hydrochloride Anacel, Pontocaine◆	*Anesthesia for tonometry, gonioscopy, removal of corneal foreign bodies, suture removal from cornea, other diagnostic and minor surgical procedures—* **Adults and children:** instill 1 to 2 drops 0.5% solution in eye just before procedure.	*Eye:* transient stinging in eye 30 seconds after initial instillation, epithelial damage in excessive or long-term use. *Other:* sensitization in repeated use (allergic skin rash, urticaria).

◆ Also available in Canada.
◆◆ Available in Canada only.
Unmarked trade names available in United States only.

INTERACTIONS	NURSING CONSIDERATIONS
None significant.	• Use cautiously in corneal abrasions, cardiac disease, hyperthyroidism. • Systemic absorption unlikely in recommended doses. • Not for long-term use. • Doesn't change pupil size, reaction to light, or accommodation. • Has slight bacteriostatic effect. • Warn patient not to rub eye while anesthetized. • Tell patient corneal reflex is restored in 1 hour. • Protective eye patch may be recommended following procedure. • For instillation instructions, see p. 801.
Epinephrine (topical): increased epinephrine effect. Use together cautiously.	• Use cautiously and sparingly in patients with known allergies, cardiac disease, hyperthyroidism, or open lesions. • Patient should be given short-acting barbiturate before administering to avoid CNS stimulation. • Solutions not commercially available; must be prepared specially by pharmacist. Rarely used. • Monitor heart rate after instillation; observe for systemic effects. • Warn patient vision will be blurred for several hours. • Warn patient not to rub eye for at least 20 minutes after instillation. • Protective eye patch recommended following procedure. • Solution should be pink-colored. Return discolored solution to pharmacy. • Doesn't require refrigeration. • For instillation instructions, see p. 801.
None significant.	• Use cautiously in cardiac diseases and hyperthyroidism. • *Not* for long-term use; may delay wound healing. • Warn patient not to rub or touch eye while cornea is anesthetized, since this may cause corneal abrasion and greater discomfort when anesthesia wears off. • Protective eye patch recommended following procedure. • Warn patient corneal pain is only relieved temporarily in abrasion. • Systemic reactions unlikely when used in recommended doses. • Topical ophthalmic anesthetic of choice in diagnostic and minor surgical procedures. • Don't use discolored solution. • Store in tightly closed container. • For instillation instructions, see p. 801.
Sulfonamides: interference with sulfonamide antibacterial activity. Wait ½ hour after anesthesia before instilling sulfonamide.	• Systemic absorption unlikely in recommended doses. • Avoid repeated use. • Does not dilate the pupil, paralyze accommodation, or increase intraocular pressure. • Protective eye patch recommended following procedure. • Don't use discolored solution. Keep container tightly closed. • For instillation instructions, see p. 801.

79

Artificial tears

artificial tears
eye irrigants

Artificial tears and external eye irrigation solutions are applied topically. Many are available without a prescription.

Major uses

• Artificial tears lubricate, remove debris, and protect against infection when normal tear production is insufficient.
• External eye irrigation solutions are sterile isotonic preparations used to irrigate the eyes following tonometry, gonioscopy, fluorescein dye examination, foreign body removal, and other procedures. They also soothe minor eye irritation and are used in large quantities for caustic chemical injury and trauma.

Mechanism of action

• Artificial tears augment insufficient tear production.
• External irrigation solutions cleanse the eye.

Absorption, distribution, and excretion

• Not applicable.

Onset and duration

• Artificial tear products with high viscosity have the longest duration of action. Those with low viscosity have a short duration of action.
• Duration of action of some artificial tear products are:
ADSORBOTEAR◆: 90 minutes or more
ISOPTO TEARS◆: 60 minutes
LIQUIFILM TEARS◆: 60 minutes
LYTEERS◆: 45 minutes
TEARISOL: 40 minutes or more
TEARS NATURALE◆: 90 minutes or more

HOW TO IRRIGATE AN EYE

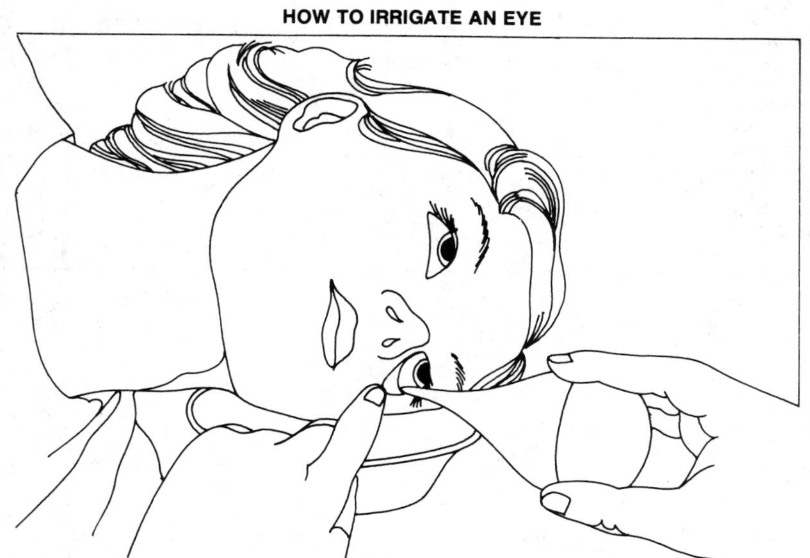

Be sure to wash your hands before instilling eye irrigation. Have the patient sit or lie with head tilted toward the affected side. Irrigating solution will then flow from the inner canthus of the affected eye toward outer canthus. Place a curved basin at the cheek on the side of the affected eye to catch irrigating solution. Use gentle force to remove secretions as you direct flow from inner to outer canthus. Do not touch any part of eye with irrigating tip. After irrigation, have patient close her eyes and wipe excess from lid and lashes.

NAME	INDICATIONS & DOSAGE	SIDE EFFECTS
artificial tears Adsorbotear◆, aqua-FLOW, Bro-Lac, Isopto Alkaline, Isopto Plain, Isopto Tears◆, Lacril◆, Liquifilm Forte, Liquifilm Tears, Lyteers, Methulose, Tearisol, Tears Naturale◆, Ultra Tears, Visculose	*Insufficient tear production*— **Adults and children:** instill 1 to 2 drops in eye t.i.d., q.i.d., or p.r.n.	*Eye:* discomfort; burning, pain on instillation; blurred vision; crust formation on eyelids and eyelashes in products with high viscosity such as Adsorbotear, Isopto Tears, and Tearisol.
eye irrigants Blinx, Collyrium Eye Lotion◆, Dacriose, EyeStream, I-Lite Eye Drops, Lauro, Lavoptik Medicinal Eye Wash, Murine Eye Drops, Neo-Flow, Sterile Normal Saline (0.9%), Zoptic Eye Lotion	*Eye irrigation*— **Adults and children:** flush eye with 1 to 2 drops t.i.d., q.i.d., or p.r.n.	None reported.

◆ Also available in Canada.
◆◆ Available in Canada only.
Unmarked trade names available in United States only.

INTERACTIONS	NURSING CONSIDERATIONS
Borate external irrigation solutions: may form gummy deposits on the lid when used with artificial tear products containing polyvinyl alcohol Liquifilm Forte, Liquifilm Tears). Keep lids clean.	• Contraindicated in hypersensitivity to active product or preservatives. • Show patient or family how to instill. For instillation instructions, see p. 801. • Warn patient not to touch tip of container to eye, surrounding tissue, or other surface, to avoid contamination of solution. • Instruct patient that product should be used by one person only.
Products containing polyvinyl alcohol: may form gel and gummy deposits on the eye. Keep lids clean.	• Contraindicated in hypersensitivity to active ingredient or preservatives. • Don't touch tip of container to eye, surrounding tissue, or other surface, to avoid contamination. • Check date of expiration to make sure solution is potent. • Store in tightly closed, light-resistant container. • Should be used by one person only. • When irrigating, have patient turn his head to side and irrigate from inner to outer canthus. Have tissues handy.

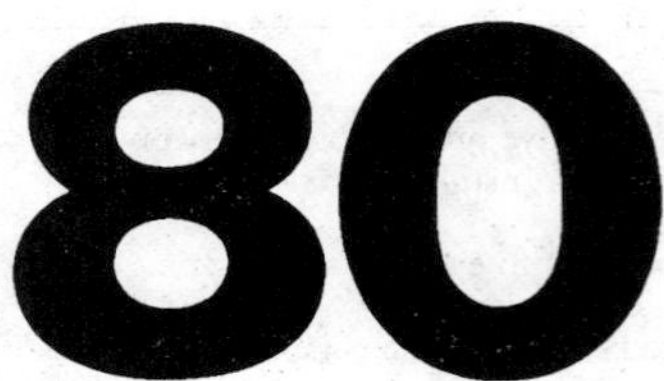

Miscellaneous ophthalmics

alpha-chymotrypsin
fluorescein sodium
glycerin-anhydrous
sodium chloride-hypertonic
timolol maleate

These drugs are used for a variety of purposes in surgical or diagnostic procedures.

Major uses

- Fluorescein is a dye used for various diagnostic procedures.
- Alpha-chymotrypsin is a fast-acting proteolytic enzyme used to dissolve the fiber system between the ciliary body and the equator of the lens in cataract surgery.
- Glycerin-anhydrous temporarily restores corneal transparency when the cornea is too edematous to permit diagnosis in ophthalmoscopy or gonioscopy.
- Sodium chloride-hypertonic reduces edema after surgery, in trauma, and in bullous keratopathy.
- Timolol reduces intraocular pressure in patients with open-angle glaucoma, ocular hypertension, aphakic glaucoma, and secondary glaucoma.

Mechanism of action

- Fluorescein produces intense green fluorescent color in alkaline solution (pH 5.0 or greater) or bright yellow if viewed under cobalt blue illumination.
- Alpha-chymotrypsin enzymatically dissolves fibers attached to the lens.
- Glycerin-anhydrous and sodium chloride-hypertonic remove excess fluid from the cornea.
- Timolol reduces aqueous formation, and possibly increases aqueous outflow. Little or no effect on pupil size.

Absorption, distribution, and excretion

- Alpha-chymotrypsin is not absorbed and must be instilled into posterior chamber. It is removed by irrigation with intraocular balanced salt solution.
- Fluorescein does not penetrate an intact corneal epithelium but is distributed to the stroma (assuming a green fluorescent color) when there is a break in the corneal epithelium. After I.V. injection, it is distributed to skin, causing a yellow discoloration, which fades in 6 to 12 hours. It is excreted in urine.
- Glycerin-anhydrous is not absorbed.
- Sodium chloride-hypertonic is not absorbed when recommended dosages are used.

Onset and duration

- Alpha-chymotrypsin and glycerin-anhydrous begin to act within 1 to 2 minutes. Glycerin-anhydrous and alpha-chymotrypsin have a very short duration of action (only minutes).
- Fluorescein begins to act immediately after topical instillation, and its duration of action is about 30 minutes. After I.V. administration, fluorescein dye appears in the retinal

vessels after 13 seconds; persists for 20 seconds.
• Sodium chloride-hypertonic has an immediate onset and duration of action up to 4 hours.
• Timolol has an onset of ½ hour. Maximum effect in 1 to 2 hours; duration of action, 24 hours.

Combination products
FLURESS: fluorescein 0.25% and benoxinate 0.4%.

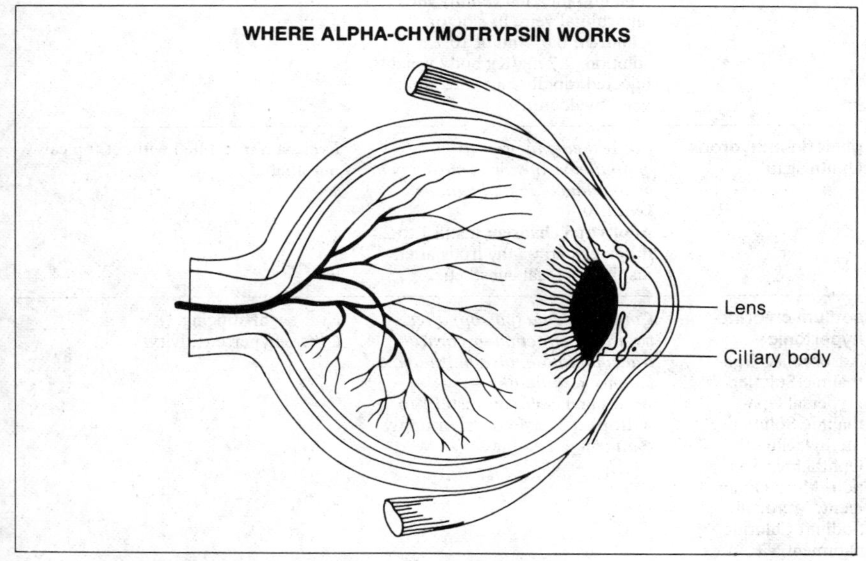

Alpha-chymotrypsin dissolves the fibers between the ciliary body and the lens in cataract surgery.

NAME	INDICATIONS & DOSAGE	SIDE EFFECTS
alpha-chymotrypsin Alpha Chymar, Alpha Chymolean••, Catarase•, Quimotrase••, Zolyse•, Zonulyn••	*Zonulysis in cataract surgery—* **Adults over 20 years:** 1 to 2 ml instilled into posterior chamber under the iris, by doctor.	*Eye:* transient increase in intraocular pressure (dose-related); moderate uveitis; corneal edema and striation.
fluorescein sodium Fluorescite, Fluor-I-Strip, Fluor-I-Strip-A.T.•, Ful-Glo Strips•, Funduscein injections	*Diagnostic in corneal abrasions and foreign bodies; fitting hard contact lenses; lacrimal patency; fundus photography; applanation tonometry—* **Topical:** Solution: instill 1 drop of 2% solution followed by irrigation or moisten strip with sterile water. Touch conjunctiva or fornix with moistened tip. Flush eye with irrigating solution. Patient should blink several times after application. *Indicated in retinal angiography—* **Adults:** 5 ml of 10% solution (500 mg) injected rapidly into antecubital vein, by doctor. **Children:** 0.077 ml of 10% solution (7.7 mg/Kg body weight) injected rapidly into antecubital vein, by doctor.	Topical use: *Eye:* stinging, burning. Intravenous use: *CNS:* headache persisting for 24 to 36 hours. *GI:* nausea, vomiting. *GU:* bright yellow urine (persists for 24 to 36 hours). *Local:* extravasation at injection site, thrombophlebitis. *Skin:* yellowish skin discoloration (fades in 6 to 12 hours). *Other:* hypersensitivity, including urticaria, cardiac arrest, and anaphylaxis.
glycerin-anhydrous Ophthalgan	*Corneal edema prior to ophthalmoscopy or gonioscopy in acute glaucoma and bullous keratitis—* **Adults and children:** instill 1 to 2 drops glycerin-anhydrous after instilling a local anesthetic.	*Eye:* pain if instilled without topical anesthetic.
sodium chloride-hypertonic Adsorbonac Ophthalmic Solution, Hypersal Ophthalmic Solution, Methylcellulose Ophthalmic Solution, Muro Ointment, Murocoll, Sodium Chloride Ointment 5%	*Corneal edema (postop) after cataract extraction or corneal transplantation; also in trauma or bullous keratopathy—* **Adults and children:** instill 1 to 2 drops q 3 to 4 hours, or apply ointment at bedtime.	*Eye:* slight stinging. *Other:* hypersensitivity.

• Also available in Canada.
•• Available in Canada only.
Unmarked trade names available in United States only.

INTERACTIONS	NURSING CONSIDERATIONS
Alcohol, surgical detergent: inactivated alpha-chymotrypsin. Rinse off all alcohol or detergents from surgical instruments and syringe with saline.	• Contraindicated in high vitreous pressure with gaping incisional wound; congenital cataract. • Solutions very unstable. Use only freshly reconstituted solution. Don't use if it is cloudy or has precipitated. Discard unused portions, including diluent, except for Zonulyn. Retains potency 1 week at room temperature, or for 1 month when refrigerated. • Remove drug by irrigating with intraocular balanced salt solution. • Don't autoclave powder or reconstituted solution; excess heat will inactivate the enzyme. • Delayed healing of incision has been reported but not confirmed.
None significant.	• Use with caution in history of allergy or bronchial asthma. • Use topical anesthetic before instilling to partially relieve burning and irritation. • Always use aseptic technique. Easily contaminated by *Pseudomonas.* • Yellow skin discoloration may persist 6 to 12 hours. • Warn patient urine will be colored bright yellow after I.V. injection. • Routine urinalysis will be abnormal within 1 hour of I.V. injection. • A water-soluble dye. • Don't freeze; store below 80° F. (26.7° C.). • Defects will appear green under normal light, or bright yellow under cobalt blue illumination. Foreign bodies are surrounded by a green ring. Similar lesions of the conjunctiva are delineated in orange-yellow. • Keep an emergency tray with antihistamine, epinephrine, and oxygen always available when giving parenterally. • For symptoms and treatment of anaphylaxis, see p. 1114.
None significant.	• Use topical tetracaine HCl or proparacaine HCl before instilling to prevent discomfort. • Don't touch tip of dropper to eye, surrounding tissues, or tear-film; glycerin will absorb moisture. • Used to temporarily restore corneal transparency when cornea is too edematous to permit diagnosis. • Store in tightly closed container.
None significant.	• An osmotic agent used to reduce corneal edema when repeated instillation is indicated. • May use a few drops of sterile irrigation solution inside bottle cap to prevent caking on tip of dropper bottle. • Store in tightly closed container. • Don't touch tip of dropper or tube to eye or surrounding tissue. • Show patient how to instill. For instillation instructions, see p. 801.

NAME	INDICATIONS & DOSAGE	SIDE EFFECTS
timolol maleate Timoptic Solution	*Chronic open-angle glaucoma, secondary glaucoma, aphakic glaucoma, ocular hypertension*—**Adults:** initially, instill 1 drop 0.25% solution in each eye b.i.d., reduce to 1 drop daily for maintenance. If patient doesn't respond, instill 1 drop 0.5% solution in each eye b.i.d. If intraocular pressure is controlled, dosage may be reduced to 1 drop in each eye daily.	*CV:* slight reduction in resting heart rate. *Eye:* minor irritation. *Other:* apnea in infants.

INTERACTIONS	NURSING CONSIDERATIONS
Propranolol HCl, metoprolol tartrate, other oral beta-adrenergic blocking agents: increased ocular and systemic effect. Use together cautiously. *MAO inhibitors, other adrenergic-augmenting psychotropic drugs:* hazardous increased effect. Use together cautiously.	• Use cautiously in bronchial asthma, sinus bradycardia, second- and third-degree heart block, cardiogenic shock, right ventricular failure resulting from pulmonary hypertension, congestive heart failure, severe cardiac disease, infants with congenital glaucoma. • Warn patient not to touch dropper to eye or surrounding tissue. • Beta-adrenergic blocking agent in ophthalmic solution. • Can be safely used in glaucoma patients wearing conventional (PMMA) hard contact lenses. • Show patient how to instill. For instillation instructions, see p. 801.

81

Otics

acetic acid
benzocaine
boric acid
carbamide peroxide
chloramphenicol
colistin B sulfate
dexamethasone sodium phosphate
hydrocortisone
methylprednisolone disodium phosphate
neomycin sulfate
oxytetracycline hydrochloride
polymyxin B sulfate
triethanolamine

Otic drugs treat infection, inflammation, and pain of ear disorders. Most of these drugs act locally and have little systemic absorption; many are combinations of two or more drugs.

Administration

Delicate ear membranes can be easily damaged by incorrect administration of otic drops. Read label carefully to determine correct temperature for instillation. Remember, extremely hot or cold drops may stimulate CNS; too hot drops may render the medication ineffective or may burn ear membranes. To warm otic drops safely, allow to stand at room temperature or roll bottle between hands for several minutes.

To administer otic drops correctly: Have patient lie on his back with affected ear uppermost. If drops are to be applied to both ears, patient should lie on one side for 5 minutes before turning onto the other side for second application. Straighten auditory canal by pulling auricle downward and backward in children; upward and backward in adults. Without touching dropper to ear, place ordered amount of drops into the affected ear. Cotton moistened with medication can be inserted. Keep patient in same position for at least 5 minutes after instillation of drops.

Major uses

- Treatment of infection, inflammation, and pain of internal or external ear disorders (swimmer's ear, perforation, otitis media) and surgical procedures (myringotomy, mastoidectomy, and fenestration).
- Softening of impacted earwax.

Mechanism of action

- Anti-infectives inhibit or destroy the bacteria present in ear canal.
- Corticosteroids control inflammation, edema, and pruritus.
- Local anesthetics produce analgesic effects.
- Cerumenolytics emulsify and disperse accumulated earwax.

Absorption, distribution, and excretion

- Long-term use of corticosteroids and certain antibiotics (gentamicin, neomycin) may result in some systemic absorption.

Onset and duration

- Most otic drugs begin to act within 1 hour, but full therapeutic effect may not be seen for 2 to 3 days.
- The short action of local anesthetics requires repeated dosage every 2 hours.

Combination products

ADRENOMYXIN•• Each ml contains neomycin SO_4 5 mg, polymyxin B SO_4 10,000 units, and hydrocortisone 10 mg.
COLY-MYCIN-S-OTIC Each ml contains neomycin SO_4 5 mg, colistin SO_4 3 mg, and hydrocortisone acetate 10 mg.
CORTISPORIN OTIC• Each ml contains neomycin SO_4 5 mg, polymyxin B SO_4 10,000 units, and hydrocortisone 10 mg.
LIDOSPORIN OTIC• Each ml contains polymyxin B SO_4 10,000 units and lidocaine HCl 50 mg.
NEO-CORT-DOME OTIC Each ml contains neomycin SO_4 5 mg, acetic acid 2%, and hydrocortisone 10 mg.
NEOCORTEF•• Each ml contains neomycin SO_4 5 mg and hydrocortisone acetate 5 mg.
NEODECADRON•• Each ml contains neomycin SO_4 5 mg and dexamethasone 1 mg.
NEOMEDROL•• Each ml contains neomycin SO_4 5 mg and methylprednisolone 1 mg.
NEOSPORIN•• Each ml contains polymyxin B SO_4 5,000 units, neomycin SO_4 2.5 mg, and gramicidin 0.025 mg.
OTIZOL HC•• Each ml contains neomycin SO_4 5 mg and hydrocortisone 10 mg.
OTOBIONE OTIC Each ml contains neomycin SO_4 3.5 mg, polymyxin B SO_4 10,000 units, and hydrocortisone 10 mg.
PENTAMYCETIN HC•• Each ml contains chloramphenicol 2 mg and hydrocortisone 10 mg.
POLYSPORIN•• Each ml contains polymyxin B SO_4 10,000 units and gramicidin 0.25 mg.
PYOCIDIN OTIC Each ml contains polymyxin B sulfate 10,000 units and hydrocortisone 5 mg.
PYOCIDIN HC OTIC• Each ml contains neomycin SO_4 5 mg, polymyxin B SO_4 10,000 units, and hydrocortisone 10 mg.
SOFRACORT•• Each ml contains framycetin 5 mg, gramicidin 50 mcg, and dexamethasone 0.5 mg.
TERRA-CORTRIL• Each ml contains oxytetracycline HC1 5 mg, polymyxin B SO_4 10,000 units, and hydrocortisone 10 mg.
TERRAMYCIN WITH POLYMYXIN B SULFATE• Each gram contains oxytetracycline HC1 5 mg and polymyxin B SO_4 10,000 units.
VOSOL HC• Each ml contains acetic acid 2% and hydrocortisone 10 mg.

NAME	INDICATIONS & DOSAGE	SIDE EFFECTS
acetic acid Domeboro Otic◆, VoSol Otic◆	*External ear canal infection—* **Adults and children:** 4 to 6 drops into ear canal t.i.d. or q.i.d. or insert saturated wick for first 24 hours, then continue with instillations. *Prophylaxis of swimmer's ear—* **Adults and children:** 2 drops in each ear b.i.d.	*Ear:* irritation or itching. *Skin:* urticaria. *Other:* overgrowth of nonsusceptible organisms.
benzocaine Americaine-Otic, Auralgan◆, Aurasol, Eardro, Myringacaine, Tympagesic	*Cerumen removal—* **Adults and children:** fill ear canal t.i.d. for 2 days. *Pain from otitis media—* **Adults and children:** fill ear canal with solution and plug with cotton. May repeat q 1 to 2 hours, p.r.n.	*Ear:* irritation or itching. *Skin:* urticaria. *Other:* edema.
boric acid Ear-Dry, Swim-Ear, Swim 'n Clear	*External ear canal infection—* **Adults and children:** fill ear canal with solution and plug with cotton. Repeat t.i.d. or q.i.d.	*Ear:* irritation or itching. *Skin:* urticaria. *Other:* overgrowth of nonsusceptible organisms.
carbamide peroxide Benadyne Ear, Debrox◆	*Impacted earwax—* **Adults and children:** 5 to 10 drops into ear canal b.i.d. for 3 to 4 days.	None reported.
chloramphenicol Chloromycetin Otic◆, Sopamycetin◆◆	*External ear canal infection—* **Adults and children:** 2 to 3 drops into ear canal t.i.d. or q.i.d.	*Ear:* itching or burning. *Local:* pruritus, burning, urticaria, vesicular or maculopapular dermatitis. *Systemic:* sore throat, angioedema. *Other:* overgrowth of nonsusceptible organisms.
colistin B sulfate available only in combination with neomycin and hydrocortisone (Coly-Mycin-S-Otic◆)	*External ear canal infection and otitis media—* **Adults and children:** 3 to 5 drops into ear canal t.i.d. or q.i.d.	*Ear:* ototoxicity in patient with a perforated eardrum and in patient undergoing tympanoplasty; irritation, itching. *Other:* overgrowth of nonsusceptible organisms.
dexamethasone sodium phosphate Decadron◆	*Inflammation of external ear canal—* **Adults and children:** 1 to 2 drops into ear canal t.i.d. or q.i.d.	*Systemic:* adrenal suppression with long-term use. *Other:* masking or exacerbation of underlying infection.
hydrocortisone **hydrocortisone acetate** Cortamed◆◆, Otall	*Inflammation of external ear canal—* **Adults and children:** 3 to 5 drops into ear canal t.i.d. or q.i.d. Available in 0.25%, 0.5%, and 1% concentrations.	*Systemic:* adrenal suppression with long-term use. *Other:* may mask or exacerbate underlying infection.

◆ Also available in Canada.
◆◆ Available in Canada only.
Unmarked trade names available in United States only.

INTERACTIONS	NURSING CONSIDERATIONS
None significant.	• Contraindicated in perforated eardrum. • Has anti-infective, anti-inflammatory, and antipruritic effects. • *Pseudomonas aeruginosa* particularly sensitive to drug. • Watch for signs of superinfection (continued pain, inflammation, fever). • Reculture persistent drainage.
None significant.	• Contraindicated in perforated eardrum. • Local anesthetic effect only. • Use with antibiotic to treat underlying cause of pain, because use alone may mask more serious condition. • Tell patient to call doctor if pain lasts longer than 48 hours. • Avoid touching ear with dropper. Do not rinse dropper. • Irrigate ear gently to remove impacted cerumen. • Keep container tightly closed and away from moisture.
None significant.	• Contraindicated in perforated eardrum or excoriated membranes in ear. • Watch for signs of superinfection (continual pain, inflammation, fever). • Weak bacteriostatic germicide; also fungistatic agent. • If cotton plug used, always moisten with medication.
None significant.	• Contraindicated in perforated eardrum. • Tell patient to call doctor if redness, pain, or swelling persists. • Cerumenolytic agent. • Irrigation of ear may be necessary to aid in removal of cerumen. • Tip of bottle should not touch ear or ear canal.
None significant.	• Avoid prolonged use. • Obtain history of past use and reaction to drug. • Watch for signs of superinfection (continued pain, inflammation, fever). • Reculture persistant drainage. • Watch for signs of sore throat (early sign of toxicity). • Bacteriostatic agent.
None significant.	• Watch for signs of superinfection (continued pain, inflammation, fever). • Reculture persistent drainage. • Observe for signs of hearing loss. • Bactericidal agent. • Avoid prolonged use. • Shake well before use.
None significant.	• Contraindicated in perforated eardrum, fungal infections, herpes or other viral infections. • Use with antibiotic to treat inflammation caused by infection. • Use alone in allergic otitis externa. • Anti-inflammatory agent.
None significant.	• Contraindicated in perforated eardrum, fungal infections, herpes or other viral infection. • Use with antibiotic to treat inflammation caused by infection. • Use alone in allergic otitis externa. • Anti-inflammatory agent.

NAME	INDICATIONS & DOSAGE	SIDE EFFECTS
methylprednisolone disodium phosphate Medrol◆◆	*Inflammation of external ear canal—* **Adults and children:** 2 to 3 drops into ear canal t.i.d. or q.i.d.	*Systemic:* adrenal suppression with long-term use. *Other:* may mask or exacerbate underlying infection.
neomycin sulfate Otobiotic	*External ear canal infection—* **Adults and children:** 2 to 5 drops into ear canal t.i.d. or q.i.d. for not longer than 10 days.	*Ear:* ototoxicity (in patients undergoing tympanoplasty). *Local:* burning, erythema, vesicular dermatitis, urticaria. *Other:* overgrowth of nonsusceptible organisms.
oxytetracycline hydrochloride available only in combination with polymyxin B sulfate (Terramycin) or polymyxin B sulfate and hydrocortisone (Terra-Cortril◆◆)	*External ear canal infection—* **Adults and children:** instill ½ inch of ointment into external ear canal t.i.d. or q.i.d.	*Ear:* irritation, itching, urticaria. *Other:* overgrowth of nonsusceptible organisms.
polymyxin B sulfate Aerosporin◆	*Acute and chronic otitis externa, otitis media if tympanic membrane perforated; otomycosis—* **Adults and children:** 3 to 4 drops t.i.d. or q.i.d.	*Ear:* irritation, itching, urticaria. *Other:* overgrowth of nonsusceptible organisms.
triethanolamine Cerumenex◆	*Impacted earwax—* **Adults and children:** fill ear canal with solution and insert cotton plug. After 15 to 30 minutes flush ear with warm water.	*Ear:* erythema, pruritus. *Skin:* severe eczema.

INTERACTIONS	NURSING CONSIDERATIONS
None significant.	• Contraindicated in perforated eardrum, fungal, herpes or other viral infections. • Use with antibiotic to treat inflammation caused by infection. • Use alone to treat seborrheic, contact, or noninfected eczematoid dermatitis. • Anti-inflammatory agent.
None significant.	• Contraindicated in perforated eardrum. • Obtain history of past use and reaction to neomycin. • Observe for signs of hearing loss. • Watch for signs of superinfection (continued pain, inflammation, fever). • Reculture persistant drainage. • Bactericidal agent. • Best used in combination with other antibiotics.
None significant.	• Obtain history of past reaction to tetracyclines. • Watch for signs of superinfection (continued pain, inflammation, fever). • Reculture persistant drainage. • Bacteriostatic agent.
None significant.	• Watch for signs of superinfection (continued pain, inflammation, fever). • Reculture persistant drainage. • Bactericidal agent. • Best used in combination. • Keep container tightly closed and away from moisture.
None significant.	• Contraindicated in perforated eardrum, otitis media, and allergies. Do patch test by placing 1 drop of drug on inner forearm; cover with small bandage. Read in 24 hours. If any reaction (redness, swelling) occurs, don't use drug. • Don't use drops more often than prescribed. Flush ear gently with warm water, using soft rubber bulb ear syringe within 30 minutes. • Cerumenolytic agent. • Moisten cotton plug with medication before insertion. • Keep container tightly closed and away from moisture.

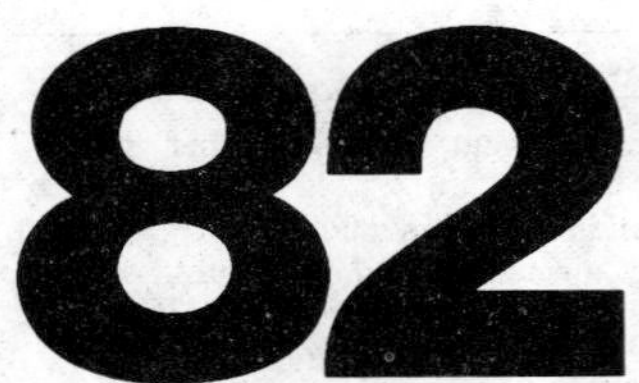

Oral and nasal agents

benzocaine
carbamide peroxide
cocaine hydrochloride
dexamethasone sodium phosphate
ephedrine sulfate
epinephrine hydrochloride
lidocaine hydrochloride
naphazoline hydrochloride
oxymetazoline hydrochloride
phenylephrine hydrochloride
piperocaine hydrochloride
tetrahydrozoline hydrochloride
triamcinolone acetonide
xylometazoline hydrochloride

Oral and nasal agents are used alone or with other drugs and therapy to treat conditions affecting the nose and mouth. Many over-the-counter products contain combinations of these drugs. Combinations for nasal use may contain antihistamines.

Major uses

- Sympathomimetic vasoconstrictors, such as ephedrine, epinephrine, naphazoline hydrochloride, oxymetazoline hydrochloride, phenylephrine hydrochloride, tetrahydrozoline hydrochloride, and xylometazoline, relieve nasal congestion resulting from the common cold, sinusitis, allergy, or chronic or vasomotor rhinitis. Epinephrine also controls local superficial bleeding.
- Local anesthetics, such as cocaine hydrochloride, piperocaine hydrochloride, benzocaine, and lidocaine hydrochloride, produce anesthesia for rhinolaryngology examinations as well as for laryngoscopy, bronchoscopy, and endotracheal intubation; they also relieve the pain of dental extractions.
- Corticosteroids, such as dexamethasone sodium phosphate and triamcinolone acetonide, reduce inflammation in allergic or inflammatory conditions, or in nasal polyps, and are also used to treat stomatitis and traumatic oral lesions.
- Carbamide peroxide cleanses and debrides, provides antimicrobial activity, and is used as an adjunct to other treatment in oral inflammation.

Mechanism of action

- Sympathomimetic agents produce local vasoconstriction of dilated arterioles to reduce blood flow and nasal congestion.
- Local anesthetics block nerve conduction through sensory nerve fibers.

• Topical corticosteroids reduce inflammation and help heal oral ulcers and lesions by a complex mechanism of action.
• Carbamide peroxide serves as a source of hydrogen peroxide to produce nascent oxygen, which aids in cleansing and debriding.

Absorption, distribution, and excretion
• All oral and nasal preparations are applied topically, but with many preparations some systemic absorption can occur.
• When systemically absorbed, sympathomimetic vasoconstrictors are metabolized in sympathetic nerve endings and in the liver and are excreted in the urine; they also cross the placenta and enter breast milk.

Onset and duration
• Varies with drug, patient response, and conditions being treated.
• In general, oral and nasal drugs begin to act quickly.
• The duration of action of local anesthetics depends on the amount of time the drug is in contact with nerve tissue.

Combination products
ALZEM NASAL SPRAY: phenylephrine hydrochloride 0.25%, combined with thenylpyramine hydrochloride 0.15% with 0.1% benzalkonium chloride.
CHLOROHIST NASAL SPRAY: phenylephrine hydrochloride 0.25% and chlorpheniramine maleate 0.25%.
4-WAY NASAL SPRAY: phenylephrine hydrochloride 5.0%, naphazoline hydrochloride 0.5%, and pyrilamine maleate 2.0%.
NAZOTOC NASAL SPRAY: phenylephrine hydrochloride 0.5% and pyrilamine maleate 0.15%, 0.04% cetyldimethylbenzylammonium chloride.
NEO-VADRIN NASAL DECONGESTANT DROPS: phenylephrine hydrochloride 0.15% and phenylpropanolamine hydrochloride 0.4%, with chlorobutanol 0.15% and benzalkonium chloride 0.005%.
NTZ NASAL DROPS: phenylephrine hydrochloride 0.5% and thenyldiamine hydrochloride 0.1%.

NAME	INDICATIONS & DOSAGE	SIDE EFFECTS
benzocaine Colrex, Dentition Syrup♦♦, Orabase with Benzocaine, Oracin, Ora-Jel, Spec-T Anesthetic, Trocaine, Tyzomint	*Pain from toothache, cold sore, canker sore, minor sore throat*— **Adults and children:** apply syrup or jelly to affected area or suck on lozenges.	*Skin:* hypersensitivity. *Other:* possible tolerance.
carbamide peroxide Cank-aid, Clear Drops, Gly-Oxide♦, Proxigel	*Canker sores, herpetic and other lesions, gingivitis, denture irritation, traumatic or surgical wounds*— **Adults, and children over 3 years:** apply, undiluted, to oral mucosa q.i.d. or p.r.n., leave for several minutes, then expectorate. Don't rinse out mouth.	None reported.
cocaine hydrochloride Controlled substance Schedule II	**Adults and children:** *Acute rhinosinusitis*—use 1% solution with nasal pack. *Diagnostic nasal examination*—apply 4% solution to nasal mucosa. *Local anesthesia of nose or throat*—apply 5% to 10% solution to oral and nasal mucosa.	*CNS:* nervousness, excitation, vasomotor collapse. *Other:* addiction with chronic use.
dexamethasone sodium phosphate Decadron Phosphate♦, Decadron Phosphate Respihaler, Turbinaire	*Allergic or inflammatory conditions, nasal polyps*— **Adults:** 2 sprays in each nostril b.i.d. or t.i.d. Maximum 12 sprays daily. **Children 6 to 12 years:** 1 or 2 sprays in each nostril b.i.d. Maximum 8 sprays daily. Each spray delivers 0.1 mg dexamethasone sodium phosphate equal to 0.084 mg dexamethasone.	*EENT:* nasal irritation, dryness, rebound nasal congestion. *Other:* hypersensitivity, systemic side effects with prolonged use (pituitary adrenal suppression, sodium retention, congestive heart failure, hypertension, hypokalemia, headaches, convulsions, peptic ulcer, ecchymoses, petechiae; masking of secondary infection).
ephedrine sulfate Ephedsol-1%, I-Sedrin Plain, Isofedrol, Nasdro	*Nasal congestion*— **Adults and children:** apply 3 to 4 drops 0.5% to 3% solution to nasal mucosa. Use no more frequently than q 4 hours.	*CNS:* nervousness, excitation. *CV:* tachycardia. *EENT:* rebound nasal congestion with long-term or excessive use. *Local:* mucosal irritation.

♦ Also available in Canada.
♦♦ Available in Canada only.
Unmarked trade names available in United States only.

INTERACTIONS	NURSING CONSIDERATIONS
None significant.	• Contraindicated in infants under 1 year. Use cautiously in children under 6 years and in severe oral trauma or sepsis. • Not intended for use in the presence of infection. • Obtain history of past reactions to local anesthetics. • Watch for allergic reactions, such as reddening or swelling. If condition persists, drug should be stopped, and doctor notified. • Show patient how to apply.
None significant.	• Use only as adjunct to regular professional care. • Don't dilute. Gently massage affected area with medication. Show patient how to apply. Tell him not to drink or rinse his mouth for 5 minutes after use. • Warn patient that drug foams in mouth when mixed with saliva. • Use after meals and at bedtime for best results. • If severe or persistent inflammation continues, patient should notify doctor or dentist. • Provides chemomechanical cleansing, debriding action, and has nonselective microbial activity. • An oxygenating agent. • Store in cool place. • Only one person should use same dropper bottle or tube.
None significant.	• Store under lock and key with other controlled drugs. • Patient should be given a short-acting barbiturate before giving cocaine HCl to prevent excess CNS stimulation or vasomotor collapse. • Nasal surgery performed with cocaine HCl anesthesia may cause a delayed capillary hemorrhage resulting from capillary dilation. Watch for postoperative nasal bleeding when effect of cocaine wears off. • Obtain history of past reactions to local anesthetics.
None significant.	• Contraindicated in cutaneous tuberculosis, fungal and herpetic lesions. Use cautiously in diabetes mellitus, peptic ulcer, or tuberculosis, as systemic absorption can activate disease. • Mothers should not breast-feed, as systemic absorption can occur. • Control underlying bacterial infection with anti-infectives. • Irritation or sensitivity may require stopping drug. • Don't break, incinerate, or store in extreme heat; contents under pressure. • Gradually reduce dose as nasal condition improves. • Fluid retention can occur as a result of systemic absorption. • Show patient how to apply. Only one person should use same nasal spray. • Hypertension and hypokalemia can occur with systemic absorption. Monitor blood pressure, serum potassium frequently. • Should not be used for prolonged periods.
MAO inhibitors: hypertensive crisis if ephedrine is absorbed. Don't use together.	• Use cautiously in hyperthyroidism, coronary artery disease, hypertension, or diabetes mellitus, as systemic absorption can occur. • Tell patient not to exceed recommended dose. Use only when needed. • Show patient how to apply. Only one person should use same dropper bottle or nasal spray. • Use only when needed.

NAME	INDICATIONS & DOSAGE	SIDE EFFECTS
epinephrine hydrochloride Adrenalin chloride	*Nasal congestion, local superficial bleeding—* **Adults and children:** apply 0.1% solution to oral or nasal mucosa.	*CNS:* nervousness, excitation. *CV:* tachycardia. *EENT:* rebound nasal congestion, slight sting upon application.
lidocaine hydrochloride Xylocaine◆, Xylocaine Viscous◆	*Local anesthesia, pain from dental extractions—* **Adults and children:** apply 2% to 5% solution, ointment or 15 ml of Xylocaine Viscous q 3 to 4 hours to oral or nasal mucosa.	*EENT:* interference with pharyngeal stage of swallowing. *Other:* hypersensitivity (CNS symptoms are excitatory or depressant; CV symptoms are depressant); systemic absorption when used repeatedly.
naphazoline hydrochloride Privine◆	*Nasal congestion—* **Adults:** apply 2 drops, or spray of 0.05% to 0.1% solution to nasal mucosa q 3 to 4 hours. **Children 6 to 12 years:** 1 to 2 drops or sprays of 0.05% solution. Repeat 3 to 6 hours, p.r.n. Use no longer than 3 to 5 days.	*EENT:* rebound nasal congestion with excessive or long-term use, sneezing, stinging, dryness of mucosa. *Other:* systemic side effects in children after excessive or long-term use; marked sedation.
oxymetazoline hydrochloride Afrin, Duration, Nafrine◆◆, St. Joseph's Decongestant for Children	*Nasal congestion—* **Adults, and children over 6 years:** apply 2 to 4 drops or spray 0.05% solution to nasal mucosa b.i.d. **Children 2 to 5 years:** apply 2 to 3 drops 0.025% solution to nasal mucosa b.i.d. Use no longer than 3 to 5 days. Dosage for younger children has not been established.	*CNS:* headache, drowsiness, dizziness, insomnia. *CV:* palpitations. *EENT:* rebound nasal congestion or irritation with excessive or long-term use, dryness of nose and throat, increased nasal discharge, stinging, sneezing. *Other:* systemic side effects in children with excessive or long-term use; possible sedation.
phenylephrine hydrochloride Alconefrin, Coricidin Nasal Mist, Coryzine, Ephrine, Isophrin, Neo-Synephrine◆, Pyracort-D, Rhinall, Sinarest Nasal Spray, Sinophen Intranasal, SuperAnahist Nasal Spray, Synasal, Vacon, Zemphrine	*Nasal congestion—* **Adults:** 2 to 3 drops or sprays 0.25% to 1% solution; apply jelly or spray to nasal mucosa. **Children 6 to 12 years:** apply 2 to 3 drops or sprays. **Children under 6 years:** apply 2 to 3 drops or sprays 0.125% solution. Drops, spray, or jelly can be given q 4 hours, p.r.n.	*CNS:* headache, tremors, dizziness, nervousness. *CV:* palpitations, tachycardia, premature ventricular contractions, hypertension, pallor. *EENT:* transient burning, stinging; dryness of nasal mucosa; rebound nasal congestion may occur with continued use. *GI:* nausea.

INTERACTIONS	NURSING CONSIDERATIONS
None significant.	• Use cautiously in hyperthyroidism, coronary artery disease, hypertension, or diabetes mellitus, as systemic absorption can occur. • Tell patient not to exceed recommended dose. Use only when needed. • Show patient how to apply. Only one person should use same dropper bottle or nasal spray.
None significant.	• Use cautiously in cardiac disease, hyperthyroidism, or severe oral or nasal trauma or sepsis, as systemic absorption can occur. • Chronic, prolonged use for oropharynx anesthesia can lead to systemic absorption and toxicity. • Instruct patient how to use. Xylocaine Viscous should be swished around in the mouth and can be swallowed. Warn patient to eat or drink cautiously within 60 minutes after oral application to avoid food aspiration. • Obtain history of past reactions to local anesthetics. • Taste can be improved by adding a drop of oil of peppermint.
None significant.	• Contraindicated in glaucoma. Use cautiously in hyperthyroidism, heart disease, hypertension, or diabetes mellitus, as systemic absorption can occur. • Use only when needed. • Warn patient not to exceed recommended dosage. • Tell patient to notify doctor if nasal congestion persists after 5 days. • Show patient how to apply. Hold container upright. Only one person should use same dropper bottle or nasal spray. • Do not shake container.
None significant.	• Use cautiously in hyperthyroidism, heart disease, hypertension, or diabetes mellitus, as systemic absorption can occur. • Tell patient not to exceed recommended dose. Use only when needed. • Show patient how to apply. Have patient bend head forward and sniff spray briskly. Only one person should use same dropper bottle or nasal spray.
None significant.	• Contraindicated in narrow-angle glaucoma. Use cautiously in hyperthyroidism, hypertension, diabetes mellitus, or ischemic heart disease, as systemic absorption may occur. • Tell patient not to exceed recommended dose. Use only when needed. • Show patient how to apply: keep head erect to minimize swallowing of medication. Only one person should use same dropper bottle or nasal spray.

NAME	INDICATIONS & DOSAGE	SIDE EFFECTS
piperocaine hydrochloride Metycaine HCl	*Anesthetic in dental procedures—* **Adults and children:** apply 5% to 10% solution as a spray or 1% to 2% solution by infiltration to oral or nasal mucosa. *Local anesthetic in rhinolaryngology exams—* **Adults and children:** apply 2% solution as a spray to oral or nasal mucosa.	*EENT:* interference with pharyngeal stage of swallowing. *Other:* hypersensitivity.
tetrahydrozoline hydrochloride Tyzine HCl, Tyzine Pediatric	*Nasal congestion—* **Adults, and children over 6 years:** apply 2 to 4 drops 0.1% solution or spray to nasal mucosa q 4 to 6 hours p.r.n. **Children 2 to 6 years:** apply 2 to 3 drops 0.05% solution to nasal mucosa q 4 to 6 hours p.r.n.	*EENT:* transient burning, stinging; sneezing, rebound nasal congestion in excessive or long-term use.
triamcinolone acetonide Kenalog in Orabase	*Stomatitis; erosive lichen planus; traumatic oral lesions, including sore denture spots—* **Adults and children:** press ¼ inch of 0.1% emollient dental paste onto affected area until thin film develops. Repeat b.i.d. or t.i.d. Don't rub in or protection of film will be lost.	*Systemic:* with prolonged use, adrenal insufficiency, altered glucose metabolism, peptic ulcer activation.
xylometazoline hydrochloride 4-Way Long Acting, Neo-Synephrine II, Otrivin◆, Sine-Off Nasal Spray, Sinex-L.A.	*Nasal congestion—* **Adults, and children over 12 years:** apply 2 to 3 drops or 2 sprays of 0.1% solution to nasal mucosa q 8 to 10 hours. **Children under 12 years:** apply 2 to 3 drops or 1 spray of 0.05% solution to nasal mucosa q 8 to 10 hours.	*EENT:* rebound nasal congestion or irritation with excessive or long-term use; transient burning, stinging; dryness or ulceration of nasal mucosa; sneezing.

INTERACTIONS	NURSING CONSIDERATIONS
None significant.	• Use cautiously in cardiac disease, hyperthyroidism, severe trauma, or sepsis of oral or nasal mucosa, as systemic absorption can occur. • Obtain history of past reaction to topical anesthetics. • Warn patient not to eat or drink within 60 minutes after oral application, to prevent possible food aspiration.
None significant.	• Contraindicated in glaucoma. Use cautiously in hyperthyroidism, hypertension, diabetes mellitus. • Don't use 0.1% solution in children under 6 years. • Tell patient not to exceed recommended dose. Use only as needed. • Show patient how to apply.
None significant.	• Contraindicated in oral herpetic or viral lesions. Use cautiously in diabetes mellitus, peptic ulcer, or tuberculosis, as systemic absorption can occur. • Apply after meals and at bedtime for best results.
None significant.	• Contraindicated in narrow-angle glaucoma. Use cautiously in hyperthyroidism, heart disease, hypertension, diabetes mellitus, and advanced arteriosclerosis, as systemic absorption can occur. • Tell patient not to exceed recommended dose. Use only as needed. • Show patient how to apply. Only one person should use same dropper bottle or nasal spray.

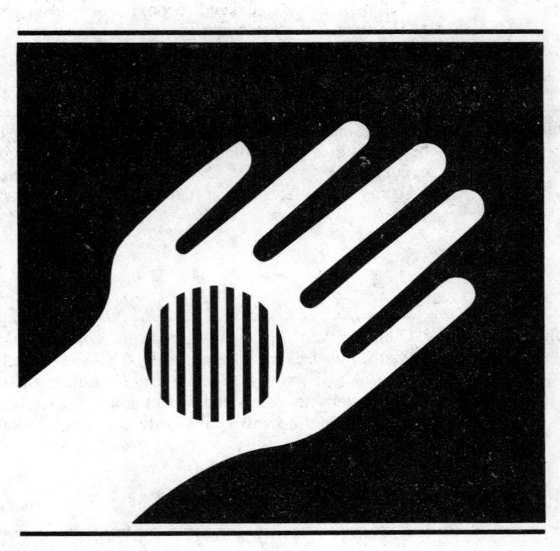

Skin and Mucous Membranes

83

Local anti-infectives

amphotericin B
bacitracin
carbol-fuchsin solution
chloramphenicol
chlortetracycline hydrochloride
clotrimazole
erythromycin
gentamicin sulfate
gentian violet
haloprogin
iodochlorhydroxyquin
mafenide acetate
miconazole nitrate 2%
neomycin sulfate
nitrofurazone
nystatin
silver sulfadiazine
tetracycline hydrochloride
tolnaftate
undecylenic acid

Local anti-infectives are popular and widely used substances and compounds that are used for treating bacterial and fungal infections. Bacteriostatic antibiotics and fungistatic agents suppress the growth of health-threatening microorganisms; bactericidal antibiotics and fungicidal agents destroy them.

Major uses

- Antibiotics are used to treat bacterial infections due to susceptible organisms and responsive to local therapy.
- Antifungal agents are used topically to treat fungal infections.

Mechanism of action

- Some antibiotics are believed to act by inhibiting cell wall synthesis; others alter membrane permeability; still others inhibit protein synthesis.
- Some antifungal agents are thought to act by altering cell permeability; others by removing diseased tissue.

Absorption, distribution, and excretion

- Most topical anti-infectives are only minimally absorbed systemically in the absence of inflammation. However, inflammation may increase the absorption of these agents.
- Applied externally, anti-infectives generally are quickly and easily absorbed into the skin.
- Long-term use of certain antibiotics, such as gentamicin and neomycin, may result in

systemic absorption.
- Many antibiotics and antifungals, when absorbed, are excreted mainly in the urine.

Onset and duration
- Most antibiotics and antifungals begin to act quickly, sometimes within minutes.
- Externally applied ointments, creams, lotions, etc. require numerous light applications because of their short action periods.
- Prolonged use of any antibiotic or antifungal may cause overgrowth of nonsusceptible organisms.

Combination products

AUREOCORT OINTMENT••: triamcinolone acetonide 0.2% and chlortetracycline HC1 3% per 15 g tube.
BACIMYCIN OINTMENT: zinc bacitracin 500 units and neomycin sulfate 5 mg per g.
BAXIMIN OINTMENT: polymyxin B sulfate 5,000 units, neomycin sulfate 5 mg, and bacitracin 400 units per g.
BIOTRES OINTMENT: polymyxin B sulfate 10,000 units and zinc bacitracin 500 units/g.
CORDRAN-N CREAM, OINTMENT: flurandrenolide 0.05% and neomycin sulfate 0.5%.
CORTISPORIN CREAM•: hydrocortisone acetate 5 mg, neomycin sulfate 5 mg, gramicidin 0.25 mg, and polymyxin B sulfate 10,000/g.
CORTISPORIN OINTMENT•: hydrocortisone 10 mg, neomycin sulfate 5 mg, bacitracin 400 units and polymyxin B sulfate 5,000 units/g.
MYCITRACIN OINTMENT: polymyxin B sulfate 5,000 units, bacitracin 500 units, and neomycin sulfate 5 mg/g.
MYCOLOG CREAM, OINTMENT: triamcinolone acetonide 0.1%, gramicidin 0.25 mg, nystatin 100,000 units and neomycin base 2.5 mg.
NEO-CORTEF CREAM: hydrocortisone acetate 1% and 2.5%, and neomycin sulfate 5 mg/g.
NEO-CORTEF LOTION, 1%: hydrocortisone acetate 10 mg and neomycin sulfate 5 mg.
NEO-CORTEF OINTMENT, 5%•: hydrocortisone acetate 5 mg, neomycin sulfate 5 mg, methylparaben 0.2 mg and propylparaben 1.8 mg.
NEODECADRON CREAM: dexamethasone phosphate 1 mg and neomycin sulfate 3.5 mg.
NEO-DELTA-CORTEF OINTMENT: prednisolone acetate 5 mg and neomycin sulfate 5 mg/g.

NEO-POLYCIN OINTMENT♦: polymyxin B sulfate 5,000 units, neomycin sulfate 5 mg, and zinc bacitracin 400 units/g.
POLYSPORIN CREAM♦♦: polymyxin B sulfate 10,000 units and gramicidin 0.25 mg/g.
POLYSPORIN OINTMENT♦: polymyxin B sulfate 10,000 units and zinc bacitracin 500 units/g.
SOFRAMYCIN OINTMENT♦♦: framycetin sulfate 15 mg, gramicidin 50 mcg and anhydrous lanolin 10%/g.
SPECTROCIN OINTMENT♦: neomycin sulfate 2.5 mg and gramicidin 0.25 mg/g.
STERISPRAY♦♦: neomycin sulfate 500 mg, polymyxin B sulfate 165,000 units and 10,000 units zinc bacitracin per 110 g container.
TERRA-CORTIL AEROSOL♦: terramycin 300 mg and hydrocortisone 100 mg/85 g.
TERRAMYCIN OINTMENT♦, POWDER: oxytetracycline 30 mg and polymyxin B sulfate 10,000 units/g.
TRI-BIOTIC OINTMENT: polymyxin B sulfate 5,000 units, bacitracin 400 units and neomycin sulfate 5 mg/g.
TRICILONE NNG CREAM: triamcinolone acetonide 1 mg, nystatin 100,000 units, neomycin sulfate 2.5 mg and gramicidin 0.25 mg/g.
VALISONE-G CREAM♦♦, OINTMENT♦♦: bethamethasone valerate NF 1.22 mg and gentamicin sulfate 1.67 mg/g.

Combination products (antifungal combinations)
CORTIN CREAM: iodochlorhydroxyquin 3% and hydrocortisone 0.5% or 1%/g.
DRENIFORM CREAM♦♦: iodochlorhydroxyquin 3% and flurandrenolide 0.0125%/20 g tube.
HYDROQUIN CREAM: iodochlorhydroxyquin 3% and hydrocortisone 1%/g.
HYSONE OINTMENT: iodochlorhydroxyquin 3% and hydrocortisone 1%.
IODOCORT CREAM♦: iodochlorhydroxyquin 3% and hydrocortisone 1%/g.
KOMED LOTION♦: sodium thiosulfate 8%, salicylic acid 1%, resorcinol 2% and isopropyl alcohol 25%/g.
LOCACORTEN-VIOFORM CREAM♦♦, OINTMENT♦♦: iodochlorhydroxyquin 3% and flumethasone pivalate 0.02%/g.
MYCOLOG CREAM, OINTMENT: gramicidin 0.25 mg, neomycin 2.5 mg, triamcinolone acetonide 1.0 mg and nystatin 100,000 units/g.
NEO-POLYCIN HC OINTMENT♦♦: neomycin sulfate 3.5 mg, polymyxin B sulfate 5,000 units, zinc bacitracin 400 units and hydrocortisone acetate 10 mg/g.
NEOSPORIN CREAM♦♦: polymyxin B sulfate 10,000 units, neomycin sulfate 5 mg, and gramicidin 0.25 mg/g.
NEOSPORIN OINTMENT♦, POWDER♦: polymyxin B sulfate 5,000 units, zinc bacitracin 400 units, and neomycin sulfate 5 mg/g.
NEOSPORIN-G CREAM: polymyxin B sulfate 10,000 units, neomycin sulfate 5 mg, and gramicidin 0.25 mg/g.
NEO-SYNALAR CREAM♦: fluocinolone acetonide 0.025% and neomycin sulfate 0.5%.
NYSTAFORM OINTMENT♦: nystatin 100,000 units and iodochlorhydroxyquin 1%.
NYSTAFORM-HC CREME♦♦, LOTION♦♦, OINTMENT♦: nystatin 100,000 units/g., iodochlorhydroxyquin 3% and hydrocortisone alcohol 0.5% or 1%.
P.B.N. OINTMENT: polymyxin B sulfate 5,000 units, neomycin sulfate 5 mg and bacitracin 400 units/g.
RACET CREAM: iodochlorhydroxyquin 3% and hydrocortisone 0.5%/g.
TINVER LOTION♦: sodium thiosulfate 25%, salicylic acid 1% and isopropyl alcohol 10%/g.
VIOFORM-HYDROCORTISONE CREAM♦, LOTION, OINTMENT♦: iodochlorhydroxyquin 3% and hydrocortisone 1%/g.
VIOFORM-HYDROCORTISONE MILD CREAM♦, OINTMENT♦: iodochlorhydroxyquin 3% and hydrocortisone 0.5%/g.
WHITFIELD'S OINTMENT: benzoic acid 12% and salicylic acid 6%/g.

TOPICAL THERAPY: MATCHING THE VEHICLE TO THE CONDITION

ACUTE

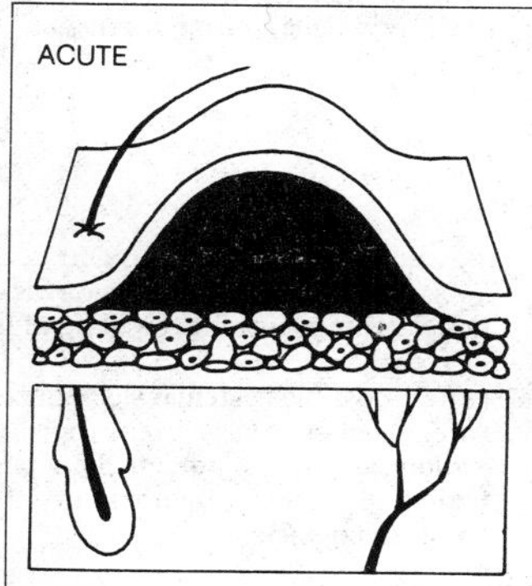

CLINICAL SIGNS	TYPE OF VEHICLE
There is marked inflammation. The lesion is erythematous, edematous, and vesicular. To the patient, these often-weepy lesions feel tender, itchy, and hot or burning.	*Apply a wet compress* as often as possible, changing it before it becomes dry. Leave the compress uncovered so as not to impede evaporation, which soothes, cools, and also helps heal through its antipruritic, anti-inflammatory actions.

SUBACUTE

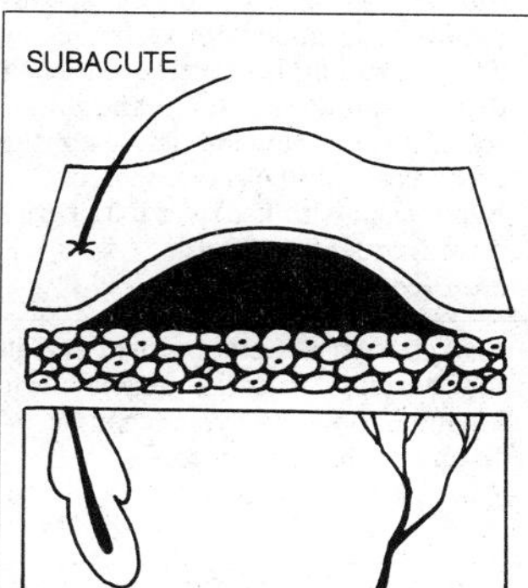

CLINICAL SIGNS	TYPE OF VEHICLE
Inflammation is still present but is often restricted to the areas immediately surrounding the lesions. The total appearance suggests a drying-out process.	*Apply lotions or creams,* which are protective and lubricating, yet not occlusive enough to stop the still-needed evaporation.

CHRONIC

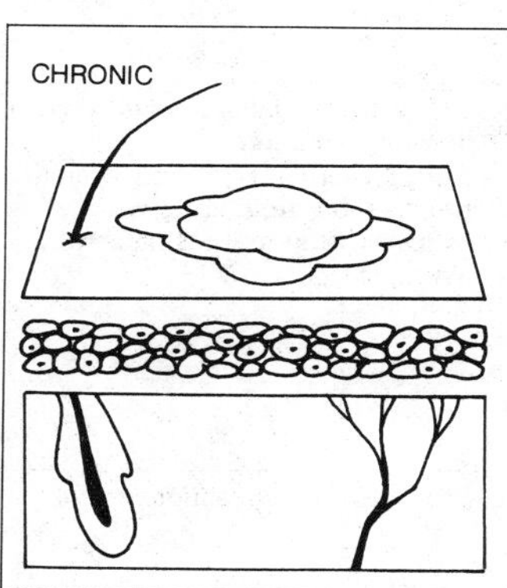

CLINICAL SIGNS	TYPE OF VEHICLE
There may still be some limited inflammation. Chronic lesions may assume a scaly, lichenified appearance.	*Apply ointments,* which are occlusive and lubricating, and help the skin to retain moisture and natural skin emollients. At this stage, active medications can be continued in the ointments.

NAME	INDICATIONS & DOSAGE	SIDE EFFECTS
amphotericin B Fungizone Cream, Lotion, Ointment (3% amphotericin B)	*Cutaneous or mucocutaneous candidal infections—* **Adults and children:** apply liberally b.i.d., t.i.d., q.i.d. for 1 to 3 weeks; up to several months for interdigital lesions, paronychias and onychomycosis (where relapses are frequent).	*Skin:* possible drying, contact sensitivity, erythema, burning, pruritus.
bacitracin Baciguent◆, Bacitin◆◆	*Primary or secondary topical infections, impetigo, abrasions, cuts, minor wounds, seborrheic dermatitis, acne, contact dermatitis, psoriasis—* **Adults and children:** apply thin film b.i.d. or t.i.d. or more often, depending on severity of condition.	*Skin:* rashes and other allergic reactions; itching, burning, swelling of lips or face. *Other:* possible systemic side effects when used over large areas for prolonged periods: potentially nephrotoxic and ototoxic, tightness in chest, hypotension.
carbol-fuchsin solution Carfusin, Castaderm, Castellani's Paint	*Tinea, dermatophytosis, skin infections—* **Adults and children:** apply liberally 1 or 2 times daily.	*Blood:* possibility of aplastic anemia, mainly associated with systemic administration; however, even when drug is applied topically, the possibility of this reaction should be considered. Possibility of bone marrow hypoplasia with use over long periods or at frequent intervals. *Skin:* contact dermatitis.
chloramphenicol Chloromycetin◆ (1% chloramphenicol)	*Superficial skin infections caused by susceptible bacteria—* **Adults and children:** after thorough cleansing, apply t.i.d. or q.i.d.	*Skin:* possible contact sensitivity; itching, burning, urticaria, angioneurotic edema in patients hypersensitive to any of the components.
chlortetracycline hydrochloride Aureomycin◆ 3%	*Superficial infections of the skin caused by susceptible bacteria—* **Adults and children:** rub into affected area b.i.d. or t.i.d.	*Skin:* rashes, dermatitis.
clotrimazole Canesten◆◆, Gyne-Lotrimin, Lotrimin (1% clotrimazole)	*Superficial fungal infections (tinea pedis, tinea cruris, tinea versicolor, candidiasis, and tinea corporis)—* **Adults and children:** apply thinly and massage into affected and surrounding area, morning and evening, 1 to 8 weeks. *Candidal vulvovaginitis—* **Adults:** insert 1 applicatorful or 1 tablet intravaginally daily for 7 to 14 days at bedtime.	*GU:* with vaginal use—mild vaginal burning, irritation. *Skin:* blistering, erythema, edema, pruritus, burning, stinging, peeling, urticaria, skin fissures, general irritation.
erythromycin Erythrocin◆◆, Ilotycin◆	*Superficial skin infections caused by susceptible organisms—* **Adults and children:** clean affected area; apply t.i.d. or q.i.d.	*Skin:* sensitivity reactions.

◆ Also available in Canada.
◆◆ Available in Canada only.
Unmarked trade names available in United States only.

INTERACTIONS	NURSING CONSIDERATIONS
None significant.	• Cream or lotion preferred for folds of groin, armpit, neck creases, etc. • Cream discolors skin slightly when rubbed in; lotion or ointment doesn't. Lotion may stain nail lesions. • Watch for and report signs of local irritation. • Avoid occlusive dressings and ointments. • Store at room temperature; avoid freezing. • Well tolerated, even by infants, for long periods. • A fungistatic agent.
None significant.	• Contraindicated in hypersensitivity to any of the components and for application in the external ear canal if the eardrum is perforated. • If used on burns that cover more than 20% of body surface, and especially if patient suffers impaired renal function, apply only once daily. • If no improvement or if condition worsens, stop using and tell doctor. • Prolonged use may result in overgrowth of nonsusceptible organisms. • Avoid excess application. • A bacteriostatic agent.
None significant.	• Do not use on large areas or on eroded skin. • Do not continue use after 1 week if no improvement shown. • Poisonous; warn against swallowing. • Clean and dry skin thoroughly before applying. • A fungicidal and bactericidal agent.
None significant.	• Contraindicated in hypersensitivity to any of the components. • If no improvement or if condition worsens, stop using and tell doctor. • Prolonged use may result in overgrowth of nonsusceptible organisms. • For all but very superficial infections, topical use of this drug should be supplemented by appropriate systemic medication. • A bacteriostatic agent.
None significant.	• Contraindicated in hypersensitivity to any of the components. • Prolonged use may result in overgrowth of nonsusceptible organisms. • If no improvement or if condition worsens, stop using and tell doctor. • A bacteriostatic agent.
None significant.	• Contraindicated in hypersensitivity to any of the components. • Not for ophthalmic use. • Watch for and report irritation or sensitivity. • Improvement usually within a week; if none in 4 weeks, review diagnosis.
None significant.	• Prolonged use may result in overgrowth of nonsusceptible organisms. • If no improvement or if condition worsens, stop using and tell doctor. • Usually a bacteriostatic agent, but in high concentrations, or against highly susceptible organisms, may be bactericidal.

NAME	INDICATIONS & DOSAGE	SIDE EFFECTS
gentamicin sulfate Garamycin◆	*Primary and secondary bacterial infections, superficial burns, skin ulcers, infected insect bites and stings, infected lacerations and abrasions, wounds from minor surgery—* **Adults, and children over 1 year:** rub in small amount gently t.i.d. or q.i.d., with or without gauze dressing.	*Skin:* small percentage of minor skin irritation; possible photosensitivity.
gentian violet (methylrosaniline chloride) Bismuth Violet solution (1% and 3%), Crystal Violet	*Superficial infections of skin, lesions, except ulcerative lesions of face particularly Candida albicans—* **Adults and children:** apply with swab b.i.d. or t.i.d. Keep affected area clean, dry, and exposed to air to prevent spread of infection.	*Skin:* permanent discoloration if applied to granulation tissue; ulceration of mucous membranes.
haloprogin Halotex◆	*Superficial fungal infections (tinea pedis, tinea cruris, tinea corporis, tinea manuum, and tinea versicolor)—* **Adults and children:** apply liberally b.i.d. for 2 to 3 weeks.	*Skin:* burning sensation, irritation, vesicle formation, increased maceration, pruritus or exacerbation of preexisting lesions.
iodochlorhydroxyquin Gentleline, Quinoform, Torofor, Vioform	*Inflamed skin conditions, including eczema, athlete's foot, other fungal infections; cutaneous or mucocutaneous mycotic infections caused by Candida species (Monilia)—* **Adults and children:** apply a thin layer b.i.d., t.i.d., q.i.d., or as directed. Continue for 1 week after clinical cure.	*Skin:* possible burning, itching, acneiform eruptions. *Systemic:* electrolyte imbalance, adrenal suppression.
mafenide acetate Sulfamylon◆	*Adjunctive treatment of second- and third-degree burns—* **Adults and children:** apply 1/16 inch daily or b.i.d. to cleansed, debrided wounds.	*Blood:* eosinophilia. *Skin:* pain, burning sensation, rash, itching, swelling, hives, blisters, erythema. *Other:* facial edema.
miconazole nitrate 2% Micatin◆	*Tinea pedis, tinea cruris, tinea corporis, cutaneous candidiasis (moniliasis), infections from common dermatophytes—* **Adults and children:** apply sparingly b.i.d. for 2 to 4 weeks.	*Skin:* isolated reports of irritation, burning, maceration.

INTERACTIONS	NURSING CONSIDERATIONS
None significant.	• Contraindicated in hypersensitivity to any of the components. • If no improvement or if condition worsens, stop using and tell doctor. • Avoid use on large skin lesions or over a wide area because of possible systemic toxic effects. • Prolonged use may result in overgrowth of nonsusceptible organisms. • May clear bacterial infections that have not responded to other antibacterial agents. • Useful for treating patients who are sensitive to neomycin. • Useful for infected skin cysts, preceded by incision and draining. • Store in cool place. • Remove crusts before application of gentamicin in impetigo contagiosa. • A bactericidal agent.
None significant.	• Contraindicated in hypersensitivity to any of the components. • Do not use on ulcerative lesions of the face. • Apply carefully to avoid undue staining.
None significant.	• Contraindicated in hypersensitivity to any of the components. • Reconsider diagnosis if no improvement in 4 weeks. • Fungistatic and fungicidal.
Systemic corticosteroids: possible increased absorption. Use together cautiously.	• Contraindicated in tuberculosis, vaccinia, and varicella. • Note all side effects and precautions of each component in the combination antifungals. • Presence in urine may cause false positive result for phenylketonuria (PKU) or inaccurate thyroid function tests. Discontinue at least 1 month before thyroid function tests. • Drug will stain fabric and hair.
None significant.	• Use with caution in acute renal failure. • Closely monitor acid-base balance, especially in the presence of pulmonary and renal dysfunction. • If acidosis occurs, discontinue use for 24 to 48 hours. • Check for pain and burning; if they occur, notify doctor. If other allergic reactions occur, treatment may have to be temporarily discontinued. • Cleanse area before applying. • Accidental ingestion may cause diarrhea. • Keep burn areas medicated at all times. • Bathe patient daily, if possible.
None significant.	• For external use only. Keep out of eyes. • Discontinue if sensitivity or chemical irritation occurs.

NAME	INDICATIONS & DOSAGE	SIDE EFFECTS
neomycin sulfate Herisan Antibiotic◆◆, Mycifradin◆◆, Myciguent◆, Neocin◆◆	*Topical bacterial infections, burns, wounds, skin grafts, following surgical procedure, lesions, pruritus, trophic ulcerations, edema—* **Adults and children:** rub in small quantity gently b.i.d., t.i.d., or as directed.	*Skin:* rashes. *Other:* possible nephrotoxicity, ototoxicity, and neuromuscular blockade; possible systemic absorption when used on extensive areas of the body.
nitrofurazone Furacin◆, Furazyme, Nisept, Nitrofurastan	*Adjunctive treatment of second- and third-degree burns (especially when resistance to other antibiotics and sulfonamides occurs); skin grafting—* **Adults and children:** apply directly to lesion daily or every few days, depending on severity of burn.	*Skin:* erythema, pruritus, burning, edema, severe reactions (vesiculation, denudation, ulceration). *Other:* overgrowth of nonsuceptible organisms.
nystatin Candex, Mycostatin◆, Nadostine◆◆, Nilstat	*Infant eczema, pruritus ani and vulvae, superficial bacterial infections, localized forms of candidiasis—* **Adults and children:** apply and rub into area b.i.d. for 2 weeks.	*Skin:* occasional contact dermatitis from preservatives present in some formulations. *Systemic:* possible nephrotoxicity or ototoxicity with prolonged or frequent use.
silver sulfadiazine Flamazine◆◆, Silvadene	*Prevention and treatment of wound infection for second- and third-degree burns—* **Adults and children:** apply 1/16 inch thickness of ointment to cleansed and debrided burn wound, then apply daily or b.i.d.	*Blood:* neutropenia (in 3% to 5%) *Skin:* pain, burning, rashes, itching. *Other:* fungal infections.
tetracycline hydrochloride Achromycin◆, Topicycline	*Superficial skin infections caused by susceptible bacteria—* **Adults and children:** rub into cleansed affected area b.i.d. or t.i.d. *Acne—* **Adults:** apply Topicycline	*Skin:* dermatitis with Achromycin; with Topicycline, temporary stinging or burning on application, slight yellowing of treated skin, especially in patients with light complexions; treated skin areas fluoresce under ultraviolet light; severe dermatitis.

INTERACTIONS	NURSING CONSIDERATIONS
None significant.	• Contraindicated in hypersensitivity to any of the components, atopy, vaccinia, varicella, fungal or other viral lesions. • If no improvement or if condition worsens, stop using and tell doctor. • If used on more than 20% of the body surface and on patient with impaired renal function, reduce application to once daily. • Prolonged use may result in overgrowth of nonsusceptible organisms. • In those combination products which contain corticosteroids, use of occlusive dressings increases the corticosteroid absorption and the likelihood of systemic effect. • Particularly absorbed on denuded or abraded areas. • A bactericidal agent.
None significant.	• Contraindicated in previous hypersensitivity to drug. • If irritation, sensitization, or infection occur, discontinue use. • When using wet dressing, protect skin around wound with zinc oxide. • Cleanse wound as indicated by doctor at each dressing change. • Remove adherent dressings by flushing with solution of nitrofurazone and sterile water, or sterile normal saline solution. • Solution should be stored in tight, light-resistant containers (brown bottles). Avoid exposure of solution at all times to direct light, prolonged heat, and alkaline materials. • Drug may discolor in light but is still usable because it retains its potency. • Discard cloudy solutions if warming to 55° to 60° C. (131° to 140° F.) does not restore clarity.
None significant.	• Contraindicated in viral diseases of the skin (vaccinia and varicella), fungal lesions (except candidiasis), and markedly impaired circulation. • Generally well tolerated by all age groups, including debilitated infants. • Preparation does not stain skin or mucous membranes. • Cream recommended for intertriginous areas, powder for very moist areas, ointment for dry areas. • Fungistatic and fungicidal.
Topical proteolytic enzymes: inactivity of enzymes when used together. Do not use together.	• Contraindicated for premature and newborn infants during first month of life. (Drug may increase possibility of kernicterus.) Use with caution in hypersensitivity to the drug or sulfonamides. • If hepatic or renal dysfunction occurs, consider discontinuing drug. • Inspect patient's skin daily, and note any changes. Notify doctor if burning or excessive pain develops. • Use only on affected areas. Keep medicated at all times. • For patients with extensive burns, monitor serum sulfa concentrations and renal function, and check urine for sulfa crystals. • Bathe patient daily, if possible. • Discard darkened cream. • Should be discontinued if infection is suspected.
None significant.	• Contraindicated in hypersensitivity to any of the components. • If no improvement or if condition worsens, stop using and tell doctor. • Prolonged use may result in overgrowth of nonsusceptible organisms. • Primarily a bacteriostatic agent. • Patient may continue normal use of cosmetics. • Store at room temperature, away from excessive heat. • Medication to be used by 1 person only. Don't share with family.

(continued on following page)

NAME	INDICATIONS & DOSAGE	SIDE EFFECTS
tetracycline hydrochloride *(continued)*	generously to affected areas b.i.d. until skin is thoroughly wet.	
tolnaftate Aftate, Tinactin◆	*Superficial fungus infections of the skin, infections due to common pathogenic fungi, tinea pedis, tinea cruris, tinea corporis, tinea manuum, tinea versicolor—* **Adults and children:** ¼- to ½-inch ribbon of cream or 1 or 3 drops of lotion to cover area of 1 hand; same amount of cream or 2 to 3 drops of lotion to cover the toes and interdigital webs of 1 foot. Apply and massage gently into skin b.i.d. for 2 or 3 weeks, up 6 weeks.	None significant.
undecylenic acid or zinc undecylenate Desenex, Ting, Unde-Jen	*Athlete's foot and ringworm of the body exclusive of nails and hairy areas—* **Adults and children:** clean thoroughly. Apply ointment liberally at night and powder during the day. Use regularly to prevent fungus infections.	*Skin:* possible irritation in hypersensitive person.

INTERACTIONS	NURSING CONSIDERATIONS
	• Apply morning and evening. Warn that drug should be used within 2 months. • Explain that floating plug in bottle of Topicycline shouldn't be removed. It's the result of proper reconstitution of the preparation. This plug is inert and harmless. • Serum levels of topical tetracycline HC1 are much lower than those for orally administered drug, so systemic effects are unlikely. • To control flow rate of solution, increase or decrease pressure of the applicator against the skin.
None significant.	• Discontinue if condition worsens. Check with doctor. • Odorless, greaseless. Won't stain or discolor skin, hair, nails, or clothing. • Only a small quantity of cream or lotion is needed; area should not be wet with solution when application is completed. • Fungistatic and fungicidal. • Commonly available product used to treat "athlete's foot" (tinea pedis).
None significant.	• Consult doctor before using on person with peripheral neuropathy and peripheral vascular diseases or diabetes.

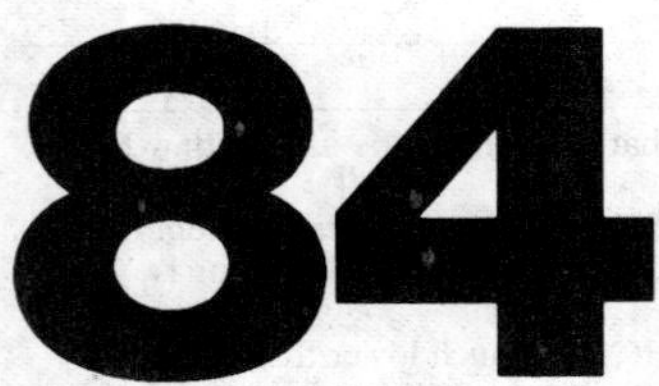

Scabicides and pediculicides

benzyl benzoate lotion
copper oleate solution
crotamiton
gamma benzene hexachloride
sulfa in petrolatum

Scabicides and pediculicides are toxic to the most common parasitic arthropods that infest man, specifically *Sarcoptes scabiei* (scabies), *Pediculus humanus* var. *capitis* (head louse), *Pediculus humanus* var. *corporis* (body louse), and *Phthirus pubis* (crab louse). One application is usually enough to eradicate active parasites, but repeated applications are sometimes necessary to destroy nits.

Major uses
• Topical treatment to eradicate infestations of parasitic arthropods such as scabies and pediculosis.

Mechanism of action
• Exact mechanism unknown.

Absorption, distribution, and excretion
• Used for their topical effect.
• Gamma benzene hexachloride is absorbed slowly and incompletely through intact skin when applied topically; through GI tract when ingested orally; and through mucous membranes when inhaled. Absorption through skin is usually greatest when drug is applied to face, scalp, neck, axillae, scrotum, or damaged skin. No information is available on systemic absorption of the other drugs.
• Gamma benzene hexachloride is stored in body fat and metabolized in the liver.
• Gamma benzene hexachloride is excreted slowly in urine and feces.

Onset and duration
• Onset immediate with all drugs.
• Duration of action limited. Must be reapplied, if necessary, according to dosage directions.

Combination products
None.

SHAMPOOING OUT SCABIES AND PEDICULOSIS

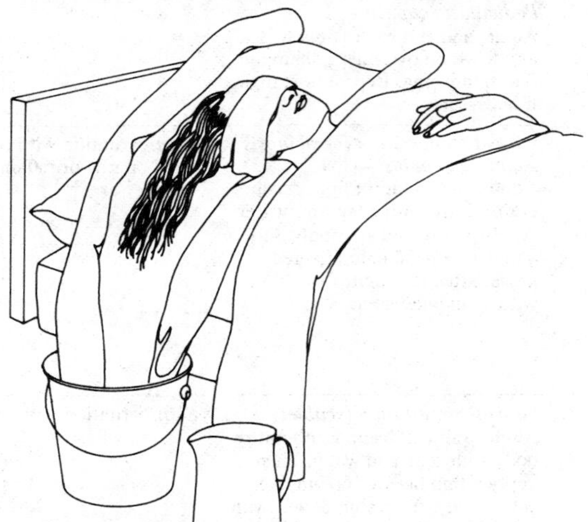

1. To wash the hair of a bedridden scabies or pediculosis patient, wear gloves and a paper gown over your uniform.
2. Thoroughly pad the patient's back and neck for comfort.
3. Arrange pillows on a slight incline to let water drain away from the patient's head.
4. Make a water-draining trough from two towels rolled in the edges of a rubber sheet leading to a bucket.
5. Produce a good lather in the hair. Rinse two or three times.
6. Dry immediately.
7. Reinspect scalp for scabies and pediculosis or other abnormalities.
8. When you are finished, discard towels and linen in a separate labeled container. With the scabies and pediculosis patient, you must pay extra attention to maintaining asepsis.

NAME	INDICATIONS & DOSAGE	SIDE EFFECTS
benzyl benzoate lotion Scabanca◆◆	*Parasitic infestation (scabies, Phthirus pubis)—* **Adults and children:** first, scrub entire body with soap and water. Then, apply the 25% lotion undiluted over entire body, except the face, while still damp. Be sure to apply around nails. Let dry. Apply second coat on the most involved areas. Bathe after 24 to 48 hours. Adults require 120 to 180 ml. Children require 60 to 90 ml. *Pediculosis capitis—* **Adults and children:** apply to scalp and leave on overnight; shampoo out in morning. Repeat next night if necessary.	*Skin:* irritation, itching; contact dermatitis with repeated applications.
copper oleate solution (with tetrahydronaphthalene) Cuprex	*Parasitic infestation (pediculosis capitis and pubis)—* **Adults and children:** first, scrub entire body with soap and water. Apply gently and sparingly 3 to 4 tablespoonsful onto affected areas; after 15 minutes wash off with soap and water.	*Skin:* irritation with repeated use, or if used on raw or inflamed skin.
crotamiton Eurax◆	*Parasitic infestation (scabies)—* **Adults and children:** scrub entire body with soap and water. Then, apply a thin layer of cream over entire body, from chin down, with special attention to folds, creases, interdigital spaces, genital areas. Apply second coat within 24 hours. Wait 48 hours, then wash off. *General itching*—apply locally b.i.d. or t.i.d.	*Skin:* irritation with repeated use.
gamma benzene hexachloride or lindane gBh◆◆, Kwell, Kwellada◆◆	*Parasitic infestation (scabies, pediculosis)—* **Adults and children:** scrub entire body with soap and water. Cream or lotion—apply thin layer over entire skin surface (with special attention to folds, creases, interdigital spaces, genital area) for scabies, or to hairy areas for pediculosis. After 8 to 12 hours wash off drug. If second application needed for scabies,	*Skin:* irritation with repeated use.

◆ Also available in Canada.
◆◆ Available in Canada only.
Unmarked trade names available in United States only.

INTERACTIONS	NURSING CONSIDERATIONS
None significant.	• Contraindicated when skin is raw or inflamed. Notify doctor immediately if skin irritation or hypersensitivity develop; tell patient to discontinue drug and to wash it off skin. • Do not apply to face, eyes, mucous membranes, or urethral meatus. If accidental contact with eyes does occur, flush with water and notify doctor. • Instruct patient to change and sterilize (boil, launder, dry clean or apply very hot iron) all clothing and bed linen after drug is washed off. • Itching may continue for several weeks; does not indicate that therapy is ineffective. To prevent acarophobia, reassure patient that itching will cease. • Tendency to overuse this drug. Estimate exact amount needed. • Topical corticosteroids may be needed if dermatitis develops from scratching. • Question other family members about possible infestation. • After application use a fine comb on hair to remove nits.
None significant.	• Contraindicated when skin is raw or inflamed, or when there is a severe infection. Notify doctor immediately if skin irritation or hypersensitivity develop; tell patient to discontinue drug and to wash it off skin. • Do not apply more than twice within 48 hours. • Do not apply to face, eyes, mucous membranes, or urethral meatus. If accidental contact with eyes does occur, flush with water and notify doctor. • Instruct patient to change and sterilize (boil, launder, dry clean or apply very hot iron) all clothing and bed linen after application. • After application use a fine comb on hair to remove nits. • Question other family members about possible infestation. • Tendency for overuse of pediculicides. Estimate exact amount needed.
None significant.	• Contraindicated when skin is raw or inflamed. Notify doctor immediately if skin irritation or hypersensitivity develop; tell patient to discontinue drug and to wash it off skin. • Do not apply to face, eyes, mucous membranes, or urethral meatus. If accidental contact with eyes does occur, flush with water and notify doctor. • Instruct patient to change and sterilize (boil, launder, dry clean or apply very hot iron) all clothing and bed linen after drug is washed off. • Topical corticosteroids may be needed if dermatitis develops from scratching. • Tendency to overuse scabicides. Estimate exact amount needed. • Question other family members about possible infestation.
None significant.	• Contraindicated when skin is raw or inflamed. Notify doctor immediately if skin irritation or hypersensitivity develop; tell patient to discontinue drug and to wash it off skin. Use cautiously in infants and small children. • Do not apply to open areas or acutely inflamed skin, or to face, eyes, mucous membranes, or urethral meatus. If accidental contact with eyes does occur, flush with water and notify doctor. • Warn parents not to let infants or children suck their fingers after drug application. • Discourage repeated use, which can lead to skin irritation and possible systemic toxicity. • Warn patient itching may continue for several weeks, particularly in scabies.

(continued on following page)

NAME	INDICATIONS & DOSAGE	SIDE EFFECTS
gamma benzene hexachloride or lindane *(continued)*	wait 1 week before repeating. For pediculosis, repeat after 24 hours, but never more than twice in a week. Shampoo—apply 30 to 60 ml onto affected area and work into lather for 4 to 5 minutes. Rinse thoroughly and rub with dry towel.	
sulfa (6%) in petrolatum	*Parasitic infestation (scabies)*— **Adults and children:** after taking a soapy bath, patient should apply drug nightly for 2 to 3 nights consecutively. He should take soapy bath 24 hours after last application.	*Skin:* may produce dermatitis if applied continuously for several days.

INTERACTIONS	NURSING CONSIDERATIONS
	• Topical corticosteroids may be needed if dermatitis develops from scratching. • Instruct patient to change and sterilize (boil, launder, dry clean or apply very hot iron) all clothing and bed linen after drug is washed off. • After application, use a fine comb on hair to remove nits. • Gamma benzene hexachloride shampoo can be used to clean comb or brushes; wash them thoroughly afterward. Warn patient not to use gamma benzene hexachloride as routine shampoo. • Question other family members about possible infestation. • Tendency for overuse. Estimate exact amount needed.
None significant.	• Instruct patient to change and sterilize (boil, launder, dry clean, or iron with a very hot iron) all clothing and bed linen after drug is washed off. • Warn patient that product has an odor, is messy, and will stain clothing. • Question other members of family about possible infestation. • Tendency to overuse scabicides. Estimate exact amount needed.

85

Anti-inflammatory agents

betamethasone
betamethasone benzoate
betamethasone dipropionate
betamethasone valerate
desonide
desoximetasone
dexamethasone
dexamethasone sodium phosphate
diflorasone diacetate
flumethasone pivalate
fluocinolone acetonide
fluocinonide
fluorometholone
flurandrenolide
halcinonide
hydrocortisone
hydrocortisone acetate
hydrocortisone valerate
methylprednisolone acetate
prednisolone
triamcinolone acetonide

Topical corticosteroids reduce inflammation, relieve itching, and constrict blood vessels. Their effectiveness depends on the potency of the drug and the amount absorbed through the skin. These agents control but do not cure dermatoses.

Major uses

• Acute and chronic inflammatory dermatoses, psoriasis, atopic eczema, infantile eczema, pruritus ani and vulvae, neurodermatitis, contact dermatitis, seborrheic dermatitis, and exfoliative dermatitis.
• Occlusive dressings used in management of psoriasis or resistant conditions such as chronic neurodermatitis, lichen planus, or lichen simplex chronicus.
• Creams are useful for wet lesions; lotions, for areas subject to chafing (axillae, feet, groin); ointments, for dry, scaly lesions.
• Tape serves as both a vehicle and an occlusive dressing. Retention of insensible perspiration by the tape results in hydration of stratum corneum and improved diffusion of medication. Tape protects the skin from scratching, rubbing, discoloration, and chemical irritation; and it acts as a mechanical splint to fissured skin and prevents removal of medication by washing or rubbing against clothing.

Mechanism of action

Exactly how these drugs work is not known. Some believe corticosteroids attach to tissue receptors, decreasing membrane permeability and inhibiting the release of toxins. They may control the rate of protein synthesis. Their action on inflammatory processes does not derive from a single action, but from the sum of discrete effects on blood vessels, leukocytes, and fibroblasts.

Corticosteroid-induced vasoconstriction decreases serum extravasation, swelling, and itching. Corticosteroids also act as an antimitotic, which may reduce cell multiplication in patches of psoriasis.

Absorption, distribution, and excretion

- Absorbed through skin. Increased absorption when skin damage exists, when drug is applied heavily, when occlusive dressings are used, or when applied over large areas. Systemic absorption leading to adrenal suppression is possible with prolonged and excessive use, especially under occlusion.
- Enter circulation and are metabolized mainly in the liver but also in extrahepatic sites.
- Excreted in urine.

Combination products

Corticosteroids for topical use are frequently combined with antibiotics, antifungals, and sulfonamides. See also Chapters 14 and 70.

A LITTLE RESTRAINT

To stop the child with eczema from scratching and further infecting inflamed face lesions, tie an elbow restraint around his arm. The child will still be able to move his arms, but he won't be able to touch his face.

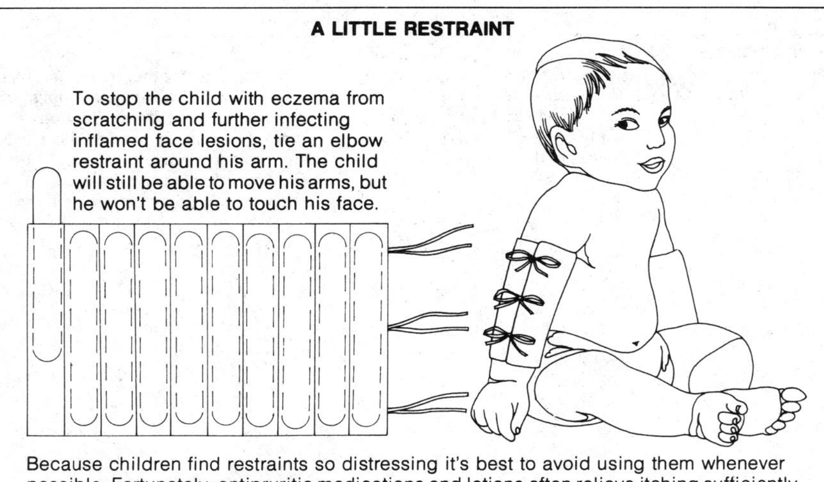

Because children find restraints so distressing it's best to avoid using them whenever possible. Fortunately, antipruritic medications and lotions often relieve itching sufficiently. When they don't, first try mild restraint such as mittens made of stockinette or an undershirt. Mitten restraints are especially effective if the child's skin lesions are on the forearm, ruling out the cuff restraint (shown above).

NAME	INDICATIONS & DOSAGE	SIDE EFFECTS
betamethasone Celestone◆	*Inflammation of corticosteroid-responsive dermatoses—* **Adults and children:** clean area; apply cream sparingly b.i.d. or t.i.d. Massage gently until it disappears. Apply thick layer with occlusive dressing to manage deep-seated dermatoses, such as neurodermatitis.	*Metabolic:* adrenal insufficiency. *Skin:* burning, itching, irritation, dryness, folliculitis, hypopigmentation, acneiform eruptions, hypertrichosis, allergic contact dermatitis. With occlusive dressings: secondary infection, maceration, skin atrophy, striae, miliaria.
betamethasone benzoate Beben◆, Benisone, Uticort	*Inflammation of corticosteroid-responsive dermatoses, including eczematous dermatosis—* **Adults and children:** clean area; apply cream, lotion, or gel sparingly daily to q.i.d.	*Metabolic:* adrenal insufficiency. *Skin:* burning, itching, irritation, dryness, folliculitis, atrophy, hypopigmentation, striae, acneiform eruptions, perioral dermatitis, hypertrichosis, allergic contact dermatitis. With occlusive dressings: secondary infection, maceration, atrophy, striae, miliaria.

◆ Also available in Canada.
◆◆ Available in Canada only.
Unmarked trade names available in United States only.

INTERACTIONS	NURSING CONSIDERATIONS
None significant.	• Contraindicated in viral diseases of skin, such as vaccinia, varicella, and herpes simplex; fungal infections; skin tuberculosis; impaired circulation. • Avoid application in or near eyes. • Systemic absorption especially likely with occlusive dressings, prolonged treatment, or extensive body-surface treatment. • Stop drug and notify doctor if patient develops signs of systemic absorption, skin irritation or ulceration, hypersensitivity, infection (if antifungals or antibacterials are being used with corticosteroids and infection does not respond immediately, corticosteroids should be stopped until infection is controlled). • Before applying, gently wash skin. To prevent damage to skin, rub medication in gently, leaving a thin coat. • Occlusive dressing: apply cream heavily, then cover with a thin, pliable, nonflammable plastic film; seal to adjacent normal skin with nonallergenic tape. Minimize adverse reactions by using occlusive dressing intermittently. • For patient with eczematous dermatitis who may develop irritation with adhesive material, hold dressing in place with gauze, elastic bandages, or stockings. • Tell doctor and remove occlusive dressing if body temperature rises. • Occlusive dressings are generally not used in presence of infection or with weeping or exudative lesions. • Change dressing as ordered by doctor. Inspect skin for infection, striae, and atrophy. Discontinue drug and notify doctor if these occur. • Treatment should be continued for a few days after clearing of lesions to prevent recurrence. • Instruct patient to report signs of drug sensitivity.
None significant.	• Contraindicated in viral diseases of skin, such as varicella, vaccinia, and herpes simplex; fungal infections; skin tuberculosis; impaired circulation. • Avoid application in or near eyes. • Due to alcohol content of vehicle, gel preparations may cause mild, transient stinging without irritation if used in or near excoriated skin. • Systemic absorption especially likely with occlusive dressings, prolonged treatment, or extensive body-surface treatment. • Stop drug and notify doctor if patient develops signs of systemic absorption, skin irritation or ulceration, signs of hypersensitivity, infection (if antifungals or antibiotics are being used with corticosteroids and infection does not respond immediately, corticosteroids should be stopped until infection is controlled). • Before applying, gently wash skin. To prevent damage to skin, rub in medication gently, leaving a thin coat. When treating hairy sites, part hair and apply directly to lesion. • Occlusive dressing: apply cream heavily, then cover with a thin, pliable, nonflammable plastic film; seal to adjacent normal skin with nonallergenic tape. Minimize adverse reactions by using occlusive dressing intermittently. • For patient with eczematous dermatitis who may develop irritation with adhesive material, hold dressing in place with gauze, elastic bandages, or stockings. • Tell doctor and remove occlusive dressing if body temperature rises. • Occlusive dressings are generally not used in presence of infections, or with weeping or exudative lesions. • Change dressings as ordered by doctor. Inspect skin for infection, striae, and atrophy. Discontinue drug and notify doctor if these occur. • Treatment should be continued for a few days after clearing of lesions to prevent recurrence. • Instruct patient to report signs of drug sensitivity.

NAME	INDICATIONS & DOSAGE	SIDE EFFECTS
betamethasone dipropionate Diprosone◆	*Inflammation of corticosteroid-responsive dermatoses*— **Adults and children:** clean area; apply cream, lotion or ointment sparingly b.i.d. Aerosol: shake can well. Direct spray onto affected area from a distance of 6 inches for only 3 seconds t.i.d.	*Metabolic:* adrenal insufficiency. *Skin:* burning, itching, irritation, dryness, folliculitis, hypopigmentation, perioral dermatitis, allergic contact dermatitis, hypertrichosis, acneiform eruptions. With occlusive dressings: maceration of skin, secondary infection, atrophy, striae, miliaria.
betamethasone valerate Betnovate◆◆, Betnovate 1/2◆◆, Celestoderm-V◆◆, Celestoderm-V/2◆◆, Valisone	*Inflammation of corticosteroid-responsive dermatoses (psoriasis, atopic and infantile eczema, nummular eczema, pruritus ani and vulvae, neurodermatitis, intertrigo, contact dermatitis, seborrheic dermatitis, exfoliative dermatitis, solar dermatitis, stasis dermatitis, and dyshidrosis)*— **Adults and children:** clean area; apply cream, lotion, ointment, or aerosol sparingly daily to q.i.d. Aerosol: shake can well. Direct spray onto affected area from a distance of 6 inches. Apply for only 3 seconds t.i.d. to q.i.d. Betnovate 1/2 and Celestoderm V/2 contain a lower amount of betamethasone.	*Metabolic:* adrenal insufficiency. *Skin:* burning, itching, irritation, dryness, folliculitis, hypopigmentation, hypertrichosis, acneiform eruptions, perioral dermatitis, allergic contact dermatitis. With occlusive dressings: maceration of skin, secondary infection, atrophy, striae, miliaria.

INTERACTIONS	NURSING CONSIDERATIONS
None significant.	• Contraindicated in viral diseases of skin, such as varicella, vaccinia, and herpes simplex; fungal infections; skin tuberculosis; impaired circulation. • Avoid application in or near eyes. • Systemic absorption especially likely with occlusive dressings, prolonged treatment, or extensive body-surface treatment. • Stop drug and notify doctor if patient develops signs of systemic absorption, skin irritation or ulceration, hypersensitivity, infection (if antifungals or antibiotics are being used with corticosteroids and infection does not respond immediately, corticosteroids should be stopped until infection is controlled). • Before applying, gently wash skin. To prevent damage to skin, rub in medication gently, leaving a thin coat. When treating hairy sites, part hair and apply directly to lesion. • Aerosol preparation contains alcohol and may produce irritation or burning in open lesions. When using about the face, cover patient's eyes and warn against inhalation of the spray. To avoid freezing tissues, do not spray longer than 3 seconds or closer than 6 inches. • For patient with eczematous dermatitis who may develop irritation with adhesive material, hold dressing in place with gauze, elastic bandages, or stockings. • Occlusive dressings are generally not used in presence of infection or with weeping or exudative lesions. • Change dressing as ordered by doctor. Inspect skin for infection, striae, and atrophy. Discontinue drug and notify doctor if these occur. • Instruct patient to report signs of drug sensitivity.
None significant.	• Contraindicated in viral diseases of skin, such as varicella, vaccinia, and herpes simplex; fungal infections; skin tuberculosis; impaired circulation. • Avoid application in or near eyes. • Systemic absorption especially likely with occlusive dressings, prolonged treatment, or extensive body-surface treatment. • Stop drug and notify doctor if patient develops signs of systemic absorption, skin irritation or ulceration, hypersensitivity, infection (if antifungals or antibiotics are being used with corticosteroids and infection does not respond immediately, corticosteroids should be stopped until infection is controlled). • Before applying, gently wash skin. To prevent damage to skin, rub in medication gently, leaving a thin coat. When treating hairy sites, part hair and apply directly to lesions. • Aerosol preparation contains alcohol and may produce irritation or burning in open lesions. When using about the face, cover patient's eyes and warn against inhalation of the spray. To avoid freezing tissues, do not spray longer than 3 seconds or closer than 6 inches. • Occlusive dressing: apply cream or ointment heavily, then cover with a thin, pliable, nonflammable plastic film; seal to adjacent normal skin with nonallergenic tape. Minimize adverse reactions by using occlusive dressing intermittently. • For patient with eczematous dermatitis who may develop irritation with adhesive material, hold dressing in place with gauze, elastic bandages, or stockings. • Tell doctor and remove occlusive dressing if body temperature rises. • Occlusive dressings are generally not used in presence of infection or with weeping or exudative lesions. • Change dressing as ordered by doctor. Inspect skin for infection, striae, and atrophy. Discontinue drug and notify doctor if these occur. • Treatment should be continued for a few days after clearing of lesions to prevent recurrence. • Instruct patient to report signs of drug sensitivity.

NAME	INDICATIONS & DOSAGE	SIDE EFFECTS
desonide Tridesilon♦	*Adjunctive therapy for inflammation in acute and chronic corticosteroid-responsive dermatoses—* **Adults and children:** clean area; apply cream, lotion, or gel sparingly b.i.d. to t.i.d.	*Metabolic:* adrenal insufficiency. *Skin:* burning, itching, irritation, dryness, folliculitis, hypopigmentation, perioral dermatitis, allergic contact dermatitis, hypertrichosis, acneiform eruptions. With occlusive dressings: maceration of skin, secondary infection, atrophy, striae, miliaria.
desoximetasone Topicort♦	*Inflammation of corticosteroid-responsive dermatoses—* **Adults and children:** clean area; apply cream sparingly b.i.d.	*Metabolic:* adrenal insufficiency. *Skin:* burning, itching, irritation, dryness, folliculitis, hypopigmentation, hypertrichosis, acneiform eruptions, perioral dermatitis, allergic contact dermatitis. With occlusive dressings: maceration of skin, secondary infection, atrophy, striae, miliaria.

INTERACTIONS	NURSING CONSIDERATIONS
None significant.	• Contraindicated in viral diseases of skin, such as varicella, vaccinia, and herpes simplex; fungal infections; skin tuberculosis; impaired circulation. • Avoid application in or near eyes. • Systemic absorption especially likely with occlusive dressings, prolonged treatment, or extensive body-surface treatment. • Stop drug and notify doctor if patient develops signs of systemic absorption, skin irritation or ulceration, hypersensitivity, infection (if antifungals or antibiotics are being used with corticosteroids and infection does not respond immediately, corticosteroids should be stopped until infection is controlled). • Before applying, gently wash skin. To prevent damage to skin, rub in medication gently, leaving a thin coat. When treating hairy sites, part hair and apply directly to lesion. • Occlusive dressing: apply cream heavily, then cover with a thin, pliable, nonflammable plastic film; seal to adjacent normal skin with nonallergenic tape. Minimize adverse reactions by using occlusive dressing intermittently. • For patient with eczematous dermatitis who may develop irritation with adhesive material, hold dressing in place with gauze, elastic bandages, or stockings. • Tell doctor and remove occlusive dressing if body temperature rises. • Occlusive dressings are generally not used in presence of infection or with weeping or exudative lesions. • Change dressing as ordered by doctor. Inspect skin for infection, striae, and atrophy. Discontinue drug and notify doctor if these occur. • Treatment should be continued for a few days after clearing of lesions to prevent recurrence. • Instruct patient to report signs of drug sensitivity.
None significant.	• Contraindicated in viral diseases of skin, such as varicella, vaccinia, and herpes simplex; fungal infections; skin tuberculosis; impaired circulation. • Avoid application in or near eyes. • Systemic absorption especially likely with occlusive dressings, prolonged treatment, or extensive body-surface treatment. • Stop drug and notify doctor if patient develops signs of systemic absorption, skin irritation or ulceration, hypersensitivity, infection (if antifungals or antibiotics are being used with corticosteroids and infection does not respond immediately, corticosteroids should be stopped until infection is controlled). • Before applying, gently wash skin. To prevent damage to skin, rub in medication gently, leaving a thin coat. When treating hairy sites, part hair and apply directly to lesions. • Occlusive dressing: apply cream heavily, then cover with a thin, pliable, nonflammable plastic film; seal to adjacent normal skin with nonallergenic tape. To minimize adverse reactions, use occlusive dressing intermittently. • For patient with eczematous dermatitis who may develop irritation with adhesive material, hold dressing in place with gauze, elastic bandages, or stockings. • Tell doctor and remove occlusive dressing if body temperature rises. • Occlusive dressings are generally not used in presence of infection or with weeping or exudative lesions. • Change dressing as ordered by doctor. Inspect skin for infection, striae, and atrophy. Discontinue drug and notify doctor if these occur. • Treatment should be continued for a few days after clearing of lesions to prevent recurrence. • Instruct patient to report signs of drug sensitivity.

NAME	INDICATIONS & DOSAGE	SIDE EFFECTS
dexamethasone Aeroseb-Dex, Decaderm, Decaspray, Hexadrol♦	*Inflammation of corticosteroid-responsive dermatoses*— **Adults and children:** clean area; apply cream, gel, or aerosol sparingly b.i.d. to q.i.d. Aerosol use on scalp: shake can well and apply to dry scalp after shampoo. Hold can upright. Slide applicator tube under hair so that it touches scalp. Spray while moving tube to all affected areas, keeping tube under hair and in contact with scalp throughout spraying, which should take about 2 seconds. Inadequately covered areas may be spot sprayed. Slide applicator tube through hair to touch scalp, press and immediately release spray button. Don't massage medication into scalp or spray forehead or eyes.	*Metabolic:* adrenal insufficiency with systemic absorption. *Skin:* burning, itching, irritation, dryness, folliculitis, hypopigmentation, hypertrichosis, acneiform eruptions, perioral dermatitis, allergic contact dermatitis. With occlusive dressings: maceration of skin, secondary infection, atrophy, striae, miliaria.
dexamethasone sodium phosphate Decadron Phosphate♦	*Inflammation of corticosteroid-responsive dermatoses*— **Adults and children:** clean area; apply cream sparingly b.i.d. to t.i.d.	*Metabolic:* adrenal insufficiency. *Skin:* burning, itching, irritation, dryness, folliculitis, hypopigmentation, hypertrichosis, acneiform eruptions, perioral dermatitis, allergic contact dermatitis. With occlusive dressings: maceration of skin, secondary infection, atrophy, striae, miliaria.

INTERACTIONS	NURSING CONSIDERATIONS
None significant.	• Contraindicated in viral diseases of skin, such as varicella, vaccinia, and herpes simplex; fungal infections; skin tuberculosis; impaired circulation. • Avoid application in or near eyes. • Systemic absorption especially likely with occlusive dressings, prolonged treatment, or extensive body-surface treatment. • Stop drug and notify doctor if patient develops signs of systemic absorption, skin irritation or ulceration, signs of hypersensitivity, infection (if antifungals or antibiotics are being used with corticosteroids and infection does not respond immediately, corticosteroids should be stopped until infection is controlled). • Before applying, gently wash skin. To prevent damage to skin, rub in medication gently, leaving a thin coat. When treating hairy sites, part hair and apply directly to lesions. • Occlusive dressing: apply cream heavily and cover with a thin, pliable, nonflammable plastic film; seal to adjacent normal skin with nonallergenic tape. To minimize adverse reactions, use occlusive dressing intermittently. • For patient with eczematous dermatitis who may develop irritation with adhesive material, hold dressing in place with gauze, elastic bandages, or stockings. • Tell doctor and remove occlusive dressing if body temperature rises. • Change dressing as ordered by doctor. Inspect skin for infection, striae, and atrophy. Discontinue drug and notify doctor if these occur. • Occlusive dressings are generally not used in presence of infection or with weeping or exudative lesions. • Aerosol preparation contains alcohol and may produce irritation or burning in open lesions. When using about the face, cover patient's eyes and warn against inhalation of the spray. To avoid freezing tissues, do not spray longer than 3 seconds or closer than 6 inches. • Treatments should be continued for a few days after clearing of lesions to prevent recurrence. • Instruct patient to report signs of drug sensitivity.
None significant.	• Contraindicated in viral diseases of skin, such as varicella, vaccinia, and herpes simplex; fungal infections; skin tuberculosis; impaired circulation. • Avoid application in or near eyes. • Systemic absorption especially likely with occlusive dressings, prolonged treatment, or extensive body-surface treatment. • Stop drug and notify doctor if patient develops signs of systemic absorption, skin irritation or ulceration, hypersensitivity, infection (if antifungals or antibiotics are being used along with corticosteroids and infection does not respond immediately, corticosteroids should be stopped until infection is controlled). • Before applying, gently wash skin. To prevent damage to skin, rub in medication gently, leaving a thin coat. When treating hairy sites, part hair and apply directly to lesions. • Occlusive dressing: apply cream heavily, then cover with a thin, pliable, nonflammable plastic film; seal to adjacent normal skin with nonallergenic tape. To minimize adverse reactions, use occlusive dressing intermittently. Occlusive dressings are generally not used in presence of infection or with weeping or exudative lesions. • For patient with eczematous dermatitis who may develop irritation with adhesive material, hold dressing in place with gauze, elastic bandages, or stockings. • Tell doctor and remove occlusive dressing if body temperature rises. • Change dressing as ordered by doctor. Inspect skin for infection, striae, and atrophy. Discontinue drug and notify doctor if these occur. • Treatment should be continued for a few days after clearing of lesions to prevent recurrence. • Instruct patient to report signs of drug sensitivity.

NAME	INDICATIONS & DOSAGE	SIDE EFFECTS
diflorasone diacetate Florone	*Inflammation of corticosteroid-responsive dermatoses, including psoriasis and the eczematous dermatoses (atopic dermatitis, neurodermatitis, contact dermatitis, nummular dermatitis, and seborrheic dermatitis)—* **Adults and children:** clean area; apply ointment daily to t.i.d.; apply cream b.i.d. to q.i.d.	*Metabolic:* adrenal insufficiency. *Skin:* burning, itching, irritation, dryness, folliculitis, hypopigmentation, perioral dermatitis, hypertrichosis, acneiform eruptions. With occlusive dressings: maceration, secondary infection, atrophy, striae, miliaria.
flumethasone pivalate Locacorten◆◆, Locorten	*Inflammation of corticosteroid-responsive dermatoses—* **Adults and children:** clean area; apply cream sparingly t.i.d. to q.i.d.	*Metabolic:* adrenal insufficiency. *Skin:* burning, itching, irritation, dryness, folliculitis, hypopigmentation hypertrichosis, acneiform eruptions, perioral dermatitis, allergic contact dermatitis. With occlusive dressings: maceration of skin, secondary infection, atrophy, striae, miliaria.

INTERACTIONS	NURSING CONSIDERATIONS
None significant.	• Contraindicated in viral diseases of skin, such as varicella, vaccinia, and herpes simplex; fungal infections; skin tuberculosis; impaired circulation. • Avoid application in or near eyes. • Systemic absorption especially likely with occlusive dressings, prolonged treatment, or extensive body-surface treatment. • Stop drug and notify doctor if patient develops signs of systemic absorption, skin irritation or ulceration, hypersensitivity, infection (if antifungals or antibiotics are being used concomitantly, corticosteroids should be stopped until infection is controlled). • Before applying, gently wash skin. To prevent damage to skin, rub in medication gently, leaving a thin coat. When treating hairy sites, part hair and apply directly to lesion. • Occlusive dressing; apply cream or ointment heavily, then cover with a thin, pliable, nonflammable plastic film; seal to adjacent normal skin with nonallergenic tape. Minimize adverse reactions by using occlusive dressing intermittently. Occlusive dressings are generally not used in presence of infection or with weeping or exudative lesions. • For patient with eczematous dermatitis who may develop irritation with adhesive material, hold dressing in place with gauze, elastic bandages, or stockings. • Tell doctor and remove occlusive dressing if body temperature rises. • Change dressing as ordered by doctor. Inspect skin for infection, striae, and atrophy. Discontinue drug and notify doctor if these occur. • Instruct patient to report signs of drug sensitivity. • Diflorasone is often effective with once daily application.
None significant.	• Contraindicated in viral diseases of skin, such as varicella, vaccinia, and herpes simplex; fungal infections; skin tuberculosis; and impaired circulation. • Avoid application in or near eyes. • Systemic absorption especially likely with occlusive dressings, prolonged treatment, or extensive body-surface treatment. • Stop drug and notify doctor if patient develops signs of systemic absorption, skin irritation or ulceration, hypersensitivity, infection (if antifungals or antibiotics are being used along with corticosteroids and infection does not respond immediately, corticosteroids should be stopped until infection is controlled). • Before applying, gently wash skin. To prevent damage to skin, rub in medication gently, leaving a thin coat. When treating hairy sites, part hair and apply directly to lesion. • Occlusive dressing: apply cream heavily, then cover with a thin, pliable, nonflammable plastic film; seal to adjacent normal skin with nonallergenic tape. To minimize adverse reactions, use occlusive dressing intermittently. Occlusive dressings are generally not used in presence of infection or with weeping or exudative lesions. • For patient with eczematous dermatitis who may develop irritation with adhesive material, hold dressing in place with gauze, elastic bandages, or stockings. • Tell doctor and remove occlusive dressing if body temperature rises. • Change dressing as ordered by doctor. Inspect skin for infection, striae, and atrophy. Discontinue drug and notify doctor if these occur. • Treatment should be continued for a few days after clearing of lesions to prevent recurrence. • Instruct patient to report signs of drug sensitivity.

NAME	INDICATIONS & DOSAGE	SIDE EFFECTS
fluocinolone acetonide Fluonid, Synalar◆, Synalar-HP◆, Synamol◆	*Inflammation of corticosteroid-responsive dermatoses*— **Adults, and children over 2:** clean area; apply cream, ointment, or solution sparingly b.i.d. to q.i.d. Treat multiple or extensive lesions sequentially, applying to only small areas at any one time.	*Metabolic:* adrenal insufficiency. *Skin:* burning, itching, irritation, dryness, folliculitis, hypopigmentation, hypertrichosis, acneiform eruptions, perioral dermatitis, allergic contact dermatitis. With occlusive dressings: maceration of skin, secondary infection, atrophy, striae, miliaria.
fluocinonide Lidemol◆◆, Lidex◆, Lidex-E, Topsyn◆	*Inflammation of corticosteroid-responsive dermatoses*— **Adults and children:** clean area; apply cream, ointment, or gel sparingly t.i.d. to q.i.d.	*Metabolic:* adrenal insufficiency. *Skin:* burning, itching, irritation, dryness, folliculitis, hypopigmentation, hypertrichosis, acneiform eruptions, perioral dermatitis, allergic contact dermatitis. With occlusive dressings: maceration of skin, secondary infection, atrophy, striae, miliaria.

INTERACTIONS	NURSING CONSIDERATIONS
None significant.	• Contraindicated in viral diseases of skin, such as varicella, vaccinia, and herpes simplex; fungal infections; skin tuberculosis; impaired circulation. • Avoid application in or near eyes. • Systemic absorption especially likely with occlusive dressings, prolonged treatment, or extensive body-surface treatment. • Stop drug and notify doctor if patient develops signs of systemic absorption, skin irritation or ulceration, hypersensitivity, infection (if antifungals or antibiotics are being used with corticosteroids and infection does not respond immediately, corticosteroids should be stopped until infection is controlled). • Before applying, gently wash skin. To prevent damage to skin, rub in medication gently, leaving a thin coat. When treating hairy sites, part hair and apply directly to lesion. • Occlusive dressing: apply gently and sparingly to the lesion until cream disappears. Then reapply, leaving a thin coat. Cover with a thin, pliable, nonflammable plastic film; seal to adjacent normal skin with nonallergenic tape. To minimize adverse reactions, use occlusive dressing intermittently. Occlusive dressings are generally not used in presence of infection or with weeping or exudative lesions. • For patient with eczematous dermatitis who may develop irritation with adhesive material, hold dressing in place with gauze, elastic bandages, or stockings. • Tell doctor and remove occlusive dressing if body temperature rises. • Change dressing as ordered by doctor. Inspect skin for infection, striae, and atrophy. Discontinue drug and notify doctor if these occur. • Instruct patient to report signs of drug sensitivity. • Fluonid solution on dry lesions may increase dryness, scaling, or itching; on denuded or fissured areas, may produce burning or stinging. If burning or stinging persists and dermatitis has not improved, solution should be discontinued.
None significant.	• Contraindicated in viral diseases of skin, such as varicella, vaccinia, and herpes simplex; untreated purulent bacterial skin infections; fungal infections; skin tuberculosis; impaired circulation. • Avoid application in or near eyes. • Systemic absorption especially likely with occlusive dressings, prolonged treatment, or extensive body-surface treatment. • Stop drug and notify doctor if patient develops signs of systemic absorption, skin irritation or ulceration, hypersensitivity, infection (if antifungals or antibiotics are being used with corticosteroids and infection does not respond immediately, corticosteroids should be stopped until infection is controlled). • Before applying, gently wash skin. To prevent damage to skin, rub in medication gently, leaving a thin coat. When treating hairy sites, part hair and apply directly to lesion. • Occlusive dressing: apply cream or ointment heavily, then cover with a thin, pliable, nonflammable plastic film; seal to adjacent normal skin with nonallergenic tape. To minimize adverse reactions, use occlusive dressing intermittently. Occlusive dressings are generally not used in presence of infection or with weeping or exudative lesions. • For patient with eczematous dermatitis who may develop irritation with adhesive material, hold dressing in place with gauze, elastic bandages, or stockings. • Tell doctor and remove occlusive dressings if body temperature rises. • Change dressing as ordered by doctor. Inspect skin for infection, striae, and atrophy. Discontinue drug and notify doctor if these occur. • Treatment should be continued for a few days after clearing of lesions to prevent recurrence. • Instruct patient to report signs of drug sensitivity.

NAME	INDICATIONS & DOSAGE	SIDE EFFECTS
fluorometholone Oxylone	*Inflammation of corticosteroid-responsive dermatoses—* **Adults and children:** clean area; apply cream sparingly daily to t.i.d.	*Metabolic:* adrenal insufficiency. *Skin:* burning, itching, irritation, dryness, folliculitis, hypopigmentation, hypertrichosis, acneiform eruptions, perioral dermatitis, allergic contact dermatitis. With occlusive dressings: maceration of skin, secondary infection, atrophy, striae, miliaria.
flurandrenolide Cordran, Cordran SP, Cordran Tape, Drenison♦♦, Drenison ¼♦♦, Drenison Tape♦♦	*Inflammation of corticosteroid-responsive dermatoses—* **Adults and children:** clean area; apply cream, lotion, or ointment sparingly b.i.d. or t.i.d. Apply tape q 12 to 24 hours. Before applying tape, cleanse skin carefully, removing scales, crust, and dried exudates. Allow skin to dry for 1 hour before applying new tape. Shave or clip hair to allow good contact with skin and comfortable removal. If tape ends loosen prematurely, trim off and replace with fresh tape. Lowest incidence of adverse reactions if tape is replaced q 12 hours but may be left in place for 24 hours if well tolerated and adheres satisfactorily. Drenison ¼: for maintenance therapy of widespread or chronic lesions.	*Metabolic:* adrenal insufficiency. *Skin:* burning, itching, irritation, dryness, folliculitis, hypopigmentation, hypertrichosis, acneiform eruptions, allergic contact dermatitis. With occlusive dressings: maceration of skin, secondary infection, atrophy, striae, miliaria. With tape: purpura, stripping of epidermis, furunculosis.

INTERACTIONS	NURSING CONSIDERATIONS
None significant.	• Contraindicated in viral diseases of skin, such as varicella, vaccinia, and herpes simplex; fungal infections; skin tuberculosis; impaired circulation. • Avoid application in or near eyes. • Systemic absorption especially likely with occlusive dressings, prolonged treatment, or extensive body-surface treatment. • Stop drug and notify doctor if patient develops signs of systemic absorption, skin irritation or ulceration, hypersensitivity, infection (if antifungals or antibiotics are being used with corticosteroids and infection does not respond immediately, corticosteroids should be stopped until infection is controlled). • Before applying, gently wash skin. To prevent damage to skin, rub in medication gently, leaving a thin coat. When treating hairy sites, part hair and apply directly to lesion. • Occlusive dressing: apply cream heavily, then cover with a thin, pliable, nonflammable plastic film; seal to adjacent normal skin with nonallergenic tape. To minimize adverse reactions, use occlusive dressing intermittently. Occlusive dressings are generally not used in presence of infection or with weeping or exudative lesions. • For patient with eczematous dermatitis who may develop irritation with adhesive material, hold dressing in place with gauze, elastic bandages, or stockings. • Tell doctor and remove occlusive dressing if body temperature rises. • Change dressing as ordered by doctor. Inspect skin for infection, striae, and atrophy. Discontinue drug and notify doctor if these occur. • Treatment should be continued for a few days after clearing of lesions to prevent recurrence. • Instruct patient to report signs of drug sensitivity.
None significant.	• Contraindicated in viral diseases of skin, such as varicella, vaccinia, and herpes simplex; fungal infections; skin tuberculosis; impaired circulation. • Tape not advised for exudative lesions or those in intertriginous areas. • Avoid application in or near eyes. • Systemic absorption especially likely with occlusive dressings, prolonged treatment, or extensive body-surface treatment. • Stop drug and notify doctor if patient develops signs of systemic absorption, skin irritation or ulceration, hypersensitivity, infection (if antifungals or antibiotics are being used with corticosteroids and infection does not respond immediately, corticosteroids should be stopped until infection is controlled). • Before applying, gently wash skin. To prevent damage to skin, rub in medication gently, leaving a thin coat. When treating hairy sites, part hair and apply directly to lesion. • Occlusive dressing: apply cream heavily, then cover with a thin, pliable, nonflammable plastic film; seal to adjacent normal skin with nonallergenic tape. To minimize adverse reactions, use occlusive dressing intermittently. Occlusive dressings are generally not used in presence of infection or with weeping or exudative lesions. • For patient with eczematous dermatitis who may develop irritation with adhesive material, hold dressing in place with gauze, elastic bandages, or stockings. • Tell doctor and remove occlusive dressing if body temperature rises. • Change dressing as ordered by doctor. Inspect skin for infection, striae, and atrophy. Discontinue drug and notify doctor if these occur. • Treatment should be continued for a few days after clearing of lesions to prevent recurrence. • Instruct patient to report signs of drug sensitivity.

NAME	INDICATIONS & DOSAGE	SIDE EFFECTS
halcinonide Halog◆	*Inflammation of acute and chronic corticosteroid-responsive dermatoses—* **Adults and children:** clean area; apply cream, ointment, or solution sparingly b.i.d. to t.i.d.	*Metabolic:* adrenal insufficiency. *Skin:* burning, itching, irritation, dryness, folliculitis, hypopigmentation, hypertrichosis, acneiform eruptions, allergic contact dermatitis. With occlusive dressings: maceration of skin, secondary infection, atrophy, striae, miliaria.
hydrocortisone Acticort, Aeroseb-HC◆, Carmol-HC, Cetacort, Cort-Dome◆, Corticreme◆◆, Cortinal, Cortril◆, Cotacort, Cremesone, Delacort, Dermacort, Durel-Cort, Ecosone, Eldecort, Emo-Cort◆◆, Epicort, HC Cream, Heb-Cort, HI-COR-2.5, Hycort, Hycortole, Hydrocortex, Hydro-Cortilean◆◆, Hytone, Ivocort, Manticor◆◆, Maso-Cort, Micro-	*Inflammation of corticosteroid-responsive dermatoses; adjunctive typical management of seborrhea dermatitis of scalp—* **Adults and children:** clean area; apply cream, lotion, ointment, or aerosol sparingly daily to q.i.d. Aerosol: shake can well. Direct spray onto affected area from a distance of 6 inches. Apply for only 3 seconds (to avoid freezing tissues). Apply to dry scalp after shampooing; no need to massage or rub medication into scalp after spraying. Apply daily until acute phase is controlled, then reduce dosage to 1 to 3 times a week as needed to maintain control.	*Metabolic:* adrenal insufficiency. *Skin:* burning, itching, irritation, dryness, folliculitis, hypopigmentation, hypertrichosis, acneiform eruptions, allergic contact dermatitis. With occlusive dressings: maceration of skin, secondary infection, atrophy , striae, miliaria.

INTERACTIONS	NURSING CONSIDERATIONS
None significant.	• Contraindicated in viral diseases of skin, such as varicella, vaccinia, and herpes simplex; fungal infections; skin tuberculosis; impaired circulation. • Avoid application in or near eyes. • Systemic absorption especially likely with occlusive dressings, prolonged treatment, or extensive body-surface treatment. • Stop drug and notify doctor if patient develops signs of systemic absorption, skin irritation or ulceration, hypersensitivity, infection (if antifungals or antibiotics are being used with corticosteroids and infection does not respond immediately, corticosteroids should be stopped until infection is controlled). • Before applying, gently wash skin. To prevent damage to skin, rub in medication gently, leaving a thin coat. When treating hairy sites, part hair and apply directly to lesion. • Occlusive dressing with cream: gently rub small amount into lesion until it disappears. Reapply, leaving a thin coating on lesion, and cover with occlusive dressing. With ointment: apply to lesion and cover with occlusive dressing. Cover with a thin, pliable, nonflammable plastic film; seal to adjacent normal skin with nonallergenic tape. To minimize adverse reactions, use occlusive dressing intermittently, or with extensive lesions occlude one part of the body at a time. • Good results have been obtained by applying occlusive dressings in the evening and removing them in the morning (i.e., 12-hour occlusion). Should then be reapplied in the morning, without using the occlusive dressings during the day. • For patient with eczematous dermatitis who may develop irritation with adhesive material, hold dressing in place with gauze, elastic bandages, or stockings. • Tell doctor and remove occlusive dressing if body temperature rises. • Occlusive dressings are generally not used in presence of infection or with weeping or exudative lesions. • Change dressing as ordered by doctor. Inspect skin for infection, striae, and atrophy. Discontinue drug and notify doctor if these occur. • Treatment should be continued for a few days after clearing of lesions to prevent recurrence. • Instruct patient to report signs of drug sensitivity.
None significant.	• Contraindicated in viral diseases of skin, such as varicella, vaccinia, and herpes simplex; fungal infections; skin tuberculosis; impaired circulation. • Avoid application in or near eyes. • Systemic absorption especially likely with occlusive dressings, prolonged treatment, or extensive body-surface treatment. • Stop drug and notify doctor if patient develops signs of systemic absorption, skin irritation or ulceration, hypersensitivity, infection (if antifungals or antibiotics are being used with corticosteroids and infection does not respond immediately, corticosteroids should be stopped until infection is controlled). • Before applying, gently wash skin. To prevent damage to skin, rub in medication gently, leaving a thin coat. When treating hairy sites, part hair and apply directly to lesions. • Occlusive dressing: apply cream heavily, then cover with a thin, pliable, nonflammable plastic film; seal to adjacent normal skin with nonallergenic tape. To minimize adverse reactions, use occlusive dressing intermittently. Occlusive dressings are generally not used in presence of infection or with weeping or exudative lesions. • For patient with eczematous dermatitis who may develop irritation with

(continued on following page)

NAME	INDICATIONS & DOSAGE	SIDE EFFECTS
hydrocortisone *(continued)* cort◆, Nutracort◆, Proctocort, Rectocort◆◆, Relecort, Rocort, Tarcortin, Ulcort, Unicort		
hydrocortisone acetate Cortifoam, Cortiprel, Cortef Acetate, Hydrocortisone Acetate, Hydrocortone Acetate, My-Cort Lotion	*Inflammation of corticosteroid-responsive dermatoses*— **Adults and children:** clean area; apply lotion, cream, ointment, or foam sparingly daily to q.i.d.	*Metabolic:* adrenal insufficiency. *Skin:* burning, itching, irritation, dryness, folliculitis, hypopigmentation, hypertrichosis, acneiform eruptions, perioral dermatitis, allergic contact dermatitis. With occlusive dressings: maceration of skin, secondary infection, atrophy, striae, miliaria.
hydrocortisone valerate Westcort Cream	**Adults and children:** massage gently 2 to 3 times daily p.r.n.	
methylprednisolone acetate Medrol Acetate◆	*Inflammation of corticosteroid-responsive dermatoses*— **Adults and children:** clean area; apply ointment daily to t.i.d.	*Metabolic:* adrenal insufficiency. *Skin:* burning, itching, irritation, dryness, folliculitis, hypopigmentation, hypertrichosis, acneiform eruptions, allergic contact dermatitis. With occlusive dressings: maceration of skin, secondary infection, atrophy, striae, miliaria.

INTERACTIONS	NURSING CONSIDERATIONS
	adhesive material, it may be helpful to hold dressing in place with gauze, elastic bandages, or stockings. • Tell doctor and remove occlusive dressing if body temperature rises. • Aerosol preparation contains alcohol, and may produce irritation or burning in open lesions. When using about the face, cover patient's eyes and warn against inhalation of the spray. To avoid freezing tissues, do not spray longer than 3 seconds, or closer than 6 inches. • Change dressing as ordered by doctor. Inspect skin for infection, striae, and atrophy. Discontinue drug and notify doctor if these occur. • Treatment should be continued for a few days following clearing of lesions to prevent recurrence. • Instruct patient to report signs of drug sensitivity.
None significant.	• Contraindicated in viral diseases of skin, such as varicella, vaccinia, and herpes simplex; fungal infections; skin tuberculosis; impaired circulation. • Avoid application in or near eyes. • Systemic absorption especially likely with occlusive dressings, prolonged treatment, or extensive body-surface treatment. • Stop drug and notify doctor if patient develops signs of systemic absorption, skin irritation or ulceration, hypersensitivity, infection (if antifungals or antibiotics are being used with corticosteroids and infection does not respond immediately, corticosteroids should be stopped until infection is controlled). • Before applying, gently wash skin. To prevent damage to skin, rub in medication gently, leaving a thin coat. When treating hairy sites, part hair and apply directly to lesion. • Occlusive dressing: apply cream or ointment heavily, then cover with a thin, pliable, nonflammable plastic film; seal to adjacent normal skin with nonallergenic tape. To minimize adverse reactions, use occlusive dressings intermittently. Occlusive dressings are generally not used in presence of infection or with weeping or exudative lesions. • For patient with eczematous dermatitis who may develop irritation with adhesive material, hold dressing in place with gauze, elastic bandages, or stockings. • Tell doctor and remove occlusive dressing if body temperature rises. • Lotions and foams are not used with occlusive dressings. • Change dressing as ordered by doctor. Inspect skin for infection, striae, and atrophy. Discontinue drug and notify doctor if these occur. • Treatment should be continued for a few days after clearing of lesions to prevent recurrence. • Instruct patient to report signs of drug sensitivity.
None significant.	• Contraindicated in viral diseases of skin, such as varicella, vaccinia, and herpes simplex; fungal infections; skin tuberculosis; impaired circulation. • Avoid application in or near eyes. • Systemic absorption especially likely with occlusive dressings, prolonged treatment, or extensive body-surface treatment. • Stop drug and notify doctor if patient develops signs of systemic absorption, skin irritation or ulceration, hypersensitivity, infection (if antifungals or antibiotics are being used with corticosteroids and infection does not respond immediately, corticosteroids should be stopped until infection is controlled). • Before applying, gently wash skin. To prevent damage to skin, rub in medication gently, leaving a thin coat. When treating hairy sites, part hair and apply directly to lesion.

(continued on following page)

NAME	INDICATIONS & DOSAGE	SIDE EFFECTS
methylprednisolone acetate *(continued)*		
prednisolone Meti-Derm	*Inflammation of corticosteroid-responsive dermatoses*— **Adults and children:** clean area; apply cream or aerosol daily to q.i.d.	*Metabolic:* adrenal insufficiency. *Skin:* burning, itching, irritation, dryness, folliculitis, hypopigmentation, hypertrichosis, acneiform eruptions, perioral dermatitis, allergic contact dermatitis. With occlusive dressings: maceration of skin, secondary infection, atrophy, striae, miliaria.

INTERACTIONS	NURSING CONSIDERATIONS
	• Occlusive dressing: apply ointment heavily, then cover with a thin, pliable, nonflammable plastic film; seal to adjacent normal skin with nonallergenic tape. To minimize adverse effects, use occlusive dressing intermittently. Occlusive dressings are generally not used in presence of infection or with weeping or exudative lesions. • For patient with eczematous dermatitis who may develop irritation with adhesive material, hold dressing in place with gauze, elastic bandages, or stockings. • Tell doctor and remove occlusive dressing if body temperature rises. • Change dressing as ordered by doctor. Inspect skin for infection, striae, and atrophy. Discontinue drug and notify doctor if these occur. • Treatment should be continued for a few days after clearing of lesions to prevent recurrence. • Instruct patient to report signs of drug sensitivity.
None significant.	• Contraindicated in viral diseases of skin, such as varicella, vaccinia, and herpes simplex; fungal infections; skin tuberculosis; impaired circulation. • Avoid application in or near eyes. • Systemic absorption especially likely with occlusive dressings, prolonged treatment, or extensive body-surface treatment. • Stop drug and notify doctor if patient develops signs of systemic absorption, skin irritation or ulceration, hypersensitivity, infection (if antifungals or antibiotics are being used with corticosteroids and infection does not respond immediately, corticosteroids should be stopped until infection is controlled). • Before applying, gently wash skin. To prevent damage to skin, rub in medication gently, leaving a thin coat. When treating hairy sites, part hair and apply directly to lesions. • Aerosol preparation contains alcohol, and may produce irritation or burning in open lesions. When using about the face, cover patient's eyes and warn against inhalation of the spray. To avoid freezing tissues, do not spray longer than 3 seconds, or closer than 6 inches. • Occlusive dressing: apply cream heavily and cover with a thin, pliable, nonflammable plastic film; seal to adjacent normal skin with nonallergenic tape. To minimize adverse reactions, use occlusive dressing intermittently. Occlusive dressings are generally not used in presence of infection or with weeping or exudative lesions. • For patient with eczematous dermatitis who may develop irritation with adhesive material, hold dressing in place with gauze, elastic bandages, or stockings. • Tell doctor and remove occlusive dressing if body temperature rises. • Change dressing as ordered by doctor. Inspect skin for infection, striae, and atrophy. Discontinue drug and notify doctor if these occur. • Treatment should be continued for a few days after clearing of lesions to prevent recurrence. • Instruct patient to report signs of drug sensitivity.

NAME	INDICATIONS & DOSAGE	SIDE EFFECTS
triamcinolone acetonide Aristocort◆, Aristocort A, Aristogel, Kenalog◆, Triamalone◆◆	*Inflammation of corticosteroid-responsive dermatoses—* **Adults and children:** clean area; apply cream, ointment, lotion, foam, or aerosol sparingly b.i.d. to q.i.d. Aerosol: shake can well. Direct spray onto affected area from a distance of approximately 6 inches, and apply for only 3 seconds.	*Metabolic:* adrenal insufficiency. *Skin:* burning, itching, irritation, dryness, folliculitis, hypopigmentation, hypertrichosis, acneiform eruptions, perioral dermatitis, allergic contact dermatitis. With occlusive dressings: maceration of skin, secondary infection, atrophy, striae, miliaria.

INTERACTIONS	NURSING CONSIDERATIONS
None significant.	• Contraindicated in viral diseases of skin, such as varicella, vaccinia, and herpes simplex; fungal infections; skin tuberculosis; impaired circulation. • Avoid application in or near eyes. • Systemic absorption especially likely with occlusive dressings, prolonged treatment, or extensive body-surface treatment. • Stop drug and notify doctor if patient develops signs of systemic absorption, skin irritation or ulceration, hypersensitivity, infection (if antifungals or antibiotics are being used with corticosteroids and infection does not respond immediately, corticosteroids should be stopped until infection is controlled). • Before applying, gently wash skin. To prevent damage to skin, rub in medication gently, leaving a thin coat. When treating hairy sites, part hair and apply directly to lesion. • Aerosol preparation contains alcohol, and may produce irritation or burning in open lesions. When using about the face, cover patient's eyes and warn against inhalation of the spray. To avoid freezing tissues, do not spray longer than 3 seconds, or closer than 6 inches. • Occlusive dressing: apply cream or ointment heavily, then cover with a thin, pliable, nonflammable plastic film; seal to adjacent normal skin with nonallergenic tape. To minimize adverse reactions, use occlusive dressing intermittently. Occlusive dressings are generally not used in presence of infection or with weeping or exudative lesions. • For patient with eczematous dermatitis who may develop irritation with adhesive material, hold dressing in place with gauze, elastic bandages, or stockings. • Tell doctor and remove occlusive dressing if body temperature rises. • Change dressing as ordered by doctor. Inspect skin for infection, striae, and atrophy. Discontinue drug and notify doctor if these occur. • Treatment should be continued for a few days after clearing of lesions to prevent recurrence. • Instruct patient to report signs of drug sensitivity.

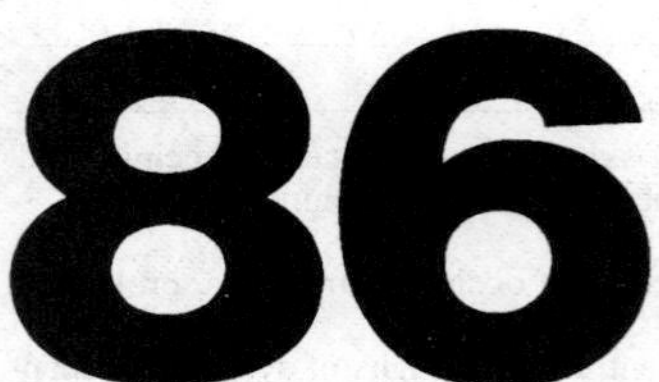

Antipruritics and local anesthetics

benzocaine
camphor
dibucaine hydrochloride
dimethisoquin hydrochloride
diperodon hydrochloride
dyclonine hydrochloride
ethyl chloride
lidocaine hydrochloride
menthol
phenol
pramoxine hydrochloride
tars
tetracaine hydrochloride

These topical preparations are used to produce local anesthesia and to relieve discomfort and pruritus. Agents in this category provide temporary relief or local anesthesia and should not be used indefinitely.

Major uses

- Relieve skin discomfort caused by minor burns, cuts, diaper rash, fungus infections, sunburn, hemorrhoids, insect bites, hives, eczema, skin ulcers, pruritus ani and vulvae.
- Provide surface anesthesia to mucous membranes and rectum. Often used before endoscopic procedures.

Mechanism of action

- Local anesthetics block conduction of nerve impulses at the sensory nerve endings.

Absorption, distribution, and excretion

- Local anesthetics may be absorbed through abraded skin, but when applied to intact skin, absorption is poor.

Onset and duration

- For most agents in this category, onset is rapid.
- Duration varies according to the chemical structure of the agent. Ethyl chloride, when used for local anesthesia, has a very short duration. Dyclonine hydrochloride has a duration of 30 to 45 minutes; dimethisoquin hydrochloride, 2 to 4 hours; benzocaine and pramoxine hydrochloride, prolonged duration.

Combination products

BALNETAR•: water-dispersible emollient tar 2.5% in lanolin fraction, mineral oil, and nonionic emulsifiers.

CARMOL-HC◆: urea 10% and hydrocortisone 1%.
CETACAINE LIQUID: benzocaine 14%, tetracaine HC1 2%, benzalkonium chloride 0.5%, butyl aminobenzoate 2%, and cetyl dimethyl ethyl ammonium bromide in a bland water-soluble base.
CETACAINE OINTMENT: benzocaine 14%, tetracaine HC1 2%, butyl aminobenzoate 2%, benzalkonium chloride 0.5%, and cetyl dimethyl ethyl ammonium bromide in a bland water-soluble base.
CHIGGERTOX LIQUID: benzocaine 2.1% and benzyl benzoate in an isopropanol base.
COR-TAR-QUIN◆: coal tar solution USP 2%, diiodohydroxyquinoline 1% with hydrocortisone ¼, ½, or 1% in an acid-mantle vehicle.
CUTAR BATH OIL EMULSION: coal tar solution 7.5% in liquid petrolatum, isopropyl myristate, acetylated lanolin, lanolin alcohols extract, and water.
DERMA-MEDICONE OINTMENT: benzocaine 2%, zinc oxide 13.7%, oxyquinoline sulfate 1.05%, ichthammol 1%, and menthol 0.48% in petrolatum and lanolin base.
DERMOPLAST SPRAY◆: benzocaine 4.5%, oxyquinoline benzoate 1.2%, benzethonium chloride 0.1% with menthol, vegetable oils, methylparaben 2%, and isopropyl alcohol 1.9%.
ESTARGEL◆: coal tar 5% and alcohol 29%.
LAVATAR◆: tar distillate 3.3% in water-miscible emulsion base.
MEDICONE DRESSING (CREAM): benzocaine 0.5%, hydroxyquinoline-sulfate 0.05%, cod-liver oil 12.5%, zinc oxide 12.5%, and menthol with petrolatum, lanolin, talcum, and paraffin.
POLYTAR BATH◆: polytar 25% (juniper, pine, and coal tars) with 25% butyl stearate 25% in water-miscible emulsion base.
PRAGMATAR OINTMENT◆: cetyl alcohol-coal tar distillate 4%, precipitated sulfur 3%, and salicylic acid 3% in an oil-in-water emulsion base.
SEBUTONE◆: tar (equivalent to 0.5% coal tar) in surface-active soapless cleansers and wetting agents, sulfur 2%, and salicylic acid 2%.
TAR-DOAK LOTION◆: tar distillate 5% and nonionic emulsifiers.
VANSEB-T◆: coal tar solution USP 5% in perfumed base.
ZETAR EMULSION◆: 3% colloidol whole coal tar in polysorbates.
ZETAR SHAMPOO◆: whole coal tar 1% in foam shampoo base.

NAME	INDICATIONS & DOSAGE	SIDE EFFECTS
benzocaine Aerocaine, Americaine, Anbesol, Ben-Caine B.B., Benzocol, Col-Vi-Nol, Dermoplast, Hurricaine, Morusan, Rhulicream, Rhulihist, Solarcaine, Urolocaine	*Local anesthetic for pruritic dermatoses and localized idiopathic pruritus—* **Adults and children:** apply locally 2 or 3 times a day. *Hemorrhoids or rectal irritation—* **Adults and children:** apply ointment 2 or 3 times a day. Suppository: insert well into rectum morning, evening, and after each bowel movement. For other uses, see pp. 852 and 858.	*Blood:* methemoglobinemia (infants). *Local:* sensitization.
camphor	*Mild antipruritic and local anesthetic; counterirritant for use in sprains and rheumatic conditions—* **Adults and children:** apply a 1% to 3% lotion or ointment of camphor as needed.	None reported.
dibucaine hydrochloride D-caine, Dulzit, Nupercainal Cream◆, Nupercainal Ointment◆, Nupercainal Suppositories, Nuporals (Troches)	*Abrasions, sunburn, hemorrhoids, and other painful conditions—* **Adults and children:** 0.5% to 1% lotion or ointment applied locally several times a day. Suppositories: insert rectally morning, evening, and after every bowel movement. Also used as a local anesthetic for the mouth and throat.	*Local:* hypersensitivity.
dimethisoquin hydrochloride Quotane Cream◆◆, Quotane Ointment	*Surface pain and itching—* **Adults and children:** 0.5% ointment or lotion applied topically up to 4 times daily or as directed.	*Skin:* sensitization and contact dermatitis can develop.
diperodon hydrochloride Diothane Cream◆◆, Diothane Ointment◆, Proctodon	*Pain caused by minor burns and cuts (cream); pain caused by anorectal disorders (ointment)—* **Adults and children:** apply 3 to 4 times a day.	None reported.
dyclonine hydrochloride Dyclone	*To relieve surface pain and itching caused by minor burns or trauma, surgical wounds, pruritus ani or vulvae, insect bites, and pruritic*	*Local:* irritation at site of application may occur.

◆ Also available in Canada.
◆◆ Available in Canada only.
Unmarked trade names available in United States only.

INTERACTIONS	NURSING CONSIDERATIONS
None significant.	• Contraindicated in hypersensitivity to procaine or other para-aminobenzoic acid (PABA) derivatives (often used in topical sun-blocking agents). • Avoid contact with eyes. • If spray preparation used, hold can 6 to 12 inches from affected area and spray liberally. Avoid inhalation. • If using rectally, cleanse and thoroughly dry rectal area before applying.
None significant.	• Extremely toxic if taken orally. • Avoid contact with eyes. • Do not apply to broken skin or mucous membranes.
None significant.	• Avoid contact with eyes. • Before applying cream or ointment rectally or inserting suppository, cleanse and thoroughly dry rectal area.
None significant.	• Don't apply to extensive areas. • Avoid contact with eyes. • Avoid prolonged use for patients with chronic conditions.
None significant.	• Before applying cream or ointment rectally, cleanse and thoroughly dry rectal area.
None significant.	• Avoid prolonged use in patients with chronic conditions. • May be useful in patients hypersensitive to other local anesthetics because it is a ketone. • Contraindicated in cystoscopic exams following an IVP. Iodine-containing

(continued on following page)

NAME	INDICATIONS & DOSAGE	SIDE EFFECTS
dyclonine hydrochloride *(continued)*	*dermatoses. Also, to anesthetize mucous membranes before endoscopic procedures—* **Adults and children:** 0.5% solution or 1% ointment applied 3 or 4 times daily. *Urethral dilation or cystourethroscopy—* **Adults:** 10 ml of 0.5% solution may be instilled into the urethra.	
ethyl chloride Ethyl Chloride Spray	*For irritation—* **Adults and children:** hold container about 24 inches from skin and spray rhythmically to cover area evenly once or twice. Application may be repeated. *As a local anesthetic in minor operative procedures; relieves pain caused by insect stings and burns, and irritation caused by myofascial and visceral pain syndromes—* **Adults and children:** dosage varies with different procedures. Use smallest dosage needed to produce desired effect. For local anesthesia, hold container about 12 inches from area to produce a fine spray. **Infants:** hold a cotton ball saturated with ethyl chloride to injection site, and make injection when site dries.	*Skin:* sensitization; frostbite and tissue necrosis may occur with prolonged spraying. *Other:* excessive cooling may increase pain and muscle spasms.
lidocaine **lidocaine hydrochloride** Lida-Mantle cream, Stanacaine, Xylocaine Jelly (2%), Xylocaine Ointment◆ (2.5%), Xylocaine Ointment◆ (5%), Xylocaine Solution◆ (4%), Xylocaine Spray◆◆ (100 mg/l gm), Xylocaine Viscous Solution (2%)	*Local anesthesia of skin or mucous membrane—* **Adults and children:** apply liberally. *In procedures involving the male or female urethra—* **Adults:** instill about 15 ml (male) or 3 to 5 ml (female) into urethra. *Pain, burning, or itching caused by burns, sunburn, or skin irritation—* **Adults and children:** apply liberally. As a local anesthetic for ear, nose, and throat, see p. 860.	*Local:* hypersensitivity.

INTERACTIONS	NURSING CONSIDERATIONS
	contrast material will cause precipitate to form with dyclonine. • Can be combined with diphenhydramine elixir to provide an effective treatment for stomatitis.
None significant.	• Do not apply to broken skin or mucous membrane. • Protect skin adjacent to area treated with petrolatum to avoid tissue sloughing. • Avoid use near eyes. • Avoid inhalation when spraying. • Highly flammable; do not use in areas where open flames or sparks are possible.
None significant.	• Use with caution on severely traumatized mucosa or where sepsis is present or for anesthesia of oropharyngeal mucosa, since gag reflex may be suppressed and aspiration may occur.

NAME	INDICATIONS & DOSAGE	SIDE EFFECTS
menthol	*As an antipruritic—* **Adults and children:** apply 0.25% to 2% lotion or ointment as needed.	None reported.
phenol	*As an antipruritic—* **Adults and children:** apply 0.5% to 2% preparations locally several times a day.	None at recommended strengths.
pramoxine hydrochloride Proctofoam, Tronothane◆	*Pain and itching caused by dermatoses, minor burns, surgical wounds, and insect bites, hemorrhoids—* **Adults and children:** apply every 3 to 4 hours.	*Local:* stinging or burning, sensitization.
tars	*As an antipruritic—* **Adults and children:** apply preparations 2 to 3 times daily.	*Skin:* irritation, folliculitis, erythema.
tetracaine **tetracaine hydrochloride** Pontocaine◆	*For relief of pain in hemorrhoids, minor burns, ulcers, and poison ivy—* **Adults and children:** apply 5% ointment or 1% cream—no more than 1 oz. for adults or ¼ oz. for children in 24 hours.	*Local:* sensitization.

INTERACTIONS	NURSING CONSIDERATIONS
None significant.	• Relieves itching by substituting a cooling effect. • Avoid contact with eyes.
None significant.	• Avoid accidental contact with normal skin. If contact occurs, remove phenol with alcohol or vegetable oil. • Tissue necrosis possible with higher concentration or extensive use. • Avoid contact with eyes.
None significant.	• Can be safely used in those allergic to other local anesthetics. • May be applied with gauze or sprayed directly on skin. Avoid contact with eyes. • Cleanse and thoroughly dry rectal area before applying ointment or cream, or inserting suppository.
None significant.	• Use caution in applying tar preparations to patients with exacerbation of psoriasis. May precipitate total body exfoliation. • Never use under occlusive dressings. • Avoid excessive exposure to sunlight. • Darkens color of blond hair when applied to scalp.
None significant.	• Contraindicated in hypersensitivity to procaine, or other para-aminobenzoic acid (PABA) derivatives (often used in topical sun-blocking agents). • Before applying cream or ointment rectally, cleanse and thoroughly dry rectal area.

87
Astringents

acetic acid lotion
aluminum acetate
aluminum sulfate
hamamelis water
tannic acid

Astringents have many purposes. Externally applied—as they almost invariably are—they are toners, tonics, and comforting agents. An astringent causes contraction, drawing together soft organic tissues, shielding skin from infection, and protecting it from such unfriendly elements as cold and heat. Astringents are not recommended for relief of long-standing or serious infections.

Major uses

- Denture and throat irritation, trench mouth, gingivitis, minor external hemorrhoidal and outer vaginal discomfort, poison ivy, poison oak, sunburn, heat rash, minor burns, insect bites. (Preparations containing astringents are also used to treat ear canal infections. See Chapter 81, Otics).

Mechanism of action

- Astringents draw together soft organic tissues which shield skin from infection.
- Some agents draw blood toward the skin, causing rubefacience and a pleasant tingling sensation.
- Some agents with analgesic properties soothe and smooth affected areas.
- Some agents assist recovery by simple cleansing.

Absorption, distribution, and excretion

- Long-term use of astringents may result in excessive skin dryness.
- Distribution is confined to affected area.
- Large amounts of tannic acid in burn treatment may cause hepatic damage.
- Most astringents penetrate only skin-deep and can be washed or wiped away.

Onset and duration

- Most astringents begin to act almost immediately, although their effects may be transient.
- Continued use or additional applications of some astringents are required.

Combination products

ASTRINGENTS WITH ANESTHETICS, e.g., PNS Suppositories, Nupercainal Suppositories.
ASTRINGENTS WITH ANTIPRURITIC/ANTIHISTAMINE, e.g., Caladryl, Dri-toxen, Peterson's Ointment, Ziradryl.
ASTRINGENTS WITH ANTIPRURITIC/ANTIHISTAMINE AND ANESTHETIC, e.g., Ivy Dry, Rhulicream, Rhulihist, Rhulispray, Zotox.
ASTRINGENTS WITH ANTISEPTICS, e.g., Tucks Pads, Tanac, Lavoris.
ASTRINGENTS WITH ANTISEPTICS AND ANESTHETICS, e.g., Rectal Medicone Suppositories and Ointment, Tanicaine Suppositories and Ointment, Wyanoid Ointment, Pazo Suppository and Ointment, Gebauer's Tannic Spray.
ASTRINGENTS WITH DEODORANTS, e.g., most common antiperspirant/deodorants available.

HOW TO APPLY TANNIC ACID

When treating burns, follow these procedures:

- First, flush the burned areas with water or saline.
- Next, apply a thick layer of tannic acid to gauze dressings. Place the dressings on burned areas.
- Later, soak loose adherent gauze with normal or slightly hypertonic saline solution.
- A dark eschar will probably form. Leave it until it loosens and peels off on its own. You may, however, trim or cut away the edges.

NAME	INDICATIONS & DOSAGE	SIDE EFFECTS
acetic acid lotion (0.1% glacial acetic acid in alcohol)	*Superficial fungal or bacterial infection to toughen skin and prevent bedsores—* **Adults and children:** apply and work into area, p.r.n.	*Skin:* burning and irritation of denuded skin and mucous membrane.
aluminum acetate (modified Burow's solution) Acid Mantle Creme and Lotion◆, Burosol, Burowets, Burow's Emulsion, Burow's Lotion, Burow's Ointment	*Mild skin irritation from exposure to soaps, detergents, chemicals, diaper rash, acne, scaly skin, eczema—* **Adults and children:** apply p.r.n. *Relieve inflammation of poison ivy, insect bites; athlete's foot—* **Adults and children:** apply as wet dressing, p.r.n. *Ulcerative skin conditions—* **Adults and children:** apply ointment, p.r.n.	*Skin:* irritation; extension of inflammation possible.
aluminum sulfate Bluboro Powder, Domeboro Powder◆ and Tablets◆, Soy-Sitz Powder	*Skin inflammation, insect bites, poison ivy, swelling, athlete's foot—* **Adults and children:** mix powder with 1 pint of water and apply every 15 to 30 minutes for 4 to 8 hours; bandage loosely.	*Skin:* irritation; extension of inflammation possible.
hamamelis water (witch hazel) Hazel-Balm, Mediconet (wipes), Tucks (Cream, Ointment, Pads)	*Anal discomfort, itching, burning, minor external hemorrhoidal or outer vaginal discomfort, diaper rash—* **Adults and children:** apply t.i.d. or q.i.d.	None.
tannic acid Amertan Jelly, Dalidyne Lotion, Tanac	*Denture irritation; trench mouth; gingivitis; throat irritation; herpes simplex; oral cavity lesions; adjunctive treatment of second- and third-degree thermal, chemical, or electrical burns—* **Adults:** apply with cotton applicator. As gargle or mouthwash, ½ teaspoon of solution in ½ glass of warm water, p.r.n. *Cold sores, throat irritation, oral cavity lesions, some second- and third-degree burns—* **Children:** apply with cotton applicator.	*GI:* large amounts in burn treatment can cause hepatic damage. *Local:* stinging.

◆ Also available in Canada.
◆◆ Available in Canada only.
Unmarked trade names available in United States only.

INTERACTIONS	NURSING CONSIDERATIONS
Heavy metals: causes precipitation of the metal acetate.	• Contraindicated under occlusive dressings. • Never confuse acetic acid solutions with *glacial* acetic acid solutions. Glacial form is a concentrate. • Keep away from eyes and mucous membranes. • Always apply to freshly cleansed area, free of other medications. • Especially good for treating topical infection due to *Pseudomonas aeruginosa.*
None significant.	• Contraindicated under occlusive dressings. • Keep away from eyes and mucous membranes. • Always apply to freshly cleansed area, free of other medications. • May be used in place of boric acid ointment. • Powder must be diluted in water to prescribed concentration. • Discontinue if irritation develops. • Clear solution may be stored at room temperature for up to 7 days.
None significant.	• Contraindicated under occlusive dressings; use open wet dressings only. • When solution is prepared, immediately decant clear portion. Discard precipitate. Use only clear solution, *not* precipitate, for soaks. Never strain or filter solutions. Decanted portion may be stored at room temperature for up to 7 days. • In general, no more than a third of the body should be treated at any one time, since excessive wet dressings may cause chilling and hypothermia. • Keep away from eyes and mucous membranes. • Discontinue if irritation develops.
None significant.	• Discontinue if irritation or itching does not improve. • Use pads or wipes after toilet tissue to help prevent pruritus ani and vulvae. • Cream can be used by nursing mother for nipple care, but wash area clean before nursing baby. • Some products contain potential allergic sensitizers. Observe for allergic reactions.
Organic salts of heavy metals: will precipitate tannate salt of heavy metal. Do not apply.	• Incompatible with organic salts of heavy metals. Apply only to surfaces free of other medication. • Produces a firm eschar on burned area that helps protect burned tissue from infection and loss of body fluids, and comforts patient. • Apply only after proper debridement of burn. • Prepare aqueous solutions freshly, as they are unstable. • Light and air cause solution to darken, which reduces potency. • Avoid extensive application and prolonged use on denuded tissue to decrease possibility of systemic toxicity from absorption. • Slight stinging on application soon subsides.

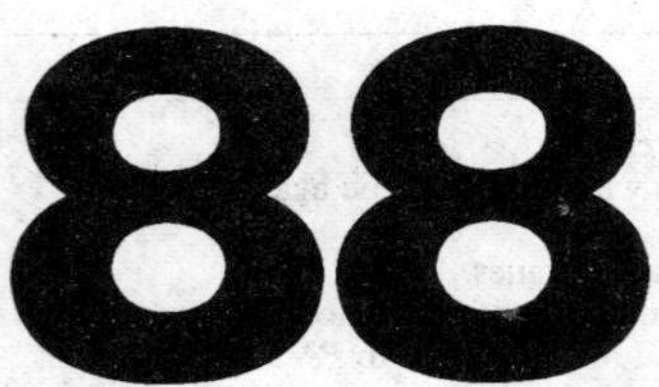

Antiseptics and disinfectants

alcohol, ethyl
alcohol, isopropyl
benzalkonium chloride
boric acid
chlorhexidine gluconate
formaldehyde
glutaraldehyde
hexachlorophene
hydrogen peroxide
iodine
merbromin
nitromersol
oxychlorosene
phenylmercuric nitrate
poloxamer iodine
potassium permanganate
povidone-iodine
silver protein, mild
sodium hypochlorite
thiomerosal

To distinguish between antiseptics and disinfectants, remember that antiseptics only inhibit microorganism growth; disinfectants destroy them. The effectiveness of these agents depends on their mechanism of action, concentration, the number of microorganisms, the length of time the organism is in contact with the agent, and the temperature and amount of organic matter present.

Major uses

- Control and prevention of infection.

Mechanism of action

- Denature protein, especially in microorganisms, changing their chemistry or structure.
- Lower surface tension, increasing cell permeability, causing lysis of cell content.
- Interfere with the metabolic processess of the cell.

Absorption, distribution, and excretion

- Not applicable.

Onset and duration

- Immediate effect on application, except with hexachlorophene, a chlorinated phenol used as a bacteriostatic cleansing agent. Antibacterial action of hexachlorophene develops only after repeated daily application.

Combination products

AMPHYL: o-phenyl phenol and potassium resinoleate.

B.F.I. POWDER: bismuth-formic-iodide, zinc phenosulfonate, amol, potassium alum, bismuth subgallate, boric acid, menthol, eucalyptol, and thymol.

MERCRESIN: secondary-amyltricresols 0.1%, o-hydroxyphenyl mercuric chloride 0.1%, acetone 10%, and alcohol 50%.

OBTUNDIA: camphor and meta-cresol in lanolin-petroleum base.

OBTUNDIA CALAMINE: camphor, meta-cresol, zinc oxide, and calamine.

S.T. 37: hexylresorcinol 0.1% in glycerin aqueous solution.

ZEASORB POWDER: parachlorometaxylenol 0.5%, aluminum 0.2%, and microporous cellulose 45%.

HOW TO WASH YOUR HANDS PROPERLY

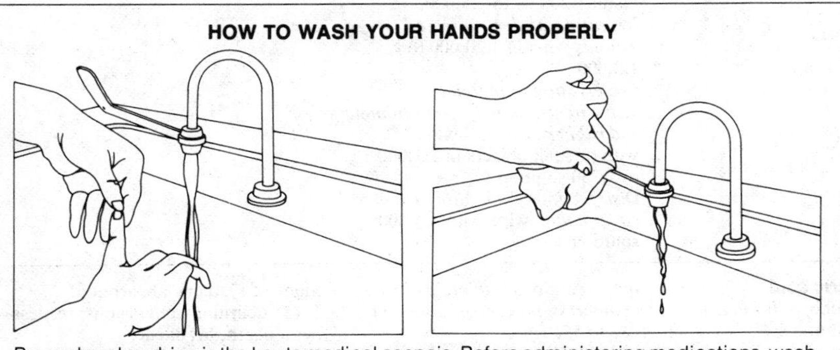

Proper handwashing is the key to medical asepsis. Before administering medications, wash your hands:

1) Using warm running water, lather well; be sure to clean your fingernails; rinse your hands and forearms; dry with a paper towel. 2) Turn faucet off with a paper towel.

NAME	INDICATIONS & DOSAGE	SIDE EFFECTS
alcohol, ethyl Alcohol, Ethanol	*To disinfect skin, instruments, and ampules*— disinfect as needed.	*Skin:* dryness.
alcohol, isopropyl isopropyl alcohol 99%, isopropyl rubbing alcohol 70%, isopropyl aqueous alcohol 75%	*To disinfect instruments and ampules*— disinfect as needed.	*Skin:* dryness.
benzalkonium chloride Benasept, Benzachlor-50◆◆, Benz-All, Drapolex◆◆, Ionax Foam◆◆, Ionax Scrub◆◆, Sabol◆◆, Spensomide, Zalkon, Zalkonium chloride, Zephiran	*Preop disinfection of unbroken skin*—apply 1:750 to 1:1,000 tincture or spray. *Disinfection of mucous membranes and denuded skin*—apply 1:10,000 to 1:5,000 aqueous solution. *Irrigation of vagina*—instill 1:5,000 to 1:2,000. *Irrigation of bladder or urethra*—instill 1:20,000 to 1:5,000. *Irrigation of deep infected wounds*—instill 1:20,000 to 1:3,000. *Preservation of metallic instruments, ampules, thermometers and rubber articles*—wipe with or soak objects in 1:1,000 to 1:750 solution. *Disinfection of operating room equipment*—wipe with 1:5,000 solution.	*Skin:* hypersensitivity.
boric acid Bluboro, Boric acid solution 5%, Borofax◆, Ting	*Skin conditions (athlete's foot) as a compress, powder, or ointment (2% to 5%)*— **Adults and children:** apply as directed.	Signs of systemic absorption: *CNS:* delirium, convulsions, restlessness, death, headache. *CV:* circulatory collapse, tachycardia. *GI:* irritation, nausea, vomiting, diarrhea. *GU:* renal damage. *Other:* hypothermia.
chlorhexidine gluconate Hibiclens Liquid	*Surgical hand scrub, hand wash, skin wound cleanser*—use p.r.n.	*EENT:* irritating to eyes. Causes deafness if instilled into middle ear through perforated eardrum.

◆ Also available in Canada.
◆◆ Available in Canada only.
Unmarked trade names available in United States only.

INTERACTIONS	NURSING CONSIDERATIONS
None signifcant.	• Effective as fat solvent germicidal, but ineffective against spore-forming organisms, tubercle bacilli, or viruses. • The only appropriate preparation for skin before venipuncture, S.C. or I.M. injections, or blood tests; do not use isopropyl alcohol. • Alcohol used as 70% solution is known commonly as "rubbing alcohol."
None significant.	• Isopropyl alcohol is slightly more effective than ethyl alcohol as an antibacterial agent, but it also tends to cause more dryness. • 75% solution for disinfection and storage of thermometers. • Not effective against spore-forming organisms, tubercle bacilli, or viruses. • Combined with formaldehyde, makes effective germicide. • Should not be used in place of ethyl alcohol as skin preparation.
Soaps: inactivate benzalkonium chloride. Remove soap traces with alcohol.	• Germicidal for some nonspore-forming organisms and fungi. No effect on tubercle bacilli. Limited viricidal use. • Used as preservative in ophthalmic solutions. • Before applying to skin, remove all traces of soap with water and apply 70% alcohol. • Don't store cotton, wool gauze, or sponges in solution. They absorb benzalkonium chloride and reduce the strength of the solution. • Don't use with occlusive dressings or vaginal packs. • Store in bottles with screw caps. • Use purified water to dilute concentrate. • Incompatible with iodine, silver nitrate, fluorescein, nitrates, peroxide, lanolin, potassium permanganate, aluminum, caramel, kaolin, pine oil, zinc sulfate, zinc oxide, and yellow oxide of mercury. • To prevent rust of metallic instruments stored in benzalkonium chloride, add sodium nitrite to final solution. Change solution weekly.
None significant.	• Mild antiseptic and astringent. • Not absorbed through intact skin, but in high concentrations, may be absorbed through abraded skin or granulating wounds. • Avoid long-term use. • Ingestion of 5 g (infants) or 20 g (adults) may be fatal.
None significant.	• Bactericidal action. Broad spectrum. • Can be used many times a day without causing irritations or dryness. • Low potential for producing skin reactions. • Rinse skin thoroughly after use. • Keep out of eyes and ears. • Action is residual. Do not cleanse skin with alcohol after application.

NAME	INDICATIONS & DOSAGE	SIDE EFFECTS
formaldehyde Formalin (37% solution of formaldehyde)	*Cold sterilization of equipment*—disinfect as needed. *Tissue preservative*—cover tissue.	*EENT:* fumes cause eye, nose, and throat irritation. *Skin:* irritation. *Other:* pungent odor.
glutaraldehyde Cidex◆	*Cold sterilization of surgical instruments*—cover instruments with 2% solution. *Fumigate hospital and operating rooms*—fog with aerosol.	*Skin:* irritation.
hexachlorophene Germa-Medica "MG," Hexamead-Ph, pHisoHex◆, pHiso-Scrub, Sept-Soft, Septisol Soy-Dome Cleanser, WescoHEX	*Surgical scrub, bacteriostatic skin cleanser*—use as directed in 0.25% to 3% concentrations.	*CNS:* systemic absorption can cause neurotoxic effects including irritability, generalized clonic muscular contractions, decerebrate rigidity, convulsions, death. *Skin:* dermatitis, mild scaling, dryness (especially when combined with excessive scrubbing).
hydrogen peroxide 3% to 6% solution	*Cleansing wound*—use 1.5% to 3% solution. *Mouth wash for Vincent's infection*—gargle with 3% solution. *Cleansing douche*—use 2% solution.	*EENT:* excessive use as mouthwash causes "hairy tongue."
iodine solution◆ (2% iodine and 2.4% sodium and iodide in water), tincture (2% iodine and 2.4% sodium iodide in diluted alcohol), Sepp Antiseptic Applicators (2% mild iodine tincture), Strong iodine tincture (7% iodine and 5% potassium iodide in diluted alcohol)	*Preop disinfection of skin (small wounds and abraded areas)*—apply p.r.n. For oral use, see Chapter 56.	*Skin:* irritation, redness, swelling (sign of hypersensitivity).
merbromin Mercurochrome (2% aqueous solution)	*General antiseptic and first aid prophylactic*— **Adults and children:** apply p.r.n. as 1% to 2% solution or tincture.	*Skin:* sensitization.

INTERACTIONS	NURSING CONSIDERATIONS
None significant.	• 0.5% solution germicidal against all forms of microorganisms, including spores, in 6 to 12 hours; 10% solution used to disinfect inanimate objects. • Not affected by organic matter. • Used with alcohol and sodium nitrite to disinfect instruments and articles that can't tolerate heat (cold sterilization). • Avoid skin or mucous membrane contact with solutions greater than 0.5%. • Always dilute 37% solution.
None significant.	• Excellent disinfectant; broad spectrum of activity against gram-positive and gram-negative bacteria (vegetative and spores), viruses, and fungi. • Use on inanimate objects only. • Comes with activator that must be mixed before use to yield active acidic glutaraldehyde. • Not affected by organic matter.
None significant.	• Use with caution in infants (especially premature infants) and burn patients. These patients tend to absorb hexachlorophene through the skin and may develop neurotoxic effects. • Bacteriostatic agent. Spectrum of activity limited to gram-positive organisms, especially staphylococcus. • Must be used preop for at least 3 days for maximum effectiveness. • After cleaning area, rinse thoroughly (especially the scrotum and perineum). Do not apply alcohol or organic solvents to cleansed area.
None significant.	• Germicidal. • Don't inject into closed body cavities or abscesses; generated gas can't escape. • Dilute concentrate with 1 to 4 parts water. • Useful to remove mucus from inner cannula of tracheostomy tube. • Store tightly capped in cool dry place. Protect from light and heat. • Do not shake bottle. This causes decomposition.
None significant.	• Microbicidal agent effective against bacteria, fungi, viruses, protozoa, and yeasts. • If skin reaction develops, remove iodine residue from skin and stop use. • To prevent skin irritation, do not cover areas treated with iodine. • Aqueous solution less irritating. • Sodium thiosulfate renders iodine colorless and is used to remove stains. It is also antidote of choice for accidental ingestion.
None significant.	• Bacteriostatic. • Least effective mercurial antiseptic. Its activity is decreased in presence of organic matter. • Cleanse injury with soap and water before applying. Let dry. • Stains may be removed with 2% permanganate solution, followed by 5% oxalic acid solution. • Never heat solution. • To prepare 1% solution dilute with equal parts water.

NAME	INDICATIONS & DOSAGE	SIDE EFFECTS
nitromersol Metaphen	*Disinfection of instruments*—soak in 0.04% solution. *Disinfection of skin*— apply 0.2 to 0.5% solution to area p.r.n. *Irrigation of mucous membranes (eye, urethra)*—instill 0.01 to 0.02% solution as directed. *Skin antiseptic for abrasions*—apply 0.290 solution to area.	*Skin:* erythematous, papular, or vesicular eruptions indicate hypersensitivity; irritation.
oxychlorosene calcium Chlorpactin XCB **oxychlorosene sodium** Clorpactin WCS-90	*Topical antiseptic for local infections, preoperative skin cleanser (sodium salt)*—apply as spray, soak, wet dressing, or irrigation as a 4% solution. *Ophthalmic and urologic irrigant (sodium salt)*— 0.1% to 0.2% solution. *Local irrigation during surgery (calcium salt)*— use 0.5% solution.	*Skin:* local irritation.
phenylmercuric nitrate Phe-Mer-Nite	*Preop disinfection*—apply p.r.n. as a 0.1% to 0.2% solution.	*Skin:* rash.
poloxamer iodine Prepodyne, SeptoDyne	*Preop skin prep and scrub, wound disinfection*—use as directed.	None reported.
potassium permanganate	*Topical antiseptic*—apply 1:10,000 to 1:500 solution. *Vaginal douche*—instill 1:5,000 to 1:1,000 solution as directed.	*Skin:* solutions greater than 1:5,000 are irritating to skin.
povidone-iodine ACU-dyne, Aerodine, Betadine♦, BPS, Bridine♦♦, Efodine, Final Step, Frepp, Frepp/Sepp, Isodine, Mallisol, Polydine, Proviodine♦♦, Sepp	*Many uses including preop skin prep and scrub, germicide for surface wounds, postop application to incisions, miscellaneous disinfection.* **Adults:** apply p.r.n.	None reported.
silver protein, mild Argyrol S.S.♦, Silvol, Solargentum	*Topical application for inflammation of eye, nose, throat*— **Adults and children:** apply p.r.n. as a 5% to 25% solution.	*Skin:* argyria in long-term use.

INTERACTIONS	NURSING CONSIDERATIONS
None significant.	• Contraindicated in nypersensitivity to mercury compounds. • Do not use when aluminum may come in contact with skin. • Incompatible with permanganates, strong acids, and heavy metal salts. • Prepare as needed. Solutions tend to precipitate on standing.
None significant.	• Effective against bacteria, fungi, viruses, mold yeast, and spores. • Powder reconstituted in saline. • Refrigerate dry crystal until reconstitution.
None significant.	• Contraindicated in hypersensitivity to mercury-containing compounds. • Antiseptic and fungicidal. • Frequent or prolonged use may cause mercury poisoning. • Orange stain removed with soap and water. • Commonly used as a preservative in ophthalmic solutions.
None significant.	• Contraindicated in hypersensitivity to iodines. • Prolonged germicidal action. • Water-soluble solution releases iodine at predetermined rate, causing prolonged action. • Relatively nonirritating to skin.
Iodine: precipitates iodine salt. Do not use together.	• Antiseptic astringent with fungicidal properties. • Germicidal effects reduced by organic matter. • Stains caused by potassium permanganate removed with dilute acids (lemon juice, oxalic acid, or dilute hydrochloric acid). • Never mix with charcoal or give charcoal as antidote. May explode.
None significant.	• Germicidal activity of iodine without irritation to skin and mucous membranes. • Thought to be superior to soap as a disinfectant; less effective than aqueous or alcoholic solutions of iodine. • Most often used for bedsores. Change dressings b.i.d. or t.i.d. Also used for leg ulcers, with hydrogen peroxide. • Treated areas may be bandaged or taped. • Germicidal activity reduced if area cleansed with alcohol or other organic solvents after application of povidone-iodine. • Prolonged, excessive use may lead to systemic absorption and toxicity.
None significant.	• Store in amber glass bottles; protect from light.

NAME	INDICATIONS & DOSAGE	SIDE EFFECTS
sodium hypochlorite 5% solution (instruments, swimming pools), 0.5% aqueous solution for wounds, Modified Dakins solution	*Athlete's foot, wound irrigation, disinfection of walls and floors*—apply as directed.	*Skin:* irritation.
thiomerosal Aeroaid thiomerosal, Merthiolate◆	*Preop disinfection of skin; antiseptic for open wounds*—apply or instill to affected area daily, b.i.d., or t.i.d. as a 0.1% solution or tincture.	*Skin:* erythematous, vesicular, papular eruptions (indicates hypersensitivity); irritation with tincture.

INTERACTIONS	NURSING CONSIDERATIONS
None significant.	• Germicidal and weakly fungicidal. • Interferes locally with thrombin formation, delaying blood clotting. Dissolves necrotic tissue. • Unstable in solution. Make fresh solution and use immediately. • Avoid contact with hair due to its bleaching properties.
None significant.	• Contraindicated in hypersensitivity to mercury-containing compounds. • Do not use when aluminum may come in contact with skin. • Incompatible with permanganate, strong acids, and salts of heavy metals. • Cleanse wound thoroughly before applying tincture. • To prevent skin irritation, allow tincture to dry completely before applying dressing. • Can be instilled into body cavities. • Store in amber glass container.

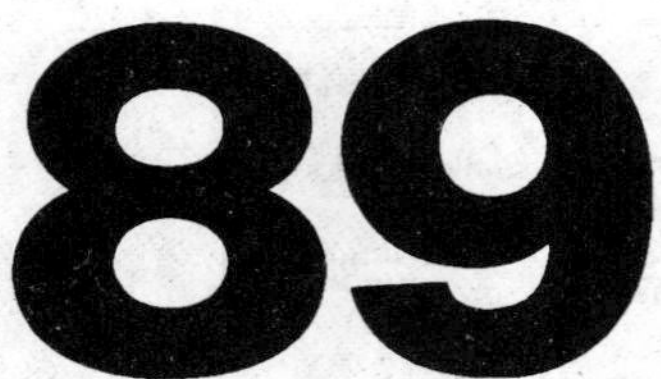

Emollients, demulcents, and protectants

aluminum paste
calamine
collodion
compound benzoin tincture
dexpanthenol
glycerin
hydrophilic lotion
hydrophilic ointment
hydrophilic petrolatum
hydrous wool fat
liquid petrolatum
methyl salicylate
oatmeal
para-aminobenzoic acid
petrolatum
silicone
starch
talc
urea or carbamide
vitamins A and D ointment
zinc gelatin

These preparations include compounds that serve as "vehicles" for other drugs, as well as some used alone for specific therapeutic actions. They are mainly applied externally. Emollients protect and soften skin and mucous membranes. Demulcents alleviate irritation and soothe. Protectants cover (occlude) and protect epithelial surfaces, ulcers, and wounds. Also included here are the basic lotions and liniments.

Major uses

- To treat burns, wounds, itching, insect bites, poison ivy, rash, skin irritation and dryness, sunburn, rheumatic pains, muscle soreness, lumbago, cutaneous ulcers, mild eczema, and varicosities.

Mechanism of action

- Protective properties to permit healing.
- Analgesic properties to soothe and cool irritation and inflammation.
- Certain agents stimulate healing process.
- Some soften dry skin; others dry skin when excessive secretions are present.

Absorption, distribution, and excretion

- Most are adsorbed to the skin; others are absorbed into the skin.
- Distribution only to affected area.
- Usually removed topically.

Onset and duration

- Relief is usually swift.
- Duration depends on agent used and time of exposure to affected areas.

Combination products

CALADRYL

Lotion: diphenhydramine hydrochloride 1%, calamine, camphor, and alcohol 2%.
Cream: diphenhydramine hydrochloride 1% with calamine.
CALAMINE LOTION, PHENOLATED: liquified phenol 1% with calamine.
CALAMINE LOTION, PHENOLATED AND MENTHOLATED: liquified phenol 1% and menthol with calamine 1%.
GER-O-FOAM, GERIATRIC: methyl salicylate 30%, benzocaine 3%, and volatile oils.
PANALGESIC: methyl salicylate 50%, aspirin 8%, menthol and camphor 4%, emollient oils 20%, alcohol 18%.

PATIENT TEACHING AID — WOUND CLEANING AND DRESSING

Dear Patient: Follow these procedures to insure the proper healing of your wound or incision.

- Change the dressing as often as your doctor suggested. But, if you notice some drainage before the next scheduled change, apply a new dressing immediately.
- Before you begin, collect all the materials you'll need and place them within reach: sterile forceps, sterile gloves, sterile dressings, nonperfumed soap, water and tape.
- If your doctor has asked you to maintain sterile technique, wear sterile gloves, use sterile equipment and avoid touching the part of the bandage that will cover the wound. In any case, wash your hands carefully before handling the dressings; then handle them carefully and as little as possible.
- Remove soiled dressings and discard carefully in a waterproof bag. Don't contaminate the outside of the bag with soiled dressings.
- If dressings stick to the wound, moisten them with sterile water or hydrogen peroxide before attempting to remove them.
- With a sterile gauze pad, clean the wound with a single circular motion; always wipe from inside to out. Use the pad only once; discard after each single circular motion.
- If an ointment was used on the wound, remove it with nonperfumed soap and water, rinse well. Again, always clean and rinse from an in-to-out direction.
- If ordered, apply ointment or other medication to dressing, then apply the dressing to the wound or incision.
- If ordered, apply a protective ointment to surrounding area.
- If wound or incision is to be covered, apply a sterile dressing, being careful to handle only the outer top surface of the dressing.
- Secure the dressing with nonallergenic tape, not adhesive tape.
- If you see any changes in the wound, such as redness, swelling, foul odors or pus, notify your doctor immediately.

NAME	INDICATIONS & DOSAGE	SIDE EFFECTS
aluminum paste (10% aluminum in zinc oxide ointment with liquid petrolatum)	*Emollient and protectant; protect colostomy area or other surgical sites*—apply p.r.n.	None.
calamine liniment (15% calamine), lotion (8% calamine), ointment (17% calamine), Rhulihist (3% calamine), Rhulispray (1% calamine)	*Topical astringent and protectant; itching, poison ivy and poison oak, nonpoisonous insect bites, mild sunburn, minor skin irritations*—apply p.r.n.	*Skin:* transient light stinging.
collodion, U.S.P. (5% pyroxylin in 1 part alcohol, 3 parts ether) **flexible collodion** (5% pyroxylin in 1 part alcohol, 3 parts ether plus 20% camphor, 30% castor oil)	*Protectant; vehicle for other medicinal agents, and used to seal small wounds*— apply to dry skin, p.r.n. or use flexible collodion when a flexible noncontracting film is desired.	None.
compound benzoin tincture (10% benzoin in alcohol mixed with glycerin and water) Benzoin Spray	*Demulcent and protectant; cutaneous ulcers, bedsores, cracked nipples, fissures of lips and anus*—apply locally once daily or b.i.d.	None.
dexpanthenol Panthoderm◆ Cream (dexpanthenol 2% in a water-miscible cream base), Panthoderm Lotion (dexpanthenol 2%, menthol 0.1%, and camphor 0.1%)	*Epithelial-bed stimulator in emollient base; itching, wounds, insect bites, poison ivy, poison oak, diaper rash, chafing, mild eczema, decubitus ulcers, dry lesions*—apply topically, p.r.n.	None.

◆ Also available in Canada.
◆◆ Available in Canada only.
Unmarked trade names available in United States only.

INTERACTIONS	NURSING CONSIDERATIONS
Topical enzymes: aluminum may inactivate preparations used to debride wounds. Don't use together.	• Zinc oxide paste can be used as an alternative. • Observe for inflammation or infection since protectants are occlusive layers that retain moisture, exclude air, and trap cutaneous bacteria. • Skin should be cleaned daily or more often as needed. • Emollients and protectants may be used alone, as vehicles for medications, or with other topical medications. Check with doctor.
None significant.	• Contraindicated in hypersensitivity to any of the components. • Watch for sensitivity reactions to calamine. Preparations containing antihistamines may cause sensitivity. • Always shake well before use. • Don't use cotton to apply; it will absorb the solute. Use gauze sponge. • Do not apply to blistered, raw, or oozing areas of the skin. • Toxic if taken internally. • Observe for inflammation or infection since protectants are occlusive layers that retain moisture, exclude air and trap skin bacteria. • Skin should be cleaned daily or more often as needed. • Emollients, demulcents, and protectants may be used alone, as vehicles for medications, or with other topical medications. Check with doctor. • Highly flammable; never use near flame. • May irritate and dry skin. • Keep container tightly closed so solvent won't evaporate.
None significant.	• Observe for inflammation or infection since protectants are occlusive layers that retain moisture, exclude air and trap cutaneous bacteria. • Skin should be cleaned daily or more often as needed. • Protectants may be used alone, as vehicles for medications, or with other topical medications. Check with doctor. • Camphor in flexible collodion is weakly antiseptic and antipruritic; may irritate and dry skin. • Highly flammable; never use near flame. • Keep container tightly closed so solvent won't evaporate. • Toxic if taken internally. • Avoid excessive inhalation of vapors.
None significant.	• Do not apply to acutely inflamed areas. • Observe for inflammation or infection since protectants are occlusive layers that retain moisture, exclude air and trap cutaneous bacteria. • Skin should be cleaned daily or more often as needed. • Protectants may be used alone, as vehicles for medications, or with other topical medications. Check with doctor. • For demulcent and expectorant action in laryngitis or croup, use in boiling water and have patient inhale vapors. • Spray is not intended for use as inhalant. • Can be mixed with magnesium-aluminum hydroxide and applied on bedsores.
None significant.	• Contraindicated in wounds of hemophilia patients. • Before each new application *always* thoroughly cleanse affected area, removing all traces of previously applied medication. Observe for inflammation or infection. • Dry lesions respond better than oozing lesions. • May heal skin lesions in mild eczema and dermatoses.

NAME	INDICATIONS & DOSAGE	SIDE EFFECTS
glycerin Corn Huskers Lotion (tragacanth 1 g, glycerin 30 ml, propylene glycol 10 ml)	*Emollient and lubricant; to lubricate rectal tubes and catheters; for dry skin, hands*—apply p.r.n.	None.
hydrophilic lotion (white petrolatum 4.2 g, stearyl alcohol 4.2 g, methylparaben 0.004 g, propylparaben 0.002 g, sodium lauryl sulfate 0.167 g, propylene glycol 2 ml, perfume q.s., purified water)	*Protectant and emollient; dry skin, irritation*—apply p.r.n.	None.
hydrophilic ointment Cetaphil, Multibase, Neobase, Unibase, Vanibase (methylparaben 0.025 g, propylparaben 0.015 g, stearyl alcohol 25 g, white petrolatum 25 g, propylene glycol 12 g, sodium lauryl sulfate 1 g, purified water)	*Protectant and emollient; dry skin, oozing lesions*—apply p.r.n.	*Local:* allergic reaction.
hydrophilic petrolatum Aquaphor, Hydrosort, Plastibase hydrophilic, Polysort (cholesterol 3 g, stearyl alcohol 3 g, white wax 8 g, white petrolatum 86 g)	*Protectant and emollient; dry skin, eczema, or psoriasis*—mix with other medicinal ingredients as ordered and apply p.r.n.	None.
hydrous wool fat Lanolin lotion (stearic acid 2 g, triethanolamine 0.8 ml, light liquid petrolatum 10 ml, propylparaben 0.2 g, rose water) **hydrous wool fat and castor oil** (hydrous wool fat 25 g, castor oil 25 g, ceresin wax 5 g, polysorbate 61 5 g, white petrolatum)	*Protectant and emollient; to soothe and lubricate*—apply hydrous wool fat p.r.n. *Protection against hydrocarbons, solvents, and cutting oils*—apply hydrous wool fat and castor oil before exposure.	*Skin:* allergic rash.

INTERACTIONS	NURSING CONSIDERATIONS
None significant.	• Applied undiluted to inflamed, dehydrated skin. Paradoxically, excessive use may dry the skin. • Diluted with rose water, glycerin is useful for irritated or dry lips.
None significant.	• Observe for inflammation or infection since protectants are occlusive layers that retain moisture, exclude air and trap skin bacteria. • Skin should be cleaned daily or more often as needed. • Emollients and protectants may be used alone, as vehicles for medications, or with other topical medications. Check with doctor.
None significant.	• Easily removed with water. • Use when little penetration of medicinal agent is desired. • Observe for inflammation or infection since protectants are occlusive layers that retain moisture, exclude air and trap skin bacteria. • Skin should be cleaned daily or more often as needed. • Emollients and protectants may be used alone, as vehicles for medications, or with other topical medications. Check with doctor.
None significant.	• Not water-soluble; greasy. • Observe for inflammation or infection since protectants are occlusive layers that retain moisture, exclude air and trap skin bacteria. • Skin should be cleaned daily or more often as needed. • Emollients and protectants may be used alone, as vechicles for medications, or with other topical medications. Check with doctor.
None significant.	• Contraindicated in hypersensitivity to lanolin. • Don't confuse with anhydrous wool fat, which will dry skin if applied alone. • Observe for inflammation or infection since protectants are occlusive layers that retain moisture, exclude air and trap skin bacteria. • Skin should be cleaned daily or more often as needed. • Emollients and protectants may be used alone, as vehicles for medications, or with other topical medications. Check with doctor.

NAME	INDICATIONS & DOSAGE	SIDE EFFECTS
liquid petrolatum Liquid Petrolatum, U.S.P., Light Liquid Petrolatum, N.F. Mineral oil	*Protectant and emollient; for protection*—apply locally, full strength or diluted.	None.
methyl salicylate Banalg, Baumodyne Gel and Ointment, Betula Oil, Gaultheria Oil, Sweet Birch Oil, Wintergreen Oil	*Counterirritant; minor pains of osteoarthritis, rheumatism, sprains, muscle and tendon soreness and tightness, lumbago, sciatica*— **Adults:** apply with gentle massage several times daily. Not recommended for children.	*Skin:* rash, irritation, burning, blistering.
oatmeal Aveeno Colloidal, Aveeno Oilated Bath (with liquid petrolatum and hypoallergenic lanolin)	*Emollient and demulcent; local irritation*—use as a lotion; 1 level tablespoon to a cup of warm water. *Skin irritation, pruritus, common dermatoses, dry skin*— **Adults and children:** mix 1 cup oatmeal with 2 cups water, put into tub of water, and soak affected area for 30 minutes. *Skin irritation pruritus, common dermatoses, dry skin*— **Adults:** 1 packet in tub of warm water. **Children:** 1 to 2 rounded tablespoons in 3" to 4" of bath water. **Infants:** 2 or 3 level teaspoons, depending on size of bath.	None.
para-aminobenzoic acid PABA◆, Pabagel◆, Pabanol◆, Pre Sun◆, Pre Sun gel, RV Paba Lipstick, Sunbrella lotion	*Topical protectant; sunburn protection, sun-sensitive skin, slow tanning*— **Adults:** apply evenly to dry skin; follow directions on various products for number and time of application, which vary from 2 to 6 hours; reapply after swimming. Not recommended for children.	*Local:* allergic reaction, irritation, sensitization. *Skin:* photocontact dermatitis.

INTERACTIONS	NURSING CONSIDERATIONS
None significant.	• Occasionally used with other drugs. • Exists in two forms: light mineral oil and heavy mineral oil. • Heavy mineral oil can be used internally as a laxative. Never use light mineral oil as a laxative. Mineral oil used as nose drops can cause lipid pneumonia. • Observe for inflammation or infection since protectants are occlusive layers that retain moisture, exclude air and trap skin bacteria. • Skin should be cleaned daily or more often as needed. • Emollients and protectants may be used alone, as vehicles for medications, or with other topical medications. Check with doctor.
None significant.	• Never apply directly, undiluted to skin. • Warning: as little as 4 ml ingested by children can cause fatal toxicity; in adults as little as 30 ml. Since GI absorption may be delayed, treat such ingestion with emetic lavage, then a saline cathartic. Continue lavage until no odor of methyl salicylate can be detected in the washings. • Absorbed through skin; prolonged increased application can cause toxicity. Toxic effects include hyperpnea leading to respiratory alkalosis, nausea, vomiting, tinnitus, hyperpyrexia, and convulsions. • Discontinue if rash or redness occurs. Consult doctor if pain or redness persists more than 10 days. • Avoid getting near eyes, open wounds, mucous membranes. • Do not use on sunburned membranes. • Do not wrap or bandage treated area. • Store in tightly closed container.
None significant.	• Not to be ingested. Don't confuse with oatmeal as food. • Instruct patient to exercise caution to avoid slipping in tub. • Avoid getting in eyes.
None significant.	• Contraindicated in hypersensitivity to any of the components and for persons with damaged or diseased skin. • Discontinue if skin rash occurs. • Encourage slow tanning and short exposure to sun. • Avoid contact with eyes and lids. • Avoid contact with open flame. • May stain clothing. • Observe for inflammation and infection since protectants produce an occlusive layer that retains perspiration, excludes air, and traps cutaneous bacteria, producing sites for anaerobic infections.

NAME	INDICATIONS & DOSAGE	SIDE EFFECTS
petrolatum Vaseline	*Topical protectant and emollient*—use alone or with other drugs, as directed.	None.
silicone Silicone and zinc oxide compound, Silon Spray	*Topical protectant; dermatoses, diaper rash, decubitus ulcers*—apply b.i.d. or t.i.d. in ointment. *Protection against water and corrosive chemicals*—apply before exposure.	None.
starch Linit	*Demulcent; minor skin irritations, pruritus associated with common dermatoses*—mix 2 cups of starch with 4 cups of water, add to tub of water, and soak affected area for 30 minutes.	None.
talc (magnesium silicate)	*Topical lubricant, protectant, drying agent, absorbent dusting powder; irritation such as intertrigo prickly heat*—sprinkle on affected areas p.r.n. for soothing and lubrication.	None.
urea or carbamide Aquacare Dry Skin Cream and Lotion◆, Aquacare/HP Cream and Lotion◆, Aqua Lacten, Artra Ashy Skin Cream, Carmol Ten, Carmol Twenty, Gormel Cream, Nutraplus◆, Rea-Lo, Ultra-Mide, Uremol◆◆, Urtex◆◆	*Emollient; hard, dry skin on hands, elbows, or knees*— **Adults:** apply to affected area b.i.d. or t.i.d., particularly after exposure to sun or wind. Not recommended for children.	*Skin:* transient stinging when applied to irritated or fissured skin.
vitamins A and D ointment A&D, Balmex, Caldesene Medicated, Clocream, Comfortine, Desitin, Primaderm	*Emollient, demulcent and epithelial-bed stimulant; superficial burns, sunburn, abrasions, slow-healing lesions, chapped skin, diaper rash, skin care of infants or bedridden patients*—apply several times a day.	*Skin:* irritation.

INTERACTIONS	NURSING CONSIDERATIONS
None significant.	• Stable, does not become rancid. • Observe for inflammation or infection since protectants are occlusive layers that retain moisture, exclude air and trap skin bacteria. • Skin should be cleaned daily or more often as needed. • Emollients and protectants may be used alone, as vehicles for medications, or with other topical medications. Check with doctor.
None significant.	• Protect eyes against spray. • Very difficult to remove from skin; resistant to water and soap. • Will not protect against oils or solvents. • Observe for inflammation or infection since protectants are occlusive layers that retain moisture, exclude air and trap cutaneous bacteria. • Skin should be cleaned daily or more often as needed. • Protectants may be used alone, as vehicles for medications, or with other topical medications. Check with doctor.
None significant.	• Instruct patient to exercise caution to avoid slipping in tub.
None significant.	• Don't use on surgical gloves; causes granulation and adhesions in open wounds. • Avoid dust entering eyes or inhalation of talc dust. • Should not be used on open, weeping surfaces; it cakes and crusts.
None significant.	• Contraindicated in viral skin diseases, or in impaired circulation. Use cautiously on face or broken skin. • Wet skin before application. If irritation persists, discontinue. • Avoid contact with eyes. • Emollients produce an occlusive layer that retains perspiration, excludes air, and traps cutaneous bacteria, producing sites for anaerobic infections. Before each new application, *always* thoroughly cleanse affected area, removing all traces of previously applied medication. Observe for inflammation or infection.
None significant.	• Discontinue if skin condition persists or irritation develops. • Observe for inflammation or infection since emollients and demulcents are occlusive layers that retain moisture, exclude air, and trap cutaneous bacteria. • Skin should be cleaned daily or more often as needed. • Emollients and demulcents may be used alone, as vehicles for medications, or with other topical medications. Check with doctor.

NAME	INDICATIONS & DOSAGE	SIDE EFFECTS
zinc gelatin Dome-Paste, Unna's Boot	*Protectant; varicosities, lesions of lower legs or arms*—heat in hot bath till liquified, clean skin, dust with talc, and apply gel with paint brush; make three layers, with gauze between each layer; retain 2 weeks. Dome-Paste, in 3- and 4-inch bandages, can be applied directly to arm or leg.	None.

INTERACTIONS	NURSING CONSIDERATIONS
None significant.	• Observe for inflammation and infection since protectants produce an occlusive layer that retains perspiration, excludes air, and traps cutaneous bacteria, producing sites for anaerobic infections. Before each new application *always* thoroughly cleanse affected area, removing all traces of previously applied medication. • If skin sensitivity, irritation, edema, or severe pain develops, discontinue and consult doctor. • Zinc gelatin boot can be removed by unwinding outer bandage and soaking leg or arm in warm water until dressing floats off. Tell patient not to shower or take tub bath with zinc gelatin boot on leg.

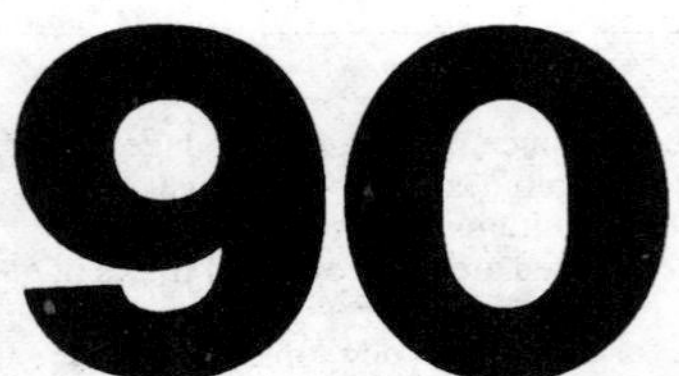

Keratolytics and caustics

cantharidin	**salicylic acid**
dichloroacetic acid	**silver nitrate**
podophyllum resin	**sulfur**
resorcinol	**sulfurated lime solution**

Keratolytic agents loosen the tightly packed layers of cell products, cell walls, and protein (keratin) that constitute the outer, protective layer (stratum corneum) of the epidermis. They are used in the treatment of benign skin growths and other dermatological disorders.

By destroying tissue at the site of application, caustic agents can treat skin problems such as moles and warts. They are used for cauterization.

Major uses

- Keratolytics are used in the treatment of dermatophytosis, warts, corns, and certain acneiform and eczematous dermatides.
- Caustics are used to destroy warts, condylomata, keratoses, certain moles, and hyperplastic tissue and have been used to control fungal infections and eczematoid dermatitis.

Mechanism of action

- Keratolytics soften keratin and loosen cornified epithelium, causing even viable cells to swell and soften.
- The most commonly used caustics precipitate cell proteins, causing formation of a scab and perhaps a scar.

Absorption, distribution, and excretion

- Not applicable.

Onset and duration

- Not applicable.

Combination products

ACNE-AID CREAM: sulfur 2.5%, resorcinol 1.25%, and parachlorometaxylenol 0.375% in a microporous cellulose base.
ACNE-DOME: colloidal sulfur 3% and resorcinol monoacetate 3% in an acid-mantle vehicle.
ACNOMEL CAKE♦: sulfur 4% and resorcinol 1% in a washable base.
ACNOMEL CREAM♦: sulfur 8%, resorcinol 2%, and alcohol 11% in a greaseless base.

BENSULFOID LOTION: bensulfoid 6%, resorcinol 2%, zinc oxide 6%, thymol 0.5%, and alcohol 12% in a greaseless base.
CLEARASIL REGULAR TINTED CREAM: sulfur 8%, resorcinol 2%, and bentonite 11.5%.
COMPOUND W WART REMOVER: salicylic acid 14%, acetic acid 11%, menthol 2%, camphor 1.5%, castor oil 22%, and alcohol 1.5% in ether and acetone.
DUOFILM•: salicylic acid 16.7% and lactic acid 16.7% in flexible collodion.
EXZIT: colloidal sulfur 3% and resorcinol monoacetate 3% in an acid-mantle vehicle.
FOSTEX CAKE•: sulfur 2% and salicylic acid 2%.
FREEZONE CORN AND CALLUS REMOVER: salicylic acid 13.59%, zinc chloride 1.9%, castor oil 3.3%, and collodion 2% in alcohol and ether.
GETS-IT-LIQUID: salicylic acid 13.9%, zinc chloride 2.7%, and collodion in ether and alcohol.
REZAMID LOTION•: microsize sulfur 5%, resorcinol 2%, parachlorometaxylenol 0.5%, and alcohol 28.5% in a hydroalcoholic lotion base.
SULFORCIN BASE CREAM: sulfur 4% and resorcinol monoacetate 1.5%.
VERRUSOL: salicylic acid 30%, podophyllin 5%, cantharidin 1% in a film-forming base.

PATIENT TEACHING AID — TREATING WARTS OR CORNS

Dear Patient:

The following tips will help you treat your warts or corns.

1. When treating warts, remember: Warts are caused by viruses and can be contagious. Therefore, wash your hands before and after treating them.
2. Gently remove any dead skin with a rough towel, callous file, or pumice stone. Do not use force.
3. Apply petroleum jelly to the healthy skin surrounding the affected area to protect it from accidental application of the corrosive wart remover.
4. Promptly report any change in size or color of a wart to the physician.
5. To prevent further irritation, make sure shoes fit properly.

NAME	INDICATIONS & DOSAGE	SIDE EFFECTS
cantharidin Cantharone	**Adults and children:** *Molluscum contagiosum*—coat each lesion. Repeat in a week on new or remaining lesions, this time covering with occlusive tape. Remove tape in 6 to 8 hours. *Palpebral warts*—apply, leave lesion uncovered. *Plantar warts*—pare away keratin, apply generously to affected area, allow to dry, apply protective padding, cover with nonporous tape for a week, then debride. Repeat 3 times, if necessary, on large lesions. *Removal of ordinary and periungual warts, and other benign epithelial growths*—apply directly to lesion and cover completely. Allow to dry, then cover with nonporous adhesive tape. Remove tape in 24 hours (or less if extreme pain) and replace with loose bandage. Reapply, if necessary.	*Skin:* annular warts, burning, tingling, extreme tenderness.
dichloroacetic acid Bichloracetic Acid	*All types verrucae; calluses, corns; xanthoma palpebrarum; ingrown toenails; cysts and benign erosion of the cervix; sebaceous adenoma; infectious granuloma; tattoo marks; epistaxis; spider nevi; tonsil tabs*— **Adults:** applied only by doctor at his discretion.	*Local:* irritation, inflammation of normal skin.
podophyllum resin Podoben	*Venereal warts and granuloma inguinale*— **Adults:** apply podophyllum resin preparation to the lesion, cover with waxed paper, and bandage. Leave covered for 8 to 12 hours, then wash lesion to remove medication. Repeat at weekly intervals.	*Blood:* thrombocytopenia, leukopenia when systemically absorbed. *Local:* irritation of normal skin. *Other:* peripheral neuropathy when systemically absorbed.

◆ Also available in Canada.
◆◆ Available in Canada only.
Unmarked trade names available in United States only.

INTERACTIONS	NURSING CONSIDERATIONS
None significant.	• If dropped on normal skin, remove immediately with acetone, alcohol, or tape remover. Scrub with warm, soapy water, and rinse well, as blistering of skin may result. • If dropped on mucous membranes or in eyes, flush well with water to remove precipitated collodion, then continue to flush with water for 15 minutes. • Treat only one or two lesions initially to test patient's sensitivity. • Stop treatment if severe inflammation develops. • If application causes burning, tenderness, or tingling, remove tape and soak area in cool water for 10 to 15 minutes; repeat, if necessary. • If annular warts develop, assure patient that lesions are superficial, and re-treat, or substitute another procedure. • Does not affect tissue layers below the epidermis, and leaves no scar. • Treatment should be supervised by a doctor.
None significant.	• Contraindicated for treatment of malignant or premalignant lesions. • Protect adjacent areas with petrolatum, especially when using 50% solutions. • Sodium bicarbonate is local antidote. • Thoroughly dry area before application. • Warn patient that once solution is applied, treated area will turn from white to red in about 4 hours. • Peeling of skin usually is noticed in 4 days and is completed in a week. • If acid comes in contact with normal skin, wipe off with cotton gauze and flush area with water.
Other keratolytics: may cause extensive damage to the skin. Do not use together.	• Resin is irritating and cytotoxic, and should not be applied to normal skin. Petrolatum can be applied to adjacent areas to protect them during treatment. • Should be applied only by a doctor because of toxicity. • Do not use on extensive areas or for prolonged therapy; may be absorbed systemically.

NAME	INDICATIONS & DOSAGE	SIDE EFFECTS
resorcinol, resorcinol monoacetate Euresol, Resorcin,	*Acute eczema, urticaria, and other inflammatory skin diseases (1% or 2% concentration in alcohol); acne or seborrhea (5% lotion or 10% soap liniment for scalp); chronic eczema, psoriasis (2% to 10% ointment); acne scarring (45% peeling paste)—* **Adults and children:** apply as directed.	*Skin:* irritation, moderate erythema or scaling. *Other:* darkening of light hair (resorcinol only).
salicylic acid Calicylic, Keralyt◆, Salactic Liquifilm, Salonil	*Superficial fungal infections, acne, psoriasis, seborrheic dermatitis, other scaling dermatoses, hyperkeratosis, calluses, warts—* **Adults and children:** apply to affected area, and place under occlusion at night.	*Skin:* irritation. *Other:* salicylism with percutaneous absorption.
silver nitrate	*Cauterization of mucous membranes, fissures, aphthous lesions (5% to 10% solution); cauterization of granulomatous tissues and warts (solid form)—* **Adults and children:** applied only by doctor at his discretion.	*Local:* argyria (permanent silver discoloration of skin).
sulfur Acne-Aid◆, Acnomead, Bensulfoid, EpiClear, Liquimat, Lotioblanc, Postacne◆, Transact, Xerac	*Acne, ringworm, psoriasis, seborrheic dermatitis, chigger infestation, scabies, favus, staphylococcal folliculitis—* **Adults and children:** apply preparation to affected areas b.i.d., t.i.d., or as directed.	*Local:* excessive drying of skin, blackheads.
sulfurated lime solution Vlem-Dome, Vleminckx	*Acne vulgaris, seborrhea—* **Adults and children:** dilute 1 packet in 1 pint hot water, and apply as hot dressing for 15 to 20 minutes daily. *Generalized furunculosis—* **Adults and children:** add 30 to 60 ml solution to bath water.	*Local:* may cause excessive drying of skin.

INTERACTIONS	NURSING CONSIDERATIONS
None significant.	• Do not use preparations on or near eyes. • If skin irritation persists, discontinue medication. • Apply lotion with cotton ball to affected area. • When applying the peeling paste, closely observe the patient and site of application until paste is removed.
None significant.	• Use with caution in diabetics or patients with peripheral vascular disease. The skin inflammation that may result is difficult to treat. Limit use for children under 12 years. (Do not exceed 1 oz in 24 hours.) • Avoid contact with eyes and mucous membranes. • If excessive skin drying or irritation occurs, apply a bland cream or lotion. • Rinse hands after application (unless they are being treated). • Skin should be hydrated for at least 5 minutes before treatment and should be washed the morning after treatment. • Most preparations are occlusive, which increases percutaneous absorption. Therefore, do not use on large surface areas for prolonged periods.
None significant.	• May cause burns. Avoid accidental contact with skin and eyes. If accidental contact with skin occurs, flush with water for at least 15 minutes; accidental contact with eyes, call doctor at once. • Not to be ingested; may cause altered respiration, coma, convulsions, paralysis, and even death. Call doctor at once. Give 1 tablespoon salt in warm water; repeat until emesis is clear. Or have patient drink milk or beaten egg whites mixed in warm water. Keep patient warm and lying down. • Warn that silver nitrate stains skin and clothing. • Silver nitrate pencils must be moistened with water before use.
None significant.	• Prolonged use may cause severe contact dermatitis. • When initiating therapy, use sparingly for patients with sensitive skin. • Avoid contact with eyes. If accidental contact occurs, flush with water. • Wash skin thoroughly before application. Tell patient that tingling sensation may be felt upon application. • Skin is more reactive to drug in cold, dry climates, so decrease frequency of application. In hot, humid climates, increase frequency of application.
None significant.	• Discontinue use if excessive drying or skin irritation develops. • Avoid contact with jewelry, metallic objects, or clothing. • Avoid getting solution in eyes, nose, or mouth. • Fumes are irritating and malodorous (rotten eggs). Ventilate adequately.

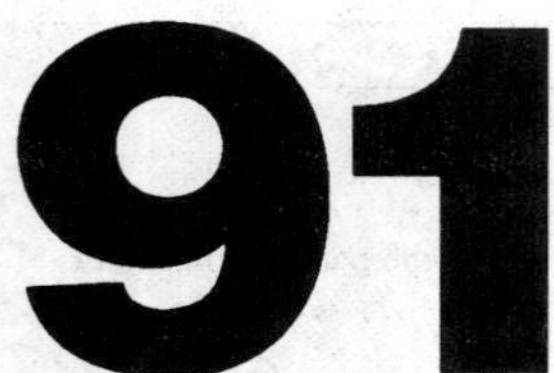

Miscellaneous

ammoniated mercury
anthralin
benzoyl peroxide
collagenase
dextranomer
fluorouracil
hydroquinone
methoxsalen
selenium sulfide
streptokinase-streptodornase
sutilains
tretinoin (vitamin A acid, retinoic acid)

Miscellaneous topical preparations include acne and burn products, irritants and rubefacients, certain enzymes, antimetabolites, antiseptics, and preparations that affect skin pigmentation.

Major uses

- Treatment of acne vulgaris.
- Treatment of psoriasis, chronic dermatitis, seborrhea, atopic dermatitis, chronic eczema, pruritus, ringworm, and other skin conditions.
- Cleansing, debridement, and healing of burns, surgical wounds, ulcerative and pyogenic lesions.
- Acceleration of pigmentation and treatment of hyperpigmentation.
- Control of dry, chapped skin and temporary relief of minor burns, irritations, sunburn, and abrasions.

Mechanism of action

- Varies with individual drugs.
- Mercuric ions inhibit sulfhydryl enzymes and combine with amino and other chemical groups.
- Some mercury compounds are effective bacteriostatic agents.
- Benzoyl peroxide has antimicrobial action and is also a keratolytic, antiseborrheic irritant.
- Collagenase is an enzymatic debriding agent that digests the undenatured collagen fibers in necrotic wound debris and removes substrates for bacterial proliferation. It permits antibodies, leukocytes, and antibiotics better access to infected areas.
- Fluorouracil acts as an antimetabolite to interfere with DNA synthesis. It also inhibits thymidylate synthetase activity.
- Hydroquinone inhibits tyrasinase and prevents the conversion of tyrosine to melanin.
- Methoxsalen is a potent photosensitizer of the skin which inhibits epidermal DNA synthesis.
- Streptokinase-streptodornase are enzymes produced during growth of certain strains of hemolytic streptococci. Streptokinase activates plasminogen activator, and streptodornase hydrolyzes deoxyribonucleo protein.
- Sutilains is a proteolytic enzyme which selectively digests necrotic tissue.
- Tretinoin has no toxic action in small doses.

Absorption, distribution, and excretion

- Most topical drugs are not absorbed systemically in appreciable amounts, but some may be absorbed systemically if used for extended periods or applied to large areas of the body.

Onset and duration

- Vary with individual drugs.
- Tretinoin (vitamin A acid) used topically is a potent irritant used for acne vulgaris.
- Methoxsalen increases skin tolerance to sunlight and facilitates repigmentation in vitiligo.

Combination products

EMERSAL: ammoniated mercury 5%, salicylic acid 2.5%, and castor oil 23%.
LOROXIDE♦: benzoyl peroxide 5.5% and chlorhydroxyquinoline 0.25%.
LOROXIDE HC♦: benzoyl peroxide 5.5%, chlorhydroxyquinoline 0.25%, and hydrocortisone 0.5%.
PERSOL♦: benzoyl peroxide 10% and colloidal sulfur 2.5%.
SULFOXYL REGULAR: benzoyl peroxide 5% and sulfur 2%.
SULFOXYL STRONG: benzoyl peroxide 10% and sulfur 5%.
VANOXIDE♦: benzoyl peroxide 5% and chlorhydroxyquinoline 0.25%.
VANOXIDE-HC: benzoyl peroxide 5%, chlorhydroxyquinoline 0.25%, and hydrocortisone 0.5%.

PLACES TO CHECK FOR DECUBITUS ULCERS

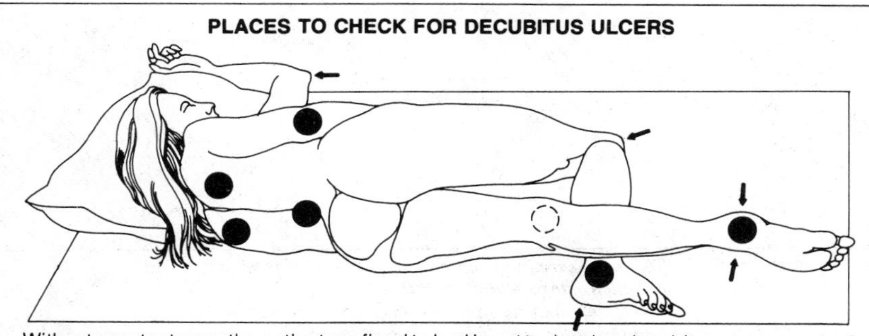

Without constant care, the patient confined to bed is apt to develop decubitus ulcers, caused by the increased pressure on tissue over bony prominences. To prevent decubitus ulcers: Regularly turn the patient. Massage areas over bony prominences. Place a flotation pad or alternating pressure mattress under key areas (illustrated above).

NAME	INDICATIONS & DOSAGE	SIDE EFFECTS
ammoniated mercury Mercuronate 5% ointment	*Psoriasis, seborrheic dermatitis, impetigo contagiosa, tinea capitis and favus—* **Adults and children:** apply to affected area b.i.d. or t.i.d.	None reported.
anthralin Anthera, Anthra-Derm◆, Lasan	*Psoriasis and chronic dermatitis—* **Adults and children:** apply thinly daily or b.i.d. Concentrations range from 0.1% to 1%; start with lowest and increase, if necessary.	*Skin:* erythema on healthy skin.
benzoyl peroxide Benoxyl◆, Benzac, Benzagel◆, Desquam-X◆◆, Dry & Clear, Epi-Clear Antiseptic, Oxy-5,-10, Panoxyl◆, Persadox, Persadox HP, Persa-Gel, Xerac BP	*Adjunctive treatment of acne—* **Adults and children:** apply once daily or b.i.d.	*Skin:* transient stinging on application, feeling of warmth, painful irritation.
collagenase Collagenase ABC, Santyl◆	*Debridement of dermal ulcers and severely burned areas—* **Adults and children:** apply ointment (250 units/g) to lesion daily or every other day.	*Skin:* slight erythema of surrounding area, especially if ointment is not confined to lesion. *Other:* hypersensitivity reactions.
dextranomer Debrisan	*To clean secreting wounds, such as venous stasis and decubitus ulcers, infected surgical wounds, and burns—* **Adults and children:** apply to affected area daily, b.i.d., or more often, p.r.n. Apply to ⅛- or ¼-inch thickness, and cover with sterile gauze pad.	*Skin:* temporary pain.

◆ Also available in Canada.
◆◆ Available in Canada only.
Unmarked trade names available in United States only.

INTERACTIONS	NURSING CONSIDERATIONS
None significant.	• Don't apply to large areas of body or use for extended periods of time. Mercury poisoning could result. • Don't apply to highly inflamed skin, sunburn, or open wounds. • Has no odor. Doesn't stain.
None significant.	• Contraindicated in renal damage. Should not be used on acute or inflammatory eruptions. • Partial excretion in urine may cause renal irritation, casts, and albuminuria. Check urine weekly. • Discontinue if allergic reaction, pustular folliculitis, or renal irritation occur. • Don't get in eyes. May cause conjunctivitis, keratitis, corneal opacity. • Wash hands thoroughly after using.
Tretinoin: reduced effectiveness of benzoyl peroxide. Do not use together.	• Contraindicated in sensitivity to any of the ingredients. • Don't use on eyelids, mucous membranes, denuded or highly inflamed skin. • Dryness, redness, and peeling should occur 3 to 4 days after starting treatment. If these common reactions cause considerable discomfort, discontinue temporarily until they subside. • If painful irritation develops, discontinue use. • Cleanser (4%) may cause bleaching of hair or colored fabric.
Detergents, hexachlorophene, antiseptics (especially those containing heavy metal ions such as mercury or silver), iodine, soaks or acidic solutions containing metal ions such as aluminum acetate, (Burow's solution): decreased enzymatic activity. Do not use together.	• Use with caution in debilitated patients, since debriding enzymes may increase risk of bacteremia; watch for signs of systemic infection. • Before application, cleanse lesion with gauze saturated in normal saline, neutral buffer solution, or hydrogen peroxide; use topical antibacterial agent (such as neomycin-bacitracin-polymyxin B) if infection is present. Apply to lesion in powder form before using collagenase. If infection does not respond, discontinue collagenase until infection is healed. Confine collagenase ointment to area of lesion (Lassar's paste may protect surrounding skin). Apply ointment in thin layers to assure contact with necrotic tissue and complete wound coverage; apply collagenase ointment with tongue depressor on deep wounds; with gauze on shallow wounds. Remove any debris that comes off easily. Remove excess ointment, and cover wound with sterile gauze pad. • Discontinue when sufficient debridement has occurred. • Observe wound to monitor progress of therapy. Appearance of granulation may indicate effectiveness. Notify doctor if inflammation or color of drainage indicates any spread of infection. • Watch for symptoms of protein sensitization (long-term therapy). • If enzymatic action must be stopped for any reason, apply Burow's solution. • Avoid getting ointment in eyes. If this occurs, flush with water at once. • Protect drug from heat.
None significant.	• Before application, cleanse wound with sterile water, saline, or other appropriate solution. Do not dry. • When saturated, medication turns gray-yellow and should be removed. • To remove, irrigate with sterile water, saline, or other cleansing solution.

NAME	INDICATIONS & DOSAGE	SIDE EFFECTS
fluorouracil Efudex◆, Fluoroplex◆	*Multiple actinic or solar keratoses; superficial basal cell carcinoma—* **Adults and children:** apply cream (5%) or solution (2% or 5%) b.i.d.	*Skin:* erythema, pain, burning, scaling, pruritus, hyperpigmentation, dermatitis, soreness, suppuration, swelling.
hydroquinone Artra Skin Tone Cream, Derma-Blanch, Eldopaque◆, Eldopaque-Forte◆, Eldoquin◆, Eldoquin Forte◆, Esoterica Medicated Cream, Golden Peacock, HQC Kit	*Bleaching of blemished skin, lentigo, chloasma, freckles, old-age spots, and other skin conditions due to melanin—* **Adults, and children 12 years and over:** apply 2% to 4% concentration daily or b.i.d.	*Skin:* mild irritation and sensitization.
methoxsalen Oxsoralen◆	*Protect against sunburn, enhance pigmentation, and induce repigmentation in vitiligo—* **Adults, and children over 12 years:** for small, well-defined lesions, apply topically weekly or less often and expose to ultraviolet light gradually, as directed. Oral dosage, see p. 1108.	*CNS:* nervousness, insomnia, depression. *GI:* discomfort, nausea, diarrhea. *Skin:* edema, erythema, painful blistering, burning, peeling.
selenium sulfide Exsel◆, Iosel 250, Selsun◆, Selsun Blue, Sul-Blue	*Dandruff, seborrheic scalp dermatitis—* **Adults and children:** massage 1 to 2 teaspoonfuls into clean, wet scalp. Leave on for 2 to 3 minutes. Rinse thoroughly, and repeat application. Apply twice weekly for 2 weeks, then once a week for 2 weeks, or as frequently as needed to maintain control.	*Skin:* oily or dry scalp and hair, hair discoloration, hair loss.

INTERACTIONS	NURSING CONSIDERATIONS
None significant.	• Wash hands immediately after handling medication. • Avoid using with occlusive dressings. • Patient should avoid prolonged exposure to sunlight or ultraviolet light. • Apply with caution near eyes, nose, and mouth. • Warn patient that treated area may be unsightly during therapy and for several weeks after therapy is stopped. Complete healing may not occur until 1 or 2 months after treatment is stopped. • Ingestion and systemic absorption may cause leukopenia, thrombocytopenia, stomatitis, diarrhea, or GI ulceration, bleeding, and hemorrhage. • Topical application to large ulcerated areas may cause systemic toxicity. • For basal cell carcinoma use 5% strength.
None significant.	• Contraindicated in patients with prickly heat, sunburn, irritated skin or as depilatory. • Don't use near eyes. • If rash or irritation develops, discontinue therapy. • Sensitivity can be tested by applying a small amount of low-concentration medication on skin before treatment is started. Allergic reactions should appear within 24 hours. • Patient should protect treated areas from ultraviolet light. • Use opaque medication during the day; cream or lotion at night. • Doesn't cause permanent depigmentation.
Photosensitizing agents: do not use together.	• Contraindicated in hepatic insufficiency, porphyria, acute lupus erythematosus, hydromorphic and polymorphic light eruptions. Use with caution in familial history of sunlight allergy, GI diseases, or chronic infection. • Monitor carefully for signs of cataracts, melanoma, or skin carcinoma. • Regulate therapy carefully. Overdosage or overexposure to light can cause serious burning or blistering. • Topical treatment should be directly supervised by a doctor. • When applied topically to face or hands, patient should protect area from light (except during treatment exposure). • Protect eyes and lips during light exposure treatments. • Monthly hepatic function tests should be done on patients with vitiligo (especially at beginning of therapy). • Significant changes require 6 to 9 months of therapy.
None significant.	• Contraindicated in sulfur hypersensitivity. • Use with caution around areas of acute inflammation or exudation to avoid increased absorption. • If sensitivity reactions occur, discontinue use. • Reduce or prevent hair discoloration by thorough rinsing after treatment. • Avoid contact with eyes. • Highly toxic if ingested. • Wash hands carefully after handling. • Protect from heat.

NAME	INDICATIONS & DOSAGE	SIDE EFFECTS
streptokinase-streptodornase Varidase◆	*Adjunctive treatment of suppurative surface tissues, including ulcers, radiation necrosis, infected wounds, burns, surgical incisions, skin grafts, and whenever clotted blood, or fibrinous or purulent accumulations are undesirable—* **Adults and children:** apply on individual basis, depending on area treated and doctor's orders. Oral dosage, see p. 1060.	*Systemic:* fever.
sutilains Travase◆	*Debridement of second- and third-degree burns, adjunctive debridement of decubitus ulcers, pyogenic wounds, or ulcers resulting from peripheral vascular disease—* **Adults and children:** apply thinly to area extending ¼ to ½ inch beyond area to be debrided. Cover with loose wet dressing t.i.d. or q.i.d.	*CNS:* local paresthesias. *Skin:* mild pain, bleeding, transient dermatitis.
tretinoin (vitamin A acid, retinoic acid) Aberel, Retin-A	*Acne vulgaris (especially grades I, II, and III)—* **Adults and children:** cleanse affected area and lightly apply solution once daily at bedtime.	*Skin:* feeling of warmth, slight stinging, local erythema, peeling at site, chapping and swelling, blistering and crusting, temporary hyperpigmentation or hypopigmentation.

INTERACTIONS	NURSING CONSIDERATIONS
Detergents, anti-infectives (such as benzalkonium chloride, hexachlorophene, iodine): decreased enzymatic activity. Do not use together.	• Contraindicated in areas of active hemorrhage. • Remove exudates carefully and frequently, especially from closed areas, to avoid pyrogenesis. • Not effective on fibrous tissue, mucoproteins, or collagens. • Refrigerated solution stable for 2 weeks. Room temperature solution stable for 24 hours. • Use rubber dams, or gauze or nylon dressing to keep medication in constant contact with lesion. • Prolonged use may result in a high antienzyme titer. Dosage may need to be increased. • Product comes as solution or jelly. Mix to dilution ordered. • To make jelly, add 5 ml sterile water for injection or sterile physiological saline to 125,000-unit vial streptokinase-streptodornase; mix with 15 ml jar of carboxymethyl cellulose (CMC) jelly 4.5%. The resulting mixure contains 5,000 IU SK and 1,250 IU SD/ml or g. • Thoroughly cleanse and irrigate wound area with sterile normal saline or water before treatment to remove antiseptics, detergents, and heavy metal antibacterials, which can decrease enzyme activity. • Moisten wound area for optimal enzymatic activity. Dress wound if necessary, but remove waste products frequently. Observe wound to monitor progress of therapy. Appearance of granulation tissue may indicate effectiveness. Notify doctor if inflammation or color of drainage indicates spread of infection. • Avoid getting solution in eyes. If this occurs, flood with water at once. • Protect drugs from heat.
Detergents, anti-infectives (such as benzalkonium chloride, hexachlorophene, iodine, and nitrofurazone), and compounds containing metallic ions (such as silver nitrate and thimerosal): adversely affected enzymatic activity. Do not use together.	• Contraindicated in wounds involving major body cavities or containing exposed nerves or nerve tissue, fungating neoplastic ulcers, wounds in women of childbearing age, persons having limited cardiac or pulmonary reserves. • Use cautiously near eyes. If accidental contact occurs, flush eyes repeatedly with large amounts of normal saline solution or sterile water. • Before application, cleanse and irrigate affected area with normal saline or sterile water solution to remove antiseptic or heavy metal antibacterial agents. • May give mild analgesic to reduce painful reactions, but discontinue if pain is severe, also discontinue if bleeding or dermatitis occur. • For best response, keep affected area moist. • In concomitant use of topical antimicrobial agent, apply sutilains first. • Store at 2° to 10° C. (35.6° to 50° F.). • Check expiration date.
None significant.	• Contraindicated in hypersensitivity to any tretinoin component. Use with caution in eczema. • If severe local irritation develops, discontinue temporarily and readjust dosage when application is resumed. • Some redness and scaling are normal reactions. • Beneficial effects should be seen within 6 weeks of treatment. • When treatment is stopped, relapses generally occur within 3 to 6 weeks. • Patient should wash face with a mild soap no more than 2 or 3 times a day. Warn against using strong or medicated cosmetics, soaps, or other skin cleansers. • Exposure to sunlight or ultraviolet rays should be minimal during treatment. If patient is sunburned, delay therapy until sunburn subsides. • Avoid contact with eyes, mouth, nose, and mucous membranes.

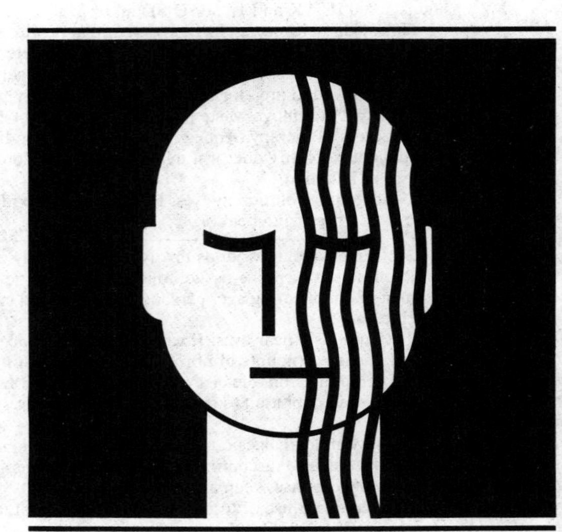

Anesthesia

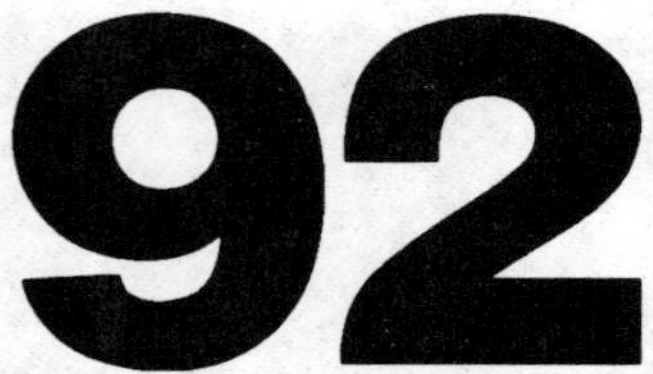

92 Local anesthetics

bupivacaine hydrochloride
chloroprocaine hydrochloride
dibucaine hydrochloride
etidocaine hydrochloride
lidocaine hydrochloride
mepivacaine hydrochloride
piperocaine hydrochloride
prilocaine hydrochloride
procaine hydrochloride
tetracaine hydrochloride

Local anesthetics cause temporary loss of feeling and motor activity by diffusing through the tissue that surrounds the nerve cell membrane, penetrating into the nerve cell, and blocking nerve impulses. Local anesthetics affect autonomic, sensory, and motor nerves. Dosage varies greatly according to the procedure to be performed, degree of anesthesia required, number of neuronal segments to be blocked, tissue vascularity, and individual patient response. The smallest dose and lowest concentration needed to produce the desired anesthesia should be used.

Major uses

- Infiltration anesthesia in dental or minor surgical procedures.
- Regional, spinal, caudal, and epidural.

Mechanism of action

- Block depolarization of nerve fiber membrane by interfering with sodium-potassium exchange across the membrane, preventing nerve impulse generation and conduction.
- When combined with epinephrine, anesthesia is prolonged because the rate of absorption into the body decreases. Vasoconstriction also helps control local bleeding.

Absorption, distribution, and excretion

- Absorption varies according to dose, site of injection, and amount of vasodilation produced by drug. Epinephrine combined with local anesthetic decreases absorption.
- Distributed to all body tissues.
- Metabolized in liver and plasma.
- Excreted in urine.

Onset and duration

- Begin to act in less than 15 minutes.
- Duration varies. Chloroprocaine and procaine have short duration of effect (30 to 60 minutes). Lidocaine, mepivacaine, piperocaine, and prilocaine have intermediate duration (1 to 3 hours). Bupivacaine, dibucaine, and tetracaine have long duration (3 to 6 hours).
- Epinephrine prolongs duration of effect.

Combination products

None, although epinephrine is added to some solutions to prolong effect.

PATIENT REACTION TO A LOCAL ANESTHETIC

After administering an anesthetic, expect your patient's sensory reactions to diminish in the following order:

- Skin veins will be dilated because of vasomotor paralysis.
- Temperature perception usually will undergo several sequential changes. First, sense of cold will disappear, followed by a sense of warmth, followed by an inability to perceive either warmth or cold.
- Slow — followed by fast — pain sensation will be blocked.
- Sense of touch will be dulled.
- Fibers carrying motor impulses will be blocked.
- Muscle, tendon, and joint sense lessen.
- Deep pressure sense is the last to weaken and may not completely disappear.

Expect sensory functions to return in the reverse order. But remember, after epidural/spinal anesthesia, sympathetic activity does not necessarily return simultaneously when sensation has returned.

NAME	INDICATIONS & DOSAGE	SIDE EFFECTS
bupivacaine hydrochloride Marcaine◆	Available with or without epinephrine. Dosages given are for drug *without* epinephrine. **Epidural:** *Sol.* / *Vol. (ml)* / *Dose (mg)* 0.75% / 10 to 20 / 75 to 150 0.50% / 10 to 20 / 50 to 100 0.25% / 10 to 20 / 25 to 50 **Caudal:** *Sol.* / *Vol. (ml)* / *Dose (mg)* 0.50% / 15 to 30 / 75 to 150 0.25% / 15 to 30 / 37.5 to 75 **Peripheral nerve block:** *Sol.* / *Vol. (ml)* / *Dose (mg)* 0.50% / 5 to 80 / 25 to 400 (max.) May repeat dose q 3 hours. Dose and interval may be increased with epinephrine. Maximum 400 mg daily.	*CNS:* excitation, depression, nervousness, dizziness, chills, drowsiness, convulsions, respiratory arrest, loss of consciousness. *CV:* myocardial depression,, hypotension, cardiac arrest, fetal bradycardia. *EENT:* blurred vision, constriction of pupils, tinnitus. *Other:* urticaria, edema as anaphylactoid reaction. *After epidural or caudal:* high or total spinal block, urinary retention, fecal incontinence, loss of perineal sensation and sexual function, paresthesia, headache, backache, slowed labor, increased incidence of forceps delivery, persistent analgesia, lower limb paralysis.
chloroprocaine hydrochloride Nesacaine (for infiltration and regional anesthesia), Nesacaine-CE (for caudal and epidural anesthesia)	Only available without epinephrine. **Infiltration and nerve block:** *Sol.* / *Vol. (ml)* / *Dose (mg)* 1% / 3 to 20 / 30 to 200 2% / 2 to 40 / 20 to 400 **Caudal and epidural:** *Sol.* / *Vol. (ml)* / *Dose (mg)* 2% to 3% / 15 to 25 / 300 to 750 May repeat with smaller doses q 40 to 50 minutes. Dose and interval may be increased with epinephrine. Maximum adult dose 800 mg, or 1 g when mixed with epinephrine.	*CNS:* excitation, depression, dizziness, nervousness, tremors, drowsiness, convulsions, respiratory arrest. *CV:* myocardial depression, hypotension, bradycardia, cardiac arrest. *EENT:* blurred vision *Skin:* lesions, urticaria. *Other:* edema.
dibucaine hydrochloride Nupercaine	Only available without epinephrine. **Spinal anesthesia:** *Perineum and lower limbs* *Sol.* / *Vol. (ml)* / *Dose (mg)* 0.5% / 0.5 to 1 / 2.5 to 5 *Lower abdomen* *Sol.* / *Vol. (ml)* / *Dose (mg)* 0.5% / 1 to 1.5 / 5 to 7.5 *Upper abdomen* *Sol.* / *Vol. (ml)* / *Dose (mg)* 0.5% / 2 / 10 *Lower extremities as high as pelvis* *Sol.* / *Vol. (ml)* / *Dose (mg)* 1;1,500 / 6 / 4	*CNS:* headache, palsies. *GI:* nausea, vomiting. *Other:* respiratory arrest, hypotension.

◆ Also available in Canada.
◆◆ Available in Canada only.
Unmarked trade names available in United States only.

INTERACTIONS	NURSING CONSIDERATIONS
Chloroform, halothane, cyclopropane, trichloroethylene, and related drugs: cardiac arrhythmias may occur when used with bupivacaine *with* epinephrine. Use with extreme caution. *MAO inhibitors, tricyclic antidepressants:* severe, sustained hypertension may occur when used with bupivacaine *with* epinephrine. Use with extreme caution.	• Contraindicated in children under 12 years and for spinal, paracervical block, or topical anesthesia. Use cautiously in debilitated, elderly, or acutely ill pattients; severe hepatic disease; drug allergies. • Use cautiously in cardiovascular disorders and in body areas with limited blood supply (ears, nose). • Keep resuscitative equipment and drugs available. • Don't use solution with preservatives for caudal or epidural block. • Onset in 4 to 17 minutes; duration 3 to 7 hours. • Causes less fetal depression than other local anesthetics. • Discard partially used vials without preservatives. 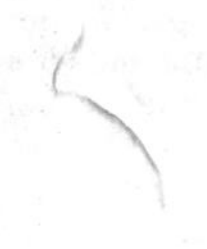
None significant.	• Contraindicated in hypersensitivity to procaine, tetracaine, or other *p*-aminobenzoic acid derivatives, and for spinal or topical anesthesia. Epidural and caudal contraindicated in CNS disease. Use cautiously in debilitated, elderly, or acutely ill patients; children; drug allergies; paracervical block; cardiovascular disease. • Use solutions with epinephrine cautiously in cardiovascular disorders and in body areas with limited blood supply (ears, nose). • A 3 ml test dose should be injected at least 10 minutes before giving total dose to check for intravascular or subarachnoid injection. Motor paralysis and extensive sensory anesthesia indicate subarachnoid injection. • Don't use solution with preservatives for caudal or epidural block. • Don't use discolored solution. • Keep resuscitative equipment and drugs available. • Onset in 12 minutes; duration 30 to 60 minutes. • Discard partially used vials without preservatives.
None significant.	• Contraindicated in cerebrospinal disease, septicemia, pernicious anemia with spinal cord symptoms, arthritis, pyogenic skin infection in puncture area. Use cautiously in hysteria, chronic backache, headache of long duration, migraine, shock, hypotension, leaking spinal fluid, cardiac decompensation, pleural effusions, increased abdominal pressure, possibility of hemorrhage. • Low spinal solution contraindicated in cesarean section or in presence of blood when doing lumbar puncture. Use low spinal solutions cautiously in cardiac or neurologic disease, back problems, uncooperative or hysterical patients. • Use solutions with epinephrine cautiously in cardiovascular disorders and in body areas with limited blood supply (ears, nose). • Keep resuscitative equipment and drugs available. • Don't use for nerve block or infiltration. • Don't use discolored solution. • Used primarily for spinal block and as topical anesthetic.

(continued on following page)

NAME	INDICATIONS & DOSAGE	SIDE EFFECTS
dibucaine hydrochloride *(continued)*	**Spinal anesthesia:** *Lower abdomen* *Sol.* / *Vol. (ml)* / *Dose (mg)* 1:1,500 / 10 to 15 / 6.67 to 10 **Spinal anesthesia:** *Upper abdomen* *Sol.* / *Vol. (ml)* / *Dose (mg)* 1;1,500 / 15 to 18 / 10 to 12	
etidocaine hydrochloride Duranest	Available with or without epinephrine. Doses cited are for drug *with* epinephrine. Dose and interval may be decreased without epinephrine. **Infiltration:** *Sol.* / *Vol. (ml)* / *Dose (mg)* 0.5% / 1 to 80 / 5 to 400 **Peripheral nerve block:** *Sol.* / *Vol. (ml)* / *Dose (mg)* 0.5% / 5 to 80 / 25 to 400 1% / 5 to 40 / 50 to 400 **Central neural block:** *Lower limbs, cesarean section, lumbar peridural* *Sol.* / *Vol. (ml)* / *Dose (mg)* 1% / 10 to 30 / 100 to 300 1.5% / 10 to 20 / 150 to 300 *Vaginal* *Sol.* / *Vol. (ml)* / *Dose (mg)* 0.5% / 10 to 30 / 50 to 150 1% / 5 to 20 / 50 to 200 **Caudal:** *Sol.* / *Vol. (ml)* / *Dose (mg)* 0.5% / 10 to 30 / 50 to 150 1% / 10 to 30 / 100 to 300	*CNS:* nervousness, tremors, dizziness, convulsions, loss of consciousness. *CV:* hypotension, bradycardia, peripheral vasodilation, myocardial depression, cardiac arrest. *Skin:* urticaria. *Other:* respiratory arrest, edema, anaphylaxis.
lidocaine hydrochloride Ardecaine, Canocaine, Dilocaine, Dolicaine, L-Caine, Nervocaine, Norocaine, Rocaine, Ultracaine, Xylocaine Hydrochloride◆	Available with or without epinephrine. Doses cited are for drug *without* epinephrine except where indicated. **Caudal** *(obstetrics)* **or epidural** *(thoracic):* *Sol.* / *Vol. (ml)* / *Dose (mg)* 1% / 20 to 30 / 200 to 300 **Caudal** *(surgery):* *Sol.* / *Vol. (ml)* / *Dose (mg)* 1.5% / 15 to 20 / 225 to 300 **Epidural** *(lumbar anesthesia):* *Sol.* / *Vol. (ml)* / *Dose (mg)* 1.5% / 15 to 20 / 225 to 300 2% / 10 to 15 / 200 to 300 Maximum dose 200 to 300 mg per hour.	*CNS:* excitation or depression, nervousness, dizziness, tremors, drowsiness, convulsions, loss of consciousness. *CV:* hypotension, bradycardia, myocardial depression, cardiac arrest. *EENT:* blurred vision. *Skin:* urticaria. *Other:* respiratory arrest, edema, anaphylaxis.

INTERACTIONS	NURSING CONSIDERATIONS
	• Onset in 10 to 15 minutes; duration 6 hours. • Discard partially used vials without preservatives.
Chloroform, halothane, cyclopropane, trichloroethylene, and related drugs: cardiac arrhythmias may occur when used with etidocaine *with* epinephrine. Use with extreme caution. *MAO inhibitors, tricyclic antidepressants, phenothiazines:* severe, sustained hypertension or hypotension may occur when used with etidocaine solution *with* epinephrine. Use with extreme caution.	• Contraindicated in inflammation or infection in puncture region, children under 14 years, septicemia, severe hypertension, spinal deformities, neurological disorders, and spinal block. Use cautiously in debilitated, elderly, or acutely ill patients; severe shock; heart block; epidural block in obstetrics; general drug allergies; hepatic and renal disease. • Use solutions with epinephrine cautiously in cardiovascular disease, and in body areas with limited blood supply (nose, ear). • Don't use solution with preservatives for caudal or epidural block. • Keep resuscitative equipment and drugs available. • Onset in 2 to 8 minutes, duration 4.5 to 13 hours. • For symptoms and treatment of anaphylaxis, see p. 1114.
Chloroform, halothane, cyclopropane, trichloroethylene, and related drugs: cardiac arrhythmias may occur when used with lidocaine *with* epinephrine. Use with extreme caution. *MAO inhibitors, tricyclic antidepressants:* severe, sustained hypertension may occur when used with lidocaine *with* epinephrine. Use with extreme caution.	• Contraindicated in inflammation or infection in puncture region, septicemia, severe hypertension, spinal deformities, neurologic disorders. Use cautiously in debilitated, elderly, or acutely ill patients; in severe shock; heart block; in obstetrics; general drug allergies; and paracervical block. • Use solutions with epinephrine cautiously in cardiovascular disorders and in body areas with limited blood supply (nose, ear). • Keep resuscitative equipment and drugs available. • A 2- to 5-ml test dose should be injected at least 5 minutes before giving total dose to check for intravascular or subarachnoid injection. Motor paralysis and extensive sensory anesthesia indicate subarachnoid injection. • Solutions containing preservatives should not be used for spinal, epidural, or caudal block. • Discard partially used vials without preservatives. • For symptoms and treatment of anaphylaxis, see p. 1114.

(continued on following page)

NAME	INDICATIONS & DOSAGE	SIDE EFFECTS
lidocaine hydrochloride *(continued)*	*For anesthesia other than spinal*—maximum single adult dose 4.5 mg/Kg or 300 mg. *With epinephrine for anesthesia other than spinal*—maximum single adult dose 7 mg/Kg or 500 mg. Don't repeat dose more often than q 2 hours. **Spinal surgical anesthesia:** *Sol.* / *Vol. (ml)* / *Dose (mg)* 5% with 7.5% dextrose / 1.5 to 2 / 75 to 100 Dose and interval may be increased with epinephrine. For antiarrhythmic doses, see p. 176.	
mepivacaine hydrochloride Carbocaine♦, Cavacaine, Isocaine	Available with or without levonordefrin (vasoconstrictor). Doses cited are for drug *without* levonordefrin. **Nerve block:** *Sol.* / *Vol. (ml)* / *Dose (mg)* 1% / 5 to 20 / 50 to 200 2% / 5 to 20 / 100 to 400 **Transvaginal block or infiltration** *(maximum dose):* *Sol.* / *Vol. (ml)* / *Dose (mg)* 1% / 40 / 400 **Paracervical block** *(obstetrics):* *Sol.* / *Vol (ml)* / *Dose (mg)* 1% / 10 / 100 Give on each side (200 mg total) per 90-minute period. **Caudal and epidural:** *Sol.* / *Vol. (ml)* / *Dose (mg)* 1% / 15 to 30 / 150 to 300 1.5% / 10 to 25 / 150 to 375 2% / 10 to 20 / 200 to 400 **Therapeutic block** *(pain management):* *Sol.* / *Vol. (ml)* / *Dose (mg)* 1% / 1 to 5 / 10 to 50 2% / 1 to 5 / 20 to 100 **Adults:** maximum single dose 7 mg/Kg up to 550 mg. Don't repeat more often than q 90 minutes. Maximum total dose 1,000 mg daily. **Children:** maximum dose 5 to 6 mg/Kg. In children under 3 years or weighing less than 14 Kg, use 0.5% or 1.5% solution only. Dose and interval may be increased with levonordefrin.	*CNS:* excitation, depression, nervousness, dizziness, drowsiness, respiratory arrest, loss of consciousness. *CV:* myocardial depression, hypotension, cardiac arrest, fetal bradycardia. *EENT:* blurred vision, constriction of pupils, tinnitus. *Skin:* urticaria. *Other:* edema. *After epidural or caudal:* high or total spinal block, urinary retention, fecal incontinence, loss of perineal sensation and sexual function, paresthesia, headache, backache, slowed labor, increased incidence of forceps delivery, persistent analgesia, lower limb paralysis.

INTERACTIONS	NURSING CONSIDERATIONS
Chloroform, halothane, cyclopropane, trichloroethylene, and related drugs: cardiac arrhythmias may occur when used with mepivacaine *with* levonordefrin. Use with extreme caution. *MAO inhibitors, tricyclic antidepressants:* severe, sustained hypertension may occur when used with mepivacaine *with* levonordefrin. Use with extreme caution.	• Contraindicated in sensitivity to methylparaben, in heart block, or for spinal anesthesia. Use cautiously in debilitated, elderly, or acutely ill patients, or for paracervical block. • Use solutions with levonordefrin cautiously in cardiovascular disease and in body areas with limited blood supply (nose, ear). • Monitor fetal heart rate when paracervical block used in delivery. • Keep resuscitative equipment and drugs available. • Don't use solutions with preservatives for caudal or epidural block. • Onset in 15 minutes; duration 3 hours. • Discard partially used vials without preservatives.

NAME	INDICATIONS & DOSAGE	SIDE EFFECTS
piperocaine hydrochloride Metycaine	**Caudal block** *(obstetrics in women with normal-sized pelvic canals):* *Sol.* *Vol. (ml)* *Dose (mg)* 1.5% 30 450 May give additional 20 ml doses (300 mg) q 30 to 40 minutes, p.r.n. **Infiltration** *(maximum dose):* *Sol.* *Vol. (ml)* *Dose (mg)* 0.5% 200 1,000 1% 80 800 For dental infiltration, use a 1% to 2% solution. For peripheral or sympathetic nerve block, use 0.5% to 2% solution.	*CNS:* excitation, depression, dizziness, nervousness, tremors, drowsiness, convulsions. *CV:* myocardial depression, hypotension, bradycardia, cardiac arrest. *EENT:* blurred vision. *Skin:* lesions, urticaria. *Other:* respiratory arrest, edema.
prilocaine hydrochloride Citanest♦, Propitocaine	**Infiltration:** *Sol.* *Vol. (ml)* *Dose (mg)* 1% to 2% 20 to 30 200 to 600 **Peripheral nerve block** *(intercostal or paravertebral):* *Sol.* *Vol. (ml)* *Dose (mg)* 1% to 2% 3 to 5 30 to 100 **Peripheral nerve block** *(sciatic [femoral or brachial plexus] or caudal nerve block [surgery]):* *Sol.* *Vol. (ml)* *Dose (mg)* 2% 20 to 30 400 to 600 3% 15 to 20 450 to 600 **Caudal nerve block** *(obstetrics):* *Sol.* *Vol. (ml)* *Dose (mg)* 1% 20 to 30 200 to 300 **Epidural:** *Sol.* *Vol. (ml)* *Dose (mg)* 1% 20 to 30 200 to 300 2% 20 to 30 400 to 600 3% 15 to 20 450 to 600 Maximum single adult dose 8 mg/Kg up to 600 mg. In continuous caudal or epidural anesthesia, don't give maximum dose more often than q 2 hours.	*CNS:* nervousness, dizziness, tremors, drowsiness, convulsions, loss of consciousness. *CV:* hypotension, myocardial depression, bradycardia, cardiac arrest. *EENT:* blurred vision. *Skin:* urticaria. *Other:* respiratory arrest, edema, anaphylaxis. *With 4% solution:* swelling and paresthesia of lips and mouth. *At maximum dose:* methemoglobinemia.

INTERACTIONS	NURSING CONSIDERATIONS
None significant.	• Contraindicated in hypersensitivity to procaine, tetracaine, or other *p*-aminobenzoic acid derivatives, CNS diseases, spinal deformity, infection at injection site, extreme obesity, profound anemia, or spinal block, in highly nervous women. • Don't use solutions with preservatives for caudal block. • Keep resuscitative equipment and drugs available. • Effect peaks in 20 to 30 minutes, then decreases over next 10 minutes. • Dilute 2% solutions to 0.5% or 1% with NaCl injection or Ringer's injection. Don't use sterile water for injection. • An 8 ml dose of anesthetic solution should be injected a few minutes before giving total dose to check for subarachnoid injection. Motor paralysis and extensive sensory anesthesia indicate subarachnoid injection. • Discard partially used vials without preservatives.
None significant.	• Contraindicated in methemoglobinemia, severe shock, heart block, infection at injection site, or for spinal block. Use cautiously in debilitated, elderly, or acutely ill patients; children under 10 years; and in general drug sensitivities. • Epidural and caudal contraindicated in CNS disease, spinal deformities, septicemia, severe hypertension, and in children. • Keep resuscitative equipment and drugs available. • Duration 1 to 3 hours. • Don't use solutions with preservatives for caudal or epidural block. • Discard partially used vials without preservatives. • A 5 ml test dose should be injected at least 5 minutes before giving total dose to check for intravascular or subarachnoid injection. Motor paralysis and extensive sensory anesthesia indicate subarachnoid injection. • For symptoms and treatment of anaphylaxis, see p. 1114.

NAME	INDICATIONS & DOSAGE	SIDE EFFECTS
procaine hydrochloride Novocain◆, Unicaine	Only available without epinephrine. **Spinal anesthesia**—before using, dilute 10% solution with 0.9% NaCl injection, sterile distilled water, or cerebrospinal fluid. For hyperbaric technique, use dextrose solution. *Perineum:* use 0.5 ml 10% solution and 0.5 ml diluent injected at fourth lumbar interspace. *Perineum and lower extremities:* use 1 ml 10% solution and 1 ml diluent injected at third or fourth lumbar interspace. *Up to costal margin:* use 2 ml 10% solution and 1 ml diluent injected at second, third, or fourth lumbar interspace. **Epidural block:** *Sol.* · *Vol. (ml)* · *Dose (mg)* 1.5% · 25 · 375 **Peripheral nerve block:** *Sol.* · *Vol. (ml)* · *Dose (mg)* 1% · 25 · 250 2% · 25 · 500 *Infiltration:* use 250 to 600 mg 0.25% to 0.5% solution. Maximum initial dose 1 g. Dose and interval may be increased with epinephrine.	*CNS:* fainting, convulsions, headache. *CV:* hypotension, weak and rapid pulse. *GI:* nausea, vomiting. *Other:* talkativeness, respiratory difficulty and paralysis.
tetracaine hydrochloride Pontocaine◆	*Low spinal (saddle block) in vaginal delivery:* give 2 to 5 mg as hyperbaric solution (in 6% dextrose). Maximum dose 15 mg. *Perineum and lower extremities:* give 5 to 10 mg. *Prolonged spinal anesthesia (2 to 3 hours):* dilute 1% solution with equal volume of cerebrospinal fluid, or dissolve 5 mg powdered drug in 1 ml cerebrospinal fluid immediately before giving. Give 1 ml/5 seconds. *Up to costal margin:* give 15 to 20 mg.	*CNS:* restlessness, meningitis, syncope, headache, vasomotor and respiratory paralysis. *CV:* hypotension, weak pulse. *GI:* nausea, vomiting. *Other:* shallow breathing, pallor, cold sweat, talkativeness.

INTERACTIONS	NURSING CONSIDERATIONS
Echothiophate iodide: reduced hydrolysis of procaine. Use together cautiously.	• Contraindicated in traumatized urethra and in hypersensitivity to chloroprocaine, tetracaine, or other *p*-aminobenzoic acid derivatives. Use cautiously in CNS diseases, infection at puncture site, shock, profound anemia, cachexia, sepsis, hypertension, hypotension, hyperexcitable patients, GI hemorrhage, bowel perforation or strangulation, peritonitis, cardiac decompensation, massive pleural effusions, and increased intra-abdominal pressure. • Contraindications to obstetric use: pelvic disproportion, placenta previa, abruptio placentae, floating fetal head, intrauterine manipulation. • Keep resuscitative equipment and drugs available. • A 1- to 5-ml test dose should be given 5 to 15 minutes before total epidural dose. Motor paralysis and extensive sensory anesthesia indicate subarachnoid injection. • Use solution without preservatives for epidural block. • Onset in 2 to 5 minutes; duration 60 minutes. • Discard partially used vials without preservatives.
None significant.	• Contraindicated in infection at injection site, serious CNS diseases, and in hypersensitivity to procaine, chloroprocaine, tetracaine, or other *p*-aminobenzoic acid derivatives. Use cautiously in shock, profound anemia, cachexia, hypertension, hypotension, peritonitis, cardiac decompensation, massive pleural effusion, increased intracranial pressure, infection, and in highly nervous patients. • Saddle block contraindicated in cephalopelvic disproportion, placenta previa, abruptio placentae, intrauterine manipulation, floating fetal head. • Don't use cloudy, discolored, or crystallized solutions. • Keep resuscitative equipment and drugs available. • 10 times as strong as procaine HCl. • Onset in 15 minutes; duration up to 3 hours. • When cerebrospinal fluid is added to powdered drug or drug solution during spinal anesthesia, solution may be cloudy. • Protect from light; store in refrigerator.

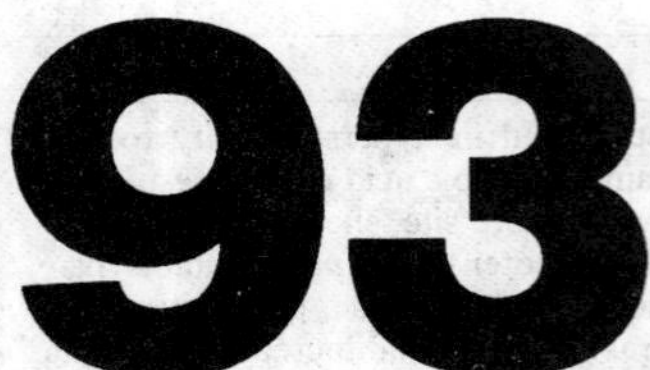

General anesthetics

fentanyl citrate with droperidol
ketamine hydrochloride
methohexital sodium
thiamylal sodium
thiopental sodium

General anesthetics are most commonly administered intravenously (or rectally when indicated for basal anesthesia; ketamine hydrochloride and fentanyl citrate with droperidol can also be administered intramuscularly). They are used for short-term procedures and with other anesthetics. With the exception of ketamine hydrochloride and fentanyl citrate with droperidol, these agents are barbiturate anesthetics with relatively weak analgesic properties.

Major uses

- As general anesthetics for short-term procedures.
- To induce anesthesia before administering other anesthetics.
- To supplement other anesthetics.
- For basal anesthesia in children.

Mechanism of action

- Barbiturate anesthetics act by depressing the central nervous system. Ketamine hydrochloride appears to interrupt association pathways of the brain, causing dissociative anesthesia, a feeling of dissociation from the environment.
- Fentanyl citrate with droperidol acts by depressing the central nervous system to produce a general calming effect, reduced motor activity, and analgesia.

Absorption, distribution, and excretion

- Exact absorption, distribution, and excretion unknown but may be absorbed in most body tissues. Excreted in urine, feces, and bile.
- Fentanyl citrate (a narcotic analgesic) with droperidol (a tranquilizer) is metabolized in the hepatic and excreted in the urine and the feces.
- Thiamylal sodium and thiopental sodium (and, to a lesser extent, methohexital sodium) accumulate in fat deposits of the body. Barbiturate anesthetics are detoxified in the hepatic and excreted in the urine.

Onset and duration

• Onset of fentanyl is within seconds; duration is 30 to 60 minutes when given intravenously.
• Onset of droperidol is within 3 to 10 minutes; duration is 2 to 4 hours.
• Onset of ketamine hydrochloride is within 30 seconds; duration is 5 to 10 minutes when administered intravenously. The duration of intramuscular induction is 12 to 25 minutes.
• Onset of the barbiturate anesthetics is within 30 to 60 seconds; duration is usually 10 to 30 minutes after last dose when given intravenously. The duration of methohexital sodium is about half as long. When administered rectally, thiamylal sodium produces maximal effects within 30 minutes; duration about 1 hour.

Combination products

None.

MANAGING RECOVERY FROM ANESTHESIA

• Immediately upon receiving patient, check airway. Usually the patient's endotracheal tube has been removed by the anesthesiologist. Watch for complications, such as laryngospasms.
• During the late stages of recovery from anesthesia, you may need to insert an oropharyngeal airway to prevent the tongue from obstructing the air passage. Leave it in place until the patient fully regains consciousness.
• Give oxygen if needed.
• Position patient so he won't aspirate vomitus or secretions into tracheobronchial passages.
• Suction patient if needed.
• Check and record vital signs at 5- to 15-minute intervals until patient is fully reactive.
• Check position and function of all drains, tubes, and intravenous fluids.

NAME	INDICATIONS & DOSAGE	SIDE EFFECTS
fentanyl citrate with droperidol Controlled substance Schedule II Innovar (each ml contains [in a 1:50 ratio] fentanyl 0.05 mg as a citrate and droperidol 2.5 mg).	Doses vary depending on application and patient. *Anesthesia—* **Adults:** *Premedication*—0.5 to 2 ml I.M. 45 to 60 minutes before to surgery. *Adjunct to general anesthesia*—Induction: 1 ml per 20 to 25 lbs. body weight by slow I.V. Maintenance: not indicated as sole agent for maintenance of surgical anesthesia. Used in combination with other measures. To prevent excessive accumulation of the relatively long-acting droperiodol component, fentanyl alone should be used in increments of 0.025 to 0.05 mg (0.5 to 1 ml) for maintenance of analgesia. However, during prolonged surgery, additional 0.5 to 1 ml amounts of Innovar may be administered with caution. *Diagnostic procedures*—0.5 to 2 ml I.M. 45 to 60 minutes before procedure. In prolonged procedure, give 0.5 to 1 ml. I.V. with caution and without a general anesthetic. *Adjunct in regional anesthesia*—1 to 2 ml I.M. or slow I.V. **Children:** Premedication—0.25 ml/20 lbs. body weight I.M. 45 to 60 minutes before surgery. *Adjunct to general anesthesia*—0.5 ml per 20 lbs. body weight (total combined dose for induction and maintenance). Following induction with Innovar, fentanyl alone in a dose of ¼ to ⅓ of adult dose should be used to avoid accumulation of droperidol. However, during prolonged surgery, additional amounts of Innovar may be administered with caution.	*CNS:* emergence delirium and hallucinations, postoperative drowsiness. *CV:* vasodilation, hypotension, decreased pulmonary arterial pressure, bradycardia, or tachycardia. *EENT:* blurred vision. *GI:* nausea, vomiting. *Other:* respiratory depression, apnea, or arrest; drug dependence; muscle rigidity; laryngospasms; chills; shivering; twitching; diaphoresis.
ketamine hydrochloride Ketaject, Ketalar♦	*Induce anesthesia for procedures, especially short-term diagnostic or surgical, not requiring skeletal muscle relaxation; before giving other general anesthetics or to supplement low-potency agents, such as nitrous oxide—* **Adults and children:** 1 to 4.5 mg/Kg I.V., administered over 60	*CNS:* tonic and clonic movements resembling convulsions. *CV:* increased blood pressure and pulse rate, hypotension, bradycardia. *EENT:* diplopia, nystagmus, slight increase in intraocular pressure, laryngospasms. *GI:* mild anorexia, nausea, vomiting. *Skin:* transient erythema, measles-

♦ Also available in Canada.
♦♦ Available in Canada only.
Unmarked trade names available in United States only.

INTERACTIONS	NURSING CONSIDERATIONS
CNS depressants (such as barbiturates, tranquilizers, narcotics, and general anesthetics): additive or potentiating effect. Dosage should be reduced. *MAO inhibitors:* severe and unpredictable potentiation of Innovar. Do not use together or within 2 weeks of MAO inhibitor therapy.	• Contraindicated in intolerance to either component. Use with caution in patients with head injuries and increased intracranial pressure, chronic obstructive pulmonary disease, hepatic and renal dysfunction, bradyarrhythmias, elderly or debilitated patients. • Hypotension is a common side effect. However, if blood pressure drops, also consider hypovolemia as a possible cause. Use appropriate parenteral fluids to help restore blood pressure. • Vital signs should be monitored frequently. • Be aware that respiratory depression, muscular rigidity of respiratory muscles, and respiratory arrest can occur. Have narcotic antagonist and CPR equipment on hand. • Maintain airway. • Postoperative EEG pattern may return to normal slowly. • Postoperatively, if narcotic analgesics are required, use initially in reduced doses, as low as ¼ to ⅓ those usually recommended. • When Innovar is given for anesthesia induction, fentanyl (Sublimaze) should be used for maintenance analgesia during the procedure. • For symptoms and treatment of toxicity, see p. 1119.
Thyroid hormones: may elevate blood pressure and cause tachycardia. Give cautiously.	• Contraindicated in history of cerebrovascular accident; patients who would be endangered by a significant rise in blood pressure; severe hypertension; severe cardiac decompensation; surgery of the pharynx, larynx, or bronchial tree, unless used with muscle relaxants. Use with caution in chronic alcoholism, alcohol-intoxicated patients, patients with cerebrospinal fluid pressure elevated before anesthesia. • Discourage giving anything orally at least 6 hours before elective surgery • Because of rapid induction, patient should be physically supported during administration.

(continued on following page)

NAME	INDICATIONS & DOSAGE	SIDE EFFECTS
ketamine hydrochloride *(continued)*	seconds; or 6.5 to 13 mg/Kg I.M. To maintain anesthesia, repeat in increments of half to full initial dose.	like rash. *Other:* dream-like states, hallucinations, confusion, excitement, irrational behavior, psychic abnormalities.
methohexital sodium Controlled substance Schedule IV Brevital Sodium, Brietal Sodium♦♦	*General anesthetic for short-term procedures (oral surgery, gynecologic and genitourinary examinations); reduction of fractures; before electroconvulsive therapy; for prolonged anesthesia when used with gaseous anesthetics—* **Adults and children:** 5 to 12 ml 1% solution (50 to 120 mg) I.V. at 1 ml/5 seconds. Dose required for induction may vary from 50 to 120 mg or more; average about 70 mg. Induction dose provides anesthesia for 5 to 7 minutes. Maintenance—intermittent injection: 2 to 4 ml 1% solution (20 to 40 mg) 4 to 7 minutes; continuous I.V. drip: administer 0.2% solution (1 drop/second).	*CNS:* muscular twitching, headache, emergence delirium, injury to nerves adjacent to injection site. *CV:* temporary hypotension, tachycardia, thrombophlebitis, circulatory depression, peripheral vascular collapse. *GI:* excessive salivation, nausea, vomiting. *Local:* pain at injection site. *Skin:* tissue necrosis with extravasation. *Other:* hiccups, coughing, acute allergic reactions, laryngospasm, bronchospasm, respiratory depression, apnea, twitching. Extended use may cause cumulative effect; may be habit-forming.
thiamylal sodium Controlled substance Schedule III Surital♦	*General anesthetic for short-term procedures; anesthetic before administering other general anesthetics (dosage individualized to patient's response)—* **Adults:** 3 to 6 ml 2.5% solution I.V. at 1 ml/5 seconds. Additional intermittent injections of 0.5 to 1 ml. Maximum dose 1 g (40 ml 2.5% solution). *Rectal administration before diagnostic procedures—* **Children:** 800 mg to 1 g 5% solution/22.5 Kg body weight. *Supplemental anesthetic—* **Adults:** 0.2% or 0.3% solution continuous I.V. drip. Recovery occurs within 20 to 30 minutes after last injection.	*CNS:* excitement, headache, injury to nerves adjacent to injection site, emergence delirium. *CV:* hypotension, circulatory depression, thrombophlebitis, hypoxia. *GI:* nausea, vomiting, excessive salivation. *Local:* pain at injection site. *Skin:* rash, urticaria, tissue necrosis with extravasation. *Other:* hiccups, laryngospasm, bronchospasm, respiratory depression, apnea. Extended use can cause cumulative effects; may be habit-forming.

INTERACTIONS	NURSING CONSIDERATIONS
	• Do not inject barbiturates and ketamine HC1 from same syringe, as they are chemically incompatible. • Monitor: vital signs before, during, and after anesthesia. • Check cardiac function for patients with hypertension or cardiac depression. • Maintain airway. • Resuscitation equipment should be available and ready for use. • Start supportive respiration if respiratory depression occurs. Use mechanical support if possible rather than administering analeptics. • Keep verbal, tactile, and visual stimulation at a minimum during recovery phase to reduce incidence of emergent reactions. • A potent hallucinogen. Abused by young adults.
None significant.	• Contraindicated in severe hepatic dysfunction, hypersensitivity to barbiturates, or porphyria; in shock or impending shock; and in patients for whom general anesthetics would be hazardous. Use with caution in debilitated patients, in patients with asthma, respiratory obstruction, severe hypertension or hypotension, myocardial disease, congestive heart failure, severe anemia, or extreme obesity. • Maintain pulmonary ventilation. • Avoid extravascular or intra-arterial injections. • Monitor vital signs before, during, and after anesthesia. • Have resuscitative equipment and drugs ready. • Reduce postoperative nausea by having patient fast before administration. • Incompatible with silicone; avoid contact with rubber stoppers or parts of syringes that have been treated with silicone. • Incompatible with lactated Ringer's solution. • Do not mix with acid solutions such as atropine sulfate. • Solvents recommended are 5% glucose solution or isotonic (0.9%) sodium chloride instead of distilled water. • Rate of flow must be individualized for each patient. • Solutions may be stored and used as long as they remain clear and colorless. Solutions cannot be heated for sterilization.
None significant.	• Contraindicated in hepatic dysfunction or disease, traumatic or impending shock, porphyria, hypersensitivity to barbiturates, and in those for whom general anesthetics would be hazardous. Use with caution in respiratory disease or obstruction, obesity, marked disturbance of arterial tension, cardiac failure, anemia, status asthmaticus, endocrine or renal dysfunction, and in debilitated patients. • Maintain airway. • Have resuscitative equipment and drugs ready. • Monitor vital signs before, during, and after anesthesia. • Avoid extravascular or intra-arterial injection. • Incompatible with lactated Ringer's solution or with solutions containing bacteriostatic or buffer agents, which tend to cause precipitation. • Don't inject air into solution; may cause cloudiness. • Sterile water is the preferred solvent for injections. For drip maintenance use 5% glucose or isotonic sodium chloride to avoid extreme hypotonicity. • Solutions of atropine sulfate, *d*-tubocurarine, or succinylcholine may be given concurrently but should not be mixed together. • Do not heat solutions for sterilization. Solutions should be stored in refrigerator and used within 6 days. If kept at room temperature, use within 24 hours.

NAME	INDICATIONS & DOSAGE	SIDE EFFECTS
thiopental sodium Controlled substance Schedule III Pentothal sodium◆ (injection and rectal suspension)	*Induce anesthesia before administering other anesthetics*— 210 to 280 mg (3 to 4 ml/Kg) usually required for average adult (70 Kg). *General anesthetic for short-term procedures*— **Adults:** 2 to 3 ml 2.5% solution (50 to 75 mg) administered I.V. only at intervals of 20 to 40 seconds, depending on reaction. Dose may be repeated with caution, if necessary. *Convulsive states following anesthesia*— 75 to 125 mg (3 to 5 ml of 2.5% solution) immediately following convulsion. *Psychiatric disorders (narcoanalysis, narcosynthesis)*— 100 mg/min (4 ml/min 2.5% solution) until confusion occurs and before sleep. Maximum dose 50 ml/min. *Basal anesthesia by rectal administration*— **Adults and children:** administer up to 1 g/22.5 Kg (50 lbs.) body weight, or 0.5 ml 10% solution/Kg body weight. Maximum 1 to 1.5 g (children weighing 75 lbs. or more) and 3 to 4 g (adults weighing 200 lbs. or more).	*CNS:* prolonged somnolence, retrograde amnesia. *CV:* myocardial depression, arrhythmias. *Local:* pain at injection site. *Skin:* tissue necrosis with extravasation. *Other:* sneezing, coughing, shivering, respiratory depression (momentary apnea following each injection is typical), bronchospasm, laryngospasm. May be habit-forming.

INTERACTIONS	NURSING CONSIDERATIONS
None significant.	• Contraindicated in absence of suitable veins for intravenous administration, hypersensitivity to barbiturates, status asthmaticus, porphyria, respiratory depression or obstruction, decompensated cardiac disease, severe anemia, hepatic cirrhosis, shock, renal dysfunction, intracranial pressure. • Give test dose (1 to 3 ml 2.5% solution) to assess reaction to drug. • When used as general anesthetic, give atropine sulfate as premedication to diminish laryngeal reflexes and to prevent spastic abduction of vocal cords. • Have resuscitative equipment and oxygen ready. • Avoid extravasation and intra-arterial injection. • Maintain airway. • Monitor vital signs before, during, and after anesthesia. • Solutions of atropine sulfate, *d*-tubocurarine, or succinylcholine may be given concurrently but should not be mixed together. • Do not heat solutions for sterilization. Solutions should be stored in refrigerator and used within 6 days. If kept at room temperature, use within 24 hours.

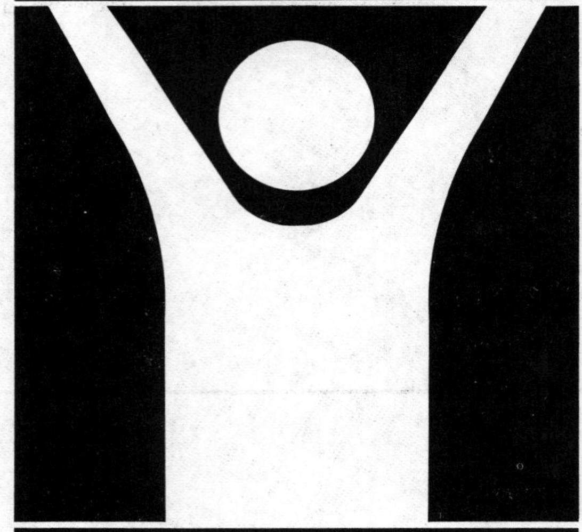

Nutrition

94
Vitamins

vitamin A
- oleovitamin A

vitamin B complex
- cyanocobalamin (B_{12})
- cyanocobalamin, hydroxocobalamin (B_{12a})
- folic acid (B_9)
- leucovorin calcium
- niacin (B_3)
- niacinamide
- pyridoxine hydrochloride (B_6)
- riboflavin (B_2)
- thiamine hydrochloride (B_1)

vitamin C
- ascorbic acid

vitamin D
- cholecalciferol (D_3)
- ergocalciferol (D_2)

vitamin E

vitamin K analogs
- menadione/menadiol sodium diphosphate (K_3)
- phytonadione (K_1)

multivitamins

trace elements
- copper
- iodine
- manganese
- zinc
- zinc sulfate

Vitamins are unrelated organic compounds the body needs for normal growth, reproduction, and homeostasis but which it cannot synthesize adequately, if at all. Trace elements, or microelements, function in several metalloenzyme systems critical for life support.

Major uses

- Vitamins are used to prevent or treat selective or multiple vitamin deficiencies and for other therapeutic purposes.
- Trace elements are used to prevent or treat dietary deficiencies and for other medical purposes that result from these deficiencies.
- Zinc sulfate is also used as adjunctive treatment for various skin disorders, rheumatoid arthritis, and a reduced sense of taste when these disorders coexist with low serum zinc levels.

Mechanism of action

- Vitamins act as coenzymes or coenzyme precursors to catalyze the metabolism of

protein, fat, and carbohydrates, and to facilitate energy-producing and anabolic reactions.
• Trace elements may act in metalloenzyme units, participating in synthesis and stabilization of proteins and nucleic acids in subcellular and membrane transport systems.

Absorption, distribution, and excretion

• Most vitamins are readily absorbed and distributed throughout the body. Excess water-soluble vitamins are rapidly excreted in urine. Fat-soluble vitamins, which require bile and adequate pancreatic secretions for absorption, are stored for longer periods. Excretion rates vary with metabolic status, stress, disease, and requirements for tissue repair.
• Trace minerals are readily absorbed after oral or parenteral administration and are distributed throughout the body. They are excreted in the urine.

Onset and duration

• Onset is usually rapid. Most vitamin and trace element deficiencies respond quickly to therapeutic doses.

Combination products

Vitamin A and D combinations
B vitamin combinations
B complex vitamins
B complex with vitamin C
Multivitamins
Multivitamins with B_{12}
Calcium and vitamin products
Fluoride with vitamins
B complex vitamins with iron
Multivitamins with iron
Miscellaneous vitamins and minerals
Geriatric supplements with multivitamins and minerals
Multivitamins and minerals with hormones

NAME	INDICATIONS & DOSAGE	SIDE EFFECTS
oleovitamin A Acon, Afaxin◆◆, Alphalin, Aquasol-A◆, Dispatabs, Natola	*Severe vitamin A deficiency with xerophthalmia—* **Adults, and children over 8 years:** 500,000 IU P.O. daily for 3 days, then 50,000 IU P.O. daily for 14 days, then maintenance with 10,000 to 20,000 IU P.O. daily for 2 months, followed by adequate dietary nutrition and RDA vitamin A supplements. *Severe vitamin A deficiency—* **Adults, and children over 8 years:** 100,000 IU P.O. or I.M. daily for 3 days, then 50,000 IU P.O. or I.M. daily for 14 days, then maintenance with 10,000 to 20,000 IU P.O. daily for 2 months, followed by adequate dietary nutrition and RDA vitamin A supplements. **Children 1 to 8 years:** 17,500 to 35,000 IU I.M. daily for 10 days. **Infants under 1 year:** 7,500 to 15,000 IU I.M. daily for 10 days. *Maintenance only—* **Children 4 to 8 years:** 15,000 IU I.M. daily for 2 months, then adequate dietary nutrition and RDA vitamin A supplements. **Children under 4 years:** 10,000 IU I.M. daily for 2 months, then adequate dietary nutrition and RDA vitamin A supplements.	Side effects are usually seen only with toxicity (hypervitaminosis A). *Blood:* hypoplastic anemia, leukopenia, elevated vitamin A levels, elevated serum lipids. *CNS:* irritability, headache, increased intracranial pressure, fatigue, lethargy, malaise. *EENT:* miosis, papilledema, exophthalmos. *GI:* anorexia, nausea, vomiting, abdominal discomfort, epigastric pain, diarrhea. *GU:* hypomenorrhea. *Skin:* alopecia; drying, cracking, scaling of skin; pruritus; lip fissures; massive desquamation; increased pigmentation; night sweating. *Other:* slow growth, decalcification of bone, fractures, hyperostosis, painful periostitis, premature closure of epiphysis, migratory arthralgia, cortical thickening over the radius and tibia, bulging fontanels, hepatomegaly, jaundice, splenomegaly.
cyanocobalamin (vitamin B_{12}) Anacobin◆◆, Bedoce, Bedoz◆◆, Berubigen, Betalin-12, Bio-12◆◆, Crystimin, Cyanabin◆◆, Cyanocobalamin, Cyano-Gel, DBH-B_{12}, Dodex, Kaybovite, Neo-Vadrin, Pernavite, Poyamin, Redisol◆, Rhodavite, Rubesol, Rubion◆◆, Rubramin◆, Ruvite, Sigamine, Sytorex, Vi-	*Vitamin B_{12} deficiency due to inadequate diet, gastrectomy, or any other condition, disorder, or disease except malabsorption related to pernicious anemia—* **Adults:** 25 mcg P.O. daily as dietary supplement, or 30 to 100 mcg S.C. or I.M. daily for 5 to 10 days, depending on severity of deficiency. Maintenance dose: 100 to 200 mcg I.M. once monthly. For subsequent prophylaxis, advise adequate nutrition and daily RDA vitamin B_{12} supplements. **Children:** 1 mcg P.O. daily as	*CV:* peripheral vascular thrombosis. *GI:* transient diarrhea. *Local:* pain, burning at S.C. or I.M. injection sites. *Skin:* itching, transitory exanthema, urticaria. *Other:* anaphylaxis, anaphylactoid reactions.

◆ Also available in Canada.
◆◆ Available in Canada only.
Unmarked trade names available in United States only.

INTERACTIONS	NURSING CONSIDERATIONS
Mineral oil, cholestyramine resin: reduced GI absorption of fat-soluble vitamins. If needed, give mineral oil at bedtime.	• Oral administration contraindicated in presence of malabsorption syndrome; if malabsorption is due to inadequate bile secretion, oral route may be used with concurrent administration of bile salts (dehydrocholic acid). Also contraindicated in hypervitaminosis A. Intravenous administration contraindicated except for special water-miscible forms intended for infusion with large parenteral volumes. Intravenous push of vitamin A of any type is also contraindicated (anaphylaxis or anaphylactoid reactions and death have resulted). • Caution: evaluate intake from fortified foods, dietary supplements, self-administered drugs, and prescription drug sources. • In pregnant women, avoid doses exceeding 6,000 IU daily. • To avoid toxicity, discourage patient self-administration of megavitamin doses without specific indications. • Watch for side effects if dosage is high. • Acute toxicity has resulted from single doses of 25,000 IU/Kg of body weight; 350,000 IU in infants, and over 2,000,000 IU in adults have also proved acutely toxic. • Chronic toxicity has resulted from doses of 25,000 IU/Kg of body weight. Chronic toxicity in infants (3 to 6 months) has resulted from doses of 18,500 IU daily for 1 to 3 months. In adults, chronic toxicity has resulted from doses of 50,000 IU daily for over 18 months; 500,000 IU daily for 2 months, and 1,000,000 IU daily for 3 days. • Monitor patient closely during vitamin A therapy for skin disorders, since high dosages may induce chronic toxicity. • Liquid preparations available if nasogastric administration is needed. • Record eating and bowel habits. Report abnormalities to doctor. • Adequate vitamin A absorption requires suitable protein intake, bile (give supplemental salts if necessary), concurrent RDA doses of vitamin E; and zinc (multivitamins usually supply zinc, but supplements may be necessary in long-term hyperalimentation). • Absorption is faster and more complete with water-miscible preparations, intermediate with emulsions, and slowest with oil suspensions. • In severe hepatic dysfunction, diabetes, and hypothyroidism, use vitamin A rather than carotenes for vitamin therapy, because the vitamin itself is more easily absorbed and the diseases adversely affect conversion of carotenes into vitamin A. If carotenes are prescribed, dosage should be doubled. • Protect from light.
Neomycin, colchicine, para-aminosalicylic acid and salts, chloramphenicol: malabsorption of vitamin B_{12}. Don't use together.	• Parenteral administration contraindicated in hypersensitivity to vitamin B_{12} or cobalt. Alternate use of large oral doses of vitamin B_{12} is controversial and should not be considered routine; combined with intrinsic factor increases risk of hypersensitive reactions and should be avoided. Therapeutic dose contraindicated before proper diagnosis; B_{12} therapy may mask folate deficiency. • I.V. administration may cause anaphylactic reactions. Use cautiously and only if other routes are ruled out. • Use cautiously in anemic patients with coexisting cardiac, pulmonary, or hypertension problems; in patients with early Leber's disease; in patients with severe B_{12} dependent deficiencies, especially those receiving cardiac glycosides (monitor closely the first 2 to 3 days for hypokalemia, fluid overload, pulmonary edema, congestive heart failure, and hypertension); and in patients with gouty conditions (monitor serum uric acid levels for hyperuricemia). • Don't mix parenteral liquids in same syringe with other medication.

(continued on following page)

NAME	INDICATIONS & DOSAGE	SIDE EFFECTS
cyanocobalamin (vitamin B_{12}) *(continued)* bedoz, Vi-Twel **cyanocobalamin, hydroxocobalamin (vitamin B_{12a})** Alpha Redisol, Alpha-uvite, Cobalpha-mead, Codroxomin, Crystallin, Droxovite, Hycobal-12, Neo-Betalin 12, Rubesol-LA, Sytobex-H	dietary supplement, or 1 to 30 mcg S.C. or I.M. daily for 5 to 10 days, depending on severity of deficiency. Maintenance: at least 60 mcg per month I.M. or S.C. For subsequent prophylaxis, advise adequate nutrition and daily RDA vitamin B_{12} supplements. *Pernicious anemia—* **Adults:** initially, 100 to 1,000 mcg I.M. daily for 2 weeks, then 100 to 1,000 mcg I.M. once monthly for life. If neurologic complications are present, follow initial therapy with 100 to 1,000 mcg I.M. once every 2 weeks before starting monthly regimen. **Children:** 1,000 to 5,000 mcg I.M. or S.C. given over 2 or more weeks as 100 mcg increments; then 60 mcg I.M. or S.C. monthly for life. *Methylmalonic aciduria—* **Neonates:** 1,000 mcg I.M. daily for 11 days with a protein-restricted diet. *Diagnostic test for vitamin B_{12} deficiency without concealing folate deficiency in patients with megaloblastic anemias—* **Adults and children:** 1 mcg I.M. daily for 10 days with low B_{12} and folate diet. Reticulocytosis between days 3 to 10 confirms diagnosis of B_{12} deficiency. *Schilling test flushing dose—* **Adults and children:** 1,000 mcg I.M. in a single dose.	
folic acid (vitamin B_9) Folvite♦, Novofolacid♦♦	*Megaloblastic or macrocytic anemia secondary to folic acid or other nutritional deficiency, hepatic disease, alcoholism, intestinal obstruction, excessive hemolysis—* **Pregnant and lactating women:** 0.8 mg P.O., S.C., or I.M. daily. **Adults, and children over 4 years:** 1 mg P.O., S.C., or I.M. daily for 4 to 5 days. After anemia secondary to folic acid deficiency is corrected, proper diet and RDA supplements are necessary to prevent recurrence.	*Skin:* allergic reactions (rash, pruritus, erythema). *Others:* allergic bronchospasms, general malaise.

INTERACTIONS	NURSING CONSIDERATIONS
	Protect from light. • Repository forms add cost without extra effectiveness and may stimulate antibody formation. • Infection, tumors, or renal, hepatic, and other debilitating diseases may reduce therapeutic response. • Deficiencies more common in strict vegetarians and their breastfed infants. • Stress need for pernicious anemia patients to return for monthly injections. Although total body stores may last 3 to 6 years, anemia will recur if not treated monthly. • May cause false positive intrinsic factor antibody test. • B_{12a} is approved for I.M. use only. Only advantage of B_{12a} over B_{12} is longer duration. • 50% to 98% of injected dose may appear in urine within 48 hours. Major portion is excreted within the first 8 hours. • Closely observe serum potassium the first 48 hours. Give potassium if necessary. • Monitor serum uric acid and CBC. • Physically incompatible with dextrose solutions, alkaline or strongly acidic solutions, oxidizing and reducing agents, and many other drugs. • For treatment of anaphylaxis, see p. 1114.
Chloramphenicol: antagonism of folic acid. Monitor for decreased folic acid effect. Use together cautiously.	• Contraindicated in normocytic, refractory, or aplastic anemias; as sole agent in treatment of pernicious anemia (since it may mask neurologic effects); in treatment of methotrexate, pyrimethamine, or trimethoprim overdose, and in undiagnosed anemia (since it may mask pernicious anemia). • Patients with small bowel resections and intestinal malabsorption may require parenteral administration routes. • Don't mix with other medications in the same syringe for I.M. injections. • Protect from light. • May use concurrent folic acid and vitamin B_{12} therapy if supported by diagnosis. • Proper nutrition is necessary to prevent recurrence of anemia. • Peak folate activity occurs in the blood in 30 to 60 minutes. • Hematologic response to folic acid in patients receiving chloramphenicol concurrently with folic acid should be carefully monitored.

(continued on following page)

NAME	INDICATIONS & DOSAGE	SIDE EFFECTS
folic acid (vitamin B_9) *(continued)*	**Children under 4 years:** up to 0.3 mg P.O., S.C., or I.M. daily. *Prevention of megaloblastic anemia of pregnancy and fetal damage—* **Women:** 1 mg P.O., S.C., or I.M. daily throughout pregnancy. *Nutritional supplement—* **Adults:** 0.1 mg P.O., S.C., or I.M. daily. **Children:** 0.05 mg P.O. daily. *Treatment of tropical sprue—* **Adults:** 3 to 15 mg P.O. daily. *Test of megaloblastic anemia patients to detect folic acid deficiency without masking pernicious anemia—* **Adults and children:** 0.1 to 0.2 mg P.O. or I.M. for 10 days while maintaining a diet low in folate and vitamin B complex. (Reticulosis, reversion to normoblastic hematopoesis, and return to normal hemoglobin indicate folic acid deficiency.)	
leucovorin calcium (citrovorum factor or folinic acid) Calcium Folinate	*Megaloblastic or macrocytic anemia secondary to folic acid or other nutritional deficiency, hepatic disease, alcoholism, intestinal obstruction, excessive hemolysis—* **Pregnant and lactating women:** 0.8 mg P.O., S.C., or I.M. daily. **Adults, and children over 4 years:** 1 mg P.O., S.C., or I.M. daily for 4 to 5 days. After anemia secondary to folic acid deficiency is corrected, proper diet and RDA supplements are necessary to prevent recurrence. **Children under 4 years:** up to 0.3 mg P.O., S.C., or I.M. daily. *Test of megaloblastic anemia patients to detect folic acid deficiency without masking pernicious anemia—* **Adults and children:** 0.1 to 0.2 mg P.O. or I.M. for 10 days while maintaining diet low in folate and vitamin B complex. *Overdose of folic acid antagonist—* **Adults and children:** P.O., I.M., or I.V. dose equivalent to the weight of the antagonist given.	*Skin:* allergic reactions (rash, pruritus, erythema). *Others:* allergic bronchospasms.

INTERACTIONS	NURSING CONSIDERATIONS
None significant.	• Contraindicated in treatment of undiagnosed anemia, since it may mask pernicious anemia. Use cautiously in pernicious anemia; a hemolytic remission may occur while neurologic manifestations remain progressive. • Do not confuse leucovorin (folinic acid) with folic acid. • Follow leucovorin rescue schedule and protocol closely to maximize therapeutic response. Generally, leucovorin should not be administered simultaneously with systemic methotrexate. • Treat overdosage of folic acid antagonists, administer within 1 hour if possible; usually ineffective after 4-hour delay. • Protect from light, especially reconstituted parenteral preparations. • Since allergic reactions have been reported with the folic acid, the possibility of allergic reactions to leucovorin should be kept in mind.

(continued on following page)

NAME	INDICATIONS & DOSAGE	SIDE EFFECTS
leucovorin calcium (citrovorum factor or folinic acid) *(continued)*	*Leucovorin rescue after high methotrexate dose in treatment of malignancy—* **Adults and children:** dose at doctor's discretion within 6 to 36 hours of last dose of methotrexate. *Toxic effects of methotrexate used to treat severe psoriasis—* **Adults and children:** 4 to 8 mg I.M. 2 hours after methotrexate dose. *Hematologic toxicity due to pyrimethamine therapy—* **Adults and children:** 5 mg P.O. or I.M. daily. *Hematologic toxicity due to trimethoprim therapy—* **Adults and children:** 400 mcg to 5 mg P.O. or I.M. daily. *Megaloblastic anemia due to congenital enzyme deficiency—* **Adults and children:** 3 to 6 mg I.M. daily, then 1 mg P.O. daily for life. *Folate deficient megaloblastic anemias—* **Adults and children:** up to 1 mg of leucovorin I.M. daily. Duration of treatment depends on hematologic response.	
niacin (vitamin B_3, nicotinic acid) **niacinamide (nicotinamide)** Diacin, Efacin, Lipo-Niacin, Niac, Nicalex, Nico400, Nicobid, Nicocap, Nicolar, Nico-Span, Ni-Span, Vasotherm, Wampocap	*Pellagra—* **Adults:** 10 to 20 mg P.O., S.C., I.M., or I.V. infusion daily, depending on severity of niacin deficiency. Maximum daily dose recommended, 500 mg, should be divided into 10 doses, 50 mg each. **Children:** up to 300 mg P.O. or 100 mg I.V. infusion daily, depending on severity of niacin deficiency. After symptoms subside, advise adequate nutrition and RDA supplements to avoid recurrence. *Hyperlipoproteinemia types III, IV, and V, and as secondary agent in type II—* **Adults:** 100 mg P.O. t.i.d. with meals, increased in 50 to 100 mg steps q 4 days until daily total is 3 to 9 g, individualized as needed to control serum lipids. *Peripheral vascular disease and circulatory disorders—* **Adults:** 250 to 800 mg P.O. daily in divided doses.	Most side effects are dose-dependent. *Blood:* hyperglycemia, hyperuricemia. *CNS:* dizziness, transient headache. *CV:* cardiac arrhythmias, excessive peripheral vasodilation, tachycardia, hypotension. *GI:* nausea, vomiting, diarrhea, possible activation of peptic ulcer, epigastric or substernal pain. *Skin:* flushing, pruritus, dryness, burning, erythema. *Others:* abnormal hepatic function, jaundice.

INTERACTIONS	NURSING CONSIDERATIONS
Antihypertensive drugs of the sympathetic blocking type: may have an additive vasodilating effect and cause postural hypotension. Use together cautiously. Warn patient about postural hypotension.	• Contraindicated in hepatic dysfunction, gallbladder disease, active severe hypotension, hemorrhaging, peptic ulcer, severe cardiac disease, polyneuritis, or cheilosis secondary to pellagra. Use with caution in diabetes or gout. • Monitor hepatic function and blood glucose early in therapy. • Give with meals to minimize GI side effects. • Use timed-release niacin or substitute amide to avoid excessive flushing effects with large doses. Give slowly I.V. Explain harmlessness of flushing syndrome to ease patient's mind. • Stress that medication used to treat hyperlipoproteinemia or to dilate peripheral vessels not "just a vitamin." Explain importance of adhering to therapeutic regimen. • Caution against excessive exposure to sun if dosage is high.

NAME	INDICATIONS & DOSAGE	SIDE EFFECTS
pyridoxine hydrochloride (vitamin B_6) Bee six, Hexa-Betalin◆, Hexacrest, Hexavibex◆	*Dietary vitamin B_6 deficiency—* **Adults:** 10 to 20 mg P.O., I.M., or I.V. daily for 3 weeks, then 2 to 5 mg daily as a supplement to a proper diet. **Children:** 100 mg P.O., I.M., or I.V. to correct deficiency, then an adequate diet with supplementary RDA doses to prevent recurrence. *Seizures related to vitamin B_6 deficiency or dependency—* **Adults and children:** 100 mg I.M. or I.V. in single dose. *Vitamin B_6 responsive anemias or dependency syndrome (inborn errors of metabolism)—* **Adults:** up to 600 mg P.O., I.M., or I.V. daily until symptoms subside, then 50 mg daily for life. **Children:** 100 mg I.M. or I.V., then 2 to 10 mg I.M. or 10 to 100 mg P.O. daily. *Prevention of B_6 deficiency during isoniazid therapy—* **Adults:** 25 to 50 mg P.O. daily. **Children:** at least 0.5 to 1.5 mg daily. **Infants:** at least 0.1 to 0.5 mg daily. If neurologic symptoms develop in pediatric patients, increase dosage as necessary. *Treatment of B_6 deficiency secondary to isoniazid—* **Adults:** 100 mg P.O. daily for 3 weeks, then 50 mg daily. **Children:** titrate dosages.	*Blood:* decreased serum folate levels. *CNS:* drowsiness, paresthesias.
riboflavin (vitamin B_2)	*Riboflavin deficiency or adjunct to thiamine treatment for polyneuritis or cheilosis secondary to pellagra—* **Adults, and children over 12 years:** 5 to 50 mg P.O., S.C., I.M., or I.V. daily, depending on severity. **Children under 12 years:** 2 to 10 mg P.O., S.C., I.M., or I.V. daily, depending on severity. For maintenance, increase nutritional intake and supplement with vitamin B complex.	*GU:* high doses make urine very yellow.

INTERACTIONS	NURSING CONSIDERATIONS
None significant.	• Contraindicated in hypersensitivity to parenteral pyridoxine and in doses larger than 5 mg for patients also receiving levodopa. Caution patient to check dosage, especially in multivitamins. • Protect from light. Do not use injection solution if it contains a precipitate. Slight darkening is acceptable. • Excessive protein intake increases daily pyridoxine requirements. • If sodium bicarbonate is required to control acidosis in isoniazid toxicity, do not mix in same syringe with pyridoxine. • If prescribed for maintainance therapy to prevent deficiency recurrence, stress importance of compliance and of good nutrition. Explain that pyridoxine in combination therapy with isoniazid has a specific therapeutic purpose and is not "just a vitamin." Emphasize need for adhering to therapeutic regimen.
None significant.	• Protect from light. • Stress proper nutritional habits to avoid recurrence of deficiency. • Riboflavin deficiency usually accompanies other B complex deficiencies and may require multivitamin therapy.

NAME	INDICATIONS & DOSAGE	SIDE EFFECTS
thiamine hydrochloride (vitamin B_1) Apatate Drops, Betalin S, Betaxin◆◆, Bewon◆, Megamin◆◆, Thia	*Beriberi—* **Adults:** 10 to 500 mg, depending on severity, I.M. t.i.d. for 2 weeks, followed by dietary correction and multivitamin supplement containing 5 to 10 mg daily thiamine for 1 month. **Children:** 10 to 50 mg, depending on severity, I.M. daily for several weeks with adequate dietary intake. *Anemia secondary to thiamine deficiency, polyneuritis secondary to alcoholism, pregnancy, or pellagra—* **Adults:** 100 mg P.O. daily. **Children:** 10 to 50 mg P.O. daily in divided doses. *Wernicke's encephalopathy—* **Adults:** up to 500 mg to 1 g I.V. for crisis therapy, followed by 100 mg b.i.d. for maintenance. *"Wet beriberi," with myocardial failure—* **Adults and children:** 100 to 500 mg I.V. emergency treatment.	*CNS:* restlessness. *CV:* hypotension after rapid I.V. injection, angioneurotic edema, cyanosis. *EENT:* tightness of throat (allergic reaction). *GI:* nausea, hemorrhage, diarrhea. *Skin:* feeling of warmth, pruritus, urticaria, sweating. *Other:* anaphylactic reactions, weakness, pulmonary edema, and death after rapid I.V. push.
ascorbic acid (vitamin C) Adenex◆◆, Ascorbajen, Ascorbicap, Ascorbineed, Ascoril◆◆, Best-C, Cecon, Cemill, Cenolate, Cetane, Cevalin, Cevi-Bid, Ce-Vi-Sol◆, Cevita, Chew-Cee, C-Ject, C-Long, C-Syrup-500, Liqui-Cee, Megascorb◆◆, Redoxon◆◆, Saro-C, Solucap C, Tega-C, Vitacee, Viterra C	*Frank and subclinical manifestations of scurvy—* **Adults:** 100 mg to 2 g, depending on severity, P.O., S.C., I.M. or I.V. daily, then at least 50 mg daily for maintenance. **Children:** 100 to 200 mg, depending on severity, P.O., S.C., I.M., or I.V. daily, then at least 35 mg daily for maintenance. **Infants:** 50 to 100 mg P.O., I.M., I.V., or S.C. daily. *Extensive burns, delayed fracture or wound healing, postoperative wound healing, and severe febrile or chronic disease states—* **Adults:** 200 to 500 mg S.C., I.M., or I.V. daily. **Children:** 100 to 200 mg P.O., S.C., I.M., or I.V. daily. *Prevention of vitamin C deficiency in those with poor nutritional habits or increased requirements—* **Adults:** at least 45 to 50 mg P.O., S.C., I.M., or I.V. daily.	*CNS:* faintness or dizziness with fast I.V. administration. *GI:* diarrhea, epigastric burning. *GU:* acid urine, oxaluria, renal stones. *Skin:* discomfort at injection site.

INTERACTIONS	NURSING CONSIDERATIONS
None significant.	• Contraindicated in hypersensitivity to thiamine products. I.V. push contraindicated, except when treating life-threatening myocardial failure in "wet beriberi." Use with caution in I.V. administration of large doses (to avoid anaphylactic reactions); skin-test patients with history of hypersensitivity before therapy. • Use parenteral administration only when P.O. route is not feasible. • Clinically significant deficiency can occur in approximately 3 weeks of totally thiamine-free diet. Thiamine deficiency usually requires concurrent treatment for multiple deficiencies. • Doses larger than 30 mg t.i.d. may not be fully utilized by body. When body tissues are saturated with thiamine, it is excreted in urine as pyrimidine. • If beriberi occurs in a breast-fed infant, both mother and child should be treated with thiamine. • Unstable in alkaline solutions; should not be used with materials that yield alkaline solutions. • For treatment of anaphylaxis, see p. 1114.
None significant.	• Use cautiously in G-6-PD deficiency to avoid possibility of hemolytic anemia. • Avoid rapid I.V. administration. • Protect solution from light. • Discourage self-administration for colds; harmful side effects possible. • May inactivate orally administered penicillin G.

(continued on following page)

NAME	INDICATIONS & DOSAGE	SIDE EFFECTS
ascorbic acid (vitamin C) *(continued)*	**Pregnant or lactating women:** at least 60 mg P.O., S.C., I.M., or I.V. daily. **Children:** at least 40 mg P.O., S.C., I.M., or I.V. daily. **Infants:** at least 35 mg P.O., S.C., I.M., or I.V. daily. *Potentiation of methenamine in urine acidification—* **Adults:** 2 g P.O. daily in divided doses. *Preop in gastrectomy patients—* **Adults:** 1 g daily for 4 to 7 days.	
vitamin D (cholecalciferol: vitamin D_3; ergocalciferol: vitamin D_2) Calciferol, Deltalin, Drisdol♦, Radiostol♦♦, Radiostol Forte♦♦	*Rickets and other vitamin D deficiency diseases—* **Adults:** 12,000 IU P.O. or I.M. daily initially, increased as indicated by response up to 500,000 IU daily in most cases and up to 800,000 IU daily for vitamin D resistant rickets. **Children:** 1,500 to 5,000 IU P.O. or I.M. daily for 2 to 4 weeks, repeated after 2 weeks, if necessary. Alternatively, a single dose of 600,000 IU. Monitor serum calcium daily to guide dosage. After correction of deficiency, maintenance includes adequate dietary nutrition and RDA supplements. *Hypoparathyroidism—* **Adults and children:** 50,000 to 200,000 IU P.O. or I.M. daily, with 4 g calcium supplement.	Side effects listed are usually seen in vitamin D toxicity only. *Blood:* hypercalcemia, hyperphosphatemia, mild acidosis, elevated SGOT, SGPT, and BUN, azotemia. *CNS:* headache, dizziness, ataxia, weakness, somnolence, decreased libido, overt psychosis, convulsions. *CV:* hypertension; calcifications of soft tissues, including the heart. *EENT:* metallic taste, rhinorrhea, conjunctivitis (calcific), photophobia, tinnitus. *GI:* anorexia, nausea, constipation, diarrhea. *GU:* polyuria, albuminuria, hypercalcuria, nocturia, impaired renal function, renal calculi. *Skin:* hyperthermia, pruritus, widespread soft-tissue calcification. *Other:* death via renal or cardiovascular failure, bone and muscle pain, bone demineralization, weight loss.
vitamin E Aquasol E♦, D-Alpha-E, Daltose♦♦, E-Ferol, Eprolin, Epsilan-M, Hy-E-Plex, Kell-E, Lethopherol, Maxi-E, Pertropin, Solucap E, Tocopher-Caps, Tokols, Viterra E	*Vitamin E deficiency in premature infants and in patients with impaired fat-absorption—* **Adults:** 5 to 30 IU, depending on severity, P.O. or I.M. daily. Maximum 400 IU daily. **Children:** 1 mg equivalent per 0.6 g of dietary unsaturated fat P.O. or I.M. daily.	None reported.

INTERACTIONS	NURSING CONSIDERATIONS
Mineral oil, cholestyramine resin: inhibited GI absorption of oral vitamin D. Space doses. Use together cautiously.	• Contraindicated in hypercalcemia, hypervitaminosis A, renal osteodystrophy with hyperphosphatemia. • If I.V. route is necessary, use only water-miscible solutions intended for dilution in large-volume parenterals. Use cautiously in cardiac patients, especially if they are receiving glycosides, and in pregnant women, since vitamin D crosses placenta and may be toxic to fetus. • Monitor eating and bowel habits for indications of toxicity. • Hyperphosphatemia patients require dietary phosphate restrictions and binding agents to avoid metastatic calcifications and renal calculi. • Dosage range between therapeutic and toxic effects is narrow. When high therapeutic doses are used, frequent serum and urinary calcium, potassium, and urea determinations should be made. • Malabsorption due to inadequate bile or hepatic dysfunction may require addition of exogenous bile salts to oral vitamin D. • Protect solution from light.
Mineral oil, cholestyramine resin: inhibited GI absorption of oral vitamin E. Space doses. Use together cautiously.	• Water-miscible forms more completely absorbed in GI tract than other forms. • Adequate bile is essential for absorption. • Requirements increase with rise in dietary polyunsaturated acids. • May protect other vitamins against oxidation. • Used for a variety of disorders with mixed successes and failures. Dosages not established. • Mega-doses can cause thrombophlebitis.

NAME	INDICATIONS & DOSAGE	SIDE EFFECTS
menadione/menadiol sodium diphosphate (vitamin K_3) Kappadione, Synkavite♦♦, Synkayvite	*Hypoprothrombinemia secondary to vitamin K malabsorption or drug therapy, or when oral administration is desired and bile secretion is inadequate—* **Adults:** 2 to 10 mg menadione P.O. or 5 to 15 mg menadiol sodium diphosphate P.O. or parenterally, titrated to patient's requirements.	*Blood:* hemolysis in G-6-PD deficiency, hyperbilirubinemia in premature infants, increased prothrombin time. *CNS:* headache, brain damage, kernicterus, death in newborn infants. *GI:* nausea, vomiting, depressed hepatic function. *Local:* pain, hematoma at injection site. *Skin:* allergic rash, pruritus, urticaria.
phytonadione (vitamin K_1) AquaMephyton♦, Konakion♦, Mephyton♦	*Hypoprothrombinemia secondary to vitamin K malabsorption drug therapy or excess vitamin A—* **Adults:** 2 to 25 mg, depending on severity, P.O. or parenterally, repeated and increased up to 50 mg, if necessary. **Children:** 5 to 10 mg P.O. or parenterally. **Infants:** 2 mg P.O. or parenterally. I.V. injection rate for children and infants should not exceed 3 mg/m²/minute or a total of 5 mg. *Hypoprothrombinemia secondary to effect of oral anticoagulants—* **Adults:** 2.5 to 10 mg P.O., S.C., or I.M., based on prothrombin time, repeated, if necessary, 12 to 48 hours after oral dose or 6 to 8 hours after parenteral dose. In emergency, give 10 to 50 mg slow I.V., rate not to exceed 1 mg/minute, repeated q 4 hours, as needed. *Prevention of hemorrhagic disease in neonates—* **Neonates:** 0.5 to 1 mg S.C. or I.M. immediately after birth, repeated in 6 to 8 hours, if needed, especially if mother received oral anticoagulants or long-term anticonvulsant therapy during pregnancy.	*Blood:* hyperbilirubinemia due to overdose and hemolytic anemia in infants, cyanosis. *CNS:* dizziness, convulsive movement. *CV:* transient hypotension after I.V. administration, rapid and weak pulse, cardiac irregularities. *GI:* nausea, vomiting. *Local:* pain, swelling, and hematoma at injection site. *Skin:* sweating, flushing, erythema. *Other:* bronchospasms, dyspnea, cramp-like pain, anaphylaxis and anaphylactoid reactions, usually after rapid I.V. administration.

INTERACTIONS	NURSING CONSIDERATIONS
Mineral oil, cholestyramine resin: inhibited GI absorption of oral vitamin K. Space doses. Use together cautiously.	• Contraindicated in treatment of oral anticoagulant overdose; in treatment for hereditary hypoprothrombinemia (because vitamin K_3 can paradoxically worsen it); in patients with hepatocellular disease, unless it is caused by biliary obstruction; or in treatment of heparin-induced bleeding. Use cautiously during last weeks of pregnancy to avoid toxic reactions in newborns and in G-6-PD deficiency to avoid hemolysis. In severe bleeding, do not delay other measures such as giving fresh frozen plasma or whole blood. Use large doses cautiously in severe hepatic disease. • Failure to respond to vitamin K_3 may indicate coagulation defects. • Excessive use of vitamin K_3 may temporarily defeat oral anticoagulant therapy. Higher doses of oral anticoagulant or interim use of heparin may be required. • Protect parenteral products from light. • When I.V. route must be used, rate shouldn't exceed 1 mg/minute. • Effects of I.V. injections more rapid but shorter lived than S.C. or I.M. injections. • Monitor prothrombin time to determine dosage effectiveness. • Observe for signs of side effects and report them to doctor. • Use caution in handling bulk menadione powder. It is irritating to the skin and respiratory tract. • Leafy vegetables are high in vitamin K content. May alter warfarin needs.
Mineral oil, cholestyramine resin: inhibited GI absorption of oral vitamin K. Use together cautiously.	• Contraindicated in hereditary hypoprothrombinemia; bleeding secondary to heparin therapy or overdose; hepatocellular disease, unless it is caused by biliary obstruction (vitamin K can paradoxically worsen the hypoprothrombinemia). Oral administration contraindicated if bile secretion is inadequate, unless supplemented with bile salts. Use cautiously, if at all, during last weeks of pregnancy to avoid toxic reactions in newborns; in G-6-PD deficiency to avoid hemolysis. Use large doses cautiously in severe hepatic disease. • Failure to respond to vitamin K may indicate coagulation defects. • In severe bleeding, don't delay other measures such as fresh frozen plasma or whole blood. • Protect parenteral products from light. Wrap containers and tubing in foil during infusion. • Effects of I.V. injections more rapid but shorter lived than S.C. or I.M. injections. • Monitor prothrombin time to determine dosage effectiveness. • Observe for signs of side effects and report them to the doctor. • Phytonadione therapy for hemorrhagic disease in infants causes fewer adverse reactions than do other vitamin K analogs. • Check brand-name labels for administration route restrictions. • Administer I.V. by slow infusion. Mix in normal saline solution, dextrose 5% in water, or dextrose 5% in normal saline. • Leafy vegetables are high in vitamin K content. May alter warfarin needs. • For treatment of anaphylaxis, see p. 1114.

(continued on following page)

NAME	INDICATIONS & DOSAGE	SIDE EFFECTS
phytonadione (vitamin K_1) *(continued)*	*Differentiation between hepatocellular disease or biliary obstruction as source of hypoprothrombinemia—* **Adults and children:** 10 mg I.M. or S.C. *Prevention of hypoprothrombinemia related to vitamin K deficiency in long-term parenteral nutrition—* **Adults:** 5 to 10 mg S.C. or I.M. weekly. **Children:** 2 to 5 mg S.C. or I.M. weekly. *Prevention of hypoprothrombinemia in infants receiving less than 0.1 mg/liter vitamin K in breast milk or milk substitutes—* **Infants:** 1 mg S.C. or I.M. monthly.	
multivitamins Available by many brand names. Contain vitamins A, B complex, C, D, and E in varying amounts.	*Prevention of vitamin deficiencies in patients with inadequate diets or increased daily requirements; treatment of multiple vitamin deficiencies and prevention of recurrence; additions to parenteral nutrition solutions to meet patient's normal or increased requirements to reduce cost and facilitate patient compliance with therapy involving multiple vitamin deficiencies—* **Adults and children:** dosage depends on nature and severity of deficiencies, and composition of multivitamin preparation.	• Multivitamin preparations with ordinary doses of each component are usually nontoxic. • Megavitamin combinations may promote significant accumulation of fat-soluble vitamins, with resultant toxicity. • Multivitamins containing therapeutic doses of folic acid may mask pernicious anemia. Unless prescribed otherwise by doctor, patient should avoid folic acid in undiagnosed but suspected pernicious anemia. • Other side effects depend on specific components and concentrations in each multivitamin preparation.
trace elements copper, iodine (as iodide), manganese, zinc	*Prevention of individual trace element deficiencies in patients receiving long-term hyperalimentation—* *Copper—* **Adults:** 2 to 5 mg P.O., or 0.5 to 1.5 mg I.V. daily. **Children:** 0.05 to 0.2 mg/Kg P.O. or I.V. daily *Iodine—* **Adults:** 1 mcg/Kg P.O. or I.V. daily. *Manganese—* **Adults:** 10 to 22 mg P.O. or 1 to 3 mg I.V. daily. *Zinc—* **Adults:** 6 to 15 mg P.O., or 2 to 4 mg I.V. daily. **Children:** 0.3 to 0.4 mg/Kg P.O. or 0.05 mg/Kg I.V. daily.	None reported.

INTERACTIONS	NURSING CONSIDERATIONS
Refer to each component of the multivitamin combination.	• A single discovered vitamin deficiency usually coexists with others. After initial deficiencies are corrected, stress need for adequate nutrition and multivitamin supplements, if appropriate. • Tell patient about possible interactions of vitamins in combinations and what precautions to take to avoid problems. • Stress need to follow doctor's orders regarding daily dosages and follow-up therapy. • Avoid excessive use of large-volume parenteral solutions of multivitamin supplements containing fat-soluble vitamins to avoid hypervitaminosis. I.V. solutions of water-soluble multivitamins may be used more freely. • Chewable flavored multivitamins available for children. Prevent use of these drugs as "candy." • Liquid preparations may contain varying percentages of alcohol. Check label and alert patient to content. • Warn against overdosing. Encourage patient to eat a well-balanced diet. • Store vitamins in a cool place in light-resistant containers to limit loss of potency.
None significant at recommended dosages.	• Check trace element serum levels of patients who have received total parenteral nutrition for 2 months or longer. Give supplement if necessary. • Serum copper and zinc levels are inversely proportional. • Normal serum levels are 0.07 to 0.15 mg/ml copper; 0.05 to 0.15 mg/100 ml zinc; 4 to 20 mcg/100 ml manganese. • Not commercially available. • Solutions of trace elements are compounded by pharmacy for addition to total parenteral nutrition solutions according to various formulas. One common trace element solution is "Shil's solution," which contains copper 1 mg/ml, iodide 0.06 mg/ml, manganese 0.4 mg/ml, and zinc 2 mg/ml.

NAME	INDICATIONS & DOSAGE	SIDE EFFECTS
zinc sulfate Orazinc	*Treatment of zinc deficiency or adjunct to treatment of disorders related to low serum zinc levels, including oral and decubitus leg ulcers, acne, granulomata of the ear, rheumatoid arthritis, and idiopathic hypogeusia; also, as adjunct to vitamin A therapy when patient fails to respond to vitamin A alone, and in acrodermatitis enteropathica.* **Adults:** 200 to 220 mg P.O. t.i.d. (equivalent to 135 to 150 mg elemental zinc daily, 9 times the adult RDA of 15 mg daily). **Children:** dosages not established. RDA is 0.3 mg/Kg daily.	*GI:* distress and irritation, nausea, vomiting with high doses.

INTERACTIONS	NURSING CONSIDERATIONS
None significant.	• Therapeutic benefits result only if patient is zinc-deficient. • Normal serum levels may not reliably show absence of zinc deficiency. • Results may not appear for 6 to 8 weeks in zinc-depleted patients. • If nausea or other GI side effects occur, decreasing dosage to 100 mg b.i.d. may help, since zinc is believed to irritate gastric mucosa. • Brown bread and dairy products may interfere with zinc absorption.

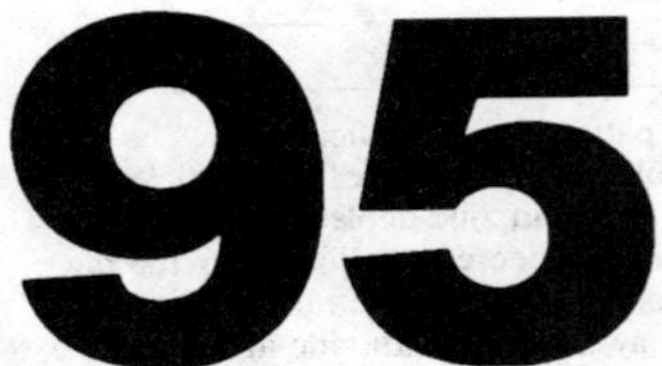

Calorics

amino acid solution
corn oil
dextrose (d-glucose)
essential crystalline amino acid solution
fat emulsions
fructose (levulose)
invert sugar
medium chain triglycerides

Calorics are nutritional substrates which furnish calories to be utilized as energy sources in metabolism.

Major uses

• Supply of calories alone or in combination with carbohydrate, fat, or protein to establish a positive nitrogen balance and stimulate anabolism in patients who cannot maintain adequate oral caloric intake.
• Partial fluid replacement.

Mechanism of action

• Provide more calories (fats provide the most; carbohydrates and proteins somewhat less) from which extra energy is produced for body repair and anabolism.

Absorption, distribution, and excretion

• Calorics are readily absorbed and rapidly utilized after intravenous administration.

Onset and duration

• Effects appear quickly. Rapid utilization usually requires daily replenishment in large amounts.

Combination products

DEXTROSE 2½%, 5%, 10% and sodium chloride 0.45%.
DEXTROSE 2½%, 5%, 10% and sodium chloride 0.9%.
DEXTROSE 3⅓% and sodium chloride 0.3%.
DEXTROSE 5% and sodium chloride 0.11%, 0.2%, 0.33%.
POTASSIUM CHLORIDE 10 mEq, 20 mEq, 27 mEq, 30 mEq, 40 mEq, in 5% dextrose in water.
POTASSIUM CHLORIDE 10 mEq, 20 mEq, 30 mEq, 40 mEq in 5% dextrose, and 0.2% sodium chloride.
POTASSIUM CHLORIDE 10 mEq, 20 mEq, 30 mEq, 40 mEq in 5% dextrose, and 0.45% sodium chloride.
DEXTROSE 5% WITH ELECTROLYTE #75: 50 g/L dextrose, 40 mEq/L Na+, 35 mEq/L K+, 40 mEq/L Cl−, 15 phosphate, and 20 lactate (mEq/L)

ISOLYTE M WITH 5% DEXTROSE: 50 g/L dextrose, 40 mEq/L Na+, 35 mEq/L K+, 40 mEq/L Cl−, 15 phosphate, and 20 mEq/L acetate.
ISOLYTE G WITH 5% DEXTROSE: 50 g/L dextrose, 63 mEq/L Na+, 17 mEq/L K+, and 150 mEq/L Cl−.
IONOSOL G IN 10% DEXTROSE: 100 g/L dextrose, 63 mEq/L Na+, 17 mEq/L K+, and 151 mEq/L Cl−.
ISOLYTE G WITH 10% DEXTROSE: 100 g/L dextrose, 63 mEq/L Na+, 17 mEq/L K+, and 150 mEq/L C1−.
DEXTROSE 2.5% IN HALF-STRENGTH RINGER'S: 25 g/L dextrose, 74 mEq/L Na+, 2 mEq/L K+, 2 mEq/L Ca++, and 78 mEq/L Cl−.
DEXTROSE 5% IN RINGER'S: 50 g/L dextrose, 147 mEq/L Na+, 4 mEq/L K+, 4 mEq/L Ca++, and 155 Cl−.
DEXTROSE 2½% IN HALF-STRENGTH LACTATED RINGER'S: 25 g/L dextrose, 65 mEq/L Na+, 2 mEq/L K+, 1 mEq/L Ca++, 54 mEq/L Cl−, and 14 mEq/L lactate.
DEXTROSE 2½% IN LACTATED RINGER'S: 25 g/L dextrose, 130 mEq/L Na+, 4 mEq/L K+, 3 mEq/L Ca++, 109 mEq/L Cl−, and 28 mEq/L lactate.
DEXTROSE 5% IN LACTATED RINGER'S: 50 g/L dextrose, 130 mEq/L Na+, 4 mEq/L K+, 3 mEq/L Ca++, 109 mEq/L C1−, and 28 mEq/L lactate.
DEXTROSE 10% IN LACTATED RINGER'S: 100 g/L dextrose, 130 mEq/L Na+, 4 mEq/L K+, 3 mEq/L Ca++, 109 mEq/L Cl−, and 28 mEq/L lactate.
DEXTROSE 5% IN ACETATED RINGER'S: 50 g/L dextrose, 130 mEq/L Na+, 4 mEq/L K+, 3 mEq/L Ca++, 109 mEq/L Cl−, and 28 mEq/L acetate.
DEXTROSE 5% WITH ELECTROLYTE #48: 50 g/L dextrose, 25 mEq/L Na+, 20 mEq/L K+, 3 mEq/L mg++, 22 mEq/L Cl−, 3 mEq/L phosphate, and 23 mEq/L lactate.
IONOSOL MB IN 5% DEXTROSE: 50 g/L dextrose, 25 mEq/L Na+, 20 mEq/L K+, 3 mEq/L Mg++, 22 mEq/L Cl−, 3 phosphate, and 23 mEq/L lactate.
ELECTROLYTE #2 WITH 5% DEXTROSE: 50 g/L dextrose, 55 mEq/L Na+, 23 mEq/L K+, 5 mEq/L Mg++, and 45 mEq/L Cl−, 12 mEq/L phosphate, and 26 mEq/L lactate.
IONOSOL B IN 5% DEXTROSE: 50 g/L dextrose, 57 mEq/L Na+, 25 mEq/L K+, 5 mEq/L Mg++, 49 mEq/L Cl−, 13 mEq/L phosphate, and [illegible] mEq/L lactate.
POLYONIC M 56 IN 5% DEXTROSE: 50 g/L dextrose, 40 mEq/L Na+, 13 mEq/L K+, 3 mEq/L Mg++, 40 mEq/L Cl−, and 16 mEq/L acetate.
PLASMA-LYTE 56 IN 5% DEXTROSE: 50 g/L dextrose, 40 mEq/L Na+, 13 mEq/L K+, 3 mEq/L Mg++, 40 mEq/L Cl−, and 16 mEq/L acetate.
ISOLYTE P WITH 5% DEXTROSE: 50 g/L dextrose, 25 mEq/L Na+, 20 mEq/L K+, 3 mEq/L Mg++, 22 mEq/L Cl−, 3 mEq/L phosphate, and 23 mEq/L acetate.
ISOLYTE S WITH 5% DEXTROSE: 50 g/L dextrose, 140 mEq/L Na+, 5 mEq/L K+, 3 mEq/L Mg++, 98 mEq/L Cl−, and 27 mEq/L acetate.

PLASMA-LYTE 148 IN 5% DEXTROSE: 50 g/L dextrose, 140 mEq/L Na+, 5 mEq/L K+, 3 mEq/L Mg++, and 98 mEq/L Cl−, and 27 mEq/L acetate.
POLYONIC R 148 IN 5% DEXTROSE: 50 g/L dextrose, 140 mEq/L Na+, 5 mEq/L K+, 3 mEq/L mg++, 98 mEq/L Cl−, and 27 mEq/L acetate.
ISOLYTE R WITH 5% DEXTROSE: 50 g/L dextrose, 40 mEq/L Na+, 16 mEq/L K+, 5 mEq/L Ca++, 3 mEq/L mg++, and 40 mEq/L Cl−, and 24 mEq/L acetate.
PLASMA-LYTE M IN 5% DEXTROSE: 50 g/L dextrose, 40 mEq/L Na+, 16 mEq/L K+, 5 mEq/L Ca++, 3 mEq/L Mg++, 40 mEq/L Cl−, 12 mEq/L lactate, and 12 mEq/L acetate.
POLYSAL WITH 5% DEXTROSE: 50 g/L dextrose, 140 mEq/L Na+, 10 mEq/L K+, 5 mEq/L Ca+, 3 mEq/L mg++, 103 mEq/L Cl−, and 55 mEq/L acetate.
PLASMA-LYTE WITH 5% DEXTROSE: 50 g/L dextrose, 140 mEq/L Na+, 10 mEq/L K+, 5 mEq/L Ca++, 3 mEq/L Mg++, 103 mEq/L Cl−, 8 mEq/L lactate, and 47 mEq/L acetate.
ISONOSOL D-CM IN 5% DEXTROSE: 50 g/L dextrose, 138 mEq/L Na+, 12 mEq/L K+, 5 mEq/L Ca++, 3 mEq/L Mg++, 108 mEq/L Cl−, and 50 mEq/L lactate.
ISOLYTE M WITH 5% FRUCTOSE: 50 g/L fructose, 40 mEq/L Na+, 35 mEq/L K+, 40 mEq/L Cl−, 15 mEq/L phosphate, and 20 mEq/L acetate.
ISOLYTE P WITH 5% FRUCTOSE: 50 g/L fructose, 25 mEq/L Na+, 26 mEq/L K+, 3 mEq/L Mg++, 23 mEq/L Cl−, and 3 mEq/L phosphate, and 23 mEq/L acetate.
POLYONIC-M 900: 150 g/L fructose, 40 mEq/L Na+, 13 mEq/L K+, 3 mEq/L Mg++, 40 mEq/L Cl−, and 16 mEq/L acetate.
NORMOSOL-M 900♦: 150 g/L fructose, 40 mEq/L Na+, 13 mEq/L K+, 3 mEq/L Mg++, 40 mEq/L Cl−, 16 mEq/L acetate.

IONOSOL G WITH 10% INVERT SUGAR: 100 g/L invert sugar, 60 mEq/L Na+, 17 mEq/L K+, and 147 mEq/L Cl−.
5% TRAVERT WITH ELECTROLYTE #4: 50 g/L invert sugar, 30 mEq/L Na+, 15 mEq/L K+, 23 mEq/L Cl−, 3 mEq/L phosphate, and 20 mEq/L lactate.
ELECTROLYTE #2 WITH 5% INVERT SUGAR: 50 g/L invert sugar, 58 mEq/L Na+, 25 mEq/L K+, 6 mEq/L Mg++, 51 mEq/L Cl−, 13 mEq/L phosphate, and 25 mEq/L lactate.
5% TRAVERT WITH ELECTROLYTE #2: 50 g/L invert sugar, 56 mEq/L Na+, 25 mEq/L K+, 6 mEq/L Mg++, 56 mEq/L Cl−, 12.5 mEq/L phosphate, and 25 mEq/L lactate.
ISONOSOL B WITH 10% INVERT SUGAR: 100 g/L invert sugar, 54 mEq/L Na+, 25 mEq/L K+, 5 mEq/L Mg++, 49 mEq/L Cl−, 13 mEq/L phosphate, and 22 mEq/L lactate.
10% TRAVERT WITH ELECTROLYTE #2: 100 g/L invert sugar, 56 mEq/L Na+, 25 mEq/L K+, 6 mEq/L Mg++, 56 mEq/L Cl−, 12.5 mEq/L phosphate, and 25 mEq/L lactate.
10% TRAVERT WITH ELECTROLYTE #1: 100 g/L invert sugar, 80 mEq/L Na+, 36 mEq/L K+, 5 mEq/L Ca++, 3 mEq/L Mg++, 64 mEq/L Cl−, and 60 mEq/L lactate.
PLASMA-LYTE WITH 10% TRAVERT: 100 g/L invert sugar, 140 mEq/L Na+, 10 mEq/L K+, 5 mEq/L Ca++, 3 mEq/L Mg++, 103 mEq/L Cl−, and 8 mEq/L lactate.

Products containing dextrose, electrolyte solutions, and vitamins are also available.

NAME	INDICATIONS & DOSAGE	SIDE EFFECTS
amino acid solution (crystalline amino acid solutions) Aminosyn, Freamine II, Travasol◆, Veinamine	*Total, supportive, or supplemental and protein-sparing parenteral nutrition when body systems must rest during healing, or when patient can't, shouldn't, or won't eat at all or eat enough for adequate nutrition—* **Adults:** 1 to 1.5 g/Kg I.V. daily. **Children:** 2 to 3 g/Kg I.V. daily. Individualize dosage to metabolic and clinical response as determined by nitrogen balance and body weight corrected for fluid balance. Add electrolyte and nonprotein caloric solutions as needed.	*CNS:* mental confusion, unconsciousness, headache, dizziness, coma (hyperosmolar syndromes). *CV:* hypervolemia related to congestive heart failure (in susceptible patients), pulmonary edema, exacerbation of hypertension (in predisposed patients), phlebitis, thrombophlebitis. *GI:* nausea, vomiting. *GU:* glycosuria, osmotic diuresis. *Local:* tissue sloughing at infusion site due to extravasation, catheter sepsis. *Metabolic:* rebound hypoglycemia (when long-term infusions are abruptly stopped), hyperglycemia, hypervolemia, metabolic acidosis, alkalosis, hypophosphatemia, hyperosmolar syndrome, hyperosmolar-hyperglycemic-nonketotic syndrome, hypo- and hypervitaminosis, hyperammonemia, electrolyte imbalances, and dehydration (if hyperosmolar solutions used). *Skin:* chills, flushing, feeling of warmth. *Other:* allergic reactions.
corn oil Lipomul◆	*As energy source—* **Adults:** 45 ml P.O. b.i.d. to q.i.d. after or between meals, alone or with proteins, milk, or other energy sources. **Children:** 30 ml P.O. daily to q.i.d. after or between meals, alone or with proteins, milk, or other energy sources.	*GI:* nausea, vomiting, diarrhea.
dextrose (d-glucose)	*Fluid replacement and caloric supplementation in patient who can't maintain adequate oral intake or is restricted from doing so—* **Adults and children:** dosage depends on fluid and caloric requirements. Use peripheral I.V. infusion of 2.5%, 5%, or 10% solutions, central I.V. infusion of 20% solution for minimal fluid needs. Use 50% solution to treat insulin-induced hypoglycemia. Solutions from 40% to 70% are used in admixtures, normally with amino acid solutions, for total central I.V. parenteral nutrition.	*CNS:* mental confusion, unconsciousness in hyperosmolar syndrome. *CV:* with fluid overload: pulmonary edema, exacerbated hypertension, and congestive heart failure in susceptible patients. Prolonged or concentrated infusions may cause phlebitis, sclerosis of vein, especially with peripheral route of administration. *GU:* glycosuria, osmotic diuresis. *Metabolic:* with rapid infusion of concentrated solution or prolonged infusion: hyperglycemia, hypervolemia, hyperosmolarity. Rapid termination of long-term infusions may cause hypoglycemia from rebound hyperinsulinemia. *Skin:* sloughing, if extravasation occurs with concentrated solutions.

◆ Also available in Canada.
◆◆ Available in Canada only.
Unmarked trade names available in United States only.

INTERACTIONS	NURSING CONSIDERATIONS
None significant.	• Contraindicated in patients with severe uncorrected electrolyte or acid/base imbalances, in hyperammonemia, and in decreased circulating blood volume. Use cautiously in renal insufficiency, or failure, cardiac disease, and hepatic impairments. Long-term use not advised for infants and children. • Monitor serum electrolytes, magnesium, glucose, BUN, renal and hepatic function. Check serum calcium levels frequently to avoid bone demineralization in children. • If long-term therapy is needed, doctor may order trace element and vitamin supplements. Avoid overuse of fat-soluble vitamins. • Refrigerate solution until ready to use. • Don't mix any medications, except electrolytes, with hyperalimentation solution without consulting pharmacist. • Control infusion rate carefully with infusion pump. • Check injection site frequently for irritation, tissue sloughing, necrosis, and phlebitis. Change I.V. sites periodically to prevent irritation; usually given by catheter into subclavian vein. • Watch closely for signs of fluid overload. Notify doctor promptly. • Some brands of crystalline amino acid solutions contain large amounts of acetates and lactates; use cautiously in alkalosis or hepatic insufficiency. • Most side effects are due to mixing amino acid with hypertonic dextrose solutions.
Griseofulvin: increased GI absorption of griseofulvin. Space doses.	• Contraindicated in gallbladder calculi or complete GI obstructions. Use cautiously in steatorrhea, partial GI obstruction, enterostomies, hepatic cirrhosis, portacaval shunts. • To minimize nausea, diarrhea, and vomiting, give more frequent, smaller doses with meals or mixed with milk.
None significant.	• Contraindicated in hyperglycemia, diabetic coma, intracranial or intraspinal hemorrhage, delirium tremens. Use cautiously in heart or pulmonary disease, hypertension, renal insufficiency, urinary obstruction, or hypovolemia. • Control infusion rate carefully. Maximal rate for dextrose infusion is 0.5 g/Kg per hour. Use infusion pump when infusing dextrose with amino acids for total parenteral nutrition. • Never infuse concentrated solutions rapidly. • Monitor serum glucose carefully. Prolonged therapy with 5% dextrose can cause depletion of pancreatic insulin production and secretion. • Never stop abruptly. If necessary, have 10% dextrose available to prevent rebound hyperinsulinemia and resulting hypoglycemia. • Take care to prevent extravasation. Check injection site frequently to prevent irritation, tissue sloughing, necrosis, and phlebitis. • Watch closely for signs of fluid overload, especially if fluid intake is restricted. • Monitor intake/output carefully, especially in impaired renal function. • Check vital signs frequently. Report side effects promptly. • Don't give dextrose solutions without saline with blood transfusions; may cause clumping of red blood cells.

NAME	INDICATIONS & DOSAGE	SIDE EFFECTS
essential crystalline amino acid solution Nephramine	*Management of potentially reversible renal decompensation—* **Adults:** 0.3 to 0.5 g/Kg I.V. up to 26 g total daily (250 ml with 500 ml 70% dextrose injection) and infuse through central I.V. line at initial rate of 20 to 30 ml/hour, increased in steps of 10 ml/ hour every 24 hours, to a maximum of 60 to 100 ml/hour. Individualize dose and infusion rate to tolerance for glucose, fluid, and nitrogen. Add electrolytes and vitamins as needed. **Children:** up to 1 g/Kg daily, individualized to patient's tolerance for glucose, fluid, and nitrogen. Add electrolytes and vitamins as needed.	*CNS:* mental confusion, dizziness, unconsciousness, headache, coma (hyperosmolar syndromes). *CV:* hypervolemia related to congestive heart failure (in susceptible patients), pulmonary edema, exacerbation of hypertension (in predisposed patients), phlebitis, thrombophlebitis. *GI:* nausea, vomiting. *GU:* glycosuria, osmotic diuresis. *Local:* tissue sloughing at infusion site due to extravasation, catheter sepsis. *Metabolic:* rebound hypoglycemia (when long-term infusions are abruptly stopped), hyperglycemia, hypervolemia, metabolic acidosis, alkalosis, hypophosphatemia, hyperosmolar syndrome, hyperosmolar-hyperglycemic-nonketotic syndrome, hypo- and hypervitaminosis, hyperammonemia, electrolyte imbalances, and dehydration (if hyperosmolar solutions used). *Skin:* chills, flushing, feeling of warmth. *Other:* allergic reactions.
fat emulsions Intralipid◆	*Source of calories adjunctive to total parenteral nutrition—* **Adults:** 1 ml/minute I.V. for 15 to 30 minutes. If no adverse reactions, increase rate to deliver 500 ml over 4 hours. Infuse only 1 500-ml unit the first day. Total daily dose should not exceed 2.5 g/ Kg (25 ml/Kg 10% emulsion). **Children:** 0.1 ml/minute for 10 to 15 minutes. If no adverse reactions, increase rate to deliver 10 ml/Kg over 4 hours. Daily dose should not exceed 4 g/Kg (40 ml/Kg 10% emulsion). Equals 60% of daily caloric intake. Protein-carbohydrate hyperalimentation should supply remaining 40%. *Fatty-acid deficiency—* **Adults and children:** 8% to 10% of total caloric intake I.V.	**Early reactions:** *Blood:* hyperlipemia, hypercoagulability, rarely thrombocytopenia in neonates. *CNS:* headache, sleepiness, dizziness. *EENT:* pressure over eyes. *GI:* nausea, vomiting. *Local:* irritation at infusion site. *Skin:* flushing, sweating. *Other:* fever, dyspnea, chest and back pains, cyanosis, allergic reactions, deposition of I.V. fat pigment. **Delayed reactions:** *Blood:* thrombocytopenia, leukopenia, leukocytosis. *CNS:* focal seizures. *CV:* shock. *Other:* fever, transient increased hepatic function test, hepatomegaly, splenomegaly.

INTERACTIONS	NURSING CONSIDERATIONS
None significant.	• Contraindicated in severe uncorrected electrolyte or acid/base imbalances, hyperammonemia, and decreased circulating blood volume. • Monitor serum electrolytes, magnesium, glucose, BUN, renal and hepatic function. Check serum calcium levels frequently to avoid bone demineralization in children. • In long-term therapy, doctor may order trace element and vitamin supplements. Avoid overuse of fat-soluble vitamins. • Refrigerate solution until ready to use. • Don't mix any medications, except electrolytes, with hyperalimentation solution without consulting pharmacist. • Control infusion rate carefully with infusion pump. • Check injection site frequently for irritation, tissue sloughing, necrosis, and phlebitis. Change I.V. sites periodically to prevent irritation; usually given by catheter into subclavian vein. • Watch closely for signs of fluid overload. Notify doctor promptly. • Essential amino acid solution is used identically to other crystalline amino acid solutions, except that it contains only the essential amino acids. By controlling amino acid content, patients with impaired renal function have decreases in blood urea nitrogen level, minimized deterioration of serum potassium, magnesium, and phosphorus balances. This may lead to earlier return of renal function in patients with potentially reversible acute renal failure and decrease morbidity associated with acute renal failure. • Most side effects are due to mixing essential crystalline amino acid solution with hypertonic dextrose solutions.
None significant.	• Contraindicated in hyperlipemia, lipoid nephrosis, and acute pancreatitis accompanied by hyperlipemia. Use cautiously in severe hepatic disease, pulmonary disease, anemia, blood coagulation disorders, or with possible danger of fat embolism. • Never mix with electrolyte or other nutrient products or dilute manufactured fat emulsions. Infusion may be piggybacked into another I.V. line, but do not place additives in the fat emulsion bottle. • Do not use an in-line filter when administering this drug. • Discard fat emulsion if it separates or becomes oily. Keep fat emulsions refrigerated until ready to use. • Avoid rapid infusion. Use an infusion pump to regulate rate. • Check injection site daily. Report signs of inflammation or infection promptly. • Watch closely for side effects, especially during first half hour of infusion. • Monitor serum lipids closely when patient's receiving fat emulsion therapy. Lipemia must clear between dosing. • Check platelet count frequently in neonates receiving fat emulsions I.V. • Monitor hepatic function carefully in long-term use.

NAME	INDICATIONS & DOSAGE	SIDE EFFECTS
fructose (levulose)	*Source of carbohydrate calories primarily when fluid replacement is also indicated and as a dextrose substitute for diabetic patients—* **Adults and children:** dosage depends on caloric needs. I.V. infusion rate should not exceed 1 g/Kg per hour. Single liter 10% solution yields 375 calories.	*CV:* increased pulse rate, precipitation or exacerbation of congestive heart failure in susceptible patients, pulmonary edema. *Local:* extravasation at infusion site may cause sloughing of skin, thrombophlebitis. *Metabolic:* metabolic acidosis, hypervolemia. *Other:* increased respiratory rate, enlarged liver.
invert sugar Travert	*Nonelectrolyte fluid replacement and caloric supplementation solution—* **Adults and children:** dosage depends on patient's age, weight, and clinical need. I.V. infusion rate should not exceed 1 g/Kg per hour. Single liter 5% invert sugar yields 375 calories.	*CNS:* mental confusion, unconsciousness. *CV:* increased pulse rate, precipitation or exacerbation of congestive heart failure in susceptible patients, pulmonary edema, increased hypertension. *GU:* glycosuria, osmotic diuresis. *Local:* extravasation at infusion site may cause sloughing of skin, thrombophlebitis. *Metabolic:* metabolic acidosis, hypervolemia, hyperglycemia, hypoglycemia. *Other:* increased respiratory rate, enlarged liver.
medium chain triglycerides M.C.T. Oil◆	*Inadequate digestion or absorption of food fats—* **Adults:** 15 ml P.O. t.i.d. to q.i.d.	*CNS:* reversible coma and precoma in susceptible patients. *GI:* nausea, vomiting, diarrhea.

INTERACTIONS	NURSING CONSIDERATIONS
None significant.	• Contraindicated in hereditary fructose intolerance or in those receiving therapy for hypoglycemia. Use cautiously in heart disease, hypertension, pulmonary disease, hypervolemia, renal insufficiency, or urinary tract obstructions. • Control infusion rate carefully. Make sure rate does not exceed 1 g/Kg per hour in infants. • Change injection sites frequently to avoid irritation with prolonged therapy. Take care to avoid extravasation. • Watch closely for signs of fluid overload, pulmonary edema, or congestive heart failure. Monitor blood pressure frequently. • May be safely used in diabetics.
None significant.	• Contraindicated in hereditary fructose intolerance, hyperglycemia, diabetic coma, intracranial or intraspinal hemorrhage, or delirium tremens. Use cautiously in heart disease, hypertension, pulmonary disease, hypervolemia, renal insufficiency, or urinary tract obstructions. • Control infusion rate carefully. Make sure rate does not exceed 1 g/Kg per hour in infants. • Change injection sites frequently to avoid irritation with prolonged therapy. Take care to avoid extravasation. • Watch closely for signs of fluid overload, pulmonary edema, or congestive heart failure. Monitor blood pressure frequently. • May be safely used in diabetics. • Monitor serum glucose closely. Prolonged therapy can cause depletion of pancreatic insulin production and secretion. • Don't stop abruptly. If necessary, have 10% dextrose available to prevent rebound hyperinsulinemia and subsequent hypoglycemia. • Monitor intake/output closely, especially if renal function is impaired. • Check vital signs frequently. Tell doctor promptly if side effects develop.
None significant.	• Contraindicated in advanced hepatic disease. • To minimize GI side effects, give smaller doses more frequently with meals or mixed with fruit juice or salad dressing. • More easily absorbed than long chain fats. • Rapid metabolism provides quick energy. • May be useful in obesity control and in lowering cholesterol levels.

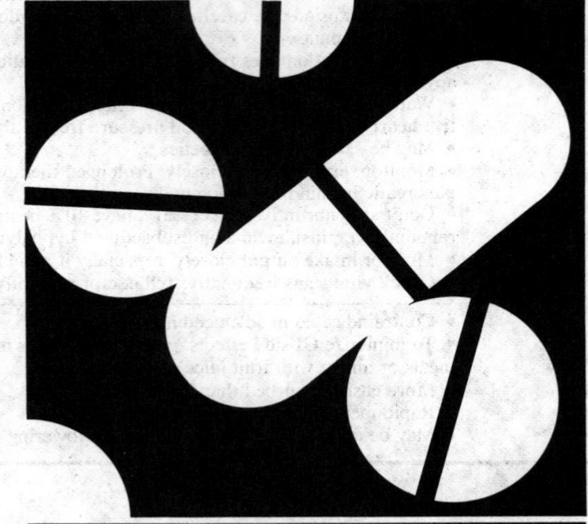

Miscellaneous Categories

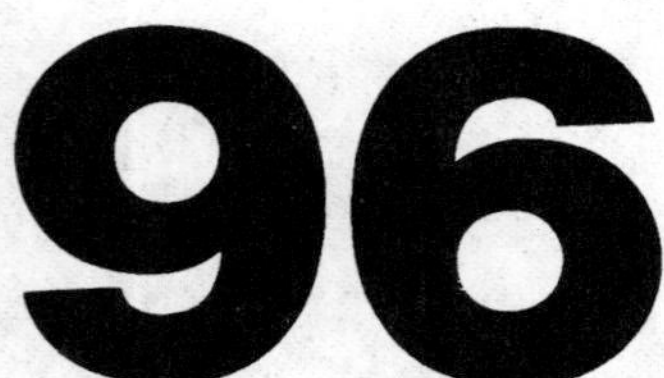

Immune serums

antirabies serum, equine
hepatitis B immune globulin, human
immune serum globulin
pertussis immune globulin, human
rabies immune globulin, human
Rho (D) immune globulin, human
tetanus immune globulin, human

Immune serums provide passive immunity against various infectious diseases or suppress antibody formation as in Rh incompatibility. Immune serum globulins are obtained from hyperimmunized donors or pooled plasma. These products are then purified and standardized. Immune serums are effective for prophylaxis. They are not effective after the onset of the disease.

Major uses

- Prevention of various infectious diseases.
- Modification of disease symptoms in patients after suspected exposure.
- Prevention of formation of active antibodies, as in Rho negative, D_u negative mothers who deliver Rho positive or D_u positive infants, or in transfusion accidents.

Mechanism of action

- Passive immunization is acquired by transfer of preformed protective substances (antibodies) from the serum of human beings or animals, especially horses.

Onset and duration

- Onset of immunity is immediate.
- Provide passive immunity of short duration (e.g., immune serum globulin, 3 to 4 weeks).

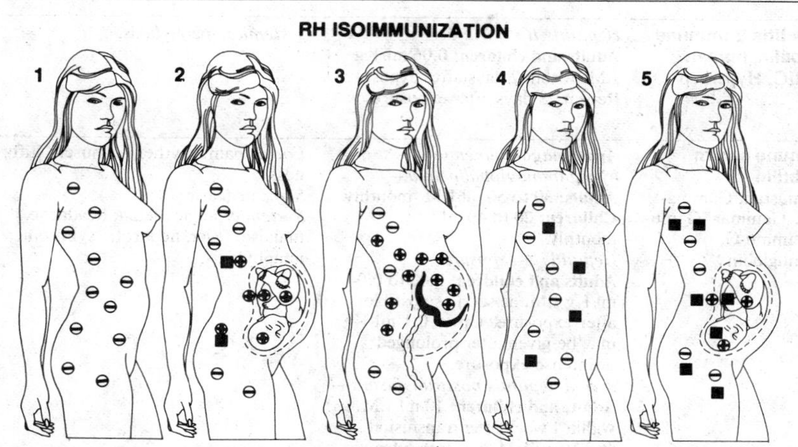

Fig. 1) Rh-negative woman prepregnancy. Fig. 2) Pregnancy with Rh-positive fetus. Fig. 3) Placental separation. 4) Postdelivery, mother becomes sensitized to Rh-positive blood and develops anti-Rh-positive antibodies (darkened squares). Fig. 5) During next pregnancy with Rh-positive fetus, maternal anti-Rh-positive antibodies enter fetal circulation, attach to Rh-positive red blood cells, and subject them to hemolysis.

NAME	INDICATIONS & DOSAGE	SIDE EFFECTS
antirabies serum, equine	*Rabies exposure—* **Adults and children:** 40 to 55 units/Kg at time of first dose of rabies vaccine. Use half dose to infiltrate wound area. Give remainder I.M. Don't give vaccine and serum in same syringe or at same site.	*Local:* pain at injection site. *Systemic:* within 6 to 12 days serum sickness occurs in 15% to 25% of patients. Symptoms are skin eruptions, arthralgia, pruritus, lymphadenopathy, fever, headache, malaise, abdominal pain, anaphylaxis.
hepatitis B immune globulin, human H-BIG, Hyperhep	*Hepatitis B exposure—* **Adults and children:** 0.06 ml/Kg I.M. within 7 days after exposure. Repeat 28 days after exposure.	*Systemic:* anaphylaxis.
immune serum globulin Gamastan, Gammagee, Gammar, Gamulin, Immu-G, Immuglobin	*Agammaglobulinemia or hypogammaglobulinemia—* **Adults:** 30 to 50 ml I.M. monthly. **Children:** 20 to 40 ml I.M. monthly. *Hepatitis A exposure—* **Adults and children:** 0.02 to 0.04 ml/Kg I.M. as soon as possible after exposure. Up to 0.1 ml/Kg may be given after prolonged or intense exposure. *Serum hepatitis posttransfusion—* **Adults and children:** 10 ml I.M. within 1 week after transfusion and 10 ml I.M. 1 month later. *Measles exposure—* **Adults and children:** 0.02 ml/Kg within 6 days of exposure. *Modification of measles—* **Adults and children:** 0.04 ml/Kg I.M. within 6 days of exposure. *Measles vaccine complications—* **Adults and children:** 0.02 to 0.04 ml/Kg I.M. *Poliomyelitis exposure—* **Adults and children:** 0.3 to 0.4 ml/Kg I.M. within 7 days after exposure. *Chickenpox exposure—* **Adults and children:** 0.2 to 1.3 ml/Kg I.M. as soon as exposed. *Rubella exposure in first trimester of pregnancy—* **Women:** 0.2 to 0.4 ml/Kg I.M. as soon as exposed.	*Local:* pain, erythema, muscle stiffness. *Skin:* urticaria. *Systemic:* angioedema, headache, malaise, fever, nephrotic syndrome, anaphylaxis.

INTERACTIONS	NURSING CONSIDERATIONS
None significant.	• In hypersensitivity, use rabies immune globulin, human, instead. If unavailable, desensitize before giving. Consult doctor or pharmacist. • Do sensitivity test on all patients before giving. Dilute serum 1:100 or 1:1,000 with 0.9% sodium chloride for injection. Inject intradermally on inner forearm. Inject other arm with 0.1 ml 0.9% sodium chloride for injection intradermally as control. Read within 20 minutes. Positive reaction: wheal 10 mm or more and erythematous flare 20 x 20 mm. • Use only when rabies immune globulin, human, not available. • Obtain history of animal bite, allergies (especially to horse serum), and past reaction to immunization. • For treatment of anaphylaxis, see p. 1114.
None significant.	• Buttocks or deltoid areas preferred injection sites. • Nurse should receive immunization if exposed to hepatitis B (e.g., needle-stick, direct contact). • Obtain history of allergies and past reaction to immunization. • For treatment of anaphylaxis, see p. 1114.
None significant.	• Obtain history of allergies and past reaction to immunization. • Have drugs available for anaphylactic reaction. • Divide dose of more than 10 ml, and inject into different sites, preferably buttocks. • Do not give for hepatitis A exposure if 6 weeks or more have elapsed since exposure, or after onset of clinical illness. • For treatment of anaphylaxis, see p. 1114.

NAME	INDICATIONS & DOSAGE	SIDE EFFECTS
pertussis immune globulin, human Hypertussis	*Pertussis therapy—* **Children and infants:** 1.25 ml I.M., repeated in 24 to 48 hours. *Pertussis prophylaxis—* **Children:** 2.5 ml I.M., repeated in 1 to 2 weeks. **Infants:** 1.25 ml I.M., repeated in 1 to 2 weeks.	*Systemic:* anaphylaxis.
rabies immune globulin, human Hyperab	*Rabies exposure—* **Adults and children:** 20 IU/Kg at time of first dose of rabies vaccine. Use half dose to infiltrate wound area. Give remainder I.M. Don't give vaccine and immune globulin in same syringe or at same site.	*Local:* pain, redness, induration at injection site. *Other:* slight fever, anaphylaxis.
Rho (D) immune globulin, human Gamulin R, HypRho D, MICRhoGAM, RhoGam	*Rh exposure—* **Women postabortion, postmiscarriage, ectopic pregnancy, or postpartum:** transfusion unit or blood bank determines fetal packed red blood cell volume entering woman's blood, then gives 1 vial I.M. if fetal packed red blood cell volume was less than 15 ml. More than 1 vial I.M. may be required if there is large fetomaternal hemorrhage. Must be given within 72 hours following delivery or miscarriage. *Transfusion accidents—* **Adults and children:** consult blood bank or transfusion unit at once. Must be given within 72 hours. *Postabortion or postmiscarriage to prevent Rh antibody formation—* **Women:** consult transfusion unit or blood bank. Must be given within 3 hours following abortion or miscarriage.	*Local:* discomfort at injection site. *Other:* slight fever.
tetanus immune globulin, human A-Tet, Homo-Tet, Hu-Tet, Hyper-Tet, Immu-Tetanus, T-I-Gammagee	*Tetanus exposure—* **Adults and children:** 250 units I.M. *Tetanus treatment—* **Adults and children:** single doses of 3,000 to 6,000 units have been used, but optimal dosage schedules not established. Do not give at same site as toxoid.	*Local:* pain, stiffness, erythema. *Other:* slight fever, allergy, anaphylaxis.

INTERACTIONS	NURSING CONSIDERATIONS
None significant.	• Obtain history of allergies and past reaction to immunization. • Of little value in preventing pertussis after exposure or for treatment. • For treatment of anaphylaxis, see p. 1114.
None significant.	• Repeated doses contraindicated once rabies vaccine started. • Use only with rabies vaccine and immediate local treatment of wound. Give regardless of interval between exposure and initiation of therapy. • Obtain history of animal bite, allergies, and past reaction to immunization. • Corticosteroids decrease resistance to infection and decrease antibody response to vaccine. Stop corticosteroids after possible rabies exposure. • For treatment of anaphylaxis, see p. 1114.
None significant.	• Contraindicated in Rho (D) positive or Du positive patients, Rho (D) negative patients who have had Rho (D) positive blood transfusions, and those previously immunized to Rho (D) blood factor. • Immediately after delivery send infant's cord blood to lab for type and crossmatch. Confirm mother is Rho (D) negative and Du negative. Infant must be Rho (D) positive or Du positive. • Give only to postpartum mother, not infant. • Obtain history of allergies and past reaction to immunization. • MicrhoGam recommended for every woman undergoing abortion or miscarriage up to 12 weeks gestation unless she is Rho (D) positive or Du positive, has Rh antibodies, or the father and/or fetus is Rh negative. • For I.M. use only. • Store at 36° to 46° F. (2° to 8° C.). Do not freeze.
None significant.	• Use tetanus immune globulin only if wound is over 24 hours old or patient has had less than 2 previous tetanus toxoid injections. • Obtain history of injury, past tetanus immunizations, last tetanus toxoid injection, allergies, and past reaction to immunization. • Thoroughly cleanse and remove all foreign matter from wound. • For treatment of anaphylaxis, see p. 1114.

97

Vaccines and toxoids

BCG vaccine
cholera vaccine
diphtheria and tetanus toxoids, combined
diphtheria and tetanus toxoids and pertussis vaccine
diphtheria toxoid, absorbed, pediatric
influenza virus vaccine, trivalent
measles, mumps, and rubella virus vaccine, live
measles (rubeola) and rubella virus vaccine, live attenuated
measles (rubeola) virus vaccine, live attenuated
meningitis vaccines
mumps vaccine, live attenuated
plague vaccine
pneumococcal vaccine, polyvalent
poliovirus vaccine, live, oral, trivalent
rabies vaccine (duck embryo), dried, killed virus
Rocky Mountain spotted fever vaccine
rubella and mumps virus vaccine, live
rubella virus vaccine, live attenuated
smallpox vaccine
staphylococcus toxoid
tetanus toxoid
typhoid vaccine
typhus vaccine
yellow fever vaccine

Vaccines and toxoids provide active immunity against certain bacterial and viral diseases. Vaccines contain killed or attenuated microorganisms that cause antibody formation. Toxoids contain exotoxins (substances formed by bacteria and secreted outside the bacterial cell). These substances are altered to make them nontoxic, but they retain the ability to stimulate antitoxin (antibody) formation.

Major uses

- Prevention of certain infectious diseases and childhood diseases such as mumps, measles, pertussis, and poliomyelitis.
- Prevention of disease transmitted through injury or animal bite, such as tetanus and rabies.

Mechanism of action

- Initiate formation of specific antibodies by stimulating antigen-antibody mechanism, providing active or acquired immunity.

Onset and duration

- Onset of active immunity is not immediate. It takes from a few days to a few weeks for antibody production to reach immunity-providing levels.
- Duration of immunity is quite long, lasting from a few years to a lifetime.

Combination products

None.

PATIENT TEACHING AID — IMMUNIZING YOUR CHILD

Dear Parent:
Consider immunizing your child an effective form of health insurance. Here is a recommended schedule for protecting your child against polio, measles, mumps, rubella, diphtheria, pertussis (whooping cough), and tetanus.

Letting your child miss one or more of these immunizations means needless risk of serious illness, perhaps with fatal complications.

VACCINATION TIME-LINE

AGE	IMMUNIZATION
2 months	First dose: diphtheria/tetanus/pertussis vaccine; polio vaccine
4 months	Second dose: diphtheria/tetanus/pertussis vaccine; polio
6 months	Third dose: diphtheria/tetanus/pertussis vaccine

AGE	IMMUNIZATION
15 months	Rubella vaccine; measles; mumps
18 months	Diphtheria/tetanus/pertussis; polio (third)
4-5 years	Diphtheria/tetanus/pertussis; polio

Fill out this form using your personal immunization records or call your doctor and ask him to check his files.

If all the blocks are not checked, contact your public health clinic or doctor for help in deciding your child's immunization needs.

IMMUNIZATION CHECKLIST
FOR YOUR CHILD'S PROTECTION

Child's Name ____________________

	1ST	2ND	3RD	4TH
POLIO	☐	☐	☐	☐
DPT	☐	☐	☐	☐

	1ST	
MEASLES	☐	(One only)
MUMPS	☐	(One only)
RUBELLA	☐	(One only)

NAME	INDICATIONS & DOSAGE	SIDE EFFECTS
BCG vaccine	*Tuberculosis exposure*— **Adults and children:** 0.1 ml intradermally. **Newborns:** 0.05 ml intradermally.	*Local:* lymphangitis, lymph node and skin abscess, ulceration at site of injection (2 to 3 weeks after injection), lupus reaction. *Other:* urticaria of trunk and limbs, anaphylaxis.
cholera vaccine	*Primary immunization*— **Adults, and children over 10 years:** 2 doses of 0.5 ml I.M. or 1 ml S.C., 1 week to 1 month before traveling in cholera area. Booster—0.5 ml q 6 months as long as protection is needed. **Children 5 to 10 years:** 0.3 ml I.M. or S.C. **Children 6 months to 4 years:** 0.2 ml I.M. or S.C. Boosters of same dose should be given q 6 months as long as protection needed.	*Systemic:* malaise, fever, flushing, urticaria, tachycardia, hypotension, headache, anaphylaxis. *Local:* erythema, swelling, pain, induration.
diphtheria and tetanus toxoids, combined	*Primary immunization*— **Adults, and children 6 years and over:** use adult strength; 0.5 ml I.M. 4 to 6 weeks apart for 2 doses and a third dose 1 year later. Booster—0.5 ml I.M. q 10 years. **Children under 6 years:** *pediatric plain toxoid:* 0.5 ml S.C. 4 to 6 weeks apart for 3 doses and a fourth dose 1 year later. *Pediatric adsorbed toxoid:* 0.5 ml I.M. 4 to 8 weeks apart for 2 doses and a third dose 6 to 12 months later. Booster: 0.5 ml when starting school.	*Systemic:* chills, fever, malaise, anaphylaxis. *Local:* stinging, edema, erythema, pain, induration.
diphtheria and tetanus toxoids and pertussis vaccine (DPT) Tri-Immunol, Triogen, Triple Antigen	*Primary immunization*— **Children 6 weeks to 6 years:** 0.5 ml I.M. 2 months apart for 3 doses and a fourth dose 1 year later. Booster: 0.5 ml I.M. when starting school. Then q 10 years. Not advised for adults or children over 6 years.	*Systemic:* slight fever, chills, malaise, encephalopathy, anaphylaxis. *Local:* soreness, redness, expected nodule remaining several weeks.

- ♦ Also available in Canada.
- ♦♦ Available in Canada only.

Unmarked trade names available in United States only.

INTERACTIONS	NURSING CONSIDERATIONS
Isoniazid (INH): inhibited multiplication of BCG. Avoid using together.	• Contraindicated in hypogammaglobulinemia, positive tuberculin reaction, corticosteroid therapy, immunosuppression, fresh smallpox vaccination, and burn patients. Use cautiously in chronic skin disease. Inject in area of healthy skin only. • Obtain history of allergies and past reaction to immunization. • Vaccine is of no value in patients with positive tuberculin test. • Keep epinephrine 1:1,000 available to treat anaphylaxis. • Recommended injection site is over insertion of deltoid muscle. • Do not shake vial after reconstitution. • Expected lesion forms in 7 to 10 days. • Live vaccine; destroy by autoclaving or formalin solution before disposal. • Patient should have tuberculin skin test 2 to 3 months after BCG vaccination to determine success of vaccine. • For treatment of anaphylaxis, see p. 1114.
None significant.	• Contraindicated in corticosteroid therapy or in immunosuppression. Defer in acute illness. • Obtain history of allergies and past reaction to immunization. • Keep epinephrine 1:1,000 available. • May be given intradermally, but I.M. and S.C. routes give higher levels of protection. • For treatment of anaphylaxis, see p. 1114.
None significant.	• Contraindicated in immunosuppression, radiation, or corticosteroid therapy. Defer in respiratory or polio outbreaks, or acute illness except in emergency. Use single antigen during polio risks. In children under 6 years, use only when diphtheria, tetanus, and pertussis toxoid combination is contraindicated because of pertussis component. • Verify strength (pediatric or adult) of toxoid used. • Don't use hot or cold compresses; may increase severity of local reaction. • Obtain history of allergies and past reaction to immunization. • Keep epinephrine 1:1,000 available. • Give in site not previously used for vaccines or toxoids. • For treatment of anaphylaxis, see p. 1114.
None significant.	• Contraindicated in corticosteroid therapy or immunosuppression. Defer in acute illness. • Obtain history of allergies and past reaction to immunization. • Keep epinephrine 1:1,000 available. • Not to be used for active infection. • Don't give subcutaneously. • Shake vial well before using. Store in refrigerator. • For treatment of anaphylaxis, see p. 1114.

NAME	INDICATIONS & DOSAGE	SIDE EFFECTS
diphtheria toxoid, adsorbed, pediatric	*Diphtheria immunization—* **Children under 6 years:** 0.5 ml I.M. 6 to 8 weeks apart for 2 doses and a third dose 1 year later. Booster: 0.5 ml I.M. at 5- to 10-year intervals. Not advised for adults, or children over 6 years; instead, adult strength of diphtheria toxoid (usually combined with tetanus toxoid).	*Systemic:* fever, malaise, urticaria, tachycardia, flushing, pruritus, hypotension, aches and pains, anaphylaxis. *Local:* erythema, pain, induration, expected nodule remaining several weeks.
influenza virus vaccine, trivalent Fluax◆◆, Fluogen◆, Fluzone-Connaught **influenza virus, trivalent types A & B**	*Brazil, Texas, and Hong Kong influenza prophylaxis—* **Adults 27 years and over:** 0.5 ml whole or split virus I.M. Use adult formula. **Youths 13 to 26 years:** 0.5 ml whole or split virus I.M. Repeat doses in 4 weeks. Those who received the 1979 vaccine require only one dose. **Children under 13 years:** give 0.5 ml split virus. Repeat dose in 4 weeks unless child received 1979 vaccine. **Children 6 to 35 months:** 0.25 ml I.M. Repeat dose in 4 weeks unless child received 1979 vaccine. Recommendations are for 1980 only. Must check yearly for new recommendations.	*Systemic:* fever, malaise, myalgia, Guillain-Barre syndrome, anaphylaxis. *Local:* erythema, induration. Side effects occur most often in children and in others not exposed to influenza viruses.
measles, mumps, and rubella virus vaccine, live M-M-R-II◆	*Immunization—* **Children over 12 months to puberty:** 1 vial (1,000 units) S.C.	*Systemic:* fever, rash, regional lymphadenopathy, urticaria, anaphylaxis. *Local:* erythema.

INTERACTIONS	NURSING CONSIDERATIONS
None significant.	• Contraindicated in immunosuppression, radiation or corticosteroid therapy, children under 12 months with cerebral damage. Defer in acute illness or polio outbreak, except in emergency. Use appropriate single or multiple fluid (plain) antigen during polio risk. • Stop immunization if CNS disorder occurs. Immunization may be continued with diphtheria and tetanus toxoids without pertussis component at doses of 0.05 to 0.1 ml. • DPT injection may be given at same time as trivalent oral polio vaccine (TOPV). • Don't use hot or cold compresses; may intensify local reaction. • Obtain history of allergies and past reaction to immunization. • Keep epinephrine 1:1,000 available to treat anaphylaxis. • Shake vial well before using. Store in refrigerator.
None significant.	• Contraindicated in egg allergy. Defer in acute respiratory or other active infection, or when there is risk of poliomyelitis infection. • Obtain history of allergies, especially to eggs, and past reaction to immunization. • Give injections into deltoid or midlateral thigh. • Keep epinephrine 1:1,000 available. • Recommended for patients with chronic disease, metabolic disorders, and those over 65 years of age. • For treatment of anaphylaxis, see p. 1114.
Immune serum globulin, whole blood, plasma: antibodies in serum may interfere with immune response. Don't use vaccine within 3 months.	• Contraindicated in immunosuppression; cancer; blood dyscrasias; corticosteroid or radiation therapy; gamma globulin disorders; fever; active, untreated tuberculosis. Use cautiously in hypersensitivity to neomycin, chickens, ducks, eggs, or feathers. Defer immunization in acute illness. • Presence of maternal antibodies may prevent response in children under 12 months. • Treat fever with antipyretics. • Store in refrigerator and protect from light. Solution may be used if red, pink, or yellow but must be clear. • Use only diluent supplied. Discard 8 hours after reconstituting. • Obtain history of allergies, especially to ducks, rabbits, and antibiotics, and past reaction to immunization. • Inject in outer aspect of upper arm. Don't give I.V. • Keep epinephrine 1:1,000 available. • For treatment of anaphylaxis, see p. 1114.

NAME	INDICATIONS & DOSAGE	SIDE EFFECTS
measles (rubeola) and rubella virus vaccine, live attenuated M-R-Vax-II	*Immunization—* **Children 15 months to puberty:** 1 vial (1,000 units) S.C.	*Systemic:* fever, rash, lymphadenopathy, anaphylaxis.
measles (rubeola) virus vaccine, live attenuated Attenuvax◆, M-Vac	*Immunization—* **Adults, and children 15 months or over:** 0.5 ml (1,000 units) S.C.	*Systemic:* fever and rash, lymphadenopathy, anaphylaxis, febrile convulsions in susceptible children, anorexia, leukopenia. *Local:* erythema, swelling, tenderness.
meningitis vaccines Meningovax-C, Menomune-A, Menomune-C, Menomune-A/C	*Meningococcal meningitis prophylaxis—* **Adults, and children over 2 years:** 0.5 ml S.C. Use vaccine group C or A, except in highly endemic areas; in these areas use A/C combination. **Children 3 months to 2 years:** 0.5 ml S.C. Use vaccine group A.	*Systemic:* headache, malaise, chills, fever, cramps, anaphylaxis. *Local:* pain, erythema, induration.
mumps vaccine, live attenuated Mumpsvax◆	*Immunization—* **Adults, and children over 15 months:** 1 vial (5,000 units) S.C.	*Systemic:* slight fever, anaphylaxis, skin rash, malaise.

INTERACTIONS	NURSING CONSIDERATIONS
Immune serum globulin, whole blood, plasma: antibodies in serum may interfere with immune response. Don't use vaccine within 3 months. *Tuberculin skin test:* may temporarily decrease response to test. Defer skin testing.	• Contraindicated in immunosuppression; cancer; blood dyscrasias; corticosteroid or radiation therapy; gamma globulin disorders; fever; active, untreated tuberculosis. Use cautiously in hypersensitivity to neomycin, chickens, ducks, eggs, or feathers, and when there is a history of febrile seizures or in cerebral injury. Defer immunization in acute illness. • Do not give within 1 month of other live virus vaccines, except oral poliovirus vaccine. • Store in refrigerator and protect from light. Solution may be used if red, pink, or yellow but must be clear (with no precipitation). • Use only diluent supplied. Discard 8 hours after reconstituting. • Inject in outer aspect of upper arm. Don't inject I.V. • For treatment of anaphylaxis, see p. 1114.
Immune serum globulin, whole blood, plasma: antibodies in serum may interfere with immune response. Don't use vaccine within 3 months. *Tuberculin skin test:* may temporarily decrease response to test. Defer skin testing.	• Contraindicated in immunosuppression; cancer; blood dyscrasias; corticosteroid or radiation therapy; gamma globulin disorders; active, untreated tuberculosis; fever. Use with caution in hypersensitivity to neomycin, chickens, eggs, or feathers. Defer in acute illness or after administration of blood or plasma. • Warn patient to avoid pregnancy for 3 months after vaccination. • Do not give I.V. • Obtain history of allergies, especially to eggs, and past reaction to immunization. • Keep epinephrine 1:1,000 available. • Store in refrigerator and protect from light. Solution may be used if red, pink, or yellow but must be clear (with no precipitation). • Use only diluent supplied. Discard 8 hours after reconstituting. • May be given with oral polio vaccine. • For treatment of anaphylaxis, see p. 1114.
None significant.	• Contraindicated in immunosuppression. Defer in acute illness. • Tell patient to avoid pregnancy for 3 months after vaccination. • Obtain history of allergies and past reaction to immunization. • Do not give I.V. • Keep epinephrine 1:1,000 available. • For treatment of anaphylaxis, see p. 1114.
Immune serum globulin, whole blood, plasma: antibodies in serum may interfere with immune response. Don't use vaccine within 3 months. *Tuberculin skin test:* may temporarily decrease response to test. Defer skin testing.	• Contraindicated in immunosuppression; cancer; blood dyscrasias; corticosteroid or radiation therapy; gamma globulin disorders; active, untreated tuberculosis. Use cautiously in hypersensitivity to neomycin, chickens, ducks, eggs, or feathers. Defer in acute illness and for 3 months after transfusions or immune serum globulin. • Stress importance of avoiding pregnancy for 3 months after immunization. If necessary, provide contraceptive information. • Treat fever with antipyretics. • Do not give within 1 month of other live virus vaccines except oral poliovirus vaccine. • Don't give I.V. • Store in refrigerator and protect from light. Solution may be used if red, pink, or yellow but must be clear. • Use only diluent supplied. Discard 8 hours after reconstituting. • Obtain history of allergies, especially to antibiotics, and past reaction to immunization. • Try to separate administration of other live virus vaccines by at least 1 month if possible. • Keep epinephrine 1:1,000 available. • For treatment of anaphylaxis, see p. 1114.

NAME	INDICATIONS & DOSAGE	SIDE EFFECTS
plague vaccine	*Primary immunization and booster—* **Adults, and children over 11 years:** 1 ml I.M. followed by 0.2 ml in 1 to 3 months, then 0.2 ml 3 to 6 months after second injection. Booster: 0.1 to 0.2 ml q 6 months while in plague area. **Children under 1 year:** 1/5 adult primary or booster dose. **Children 1 to 4 years:** 2/5 adult primary or booster dose. **Children 5 to 10 years:** 3/5 adult primary or booster dose.	*Systemic:* malaise, headache, slight fever, lymphadenopathy, anaphylaxis. *Local:* swelling, induration, erythema.
pneumococcal vaccine, polyvalent Pneumovax◆, Pnu-Imune	*Pneumococcal immunization—* **Adults, and children 2 years or over:** 0.5 ml I.M. or S.C. Not recommended for children under 2 years.	*Systemic:* slight fever, anaphylaxis. *Local:* severe local reaction can occur when revaccination takes place within 3 years.
poliovirus vaccine, live, oral, trivalent Diplovax, Orimune	*Poliovirus immunization—* **Adults, and children over 6 weeks:** 2 drops or 0.5 ml P.O. in 5 ml water or simple syrup, or on sugar cube. Repeat dose in 8 weeks. Give third dose at 18 months. Booster: 2 drops or 0.5 ml P.O.	None reported.
rabies vaccine (duck embryo), dried, killed virus	*Postexposure immunization for domestic animal bite—* **Adults and children:** 1 ml S.C. daily for 14 days in the abdomen on alternate sides. *Postexposure immunization for wild animal bite—* **Adults and children:** 2 ml S.C. daily for 7 days, then 1 ml daily for 7 more days. Supplemental doses may be needed after initial therapy. *Preexposure immunization (for patients constantly exposed to rabies)—* **Adults and children:** 1 ml S.C. weekly for 3 weeks, then fourth dose 6 months later; or 1 ml S.C. 1 month apart for 2 doses, then third dose 7 months after second. Booster (for patients constantly exposed to rabies): 1 ml q 1 to 2 years.	*Systemic:* peripheral neuritis, dorsolumbar myelitis, acute idiopathic polyneuritis, acute encephalomyelitis, fever, weakness, stiff neck, respiratory distress, anaphylaxis. *GI:* nausea, vomiting, diarrhea, abdominal cramps. *Skin:* urticaria. *Local:* stinging, pain, erythema, induration, lymphadenopathy.

INTERACTIONS	NURSING CONSIDERATIONS
None significant.	• Contraindicated in immunosuppression. Defer in respiratory infection. • Deltoid area preferred injection site. • Obtain history of allergies and past reaction to immunization. • Keep epinephrine 1:1,000 available. • For treatment of anaphylaxis, see p. 1114.
None significant.	• Check immunization history carefully to avoid revaccination within 3 years. • Inject in deltoid or midlateral thigh. Don't inject I.V. • Keep refrigerated. Reconstitution or dilution not necessary. • Treat fever with mild antipyretics. • Protects against 14 pneumococcal types, which account for 80% of pneumococcal disease. • Obtain history of allergies and past reaction to immunization. • Keep epinephrine 1:1,000 available. • For treatment of anaphylaxis, see p. 1114.
Immune serum globulin, whole blood, plasma: antibodies in serum may interfere with immune response. Don't use vaccine within 3 months.	• Contraindicated in immunosuppression, cancer, immunoglobulin abnormalities, radiation or corticosteroid therapy. Defer in acute illness, vomiting, or diarrhea. • Keep frozen until used. Once thawed, if unopened, may store refrigerated up to 30 days. Opened vials may be refrigerated up to 7 days. • Discard if vaccine color changes from red or pink to yellow. • Obtain history of allergies and past reaction to immunization. • Not for parenteral use. • Try to separate administration of other live virus vaccines by at least 1 month if possible.
None significant.	• Contraindicated in corticosteroid therapy. Stop corticosteroids during immunization period. • When postexposure immunization is indicated, pregnancy is not a contraindication. • Immediate, thorough cleaning of wound is best way to prevent rabies. • In serious reaction to duck embryo component, state health department and Center for Disease Control in Atlanta, Georgia, can advise on experimental alternatives. • Rabies immune globulin may be given at time of first vaccine dose to provide immediate protection. • Use 23- or 24-gauge, ½- to ¾-inch needle. • Obtain history of allergies, especially to eggs, ducks, or proteins, and past reaction to immunization. • Keep epinephrine 1:1,000 available. • For treatment of anaphylaxis, see p. 1114.

NAME	INDICATIONS & DOSAGE	SIDE EFFECTS
Rocky Mountain spotted fever vaccine	*Rocky Mountain spotted fever (tick typhus) primary immunization—* **Adults, and children over 12 years:** 1 ml S.C. q 7 to 10 days for 3 doses. Booster: 1 ml S.C. q 2 years. **Children under 12 years:** 0.5 ml S.C. q 7 to 10 days for 3 doses. Booster: 0.5 ml S.C. q year. Not recommended for children under 6 months.	*Systemic:* hypersensitivity.
rubella and mumps virus vaccine, live Biavax-II	*Measles and mumps immunization—* **Adults, and children over 12 months:** 1 vial (1,000 units) S.C.	*Systemic:* fever, rash, thrombocytopenic purpura, urticaria, arthritis, arthralgia, polyneuritis, anaphylaxis. *Local:* pain, erythema, induration, lymphadenopathy.
rubella virus vaccine, live attenuated Meruvax-II◆	*Measles immunization—* **Adults, and children over 12 months:** 1 vial (1,000 units) S.C. or I.M.	*Systemic:* fever, rash, thrombocytopenic purpura, urticaria, arthritis, arthralgia, polyneuritis. *Local:* pain, erythema, induration, lymphadenopathy.

INTERACTIONS	NURSING CONSIDERATIONS
None significant.	• Contraindicated in immunosuppression, allergy to chickens, eggs, or feathers. • For prevention, not treatment, of disease. • Obtain history of allergies, especially to eggs or chickens, and past reaction to immunization. • Don't use within 1 month of other live virus vaccines. • Keep epinephrine 1:1,000 available. • For treatment of anaphylaxis, see p. 1114.
Immune serum globulin, whole blood, plasma: antibodies in serum may interfere with immune response. Don't give vaccine within 3 months. *Tuberculin skin test:* may temporarily decrease response to test. Defer skin testing.	• Contraindicated in immunosuppression; cancer; blood dyscrasias; corticosteroid or radiation therapy; gamma globulin disorders; active, untreated tuberculosis; fever, pregnancy. Use with caution in hypersensitivity to neomycin, chickens, ducks, eggs, or feathers. Defer in acute illness and after administration of immune serum globulin, blood, or plasma. • Stress importance of avoiding pregnancy for 3 months after immunization. If necessary, provide contraceptive information. • Store in refrigerator and protect from light. Solution may be used if red, pink, or yellow but must be clear. • Use only diluent supplied. Discard 8 hours after reconstituting. • Obtain history of allergies, especially to ducks, rabbits, and antibiotics, and past reaction to immunization. • Inject into outer aspect of upper arm. Don't inject I.V. • Keep epinephrine 1:1,000 available. • For treatment of anaphylaxis, see p. 1114.
Immune serum globulin, whole blood, plasma: antibodies in serum may interfere with immune response. Don't use vaccine within 3 months. *Tuberculin skin test:* may temporarily decrease response to test. Defer skin testing.	• Contraindicated in immunosuppression; cancer; blood dyscrasias; corticosteroid or radiation therapy; gamma globulin disorders; active, untreated tuberculosis; fever. Use cautiously in hypersensitivity to neomycin, chickens, ducks, eggs, or feathers. Also, use Cendevax cautiously in hypersensitivity to rabbits. Defer in acute illness and after administration of human immune serum globulin, blood, or plasma. • Stress importance of avoiding pregnancy for 3 months after immunization. If necessary, provide contraceptive information. • Store in refrigerator and protect from light. Solution may be used if red, pink, or yellow but must be clear. • Use only diluent supplied. Discard 8 hours after reconstituting. • Obtain history of allergies, especially to ducks and rabbits, and past reaction to immunization. • Inject into outer aspect of upper arm. Don't inject I.V. • Keep epinephrine 1:1,000 available. • For treatment of anaphylaxis, see p. 1114.

NAME	INDICATIONS & DOSAGE	SIDE EFFECTS
smallpox vaccine Dryvax	*Immunization—* **Adults and children:** deposit drop of vaccine onto cleansed site and make series of multiple pressures with sharp needle through drop. Use only for lab personnel working with virus.	*Systemic:* encephalopathy, transverse myelitis, acute infection, polyneuritis, eczema vaccinatum, eye infection, rash, anaphylaxis, fever. *Local:* necrosis, pustule (expected), infection.
staphylococcus toxoid	*Prophylaxis and treatment of recurrent boils, carbuncles, pustular acne (when combined with antibiotics)—* **Adults and children:** administer a graded series of I.M. or S.C. injections based on sensitivity testing results. Give injections q 2 to 7 days, utilizing two dilutions supplied.	*Systemic:* hypersensitivity, anaphylaxis.
tetanus toxoid, adsorbed◆ Tet Tox Adsorbed **tetanus toxoid fluid** Tet Tox Fluid	*Primary immunization—* **Adults and children:** 0.5 ml (adsorbed) I.M. 4 to 6 weeks apart for 2 doses, then third dose 1 year after the second. *Primary immunization—* **Adults and children:** 0.5 ml (fluid) I.M. or S.C. 4 to 8 weeks apart, for 3 doses, then fourth dose of 0.5 ml 6 to 12 months after third dose. Booster: 0.5 ml I.M. at 10-year intervals.	*Systemic:* slight fever, chills, malaise, aches and pains, flushing, urticaria, pruritus, tachycardia, hypotension, anaphylaxis. *Local:* erythema, induration, nodule.
typhoid vaccine	*Primary immunization—* **Adults, and children over 10 years:** 0.5 ml S.C.; repeat in 4 weeks. Booster: same dose as primary immunization q 3 years. **Children 6 months to 10 years:** 0.25 ml S.C.; repeat in 4 weeks. Booster: same dose as primary immunization q 3 years.	*Systemic:* fever, malaise, headache, nausea, anaphylaxis. *Local:* swelling, pain, inflammation.

INTERACTIONS	NURSING CONSIDERATIONS
Immune serum globulin, whole blood, plasma: antibodies in serum may interfere with immune response. Don't use vaccine within 3 months. *Methotrexate:* may interfere with immune response. Don't use together.	• Contraindicated in infants failing to thrive, wounds or burns, skin disorders, patients with direct contact with smallpox virus, immunosuppression, antimetabolite and radiation therapy. Weigh risks against benefits. Use cautiously in hypersensitivity to eggs, chickens, or feathers or to neomycin or other antibiotic preservatives in this vaccine (polymyxin B, streptomycin, chlortetracycline). • Don't expose site to direct sunlight for several days, or water for 2 hours. Don't cover site initially. In pustular stage, loose dressing may be applied. Warn against touching site. May spread lesion and cause secondary infection. • Obtain history of allergies, especially to chickens or beef, antibiotics, and past reaction to immunization. • Do not inject. • Reconstituted solution may be kept for 3 months under refrigeration. • Keep epinephrine 1:1,000 available. • For treatment of anaphylaxis, see p. 1114.
None significant.	• Use with antibiotics. • Give test dose first. • Obtain history of allergies and past reaction to immunization. • Keep epinephrine 1:1,000 available. • For treatment of anaphylaxis, see p. 1114.
None significant.	• Contraindicated in immunosuppression and immunoglobulin abnormalities. Defer in acute illness and polio outbreaks, except in emergencies. • For prevention, not treatment, of tetanus infections. • Determine date of last tetanus immunization. • Don't use hot or cold compresses; may increase severity of local reaction. • Obtain history of allergies and past reaction to immunization. • Keep epinephrine 1:1,000 available.
None significant.	• Contraindicated in corticosteroid therapy. Defer in acute illness. • Treat fever with antipyretics. • Do not give intradermally. • Obtain history of allergies and past reaction to immunization. • Keep epinephrine 1:1,000 available. • Store at 2° to 10° C. (35.6° to 50° F.). • Shake thoroughly before withdrawal from vial. • For treatment of anaphylaxis, see p. 1114.

NAME	INDICATIONS & DOSAGE	SIDE EFFECTS
typhus vaccine	*Immunization against louse-borne epidemic typhus—* **Adults:** 0.5 ml Lederle vaccine or 1 ml Lilly vaccine S.C.; repeat in 4 weeks. **Children under 10 years:** 0.25 ml Lederle vaccine or 0.5 ml Lilly vaccine S.C.; repeat in 4 weeks.	*Systemic:* fever, malaise, anaphylaxis. *Local:* pain, induration, erythema.
yellow fever vaccine	*Primary vaccination—* **Adults, and children over 6 months:** 0.5 ml S.C. Booster: repeat 0.5 ml S.C. q 10 years.	*Systemic:* fever, malaise, anaphylaxis.

INTERACTIONS	NURSING CONSIDERATIONS
None significant.	• Contraindicated in corticosteroid therapy and in egg hypersensitivity. Defer in acute illness. • Use for classical epidemic typhus, not endemic forms. • Obtain history of allergies, especially to eggs, and past reaction to immunization. • Keep epinephrine 1:1,000 available. • For treatment of anaphylaxis, see p. 1114.
None significant.	• Contraindicated in gamma globulin deficiency, immunosuppression, cancer, corticosteroid or radiation therapy, allergies to chickens or eggs, and in pregnancy and in infants under 6 months except in high-risk areas. • Reconstitute with sodium chloride injection that contains no preservatives (preservatives decrease potency of vaccine). • Must be kept frozen. Shake well before using. Use within 1 hour following reconstitution. Discard remainder. • Obtain history of allergies, especially to eggs, and past reaction to immunization. • Don't give within 1 month of other live virus vaccines. • Keep epinephrine 1:1,000 available. • For treatment of anaphylaxis, see p. 1114.

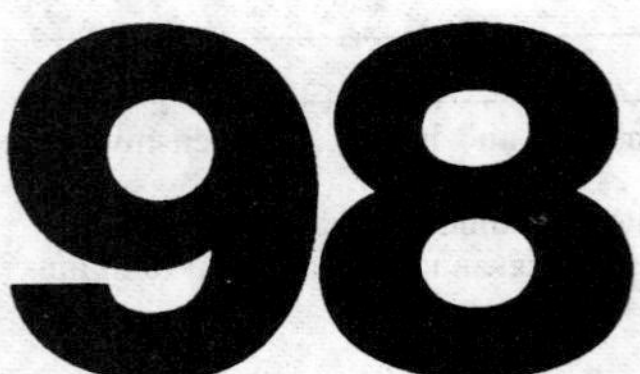

Antitoxins and antivenins

black widow spider antivenin
botulism antitoxin, bivalent equinine
crotaline antivenin, polyvalent
diphtheria antitoxin, equine
Micrurus fulvius antivenin
tetanus antitoxin, equine

Antitoxins and antivenins provide passive immunity to patients exposed to various toxins and venoms. These preparations are made from blood extracted from horses inoculated with specific toxins.

Major uses

- Prevention and treatment of bacterial toxin infections.
- Treatment of symptoms caused by insect, spider, and snake bites.

Mechanism of action

- Passive immunity is acquired by transfer of antibodies formed in blood of horses inoculated with specific toxins.
- Unbound toxins and venoms are bound and neutralized by the specific antitoxin or antivenin.

Onset and duration

- Onset of action is immediate. Immunity is undetermined.

Special information

These preparations frequently cause hypersensitivity. All patients, therefore, should receive a test dose of the drug either intradermally or ophthalmically regardless of past history of negative sensitivity.

Intradermal test: Dilute serum 1:10 with 0.9% sodium chloride for injection. Inject 0.02 ml of diluted serum intradermally on inner surface of forearm. As a control, inject other arm with 0.02 ml of 0.9% sodium chloride for injection. Observe for 20 minutes. If a wheal 10 mm or more develops at the test site, surrounded by an erythematous flare 20 mm by 20 mm, the test is positive for hypersensitivity. If skin test is positive, give a conjunctival test.

Ophthalmic test: Dilute serum 1:10 with 0.9% sodium chloride for injection. Instill 1 drop of dilution into conjunctival sac. Observe for 20 minutes. Hyperemia and injection of the mucous membranes is a positive test for hypersensitivity. If skin test is positive and eye test is negative, patient may be desensitized before antitoxin is administered.

- Have epinephrine 1:1,000 available to treat anaphylaxis.

Combination products
None.

RECOGNIZE AND TREAT SPIDER BITES

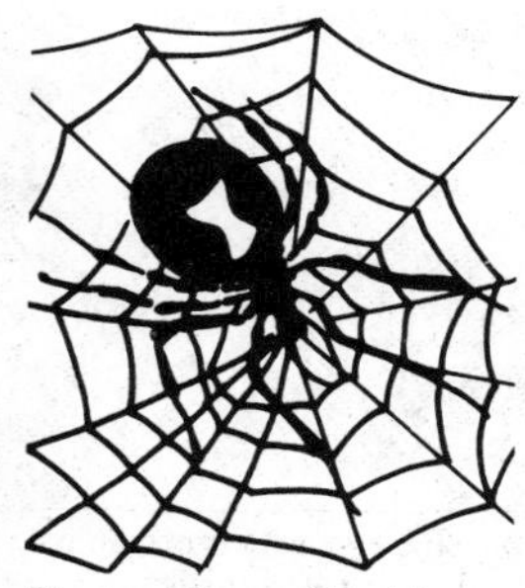

Black widow spider bites may go unnoticed until severe pain at the puncture site and intense cramping abdominal pain strike the victim 10 to 14 minutes later.

Since no lab test can detect the cause, a diagnosis must be made clinically. When taking a history, ask the patient if he's recently been in a lumber or junk pile, an outdoor privy, or an old barn, garage, or basement. Black widow spiders may inhabit any of these places.

Here's how to recognize and treat symptoms of spider bites.

Spider bite victims may suffer spasmodic muscle pain in the legs, chest, and back. At the puncture site you'll see two tiny red spots and slight swelling or urticaria. The patient will experience weakness, nausea, fever, chills, and a rigid abdomen with diminished bowel sounds. He'll have elevated blood pressure, labored breathing, profuse sweating, and numb or tingling feet. Small children may suffer delirium and convulsions.

Keep the patient quiet and the affected part immobile. If a tourniquet is in place, check his pulse regularly. Don't release the tourniquet as this would also release toxins into the circulatory system. Apply cold packs to relieve pain and swelling and to slow circulation.

NAME	INDICATIONS & DOSAGE	SIDE EFFECTS
black widow spider antivenin Antivenin (Latrodectus Mactans)◆	*Black widow spider bite—* **Adults and children:** 2.5 ml I.M. in deltoid. Second dose may be needed.	*Systemic:* hypersensitivity, anaphylaxis.
botulism antitoxin, bivalent equine	*Botulism—* **Adults and children:** 1 vial I.V. stat and q 4 hours, p.r.n., until patient's condition improves. Dilute antitoxin 1:10 in 5% or 10% dextrose in water or normal saline solution before giving. Give first 10 ml of dilution over 5 minutes; after 15 minutes, rate may be increased.	*Systemic:* hypersensitivity, anaphylaxis, serum sickness (urticaria, pruritus, fever, malaise, arthralgia) may occur in 5 to 13 days.
crotaline antivenin, polyvalent	*Crotalid (rattlesnake) bites—* **Adults and children:** initially, 10 to 50 ml or more I.M. or S.C., depending on severity of bite and patient's response. If large amount of venom, 70 to 100 ml I.V. directly into superficial vein. Subsequent doses based on patient's response; may give 10 ml q ½ to 2 hours, p.r.n. If bite is in extremity, inject part of initial dose at various sites around limb above swelling; don't inject in finger or toe. The smaller the body, the larger the initial dose.	*Systemic:* hypersensitivity, anaphylaxis.
diphtheria antitoxin, equine	*Diphtheria prevention—* **Adults and children:** 1,000 to 5,000 units I.M. *Diphtheria treatment—* **Adults and children:** 20,000 to 80,000 units or more slow I.V. Additional doses may be given in 24 hours. I.M. route may be used in mild cases.	*Systemic:* hypersensitivity, anaphylaxis, serum sickness (urticaria, pruritus, fever, malaise, arthralgia) may occur in 7 to 12 days.

INTERACTIONS	NURSING CONSIDERATIONS
None significant.	• If possible, hospitalize patient. • Test for sensitivity before giving. Test described on pp. 1036-1037. • Epinephrine should be available in case of adverse reaction. • Venom is neurotoxic and may cause respiratory paralysis and convulsions. Watch patient carefully for 2 to 3 days. • Obtain accurate patient history of allergies, especially to horses, and past reaction to immunization. • Earliest possible use of the antivenin is recommended for best results. • For treatment of anaphylaxis, see p. 1114.
None significant.	• Test for sensitivity before giving. Test described on pp. 1036-1037. • Epinephrine should be available in case of adverse reaction. Bivalent antitoxin contains antibodies against types A and B *Clostridium botulinum*. Antitoxins against other types available only from Center for Disease Control in Atlanta, Georgia. • Obtain accurate patient history of allergies, especially to horses, and past reaction to immunization. • Earliest possible use of the antitoxin is recommended for best results. • For treatment of anaphylaxis, see p. 1114.
Antihistamines: enhanced toxicity of crotaline venoms. Don't use together.	• Test for sensitivity before giving. Test described on pp. 1036-1037. • Immobilize patient immediately. Splint bitten extremity. • Epinephrine should be available in case of adverse reaction. • Type and crossmatch as soon as possible since hemolysis from venom prevents accurate crossmatching. • Early use of antivenin recommended for best results. • Watch patient carefully for delayed allergic reaction or relapse. • Because children have less resistance and less body fluid to dilute venom, they may need twice the adult dose. • Obtain accurate patient history of allergies, especially to horses, and past reaction to immunization. • Discard unused reconstituted drug. • For treatment of anaphylaxis, see p. 1114.
None significant.	• Test for sensitivity before giving. Test described on pp. 1036-1037. • Epinephrine should be available in case of adverse reaction. • Obtain accurate patient history of allergies, especially to horses, and past reaction to immunization. • Therapy should be started immediately, without waiting for culture and sensitivity reports, if patient has clinical symptoms of diphtheria (sore throat, fever, tonsillar membrane). • Refrigerate antitoxin at 35.6° to 50° F. (2° to 10° C.). May be warmed 90° to 95° F. (32.2° to 35° C.) never higher. • For treatment of anaphylaxis, see p. 1114.

NAME	INDICATIONS & DOSAGE	SIDE EFFECTS
Micrurus fulvius antivenin	*Eastern and Texas coral snake bite—* **Adults and children:** 3 to 5 vials slow I.V. through running I.V. of 0.9% normal saline solution. Give first 1 to 2 ml over 3 to 5 minutes and watch for signs of allergic reaction. If no signs develop, continue injection. Up to 10 vials may be needed. Not effective for Sonoran or Arizona coral snake bites.	*Systemic:* hypersensitivity, anaphylaxis.
tetanus antitoxin (TAT), equine	*Tetanus prophylaxis—* **Patients over 65 lbs:** 3,000 to 5,000 units I.M. or S.C. **Patients under 65 lbs:** 1,500 to 3,000 units I.M. or S.C. *Tetanus treatment—* **All patients:** 10,000 to 20,000 units injected into wound. Give additional 40,000 to 200,000 units I.V. Start tetanus toxoid at same time but at different site and with a different syringe.	*Local:* pain, numbness, skin eruptions. *Systemic:* joint pain, hypersensitivity, anaphylaxis.

INTERACTIONS	NURSING CONSIDERATIONS
None significant.	• Test for sensitivity before giving. Test described on pp. 1036-1037. • Immobilize patient or splint bitten limb to prevent spread of venom. • Hospitalize patient if possible. • Early use of antivenin recommended for best results. • Venom is neurotoxic and may cause respiratory paralysis. Watch patient carefully for 24 hours. Be ready to take supportive measures. Epinephrine should be available in case of adverse reaction. • Obtain accurate patient history of allergies, especially to horses, and past reaction to immunization. • For treatment of anaphylaxis, see p. 1114.
None significant.	• Test for sensitivity before giving. Test described on pp. 1036-1037. • Use only when tetanus immune globulin (human) not available. • Obtain accurate patient history of allergies, especially to horses, and past reaction to immunization. If respiratory difficulty develops, give 0.4 ml of 1:1,000 solution epinephrine HC1. • Preventative dose should be given to those who have had 2 or fewer injections of tetanus toxoid and who have tetanus-prone injuries more than 24 hours old. • For treatment of anaphylaxis, see p. 1114.

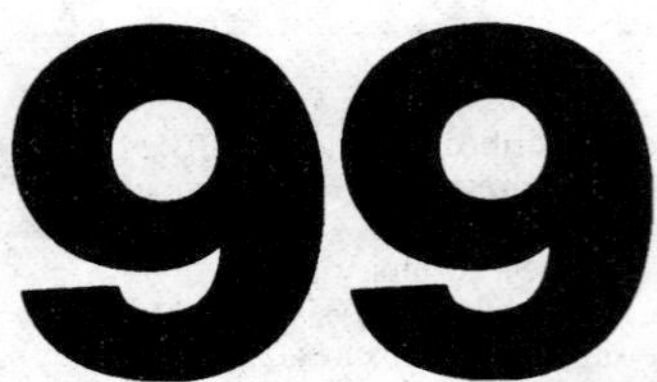

Acidifiers and alkalinizers

Acidifiers:
ammonium chloride
dilute hydrochloric acid

Alkalinizers:
sodium bicarbonate
sodium lactate
tromethamine

Acidifiers and alkalinizers are used to correct acid-base imbalance in metabolic disorders. In severe metabolic alkalosis, acidifiers may be given to lower blood pH. Conversely, alkalinizers, which raise blood pH, may be given to treat metabolic acidosis. Sodium bicarbonate, an alkalinizer, may be used to increase other drugs' effectiveness by decreasing excretion. It's also used to treat acid toxicity by increasing fixation of acidic drugs.

Major uses

- Acidifiers: treatment of metabolic alkalosis; and acidification of urine (ammonium chloride).
- Alkalinizers: treatment of metabolic acidosis.

Mechanism of action

- Alkalinizers decrease free $H+$ concentration.
- Acidifiers increase free $H+$ concentration.

Absorption, distribution, and excretion

- Ammonium chloride and sodium bicarbonate are rapidly and well absorbed orally. All others are administered parenterally.
- Ammonium chloride and sodium lactate are metabolized in liver. Tromethamine is not metabolized and is excreted in the urine.
- Ammonium chloride is excreted by the kidneys.

Onset and duration

- Onset of drugs given orally is rapid. Intravenous administration has immediate onset.
- Duration of effect is variable, depending on use and underlying disease state.

Combination products
None.

RECOGNIZE ACIDOSIS AND ALKALOSIS

CONDITION	NORMAL	RESPIRATORY ACIDOSIS	RESPIRATORY ALKALOSIS	METABOLIC ACIDOSIS	METABOLIC ALKALOSIS
POSSIBLE CAUSES		Impaired alveolar ventilation, respiratory depressant drugs, intracranial tumors	Ventilatory support, hyperventilation, CNS disease, anxiety, persistent fever, liver disease, CHF, pulmonary embolism	Aspirin, renal disease, diabetes, lactic acidosis, diarrhea, biliary fistulae	Vomiting, diuretics, hyperadrenocorticism, alkali, hyperaldosteronism, nasogastric suction
SYMPTOMS		Lethargy, shallow irregular respirations, disorientation	Hyperactive reflexes, blurred vision, tetany, vertigo, muscle cramps, sighing, diaphoresis	Kussmaul respiration, restlessness, disorientation	Weakness, paralysis, leg cramps, paresthesias
SIGNS		Hypoventilation, asterixis	Hyperventilation, latent tetany	Shock, coma, tachypnea, almond odor from mouth	Signs of potassium depletion, latent tetany
pH	7.35 to 7.45	Normal or decreased	Increased	Decreased	Increased
PO_2	90 to 95 mmHg	Decreased	Altered	Normal or increased	Normal or decreased
PCO_2	34 to 46 mmHg	Increased	Decreased	Decreased	Increased
HCO_3	24 to 26 mEq/L	Increased	Decreased	Decreased	Increased
RESPIRATORY RATE	10 to 20/mm	Irregular	Altered	Increased	Decreased

NAME	INDICATIONS & DOSAGE	SIDE EFFECTS
ammonium chloride	*Metabolic alkalosis*— **Adults and children:** 4 mEq/Kg slow I.V. or calculated by amount of chloride deficit. Infusion rate: 0.9 to 1.3 ml/min 2.14% solution. Do not exceed 2 ml/min. Hypodermoclysis has been used in infants and young children. One half calculated volume should be given and then patient reassessed. See also Chapter 40, Expectorants and Antitussives.	Side effects usually result from ammonia toxicity or too rapid I.V. administration. *CNS:* headache, confusion, progressive drowsiness, excitement alternating with coma, hyperventilation, jerky respirations with apneic periods, calcium-deficient tetany, twitching, hyperreflexia, EEG abnormalities. *CV:* bradycardia. *GI* (with oral dose): gastric irritation, nausea, vomiting, thirst, anorexia, retching. *GU:* glycosuria. *Local:* pain at injection site. *Metabolic:* acidosis, hyperchloremia, hypokalemia, hyperglycemia. *Skin:* rash, pallor.
dilute hydrochloric acid	*Metabolic alkalosis*— pharmacy prepares (0.1 normal HCl solution in sterile water) 100 mEq hydrogen and 100 mEq chloride per liter.	None confirmed.
sodium bicarbonate	*Cardiac arrest*— **Adults and children:** as a 7.5% or 8.4% solution 1 to 3 mEq/Kg I.V. initially; may repeat in 10 minutes. Further doses based on blood gases. If blood gases unavailable, use 0.5 mEq/Kg q 10 minutes until spontaneous circulation returns. **Infants up to 2 years:** 4.2% solution, I.V. infusion. Rate not to exceed 8 mEq/Kg/day. *Metabolic acidosis*— **Adults and children:** dose depends on blood CO_2 content, pH, and patient's clinical condition. Generally 2 to 5 mEq/Kg; I.V. required over 4- to 8-hour period. *Systemic or urinary alkalinization*— **Adults:** 325 mg to 2 g P.O. q.i.d.	*GI:* gastric distention, belching, flatulence. *GU:* renal calculi or crystals. *Metabolic:* with overdose: alkalosis, hypernatremia, hyperosmolarity.
sodium lactate	*Alkalinize urine*— **Adults:** 30 ml of a 1/6 molar solution/Kg of body weight given in divided doses over 24 hours. *Metabolic acidosis*— **Adults:** usually given as 1/6 molar injection (167 mEq lactate per liter). Dosage depends on degree of bicarbonate deficit.	*Metabolic:* with overdose: alkalosis, hypernatremia, hyperosmolarity.

• Also available in Canada.
•• Available in Canada only.
Unmarked trade names available in United States only.

INTERACTIONS	NURSING CONSIDERATIONS
Spironolactone: systemic acidosis. Use together cautiously.	• Contraindicated in severe hepatic or renal dysfunction. Use cautiously in pulmonary insufficiency or cardiac edema and in infants. • Give after meals to decrease GI side effects. Enteric-coated tablets may also minimize GI symptoms but are absorbed erratically. • Pain of I.V. injection may be lessened by decreasing rate of infusion. • Determine CO_2 combining power and serum electrolytes before and during therapy. • Monitor BUN for urea formation. Monitor urine pH and output. Diuresis normal for first 2 days. • Dilute concentrated solutions (21.4%, 26.75%) to 2.14% before giving. • Monitor rate and depth of respiration frequently. • Hypodermoclysis should be into lateral aspect of thigh. Stop infusion immediately if pain occurs.
None significant.	• Not available commercially; prepared in pharmacy. • Administer I.V. solution slowly through a central venous line. • Monitor pH, blood gases, and electrolytes at 4- to 6- hour intervals.
None significant.	• No contraindications for use in life-threatening emergencies. Contraindicated in hypertension; in patients with tendency toward edema; in patients who are losing chlorides by vomiting or from continuous GI suction; in patients receiving diuretics known to produce hypochloremic alkalosis, and in patients on salt restriction or with renal disease. • May be added to other I.V. fluids. • Parenteral bicarbonate solutions will precipitate calcium salts. Do not mix in same infusion fluid. I.V. bolus injections should be given only through running I.V. lines free of calcium salts. • To avoid risk of alkalosis, determine blood pH, PO_2, PCO_2, and electrolytes. Keep doctor informed of lab results. • Tell patient not to take with milk. May cause hypercalcemia, alkalosis, and possibly renal calculi. • Because sodium bicarbonate inactivates catecholamines such as epinephrine and levarterenol, do not mix with I.V. solutions of these agents.
None significant.	• Contraindicated in respiratory alkalosis and in acidosis associated with congenital heart disease with persistent cyanosis.

NAME	INDICATIONS & DOSAGE	SIDE EFFECTS
tromethamine THAM◆	*Metabolic acidosis (associated with cardiac bypass surgery or with cardiac arrest)*— **Adults:** dose depends on bicarbonate deficit. Calculate as follows: ml of 0.3 M tromethamine solution required = wt in Kg x bicarbonate deficit (mEq/L). Additional therapy based on serial determinations of existing bicarbonate deficit. **Children:** calculate dose as above. Give ¼ dose over 2 to 5 minutes; ¼ dose slowly over 3 to 6 hours. Additional therapy based on degree of acidosis. Total 24-hour dose should not exceed 33 to 40 ml/Kg.	*Blood:* possible increase in coagulation time (shown in animal studies). *CNS:* respiratory depression. *Local:* venospasm; intravenous thrombosis; inflammation, necrosis, and slough if extravasation occurs. *Metabolic:* hypoglycemia, hyperkalemia (with decreased urinary output).

INTERACTIONS	NURSING CONSIDERATIONS
None significant.	• Contraindicated in anuria, uremia, chronic respiratory acidosis, pregnancy (except acute, life-threatening situations). Use cautiously in renal disease or poor urinary output. Monitor EKG and serum K+ in these patients. • To prevent blood pH from rising above normal, adjust dose carefully. • Give slowly through large needle (18G to 20G) into largest antecubital vein or by indwelling catheter. • Before, during, and after therapy, make these following determinations: blood pH; carbon dioxide tension; bicarbonate, glucose, and electrolyte levels. • Mechanical ventilation should be available. Use when giving drug to patient with associated respiratory acidosis. • Except in life-threatening situations, do not use longer than 1 day. • If I.V. extravasates, infiltrate area with 1% procaine and hyaluronidase 150 units; may reduce vasospasm and dilute remaining drug in local area. • Concentration of tromethamine should not exceed 0.3 M.

100

Uricosurics

probenecid
sulfinpyrazone

Uricosuric drugs are renal tubular blocking agents. They inhibit active reabsorption of uric acid at the proximal renal tubule, allowing excretion of uric acid in the urine, and also lowering the level of serum uric acid. Sulfinpyrazone also inhibits platelet aggregation. For information on allopurinol and colchicine, which are not uricosuric agents, but are used in gout, see Chapter 106.

Major uses

- For maintenance therapy in chronic gouty arthritis and tophaceous gout.
- As adjunct to antibiotic therapy to increase antibiotic concentrations.

Mechanism of action

- Block renal tubular reabsorption of uric acid, increasing excretion.
- Inhibit secretion of many weak organic acids.

Absorption, distribution, and excretion

- Rapidly and completely absorbed from GI tract after oral administration.
- Bound to plasma protein.
- Metabolized in the liver and excreted in urine, with small amounts excreted in the stools.

Onset and duration

- Onset (appearance in plasma and uric acid clearance) begins 30 minutes after oral administration. Probenecid's effect on penicillin begins after 2 hours.
- Peak occurs at about 2 to 4 hours.
- Duration of action is 4 to 10 hours.

Combination products

COLBENEMID: probenecid 500 mg and colchicine 0.5 mg.
COLBENI-MOR: probenecid 500 mg and colchicine 0.5 mg.
PROBEN-C: probenecid 500 mg and colchicine 0.5 mg.
ROBENECOL: probenecid 500 mg and colchicine 0.5 mg.

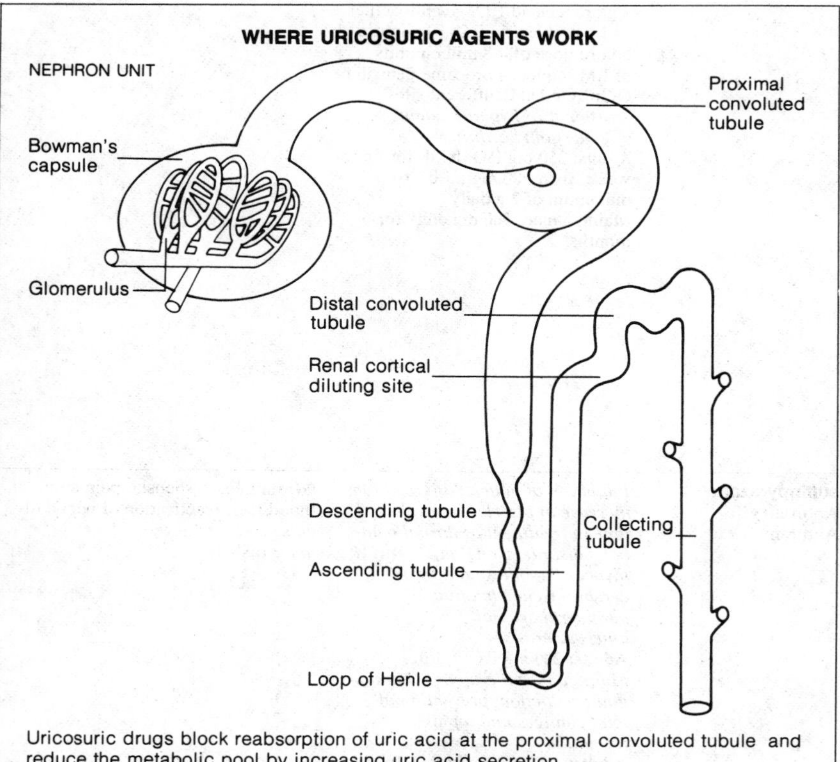

Uricosuric drugs block reabsorption of uric acid at the proximal convoluted tubule and reduce the metabolic pool by increasing uric acid secretion.

NAME	INDICATIONS & DOSAGE	SIDE EFFECTS
probenecid Benemid♦, Benn, Benuryl♦♦, Probalan, Probenimead, Robenecid	*Adjunct to penicillin or cephalosporin therapy—* **Adults, and children over 50 Kg:** 500 mg P.O. q.i.d. **Children 2 to 14 years (under 50 Kg):** initially, 25 mg/Kg P.O., then 40 mg/Kg divided q.i.d. *Single-dose treatment of gonorrhea—* **Adults:** 3.5 g ampicillin P.O. with 1 g probenecid P.O. given together; or 1 g probenecid P.O. 30 minutes before dose of 4.8 million units of I.M. aqueous procaine penicillin G, injected at 2 different sites. *Treatment of hyperuricemia of gout, gouty arthritis—* **Adults:** 250 mg P.O. b.i.d. for first week, then 500 mg b.i.d., to maximum of 2 g daily. Maintenance: 500 mg daily for 6 months.	*Blood:* hemolytic anemia. *CNS:* headache, dizziness. *CV:* hypotension. *GI:* anorexia, nausea, and vomiting. *GU:* urinary frequency. *Skin:* dermatitis, pruritus. *Other:* flushing, sore gums, fever, sweating, anaphylaxis.
sulfinpyrazone Anturan♦♦, Anturane	*Inhibition of platelet aggregation, increase of platelet survival time in treatment of thromboembolic disorders, angina, myocardial infarction, transient cerebral ischemic attacks, peripheral arterial atherosclerosis—* **Adults:** 200 mg P.O. q.i.d. *Maintenance therapy of common gout: reduction, prevention of joint changes and tophi formation—* **Adults:** 100 to 200 mg P.O. b.i.d. first week, then 200 to 400 mg P.O. b.i.d. Maximum 800 mg daily.	*GI:* nausea, dyspepsia, pain and blood loss, reactivation of peptic ulcers. *Skin:* rash.

♦ Also available in Canada.
♦♦ Available in Canada only.
Unmarked trade names available in United States only.

INTERACTIONS	NURSING CONSIDERATIONS
Salicylates: inhibited uricosuric effect of probenecid, causing urate retention. Do not use together.	• Contraindicated in blood dyscrasias; acute gout attack; penicillin therapy in presence of known renal impairment; gouty nephropathy; urinary tract stones or obstruction; azotemia; hyperuricemia secondary to cancer chemotherapy, radiation, or myeloproliferative neoplastic diseases. Use cautiously with peptic ulcer or renal impairment. • Usually preferred over sulfinpyrazone because probenecid produces fewer, less severe GI and hematological side effects. • Contains no analgesic or anti-inflammatory agent and is of no value during acute gout attacks. • Suitable for long-term use; no cumulative effects or tolerance. • Not effective with chronic renal insufficiency (glomerular filtration rate less than 30 ml/min). • Periodic BUN and renal function tests recommended (long-term therapy). • May increase frequency, severity, and length of acute gout attacks during first 6 to 12 months of therapy. Prophylactic colchicine is given during first 3 to 6 months. • Avoid alcohol; increases urate level. • Force fluids to maintain daily output of 2 to 3 liters minimum. Alkalize urine with sodium bicarbonate or other agent ordered by doctor. • Give with milk, food, or antacids to minimize GI distress. Continued disturbances might indicate need to lower dose. • Restrict foods high in purine: anchovies, liver, sardines, kidneys, sweetbreads, peas, lentils. • Watch for signs of hyperglycemia. • Instruct patient and family that drug must be taken regularly as ordered or gout attacks may result. Tell him to visit doctor regularly so blood levels can be monitored and dosage can be adjusted if necessary. • May have false positive glucose tests with Benedict's solution or Clinitest, but not with the glucose oxidase method (Clinistix, Diastix, Tes-Tape). • Decreases urinary excretion of 17-ketosteroids, PSP, BSP, aminohippuric acid, iodine-related organic acids, interfering with laboratory procedures. • For symptoms and treatment of anaphylaxis, see p. 1114.
Probenecid: inhibited renal excretion of sulfinpyrazone. Use together with caution. *Salicylates:* inhibited uricosuric effect of sulfinpyrazone. Do not use together.	• Contraindicated in hypersensitivity to pyrazole derivatives (including oxyphenbutazone, phenylbutazone); active peptic ulcer; during or within 2 weeks after gout attack; gouty nephropathy; urolithiasis, or urinary obstruction; bone marrow depression; azotemia; hyperuricemia secondary to cancer chemotherapy, radiation, or myeloproliferative neoplastic diseases. Use cautiously with diminished hepatic or renal dysfunction. • Use for treating thromboembolic conditions is investigatory and is most often directed at prevention of myocardial infarction recurrence. • Recommended for patients unresponsive to other uricosurics. Suitable for long-term use; no cumulative effects or tolerance. • Contains no analgesic or anti-inflammatory agent and is of no value during acute gout attacks. • Periodic BUN and renal function studies advised (long-term use). • May increase frequency, severity, and length of acute gout attacks during first 6 to 12 months of therapy; prophylactic colchicine is given during first 3 to 6 months.

(continued on following page)

NAME	INDICATIONS & DOSAGE	SIDE EFFECTS
sulfinpyrazone *(continued)*		

INTERACTIONS	NURSING CONSIDERATIONS
	• Therapy, especially at start, may lead to renal colic and formation of uric acid stones. Until acid levels are normal (about 6 mg/100 ml), monitor intake and output closely. • Force fluids to maintain daily output of 2 to 3 liters minimum. Alkalize urine with sodium bicarbonate or other agent ordered by doctor. • Give with milk, food, or antacids to minimize GI disturbances. • Restrict foods high in purine: anchovies, liver, sardines, kidneys, sweetbreads, peas, lentils. • Instruct patient and family that drug must be taken regularly as ordered or gout attacks may result. Tell him to visit doctor regularly so blood levels can be monitored and dosage adjusted if necessary. • Decreases urinary excretion of aminohippuric acid and PSP, interfering with laboratory procedures. • Alkalinizing agents are used therapeutically to increase sulfinpyrazone activity, preventing urolithiasis.

101

Enzymes

bromelains	**hyaluronidase**
chymotrypsin	**papain**
fibrinolysin	**streptokinase-streptodornase**
fibrinolysin and desoxyribonuclease	**trypsin**

Enzymes are complex proteins that induce chemical changes without being changed themselves. Several groups of enzymes are used therapeutically, but only those with proteolytic, anti-inflammatory, or debridement properties are included in this chapter. Some are used systemically for anti-inflammatory action. Enzymes are most useful, however, in the debridement of wounds and other injuries. They are given orally, topically, locally, subcutaneously, or intramuscularly; they work best in a moist environment; are destroyed by heat or cold; are inactivated by detergents, antiseptics, and heavy metal compounds. Enzyme treatment is adjunctive therapy and must be accompanied by management of the underlying causes of illness or inflammation.

Major uses

- Biochemical debridement of wounds and burns.
- Reduction of inflammation and edema after surgery.
- Reduction of inflammation in chronic or recurrent inflammatory conditions.
- Increase absorption and dispersion of fluids, locally injected drugs, local anesthetics, anti-infectives, and contrast media (hyaluronidase).
- Dissolution of clotted blood and purulent material from wounds and infections.

Mechanism of action

- Not completely established.
- May reverse decreased tissue permeability that occurs with inflammation and edema, thus restoring flow of blood and other fluids and facilitating drainage and tissue repair.
- Degrades protein of blood clots, necrotic tissue, and purulent exudates which may block free flow of body fluids and impede resolution of inflammation and edema.
- Digests protein matter, cleansing wounds by liquefaction and dissolution.

Absorption, distribution, and excretion

- Information not established for majority of compounds.
- Vary with each drug.
- Bromelains absorbed from gastrointestinal tract.
- Papain not orally absorbed; systemic effects may be caused by indirect activation of plasminogen precursors.

Onset and duration

- Unknown.

Combination products

BIOZYME OINTMENT: 10,000 units enzymatic activity; mixture of trypsin and chymotrypsin.
CHYMORAL ENTERIC-COATED TABLETS: 50,000 units enzymatic activity; trypsin and chymotrypsin in ratio of 6:1.
CHYMORAL-100: 100,000 units enzymatic activity; trypsin and chymotrypsin in ratio of 6:1.
GRANULEX-AEROSOL: trypsin 0.1 mg, balsam peru 72.5 mg, and castor oil 650 mg.
NEOMYCIN PALMITATE: 3.5 mg.
ORENZYME BITABS ENTERIC-COATED TABLETS: 100,000 units trypsin and 8,000 units chymotrypsin.
ORENZYME ENTERIC-COATED TABLETS•: 50,000 units trypsin and 4,000 units chymotrypsin.

ENZYME THERAPY FOR DECUBITUS ULCERS

Proteolytic enzymes are used primarily for debridement of necrotic tissue from wounds of decubitus ulcers. Their main effect is a gradual appearance of granulation tissue around the site and gradual decrease in the depth of the crater as deeper tissue generates new cells.

Enzyme therapy has many limitations. Because enzymes are proteins, they need a high degree of purification before administration. Even then, they may be antigenic and cause toxic reactions. Another drawback is that protein-digesting enzymes of the gastrointestinal tract tend to inhibit proteolytic enzyme activity. Despite these limitations, enzymes have been proven useful.

However, effective treatment with enzymes requires certain supportive measures, depending on the underlying cause: stasis, trauma, or infection.

— Use sterile technique in caring for the decubitus ulcer.

— Use a heat lamp and air exposure between dressings to promote drying and increase the blood supply to the ulcerated area.

— Provide oxygen saturation by inserting an oxygen catheter through a paper cup tent over decubiti. This will promote healing by producing a drying effect.

— Use enzymes carefully according to the progress of the wound or decubitus area. Remember that denuding necrotic areas may expose capillaries and cause bleeding at the site.

— Place patient on a flotation pad to protect pressure points on the body.

— Turn the patient frequently.

— Give regular back rubs and gently massage all pressure areas of the body.

— Monitor adequate food and fluid intake to speed recovery.

NAME	INDICATIONS & DOSAGE	SIDE EFFECTS
bromelains Ananase	*Adjunct to reduce inflammation and edema, ease pain, and speed tissue repair of traumatic injuries (contusions, sprains, strains, dislocations), cellulitis, furunculosis, ulcerations—* **Adults:** initially, 100,000 units P.O., q.i.d. then 50,000 units t.i.d. or q.i.d. for maintenance.	*Blood:* bleeding tendencies. *GI:* mild diarrhea, nausea, vomiting. *GU:* menorrhagia, metrorrhagia. *Other:* elevated temperature, hypersensitivity reactions (rash, urticaria).
chymotrypsin	*Adjunct in general, rectal, oral, and dental surgery—* **Adults:** preoperatively, 2,500 units I.M., then 2,500 units once or twice daily, as indicated. *Adjunct in treatment of respiratory conditions (asthma, bronchitis, rhinitis, sinusitis)—* **Adults:** 2,500 to 5,000 units I.M. once or twice weekly; more often if needed. **Children:** ½ adult dose. *Chronic or recurrent inflammation (peptic ulcer, ulcerative colitis, phlebitis, thrombophlebitis, dermatologic conditions)—* **Adults:** 2,500 to 5,000 units I.M. once or twice weekly. Tablet containing 10,000 units may be given buccally q.i.d. alone or in conjunction with I.M. therapy. *Relief of episiotomy symptoms—* **Adults:** 5,000 units I.M. repeated twice at 12-hour intervals. *Pelvic inflammatory diseases—* **Adults:** 2,500 units daily for 7 days; repeat course if needed.	*Blood:* increased bleeding tendency. *GI:* nausea and vomiting, diarrhea with oral administration. *GU:* hematuria, albuminuria, menorrhagia, metrorrhagia. *Local:* pain, induration at injection site. *Other:* chills, dizziness, fever, rapid dissolution of animal-origin sutures, hypersensitivity (rash, urticaria, itching, anaphylaxis).
fibrinolysin Thrombolysin	*Thrombophlebitis, phlebothrombosis, pulmonary embolism, thrombosis of arteries (excluding cerebral and coronary arteries)—* **Adults:** 50,000 to 100,000 units per hour by I.V. drip in dextrose 5% in water for 1 to 6 hours each day. Repeat for 3 or 4 consecutive days if indicated. Extensive venous thrombi may require 250,000 to 400,000 units.	*CNS:* dizziness, headache. *CV:* hypotension, hypertension, tachycardia. *GI:* nausea, vomiting, abdominal pain. *GU:* proteinuria. *Other:* chills, muscle, chest or back pain, fever, angioneurotic edema.

• Also available in Canada.
•• Available in Canada only.
Unmarked trade names available in United States only.

INTERACTIONS	NURSING CONSIDERATIONS
Alkaline solutions, antacids: dissolved enteric coating of tablet. Do not use within 1 hour of bromelains.	• Contraindicated in hypersensitivity to pineapple or pineapple products. Use cautiously with anticoagulant therapy and in patients with blood-clotting abnormalities, including hemophilia, hepatic or renal disease, and systemic infection. • Obtain history of previous allergies. Watch for hypersensitivity reactions. • Destruction of enteric coating may decrease effectiveness. Tablets must be swallowed whole; do not crush or break. • Observe wound to monitor progress of therapy. Appearance of granulation tissue may indicate effectiveness. Notify doctor if inflammation or color of drainage indicates spread of infection. • Protect from heat.
Alkaline solutions, antacids: dissolved enteric coating of tablet. Do not use within 1 hour of oral administration of chymotrypsin.	• Contraindicated in hypersensitivity to trypsin or to sesame oil (injectable form), septicemia, severe generalized or localized infection, and blood coagulation disorders such as hemophilia. Use with caution in severe hepatic or renal disease. • Parenteral administration: Do not give I.V. Test for sensitivity before giving. Inject deep into gluteal muscle; rotate sites. Watch for hypersensitivity reactions, including changes in blood pressure and pulse. Watch for pain, induration at injection site. Stop if reaction occurs. • Avoid getting in eyes. If it does get into eyes, flood with water immediately. • Protect from heat. • For treatment of anaphylaxis, see p. 1114.
None significant.	• Contraindicated in hemorrhagic diathesis, severe hepatic dysfunction, or hypofibrinogenemia. Use with caution after massive hemorrhage, serious myocardial disease, anesthesia, or surgery. • Incompatible with sodium chloride injection. • Reconstitute in 25 ml sterile water for injection and add to dextrose 5% in water for infusion. Use within 2 hours after reconstitution. Do not shake.

NAME	INDICATIONS & DOSAGE	SIDE EFFECTS
fibrinolysin and desoxyribonuclease Elase◆	*Debridement of inflammatory and infected lesions (surgical wounds; ulcerative lesions, second- and third-degree burns, circumcision, episiotomy; cervicitis; vaginitis, abscesses, fistulas and sinus tracts)*— **Intravaginally:** 5 ml ointment may be inserted using applicator supplied, once daily for vaginitis or cervicitis. *Topical use*—apply ointment 30 units fibrinolysin, 20,000 units desoxyribonuclease/30 g at intervals as long as enzyme action is desired. *Irrigating agent for infected wounds, empyema cavities, abscesses, otorhinolaryngologic wounds, subcutaneous hematomas*—dilution for irrigation depends on extent and severity of wound: 25 units fibrinolysin powder, 15,000 units desoxyribonuclease per 30 ml vial.	*Local:* hyperemia with high doses.
hyaluronidase Hyazyme, Wydase◆	*Adjunct to increase absorption and dispersion of other injected drugs*— **Adults and children:** 150 units to injection medium containing other medication. *Hypodermoclysis*— **Adults, and children over 3 years:** 150 units injected S.C. before clysis, or injected into clysis tubing near needle for each 1,000 ml clysis solution. *Subcutaneous urography*— **Adults and children:** with patient prone, give 75 units S.C. over each scapula, followed by injection of contrast medium at same sites.	*Skin:* rash, urticaria.
papain Panafil, Papase◆	*Prevention of inflammation and edema in surgical procedures*— **Adults and children:** 10,000 to 20,000 units P.O. or buccal 1 to 2 hours before surgery, then 20,000 units q.i.d. for up to 5 days. *Treatment of inflammation and burns, enzymatic debridement, promotion of normal healing and deodorization of surface lesions, particularly in local*	*Blood:* increased bleeding tendencies. *GI:* nausea, vomiting, diarrhea with oral administration. *Local:* tenderness after buccal administration, occasional itching or stinging with first application of ointment. *Other:* fever, hypersensitivity reactions (rash, urticaria, pruritus).

INTERACTIONS	NURSING CONSIDERATIONS
None significant.	• Contraindicated for parenteral use. • Dense, dry eschar must be removed surgically before enzymatic debridement. Enzyme must be in constant contact with substrate. Accumulated necrotic debris must be removed periodically. • Clean wound with water or peroxide and dry gently; cover with thin layer of Elase. Cover with nonadhering dressing. • Change dressing at least once a day. Flush away necrotic debris and reapply ointment. • Solution as wet dressing: Mix 1 vial of Elase powder with 10 to 50 ml saline solution; saturate strips of fine gauze with solution. Pack ulcerated area with Elase gauze. Allow gauze to dry in contact with ulcerated lesion for about 6 to 8 hours. Remove dried gauze and repeat 3 to 4 times daily. • Solution as irrigant: Drain cavity and replace Elase every 6 to 10 hours to reduce amount of by-product accumulation and to minimize loss of enzyme activity. Although parenteral use is contraindicated, Elase is used as an irrigant in certain specific conditions. • Prepare solution just before use. Discard after 24 hours.
Local anesthetics: increased potential for toxic local reaction. Use together cautiously.	• Use with caution in blood-clotting abnormalities, severe hepatic or renal disease. • Do not inject into acutely inflamed or cancerous areas. • In hypodermoclysis, adjust dose, rate of injection, and type of solution to patient response. • Administration precautions: Skin-test for sensitivity. Avoid injecting into diseased areas (may spread infection). Observe injection site for local reactions. • Avoid getting solution in eyes. If it does get into eyes, flood with water at once. • Protect from heat. Do not use cloudy or discolored solution.
With topical use, detergents and antiseptics (benzalkonium chloride, hexachlorophene, iodine, hydrogen peroxide): decreased enzymatic activity. Do not use together.	• Contraindicated in hypersensitivity to papaya fruit. Oral administration contraindicated in anticoagulant therapy; blood-clotting abnormalities, including hemophilia; and systemic infections. Use cautiously in severe hepatic or renal disease. • Instruct patient on proper route to be used. Oral tablets may be swallowed with water or chewed. • Before treatment, thoroughly cleanse and irrigate wound area with sterile normal saline or water to remove antiseptics, detergents, and heavy metal antibacterials, which can decrease enzyme activity. Don't use hydrogen peroxide. Moisten area for optimal enzymatic activity. Apply ointment in thin layers to assure contact with necrotic tissue. Cover with gauze.

(continued on following page)

NAME	INDICATIONS & DOSAGE	SIDE EFFECTS
papain (continued)	*infection, necrosis, fibrinous or purulent debris, sloughing—* **Adults and children:** apply ointment 10% directly to lesion 1 to 2 times daily. Cover with gauze.	
streptokinase-streptodornase Varidase♦	*Anti-inflammatory agent to relieve pain, swelling, tenderness, erythema; management of edema and localized extravasation of blood from infection, trauma, certain dental conditions—* Dose, route of administration are determined by patient's response, location of lesion, ease of drainage or aspiration, size of cavity, and ability of cavity to expand. Higher doses than those stated may be advisable in severe cases. **Adults and children:** 1 tablet P.O. containing 10,000 IU streptokinase (SK) and 2,500 IU streptodornase (SD) q.i.d. for 4 to 6 days; 0.5 ml I.M. of injectable solution (5,000 IU SK, b.i.d.). For local or topical use, see p. 954.	*GI:* nausea, vomiting, diarrhea with oral administration. *Skin:* rash, urticaria.
trypsin Tryptar	*In general and oral surgical procedures to reduce inflammation, accelerate reabsorption of attendant edema, facilitate restoration of local tissue circulation; to reduce inflammation and edema of bronchial mucosa; as adjunct in treatment of phlebothrombosis, thrombophlebitis, iritis, iridocyclitis, chorioretinitis, cutaneous ulcerative conditions—* **Adults:** 50,000 to 100,000 units P.O. q.i.d.; or 12,500 units I.M. daily or for severe conditions b.i.d. for 1 to 2 days then 12,500 units daily. Solution for wet dressings: 10,000 units in each ml normal saline solution or water for injection. Apply new dressings when dry. Ointment: 5,000 units/g once daily or b.i.d. Inhalation: 125,000 units dissolved in 3 ml saline solution or water inhaled at least once daily.	*Blood:* increased tendency to bleed. *CNS:* dizziness, fainting. *EENT:* rhinorrhea, sneezing, with aerosol inhalation. *GI:* nausea, vomiting, diarrhea, abdominal pain. *GU:* albuminuria, hematuria. *Local:* pain and induration, local irritations. *Skin:* rash, pruritus, urticaria. *Other:* febrile reactions, angioneurotic edema, rapid dissolution of sutures of animal origins.

INTERACTIONS	NURSING CONSIDERATIONS
	• Irrigate lesion with mild cleansing solution (not hydrogen peroxide) at each redressing. • Observe wound to monitor progress of therapy. Appearance of granulation tissue may indicate effectiveness. Notify doctor if inflammation or color of drainage indicates spread of infection. • Avoid getting ointment in eyes. If it does get into eyes, flood with water at once. • Protect drug from heat.
None significant.	• Contraindicated in active hemorrhage; decreased level of fibrinogen; acute cellulitis without suppuration; or risk of reopening preexisting bronchopleural fistulas, especially in active tuberculosis. Use oral and I.M. forms with caution in severe renal disease, depressed hepatic function or hepatic disease, or abnormalities of blood-clotting mechanism. • Do not give I.V. • If infection is present, consider concomitant antimicrobial therapy with compatible agent, such as tetracycline, penicillin, streptomycin. • I.M. use: Add 2 ml sterile water for injection or sterile physiologic saline solution to 25,000-unit vial streptokinase-streptodornase (result is solution of 5,000 IU SK per 0.5 ml). Inject deep I.M., preferably into gluteal muscle. Store remaining solution for 2 weeks in refrigerator or 24 hours at room temperature. • Avoid getting solution in eyes. If it does get into eyes, flood with water at once. • Protect from heat. • Streptokinase and streptodornase are antigenic; antienzymes may develop following prolonged therapy or acute hemolytic streptococcal infections. High antienzyme titer apparently not harmful, but dosage may have to be increased to overcome its effect.
With topical use, detergents and antiseptics (benzalkonium chloride, hexachlorophene, iodine, hydrogen peroxide): decreased enzymatic activity. Do not use together.	• Contraindicated in history of allergic reactions to parenteral enzyme therapy. Use with extreme caution in severe hepatic or renal disease, abnormalities of blood-clotting mechanism. • Test for possible hypersensitivity reactions before I.M. administration. Observe for 30 minutes after I.M. administration. Have epinephrine 1:1,000 available. • Do not apply to actively bleeding areas, ocular lesions, or to ulcerated carcinomas. • Do not give I.V. • Enteric-coated tablets must be swallowed whole; do not crush or break. • Give deep I.M. in gluteal muscle, alternating sites. Do not use I.M. route in infants or children. • Follow nasal inhalation with water or saline spray. Have patient take several swallows of water to remove large droplets from oropharynx. • Store in tight container. Protect from heat.

102

Oxytocics

dinoprost tromethamine	**oxytocin citrate, buccal**
dinoprostone	**oxytocin, synthetic injection**
ergonovine maleate	**oxytocin, synthetic nasal**
methylergonovine maleate	**sodium chloride 20% solution**

Oxytocics stimulate the smooth muscle of the uterus and are used for a variety of obstetrical purposes.

Major uses

- To induce labor or improve uterine contraction at term.
- To correct postpartum uterine atony.
- To induce therapeutic abortion in second trimester.
- To overcome prolonged uterine inertia.
- To control postpartum bleeding or hemorrhage.
- To stimulate contraction of myoepithelium in mammary glands, facilitating milk ejection in lactating females.
- May have some limited usefulness in relieving postpartum breast engorgement.

Mechanism of action

- Dinoprost and dinoprostone (prostaglandins) produce strong and prompt uterine contractions, possibly mediated by calcium and cyclic 3',5'-adenosine monophosphate. Contractile response are also affected by endocrine levels. They produce cervical dilation and softening, and exert uterine effects via direct myometrial stimulation.
- Ergonovine maleate and methylergonovine (ergot alkaloids) increase motor activity of the uterus by direct stimulation. Gravid uterus responds markedly to even small dose.
- Oxytocin may act as a hormone in potent and selective stimulation of smooth muscle of uterus and mammary gland and produces uterine contraction indistinguishable in amplitude, duration, and frequency from those of spontaneous labor. Oxytocin may stimulate contraction of uterine smooth muscle by increasing sodium permeability of uterine myofibrils.
- Sodium chloride hypertonic solution may damage decidual cells, causing the release of prostaglandins, and resulting in fetal death and abortion.

Absorption, distribution, and excretion

- Dinoprost and dinoprostone (prostaglandins): dinoprost diffuses slowly into maternal blood following administration and is widely distributed in mother and fetus. It concentrates in fetal liver, is rapidly metabolized in maternal lungs and liver, and is excreted within 24 hours, mainly in the urine, but about 5% excreted in feces. Dinoprostone distributes widely in mother and is rapidly metabolized in maternal lungs, kidneys, spleen, and other tissue.

• Ergonovine maleate and methylergonovine maleate (ergot alkaloids) are rapidly absorbed following oral or intramuscular administration and are slowly metabolized, possibly in the liver. Metabolism may be prolonged in neonates. Sensitivity varies with degree of maturity and stage of gestation.

• Oxytocin is inactivated by trypsin in the GI tract; tissue peptidases inactivate most of drug when administered buccally. Oxytocin is distributed throughout extracellular fluid, and small amounts may reach fetal circulation. Short half-life of drug (3 to 5 minutes) is reduced late in pregnancy and during lactation. Liver and kidneys destroy most of drug; only small amounts are excreted unchanged in the urine.

• Sodium chloride has little or no systemic absorption. It appears to concentrate in the decidual and fetal part of the placenta. Some of the drug diffuses into the maternal blood. It is excreted by kidneys.

Onset and duration

• Dinoprost and dinoprostone (prostaglandins) begin to act promptly. Their effect is dose-dependent, with sensitivity increasing at term. Contractions usually begin within 10 to 15 minutes and may continue 10 to 30 minutes after drug is stopped. Abortion occurs within 30 hours in most patients.

• Ergonovine maleate and methylergonovine maleate produce uterine contractions within 5 to 15 minutes of oral or intramuscular administration, and immediately following intravenous administration. They may continue for 3 hours or more after oral or intramuscular administration, and 45 minutes following intravenous. Small doses produce increased contractions followed by normal degree of relaxation; larger doses produce more forceful contractions but increase resting tonus.

• Oxytocin produces uterine response within several minutes which continues for 2 to 3 hours.

• Sodium chloride 20% injection. An amniotic fluid sodium concentration of at least 2.2 mEq/ml usually induces abortion within 50 hours. Instillation may be repeated in 48 hours, but patients who fail to respond to second dose should be considered for other methods.

Combination products

None.

NAME	INDICATIONS & DOSAGE	SIDE EFFECTS
dinoprost tromethamine Prostin F_2 Alpha	*Abort second trimester pregnancy*—amniotic fluid 1 ml is withdrawn via transabdominal intra-amniotic catheter. If no blood is present in tap, dinoprost 40 mg is injected directly into amniotic sac. Initially, 5 mg is given very slowly (1 mg/min) and patient watched for adverse reactions. Then, remainder is injected. If abortion not completed in 24 hours, another 10 to 40 mg may be given. Uterine activity may continue 10 to 30 minutes after drug is stopped.	*CNS:* dizziness, fainting. *CV:* bradycardia, hyper- or hypotension, arrythmias. *GI:* nausea, vomiting, diarrhea, abdominal cramps, epigastric pain. *Other:* bronchospasm, wheezing, dyspnea.
dinoprostone Prostin E_2♦	*Abort second trimester pregnancy, evacuate uterus in cases of missed abortion, intrauterine fetal deaths up to 28 weeks of age, benign hydatidiform mole*—insert 20 mg suppository high into posterior vaginal formix. Repeat q 3 to 5 hours until abortion is complete.	*CNS:* headache. *CV:* hypotension (in large doses), arrhythmias. *GI:* nausea, vomiting, diarrhea. *GU:* vaginal pain, vaginitis, vulvitis. *Other:* fever, shivering, chills.
ergonovine maleate Ergotrate Maleate♦	*Prevent or treat postpartum and postabortion hemorrhage due to uterine atony or subinvolution*—0.2 mg I.M. q 2 to 4 hours, maximum 5 doses; or 0.2 mg I.V. (only for severe uterine bleeding or other life-threatening emergency) over 1 minute while blood pressure and uterine contractions are monitored. I.V. dose may be diluted to 5 ml with 0.9% sodium chloride injection. Following initial I.M. or I.V. dose, may give 0.2 to 0.4 mg P.O. q 6 to 12 hours for 2 to 7 days. Decrease dose if severe uterine cramping occurs.	*CNS:* dizziness, headache. *CV:* hypertension. *EENT:* tinnitus. *GI:* nausea, vomiting. *GU:* uterine cramping. *Other:* sweating, chest pain, dyspnea, hypersensitivity.

♦ Also available in Canada.
♦♦ Available in Canada only.
Unmarked trade names available in United States only.

INTERACTIONS	NURSING CONSIDERATIONS
Alcohol (I.V. infusions of 500 ml of 10% over 1 hour): inhibited uterine activity. *I.V. oxytocin:* cervical perforation, especially in primigravida patients or in those with inadequately dilated cervices. Use with caution.	• Contraindicated in those with pelvic inflammatory disease. Use with caution in cardiovascular, renal, or hypertensive disease; asthma; glaucoma; or epilepsy. • Observe and record character and amount of vaginal bleeding. • Live birth may result. • Other measures may be needed if dinoprost fails to terminate pregnancy completely. Utilization of hypertonic saline should be delayed until uterine contractions stop. • Monitor vital signs. Report rapid fall in blood pressure or hypertonic uterine contractions. • Instruct patient to remain in prone position. • After abortion, observe patient frequently for cervical injuries. • Store at 2° to 8° C. (35.6° to 46.4° F.). Discard 24 months after manufacture date. • Should be used only in hospital setting.
None significant.	• Contraindicated in those with pelvic inflammatory disease or history of pelvic surgery, incisions, uterine fibroids, or cervical stenosis. Use with caution in asthma, epilepsy, anemia, diabetes, hyper- or hypotension, jaundice, or cardiovascular, renal, or hepatic disease. • Live birth may result. • Warm dinoprostone suppositories in their wrapping to room temperature. • After insertion, patient should stay supine for 10 minutes. • Store suppositories at temperature no higher than −20° C. (−4° F.). • Should only be used when critical care facilities are readily available. • Dinoprostone-induced fever is self-limiting and transient. Treat with water or alcohol sponging and increased fluid intake rather than with aspirin, which has not proved effective. • Abortion should be complete within 30 hours.
Regional anesthetics, dopamine, I.V. oxytocin: excessive vasoconstriction. Use together cautiously.	• Contraindicated for induction or augmentation of labor; before delivery of placenta; in threatened spontaneous abortion; in patients with allergy or sensitivity to ergot preparations. Use cautiously in hypertension, heart disease, venoatrial shunts, mitral valve stenosis, obliterative vascular disease, sepsis, or hepatic or renal impairment. • Monitor blood pressure, pulse, uterine response, and report any sudden changes in vital signs or frequent periods of uterine relaxation, and character and amount of vaginal bleeding. • Hypocalcemia may decrease patient response. If patient is not also taking digitalis, cautious administration of calcium gluconate I.V. may produce desired oxytocic action. • Contractions begin 5 to 15 minutes after P.O. administration; immediately following I.V. injection. May continue 3 hours or more after P.O. or I.M. administration; 45 minutes after I.V. injection. • Store in tightly closed, light-resistant containers. Discard if discolored. • Store I.V. solutions below 8° C. (46.4° F.). Daily stock may be kept at cool room temperature for 60 days. • Keep patient warm. • Have drug ready for immediate use if it is to be given postpartum.

NAME	INDICATIONS & DOSAGE	SIDE EFFECTS
methylergonovine maleate Methergine	*Prevent and treat postpartum hemorrhage due to uterine atony or subinvolution*—0.2 mg I.M. q 2 to 5 hours for maximum of 5 doses; or I.V. (excessive uterine bleeding or other emergencies) over 1 minute while blood pressure and uterine contractions are monitored. I.V. dose may be diluted to 5 ml with 0.9% sodium chloride injection. Following initial I.M. or I.V. dose, may give 0.2 to 0.4 mg P.O. q 6 to 12 hours for 2 to 7 days. Dose may be decreased if severe cramping occurs.	*CNS:* dizziness, headache. *CV:* hypertension, transient chest pain, dyspnea, palpitation. *EENT:* tinnitus. *GI:* nausea, vomiting. *Other:* sweating, hypersensitivity.
oxytocin citrate, buccal Pitocin Citrate◆	*Induction of labor*—1 tablet (200 U.S.P. units) in alternate cheeks until firm, regular uterine contractions, 40 to 60 seconds long, q 3 minutes, are achieved. Repeat q 30 minutes until 15 tablets (3,000 units) have been given over 24 hours, or until delivery is imminent or anesthetic is administered. Average dose to complete labor, 1,700 units; same number of tablets are used to maintain labor once induced.	**Maternal:** *CV:* hypertension; premature ventricular contractions; hypotension; increase in heart rate, venous return, cardiac output; arrhythmias in large doses. *GI:* nausea, vomiting. *Local:* parabuccal irritation. *GU:* uterine hypertonicity, spasm, tetanic contraction or rupture, postpartum hemorrhage. *Other:* anaphylaxis. **Fetal:** *CV:* bradycardia, cardiac arrhythmias. *Other:* anaphylaxis, birth canal trauma, jaundice.

INTERACTIONS	NURSING CONSIDERATIONS
Regional anesthetics, dopamine, I.V. oxytocin: excessive vasoconstriction. Use together cautiously.	• Contraindicated for induction of labor; before delivery of placenta; in patients with hypertension, toxemia, or sensitivity to ergot preparations; in threatened spontaneous abortion. Use with caution in sepsis, obliterative vascular disease, hepatic or renal problems, hypertension, heart disease, venoatrial shunts, mitral valve stenosis. • Monitor and record blood pressure, pulse, uterine response, and report any sudden change in vital signs or frequent periods of uterine relaxation, and character and amount of vaginal bleeding. • Contractions begin 5 to 15 minutes after P.O. administration; 2 to 5 minutes after I.M. injection; immediately following I.V. injection. May continue 3 hours or more after P.O. or I.M. administration; 45 minutes after I.V. injection. • Store in tightly closed, light-resistant containers. Discard if discolored. • Store below 8° C. (46.4° F.). Daily stock may be kept at room temperature for 60 to 90 days.
Cyclopropane anesthesia: increased risk of hypotension or bradycardia. Use together cautiously. *Thiopental anesthesia:* delayed induction time. Adjust dose. *Vasoconstrictors (vasopressors):* severe hypertension if oxytocin is used within 3 to 4 hours of vasoconstrictor. Monitor patient closely.	• Contraindicated in control and management of third stage of labor; to expel placenta; to control postpartum bleeding; in unconscious or postpartum patients; in management of inevitable, incomplete, or missed abortion, abruptio placenta, placenta previa, fetal distress, or other obstetrical emergencies. Use cautiously in prematurity, previous major cervical or uterine surgery (including C-section), grand multiparity, invasive cervical carcinoma, overdistention of uterus, history of uterine sepsis. • In eclampsia, if delivery isn't imminent within 12 hours after oxytocin is started, C-section is recommended. • Used to induce or reinforce labor only when pelvis is known to be adequate, when fetal maturity is assured, when fetal position is favorable and vaginal delivery is indicated. • May be hazardous in patients with heart disease or in those receiving spinal or epidural anesthesia. • Should be given only in hospital setting under qualified supervision. • Buccal administration is more difficult to control than I.M. or I.V. route; can be given by different routes sequentially but never at same time. • Monitor uterine contractions, heart rate, blood pressure, intrauterine pressure, and character and volume of blood loss. • Monitor and record fetal heart beat. • Observe character and volume of blood loss. • Patient may rinse mouth with cold water before tablet is placed in parabuccal space. For maximum buccal absorption, patient should avoid disturbing tablet. A tablet swallowed accidentally is not harmful, but the digestive process destroys its oxytocic action. • Store at temperature lower than 25° C. (77° F.). • For treatment of anaphylaxis, see p. 1114.

NAME	INDICATIONS & DOSAGE	SIDE EFFECTS
oxytocin, synthetic injection Oxytocin◆, Pitocin◆, Syntocinon◆, Utera-con	*Induction of or stimulation of labor*—initially, 1 ml (10 units) ampule in 1,000 ml 5% dextrose injection or 0.9% sodium chloride I.V. infused at 1 ml (10 milliunits) to 2 ml/minute. Increase rate at 15- to 30-minute intervals until normal contraction pattern is established. Maximum 1 to 2 ml (20 milliunits)/minute. Decrease rate when labor is firmly established. *Reduction of postpartum bleeding after expulsion of placenta*—10 to 40 units added to 1,000 ml 5% dextrose in water or 0.9% sodium chloride infused at rate necessary to control bleeding. *Facilitate threatened abortion*—10 to 40 units (1 to 4 ml) oxytocin added to 1,000 ml dextrose 5% in water, normal saline solution, or other nonhydrating solution; infused at rate necessary to control uterine atony.	**Maternal:** *Blood:* afibrinogenemia; may be related to increase in postpartum bleeding. *CNS:* subarachnoid hemorrhage resulting from hypertension; convulsions or coma resulting from water intoxication. *CV:* hypotension, increased heart rate, systemic venous return and cardiac output; arrhythmia. *GI:* nausea, vomiting. *Other:* hypersensitivity, tetanic contractions, abruptio placenta, impaired uterine blood flow and increased uterine motility. **Fetal:** *Blood:* increased risk of hyperbilirubinemia. *CV:* bradycardia, tachycardia, premature ventricular contractions, anoxia, asphyxia.
oxytocin, synthetic nasal	*To promote initial milk ejection; may be useful in relieving postpartum breast engorgement*—1 spray or 3 drops into 1 or both nostrils 2 or 3 minutes before nursing or pumping breasts.	None reported.
sodium chloride 20% solution	*To induce fetal death and abortion in second trimester of pregnancy (beyond 16th week of gestation)*—following transabdominal tap of amniotic sac, at least 1 ml fluid is withdrawn and examined. If no blood is found, 250 ml of amniotic fluid may be aspirated and 250 ml (maximum dose) of sodium chloride instilled over 20 to 30 minutes, while patient is observed for adverse reactions. Sodium chloride instillation may be repeated in 48 hours if membranes are still intact. I.V. infusion of oxytocin or intra-amniotic dinoprost tromethamine may be given to patients who fail to respond to second dose after oxytocic action of saline has ceased.	*Blood:* mild, self-limiting disseminated intravascular coagulation; coagulation changes, including decreased platelet count, hemocrit, fibrinogen, and Factors V and VIII; increased plasma volume, fibrin levels and thrombin, PT and PTT times. Occur within first 12 to 24 hours. *CV:* pulmonary embolism, pneumonia. *GU:* cortical necrosis of kidneys, cervical laceration and perforation, cervico-vaginal fistula, and uterine rupture reported in primigravida patients receiving concomitant I.V. oxytocin before cervix is adequately dilated. *Local:* infection at injection site. *Other:* fever, flushing.

INTERACTIONS	NURSING CONSIDERATIONS
Cyclopropane anesthesia: less pronounced bradycardia; more severe hypotension than occurs with oxytocin alone. Use together cautiously. *Thiopentol anesthesia:* delayed induction reported. May require dosage adjustment. *Vasoconstrictors:* severe hypertension if oxytocin is given within 3 to 4 hours of vasoconstrictor in patient receiving caudal block anesthesia. Monitor patient closely.	• Contraindicated in cases of cephalo-pelvic disproportion or where delivery requires conversion, as in transverse lie; fetal distress, when delivery isn't imminent, severe toxemia, and other obstetrical emergencies. Use cautiously in history of cervical or uterine surgery, grand multiparity, uterine sepsis, traumatic delivery, or overdistended uterus and primipara over 35 years. Use with extreme caution during first and second stages of labor, since cervical laceration, uterine rupture, and maternal and fetal death are reported. • Used to induce or reinforce labor only when pelvis is known to be adequate, when vaginal delivery is indicated, when fetal maturity is assured, and when fetal position is favorable. Should be used only in hospital critical care facilities and doctor are immediately available. • Oxytocin should never be given simultaneously by more than one route. • Incompatible with fibrinolysis, levarterenol bitartrate, prochlorperazine edisylate, protein hydrolysate, and warfarin sodium. Compatibility with other I.V. infusion fluids may be influenced by drug concentration, temperature, pH, and other factors. Rotate bottle gently to distribute drug in diluted solution. • Monitor and record uterine contractions, heart rate, blood pressure, intrauterine pressure, fetal heart rate, and character and volume of blood loss. • Store at temperature below 25° C. (77° F.), but do not freeze. • Oxytocin may produce antidiuretic effect; monitor fluid intake/output. • If contractions occur less than 2 minute apart and if contractions above 50 mm Hg are recorded, or if contractions last 90 seconds or longer, stop infusion, turn patient on her side, and notify doctor. • Oxygen administration may be necessary. • Not recommended for I.M. use.
None significant.	• Instruct patient to clear nasal passages first. With patient's head in vertical position, hold squeeze bottle upright and eject solution into patient's nostril. • Support patient's wish to breast-feed with quiet nonstressful environment and encouragement.
Indomethacin: may prolong abortion if used within 4 to 6 hours after intra-amniotic instillation of sodium chloride. Defer indomethacin dose. *Oxytocin:* intense uterine contractions and increased risk of uterine rupture or cervical laceration. Don't use together.	• Contraindicated in blood disorders or in actively contracting or hypertonic uterus. Use with extreme caution in heart disease, hypertension, epilepsy, renal impairment, uterine incision, or pelvic adhesions or in history of pelvic surgery. • Should be done only by doctors trained in amniocentesis when critical care facilities are immediately available. • Monitor constantly for signs of accidental intravascular, endometrial, or intraperitoneal injection. Procedure usually painless. If patient complains of pain, burning, feeling of heat, thirst, severe headache, mental confusion, distress, tinnitus, numbness of fingertips, or anxiety, stop instillation at once. Inadvertent I.V. injection can cause hypernatremia, myometrial necrosis, with secondary vomiting, cerebral blood clots, cardiovascular collapse, and death. • Patient should drink at least 2 liters of water on day of procedure to improve salt excretion. • General anesthetics or sedatives should not be used during administration of hypertonic saline.

103 Spasmolytics

aminophylline
dyphylline
flavoxate hydrochloride
oxtriphylline
oxybutynin chloride
theophylline
theophylline monoethanolamine
theophylline sodium glycinate

Xanthine derivatives (theophylline and its salts, and dyphylline) are spasmolytic agents that have bronchodilating effects, increase cardiac output and coronary blood flow, and exert mild diuretic action. Flavoxate hydrochloride, and oxybutynin chloride directly relax most smooth muscles. All produce central nervous system effects.

Major uses

- To relieve acute bronchial asthma and treat reversible bronchospasm associated with bronchitis and emphysema (theophyllines).
- May be useful in treatment of Cheyne-Stokes respiration.
- To relieve symptoms of some bladder disorders (flavoxate, oxybutynin).
- May also relieve visceral spasm.

Mechanism of action

- Xanthine derivatives competitively inhibit phosphodiesterase, producing an increase in cyclic AMP that may potentiate the actions of catecholamines.
- Xanthine derivatives may also affect neuromuscular transmission as a result of intracellular translocation of ionized calcium.
- Flavoxate hydrochloride exerts direct spasmolytic action on smooth muscles; it also has some local anesthetic and analgesic action.
- Oxybutynin chloride exerts a direct spasmolytic action and an atropine-like action on smooth muscles; has little or no effect on smooth muscles of blood vessels; increases urinary bladder capacity; has some local anesthetic and mild analgesic action.

Absorption, distribution, and excretion

• Xanthine derivatives are distributed throughout extracellular fluids and body tissues; cross the placenta; are metabolized in the liver; and are excreted by the kidneys. Plasma clearance decreases in patients with congestive heart failure, hepatic dysfunction, cor pulmonale, and in the elderly. Absorption is delayed by the presence of food in the stomach and when given by I.M. injection or rectal suppository.

• Fate of flavoxate hydrochloride in the body has not been determined, but it is excreted by the kidneys.

• Fate of oxybutynin chloride in the body has not been determined, but it may be metabolized by the liver and excreted by the kidneys.

Onset and duration

• Because xanthine derivatives produce a wide variation in onset and duration, individual responses must be carefully observed. Serum levels of 10 to 20 mcg/ml are usually needed to produce optimum bronchodilator response. Intravenous administration produces highest and most rapid concentrations. Serum concentrations usually peak about 1 to 2 hours following oral administration of capsules or uncoated tablets. Coated tablets require about 5 hours to reach peak levels; extended-release forms about 4 hours; retention enemas, 1 to 2 hours; rectal suppositories, 3 to 5 hours.

• Onset and duration of flavoxate hydrochloride not determined.

• Onset of oxybutynin, 30 minutes to 1 hour; peak, 3 to 6 hours; duration, 6 to 10 hours.

Combination products

• Xanthine derivatives are commercially available in combination with sympathomimetics, sedatives, expectorants, antitussives, antacids, mercurial diuretics, and alcohol.

NAME	INDICATIONS & DOSAGE	SIDE EFFECTS
aminophylline or theophylline ethylenediamine Aminodur Dura-Tab, Aminophyl◆◆, Aminophyllin, Corophyllin◆◆, Lixaminol, Mini-Lix, Somophyllin	*For treatment of acute and chronic bronchial asthma, bronchospasm; also used for Cheyne-Stokes respiration, pulmonary vasodilator—* Oral: **Adult:** 500 mg stat; then 250 to 500 mg q 6 to 8 hours. **Children:** 7.5 mg/Kg stat; then 3 to 6 mg/Kg q 6 to 8 hours. I.V.: inject very slowly, minimum time of 4 to 5 minutes; do not exceed 25 mg/min infusion rate. Loading dose: 5.6 mg/Kg over 30 minutes; maintenance dose: **Adults:** 0.6 to 0.9 mg/Kg/hr I.V. by continuous infusion. **Children less than 9 years:** 1 mg/Kg/hour. I.M.: **Adult:** 500 mg. Painful. Not recommended. Rectal: **Adult:** 500 mg suppository or by retention enema q 6 to 8 hours.	*CNS:* restlessness, dizziness, headache, insomnia, light-headedness. *CV:* palpitation, sinus tachycardia, extrasystoles, flushing, marked hypotension, increase in respiratory rate. *GI:* nausea, vomiting, anorexia, bitter aftertaste, dyspepsia, heavy feeling in stomach. *Local:* rectal suppositories may cause irritation. *Skin:* urticaria.
dyphylline Airet, Air-Tabs, Brophylline, Coeurophylline◆◆, Dilin◆, Dilor, Dyflex, Dylline, Emfabid, Lufyllin, Neothylline, Protophylline◆◆	*For relief of acute and chronic bronchial asthma and reversible bronchospasm associated with chronic bronchitis and emphysema—* **Adults:** 200 to 800 mg P.O. q 6 hours; or 250 to 500 mg I.M. injected slowly at 6-hour intervals. **Children over 6 years:** 4 to 7 mg/Kg P.O. daily, in divided doses.	*CNS:* stimulation, restlessness, irritability, insomnia, agitation, convulsions, headache. *CV:* palpitations, tachycardia, hypotension, extrasystoles, circulatory failure. *GI:* irritation, nausea, vomiting, epigastric pain, diarrhea. *GU:* albuminuria. *Other:* respiratory arrest, fever, dehydration.

◆ Also available in Canada.
◆◆ Available in Canada only.
Unmarked trade names available in United States only.

INTERACTIONS	NURSING CONSIDERATIONS
Alkali-sensitive drugs: reduced activity. Do not add to I.V. fluids containing aminophylline. *Propranolol:* antagonism. Propranolol weakened effects of aminophylline. Use together cautiously. *Troleandomycin, erythromycin:* decreased hepatic clearance of theophylline; elevated theophylline levels. Monitor for signs of toxicity. *Barbiturates:* enhanced metabolism and decreased theophylline blood levels. Monitor for decreased aminophylline effect.	• Contraindicated in hypersensitivity to xanthine compounds (caffeine, theobromine). Use cautiously in young children; in elderly patients with congestive heart failure or other cardiac or circulatory impairment, cor pulmonale, hepatic disease; in patients with active peptic ulcer, since it may increase volume and acidity of gastric secretions; and in hyperthyroidism, glaucoma, or diabetes mellitus. • Individuals metabolize xanthines at different rates. Adjust dose by monitoring response, tolerance, pulmonary function, and theophylline plasma levels: therapeutic level = 10 to 20 mcg/ml; toxicity seen over 20 mcg/ml. • Plasma clearance may be decreased in patients with congestive heart failure, hepatic dysfunction, or pulmonary edema. Smokers show accelerated clearance. Dose adjustments necessary. • Monitor vital signs; measure and record intake/output. Expected clinical effects include improvement in quality of pulse and respiration. • Warn elderly patient of dizziness, common side effect at start of therapy. • May cause elevation in serum uric acid, urinary catecholamines, or plasma-free fatty acids. • GI symptoms may be relieved by taking oral drug with full glass of water at meals, although food in stomach delays absorption. Enteric-coated tablets may also delay and impair absorption. No evidence that antacids reduce GI side effects. • Suppositories slowly and erratically absorbed; retention enemas may be absorbed more rapidly. Rectally administered preparations can be given when patient cannot take drug orally. Schedule following evacuation, if possible; may be retained better if given before meal. Advise patient to remain recumbent 15 to 20 minutes following insertion. • Question patient closely about other drugs used. Warn that over-the-counter remedies may contain ephedrine in combination with theophylline salts; excessive CNS stimulation may result. Tell him to check with doctor before taking *any* other medications. • Before giving loading dose, check that patient has not had recent theophylline therapy. • Supply instructions for home care and dosage schedule. Some patients may require round-the-clock dosage schedule. • Avoid major changes in protein or carbohydrate intake. • For symptoms of toxicity and treatment, see p. 1123.
None significant.	• Contraindicated in hypersensitivity to xanthine compounds (caffeine, theobromine); preexisting cardiac arrythmias, especially tachycardias. Use cautiously in young children; in elderly patients with congestive heart failure, any impaired cardiac or circulatory function, cor pulmonale, renal or hepatic disease; in patients with peptic ulcer, hyperthyroidism, glaucoma, or diabetes mellitus. • I.V. use not recommended. • Plasma clearance may be decreased in patients with congestive heart failure, hepatic dysfunction, or pulmonary edema. Adjust dosage by monitoring response, tolerance, pulmonary function, and dyphylline plasma levels: therapeutic level = 10 to 20 mcg/ml; toxicity seen above 20 mcg/ml. • Dyphylline is metabolized faster than theophylline; dosage intervals may have to be decreased to ensure continual therapeutic effect. Higher daily doses may be needed. • Dose should be decreased in renal insufficiency. • Monitor vital signs; measure and record intake/output. Expected clinical effects include improvement in quality of pulse and respiration. • Warn elderly patient of dizziness, a common side effect.

(continued on following page)

NAME	INDICATIONS & DOSAGE	SIDE EFFECTS
dyphilline *(continued)*		
flavoxate hydrochloride Urispas	*Symptomatic relief of dysuria, frequency, urgency, nocturia, incontinence, and suprapubic pain associated with urologic disorders—* **Adults, and children over 12 years:** 100 to 200 mg P.O. q.i.d.	*CNS:* mental confusion (especially in elderly), nervousness, dizziness, headache, drowsiness, difficulty with concentration. *CV:* tachycardia, palpitations. *EENT:* dry mouth and throat, blurred vision, increased ocular tension, disturbed eye accommodation. *GI:* abdominal pain, constipation (with high doses), nausea, vomiting. *GU:* dysuria. *Skin:* urticaria, dermatoses. *Other:* fever.
oxtriphylline Choledyl♦, Theophylline Choline♦♦	*To relieve acute bronchial asthma and reversible bronchospasm associated with chronic bronchitis and emphysema—* **Adults, and children over 12 years:** 200 mg P.O. q 6 hours. **Children 2 to 12 years:** 4 mg/Kg P.O. q 6 hours. Increase as needed to maintain therapeutic levels of theophylline (10 to 20 mcg/ml).	*CNS:* stimulation. *CV:* palpitations. *GI:* gastric distress.
oxybutynin chloride Ditropan	*Antispasmodic for neurogenic bladder—* **Adults:** 5 mg P.O. b.i.d. to t.i.d. to maximum of 5 mg q.i.d. **Children over 5 years:** 5 mg P.O. b.i.d. to maximum of 5 mg t.i.d.	*CNS:* drowsiness, dizziness, insomnia, dry mouth, flushing. *CV:* palpitations, tachycardia. *EENT:* transient blurred vision, mydriasis, cycloplegia, increased ocular tension. *GI:* nausea, vomiting, constipation, bloated feeling. *GU:* impotence, suppression of lactation, urinary hesitance or retention. *Skin:* urticaria, severe allergic reactions in patients sensitive to anticholinergics. *Other:* decreased sweating, fever.

INTERACTIONS	NURSING CONSIDERATIONS
	• Has low incidence of gastric irritation, which may be relieved by taking oral drug after meals; no evidence that antacids reduce this side effect. May produce less gastric discomfort than theophylline. • Discard dyphylline ampule if precipitate is present. Protect from light. • Question patient closely about other drugs used. Warn that over-the-counter remedies may contain ephedrine in combination with theophylline salts; excessive CNS stimulation may result. Tell him to check with doctor before taking *any* other medications. • Supply instructions for home care and dosage schedule. • Analogue of theophylline; equivalent to 70% anhydrous theophylline. • For symptoms of toxicity and treatment, see p. 1123.
None significant.	• Contraindicated in pyloric or duodenal obstruction, obstructive intestinal lesions or ileus, achalasia, GI hemorrhage, obstructive uropathies of lower urinary tract. Use cautiously in patients with glaucoma. • Check history for other drug use before giving drugs with anticholinergic side effects.. • Warn about possible drowsiness, mental confusion, and blurred vision. • Tell patient to report adverse effects or lack of response to drug. • For symptoms and treatment of toxicity, see p. 1115.
Erythromycin, troleandomycin: decreased hepatic clearance of theophylline; increased plasma level. Monitor for signs of toxicity. *Barbiturates:* enhanced metabolism and decreased theophylline blood levels. Monitor for decreased effect. *Propranolol;* antagonism. Weakened effects of theophylline. Use together cautiously.	• Contraindicated in hypersensitivity to xanthines (caffeine, theobromine). • Tell patient to report GI distress, palpitations, irritability, restlessness, nervousness, or insomnia; may indicate excessive CNS stimulation. • Administer drug after meals and at bedtime. • Store at 15° to 30° C. (59° to 86° F.). Protect elixir from light, tablets from moisture. • Equivalent to 80% anhydrous theophylline. • Monitor therapy carefully. • Combination products that contain ephedrine not recommended; excessive CNS stimulation may result. • For symptoms and treatment of toxicity, see p. 1123.
None significant.	• Contraindicated in glaucoma, myasthenia gravis, GI obstruction, adynamic ileus, megacolon, severe or ulcerative colitis; in elderly or debilitated patients with intestinal atony; and in patients with obstructive uropathy. Use cautiously in elderly patients; in patients with autonomic neuropathy, reflex esophagitis, or hepatic or renal disease. • May aggravate symptoms of hyperthyroidism, coronary heart disease, congestive heart failure, cardiac arrhythmias, tachycardia, hypertension, or prostatic hypertrophy. • Therapy should be stopped periodically to determine whether patient can get along without it. Minimizes tendency toward tolerance. • Rapid onset of action, peaks at 3 to 4 hours, lasts 6 to 10 hours. • Neurogenic bladder should be confirmed by cystometry before oxybutynin is given. Evaluate patient response to therapy periodically by cystometry.

(continued on following page)

NAME	INDICATIONS & DOSAGE	SIDE EFFECTS
oxybutynin chloride *(continued)*		
theophylline Accurbron, Adophyllin, Aerolate, Aqualin, Asthmophylline♦♦, Bronkodyl, Elixicon, Elixophyllin♦, Lanophyllin, Liquophylline, Norophylline, Optiphyllin, Oralphyllin, Physpan, Slo-Phyllin, Somophyllin♦, Theo-dur, Theo-Lix, Theo II, Theobid, Theocap, Theoclear, Theolair♦, Theolixir♦, Theolline, Theon, Theophyl♦, Theo-Span, Theotal	*Prophylaxis and symptomatic relief of bronchial asthma, bronchospasm of chronic bronchitis and emphysema*— **Adults:** 100 to 200 mg P.O. q 6 hours; or 250 to 500 mg rectally q 8 to 12 hours. **Children:** 50 to 100 mg P.O. q 6 hours, not to exceed 10 to 12 mg/Kg/24 hours, in divided doses q 8 to 12 hours. Oral timed-release form given q 8 to 12 hours.	*CNS:* irritability, restlessness, headache, insomnia, hyperexcitability, dizziness, muscle twitching, clonic and tonic generalized convulsions. *CV:* palpitations, tachycardia, extrasystoles, flushing, decreased pulmonary vascular resistance, marked hypotension, circulatory failure. *GI:* nausea, anorexia, vomiting, epigastric pain, diarrhea, abdominal pain, activation of peptic ulcer. *GU:* albuminuria, transient urinary frequency, dehydration, kidney irritation. *Local:* rectal irritation or strictures with continued use of suppositories. *Other:* false positive serum uric acid, fever, hyperglycemia, inappropriate ADH syndrome, tachypnea, respiratory arrest.
theophylline monoethanolamine Fleet Theophylline Rectal Unit	*Relief of acute bronchial asthma and of reversible bronchospasm associated with chronic bronchitis and emphysema*— **Adult:** 250 to 500 mg rectally once, or twice daily. Do not repeat in less than 8 hours nor exceed 2 doses in 24 hours; or 250 to 500 mg once daily rectally as retention enema q 12 hours. Not recommended for children; deaths have been reported.	
theophylline sodium glycinate Acet-Am♦♦, Glynazan, Panophylline Forte, Synophylate, Theocyne♦♦, Theotort	*Symptomatic relief of bronchial asthma, pulmonary emphysema, and chronic bronchitis*— **Adults:** 330 to 660 mg P.O. q 6 to 8 hours, after meals. **Children over 12 years:** 220 to 330 mg P.O. q 6 to 8 hours. **Children 6 to 12 years:** 330 mg P.O. q 6 to 8 hours. **Children 3 to 6 years:** 110 to 165 mg P.O. q 6 to 8 hours; **Children 1 to 3 years:** 55 to 110 mg P.O. q 6 to 8 hours.	

INTERACTIONS	NURSING CONSIDERATIONS
	• Rule out partial intestinal obstruction in patients with diarrhea, especially those with colostomy or ileostomy, before giving oxybutynin. • If urinary tract infection is present, patient should receive antibiotics concomitantly. • Warn patient that drug may impair alertness or vision. • Since oxybutynin suppresses sweating, its use during very hot weather may precipitate fever or heat stroke. • Store in tightly closed containers at 15° to 30° C. (59° to 86° F.). • For symptoms and treatment of toxicity, see p. 1115.
Erythromycin, troleandomycin: decreased hepatic clearance of theophylline; increased plasma levels. Monitor for signs of toxicity. *Barbiturates:* enhanced metabolism and decreased theophylline blood levels. Monitor for decreased effect. *Propranolol:* weakened effect of aminophylline. Use together cautiously.	• Contraindicated in hypersensitivity to xanthine compounds (caffeine, theobromine). Use cautiously in young children; in elderly patients with congestive heart failure or other circulatory impairment, cor pulmonale, renal or hepatic disease; and in patients with peptic ulcer, hyperthyroidism, glaucoma, or diabetes mellitus. • Individuals metabolize xanthines at different rates; determine dose by monitoring response, tolerance, pulmonary function, and theophylline plasma levels: therapeutic level = 10 to 20 mcg/ml. • Monitor vital signs; measure and record intake/output. Expected clinical effects include improvement in quality of pulse and respiration. • Warn elderly patients of dizziness, common side effect at start of therapy. • GI symptoms may be relieved by taking oral drug with full glass of water after meals, although food in stomach delays absorption. • Rectal preparations can be ordered when patient cannot take drug orally. Schedule dose following evacuation, if possible; may be retained better if preparation can be given before meal. Advise patient to remain recumbent 15 to 20 minutes following insertion. Toxicity may occur with rectal administration because of erratic rate of absorption; children appear to absorb drug faster than adults. Instruct patient to report rectal irritation promptly. • Question patient closely about other drugs used. Warn that over-the-counter remedies may contain ephedrine in combination with theophylline salts; excessive CNS stimulation may result. Tell him to check with doctor before taking *any* other medications. • Supply instructions for home care and dosage schedule. • Decrease daily dosage in congestive heart failure, hepatic disease, or in elderly patients, since metabolism and excretion may be decreased. Monitor carefully, using serum levels, observation, examination, and interview. Give drug around the clock, using sustained-release product at bedtime. • Drug of choice for long-term use; low incidence of tolerance. • Avoid major changes in protein or carbohydrate intake. • Theophylline sodium glycinate products available as elixir.

104

Heavy metal antagonists

deferoxamine mesylate
dimercaprol
edetate calcium disodium
edetate disodium
d-penicillamine

Heavy metals such as antimony, arsenic, cadmium, lead, mercury, and thallium form insoluble metal complexes with organic compounds in the body. These complexes interfere with normal physiological function and produce toxic effects in the central nervous and skeletal systems, gastrointestinal tract, and various organs, especially the kidneys. Heavy metal antagonists prevent or reverse the formation of these complexes and lower toxic tissue levels of the metals to less toxic or nontoxic levels.

Major uses

- To treat acute and chronic heavy metal and iron poisoning.
- To treat hypercalcemia, iron storage diseases, and Wilson's disease.
- To treat rheumatoid arthritis.
- To prevent stone formation in cystinuria.

Mechanism of action

- Heavy metals, calcium, cysteine, and metals such as iron and copper bind more easily to heavy metal antagonists than to body tissues. The resulting complex (chelate) is stable, soluble, and easily excreted by the kidneys.

Absorption, distribution, and excretion

- Good oral absorption occurs only with d-penicillamine. Others must be given parenterally.
- Most are distributed to all body tissues, except edetate calcium disodium, which doesn't penetrate cerebrospinal fluid or erythrocytes.
- Excreted primarily in urine.

Onset and duration

- Onset in 30 to 60 minutes (slightly delayed by I.M. route).
- Duration of action varies with ratio of heavy metal antagonist to metal present and also with renal function.

Combination products

None.

SUPPORTIVE CARE OF POISONED PATIENT

After poison has been removed from the poisoned patient, the patient's survival depends on the quality of the nursing care he receives. Give him the same care you would give any critically ill patient.

- Mainly support his vital functions — respirations, circulation, and kidney function.
- Carefully observe the patient's breathing response. Periodically report changes in breath rate, depth and quality to the physician.
- Maintain adequate respiration by every available means from mouth-to-mouth breathing to mechanical ventilation of the lungs.
- Clear the patient's airway of secretions. Insert an endotracheal tube to ease suctioning and mechanical ventilation, if required.
- Watch patients poisoned with depressant drugs who are receiving intravenous fluids for signs of acute pulmonary edema.
- Position semicomatose patients to help them cough and expel secretions.
- To maintain circulatory function, start a slow intravenous infusion of saline which will make up for the loss of salt and water that usually accompanies poisoning.
- If the patient has gastrointestinal bleeding from drug-damaged mucosa, give a whole blood transfusion to prevent shock. Usually, administration of plasma or a plasma expander will suffice.
- When administering blood-volume expanders, monitor both blood and central nervoús pressures. Pressure abnormalities could lead to reduced cardiac output.
- Patients in shock who do not respond to fluid, plasma, or blood replacement may require treatment with vasopressor drugs. After administering a vasopressor, stay with the patient and frequently check his blood pressure to monitor his reaction to the drug.
- Have potent resuscitative drugs and equipment available.
- In a patient with oliguria: Measure daily urinary output; encourage patient to sip small amounts of fluid; carefully monitor intravenous infusions of fluids and electrolytes ordered by the doctor.
- Watch for signs of complications: drug-induced coma, convulsions, pain and delirium.
- Throughout, provide general supportive care aimed at: hastening the patient's recovery, reducing his pain, and seeing to his comfort.

You can help in poison detection by observing emergency room patients for suspicious signs of poisoning: abdominal pain, dyspnea, alteration of vital signs, restlessness, and agitation. To confirm your suspicions, take a meticulously detailed recent history. (What foods did he eat? Where does he work?)

NAME	INDICATIONS & DOSAGE	SIDE EFFECTS
deferoxamine mesylate Desferal◆	*Acute iron intoxication—* **Adults and children:** 1 g I.M. or I.V. followed by 500 mg I.M. or I.V. for 2 doses, q 4 hours; then 500 mg I.M. or I.V. q 4 to 12 hours. Infusion rate shouldn't exceed 15 mg/Kg/hour. *Chronic iron overload—* **Adults and children:** 500 mg to 1 g I.M. daily and 2 g slow I.V. infusion in separate solution along with each unit blood transfused. Maximum dose 6 g daily. I.V. infusion rate shouldn't exceed 15 mg/Kg/hour. S.C.: 1 to 2 g administered over 8 to 24 hours.	*GU:* colors urine red. *Local:* pain and induration at injection site. After rapid I.V. administration: erythema, urticaria, hypotension. *With long-term use:* sensitivity reaction (cutaneous wheal formation, pruritus, rash, anaphylaxis), diarrhea, leg cramps, fever, tachycardia, blurred vision, dysuria, abdominal discomfort.
dimercaprol BAL in Oil◆	**Adults and children:** *Severe arsenic or gold poisoning*—3 mg/Kg deep I.M. q 4 hours for 2 days, then q.i.d. on 3rd day, then b.i.d. for 10 days. *Mild arsenic or gold poisoning—* 2.5 mg/Kg deep I.M. q.i.d. for 2 days, then b.i.d. on 3rd day, then once daily for 10 days. *Mercury poisoning*—5 mg/Kg deep I.M. initially, then 2.5 mg/Kg daily or b.i.d. for 10 days. *Acute lead encephalopathy or lead level more than 100 mcg/ml—* 4 mg/Kg deep I.M. injection, then q 4 hours with edetate calcium disodium (12.5 mg/Kg I.M.). Use separate sites. Maximum dose 5 mg/Kg per dose.	*CNS:* pain or tightness in throat, chest, or hands; headache, paresthesias, muscle pain or weakness. *CV:* transient increase in blood pressure, returns to normal in 2 hours; tachycardia. *EENT:* blepharal spasm, conjunctivitis, lacrimation, rhinorrhea, excessive salivation. *GI:* halitosis; nausea; vomiting; burning sensation in lips, mouth, and throat. *GU:* renal damage if alkaline urine not maintained. *Metabolic:* decreased iodine uptake. *Local:* sterile abscess, pain at injection site. *Other:* fever (especially in children), sweating, pain in teeth.
edetate calcium disodium Calcium Disodium Versenate◆	*Lead poisoning—* **Adults:** 1 g/250 to 500 ml 5% dextrose in water or 0.9% normal saline solution I.V. over 1 to 2 hours daily or q 12 hours for 3 to 5 days; repeat after 2 days if indicated. Maximum dose 50 mg/Kg daily. **Children:** 35 mg/Kg I.M. daily divided q 8 to 12 hours. Maximum dose 50 mg/Kg daily. *Acute lead encephalopathy or lead levels more than 100 mcg/ml—* **Adults and children:** 12.5 mg/Kg with dimercaprol 4 mg/Kg deep I.M. after initial dose of dimercaprol 4 mg deep I.M. Use separate sites. After first dose reduce to 3 mg/Kg for 2 to 7 days.	*CNS:* headache, paresthesias, numbness. *CV:* cardiac arrhythmias, hypotension. *GI:* anorexia, nausea, vomiting. *GU:* proteinuria, hematuria; nephrotoxicity with renal tubular necrosis leading to fatal nephrosis in excessive dose. *Other:* arthralgia, myalgia, hypercalcemia. *4 to 8 hours after infusion:* sudden fever and chills, fatigue, excessive thirst, sneezing, nasal congestion.

◆ Also available in Canada.
◆◆ Available in Canada only.
Unmarked trade names available in United States only.

INTERACTIONS	NURSING CONSIDERATIONS
None significant.	• Contraindicated in severe renal disease or anuria. Use cautiously in impaired renal function. • Monitor intake/output carefully. • I.M. route preferred. • Use I.V. only when patient has cardiovascular collapse or shock. For I.V. use, dissolve as for I.M. use; dilute in normal saline, 5% dextrose in water, or lactated Ringer's solution. • If giving I.V., change to I.M. as soon as possible. • For reconstitution, add 2 ml sterile water for injection to each ampule. Make sure drug is completely dissolved. Reconstituted solution good for 1 week at room temperature. Protect from light. • For symptcms and treatment of anaphylaxis, see p. 1114.
^{131}I uptake thyroid tests decreased: don't schedule patient for this test during course of dimercaprol therapy. *Iron:* formed toxic metal complex; concurrent therapy contraindicated.	• Contraindicated in hepatic dysfunction (except postarsenical jaundice), acute renal insufficiency. • Don't use for iron, cadmium, or selenium toxicity. Complex formed is highly toxic, even fatal. • Ephedrine or antihistamine may prevent or relieve mild side effects. • Ineffective in arsine gas poisoning. • Solution with slight sediment is usable. • Keep urine alkaline to prevent renal damage. Oral $NaHCO_3$ may be ordered. • Don't give I.V.; give by deep I.M. route only.
None significant.	• Contraindicated in severe renal disease or anuria. Use cautiously in active tuberculosis or healed calcified tubercular lesions. • I.V. use contraindicated in lead encephalopathy; may increase intracranial pressure. Use I.M. route instead. • Force fluids in all patients except those with lead encephalopathy. • Monitor intake/output, urinalysis, BUN, and EKGs. • To avoid toxicity, use with dimercaprol. • Oral form available but ineffective because of poor GI absorption; often used ineffectively as prophylaxis against lead exposure; can even increase lead absorption from GI tract. • Procaine HCl may be added to I.M. solutions to minimize pain. Watch for local reactions. • Avoid rapid I.V. infusions. I.M. route preferred.

NAME	INDICATIONS & DOSAGE	SIDE EFFECTS
edetate disodium Disotate, Endrate, Sodium Versenate	*Hypercalcemic crisis—* **Adults and children:** 15 to 50 mg/Kg daily slow I.V. infusion for 5 days, followed by 2 days without medication; repeat cycle if indicated up to 15 days. Dilute in 500 ml 5% dextrose in water or 0.9% normal saline solution. Give over 3 to 4 hours. Maximum adult dose 3 g/day. Maximum children's dose 70 mg/Kg/day.	*CNS:* circumoral parethesias, numbness, headache, malaise, fatigue, muscle pain or weakness. *CV:* hypertension, thrombophlebitis. *GI:* nausea, vomiting, diarrhea, anorexia, abdominal cramps. *GU:* in excessive doses—toxicity with urgency, nocturia, dysuria, polyuria, proteinuria, renal insufficiency and failure, tubular necrosis. *Local:* pain at site of infusion, erythema, dermatitis. *Metabolic:* hypocalcemia, decreased magnesium.
d-penicillamine Cuprimine◆	*Wilson's disease—* **Adults:** 250 mg P.O. q.i.d. before meals. Adjust dose to achieve urinary copper excretion of 0.5 to 1 mg daily. **Children:** 20 mg/Kg daily P.O. divided q.i.d. before meals. Adjust dose to achieve urinary copper excretion of 0.5 to 1 mg daily. *Cystinuria—* **Adults:** 250 mg P.O. q.i.d. before meals. Adjust dose to achieve urinary cystine excretion of less than 100 mg daily when renal calculi present, or 100 to 200 mg daily when no calculi present. Maximum adult dose is 5 g daily. **Children:** 30 mg/Kg daily P.O. divided q.i.d. before meals. Adjust dose to achieve urinary cystine excretion of less than 100 mg daily when renal calculi present, or 100 to 200 mg daily when no calculi present. *Rheumatoid arthritis—* **Adults:** 250 mg P.O. daily initially, with increases of 250 mg q 3 months if necessary. Maximum dose 1 g daily.	*Blood:* leukopenia, eosinophilia, thrombocytopenia, monocytosis, granulocytopenia, elevated sedimentation rate, lupus erythematosus-like syndrome. *EENT:* tinnitus. *GU:* nephrotic syndrome, glomerulonephritis. *Metabolic:* decreased pyridoxine (may cause optic neuritis), decreased zinc and mercury. *Skin:* friability, especially at pressure spots; wrinkling, erythema, urticaria, ecchymoses. *Other:* reversible taste impairment, especially of salts and sweets, hair loss. About ⅓ of patients develop allergic reactions (rash, pruritus, fever), arthralgia, lymphadenopathy. With long term use, myasthenia gravis syndrome.

INTERACTIONS	NURSING CONSIDERATIONS
None significant.	• Contraindicated in anuria, known or suspected hypocalcemia, or significant renal disease; active or healed tubercular lesions; history of seizures or intracranial lesions; generalized arteriosclerosis associated with aging. Use cautiously in limited cardiac reserve, incipient congestive failure, hypokalemia, diabetes. • Avoid rapid I.V. infusion; profound hypocalcemia may occur. • Monitor EKG and test renal and hepatic function frequently. • Measure blood, urine glucose, and serum potassium frequently. Obtain serum calcium levels after each dose. • Keep I.V. calcium available. • Keep patient in bed for 15 minutes after infusion to avoid postural hypotension. • Don't use to treat lead toxicity; use edetate calcium disodium instead. • Edetate disodium not currently drug of choice for treatment of hypercalcemia; other treatments are safer and more effective.
Oral iron: decreased effectiveness of d-penicillamine. If used together, give at least 2 hours apart.	• Contraindicated in pregnant women with cystinuria. Use cautiously in penicillin allergy; cross sensitivity may occur. • Report to doctor if fever or other allergic reactions occur. • Patient should receive pyridoxine daily. • Handle patients carefully to avoid skin damage. • Dose should be given on empty stomach. • Patient should drink large amounts of fluid, especially at night. • Sulfurated potash taken with each meal can block copper absorption. • If impaired taste persists, restore with 5 to 10 drops 4% copper sulfate daily in fruit juice, except in Wilson's disease. • Tell patient that therapeutic effect may be delayed up to 3 months. • Monitor CBC, renal and hepatic function. • Recently approved for treatment of rheumatoid arthritis.

105

Gold compounds

aurothioglucose
gold sodium thiomalate

Gold, the precious metal, has been used to treat arthritis since 1929. During the last 20 years, gold therapy (also known as chrysotherapy) has become more popular as numerous studies have confirmed its effectiveness. These drugs are gold *salts* in which the gold is attached to a sulfur molecule; they contain about 50% gold. Gold salts stop the progression of rheumatoid arthritis but have little value in advanced disease. Unfortunately, gold salts often produce serious side effects that require discontinuation of treatment. In patients who can tolerate gold treatment without severe toxicity, about 75% experience symptomatic improvement; 20% to 25% experience remission; the remainder show minor improvement.

Major uses

- To treat rheumatoid arthritis.

Mechanism of action

- The exact mechanism of action of gold is unknown. Anti-inflammatory effects in the active stage of rheumatoid arthritis are probably due to inhibition of sulfhydryl systems that alters cellular metabolism. Gold salts may also alter enzyme function and immune response, and suppress phagocytic activity.

Absorption, distribution, and excretion

- Rapidly absorbed after I.M. injection, gold sodium thiomalate solution has a peak serum concentration in 3 to 6 hours. The oil suspension of aurothioglucose is absorbed more slowly and irregularly.
- Gold salts are widely distributed throughout body tissues. Arthritic joints contain 2 to 2.5 times as much gold as uninvolved joints.
- Gold salts are excreted slowly, mostly via the kidneys. A small amount is eliminated through the feces. After a cumulative dose of 1 g, urinary excretion of gold can be detected for as long as 1 year.

Onset and duration

- Beneficial effects may not occur for 8 to 12 weeks and may persist long after therapy has been stopped.

Combination products

None.

RHEUMATOID ARTHRITIS

Rheumatoid arthritis (RA), which is often treated with gold compounds, is a chronic systemic disease characterized by a fluctuating, progressive inflammation of the joints.

TYPICAL CLINICAL AND DIAGNOSTIC FEATURES

- History of persistent painful morning stiffness that may last for hours (in other forms of arthritis, stiffness may last only a few minutes)
- Spindle-shaped joint swelling
- Subcutaneous nodules (small nontender masses over pressure points)
- Swelling of ulnar side of the wrist
- Signs of muscle wasting, weight loss, erythema of palms, malaise
- Fatigue occurring at same time each day regardless of previous activity
- Elevated erythrocyte sedimentation rate
- Presence of rheumatoid factor in the serum (in about 30% of patients with RA)

TREATMENT AND PATIENT TEACHING

Long-term management aims to relieve pain, arrest inflammatory process, and prevent further joint damage via....

- *Team evaluation* (nurse, doctor, physical therapist, social worker, dietitian)
- *Drug therapy:* Teach patient to watch for and report side effects of salicylates, anti-inflammatory agents, corticosteroids, antimalarial agents, cytotoxic and immunosuppressive agents, chelating agents, and gold compounds.
- *Specialized physical and occupational therapy:* Teach the importance of continuing prescribed range of motion and specialized exercises. Assess tolerance for physical activities, including activities of daily living.
- *Prescribed rest:* 8 to 12 hours of sleep a night and a rest period during the day (total body rest or rest of the involved joints). To achieve correct resting and sleeping positions, patient should use a firm mattress; a small pillow, to avoid flexion contractures of neck; and a footboard, to avoid footdrop. He should avoid using pillows under the knees.
- *Diets:* For weight reduction or increased protein intake
- *Orthopedic appliances:* Special shoes, splints, and soft collars can ease pain, prevent fatigue, and provide proper alignment.

Some specific advice for RA patients:

- Avoid fatigue: Try to rest 5 to 10 minutes out of each hour. Plan your work. Work slowly but at an even pace. Sit whenever possible. Alternate sitting and standing tasks. Use good posture.
- Avoid undue stress on the joints: Use the largest joint available for a given task. Support weak or painful joints. Avoid holding objects for long periods; hold objects parallel to knuckles. Use hands toward the center of the body. Slide—don't lift—objects. Avoid bending and climbing.
- Use aids for dressing: long-handled shoehorn, reacher, elastic shoelaces. Whenever possible, sit to dress. Use a zipper-pull for long or difficult zippers; avoid back zippers. Use a buttonhook for manipulating buttons. Arrange closets efficiently. Keep like items and items usually worn together, hanging together.

NAME	INDICATIONS & DOSAGE	SIDE EFFECTS
aurothioglucose Solganal	*Rheumatoid arthritis*— **Adults:** initially 10 mg I.M. followed by 25 mg for second and third dose at weekly intervals. Then, 50 mg weekly until 1 g has been given. If improvement occurs without toxicity, continue 25 to 50 mg at 3-to 4-week intervals indefinitely. **Children 6 to 12 years:** ¼ usual adult dose. Alternatively, 1 mg/Kg I.M. once weekly for 20 weeks.	Adverse reactions to gold are considered severe and potentially life-threatening. Report any side effect to the doctor at once. *Blood:* thrombocytopenia (with or without purpura), aplastic anemia, agranulocytosis, leukopenia, eosinophilia. *CV:* bradycardia. *EENT:* corneal gold deposition. *GU:* albuminuria, proteinuria, nephrotic syndrome, nephritis, acute tubular necrosis. *Skin:* rash and dermatitis in 20%. (If drug is not stopped, may lead to fatal exfoliative dermatitis.) *Other:* anaphylaxis, angioneurotic edema, hepatitis, jaundice, metallic taste, stomatitis.
gold sodium thiomalate Myochrysine◆	*Rheumatoid arthritis*— **Adults:** initiallly 10 mg I.M. followed by 25 mg in 1 week. Then, 50 mg weekly until 14 to 20 doses have been given. If improvement occurs without toxicity, continue 50 mg q 2 weeks for 4 doses; then, 50 mg q 3 weeks for 4 doses; then, 50 mg q month indefinitely. If relapse occurs during maintenance therapy, resume injections at weekly intervals. **Children:** 1 mg/Kg I.M. per week for 20 weeks. If good response occurs, may be given q 3 to 4 weeks indefinitely.	

◆ Also available in Canada.
◆◆ Available in Canada only.
Unmarked trade names available in United States only.

INTERACTIONS	NURSING CONSIDERATIONS
None significant.	• Contraindicated in severe uncontrollable diabetes, renal disease, hepatic dysfunction, marked hypertension, heart failure, systemic lupus erythematosus, Sjögren's syndrome. Use cautiously with other drugs that cause blood dyscrasias. • Indicated only in active rheumatoid arthritis that has not responded adequately to salicylates, penicillamine, rest, and physical therapy. • Should be administered only under constant supervision of a doctor who is thoroughly familiar with its toxicities and benefits. • Most side effects are readily reversible if drug is stopped immediately. • Administer all gold compounds intramuscularly, preferably intragluteally. • Observe patient for 30 minutes after administration because of possibility of anaphylactic reaction. • Reassure patient that benefits of therapy may not appear for 6 to 8 weeks. • Aurothioglucose is a suspension. Immerse vial in warm water and shake vigorously before injecting. • When giving gold sodium thiomalate, advise patient to lie down and to remain recumbent for 10 minutes following injection. • Complete blood counts should be performed at 2- to 4-week intervals. • If side effects are mild, some rheumatologists resume gold therapy after 2 to 3 weeks' rest. • Dimercaprol (BAL) should be kept on hand to treat acute toxicity.

106

Diagnostic skin tests

histoplasmin
Old Tuberculin
tuberculin purified protein derivative, Mantoux

Diagnostic skin tests contain products that act as antigens. When injected intradermally, these antigens combine with previously formed antibodies to cause an antigen-antibody response, producing inflammation at the injection site. Reactions are read as positive or negative according to size of induration (varies with specific test). Positive reactions show past or possibly active infection. Negative reactions mean active infection is highly unlikely. False positive and false negative reactions may occur, so skin tests alone are not diagnostic.

Major uses

- Diagnosis and differentiation of infectious diseases.
- Detection of immunity.

Mechanism of action

- Cause antigen-antibody reaction.

Absorption, distribution, and excretion

- Not applicable.

Onset and duration

- Not applicable.

Combination products

None.

MANTOUX TEST FOR TUBERCULOSIS

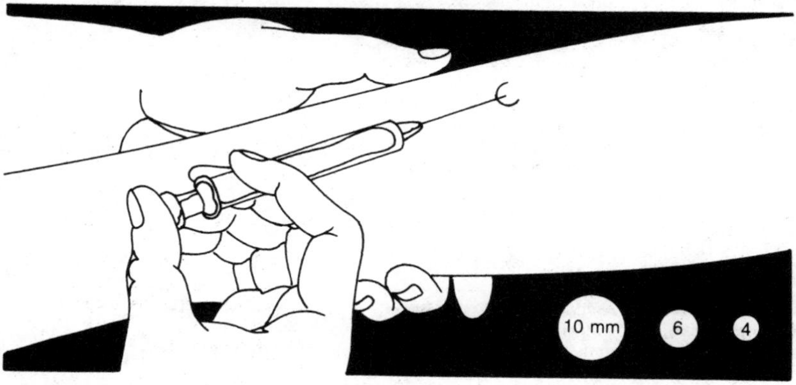

10 mm
6
4

As illustrated, give the intradermal injection in the upper third of the forearm. Stretch the skin tightly — a wheal 6 mm in diameter should appear. Read the results 48 to 72 hours later in a good light. Be sure to palpate the area of induration and record its diameter accurately in millimeters. Measure erythema if present.

Erythema without induration is not significant. Induration of 10 mm or more is a positive result; 5 to 9 is considered doubtful, indicating the need for further testing; and 4 mm or less is negative.

NAME	INDICATIONS & DOSAGE	SIDE EFFECTS
histoplasmin◆	*Suspected histoplasmosis*— **Adults and children:** 0.1 ml of 1:100 dilution intradermally on inner forearm. Use tuberculin syringe with 26- or 27-gauge, ⅜-inch needle.	*Local:* urticaria, ulceration or necrosis in highly sensitive patients. *Other:* shortness of breath, sweating, anaphylaxis.
Old Tuberculin Old Tuberculin Test◆; Tuberculin, Mono-Vacc Test; Tuberculin Tine Test	*Diagnosis of tuberculosis*— **Adults and children:** 10 tuberculin units (0.1 ml of 1:1,000) Old Tuberculin intradermally on inner forearm. In suspected tuberculosis, use 1 tuberculin unit first. Use tuberculin syringe with 26- or 27-gauge, ⅜-inch needle. Multiple-puncture test: cleanse skin thoroughly with alcohol; make skin taut on inner forearm; press points firmly into selected site.	*Local:* hypersensitivity (vesiculation, ulceration, necrosis). *Other:* anaphylaxis.
tuberculin purified protein derivative, Mantoux Aplisol, Aplitest, Sclavo test-PPD, Ster-needle, Tuberculin PPD-Heaf, Tuberculin PPD-Stabilized, Tubersol	*Diagnosis of tuberculosis*— **Adults and children:** 5 tuberculin units (0.1 ml) intradermally on inner forearm. Suspected sensitivity dose is 1 tuberculin unit. Patients failing to react to 5 tuberculin units should be tested with 250 tuberculin units. First strength equals 1 tuberculin unit/ 0.1 ml; intermediate strength, 5 tuberculin units/0.1 ml. Second strength equals 250 tuberculin units/0.1 ml. Use tuberculin syringe with 26- or 27-gauge, ⅜-inch needle. Multiple-puncture test: cleanse skin thoroughly with alcohol; make skin taut on inner forearm; press points firmly into selected site.	*Local:* pain, pruritus, ulceration, necrosis. *Other:* anaphylaxis.

◆ Also available in Canada.
◆◆ Available in Canada only.
Unmarked trade names available in United States only.

INTERACTIONS	NURSING CONSIDERATIONS
None significant.	• Read test at 24 to 48 hours. Induration of 5 mm or more is positive. • Reaction may be depressed in malnutrition or in immunosuppression. • Crossreaction may occur with other fungi (e.g., *Candida albicans, Blastomyces dermatitides).* • Obtain accurate history of allergies and past reactions to skin tests. • Keep epinephrine 1:1,000 available. • Cold packs or topical corticosteroids may relieve pain and itching if severe reaction occurs. • For treatment of anaphylaxis, see p. 1114.
None significant.	• Use cautiously in active tuberculosis. • False positive reaction can occur in sensitive patients. • Reaction may be depressed in malnutrition or in immunosuppression. • Read test in 48 to 72 hours. Induration of 10 mm or more is positive; 5 to 9 mm, doubtful; less than 5, negative. • Multiple-puncture test: 1 to 2 mm induration is positive. • Old Tuberculin Tine Test equals 5 tuberculin units purified protein derivatives. • Obtain accurate history of allergies, especially to acacia (contained in tine test as stabilizer), and past reactions to skin tests. • Keep epinephrine 1:1,000 available. • S.C. injection invalidates test results. Bleb must form on skin upon injection. • Corticosteroids and other immunosuppressants may suppress skin test reaction. • Cold packs or topical corticosteroids may relieve pain and itching if severe reaction occurs. • For treatment of anaphylaxis, see p. 1114.
None significant.	• Contraindicated in known tuberculin-positive reactors; severe reactions may occur. Use cautiously with active tuberculosis. • Read test in 48 to 72 hours. Induration of 10 mm or more is positive; 5 to 9 mm, doubtful; less than 5 mm, negative. • Multiple-puncture test: vesiculation is positive reaction; induration of less than 2 mm without vesiculation is negative. • 1 tuberculin unit may give false negative test; 250 tuberculin units may give false positive test. • Obtain accurate history of allergies and past reactions to skin tests. • Reaction may be depressed in malnutrition, immunosuppression, or viral infections (up to 4 weeks postinfection). • Solution adsorbed by plastic. Use at once after drawing into plastic syringe. • Keep epinephrine 1:1,000 available. • S.C. injection invalidates test results. Bleb must form on skin upon injection. • Cold packs or topical corticosteroids may relieve pain and itching if severe reaction occurs. • Never give initial test with second test strength (250 tuberculin units). • A tine test is available for rapid screening. • Corticosteroids and other immunosuppressants may suppress skin test reaction. • For treatment of anaphylaxis, see p. 1114.

107

Uncategorized agents

adenosine phosphate
allopurinol
amantadine hydrochloride
bromocriptine mesylate
clomiphene citrate
colchicine
cromolyn sodium
diazoxide, oral
dimethyl sulfoxide 50%
disulfiram
lactulose
levodopa
levodopa-carbidopa
methoxsalen
pralidoxime chloride

These drugs, used for a variety of indications, do not fall into the classes of drugs summarized in the preceding chapters.

Major uses

- Adenosine phosphate: adjunctive therapy in the treatment of varicose veins and thrombophlebitis; also used in symptomatic treatment of bursitis, tendonitis, tenosynovitis, intractable pruritus, multiple sclerosis.
- Allopurinol: to lower serum and urinary uric acid levels in the treatment of primary gout.
- Amantadine hydrochloride: used in the treatment of idiopathic parkinsonism, parkinsonian syndrome, and drug-induced extrapyramidal reactions; chemoprophylaxis against influenza A virus.
- Bromocriptine mesylate: for short-term treatment of amenorrhea/galactorrhea associated with hyperprolactinemia, prevention of postpartum galactorrhea.
- Clomiphene citrate: to induce ovulation in anovulatory women desiring pregnancy.
- Colchicine: to relieve attacks of acute gouty arthritis.
- Cromolyn sodium: as an adjunct in the treatment of patients with severe, perennial, bronchial asthma.
- Oral diazoxide: used in the treatment of hypoglycemia.
- Dimethyl sulfoxide: instilled into the bladder for symptomatic relief of interstitial cystitis.
- Disulfiram: used as an alcohol deterrent in the treatment of chronic alcoholism.
- Lactulose: for the prevention and treatment of portal-systemic encephalopathy, including stages of hepatic coma and precoma.
- Levodopa and levodopa/carbidopa: used in the symptomatic treatment of idiopathic parkinsonism and parkinsonian syndrome resulting from lethargica encephalitis, carbon monoxide intoxication, chronic manganese intoxication, or cerebral arteriosclerosis.
- Methoxsalen: repigmentation of idiopathic vitiligo.
- Pralidoxime chloride: as an antidote for poisoning by pesticides and organophosphate

chemicals; to treat overdosage with anticholinesterase drugs given in myasthenia gravis.

Mechanism of action

• Adenosine phosphate: clinical benefit may result from correction of biochemical imbalance or deficiency at cellular level; therapeutic effects may also result from drug's vasodilating action and ability to reduce tissue edema and inflammation.
• Allopurinol: reduces production of uric acid by inhibiting the biochemical reactions preceding its formation.
• Amantadine: increases dopamine release in animal brain but exact mechanism of action in humans is not known.
• Bromocriptine mesylate: inhibits secretion of prolactin in humans; acts as a dopamine receptor antagonist by activating postsynaptic dopamine receptors.
• Clomiphene citrate: appears to stimulate release of pituitary gonadotropins, follicle-stimulating hormone (FSH) and luteinizing hormone (LH), which results in maturation of ovarian follicle, ovulation and development of corpus luteum.
• Colchicine: inhibits migration of granulocytes to inflammatory area; decreases lactic acid production associated with phagocytosis, thus interrupts the cycle of urate crystal deposition and inflammatory response.
• Cromolyn sodium: inhibits the degranulation of sensitized mast cells which occurs after exposure to specific antigens; also inhibits release of histamine and slow-reacting substance of anaphylaxis (SRS-A).
• Oral diazoxide inhibits release of insulin from the pancreas and decreases peripheral utilization of glucose.
• Dimethyl sulfoxide acts nonspecifically as an anti-inflammatory agent.
• Disulfiram: blocks oxidation of alcohol at acetaldehyde stage; accumulation of acetaldehyde produces highly unpleasant reaction in presence of even small amounts of alcohol.
• Lactulose: a nonabsorbable disaccharide which is degraded by colon bacteria, acidifying colon contents. Causes a decrease in blood ammonia concentration and reduces degree of portal-systemic encephalopathy.
• Levodopa and levodopa/carbidopa: may be rapidly decarboxylated to dopamine, countering the depletion of striatal dopamine in extrapyramidal centers thought to produce symptoms of parkinsonism.
• Methoxsalen: may enhance melanogenesis directly, or secondary to an inflammatory process.
• Pralidoxime chloride: reactivates cholinesterase which has been inactivated by organophosphate pesticides and related compounds. Allows degradation of accumulated acetylcholine to proceed and neuromuscular junctions to function normally.

Drug	Absorption	Distribution	Excretion
adenosine phosphate	Information not available	Information not available	Information not available
allopurinol	Approximately 80% of oral dose is absorbed	All extracellular fluid except brain	Rapidly cleared from plasma, small portion unchanged in urine. Metabolite is excreted slowly; may accumulate in chronic use
amantadine hydrochloride	Rapidly absorbed from GI tract	Information not available	Approximately 90% of dose excreted unchanged in urine
bromocriptine mesylate	28% of oral dose absorbed from GI tract; drug is bound mostly to serum albumin	Completely metabolized before excretion	Excreted via bile; almost all excreted in feces in 120 hours; small amount excreted in urine
clomiphene citrate	Readily absorbed from GI tract	Detoxified in liver	50% of dose is excreted in feces in 5 days; remaining drug and metabolites excreted from enterohepatic pool or stored in body fat
colchicine	Absorbed from GI tract after oral dose	Drug and metabolites recycled to intestinal tract via biliary and intestinal secretions; concentrates in liver, kidneys, spleen, intestines	Excreted primarily in feces; 10% to 20% in urine
cromolyn sodium	Following inhalation, about 8% of dose reaching lungs is absorbed into systemic circulation	Distributes in plasma; doesn't cross most biological membranes	Rapidly excreted unchanged in bile and urine; small amount is exhaled; drug swallowed excreted in feces

Drug	Absorption	Distribution	Excretion
diazoxide	Readily absorbed from GI tract	Widely distributed	90% excreted unchanged in urine
dimethyl sulfoxide	Unknown	Unknown	Excreted through breath and skin
disulfiram	Rapidly but incompletely absorbed from GI tract	Accumulates in body fat depots	Most of drug is oxidized, probably by liver, excreted slowly in urine. About 20% of drug remains in body 1 to 2 weeks
lactulose	Not absorbed; used for local action in colon	Used for local action in colon	Metabolized in colon; excreted in feces
levodopa and levodopa-carbidopa	Rapidly and completely absorbed in GI tract	Converted to dopamine in liver and GI tract; small amount reaches CNS	85% of dose is excreted in urine in 24 hours; small amount eliminated in feces
methoxsalen	Rapidly absorbed from GI tract	Information not available	80% of dose excreted within 24 hours
pralidoxime chloride	Not bound to plasma proteins	Distributed throughout extracellular water; metabolized mostly in liver	Rapidly excreted in urine; unchanged and partly as a metabolite produced by the liver

Drug	Onset	Duration
adenosine phosphate	Information not available	1 to 2 hours
allopurinol	Appears in plasma in 30 to 60 minutes; peaks in 2 to 4 hours	Serum and urinary uric acid fall within 2 to 3 days, but week may be needed for full effect; uric acid returns to pretreatment levels slowly
amantadine hydrochloride	Peak blood levels appear within hours; readily absorbed following oral administration	Acidification of urine increases rate of excretion; has relatively long duration of action
bromocriptine mesylate	2 hours	Information not available
clomiphene citrate	Information not available	Information not available
colchicine	Pain alleviated within 12 hours after P.O. administration; usually is completely gone within 24 to 48 hours after P.O. and 4 to 12 hours after I.V. therapy	Plasma levels decline 1 to 2 hours after oral dose, then increase due to recycling; drug concentrations found in leukocytes 9 days after single I.V. dose
cromolyn sodium	Immediately upon inhalation of drug	3 to 4 hours
diazoxide	Within 1 hour	8 hours

Drug	Onset	Duration
dimethyl sulfoxide	Unknown	Unknown
disulfiram	Rapidly absorbed from GI tract, but 12 hours may be needed for full effect	Slowly eliminated; about 1/5 remains in body after 1 week; sensitization to alcohol may last for 6 to 12 days following last dose of drug
lactulose	Clinical improvement may be noted within 24 hours	24 hours
levodopa and levodopa-carbidopa	Rapidly absorbed, especially when stomach is empty	5 to 24 hours
methoxsalen	Increased sensitivity in 1 hour; peaks in 2 hours	8 hours
pralidoxime chloride	Immediate	Short-acting; repeated doses may be needed

Combination products

APCOGESIC: sodium salicylate 300 mg, colchicine 0.2 mg, calcium carbonate 60 mg, dried aluminum hydroxide gel 120 mg, and phenobarbital 8 mg.
BENN-C: probenecid 500 mg and colchicine 0.5 mg.
COLBENEMID: probenecid 500 mg and colchicine 0.5 mg.
COLSALIDE: sodium salicylate 300 mg, potassium iodide 30 mg, and colchicine 0.4 mg.
DOLORAL: colchicine salicylate 0.1 mg, phenobarbital 8 mg, sodium *p*-aminobenzoate 15 mg, vitamin B_1 25 mg, and aspirin 325 mg.
PROBENECID WITH COLCHICINE: probenecid 500 mg and colchicine 0.5 mg.
SALCOCE: sodium salicylate 500 mg and colchicine 0.54 mg.

NAME	INDICATIONS & DOSAGE	SIDE EFFECTS
adenosine phosphate Adenocrest, Adenyl, Cobalasine, My-B-Den	*To relieve edema, pruritus, dermatitis, and erythema of varicose veins; symptomatic treatment of bursitis, tendonitis, intractable pruritus—* **Adults:** 20 to 100 mg I.M. (extended-release) daily for 3 or 4 days, reduced to same dosage every other day. Depending on patient response, reduce dose to 20 mg once or twice weekly; or 20 mg I.M. daily to t.i.d. (simple aqueous solution); or every hour for 5 doses for first 3 days, followed by 20 mg daily as needed; or 100 mg in aqueous solution injected as single dose daily for 3 days, followed by 100 mg on alternate days thereafter as needed. *Sublingual dose to supplement I.M. injection—* **Adults:** 20 mg sublingually q hour, 5 to 7 doses per day for 4 to 7 days. Maintenance dose: 40 to 100 mg daily sublingually, adjusted to patient response.	*CNS:* dizziness. *CV:* palpitations, hypotension, dyspnea. *GI:* epigastric discomfort, nausea. *Skin:* erythema, flushing.
allopurinol Zyloprim◆	*Gout, primary, or secondary to hyperuricemia; secondary to diseases such as acute or chronic leukemia, polycythemia vera, multiple myeloma, and psoriasis—* Dosage varies with severity of disease; can be given as single dose or divided, but doses larger than 300 mg must be divided. **Adults:** mild gout, 200 to 300 mg P.O. daily; severe gout, 400 to 600 mg P.O. daily. Same dose for maintenance in secondary hyperuricemia. *Hyperuricemia secondary to malignancies—* **Children 6 to 10 years:** 300 mg P.O. daily. **Children under 6 years:** 150 mg P.O. daily.	*Blood:* agranulocytosis, anemia, aplastic anemia, bone marrow depression, leukopenia, pancytopenia, thrombocytopenia (usually in connection with other drug use). *CNS:* drowsiness. *EENT:* cataracts, retinopathy. *GI:* nausea, vomiting, diarrhea, abdominal pain. *Skin:* rash, usually maculopapular; exfoliative, urticarial, and purpuric lesions; erythema multiforme; severe furunculosis of nose; ichthyosis, toxic epidermal necrolysis. *Other:* altered hepatic function tests.

◆ Also available in Canada.
◆◆ Available in Canada only.
Unmarked trade names available in United States only.

INTERACTIONS	NURSING CONSIDERATIONS
None significant.	• Contraindicated in myocardial infarction and cerebral hemorrhage. Use cautiously in patients with history of allergy; have treatment available. Obtain adequate history of allergies before giving first dose. • Anaphylactoid reactions have occurred following use of gelatin I.M. solution. Discontinue if patient complains of dyspnea or tightness in chest. • Don't give I.V. • Place sublingual tablets under tongue. Warn patient not to mix with food or water, or to swallow excessively until dissolved. • I.M. extended-release in gelatin vehicle: warm solution before using. Inject into gluteal muscle, using 22G to 20G needle, 1 to 1½ inches long.
Uricosuric agents: additive effect; may be used to therapeutic advantage.	• Contraindicated in hypersensitive individuals or those with idiopathic hemocromatosis; and in patients who have developed reactions to it. Use cautiously in hepatic or renal disease. • Obtain accurate patient history; note possible allergies with other drug use before first dose. • Discontinue at first sign of skin rash, which may precede severe hypersensitivity reaction, or any other adverse reaction. Warn patient to report all side effects immediately. • Monitor intake/output; daily urinary output of at least 2 liters and maintenance of neutral or slightly alkaline urine are desirable. • Periodically check CBC, hepatic and renal function, especially at start of therapy. • Acute gouty attacks may occur in first 6 weeks of therapy; concurrent use of colchicine may be prescribed prophylactically. • Warn patient that allopurinol may cause drowsiness. • Minimize GI side effects by giving with meals or immediately after. • Evaluate effectiveness, using serum uric acid levels. Goal is to lower serum level to 6 mg/100 ml, usually within 7 to 10 days; to gradually reduce size of tophi, with no new deposits within 6 months; and to relieve joint pain and increase mobility. • Allopurinol may predispose patient to ampicillin-induced skin rash.

(continued on following page)

NAME	INDICATIONS & DOSAGE	SIDE EFFECTS
allopurinol *(continued)*	*In patients with impaired renal function—* **Adults:** 200 mg daily if creatinine clearance is 10 to 20 ml/min; 100 mg daily if creatinine is less than 10 ml/min; 100 mg more than 24 hours apart if clearance is less than 3 ml/min. *To prevent acute gouty attacks—* **Adults:** 100 mg daily; increase at weekly intervals by 100 mg without exceeding maximum (800 mg) until serum uric acid level falls to 6 mg/100 ml or less. *To prevent uric acid nephropathy during cancer chemotherapy—* **Adults:** 600 to 800 mg P.O. daily for 2 to 3 days, with high fluid intake.	
amantadine hydrochloride Symmetrel◆	*Drug-induced extrapyramidal reactions—* **Adults:** 100 mg P.O. b.i.d. up to 300 mg daily in divided doses. Patients may benefit from as much as 400 mg daily, but doses over 200 mg must be closely supervised. *Prophylaxis and symptomatic management of influenza A virus, respiratory tract illness—* see p.146. *To treat idiopathic parkinsonism, parkinsonian syndrome—* **Adults:** 100 mg P.O. b.i.d.; in patients who are seriously ill or receiving other antiparkinsonism drugs, 100 mg daily for at least 1 week, then 100 mg b.i.d., p.r.n.	*CNS:* confusion, depression, fatigue, psychosis, dizziness, headache, light-headedness, insomnia, nervous excitement, difficulty in concentrating, tremors, slurred speech, lethargy, drowsiness, ataxia, psychic disturbances, convulsions (with high dosage). *CV:* congestive heart failure, orthostatic hypotension, dyspnea, peripheral edema. *EENT:* blurring or loss of vision, oculogyric episodes. *GI:* dry mouth, mild indigestion, anorexia, nausea, vomiting, constipation. *GU:* urinary retention. *Skin:* livedo reticularis, dermatitis.
bromocriptine mesylate Parlodel◆	*To treat amenorrhea and galactorrhea associated with hyperprolactinemia and to prevent or suppress lactation—* **Women:** 2.5 mg P.O. b.i.d. or t.i.d. with meals for 14 days; and for no more than 6 months.	*CNS:* dizziness, headache, fatigue, nervousness. *EENT:* nasal congestion, tinnitus, blurred vision. *GI:* nausea, vomiting, abdominal cramps, constipation, diarrhea.

INTERACTIONS	NURSING CONSIDERATIONS
None significant.	• Use cautiously in epilepsy or "seizures," with congestive heart failure, renal impairment, peripheral edema, hepatic disease, eczematoid dermatitis, uncontrolled psychosis, or severe psychoneurosis. • Don't stop abruptly, since this might precipitate a parkinsonian crisis; taper off gradually. • Warn elderly patients about orthostatic hypotension. Suggest that they change position slowly, dangle legs before getting up, and lie down if they feel faint or dizzy. Advise elderly males to sit down to urinate, especially at night. Patient should be careful not to fall asleep in a sitting position. • Last daily dose should be given as early as possible to avoid insomnia. • Warn that drug may produce dizziness, blurred vision, and impaired coordination; activities requiring mental alertness should be resumed gradually. • Advise patient to report any decrease in drug's effectiveness to doctor.
None significant.	• Contraindicated in hypersensitivity to ergot derivatives. • Patient should be examined carefully for pituitary tumor (Forbes-Albright syndrome). • May lead to early postpartum conception. Test for pregnancy every 4 weeks or whenever period is missed once menses are reinitiated. • Advise patient to use contraceptive methods other than oral contraceptive during treatment. • "First-dose phenomenon" occurs in 1% of patients. Sensitive patients may collapse for 15 to 60 minutes but can usually tolerate subsequent treatment without ill effects. • Should be given with meals.

NAME	INDICATIONS & DOSAGE	SIDE EFFECTS
clomiphene citrate Clomid◆	*To induce ovulation—* **Women:** 50 to 100 mg P.O. daily for 5 days, starting any time; or 50 to 100 mg P.O. daily starting on day 5 of menstrual cycle (first day of menstrual flow is day 1). Repeat until conception occurs or until 3 courses of therapy are completed.	*CNS:* headache, restlessness, insomnia, dizziness, light-headedness, depression, fatigue, tension. *EENT:* blurred vision, diplopia, scotomata, photophobia (signs of impending visual toxicity). *GI:* nausea, vomiting, bloating, distention, increased appetite, weight gain. *GU:* urinary frequency and polyuria; ovarian enlargement and cyst formation which regress spontaneously when drug is stopped. *Skin:* urticaria, rash, dermatitis. *Other:* hot flashes, reversible alopecia, breast discomfort.
colchicine Colchicine, Novocolchine◆◆	*To prevent acute attacks of gout as prophylactic or maintenance therapy—* **Adults:** 0.5 or 0.6 mg P.O. daily, 3 or more times weekly for patients with less than 1 attack yearly; 0.5 to 0.6 mg P.O. daily for patients with more than 1 attack yearly; or 1 to 1.8 mg P.O. daily for more severe cases. Or 0.5 to 1 mg I.V. once or twice daily. *To prevent attacks of gout in patients undergoing surgery—* **Adults:** 0.5 to 0.6 mg P.O. t.i.d. 3 days before and 3 days after surgery. *To treat gout, acute gouty arthritis—* **Adults:** initially, 1 to 1.2 mg P.O., then 0.5 or 0.6 mg q hour, or 1 to 1.2 mg q 2 hours until pain is relieved or until nausea, vomiting, or diarrhea ensues. After initial dose, 0.5 to 0.6 mg q 2 or 3 hours; or 2 mg I.V. followed by 0.5 mg q 6 hours. Total I.V. dose over 24 hours not to exceed 4 mg. *Note:* Give I.V. by slow I.V. push over 1 to 2 minutes, or I.V. infusion (drip chamber) in 50 to 100 ml normal saline solution over 15 to 20 minutes.	*Blood:* aplastic anemia and agranulocytosis with prolonged use; nonthrombocytopenic purpura. *CNS:* peripheral neuritis. *GI:* nausea, vomiting, abdominal pain, diarrhea. *Skin:* urticaria, dermatitis. *Local:* severe local irritation if extravasation of injection occurs. *Other:* alopecia.

INTERACTIONS	NURSING CONSIDERATIONS
None significant.	• Contraindicated in thrombophlebitis, thromboembolic disorders, or past history of these conditions; cancer of breast or reproductive organs; undiagnosed abnormal genital bleeding; ovarian cyst; hepatic disease or dysfunction. Use cautiously in hypertension, mental depression, migraines, seizures, diabetes mellitus, or gonadotropin sensitivity. Report development or worsening of these conditions to doctor. May require stopping drug. • Warn patient to report immediately abdominal pain, numbness or stiffness in legs or buttocks, pressure or pain in chest, shortness of breath, severe headaches, undiagnosed vaginal bleeding or discharge, breast lumps, swelling of hands or feet. • Patient with visual disturbances should stop drug and tell doctor at once. Complete ophthalmic exam should precede resumption of therapy. • Majority of patients ovulate and a large percentage become pregnant after clomiphene citrate therapy. • Tell patient that possibility of multiple births exists with this drug. Risk increases with higher doses.
None significant.	• Use cautiously in hepatic dysfunction, heart disease, renal disease, GI disorders, and in aged or debilitated patients. • Reduce dosage if weakness, anorexia, nausea, vomiting, or diarrhea appear. First sign of acute overdosage may be GI symptoms, followed by vascular damage, muscle weakness, ascending paralysis. Delirium and convulsions may occur without patient losing consciousness. • Do not administer I.M. or S.C.; severe local irritation occurs. • Give with meals to reduce GI effects. May be used with uricosuric agents. • Baseline lab studies including CBC should precede therapy and be repeated periodically. • Monitor fluid intake/output. Keep output at 2,000 ml daily. • Tell patient on prophylactic use to increase dose at first sign of impending attack and to notify doctor. • Store in tightly closed, light-resistant container. • Change needle before making direct I.V. injection.

NAME	INDICATIONS & DOSAGE	SIDE EFFECTS
cromolyn sodium Aarane, Intal♦, Rynacrom♦♦	*Adjunct in treatment of severe perennial bronchial asthma—* **Adults, and children over 5:** contents of 20 mg capsule inhaled q.i.d. at regular intervals.	*CNS:* dizziness, headache. *EENT:* irritation of the throat and trachea, cough, bronchospasm following inhalation of dry powder; nasal congestion; pharyngeal irritation; wheezing. *GI:* nausea. *GU:* dysuria, urinary frequency. *Skin:* rash, urticaria. *Other:* joint swelling and pain, lacrimation, swollen parotid gland, angioedema.
diazoxide, oral Proglycem	*Management of hypoglycemia due to a variety of conditions resulting in hyperinsulinism—* **Adults and children:** 3 to 8 mg/Kg/day P.O., divided into 3 equal doses q 8 hours. **Infants and newborns:** 8 to 15 mg/Kg/day P.O., divided into 2 or 3 equal doses q 8 to 12 hours.	*Blood:* leukopenia, thrombocytopenia. *CV:* cardiac arrhythmias, hypotension. *EENT:* diplopia. *GI:* nausea, vomiting. *Metabolic:* sodium and fluid retention, ketoacidosis and hyperosmolar nonketotic coma, hyperuricemia. *Other:* severe hypertrichosis (hair growth) in 25% of adults and higher percentage of children.
dimethyl sulfoxide 50% (DMSO) Rimso-50	*Symptomatic relief of interstitial cystitis—* **Adults:** instill 50 ml directly into bladder with catheter or syringe, allow to remain for 15 minutes. Repeat every 2 weeks until maximum symptomatic relief is obtained. Thereafter, time intervals between therapy may be increased.	*Other:* garlic-like taste in mouth, hypersensitivity.
disulfiram Antabuse♦, Cronetal, Ro-Sulfiram	*Adjunct in management of chronic alcoholism—* **Adults:** maximum of 500 mg q morning for 1 to 2 weeks. Can be taken in evening if drowsiness occurs. Maintenance: 125 to 500 mg daily (average dose 250 mg) until permanent self-control is established. Treatment may continue for months or years.	*CNS:* drowsiness, headache, fatigue, neuritis. *EENT:* optic neuritis. *GI:* metallic or garlic-like aftertaste. *GU:* impotence. *Skin:* acneiform or allergic dermatitis.

INTERACTIONS	NURSING CONSIDERATIONS
None significant.	• Contraindicated in acute asthma attacks, status asthmaticus. • Not to be taken orally; insert capsule into inhaler provided; follow manufacturer's directions. • Watch for recurrence of asthmatic symptoms when dosage is decreased, especially when corticosteroids are also used. • Use only when acute episode has been controlled, airway is cleared, and patient is able to inhale. • Gradually reduce dose from 4 to 3 capsules daily after patient is stabilized. • Monitor patient closely, especially if he's also taking corticosteroids. • Patient considered for cromolyn therapy should have pulmonary function tests to show significant bronchodilator-reversible component to his airway obstruction. • Teach correct use of inhaler: exhale completely before placing mouthpiece between lips, then inhale deeply and rapidly with steady, even breath; remove inhaler from mouth, hold breath a few seconds, and exhale. Repeat until all powder has been inhaled. • Store capsules at room temperature in tightly closed containers; protect from moisture and temperatures higher than 40° C. (104° F.). • Instruct patient to avoid excessive handling of capsule.
Thiazide diuretics: may potentiate hyperglycemic, hyperuricemic, and hypotensive effects. Monitor appropriate lab values.	• Contraindicated in thiazide hypersensitivity and functional hypoglycemia. • Oral diazoxide does not significantly lower blood pressure. • A nondiuretic congener of thiazide diuretics. • Most important use is in management of hypoglycemia due to hyperinsulinism in infants and children. • Monitor urine regularly for glucose and ketones; report any abnormalities to doctor. • If not effective after 2 or 3 weeks, drug should be stopped. • Hair growth on arms and forehead is a common side effect that will subside when drug treatment is completed. Reassure patient. • Available in capsules and oral suspension.
None significant.	• Chronic use of DMSO may produce ophthalmic changes. Eyes should be examined periodically. • After retention of Rimso-50 for 15 minutes, it's expelled by spontaneous voiding. • Administration of oral analgesics before instillation can reduce bladder spasm in sensitive patients. • Lidocaine jelly or similar local anesthetic should be applied to urethra before insertion of catheter to avoid spasm. • Not for I.M. or I.V. injection.
Isoniazid (INH): ataxia or marked change in behavior. Avoid use. *Metronidazole (Flagyl):* psychotic reaction. Do not use together. *Paraldehyde:* toxic levels of the acetalde-	• Contraindicated in alcohol intoxication, psychoses, myocardial disease, coronary occlusion, or those receiving metronidazole, paraldehyde, alcohol, or alcohol-containing preparations. Use cautiously in diabetes mellitus, hypothyroidism, epilepsy, cerebral damage, nephritis, hepatic cirrhosis or insufficiency, abnormal EEG, multiple drug dependence. • Used only under close medical and nursing supervision. Patient should clearly understand consequences of disulfiram therapy and give permission. Drug should be used only in patients who are cooperative, well motivated, and are receiving supportive psychiatric therapy. • Complete physical exam and lab studies, including CBC, SMA-12, and

(continued on following page)

NAME	INDICATIONS & DOSAGE	SIDE EFFECTS
disulfiram *(continued)*		
lactulose Cephulac♦, Chronulac♦♦, Duphalac	*To prevent and treat portal-systemic encephalopathy, including hepatic precoma and coma in patients with severe hepatic disease*— **Adults:** initially, 20 to 30 g P.O. (30 to 45 ml) t.i.d. or q.i.d., until 2 or 3 soft stools are produced daily. Usual dose is 60 to 100 g daily in divided doses. Can also be given by retention enema in at least 100 ml of fluid.	*GI:* abdominal cramps, belching, diarrhea, gaseous distention, flatulence.
levodopa Bendopa, Bio Dopa, Dopar, Larodopa♦, Levopa♦, Parda, Rio-Dopa	*Treatment of idiopathic parkinsonism and parkinsonian syndrome resulting from lethargica encephalitis; carbon monoxide and chronic manganese intoxication; and cerebral arteriosclerosis*—administered orally with food in dosages carefully adjusted to individual's requirements, tolerance, response. **Adults:** initially, 0.5 to 1 g P.O. b.i.d., t.i.d., q.i.d. with food; increase by no more than 0.75 g daily q 3 to 7 days, until usual maximum of 8 g is reached. Larger dose requires close supervision.	*Blood:* hemolytic anemia. *CNS:* choreiform; dystonic, dyskinetic movements; involuntary grimacing, head movements, myoclonic body jerks, ataxia, tremors, muscle twitching; bradykinetic episodes; psychiatric disturbances, memory loss, nervousness, anxiety, disturbing dreams, euphoria, malaise, fatigue; severe depression, suicidal tendencies, dementia, delirium, hallucinations (may necessitate reduction or withdrawal of drug). *CV:* orthostatic hypotension, cardiac irregularities, flushing, hypertension; hyperventilation, phlebitis. *EENT:* blepharospasm, blurred vision, diplopia, mydriasis or miosis, widening of palpebral fissures, activation of latent Horner's syndrome, oculogyric crises, nasal discharge. *GI:* nausea, vomiting, anorexia, weight loss may occur at start of therapy; constipation; flatulence; diarrhea; epigastric pain; hiccups; sialorrhea; dry mouth; bitter taste.

INTERACTIONS	NURSING CONSIDERATIONS
hyde. Do not use together.	transaminase, should precede therapy and be repeated regularly. • If compliance is questionable, crush tablets and mix with juice or other liquid; observe patient. • Warn patient to avoid all sources of alcohol: sauces, cough syrups. Even external application of liniments, shaving lotion, back-rub preparations may precipitate disulfiram reaction! Tell him that alcohol reaction may occur as long as 2 weeks after single dose of disulfiram; the longer patient remains on drug, the more sensitive he will become to alcohol. • Patient should wear a bracelet or carry a card supplied by drug manufacturer identifying him as disulfiram user. Note: Mild reactions may occur in sensitive patients with blood alcohol level of 5 to 10 mg/100 ml; symptoms are fully developed at 50 mg/100 ml; unconsciousness usually occurs at 125 to 150 mg/100 ml level. Reaction may last ½ hour to several hours, or as long as alcohol remains in blood. Caution: Warn patient to ingest no alcohol or alcohol-containing products for at least 12 hours before administering.
None significant.	• Contraindicated in patients who need low-galactose diet. Use cautiously in diabetes mellitus. • Reduce dosage if diarrhea occurs. Replace fluid loss. • Minimize drug's sweet taste by diluting with water or fruit juice or giving with food. • Store at room temperature, preferably below 30° C. (86° F.) Don't freeze. • Underlying hepatic disease must be treated. • Can also be used as a laxative to treat chronic constipation.
Anticholinergic drugs, tricyclic antidepressants, benzodiazepines, clonidine, papaverine, phenothiazines and other antipsychotics, phenytoin: watch for decreased levodopa effect. *Pyridoxine:* reduced efficacy of levodopa. Examine vitamin preparations for content of vitamin B_6 (pyridoxine). *Antacids, propranolol:* may increase levodopa effect. Use together cautiously.	• Contraindicated in narrow-angle glaucoma, melanoma or undiagnosed skin lesions. Use cautiously in cardiovascular, renal, hepatic, pulmonary disorders; in those with peptic ulcer, psychiatric illness, myocardial infarction with residual arrhythmias; and in patients with bronchial asthma, emphysema, and endocrine disease. • Carefully monitor patients also receiving antihypertensive medication, hypoglycemic agents. Stop MAO inhibitors at least 2 weeks before therapy is begun. • Adjust dosage according to patient's response and tolerance. Observe and monitor vital signs, especially while adjusting dose. Report significant changes. • Instruct patient to report adverse reactions and therapeutic effects. • Warn of possible dizziness and orthostatic hypotension, especially at start of therapy. Patient should change position slowly and dangle legs before getting out of bed. Elastic stockings may control this side effect in some patients. • Muscle twitching and blepharospasm (twitching of eyelids) may be an early sign of drug overdosage; report immediately. • Patients on long-term use should be tested regularly for diabetes and acromegaly; repeat blood tests, hepatic and renal function studies periodically. • Multivitamin preparations, fortified cereals, and certain over-the-counter medications may contain pyridoxine (vitamin B_6), which can reverse the effects of levodopa. • If therapy is interrupted for long period, drug should be adjusted gradually to previous level.

(continued on following page)

NAME	INDICATIONS & DOSAGE	SIDE EFFECTS
levodopa *(continued)*		*GU:* urinary frequency, retention, incontinence, darkened urine, excessive and inappropriate sexual behavior, priapism. *Other:* dark perspiration.
levodopa-carbidopa (combination) Sinemet♦	*Treatment of idiopathic Parkinson's disease, postencephalitic parkinsonism, and symptomatic parkinsonism; and carbon monoxide and manganese intoxication*— **Adults:** 3 to 6 tablets of 25 mg carbidopa/250 mg P.O. levodopa daily given in divided doses. Do not exceed 8 tablets of 25 mg carbidopa/250 mg levodopa a day. Optimum daily dosage must be determined by careful titration for each patient.	*Blood:* hemolytic anemia. *CNS:* choreiform; dystonic, dyskinetic movements; involuntary grimacing, head movements, myoclonic body jerks, ataxia, tremors, muscle twitching; bradykinetic episodes; psychiatric disturbances, memory loss, nervousness, anxiety, disturbing dreams, euphoria, malaise, fatigue; severe depression, suicidal tendencies, dementia, delirium, hallucinations (may necessitate reduction or withdrawal of drug). *CV:* orthostatic hypotension, cardiac irregularities, flushing, hypertension; hyperventilation, phlebitis. *EENT:* blepharospasm, blurred vision, diplopia, mydriasis or miosis, widening of palpebral fissures, activation of latent Horner's syndrome, oculogyric crises, nasal discharge. *GI:* nausea, vomiting, anorexia, weight loss may occur at start of therapy; constipation; flatulence; diarrhea; epigastric pain; hiccups; sialorrhea; dry mouth; bitter taste. *GU:* urinary frequency, retention, incontinence, darkened urine, excessive and inappropriate sexual behavior, priapism. *Other:* dark perspiration.
methoxsalen Oxsoralen♦	*Protect against sunburn, enhance pigmentation, and induce repigmentation in vitiligo*— **Adults, and children over 12 years:** 20 mg P.O. daily, 2 to 4 hours before carefully timed exposure to ultraviolet light.	*CNS:* nervousness, insomnia, depression. *GI:* discomfort, nausea, diarrhea. *Skin:* edema, erythema, painful blistering, burning, peeling.

INTERACTIONS	NURSING CONSIDERATIONS
	• Therapeutic response usually occurs after each dose and disappears within 5 hours but varies considerably. • Patient who must undergo surgery should continue levodopa as long as oral intake is permitted, generally 6 to 24 hours before surgery. Drug should be resumed as soon as patient is able to take oral medication. • Protect from heat, light, moisture. If preparation darkens, it has lost potency and should be discarded. • Coombs test occasionally becomes positive during extended use. Expect uric acid elevations with colorimetric method, but not with uricase method. • Alkaline phosphatase, SGOT, SGPT, LDH, bilirubin, BUN, and PBI show transient elevations in patients receiving levodopa; WBC, hemoglobin, and hematocrit show occasional reduction. • Combination of levodopa-carbidopa usually reduces amount of levodopa needed by 75%, thereby reducing incidence of side effects.
Papaverine, diazepam, clonidine, phenothiazines: may antagonize antiparkinson actions. Use together cautiously.	• Contraindicated in narrow-angle glaucoma, melanoma or undiagnosed skin lesions. Use cautiously in cardiovascular, renal, hepatic, pulmonary disorders; in history of peptic ulcer, psychiatric illness, myocardial infarction with residual arrhythmias; and in bronchial asthma, emphysema, and endocrine disease. • Carefully monitor patients also receiving antihypertensive medication, hypoglycemic agents. Discontinue MAO inhibitors at least 2 weeks before therapy is begun. • Dosage is adjusted according to patient's response and tolerance to drug. Therapeutic and adverse reactions occur more rapidly with levodopa-carbidopa than with levodopa alone. Observe and monitor vital signs, especially while dosage is being adjusted; report significant changes. • Instruct patient to report adverse reactions and therapeutic effects. • Warn patient of possible dizziness and orthostatic hypotension, especially at start of therapy. Patient should change position slowly and dangle legs before getting out of bed. Elastic stockings may control this side effect in some patients. • Muscle twitching and blepharospasm (twitching of eyelids) may be an early sign of drug overdosage; report immediately. • Patients on long-term therapy should be tested regularly for diabetes and acromegaly; blood tests, hepatic and renal function studies should be repeated periodically. • If patient is being treated with levodopa, discontinue at least 8 hours before starting Sinemet. • This combination drug usually reduces the amount of levodopa needed by 75%, thereby reducing the incidence of side effects. • Pyridoxine (B_6) does not reverse the beneficial effects of Sinemet. Multivitamins can be taken without fear of losing control of symptoms. • If therapy is interrupted temporarily, the usual daily dosage may be given as soon as patient resumes oral medication. • Available as tablets with carbidopa-levodopa in a 1 to 10 ratio (Sinemet 10/100 and Sinemet 25/250).
Photosensitizing agents: do not use together.	• Contraindicated in hepatic insufficiency, porphyria, acute lupus erythematosus, hydromorphic and polymorphic light eruptions. Use with caution in familial history of sunlight allergy, GI diseases, or chronic infection. • Carefully check for signs of cataracts, melanoma, or skin carcinoma. • Regulate therapy carefully. Overdosage or overexposure to light can cause serious burning or blistering. • Drug should be taken orally with meals or milk. • During light exposure treatments, protect eyes and lips. • Monthly liver function tests should be done on patients with vitiligo (especially at beginning of therapy).

NAME	INDICATIONS & DOSAGE	SIDE EFFECTS
pralidoxime chloride Protopam◆	*Antidote for organophosphate poisoning—* **Adults:** I.V. infusion of 1 to 2 g in 100 ml saline over 15 to 30 minutes. If pulmonary edema is present, give drug by slow I.V. push over 5 minutes. Repeat in 1 hour if muscle weakness persists. Additional doses may be given cautiously. I.M. or S.C. injection can be used if I.V. is not feasible; or 1 to 3 g P.O. q 5 hours. **Children:** 20 to 40 mg/Kg I.V. *To treat cholinergic crisis in myasthenia gravis—* **Adults:** 1 to 2 g I.V., followed by increments of 250 mg I.V. q 5 minutes.	*CNS:* dizziness, headache, drowsiness, excitement, and manic behavior following recovery of consciousness. *CV:* tachycardia. *EENT:* blurred vision, diplopia, impaired accommodation, laryngospasm. *GI:* nausea. *Other:* muscular weakness, muscle rigidity, hyperventilation.

INTERACTIONS	NURSING CONSIDERATIONS
None significant.	• Contraindicated in poisoning with Sevin, a carbamate insecticide, since it increases drug's toxicity. Use with extreme caution in renal insufficiency or myasthenia gravis (overdosage may precipitate myasthenic crisis). • Use in hospitalized patients only; have respiratory and other supportive measures available. Obtain accurate medical history and chronology of poisoning if possible. Give as soon as possible after poisoning. • I.V. preparation should be given slowly, as dilute solution. • Initial measures should include removal of secretions, maintenance of patient airway, artificial ventilation if needed. • Drug relieves paralysis of respiratory muscles but is less effective in relieving depression of respiratory center. • Atropine along with pralidoxime should be given I.V., 2 to 4 mg, if cyanosis is not present. If cyanosis is present, atropine should be given I.M. Give atropine every 5 to 10 minutes until signs of atropine toxicity appear; maintain atropinization for at least 48 hours. • Dilute with sterile water without preservative. • Not effective against poisoning due to phosphorus, inorganic phosphates, or organophosphates with no anticholinesterase activity. • Difficult to distinguish toxic effects produced by atropine, or organophosphate compounds, from pralidoxime. Observe patient for 48 to 72 hours if poison ingested. Delayed absorption may occur from lower bowel.

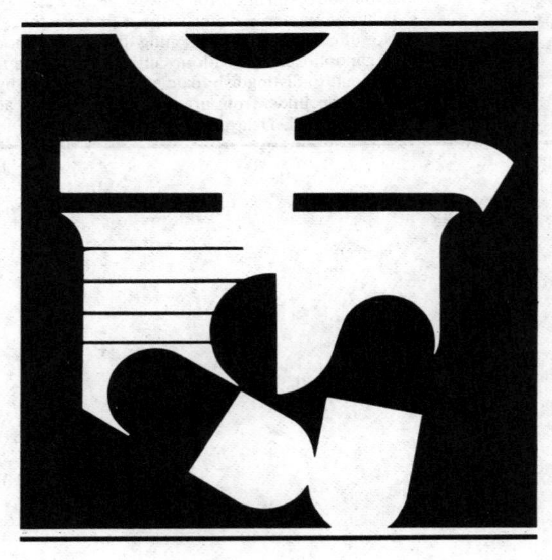

Appendices

Drug toxicities

Drug toxicity—unlike anaphylaxis, which depends on hypersensitivity—results from overdosage, or from ingestion of a drug meant for external use. Cumulative toxicity may result from long-term use of a drug which is not rapidly excreted. This section tells you how to identify and treat such toxic reactions; how to reverse them with specific antidotes; and how to relieve their symptoms with other drugs or with supportive measures. Generally, doses given are for adults. With some exceptions, children's doses should be calculated individually. (If treatment of toxicity is purely supportive, this is covered in the tabular information for that drug.)

ANAPHYLAXIS

Anaphylaxis (anaphylactoid shock) is an immediate allergic reaction that occurs within 1 hour—though usually within minutes—after administration of a drug to a patient who is hypersensitive to it. Anaphylaxis is theoretically possible after the administration of almost any drug but is most likely with certain ones, such as antibiotics (especially penicillin), immune serums, vaccines, toxoids, antitoxins, antivenins, sulfonamides, insulin, iodinated contrast media, dextran, dextran with iron, and drugs used in diagnostic skin tests.

Symptoms to watch for:

- CNS: loss of consciousness, agitation.
- CV: rapid pulse, hypotension, fainting, arrhythmias, shock, cardiac arrest.
- EENT: conjunctivitis, ocular itching, tearing, rhinitis; nasal congestion and itching.
- GI: nausea, vomiting, abdominal pain, diarrhea.
- Skin: flushing, urticaria, pruritus, angioedema; nonpruritic swelling of an extremity, or of the perioral or periorbital region.
- Other: sense of uneasiness, laryngeal edema, dyspnea, bronchospasm, cough, wheezing, sensation of retrosternal oppression.

What to do:

- Stop drug.
- Maintain airway and respirations.
- Inject 0.2 to 1 ml epinephrine 1:1000 S.C.
- Inject 10 to 50 mg diphenhydramine hydrochloride I.V. May use other antihistamines instead.
- For bronchospasm, administer oxygen, and give aminophylline 5.6 mg/Kg I.V. over 30 minutes, then 0.6 to 0.9 mg/Kg/hour; and hydrocortisone sodium succinate I.V. 100 mg/q 1 to 2 hours, until symptoms are controlled, then q 2 to 4 hours for 24 hours. Monitor blood gases.
- For hypotension, give 15 to 100 mg metaraminol bitartrate I.V. diluted in 1000 ml 5% dextrose in water, and isoproterenol 1 mg diluted in 5% dextrose in water (infused at a rate of 0.5 to 1 ml/min.) for low cardiac output. May also give I.V. normal saline solutions. Monitor blood pressure and watch for renal failure or cardiac arrhythmias.
- Have emergency resuscitative equipment available.

Avoid anaphylaxis by obtaining a history of past reactions to the drugs before giving any drug, and by skin testing before administering horse serums and penicillins.

ACETAMINOPHEN

Symptoms to watch for:

- In the first 3 to 4 hours after ingestion: nausea, vomiting, anorexia, and sweating are likely, but some patients have no symptoms.
- Later, 24 to 36 hours after ingestion, the patient may still be asymptomatic; or liver enzymes may begin to rise.
- Hepatic toxicity may develop 2 to 5 days after ingestion. Watch for vomiting, right upper quadrant tenderness, elevated SGOT and SGPT, elevated serum bilirubin, and increased prothrombin time. Hypoglycemia is possible.

How to confirm toxicity:

- Monitor SGOT, SGPT, serum bilirubin, and PT.
- Monitor serum acetaminophen levels. Levels more than 300 mcg/ml 4 hours after ingestion are associated with severe hepatic damage; levels under 120 mcg/ml 4 hours after ingestion usually mean hepatic damage is unlikely.

What to do:

- Induce emesis with 15 to 30 ml of ipecac syrup or do gastric lavage.
- Give activated charcoal (5 to 50 g, or 5 to 10 times estimated weight of ingested drug) only within first ½ hour after ingestion. After this time, activated charcoal is not effective.
- Supportive measures include parenteral fluids, fresh frozen plasma, or clotting factors.
- Immediately begin therapy with acetylcysteine (Mucomyst), the direct antidote to acetaminophen overdose: Give 140 mg/Kg P.O. of the 20% acetylcysteine (Mucomyst) solution; then give 70 mg/Kg P.O. q 4 hours for a total of 17 doses. Total dose is 133 mg/Kg. Acetylcysteine solution may be diluted to a 5% concentration with a soft drink (cola, ginger ale, etc.) to make it more palatable.

ANTICHOLINERGICS

Anisotropine methylbromide, atropine sulfate, belladonna leaf, benztropine mesylate, biperiden hydrochloride, biperiden lactate, chlorphenoxamine hydrochloride, clidinium bromide, cycrimine hydrochloride, dicyclomine hydrochloride, diphemanil methylsulfate, ethopropazine hydrochloride, flavoxate hydrochloride, glycopyrrolate, hexocyclium methylsulfate, homatropine methylbromide, hyoscyamine sulfate, isopropamide iodide, mepenzolate bromide, methantheline bromide, methixene hydrochloride, methscopolamine bromide, orphenadrine hydrochloride, oxybutynin chloride, oxyphencyclimine hydrochloride, oxyphenonium bromide, procylidine hydrochloride, propantheline bromide, scopolamine hydrobromide, thiphenamil hydrochloride, tridihexethyl chloride, trihexyphenidyl hydrochloride. Diphenoxylate hydrochloride with atropine sulfate may cause anticholinergic toxicity as well as narcotic-like toxicity. Keep in mind that other drugs, such as tricyclic antidepressants, antihistamines, and phenothiazines also have secondary anticholinergic actions.

Symptoms to watch for:

CNS: confusion, excitement, convulsions, coma.

CV: increased heart rate (may occur with therapeutic doses).

EENT: dilated pupils, blurred vision, and increased intraocular tension, dry mouth (all may occur with therapeutic doses).

GI: dysphagia.

GU: urinary retention.

Skin: hot, dry, red.

Other: rapid respirations, muscle stiffness, fever.

What to do:

- Maintain airway and respirations
- Remove drug by gastric lavage and give activated charcoal 5 to 50 g, or 5 to 10 times estimated weight of ingested drug.
- Give saline laxative (e.g., 200 ml magnesium citrate).
- Give antidote: physostigmine salicylate can reverse life-threatening central and peripheral effects of anticholinergics. Dilute each 1 mg in 5 ml normal saline. Give 0.5 to 4 mg I.M. or I.V. slowly every 2 hours. Keep atropine sulfate available for treating possible physostigmine salicylate toxicity (symptoms are bradycardia, convulsions, severe bronchoconstriction). Remember that physostigmine is contraindicated in hypotension.
- Monitor ECG.
- If patient has fever, sponge with wet towels.
- If patient shows excitement, delirium, or convulsions, give small doses of short-acting barbiturate (sodium pentobarbital).
- Catheterize patient unable to void.
- Darken patient's room, or use pilocarpine eye drops for dilated pupils.

BARBITURATES AND PRIMIDONE

Amobarbital, amobarbital sodium, aprobarbital, barbital, butabarbital sodium, hexobarbital, mephobarbital, metharbital, pentobarbital, pentobarbital sodium, phenobarbital, phenobarbital sodium, secobarbital, secobarbital sodium, talbutal. Primidone is not a barbiturate, but symptoms and treatment of primidone toxicity are similar to those for barbiturate toxicity.

Symptoms to watch for: (All signs of acute toxicity)

CNS: headache, confusion, ataxia, CNS depression ranging from sleepiness to coma, (may be

preceded by excitement and hallucinations).
CV: hypotension.
GU: crystalluria (in primidone toxicity), low urinary output.
EENT: ptosis of eyelids, miosis, mydriasis in severe poisoning.
Skin: cyanosis, especially in skin of ear lobes, nose, or fingers; occasional blisters or bullous lesions.
Other: slow, shallow breathing; flaccid muscles; hypothermia, hyperthermia; shock.
How to confirm toxicity:
• Positively identify ingested drug.
• Measure and identify barbiturates in blood or urine.
• Monitor for potentially lethal blood levels:
—phenobarbital, 80 mcg/ml or higher
—amobarbital and butabarbital, 50 mcg/ml or higher
—secobarbital and pentobarbital, 30 mcg/ml or higher
What to do:
• Stop drug.
• Maintain adequate airway. Perform endotracheal suction every hour unless pulmonary edema develops (then endotracheal suction contraindicated).
• Maintain adequate oxygen intake and carbon dioxide removal.
• Begin gastric lavage; most effective when started within 2 hours of ingestion. Use cuffed endotracheal tube. Lavage solution may be charcoal slurry, sodium sulfate 50% solution, or Phospho-Soda.
• Delay absorption with activated charcoal. Dose: 5 to 10 times estimated weight of drug ingested.
• Barbiturate toxicity has no specific antidote. Don't give analeptic drugs such as caffeine, bemegride, or ethamivan.
• Maintain blood pressure by giving 5% plasma or low molecular weight dextran I.V. Monitor central venous pressure. If fluid infusion doesn't maintain pressure, give metaraminol or levarterenol.
• Elevate patient's head 15 degrees to help prevent cerebral edema.
• Turn patient at least every 2 hours.
• Give up to 40 ml/Kg fluids daily if renal function is adequate. Maintain daily urine output 15 to 30 ml/Kg.
• Monitor sodium, potassium, and chloride daily.
• In phenobarbital toxicity, forced alkaline diuresis with sodium bicarbonate and osmotic diuretic may be useful.
• Treat hypothermia by applying blankets. Avoid too-rapid warming.
• Dialysis is indicated in severe barbiturate poisoning or if renal function is inadequate.
• Frequently monitor patient's pulse rate, temperature, color of skin, reflexes, and response to painful stimuli.

CARDIOTONIC GLYCOSIDES:
Acetyldigitoxin, deslanoside, digitalis leaf, digitoxin, digoxin, gitalin, lanatoside, ouabain.
Symptoms to watch for:
CNS: headache, weakness, lassitude, fatigue, somnolence, drowsiness, memory loss, dizziness, ataxia, confusion, aphasia, neuralgias, paresthesias, muscle pain and weakness, fainting, seizures, stupor, coma, apathy, depression, personality changes, irritability, restlessness, insomnia, nightmares, euphoria, mania, giddiness, excitement, agitation, belligerence, violent behavior, delusions, hallucinations, psychosis, delirium.
CV: ventricular premature beats (most common in adults), paroxysmal and nonparoxysmal nodal rhythms, atrioventricular dissociation; paroxysmal atrial tachycardia with AV block (most common in children).
How to confirm toxicity:
• Monitor EKG. Watch for premature ventricular contractions, paroxysmal atrial tachycardia with AV block, nonparoxysmal AV nodal tachycardia, sinus bradycardia, atrial fibrillation, ventricular tachycardia or fibrillation, sinus arrest, SA block, premature atrial contraction, premature AV nodal contraction, junctional tachycardia with escape rhythms.
• Monitor blood levels: 2 ng/ml of digoxin and 35 ng/ml of digitoxin may indicate toxicity.
What to do:
• Withhold drug.

• Treat arrhythmias. If patient has marked hypokalemia and atrial, junctional, or ventricular tachycardia, give potassium chloride: adults 40 mEq/1000 ml of 5% dextrose in water, maximum 20 mEq/hour; children, potassium chloride 0.5 mEq/Kg in 5% dextrose in water. Don't use potassium in patients with hyperkalemia, impaired kidney function, second and third degree AV block, or SA block. Throughout, monitor EKG to end the infusion promptly when hypokalemia is corrected and to avoid overcorrection to hyperkalemia by watching for signs of potassium toxicity (peaking T-waves).

If patient is not hypokalemic, use *phenytoin*. The loading dose is up to 15 mg/Kg I.V. at 50 mg/minute; maintenance, 5 to 7 mg/Kg I.V. q12 hours at rate not to exceed 50 mg/minute. Don't use phenytoin in patients with second and third degree AV block, SA block, or marked sinus bradycardia. If phenytoin is contraindicated, infuse 1 mg/Kg lidocaine hydrochloride as an I.V. bolus, at 25 to 50 mg/minute followed by constant infusion of 1 to 4 mg/minute. Use lidocaine hydrochloride with caution in patients with congestive heart failure. Lidocaine is contraindicated in patients with second and third degree AV block, SA block, and marked sinus bradycardia.

In patients with atrial tachycardia with AV block and premature ventricular contractions, give 1 to 3 mg propranolol by slow I.V. infusion (1 mg/minute). May repeat after 2 minutes. Wait 4 hours before giving subsequent doses. Propranolol is contraindicated in patients with asthma, marked sinus bradycardia, SA block, second and third degree AV block, cardiogenic shock, heart failure, or pulmonary hypertension. Occasionally, quinidine and procainamide are also useful. If the patient has second or third degree AV block, SA block, and marked sinus bradycardia, he may need an artificial pacemaker.

• Remember, all patients with cardiotonic glycoside toxicity need constant EKG monitoring.

• Keep in mind that many of the arrhythmias that cardiotonic glycosides are used to treat closely resemble the arrhythmias caused by cardiotonic glycoside toxicity, and that patients with congestive heart failure often complain of nausea and vomiting. So whenever you see these symptoms in a patient receiving cardiotonic glycosides, and you can't positively rule out toxicity, withhold the drug temporarily if the patient's clinical condition permits.

CHOLINERGIC (PARASYMPATHETIC) DRUGS:
Ambenonium chloride, edrophonium chloride, neostigmine bromide, neostigmine methylsulfate, physostigmine salicylate, pyridostigmine bromide.
Symptoms to watch for: (All signs of cholinergic crisis)
CNS: incoordination, blurred vision, weakness, fasciculation, paralysis; agitation and restlessness with extreme overdosage of neostigmine bromide, neostigmine methylsulfate, and pyridostigmine bromide; agitation, restlessness, dizziness, and mental confusion with extreme overdosage of ambenonium chloride.
CV: hypotension, cardiospasm, bradycardia, tachycardia.
EENT: miosis, lacrimation.
GI: nausea, vomiting, diarrhea.
Other: salivation, sweating, muscle cramps, bronchospasm, dyspnea, death.
What to do:

• Stop drug immediately.

• Maintain adequate respirations; if necessary, use mechanical ventilation with repeated bronchial aspiration.

• Give atropine sulfate I.V. For overdose with edrophonium chloride, give 0.4 to 0.5 mg initial dose followed by additional doses q 3 to 10 minutes p.r.n.; for overdose with physostigmine salicylate, give 2 to 4 mg atropine q 3 to 10 minutes; for overdose with neostigmine bromide, neostigmine methylsulfate or pyridostigmine bromide, give 1 to 4 mg atropine repeated every 5 to 30 minutes; and for overdose with ambenonium chloride give 0.5 to 1 mg atropine repeated every 5 to 30 minutes p.r.n.

• To reduce ganglionic and skeletal side effects of physostigmine salicylate, may give slow infusion of pralidoxime chloride I.V.: 1 to 2 g in 100 ml normal saline over 15 to 30 minutes, for adults; 20 to 40 mg/Kg for children.

BETHANECHOL CHLORIDE
Symptoms to watch for:
CNS: headache.
CV: circulatory collapse, hypotension, and cardiac arrest after I.M. or I.V. administration; substernal pressure or pain, transient complete heart block, orthostatic hypotension.

GI: bloody diarrhea after I.M. or I.V. administration; abdominal cramps, nausea, vomiting.
Skin: flushing.
Other: shock after I.M. or I.V. administration; salivation, sweating, fainting, bronchoconstriction.
What to do:
- Stop drug immediately.
- Give 0.4 to 0.6 mg atropine sulfate S.C. or I.V. every 4 to 6 hours.
- For severe CV reactions or bronchoconstriction, give 0.2 to 1 ml epinephrine 1:1000.

HEPARIN SODIUM
Symptoms to watch for:
- Bleeding, especially in elderly females, postoperative patients, or patients undergoing recent trauma.

How to recognize it:
- Watch for partial thromboplastin time or activated clotting time greater than 2 1/2 times control value.
- Monitor for decreased red blood cell count, hematocrit, or hemoglobin.

What to do:
- Stop heparin immediately.
- If necessary, give heparin antagonist protamine sulfate by slow I.V. injection over 1 to 3 minutes. Usually, 1 mg protamine sulfate will neutralize 90 units of heparin.
- Protamine sulfate doses may have to be repeated, based on clotting tests.

However, repeat doses cautiously, because large doses of protamine sulfate may act as an anticoagulant. Don't give more than 50 mg protamine sulfate in a 10-minute period.

INSULIN AND ORAL HYPOGLYCEMIC AGENTS (ANTIDIABETIC DRUGS)
Acetohexamide, chlorpropamide, insulin (all forms), phenformin hydrochloride, tolazamide, tolbutamide.
Symptoms to watch for: (All signs of hypoglycemia)
- Parasympathetic phase—hunger, nausea, belching, bradycardia, mild hypotension.
- Decreased cerebral function phase—lethargy, frequent yawning, decreased spontaneity of conversation, inability to do simple calculations.
- Sympathetic phase—increased systolic and mean blood pressure, sweating, tachycardia.
- Coma, with or without convulsions.

Confirming diagnostic measures:
- Monitor blood for hypoglycemia: (serum glucose level less than 50 mg/100 ml).

What to do:
- For mild hypoglycemia, if patient is alert, give 120 ml (4 oz.) of an oral carbohydrate such as orange juice or other juices, cola, or ginger ale q 5 to 10 minutes until signs of hypoglycemia disappear. Alternately, may give 0.5 to 2 mg glucagon I.M.
- For comatose patients or those not responding to or refusing oral carbohydrates, give 50 ml of 50% dextrose I.V., or 0.5 to 2 mg glucagon I.M. if not used previously. Keep airway open. Prevent tongue-biting.
- If patient doesn't respond to above treatment, repeat 50% dextrose dose twice; then start 10% dextrose by continuous I.V. infusion (at rate of 20 drops/minute). Monitor blood glucose.

LITHIUM CARBONATE, LITHIUM CITRATE
Symptoms to watch for:
CNS: seizures, impaired consciousness, transitory neurologic asymmetries similar to those produced by cerebral hemorrhage; tremors, fasciculations, stiff neck, ataxia, seizures, restlessness, confusion, stupor, coma.
CV: arrhythmias, pulse deficit, hypotension.
EENT: widely opened eyes, transient vertical nystagmus, tinnitus.
GI: dry mouth.
GU: urinary incontinence
Other: irregular or deep respirations; gasping and grunting with hyperextension of arms and legs, allergic vasculitis, fecal incontinence.
What to do:
- Reduce dosage or stop drug.
- Use gastric suction.

- Monitor lithium serum levels (should not exceed 2 mEq/L in acute treatment phase; or 1.5 mEq/L in maintenance phase).
- Replace fluids and electrolytes as necessary.
- Increase lithium excretion by:
  —forced osmotic diuresis, using up to 200 g mannitol I.V. (5% to 10% solution). Maintain urinary output of 100 to 500 ml/hour and a positive fluid balance.
  —alkalization of urine with 325 mg to 2 g sodium bicarbonate P.O. q.i.d., or 30 ml/Kg sodium lactate by slow I.V. infusion daily.
  —administration of caffeine, aminophylline, and sometimes acetazolamide.

METHAQUALONE

Symptoms to watch for:

Blood: nasal or GI bleeding.
CNS: hypertonia, hyperreflexia, muscle twitching, convulsions, coma, delirium.
CV: tachycardia.
EENT: dilated pupils.
GI: vomiting.
GU: renal insufficiency.
Other: pulmonary and cutaneous edema, shock, hepatic damage.

What to do:

- Stop drug.
- If patient is not convulsing, use gastric lavage.
- Use supportive measures.
- Adults: For prolonged convulsions, give a neuromuscular blocker such as tubocurarine 1 unit/Kg of body weight I.V. slowly over a period of 60 to 90 seconds. Initial dose should be 20 units (3 mg) less than dose calculated by body weight. Assist respirations.
- Hemodialysis may be useful.

METHYPRYLON

Symptoms to watch for:

CNS: coma, excitation, convulsions, delirium, hallucinations, somnolence, confusion.
CV: hypotension.
EENT: constricted pupils.
Other: fever, hypothermia, respiratory depression.

What to do:

- Stop drug.
- Gastric lavage.
- Supportive measures.
- Give levarterenol 8 to 12 mcg/minute by I.V. infusion adjusted to maintain normal blood pressure. To dilute, add 4 mg levarterenol to 1000 ml 5% dextrose in water.
- To treat convulsions and excitation, give short-acting barbiturate such as thiopental sodium 75 to 124 mg I.V.
- In severe overdosage, hemodialysis may be needed.

NARCOTICS

Phenanthrene derivatives: codeine, codeine phosphate, codeine sulfate, hydrocodone bitartrate, hydromorphone hydrochloride, hydromorphone sulfate, levorphanol tartrate, morphine sulfate, opium alkaloids (concentrated), oxycodone, oxymorphone hydrochloride. Morphine sulfate is the prototype of this class.
Phenylpiperidine derivatives: alphaprodine hydrochloride, anileridine hydrochloride, fentanyl citrate, meperidine hydrochloride. Meperidine hydrochloride is the prototype of this class.
Diphenoxylate hydrochloride with atropine sulfate may cause meperidine-like toxicity as well as anticholinergic toxicity.

Symptoms to watch for:

CNS: respiratory depression which may progress to Cheyne-Stokes; apnea, CNS depression ranging from stupor to profound coma; muscle tremors and twitches, delirium, disorientation, hallucinations, and occasionally grand mal seizures (with meperidine derivatives).
CV: bradycardia, hypotension, cyanosis, circulatory collapse, cardiac arrest, possibly tachycardia (with meperidine derivatives).

EENT: miosis (with morphine derivatives and methadone), mydriasis (with meperidine derivatives).
GI: dry mouth (with meperidine derivatives).
Other: cold, clammy skin; hypothermia; flaccid skeletal muscles.
Confirming diagnostic measures:
- Make a positive identification of ingested drug if possible.
- Note symptoms:
  —coma, pinpoint pupils, depressed respirations indicative of morphine derivative and methadone toxicity. Keep in mind that in terminal narcosis or severe hypoxia, mydriasis may occur in morphine and methadone toxicity.
  —coma, dilated pupils, depressed respirations indicative of meperidine derivative toxicity.
- Analyze urine, blood, and/or gastric contents for presence of narcotics.

What to do:
- Stop drug.
- Establish airway; ventilate as needed.
- If patient is fully conscious, do gastric lavage or induce emesis, especially within first 2 hours of ingestion; gastric lavage contraindicated if patient is unconscious or shows signs of CNS depression.
- Give naloxone (Narcan): in adults, 0.4 mg I.V., I.M., or S.C. repeated after 2 to 3 minutes up to 3 times if needed; in children, 0.1 mg/Kg. I.V., I.M., or S.C. repeated after 2 to 3 minutes up to 3 times if needed.
- Keep in mind that a narcotic antagonist (naloxone) may precipitate acute withdrawal syndrome in patients physically addicted to narcotics.
- Maintain body warmth.
- Maintain adequate fluid intake.
- Treat shock with oxygen, intravenous fluids, and vasopressors as needed.
- Monitor vital signs and level of consciousness frequently.

ORAL ANTICOAGULANTS
Acenocoumarol, anisindione, dicumarol, diphenadione, phenindione, phenprocoumon, warfarin potassium, warfarin sodium.
Symptoms to watch for:
- Minor bleeding, such as purpura, hematoma, epistaxis, or hematuria. Red-orange discoloration of urine with phenindione, diphenadione, and anisindione may be mistaken for hematuria.
- Major bleeding, such as gastrointestinal or intracranial bleeding. Intrapulmonary, adrenal, or retroperitoneal bleeding, hemarthroses, and bleeding into pericardial space are also possible but less common.
- Skin necrosis and the sudden onset of painful ecchymoses, usually on the lower half of the body or on the breast, with coumarin derivatives.

How to confirm toxicity:
- Watch for prothrombin time greater than 2 times control value.
- Monitor for decreased red blood cell count, hematocrit, or hemoglobin.
- Test for blood in stools (Hematest, Hemoccult).

What to do:
- Stop anticoagulant and control bleeding immediately.
- Give antidote, vitamin K1 (phytonadione) 2.5 to 10 mg I.M., S.C., or slow I.V. injection. Repeat in 6 to 8 hours if necessary. If patient is not bleeding but has elevated prothrombin time, may give 2.5 to 10 mg phytonadione P.O. Repeat in 12 to 48 hours, if necessary. In emergency, may give 10 to 50 mg by slow I.V.; maximum rate 1 mg/minute. Repeat q 4 hours, p.r.n.
- May give fresh frozen plasma or fresh whole blood to replace clotting factors. In major bleeding, fresh frozen plasma is necessary since onset of phytonadione action begins after 6 to 8 hours.

PHENOTHIAZINES
Acetophenazine maleate, butaperazine maleate, carphenazine maleate, chlorpromazine hydrochloride, dimethothiazine mesylate, fluphenazine decanoate, fluphenazine enanthate,

fluphenazine hydrochloride, mesoridazine besylate, methdilazine hydrochloride, perphenazine, piperacetazine, prochlorperazine, prochlorperazine edisylate, prochlorperazine maleate, promazine hydrochloride, promethazine hydrochloride, thiethylperazine maleate, thiopropazate hydrochloride, thioridazine, trifluoperazine, triflupromazine, trimeprazine tartrate.

Symptoms to watch for:

CNS: restlessness, confusion, excitement in early or mild intoxication; convulsions; depression ranging from drowsiness to coma; areflexia; parkinsonian-like extrapyramidal symptoms (tremors, rigidity, akinesia, shuffling gait, postural abnormalities, pill-rolling movements, mask-like facies, excessive salivation); dystonic and dyskinesic extrapyramidal symptoms (dystonia occurs most frequently in children; dyskinesia most commonly in adults (disordered tonicity of muscles and torsion spasms, opisthotonos, drooping of the head, protrusion of tongue, mandibular tics, stiff neck.) difficulty swallowing and breathing. (accompanied by profuse sweating, pallor, fever); akathisia (extreme motor restlessness, continual moving of hands, mouth, and body).

CV: hypotension, tachycardia, EKG changes, cardiac arrhythmias, cyanosis, vasomotor collapse.

EENT: miosis.

GI: dry mouth.

Other: hypothermia, sudden apnea.

What to do:

- Stop drug.
- Maintain airway; promote adequate oxygen uptake and carbon dioxide removal.
- Gastric lavage is effective up to several hours after drug is ingested.
- Don't induce emesis; dystonic reactions may cause aspiration of vomitus.
- Treat severe dystonia and dyskinesia with 2 mg benztropine mesylate I.V. followed by 1 to 2 mg P.O. b.i.d. to prevent recurrence; or diphenhydramine hydrochloride 25 to 50 mg deep I.M. or I.V.
- Treat parkinsonian reactions with benztropine mesylate 0.5 to 6 mg P.O. daily; trihexyphenidyl hydrochloride 2.5 mg P.O. daily to t.i.d.; biperiden hydrochloride or lactate 2 mg t.i.d. to q.i.d.; or 2 to 2.5 mg procyclidine hydrochloride P.O. t.i.d.; may increase up to 60 mg daily. Don't use levodopa.
- Attempt to treat akathisia with antiparkinson drugs as above; treatment often ineffective.
- If stimulants are needed, use amphetamines, ephedrine, or caffeine and sodium benzoate. Don't use picrotoxin, pentylenetetrazol or other stimulants which may cause convulsions.
- Observe patient for orthostatic hypotension; monitor blood pressure in lying and standing positions. If patient is ambulatory, instruct him to rise from bed slowly, dangle feet for a few minutes before standing.
- Treat severe hypotension with slow I.V. infusion of levarterenol 8 to 12 mcg/minute. Adjust to maintain normal blood pressure. To dilute, add 4 mg levarterenol to 1000 ml of 5% dextrose in water. Or use phenylephrine hydrochloride 0.1 to 0.5 mg added to 500 ml of 5% dextrose in water, at a rapid rate initially, then slowed to maintain blood pressure at desired level. Do not use epinephrine; may paradoxically lower blood pressure.
- Stay with patient and give reassurance that symptoms will subside.

PROPOXYPHENE HYDROCHLORIDE OR NAPSYLATE

Symptoms to watch for:

CNS: stupor, coma, convulsions.

CV: EKG abnormalities, circulatory collapse.

EENT: miosis.

Metabolic: nephrogenic diabetes insipidus.

Other: respiratory depression, pulmonary edema, cyanosis.

Confirming diagnostic measures:

- Watch for EKG abnormalities.

What to do:

- Stop drug.
- Maintain airway.
- Give antidote, naloxone hydrochloride (Narcan): in adults, 0.4 mg I.V., I.M., or S.C.; in children, 0.01 mg/Kg I.V. or I.M. Doses may be repeated in 2 to 3 minutes.

- Induce emesis or use gastric lavage.
- Give 10 g activated charcoal (or 5 to 10 times the estimated weight of drug ingested).
- Use supportive measures as needed (oxygen, intravenous fluids, and vasopressors).

SALICYLATES

Aluminum aspirin, aspirin, calcium carbaspirin, choline salicylate, methyl salicylate, magnesium salicylate, salicylamide, salsalate, sodium salicylate, sodium thiosalicylate.

Symptoms to watch for:

- Mild toxicity—burning pain in mouth, throat, or abdomen; slight to moderate hyperpnea; lethargy, vomiting, tinnitus, hearing loss, dizziness.
- Moderate toxicity—ecchymoses, restlessness, incoordination, dehydration, fever, sweating, delirium, excitability, marked lethargy, severe hyperpnea.
- Severe toxicity—sodium, potassium, and bicarbonate loss, and metabolic acidosis in young children; coma, convulsion, cyanosis, oliguria, uremia, pulmonary edema, respiratory failure, severe hyperpnea.
- Small doses of methyl salicylate are potentially fatal in children.

Confirming diagnostic measures:

- Monitor blood salicylate levels for 6 hours after ingestion. Look for the following levels in adults:
  - —no intoxication: less than 45 mg/100 ml
  - —mild intoxication: 45 to 65 mg/100 ml
  - —moderate intoxication: 65 to 90 mg/100 ml
  - —severe intoxication: 90 to 120 mg/100 ml

Blood levels of 120 mg/100 ml or more are usually fatal.

- Blood levels may continue to rise for 6 to 10 hours after overdose.

What to do:

- Induce emesis with 15 ml to 30 ml of ipecac syrup.
- If patient shows CNS depression, use gastric lavage and protect airway.
- Give activated charcoal up to 10 times the amount of salicylate ingested.
- Give a saline cathartic (e.g., magnesium citrate 200 ml).
- For hypotension, give I.V. fluids according to the patient's acid/base and electrolyte status.
- For respiratory depression, give artificial respiration with oxygen.
- For hypoglycemia, give dextrose I.V.
- Maintain fluid balance with 5% dextrose in water with sodium chloride. The following dosages are for initial management and should be adjusted according to results of physical and lab exams.
  - —in mild salicylate intoxication, give 100 ml/Kg fluids P.O.
  - —in severe intoxication, give 400 ml 5% dextrose in water/m² body surface area, with 5 mEq sodium chloride/100 ml and 2.5 mEq sodium bicarbonate/100 ml.
  - —when adequate urine flow is established, decrease sodium dose by 50% and add potassium chloride.
- For acidosis, initially give 2 to 5 mEq sodium bicarbonate/Kg by slow I.V. infusion over 24 to 48 hours.

- For bleeding due to hypoprothrombinemia give phytonadione (vitamin K) 25 mg/day I.M. or I.V
- For impaired renal function, use dialysis to remove salicylates.
- For hyperpyrexia, sponge patient with tepid water. Don't use alcohol.
- Continue monitoring patient's serum sodium, potassium, glucose, blood gases, and salicylate levels.

SPASMOLYTICS

Aminophylline, dyphilline, oxtriphylline, papaverine, theophylline, theophylline monoethanolamine, theophylline sodium glycinate.

Symptoms to watch for:

CNS: headache, insomnia, irritability, restlessness, convulsions (especially in infants and small children), hyperreflexia, fasciculations, coma, fainting.
CV: tachycardia, marked hypotension, circulatory failure.
EENT: tinnitus, flashing lights.
GI: nausea, vomiting, epigastric pain, hematemesis, diarrhea.
GU: albuminuria, microhematuria.
Skin: cyanosis.
Other dehydration, extreme thirst, tachypnea, respiratory arrest, fever.

What to do:

- Stop drug.
- Use gastric lavage.
- If patient is conscious, may induce emesis.
- Give intravenous fluids and oxygen and use additional supportive measures to prevent hypotension and maintain fluid and electrolyte balance.
- Monitor serum levels until drug level below 20 mcg/ml.
- No known specific antidote.

TRANQUILIZERS

Chlordiazepoxide hydrochloride, diazepam, lorazepam, prazepam, oxazepam.

Symptoms to watch for:

CNS: confusion, coma, somnolence, diminished reflexes.
CV: possible hypotension.
Other: possible depression.

What to do:

- Stop drug.
- Maintain airway; promote oxygen intake and carbon dioxide removal.
- Monitor respirations, pulse, and blood pressure.
- If patient is conscious, induce vomiting with ipecac syrup, 15 ml.
- Apply tourniquet and ice pack after diazepam injection to delay absorption.
- After oral ingestion, do gastric lavage immediately.
- Use caffeine or sodium benzoate to reduce CNS and respiratory depression.

For chlordiazepoxide hydrochloride or diazepam toxicity, may also use methylphenidate.

Intravenous Solution Compatibilities

Caution: Avoid mixing multiple drugs in I.V. solutions whenever possible; physical compatibility does not exclude the possibility of therapeutic incompatibility. (See tabular material, Interactions.)

	amikacin	aminophylline	amino acid injection	amphotericin B	ampicillin	calcium gluconate	carbenicillin	cefazolin	cephalothin	chloramphenicol	cimetidine	corticotropin (ACTH)	dexamethasone	Dextrose 5% in water	Dextrose 5% in Lactated Ringers	Dextrose 5% in 0.45% NaCl	Dextrose 5% in 0.9% NaCl	diazepam	diazoxide	diphenhydramine	dopamine	epinephrine	erythromycin I.V.
amikacin		24	NR	●	NR	24	24	8	●	24	NR		24	24	24	24	24	●	●	24	NR	24	24
aminophylline	24				●	C		C	●	●	●	●	C	C	C	C	C	●	●	C		●	C
amino acid injection	NR			NR	NR	C	NR	NR	NR	NR		NR	NR	C	C	C	C	●	●		NR	NR	NR
amphotericin B	●		NR							T	O			B	E			P	R	E	P	A	R
ampicillin	NR	●	NR			●	NR	NR	NR	●	NR	NR		4	4	4	4	●	●	NR	●	●	●
calcium gluconate	24	C	C		●			●	●	●		C	C	C	C	C	C	●	●	C		●	C
carbenicillin	24		NR		NR			●		●				24	24	24	24	●	●		24	●	NR
cefazolin	8	C	NR		NR	●	●			24	C	C	C	96	96	96	96	●	●				●
cephalothin	●	●	NR		NR	●				●	C			24	24	24	24	●	●	●	6	●	●
chloramphenicol	24	●	NR	T	●	●	●	24	●			●	C	24	24	24	24	●	●	C	24	●	●
cimetidine	NR	●		O	NR			C	C					C	C	C	C	●	●				NR
corticotropin (ACTH)		●	NR		NR	C		C		●				C	C	C	C	●	●				NR
dexamethasone	24	C	NR			C		C		C				C	C	C	C	●	●	●			
dextrose 5% in water	24	C	C	B	4	C	24	96	24	24	C	C	C					●	●	C	48	C	6
dextrose 5% in lactated Ringer's	24	C	C	E	4	C	24	96	24	24	C	C	C					●	●	C	48	C	6
dextrose 5% in 0.45% NaCl	24	C	C		4	C	24	96	24	24	C	C	C					●	●	C	48	C	6
dextrose 5% in 0.9% NaCl	24	C	C		4	C	24	96	24	24	C	C	C					●	●	C	48	C	6
diazepam	●	●	●	P	●	●	●	●	●	●	●	●	●	●	●	●	●		●	●	●	●	●
diazoxide	●	●	●	R	●	●	●	●	●	●	●	●	●	●	●	●	●	●		●	●	●	●
diphenhydramine	24	C		E	NR	C			●	C			●	C	C	C	C	●	●				C
dopamine	NR		NR	P	●		24		6	24				48	48	48	48	●	●				NR
epinephrine	24	●	NR	A	●	●	●		●	●				C	C	C	C	●	●				NR
erythromycin I.V.	24	C	NR	R	●	C	NR	●	●	●	NR	NR		6	6	6	6	●	●	C	NR	NR	
fat emulsion 10%	NR	NR	NR	E	NR	●	NR	NR	NR	NR	NR	NR	NR	NR	NR	NR	NR	●	●	NR	NR	NR	NR
gentamicin	NR		NR	D	●		●	●	●	●	C			48	24	24	24	●	●		6		NR
heparin sodium	●	●	C		NR	C			8	●		C	C	24	C	24	24	●	●				●
hydrocortisone sodium succinate	24	C	C		●	C	C		C	C		C	C		C		C	●	●	●			C
insulin	NR	●	C	B	NR				8		C			C	C	C	C	●	●				NR
isoproterenol	NR	●	NR	Y	NR	C			C					24	24	24	24	●	●				NR
kanamycin	NR	C	NR		●	●	●	●	●	C	C		C	24	24	24	24	●	●		24		NR
lactated ringers	24	C	C		C	C	24	96	24	24	C	C						●	●	C	48	C	6
levarterenol	24	●	NR	P	●	C		24	●	●		C		C	C	C	C	●	●			●	NR
lidocaine	NR	C	●	H	C		C		●	C			C	C	C	C	C	●	●	C		●	C
metaraminol	24		NR	A	●	C			●	C		C	●	24	24	24	24	●	●	C		C	●
methicillin	8	●	24	R	NR	C	NR		●	●		C	C	24	24	24	24	●	●	C	NR		C
methylprednisolone	NR	●	NR	M	NR	C	C		●	●				C	C	C	C	●	●	●			NR
multiple vitamin infusion (MVI)	NR		C	A	NR									C	C	C	C	●	●				NR
nafcillin	NR	C	NR	C	NR					C			C	24	24	24	24	●	●	C			NR
nitroprusside	NR	NR	NR	Y	NR	NR	NR	NR	NR	NR	NR	NR	NR	C	NR	●	NR	●	●	NR	NR	NR	NR
0.9% NSS	24	C	C		8	C	24	96	24	24	C	C	C					●	●		48	C	8
oxacillin	24	●	NR		NR	C	C	C	●	●				24	24	24	24	●	●			●	NR
oxytocin	NR			O				C		C				C	C	C	C	●	●				NR
penicillin G	24	●	NR	N	●	C		C	●	C	C	C	C	24	24	24	24	●	●	C	12	●	C
phenytoin	●	●	●	L	●	●	●	●	●	●	●	●	●	●	●	●	●	●	●	●	●	●	●
phytonadione	24	●		Y	●	C			●	●			C	C	C	C	C	●	●	C		●	NR
polymyxin B	24	C	NR		NR		●	●	●	●				C	NR	C	C	●	●	C			C
potassium chloride	24	C	C		NR	C	C	C	C	C	C	C		C	C	C	C	●	●			●	C
procainamide	NR	C				C				C								●	●	C			NR
sodium bicarbonate	24	C	C		NR	●	24		●	C		●		C	C	C	C	●	●		●	●	C
tetracycline	24	●	NR		●	●	●	●	●	●		C	C	24	24	24	24	●	●	C	24	●	●
thiamine	NR		C		NR									C	C	C	C	●	●				NR
ticarcillin	NR	●	NR		NR									72	C	72	C	●	●				NR
tobramycin	NR		NR		NR	●	●	●	●					24	24	24	24	●	●				NR
vancomycin	24	●	NR		NR	●				●		C	●	C				●	●	C		●	NR
vitamin B complex with C	●	●	C		●	C	24	●	C	●		C	8	24	24	24	24	●	●	C		●	●

KEY: **C** = Compatible ● = Incompatible **NR** = Not recommended by the manufacturer

fat emulsion 10%	gentamicin	heparin sodium	hydrocortisone sodium succinate	insulin	isoproterenol	kanamycin	lactated Ringer's	levarterenol	lidocaine	metaraminol	methicillin	methylprednisolone	multiple vitamin infusion (MVI)	nafcillin	nitroprusside	0.9% NSS	oxacillin	oxytocin	penicillin G	phenytoin	phytonadione	polymyxin B	potassium chloride	procainamide	sodium bicarbonate	tetracycline	thiamine	ticarcillin	tobramycin	vancomycin	vitamin B complex with C
NR	NR	●	24	NR	NR	NR	24	24	NR	24	8	NR	NR	NR	NR	24	24	NR	24	●	24	24	24	NR	24	24	NR	NR	NR	24	●
NR		●	C	●	●	C	C	●	C		●	●		C	NR	C	●		●	●	●	C	C	C	C	●		●		●	●
NR	NR	C	C	C	NR	NR	C	NR	●	NR	24	NR	C	NR	NR	C	NR		NR	●		NR	C		C	NR	C	NR	NR	NR	C
E	D			B	Y			P	H	A	R	M	A	C	Y			O	N	L	Y										
NR	●	NR	●	NR	NR	●	C	●	C	●	NR	NR	NR	NR	NR	8	NR		●	●	●	NR	NR		NR	●	NR	NR	NR	NR	●
●		C	C		C	●	C	C		C	C	C			NR	C	C		C	●	C		C	C	●	●			●	●	C
NR	●		C			●	24		C		NR	C			NR	24	C			●		●	C		24	●			●		24
NR	●					●	96	24							NR	96	C	C	C	●		●	C			●			●		●
NR	●	8	C	8	C	●	24	●	●	●	●	●			NR	24	●		●	●	●	●	C		●	●			●		C
NR	●	●	C			C	24	●	C	C	●	●		C	NR	24	●	C	C	●	●	●	C	C	C	●				●	●
NR	C			C		C	C								NR	C			C	●			C								
NR		C	C				C	C		C	C				NR	C			C	●			C		●	C				C	C
NR		C	C			C			C	●	C			C	NR	C			C	●	C					C				●	8
NR	48	24		C	24	24		C	C	24	24	C	C	24	C		24	C	24	●	C	C	C		C	24	C	72	24	C	24
NR	24	C	C	C	24	24		C	C	24	24	C	C	24	NR		24	C	24	●	C	NR	C		C	24	C	C	24		24
NR	24	24		C	24	24		C	C	24	24	C	C	24	●		24	C	24	●	C	C	C		C	24	C	72	24		24
NR	24	24	C	C	24	24		C	C	24	24	C	C	24	NR		24	C	24	●	C	C	C		C	24	C	C	24		24
●	●	●	●	●	●	●	●	●	●	●	●	●	●	●	●	●	●	●	●	●	●	●	●	●	●	●	●	●	●	●	●
●	●	●	●	●	●	●	●	●	●	●	●	●	●	●	●	●	●	●	●	●	●	●	●	●	●	●	●	●	●	●	●
NR			●				C		C	C	C	●		C	NR				C	●	C	C		C		C				C	C
NR	6					24	48				NR				NR	48			12	●					●	24					
NR							C	●	●	C					NR	C	●		●	●	●		●		●	●				●	●
NR	NR	●	C	NR	NR	NR	6	NR	C	●	C	NR	NR	NR	NR	8	NR	NR	C	●	NR	C	C	NR	C	●	NR	NR	NR	NR	●
■	NR	NR	NR	NR	NR	NR	NR	NR	NR	NR	NR	NR	NR	NR	NR	NR	NR	NR	NR	NR	NR	NR	NR	NR	NR	NR	NR	NR	NR	NR	NR
NR	■	●				NR	24				24			●	NR	48	●		24	●								●			
NR	●	■	●	●	C	●	24	●	C	●	●			C	NR	24			●	●	●	●	C	C		●			●	●	C
NR		●	■	8		●	C	C	C	●	●	C		●	NR	C			C	●		C	C	C	C	●				●	C
NR		●	8	■					●						NR	C			●	●			C		●						C
NR		C			■		24		●		NR		C		NR	24				●			C		●	C					C
NR	NR	●	●			■	24			C	●			NR	NR	24	NR		C	●	C	C			●	C		NR	NR	NR	C
NR	24	24	C		24	24	■	C	24	24	24	C	C	24	NR		24	C	24	●	C	NR	C		C	24	C	48	24	C	24
NR		●	C				C	■	●	●	●	C	C	24	NR	NR	●	●	●	●			C		●	●					C
NR		C	C	●	●		24	●	■	C	NR				NR	24			C	●			C		●	C					C
NR		●	●			C	24	●	C	■	●	●	●	●	NR	24	●	C	●	●	●		C	C	C	C				C	C
NR	24	●	●		NR	●	24	●	NR	●	■	NR	NR	NR	NR	24	NR	NR	C	●	NR	C	C	NR	NR	●	NR	NR	NR	●	●
NR			C				C	C		●	NR	■			NR	C			C	●			C			●					●
NR					C		C	C		●	NR		■	●	NR	C				●			C			●					
NR	●	C	●			NR	24	24		●	NR		●	■	NR	24	NR			●			24		C	●	●		●		●
NR	NR	NR	NR	NR	NR	NR	NR	NR	NR	NR	NR	NR	NR	NR	■	NR	NR	NR	NR	NR	NR	NR	NR	NR	NR	NR	NR	NR	NR	NR	NR
NR	48	24	C	C	24	24		NR	24	24	24	C	C	24	NR	■	24	C	24	●	C	C	C		C	24	C	72	24		24
NR	●					NR	24	●		●	NR			NR	NR	24	■		●	●	●		C			●			●		●
NR							C	●		C	NR				NR	C		■	C	●	C					C					
NR	24	●	C	●		C	24	●	C	●	C	C			NR	24	●	C	■	●	C	●	C	C	●	●			●	●	
NR	●	●	●	●	●	●	●	●	●	●	●	●	●	●	NR	●	●	●	●	■	●	●	●	●	●	●	●	●	●	●	●
NR		●				C	C			●	NR				NR	C	●	C	C	●	■		C			C				●	
NR		●	C			C	NR				C				NR	C			●	●		■				●					C
NR		C	C	C	C		C	C	C	C	C	C	C	24	NR	C	C		C	●	C		■			C				C	C
NR		C	C							C	NR				NR				C	●				■		C				C	C
NR			C	●	●	●	C	●	●	C	NR			C	NR	C			●	●					■	●				●	●
NR		●	●		C	C	24	●	C	C	●	●	●	●	NR	24	●	C	●	●	C	●	C	C	●	■				C	C
NR							C				NR			●	NR	C				●							■				C
NR	●					NR	48				NR				NR	72				●								■			
NR		●				NR	24				NR			●	NR	24	●		●	●									■		
NR		●	●			NR	C			C	●				NR				●	●	●		C	C	●	C				■	●
NR		C	C	C	C	C	24	C	C	C	●	●		●	NR	24	●			●		C	C	C	●	C	C			●	■

4, 6, 8, 24, 48, 96 = Compatible only for the number of hours indicated   □ = Blank space data unavailable

Table of equivalents

PENICILLIN UNITS

1 unit=0.6 mcg penicillin G
1 mg penicillin=1667 units

WEIGHTS

APOTHECARY		METRIC	APOTHECARY		METRIC
1 ounce	=	31.1 g	1/150 grain	=	0.4 mg
15.43 grains	=	1 g	1/200 grain	=	0.3 mg
1 grain	=	60 mg	1/250 grain	=	0.25 mg
1/60 grain	=	1.0 mg	1/300 grain	=	0.2 mg
1/80 grain	=	0.8 mg	1/400 grain	=	0.15 mg
1/100 grain	=	0.6 mg	1/500 grain	=	0.12 mg
1/120 grain	=	0.5 mg	1/600 grain	=	0.1 mg

LIQUID MEASURE

HOUSEHOLD		APOTHECARY		APPROXIMATE METRIC
1 teaspoonful	=	1 fluid dram	=	5 ml
1 tablespoonful	=	4 fluid drams	=	15 ml
2 tablespoonsful	=	1 fluid ounce	=	30 ml
1 measuring cupful	=	8 fluid ounces	=	240 ml
1 pint	=	16 fluid ounces	=	500 ml
1 quart	=	32 fluid ounces	=	1000 ml

TEMPERATURE

9C.°=5F.°−160

Centigrade Fahrenheit
(C.°x9/5)+32=F.°

Fahrenheit Centigrade
(F.°−32)x5/9=C.°

METRIC WEIGHT EQUIVALENTS

1 Kg	=	1000 g
1 g	=	1000 mg
1 mg	=	0.001 g
1 mcg or μg	=	0.001 mg

CONVERSIONS

1 oz	=	30 g
1 lb	=	453.6 g
2.2 lb	=	1 Kg

METRIC VOLUME EQUIVALENTS

1 liter	=	1000 ml
1 deciliter	=	100 ml

Nomogram for estimating surface area in children

The surface area is indicated where a straight line which connects the height and weight levels intersects the surface area column; or if the patient is roughly of average size, from the weight alone (enclosed area).

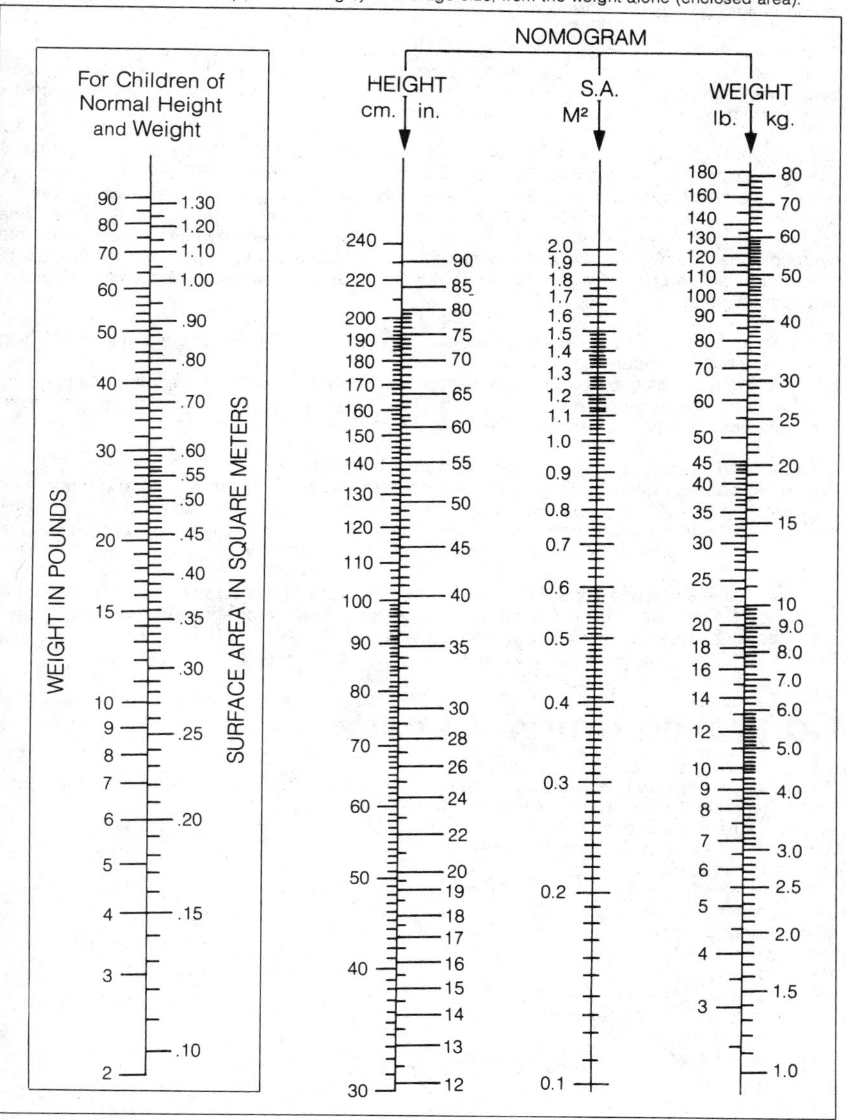

Nelson *Textbook of Pediatrics*, 10th edition, W. B. Saunders Co., Phila., Pa.

Schedules of controlled substances, USA

Drugs that are regulated under the jurisdiction of the Controlled Substances Act of 1970 are divided into 5 groups or schedules:

Schedule I: No accepted medical use in the United States, with high potential for abuse.
Examples: heroin, marijuana, LSD, peyote, mescaline, psilocybin, tetrahydrocannabinols, ketobemidone, levomoramide, racemoramide, benzylmorphine, dihydromorphine, methysulfonate, nicocodeine, nicomorphine, etorphine, and others.

Schedule II: High potential for abuse, with severe psychic or physical dependence possible.
Examples: alphaprodine, amobarbital, amphetamine sulfate/hydrochloride, anileridine, apomorphine, cocaine hydrochloride, codeine, codeine phosphate/glucuronidine, desoxyephedrine hydrochloride, dextro-amphetamine sulfate, fentanyl, hydromorphone, levorphanol, meperidine hydrochloride, methadone hydrochloride, methamphetamine, methaqualone, methylphenidate hydrochloride, methylphenidyl acetate, morphine phosphate/sulfate, opium (gum or extract), oxycodone, oxymorphone hydrochloride, pentobarbital sodium, phenmetrazine, phenobarbital, secobarbital, secobarbital sodium.

Schedule III: Less abuse potential than drugs in Schedule II, and include compounds containing certain narcotic and nonnarcotic drugs.
Examples: derivatives of barbituric acid (except those listed in another schedule), glutethimide, methyprylon, chlorhexadol, phencyclidine, sulfondiethylmethane, sulfonmethane, benzphetamine, chlorpentermine, clortermine, mazindol, phendimetrazine, and paregoric.

Schedule IV: Less abuse potential than drugs in Schedule III.
Examples: barbital, phenobarbital, methylphenobarbital, chloral betaine, chloral hydrate, ethchlorvynol, ethinamate, meprobamate, paraldehyde, methohexital, fenfluramine, diethylpropion, phentermine, chlordiazopoxide, diazepam, oxazepam, chlorazepate, flurazepam, clonazepam, and mebutamate, pentazocine, propoxyphene, and pemoline.

Schedule V: Less potential for abuse than the drugs in Schedule IV and consist of preparations containing limited quantities of certain narcotic drugs generally for antitussive or antidiarrheal purposes which may be distributed without a prescription.
Examples: APC with codeine tablets and expectorants with codeine.

Controlled drugs, Canada

Drugs that are regulated under the jurisdiction of the Food and Drugs Act and regulations issued by the Health Protection Branch, Ottawa, Canada:
Amphetamine and its salts
Barbituric acid and its salts and derivatives
Benzphetamine and its salts
Butorphanol and its salts
Diethylpropion and its salts
Methamphetamine and its salts
Methaqualone and its salts
Methylphenidate and its salts
Pentazocine and its salts
Phendimetrazine and its salts
Phenmetrazine and its salts
Thiobarbituric acid and its salts and derivatives

MEDICAL ABBREVIATIONS

a.c. — before meals
ACTH — adrenocorticotropic hormone
A-V — arteriovenous
b.i.d. — twice a day
BP — blood pressure
BSP — bromsulphalein
BUN — blood urea nitrogen
Ca — calcium
CBC — complete blood count
CNS — central nervous system
CSF — cerebrospinal fluid
EEG — electroencephalogram
EENT — eyes, ears, nose, and throat
EKG — electrocardiogram
FBS — fasting blood sugar
G6PD — glucose 6 phosphate dehydrogenase
GI — gastrointestinal
gtts. — drops
GU — genitourinary (urogenital)
HCl — hydrochloride
h.s. — at bedtime
IM — intramuscular
I & O — intake and output
I.U. — international units
I.V. — intravenous
Kg — kilogram
L — liter
LDH — lactic acid dehydrogenase
mEq/L — milliequivalents per liter
MI — myocardial infarction
p.c. — after meals
Pco_2 — arterial carbon dioxide content
pH — hydrogen ion concentration
P.O. — by mouth
Po_2 — arterial oxygen content
Postop — postoperative
Preop — preoperative
p.r.n. — whenever necessary
PSP — phenolsulfonphthalein
q. — every
RBC — red blood cells; red blood count
SGOT — serum glutamic oxaloacetic transaminase
SGPT — serum glutamic pyruvic transaminase
SL — sublingual
SC — subcutanous
t.i.d. — three times a day
U.S.P. — United States Pharmacopeia
WBC — white blood cells; white blood count

Notes

Notes

Notes

Notes

Index

When drugs are indexed on more than one page, primary entry is in bold type.

B

B

C

E

H

I

M

N

O

P

P

Q

S

S

T